MCAT®

BIOLOGY

2009–2010 EDITION

The Staff of Kaplan

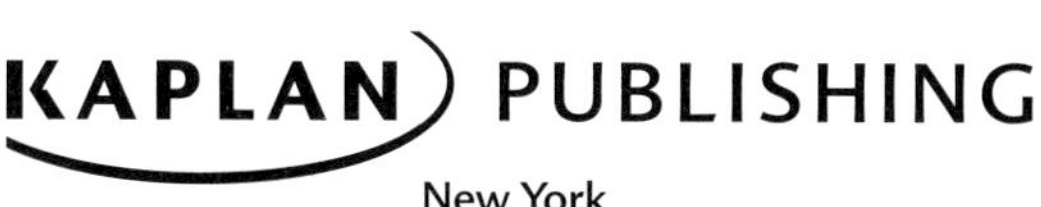

New York

Published by Kaplan Publishing, a division of Kaplan, Inc.
1 Liberty Plaza, 24th Floor
New York, NY 10006

Printed in the United States of America

10 9 8 7 6 5 4 3 2 1

ISBN: 978-1-4277-9872-5

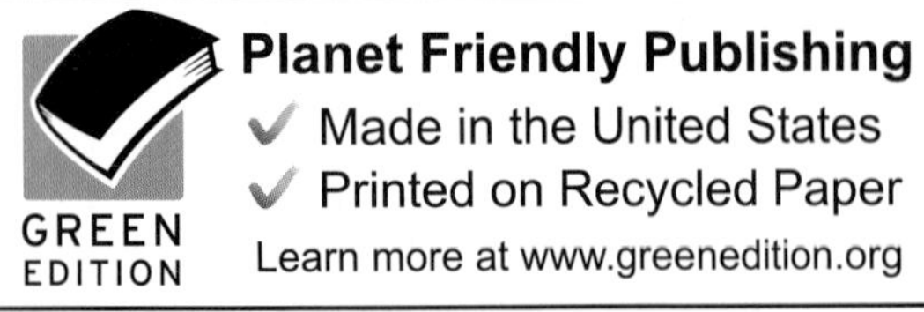

- Manufacturing books in the United States ensures compliance with strict environmental laws and eliminates the need for international freight shipping, a major contributor to global air pollution. Printing on recycled paper helps minimize our consumption of trees, water and fossil fuels.
- Trees Saved: 66 • Air Emissions Eliminated: 5,843 pounds
- Water Saved: 25,595 gallons • Solid Waste Eliminated: 2,605 pounds

Contents

How to Use this Book

Kaplan MCAT Biology, along with the other four books in our MCAT subject review series, brings the Kaplan classroom experience right into your home!

Kaplan has been preparing premeds for the MCAT for more than 40 years in our comprehensive courses. In the past 15 years alone, we've helped over 400,000 students prepare for this important exam and improve their chances of medical school admission.

TEACHER TIPS

Think of Kaplan's five MCAT subject books as having a private Kaplan teacher right by your side! We've created a team of the **top MCAT teachers in the country,** who have read through these comprehensive guides. On every page, they offer the same tips, advice, and Test Day insight as in their Kaplan classroom.

Pay close attention to **Teacher Tip** sidebars like this:

TEACHER TIP

Hyper- and hypotonicity are commonly tested using an RBC and the Na/K ATPase, which can control the volume of a RBC placed in a stressful environment.

When you see these, you know what you're getting the same insight and knowledge that students in Kaplan MCAT classrooms across the country receive.

HIGH-YIELD MCAT REVIEW

At the end of several chapters, you'll find a special **High-Yield Questions** spread. These questions tackle the most frequently tested topics found on the MCAT. For each type of problem, you will be provided with a stepwise technique for solving the question and key directional points on how to solve for the MCAT specifically. Included on each spread are two icons: the first, a sideways hand pointing toward equations, notes equations that you should memorize for the MCAT. The second, an open hand, indicates where in a problem you can stop without doing further calculation.

At the end of each topic you will find a "Takeaways" box, which gives a concise summary of the problem-solving approach; and a "Things to watch out for" box, which points out any caveats to the approach discussed above that usually lead to wrong answer choices. Finally, there is a "Similar Questions" box at the end so you can test your ability to apply the stepwise technique to analogous questions. You can find the answers in the Answers and Explanations section of this book.

We're confident that this guide, and our award-wining Kaplan teachers, can help you achieve your goals of MCAT success and admission into medical school!

Good luck!

EXPERT KAPLAN MCAT TEAM

Marilyn Engle

MCAT Master Teacher; Teacher Trainer; Kaplan National Teacher of the Year, 2006; Westwood Teacher of the Year, 2007; Westwood Trainer of the Year, 2007; Encino Trainer of the Tear, 2005

John Michael Linick

MCAT Teacher; Boulder Teacher of the Year, 2007; Summer Intensive Program Faculty Member

Dr. Glen Pearlstein

MCAT Master Teacher; Teacher Trainer; Westwood Teacher of the Year, 2006

Matthew B. Wilkinson

MCAT Teacher; Teacher Trainer; Lone Star Trainer of the Year, 2007

Introduction to the MCAT

THE MCAT

The Medical College Admission Test, affectionately known as the MCAT, is different from any other test you've encountered in your academic career. It's not like the knowledge-based exams from high school and college, whose emphasis was on memorizing and regurgitating information. Medical schools can assess your academic prowess by looking at your transcript. The MCAT isn't even like other standardized tests you may have taken, where the focus was on proving your general skills.

TEST TIP

The MCAT places more weight on your thought process. However, you must have a strong hold of the required core knowledge. The MCAT may not be a perfect gauge of your abilities, but it is a relatively objective way to compare you with students from different backgrounds and undergraduate institutions.

Medical schools use MCAT scores to assess whether you possess the foundation upon which to build a successful medical career. Though you certainly need to know the content to do well, the stress is on thought process, because the MCAT is above all else a thinking test. That's why it emphasizes reasoning, critical and analytical thinking, reading comprehension, data analysis, writing, and problem-solving skills.

The MCAT's power comes from its use as an indicator of your abilities. Good scores can open doors. Your power comes from preparation and mindset, because the key to MCAT success is knowing what you're up against. That's where this section of this book comes in. We'll explain the philosophy behind the test, review the sections one by one, show you sample questions, share some of Kaplan's proven methods, and clue you in to what the test makers are really after. You'll get a handle on the process, find a confident new perspective, and achieve your highest possible scores.

ABOUT THE MCAT

Information about the MCAT CBT is included below. For the latest information about the MCAT, visit www.kaptest.com/mcat.

MCAT CBT

Format	U.S.—All administrations on computer International—Most on computer with limited paper and pencil in a few isolated areas
Essay Grading	One human and one computer grader
Breaks	Optional break between each section
Length of MCAT Day	Approximately 5.5 hours
Test Dates	Multiple dates in January, April, May, June, July, August, and September Total of 24 administrations each year.
Delivery of Results	Within 30 days. If scores are delayed notification will be posted online at www.aamc.org/mcat Electronic and paper
Security	Government-issued ID Electronic thumbprint Electronic signature verification
Testing Centers	Small computer testing sites

PLANNING FOR THE TEST

As you look toward your preparation for the MCAT consider the following advice:

Complete your core course requirements as soon as possible. Take a strategic eye to your schedule and get core requirements out of the way now.

Take the MCAT once. The MCAT is a notoriously grueling standardized exam that requires extensive preparation. It is longer than the graduate admissions exams for business school (GMAT, 3½ hours), law school (LSAT, 3¼ hours) and graduate school (GRE, 2½ hours). You do not want to take it twice. Plan and prepare accordingly.

KAPLAN EXCLUSIVE

Go online and sign up for a local Kaplan Pre-Med Edge event to get the latest information on the test.

THE ROLE OF THE MCAT IN ADMISSIONS

More and more people are applying to medical school and more and more people are taking the MCAT. It's important for you to recognize that while a high MCAT score is a critical component in getting admitted to top med schools, it's not the only factor. Medical school admissions officers weigh grades, interviews, MCAT scores, level of involvement in extracurricular activities, as well as personal essays.

In a Kaplan survey of 130 pre-med advisors, 84 percent called the interview a "very important" part of the admissions process, followed closely by college grades (83 percent) and MCAT scores (76 percent). Kaplan's college admissions consulting practice works with students on all these issues so they can position themselves as strongly as possible. In addition, the AAMC has made it clear that scores will continue to be valid for three years, and that the scoring of the computer-based MCAT will not differ from that of the paper and pencil version.

REGISTRATION

The only way to register for the MCAT is online. The registration site is: www.aamc.org/mcat.

You will be able to access the site approximately six months before your test date. Payment must be made by MasterCard or Visa.

Go to www.aamc.org/mcat/registration.htm and download *MCAT Essentials* for information about registration, fees, test administration, and preparation. For other questions, contact:

MCAT Care Team
Association of American Medical Colleges
Section for Applicant Assessment Services
2450 N. St., NW
Washington, DC 20037
www.aamc.org/mcat
Email: mcat@aamc.org

You will want to take the MCAT in the year prior to your planned start date. For example, if you want to start medical school in Fall 2010, you will need to take the MCAT and apply in 2009. Don't drag your feet gathering information. You'll need time not only to prepare and practice for the test, but also to get all your registration work done.

ANATOMY OF THE MCAT

Before mastering strategies, you need to know exactly what you're dealing with on the MCAT. Let's start with the basics: The MCAT is, among other things, an endurance test.

TEST TIP

The MCAT should be viewed just like any other part of your application: as an opportunity to show the medical schools who you are and what you can do. Take control of your MCAT experience.

If you can't approach it with confidence and stamina, you'll quickly lose your composure. That's why it's so important that you take control of the test.

The MCAT consists of four timed sections: Physical Sciences, Verbal Reasoning, Writing Sample, and Biological Sciences. Later in this section we'll take an in-depth look at each MCAT section, including sample question types and specific test-smart hints, but here's a general overview, reflecting the order of the test sections and number of questions in each.

Physical Sciences

Time	70 minutes
Format	• 52 multiple-choice questions: approximately 7–9 passages with 4–8 questions each • approximately 10 stand-alone questions (not passage-based)
What it tests	basic general chemistry concepts, basic physics concepts, analytical reasoning, data interpretation

Verbal Reasoning

Time	60 minutes
Format	• 40 multiple-choice questions: approximately 7 passages with 5–7 questions each
What it tests	critical reading

Writing Sample

Time	60 minutes
Format	• 2 essay questions (30 minutes per essay)
What it tests	critical thinking, intellectual organization, written communication skills

Biological Sciences

Time	70 minutes
Format	• 52 multiple-choice questions: approximately 7–9 passages with 4–8 questions each • approximately 10 stand-alone questions (not passage-based)
What it tests	basic biology concepts, basic organic chemistry concepts, analytical reasoning, data interpretation

TEACHER TIP

There's no penalty for a wrong answer on the MCAT, so NEVER LEAVE ANY QUESTION BLANK, even if you have time only for a wild guess.

The sections of the test always appear in the same order:

Physical Sciences

[optional 10-minute break]

Verbal Reasoning

[optional 10-minute break]

Writing Sample

[optional 10-minute break]

Biological Sciences

SCORING

Each MCAT section receives its own score. Physical Sciences, Verbal Reasoning, and Biological Sciences are each scored on a scale ranging from 1–15, with 15 as the highest. The Writing Sample essays are scored alphabetically on a scale ranging from J to T, with T as the highest. The two essays are each evaluated by two official readers, so four critiques combine to make the alphabetical score.

The number of multiple-choice questions that you answer correctly per section is your "raw score." Your raw score will then be converted to yield the "scaled score"—the one that will fall somewhere in that 1–15 range. These scaled scores are what are reported to medical schools as your MCAT scores. All multiple-choice questions are worth the same amount—one raw point—and *there's no penalty for guessing*. That means that *you should always select an answer for every question, whether you get to that question or not!* This is an important piece of advice, so pay it heed. Never let time run out on any section without selecting an answer for every question.

Your score report will tell you—and your potential medical schools—not only your scaled scores, but also the national mean score for each section, standard deviation, national scoring profile for each section, and your percentile ranking.

WHAT'S A GOOD SCORE?

There's no such thing as a cut-and-dry "good score." Much depends on the strength of the rest of your application (if your transcript is first rate, the pressure to strut your stuff on the MCAT isn't as intense) and on where you want to go to school (different schools have different score expectations). Here are a few interesting statistics:

For each MCAT administration, the average scaled scores are approximately 8s for Physical Sciences, Verbal Reasoning, and Biological Sciences, and N for the Writing Sample. You need scores of at least 10–11s to be considered competitive by most medical schools, and if you're aiming for the top you've got to do even better, and score 12s and above.

You don't have to be perfect to do well. For instance, on the AAMC's Practice Test 5R, you could get as many as 10 questions wrong in Verbal Reasoning, 17 in Physical Sciences, and 16 in Biological Sciences and still score in the 80th percentile. To score in the 90th percentile, you could get as many as 7 wrong in Verbal Reasoning, 12 in Physical Sciences, and 12 in Biological Sciences. Even students who receive perfect scaled scores usually get a handful of questions wrong.

It's important to maximize your performance on every question. Just a few questions one way or the other can make a big difference in your scaled score. Here's a look at recent score profiles so you can get an idea of the shape of a typical score distribution.

TEST TIP

The percentile figure tells you how many other test takers scored at or below your level. In other words, a percentile figure of 80 means that 80 percent did as well or worse than you did, and that only 20 percent did better.

TEST TIP

The raw score of each administration is converted to a scaled score. The conversion varies with administrations. Hence, the same raw score will not always give you the same scaled score.

Physical Sciences		
Scaled Score	Percent Achieving Score	Percentile Rank Range
15	0.1	99.9–99.9
14	1.2	98.7–99.8
13	2.5	96.2–98.6
12	5.1	91.1–96.1
11	7.2	83.9–91.0
10	12.1	71.8–83.8
9	12.9	58.9–71.1
8	16.5	42.4–58.5
7	16.7	25.7–42.3
6	13.0	12.7–25.6
5	7.9	04.8–12.6
4	3.3	01.5–04.7
3	1.3	00.2–01.4
2	0.1	00.1–00.1
1	0.0	00.0–00.0
Scaled Score Mean = 8.1 Standard Deviation = 2.32		

Verbal Reasoning		
Scaled Score	Percent Achieving Score	Percentile Rank Range
15	0.1	99.9–99.9
14	0.2	99.7–99.8
13	1.8	97.9–99.6
12	3.6	94.3–97.8
11	10.5	83.8–94.2
10	15.6	68.2–83.7
9	17.2	51.0–68.1
8	15.4	35.6–50.9
7	10.3	25.3–35.5
6	10.9	14.4–25.2
5	6.9	07.5–14.3
4	3.9	03.6–07.4
3	2.0	01.6–03.5
2	0.5	00.1–01.5
1	0.0	00.0–00.0
Scaled Score Mean = 8.0 Standard Deviation = 2.43		

Writing Sample		
Scaled Score	Percent Achieving Score	Percentile Rank Range
T	0.5	99.9–99.9
S	2.8	94.7–99.8
R	7.2	96.0–99.3
Q	14.2	91.0–95.9
P	9.7	81.2–90.9
O	17.9	64.0–81.1
N	14.7	47.1–63.9
M	18.8	30.4–47.0
L	9.5	21.2–30.3
K	3.6	13.5–21.1
J	1.2	06.8–13.4
		02.9–06.7
		00.9–02.8
		00.2–00.8
		00.0–00.1
75th Percentile = Q 50th Percentile = O 25th Percentile = M		

Biological Sciences		
Scaled Score	Percent Achieving Score	Percentile Rank Range
15	0.1	99.9–99.9
14	1.2	98.7–99.8
13	2.5	96.2–98.6
12	5.1	91.1–96.1
11	7.2	83.9–91.0
10	12.1	71.8–83.8
9	12.9	58.9–71.1
8	16.5	42.4–58.5
7	16.7	25.7–42.3
6	13.0	12.7–25.6
5	7.9	04.8–12.6
4	3.3	01.5–04.7
3	1.3	00.2–01.4
2	0.1	00.1–00.1
1	0.0	00.0–00.0
Scaled Score Mean = 8.2 Standard Deviation = 2.39		

WHAT THE MCAT REALLY TESTS

It's important to grasp not only the nuts and bolts of the MCAT, so you'll know *what* to do on Test Day, but also the underlying principles of the test so you'll know *why* you're doing what you're doing on Test Day. We'll cover the straightforward MCAT facts later. Now it's time to examine the heart and soul of the MCAT, to see what it's really about.

THE MYTH

Most people preparing for the MCAT fall prey to the myth that the MCAT is a straightforward science test. They think something like this:

> *"It covers the four years of science I had to take in school: biology, chemistry, physics, and organic chemistry. It even has equations. OK, so it has Verbal Reasoning and Writing, but those sections are just to see if we're literate, right? The important stuff is the science. After all, we're going to be doctors."*

Well, here's the little secret no one seems to want you to know: The MCAT is not just a science test; it's also a thinking test. This means that the test is designed to let you demonstrate your thought process, not only your thought content.

The implications are vast. Once you shift your test-taking paradigm to match the MCAT modus operandi, you'll find a new level of confidence and control over the test. You'll begin to work with the nature of the MCAT rather than against it. You'll be more efficient and insightful as you prepare for the test, and you'll be more relaxed on Test Day. In fact, you'll be able to see the MCAT for what it is rather than for what it's dressed up to be. We want your Test Day to feel like a visit with a familiar friend instead of an awkward blind date.

THE ZEN OF MCAT

Medical schools do not need to rely on the MCAT to see what you already know. Admission committees can measure your subject-area proficiency using your undergraduate coursework and grades. Schools are most interested in the potential of your mind.

In recent years, many medical schools have shifted pedagogic focus away from an information-heavy curriculum to a concept-based curriculum. There is currently more emphasis placed on problem solving, holistic thinking, and cross-disciplinary study. Be careful not to dismiss this important point, figuring you'll wait to worry about academic trends until you're actually in medical school. This trend affects you right now, because it's reflected in the MCAT. Every good tool matches its task. In this case the tool is the test, used to measure you and other candidates, and the task is to quantify how likely it is that you'll succeed in medical school.

Your intellectual potential—how skillfully you annex new territory into your mental boundaries, how quickly you build "thought highways" between ideas, how confidently and creatively you solve problems—is far more important to admission committees than your ability to recite Young's modulus for every material known to man. The schools assume they can expand your knowledge base. They choose applicants carefully because expansive knowledge is not enough to succeed in medical school or in the profession. There's something more. It's this "something more" that the MCAT is trying to measure.

Every section on the MCAT tests essentially the same higher-order thinking skills: analytical reasoning, abstract thinking, and problem solving.

Most test takers get trapped into thinking they are being tested strictly about biology, chemistry, etc. Thus, they approach each section with a new outlook on what's expected. This constant mental gear-shifting can be exhausting, not to mention counterproductive. Instead of perceiving the test as parsed into radically different sections, you need to maintain your focus on the underlying nature of the test: It's designed to test your thinking skills, not your information-recall skills. Each test section thus presents a variation on the same theme.

TEST TIP

Don't think of the sections of the MCAT as unrelated timed pieces. Each is a variation on the same theme, because the underlying purpose of each section and of the test as a whole is to evaluate your thinking skills. Memorizing formulas won't boost your score. Understanding fundamental scientific principles will.

WHAT ABOUT THE SCIENCE?

With this perspective, you may be left asking these questions: "What about the science? What about the content? Don't I need to know the basics?" The answer is a resounding "Yes!" You must be fluent in the different languages of the test. You cannot do well on the MCAT if you don't know the basics of physics, general chemistry, biology, and organic chemistry. We recommend that you take one year each of biology, general chemistry, organic chemistry, and physics before taking the MCAT, and that you review the content in this book thoroughly. Knowing these basics is just the beginning of doing well on the MCAT. That's a shock to most test takers. They presume that once they recall or relearn their undergraduate science, they are ready to do battle against the MCAT. Wrong! They merely have directions to the battlefield. They lack what they need to beat the test: a copy of the test maker's battle plan!

You won't be drilled on facts and formulas on the MCAT. You'll need to demonstrate ability to reason based on ideas and concepts. The science questions are painted with a broad brush, testing your general understanding.

TAKE CONTROL: THE MCAT MINDSET

In addition to being a thinking test, as we've stressed, the MCAT is a standardized test. As such, it has its own consistent patterns and idiosyncrasies that can actually work in your favor. This is the key to why test preparation works. You have the opportunity to familiarize yourself with those consistent peculiarities, to adopt the proper test-taking mindset.

TEST TIP

Those perfectionist tendencies that make you a good student and a good medical school candidate may work against you in MCAT Land. If you get stuck on a question or passage, move on. Perfectionism is for medical school—not the MCAT. Moreover, you don't need to understand every word of a passage before you go on to the questions—what's tripping you up may not even be relevant to what you'll be asked.

The following are some overriding principles of the MCAT Mindset that will be covered in depth in the chapters to come:

- Read actively and critically.
- Translate prose into your own words.

- Save the toughest questions for last.
- Know the test and its components inside and out.
- Do MCAT-style problems in each topic area after you've reviewed it.
- Allow your confidence to build on itself.
- Take full-length practice tests a week or two before the test to break down the mystique of the real experience.
- Learn from your mistakes—get the most out of your practice tests.
- Look at the MCAT as a challenge, the first step in your medical career, rather than as an arbitrary obstacle.

That's what the MCAT Mindset boils down to: Taking control. Being proactive. Being on top of the testing experience so that you can get as many points as you can as quickly and as easily as possible. Keep this in mind as you read and work through the material in this book and, of course, as you face the challenge on Test Day.

Now that you have a better idea of what the MCAT is all about, let's take a tour of the individual test sections. Although the underlying skills being tested are similar, each MCAT section requires that you call into play a different domain of knowledge. So, though we encourage you to think of the MCAT as a holistic and unified test, we also recognize that the test is segmented by discipline and that there are characteristics unique to each section. In the overviews, we'll review sample questions and answers and discuss section-specific strategies. For each of the sections—Verbal Reasoning, Physical/Biological Sciences, and the Writing Sample—we'll present you with the following:

- **The Big Picture**
  You'll get a clear view of the section and familiarize yourself with what it's really evaluating.
- **A Closer Look**
  You'll explore the types of questions that will appear and master the strategies you'll need to deal with them successfully.
- **Highlights**
  The key approaches to each section are outlined, for reinforcement and quick review.

TEST EXPERTISE

The first year of medical school is a frenzied experience for most students. In order to meet the requirements of a rigorous work schedule, students either learn to prioritize and budget their time or else fall hopelessly behind. It's no surprise, then, that the MCAT, the test specifically designed to predict success in the first year of medical school, is a high-speed, time-intensive test. It demands excellent time-management skills as well as that sine qua non of the successful physician—grace under pressure.

It's one thing to answer a Verbal Reasoning question correctly; it's quite another to answer several correctly in a limited time frame. The same goes for Physical and Biological Sciences—it's a whole new ball game once you move from doing an individual passage at your leisure to handling a full section under actual timed conditions. You also need to budget your time for the Writing Sample, but this section isn't as time sensitive. Nevertheless when it comes to the multiple-choice sections, time pressure is a factor that affects virtually every test taker.

TEST TIP

For complete MCAT success, you've got to get as many correct answers as possible in the time you're allotted. Knowing the strategies is not enough. You have to perfect your time-management skills so that you get a chance to use those strategies on as many questions as possible.

So when you're comfortable with the content of the test, your next challenge will be to take it to the next level—test expertise—which will enable you to manage the all-important time element of the test.

THE FIVE BASIC PRINCIPLES OF TEST EXPERTISE

On some tests, if a question seems particularly difficult you'll spend significantly more time on it, as you'll probably be given more points for correctly answering a hard question. Not so on the MCAT. Remember, every MCAT question, no matter how hard, is worth a single point. There's no partial credit or "A" for effort. Moreover because there are so many questions to do in so little time, you'd be a fool to spend 10 minutes getting a point for a hard question and then not have time to get a couple of quick points from three easy questions later in the section.

TEST TIP

In order to meet the stringent time requirements of the MCAT, you have to cultivate the following elements of test expertise:

- Feel free to skip questions.
- Learn to recognize and seek out questions you can do.
- Use a process of answer elimination.
- Remain calm.
- Keep track of time.

Given this combination—limited time, all questions equal in weight—you've got to develop a way of handling the test sections to make sure you get as many points as you can as quickly and easily as you can. Here are the principles that will help you do that:

1. FEEL FREE TO SKIP AROUND

One of the most valuable strategies to help you finish the sections in time is to learn to recognize and deal first with the questions that are easier and more familiar to you. That means you must temporarily skip those that promise to be difficult and time-consuming, if you feel comfortable doing so. You can always come back to these at the end, and if you run out of time, you're much better off not getting to questions you may have had difficulty with, rather than not getting to potentially feasible material. Of course, because there's no guessing penalty, always put an answer to every question on the test, whether you get to it or not. (It's not practical to skip passages, so do those in order.)

TEST TIP

Every question is worth exactly one point, but questions vary dramatically in difficulty level. Given a shortage of time, work on easy questions and then move on to the hard ones.

This strategy is difficult for most test takers; we're conditioned to do things in order. But give it a try when you practice. Remember, if you do the test in the exact order given, you're letting the test makers control you. But you control how you take this test. On the other hand, if skipping around goes against your moral fiber and makes you a nervous wreck—don't do it. Just be mindful of the clock, and don't get bogged down with the tough questions.

2. LEARN TO RECOGNIZE AND SEEK OUT QUESTIONS YOU CAN DO

Another thing to remember about managing the test sections is that MCAT questions and passages, unlike items on the SAT and other standardized tests, are not presented in order of difficulty. There's no rule that says you have to work through the sections in any particular order; in fact, the test makers scatter the easy and difficult questions throughout the section, in effect rewarding those who actually get to the end. Don't lose sight of what you're being tested for along with your reading and thinking skills: efficiency and cleverness.

Don't waste time on questions you can't do. We know that skipping a possibly tough question is easier said than done; we all have the natural instinct to plow through test sections in their given order. But it just doesn't pay off on the MCAT. The computer won't be impressed if you get the toughest question right. If you dig in your heels on a tough question, refusing to move on until you've cracked it, well, you're letting your ego get in the way of your test score. A test section (not to mention life itself) is too short to waste on lost causes.

TEST TIP

Don't let your ego sabotage your score. It isn't easy for some of us to give up on a tough, time-consuming question, but sometimes it's better to say "uncle." Remember, there's no point of honor at stake here, but there are MCAT points at stake.

3. USE A PROCESS OF ANSWER ELIMINATION

Using a process of elimination is another way to answer questions both quickly and effectively. There are two ways to get all the answers right on the MCAT. You either know all the right answers, or you know all the wrong answers. Because there are three times as many wrong answers, you should be able to eliminate some if not all of them. By doing so you either get to the correct response or increase your chances of guessing the correct response. You start out with a 25 percent chance of picking the right answer, and with each eliminated answer your odds go up. Eliminate one, and you'll have a $33\frac{1}{3}$ percent chance of picking the right one, eliminate two, and you'll have a 50 percent chance, and, of course, eliminate three, and you'll have a 100 percent chance. Increase your efficiency by actually crossing out the wrong choices on the screen using the strikethrough feature. Remember to look for wrong-answer traps when you're eliminating. Some answers are designed to seduce you by distorting the correct answer.

4. REMAIN CALM

It's imperative that you remain calm and composed while working through a section. You can't allow yourself to become so rattled by one hard reading passage that it throws off your performance on the rest of the section. Expect to find at least one killer passage in every section, but remember, you won't be the only one to have trouble with it. The test is curved to take the tough material into account. Having trouble with a difficult question isn't going to ruin your score—but getting upset about it and letting it throw you off track will. When you understand that part of the test maker's goal is to reward those who keep their composure, you'll recognize the importance of not panicking when you run into challenging material.

5. KEEP TRACK OF TIME

Of course, the last thing you want to happen is to have time called on a particular section before you've gotten to half the questions. Therefore, it's essential that you pace yourself, keeping in mind the general guidelines for how long to spend on any individual question or passage. Have a sense of how long you have to do each question, so you know when you're exceeding the limit and should start to move faster.

So, when working on a section, always remember to keep track of time. Don't spend a wildly disproportionate amount of time on any one question or group of questions. Also, give yourself 30 seconds or so at the end of each section to fill in answers for any questions you haven't gotten to.

SECTION-SPECIFIC PACING

Let's now look at the section-specific timing requirements and some tips for meeting them. Keep in mind that the times per question or passage are only averages; there are bound to be some that take less time and some that take more. Try to stay balanced. Remember, too, that every question is of equal worth, so don't get hung up on any one. Think about it: If a question is so hard that it takes you a long time to answer it, chances are you may get it wrong anyway. In that case, you'd have nothing to show for your extra time but a lower score.

VERBAL REASONING

Allow yourself approximately eight to ten minutes per passage and respective questions. It may sound like a lot of time, but it goes quickly. Keep in mind that some passages are longer than others. On average, give yourself about three or four minutes to read and then four to six minutes for the questions.

> **TEST TIP**
>
> For Verbal Reasoning, here are some of the important time techniques to remember:
>
> - Spend eight to ten minutes per passage
> - Allow about three to four minutes to read and four to six minutes for the questions

PHYSICAL AND BIOLOGICAL SCIENCES

Averaging over each section, you'll have about one minute and 20 seconds per question. Some questions, of course, will take more time, some less. A science passage plus accompanying questions should take about eight to nine minutes, depending on how many questions there are. Standalone questions can take anywhere from a few seconds to a minute or more. Again, the rule is to do your best work first. Also, don't feel that you have to understand everything in a passage before you go on to the questions. You may not need that deep an understanding to answer questions, because a lot of information may be extraneous. You should overcome your perfectionism and use your time wisely.

> **TEST TIP**
>
> Some suggestions for maximizing your time on the science sections:
>
> - Spend about eight to nine minutes per passage
> - Maximize points by doing the questions you can do first
> - Don't waste valuable time trying to understand extraneous material

WRITING SAMPLE

You have exactly 30 minutes for each essay. As mentioned in discussion of the 7-step approach to this section, you should allow approximately five minutes to prewrite the essay, 23 minutes to write the essay, and two minutes to proofread. It's important that you budget your time, so you don't get cut off.

COMPUTER-BASED TESTING STRATEGIES

ARRIVE AT THE TESTING CENTER EARLY

Get to the testing center early to jump-start your brain. However, if they allow you to begin your test early, decline.

USE THE MOUSE TO YOUR ADVANTAGE

If you are right-handed, practice using the mouse with your left hand for Test Day. This way, you'll increase speed by keeping the pencil in your right hand to write on your scratch paper. If you are left-handed, use your right hand for the mouse.

KNOW THE TUTORIAL BEFORE TEST DAY

You will save time on Test Day by knowing exactly how the test will work. Click through any tutorial pages and save time.

PRACTICE WITH SCRATCH PAPER

Going forward, always practice using scratch paper when solving questions because this is how you will do it on Test Day. Never write directly on a written test.

GET NEW SCRATCH PAPER

Between sections, get a new piece of scratch paper even if you only used part of the old one. This will maximize the available space for each section and minimize the likelihood of you running out of paper to write on.

REMEMBER YOU CAN ALWAYS GO BACK

Just because you finish a passage or move on, remember you can come back to questions about which you are uncertain. You have the "marking" option to your advantage. However, as a general rule minimize the amount of questions you mark or skip.

MARK INCOMPLETE WORK

If you need to go back to a question, clearly mark the work you've done on the scratch paper with the question number. This way, you will be able to find your work easily when you come back to tackle the question.

LOOK AWAY AT TIMES

Taking the test on computer leads to faster eye-muscle fatigue. Use the Kaplan strategy of looking at a distant object at regular intervals. This will keep you fresher at the end of the test.

PRACTICE ON THE COMPUTER

This is the most critical aspect of adapting to computer-based testing. Like anything else, in order to perform well on computer-based tests you must practice. Spend time reading passages and answering questions on the computer. You often will have to scroll when reading passages.

Part I
Subject Review

CHAPTER 1

THE CELL

The cell is the fundamental unit of all living things. Every function in biology involves a process that occurs within cells or at the interface between cells. Therefore, to understand biology, you need to appreciate the structure and function of the different parts of the cell (the organelles) as well as the properties that define the plasma membrane that surrounds the cell.

CELL THEORY

The cell was not discovered or studied in detail until the development of the microscope in the 17 century. Since then much more has been learned, and a unifying theory known as the **Cell Theory** has been proposed.

TEACHER TIP

Know these points: The MCAT likes to test what sorts of systems could be considered "cells."

The Cell Theory may be summarized as follows:

- All living things are composed of cells.
- The cell is the basic functional unit of life.
- Cells arise only from pre-existing cells.
- Cells carry genetic information in the form of **DNA.** This genetic material is passed from parent cell to daughter cell.

METHODS AND TOOLS

There are many tools available to study the cell and its structures. Three primary methods are **microscopy, autoradiography,** and **centrifugation.**

A. MICROSCOPY

Of the many tools used by scientists to study cells, the microscope is the most basic. **Magnification** is the increase in apparent size of an object. **Resolution** is the differentiation of two closely situated objects.

Teacher Tip

Although the power of a microscope is a physics concept, it is commonly also tested in biology.

1. Compound Light Microscope

A compound light microscope uses two lenses or lens systems to magnify an object. The total magnification is equal to the product of the eyepiece magnification (usually 10×) and the magnification of the selected objective lens (usually 4×, 10×, 20×, or 100×). The chief components of the microscope are the **diaphragm,** the **coarse adjustment knob,** and the **fine adjustment knob** (see Figure 1.1).

- The diaphragm controls the amount of light passing through the specimen.
- The coarse adjustment knob roughly focuses the image.
- The fine adjustment knob sharply focuses the image.

In general, the compound light microscope is used in the observation of nonliving specimens. Light microscopy requires contrast between cells and cell structures; such contrast is obtained through staining techniques that result in cell death. Various stains and dyes may be used for light microscopy. For example, the dye hematoxylin reveals the distribution of **DNA** and **RNA** within a cell due to its affinity for negatively charged molecules.

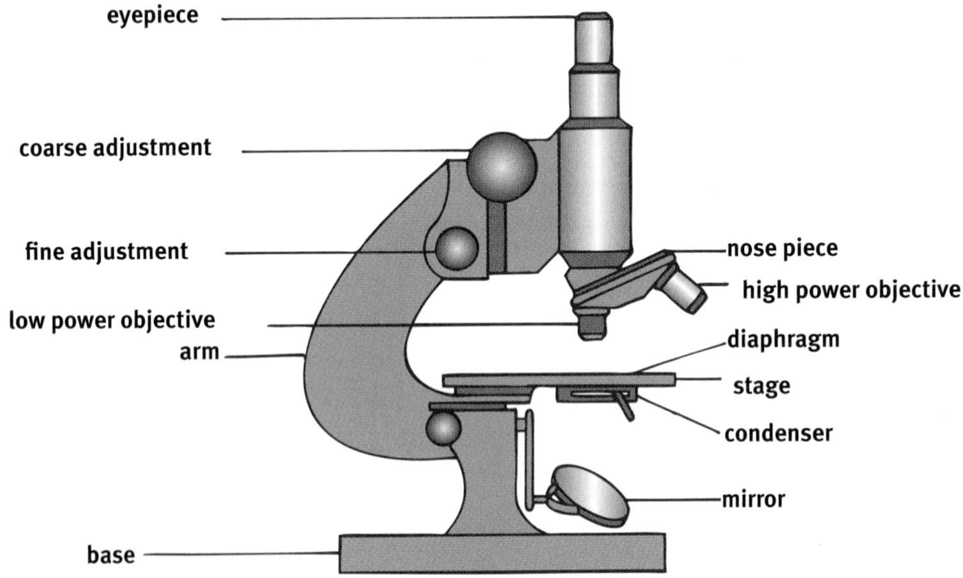

Figure 1.1. Compound Light Microscope

2. Phase Contrast Microscope

A phase contrast microscope is a special type of light microscope that permits the study of living cells. Differences in refractive index are used to produce contrast between cellular structures. This technique does not kill the specimen.

TEACHER TIP

Don't overfocus on the physics here; concepts like refraction are much more likely to be tested in the Physical Sciences section rather than here.

3. Electron Microscope

An electron microscope uses a beam of electrons to allow a thousand-fold higher magnification than is possible with light microscopy. Unfortunately, examination of living specimens is not possible because of the preparations necessary for electron microscopy; tissues must be fixed and sectioned and, sometimes, stained with solutions of heavy metals.

B. AUTORADIOGRAPHY

This technique uses radioactive molecules to trace and identify cell structures and biochemical activity. Cells are exposed to a radioactive compound for a brief, measured period of time (enough time for it to be incorporated into the cell). They are incubated, fixed at various intervals, and processed for microscopy. Each preparation is covered with a film of photographic emulsion. The preparations must be kept in the dark for several days while the radioactive compound decays. The emulsion is then developed; dark silver grains reveal the distribution of radioactivity within the specimen. Autoradiography can be used to study protein synthesis: Labeling amino acids with radioactive isotopes allows the pathways of protein synthesis to be examined. Similar techniques are used to study the mechanisms of DNA and RNA synthesis.

TEACHER TIP

While concepts like these may seem very basic, a simple understanding is often all that is necessary to result in a higher score.

C. CENTRIFUGATION

Differential centrifugation can be used to separate cells or mixtures of cells without destroying them in the process. At lower speeds, cell mixtures separate into layers on the basis of cell type. Spinning fragmented cells at high speeds in the centrifuge will cause their components to sediment at different levels in the test tube on the basis of their respective densities. For example, centrifugation of a **eukaryotic** cell sediments high-density **ribosomes** at the bottom of the test tube, while low-density **mitochondria** and **lysosomes** remain at the top.

TEACHER TIP

Although viruses cannot replicate independently, they do contain a genome in the form of RNA or DNA.

TEACHER TIP

KEY POINT: The regulation of prokaryotic genomes is distinct from that of eukaryotic ones.

MCAT SYNOPSIS

Prokaryotes	Eukaryotes
Bacteria	Protists, fungi, plants, animals
Cell wall present in all prokaryotes	Cell wall present in fungi and plants only
No nucleus	Nucleus
Ribosomes (subunits = 30S and 50S)	Ribosomes (subunits = 40S and 60S)
No membrane-bound organelles	Membrane-bound organelles

PROKARYOTES VS. EUKARYOTES

Cells can be structurally categorized into two distinct groups, **prokaryotic** and **eukaryotic. Viruses** occupy a unique category and are not technically considered cells because they are not capable of living independently.

A. PROKARYOTES

Prokaryotes, which include **bacteria** and **cyanobacteria** (blue-green algae), are unicellular organisms with a simple cell structure. Prokaryotic cells have an outer cell membrane but do not contain any membrane-bound organelles. There is no true nucleus; the genetic material consists of a single circular molecule of DNA concentrated in an area of the cell called the **nucleoid** region. In addition, there may be smaller rings of DNA called **plasmids,** consisting of just a few genes. Plasmids replicate independently of the main chromosome, and often contain genes that allow the prokaryote to survive adverse conditions. Plasmids are one mechanism, for example, of imparting resistance to antibiotics.

Bacteria have a **cell wall,** a **cell membrane, cytoplasm,** ribosomes (somewhat different from those found in eukaryotes), and sometimes **flagella** (also different from those in eukaryotes) that are used for locomotion. Respiration occurs at the cell membrane (see Figure 1.2).

B. EUKARYOTES

All multicellular organisms and all nonbacteria unicellular organisms are composed of eukaryotic cells. A typical eukaryotic cell is bounded by a cell membrane and contains cytoplasm. Cytoplasm contains **organelles** suspended in a semifluid medium called the **cytosol.** The genetic material consists of linear strands of DNA organized into **chromosomes** and located within a membrane-enclosed organelle called the **nucleus.** Although both animal and plant cells are eukaryotic, they differ from each other. **Centrioles,** located in the centrosome area, are found in animal cells but not in plant cells (see Figure 1.3).

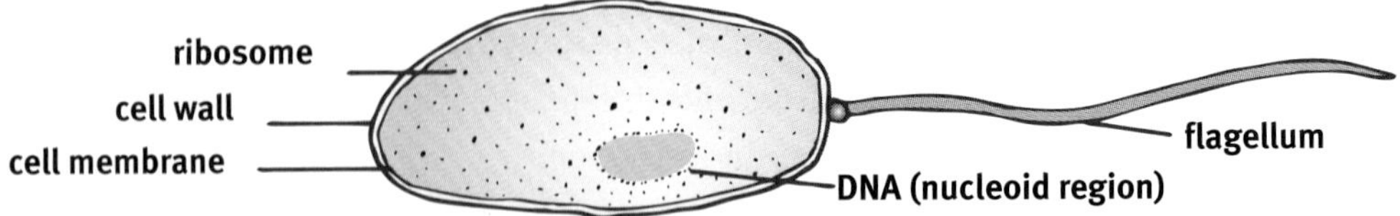

Figure 1.2. Prokaryotic Cell

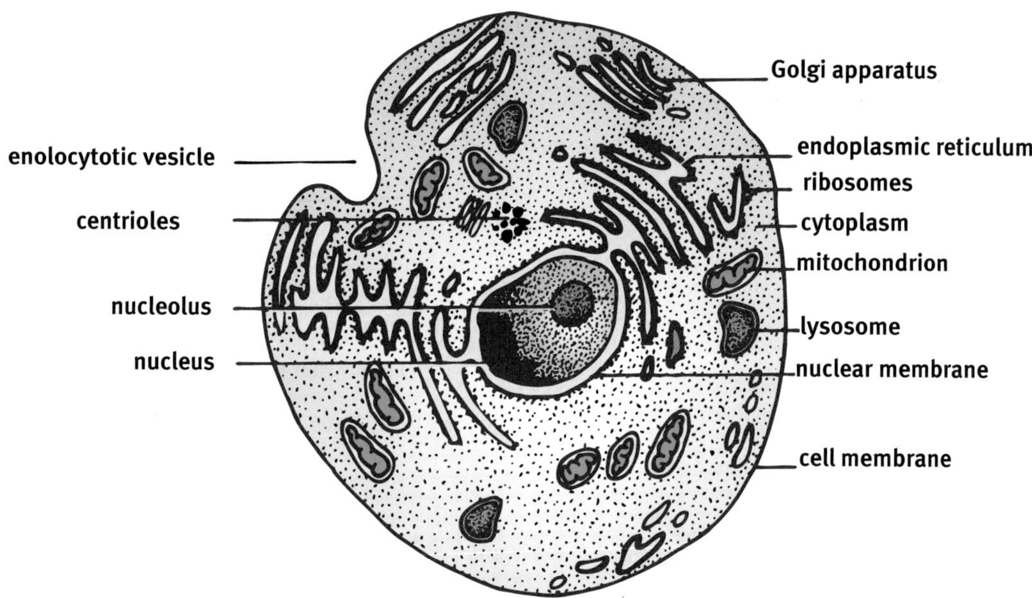

Figure 1.3. Eukaryotic Cell

EUKARYOTIC ORGANELLES

Cytosol is the fluid component of the cytoplasm and consists of an aqueous solution containing free proteins, nutrients, and other solutes. The **cytoskeleton,** which is composed of **microtubules, microfilaments, intermediate fibers,** and other accessory proteins, is also found in the cytosol. These proteinaceous filaments give the cell its shape and anchor the organelles. They also function in cell maintenance and aid in intracellular transport. The cell membrane surrounds the cell and regulates passage of materials in both directions.

The organelles are specialized structures of unique form and function. They include the nucleus, ribosomes, **endoplasmic reticulum, Golgi apparatus, vesicles, vacuoles,** lysosomes, **microbodies,** mitochondria, chloroplasts, and centrioles.

A. CELL MEMBRANE

The cell membrane (plasma membrane) encloses the cell and is composed of a **phospholipid bilayer.** Phospholipids have both a hydrophilic (polar) phosphoric acid and a hydrophobic (nonpolar) fatty acid region. In a lipid bilayer, the hydrophilic regions are found on the exterior surfaces of the membrane whereas the hydrophobic regions are found on the interior of the membrane (see Figure 1.4).

Teacher Tip

The ability of different molecules to traverse a membrane is critical to cells. The cell must be able to allow nutrients and required compounds in, while preventing bacteria, viruses, and harmful compounds from entering.

MCAT FAVORITE

1) Nonpolar (hydrophobic) compounds pass through plasma membrane easily.
2) Polar (hydrophilic) compounds do NOT pass through plasma membrane easily. They may require the use of carrier proteins.

This phospholipids bilayer structure allows the cell membrane to regulate the passage of material and molecules in and out of the cell and exhibits **selective permeability.** Selective permeability means that the cell membrane allows some compounds/molecules to pass through freely, where others are prohibited or regulated. Specifically, small nonpolar (hydrophobic) molecules generally pass through freely (diffuse) across the cell membrane. In contrast, charged ions and large molecules such as proteins and complex carbohydrates do not diffuse freely. They may require carrier proteins to help carry them across the cell membrane.

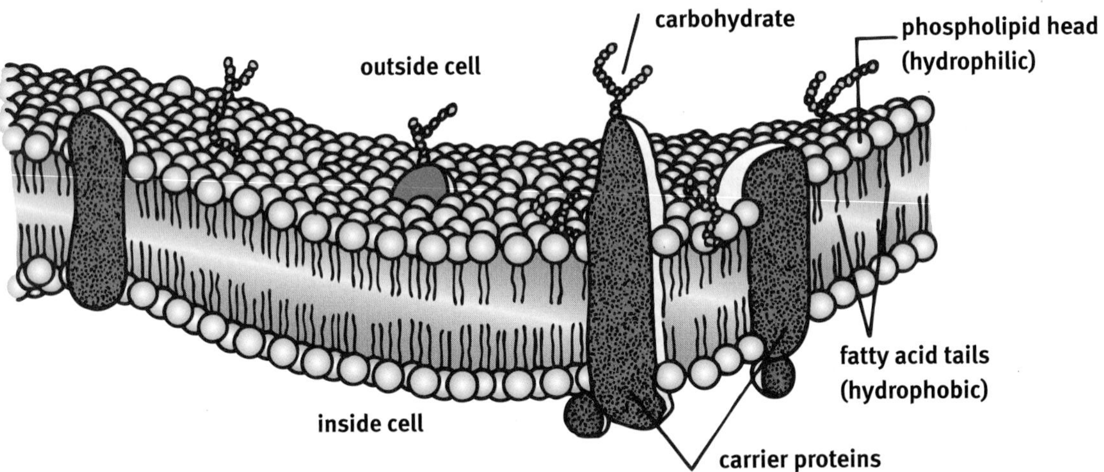

Figure 1.4. Fluid Mosaic Model

According to the generally accepted fluid mosaic model, the cell membrane consists of a phospholipids bilayer with proteins embedded throughout. The lipids and many of the proteins can move freely within the membrane. Cholesterol molecules are often embedded in the hydrophobic interior and contribute to the cell membrane's fluidity. Proteins interspersed throughout the membrane may be partially or completely embedded in the bilayer; one or both ends of the protein may extend beyond the membrane on either side. Such proteins can play a role in cell adhesion by forming junctions with proteins on adjacent cells. Transport proteins are membrane-spanning proteins that allow certain ions and polar molecules to pass through the lipid bilayer. Cell adhesion molecules (CAMs) are proteins that contribute to cell recognition and adhesion, and are particularly important during development.

Receptors are complex proteins or glycoproteins generally embedded in the membrane with sites that bind to specific molecules in the cell's external environment. The receptor may carry the molecule into the cell via **pinocytosis** or it may signal across the membrane and into the cell via a second messenger (see chapter 11).

TEACHER TIP

We will have more to say about receptors later; they may be tested in many ways including membrane trafficking, isomerism, specificity, and binding kinetics.

B. NUCLEUS

The nucleus controls the activities of the cell, including cell division. It is surrounded by a **nuclear membrane, or envelope,** which is a double membrane that maintains a nuclear environment distinct from that of the cytoplasm. Interspersed throughout the nuclear membrane are **nuclear pores** that allow selective two-way exchange of materials between the nucleus and the cytoplasm. The nucleus contains the DNA, which is complexed with structural proteins called **histones** to form chromosomes. The **nucleolus** is a dense structure in the nucleus where ribosomal RNA (rRNA) synthesis occurs.

C. RIBOSOMES

Ribosomes are the sites of protein production and are synthesized by the nucleolus (see chapter 14). Ribosomes consist of two subunits, one large and one small; each subunit is composed of rRNA and proteins. **Free ribosomes** are found in the cytoplasm, while **bound ribosomes** line the outer membrane of the endoplasmic reticulum.

D. ENDOPLASMIC RETICULUM

The endoplasmic reticulum **(ER)** is a network of membrane-enclosed spaces connected at points with the nuclear membrane. ER with ribosomes lining its outer surface is known as **rough ER (RER)** and ER without ribosomes is known as **smooth ER.**

KAPLAN EXCLUSIVE

Rough ER—makes protein for secretion and intracellular transport.

Smooth ER—lipid synthesis and detoxification.

In general, ER is involved in the transport of materials throughout the cell, especially those materials destined to be secreted from the cell. Smooth ER is involved in lipid synthesis and the detoxification of drugs and poisons, while rough ER is involved in protein synthesis. Proteins synthesized by the bound ribosomes cross into the cisternae of the RER, where they undergo chemical modification. The proteins then cross into smooth ER, where they are secreted into cytoplasmic vesicles and transported to the Golgi apparatus.

TEACHER TIP

The ER is like a factory. It produces all the products that the cell puts out.

TEACHER TIP

The Golgi is packaging central. It directs the packages where to go within the cell.

E. GOLGI APPARATUS

The Golgi apparatus consists of a stack of membrane-enclosed sacs. The Golgi receives vesicles and their contents from smooth ER, modifies them (e.g., glycosylation), repackages them into vesicles, and distributes them. The Golgi is particularly active in the distribution of newly synthesized materials to the cell surface. **Secretory vesicles,** produced by the Golgi, release their contents to the cell's exterior by the process of **exocytosis.**

F. VESICLES AND VACUOLES

Vesicles and vacuoles are membrane-bound sacs involved in the transport and storage of materials that are ingested, secreted, processed, or digested by the cell. Vacuoles are larger than vesicles and are more likely to be found in plant cells.

G. LYSOSOMES

Lysosomes are membrane-bound vesicles that contain hydrolytic enzymes involved in intracellular digestion. These enzymes are maximally effective at a pH of 5 and therefore need to be enclosed within the lysosome—an acidic environment distinct from the neutral pH of the cytosol. Lysosomes fuse with endocytotic vacuoles, thereby breaking down the material ingested by the cell. Lysosomes also aid in renewing a cell's own components by breaking down the old ones and releasing their molecular building blocks into the cytosol for reuse. A cell in an injured or dying tissue may "commit suicide" by rupturing the lysosome membrane and releasing its hydrolytic enzymes, which will digest cellular contents; this process is referred to as **autolysis.**

H. MICROBODIES

Microbodies are membrane-bound organelles specialized as containers for metabolic reactions. Two important types of microbodies are **peroxisomes** and **glyoxysomes.** Peroxisomes contain oxidative enzymes that catalyze a class of reactions in which hydrogen peroxide is produced by the transfer of hydrogen from a substrate to oxygen. Peroxisomes break fats down into smaller molecules that can be used for fuel, and are also used in the liver to detoxify compounds harmful to the body, such as alcohol. Glyoxysomes are usually found in fat tissue of germinating seedlings. They are used by the seedling to convert fats into sugars until the seedling is mature enough to produce its own supply of sugars by photosynthesis.

I. MITOCHONDRIA

Mitochondria are the sites of aerobic respiration within the cell and hence the suppliers of energy. Each mitochondrion is bound by an outer and an inner phospholipid bilayer membrane. The outer membrane is smooth and acts as a sieve, allowing molecules through on the basis of size. The area between the inner and outer membranes is known as the **intermembrane space.** The inner membrane has many convolutions called **cristae** and a high protein content that includes the proteins of the electron transport chain. The area bounded by the inner membrane is known as the mitochondrial **matrix** and is the site of many of the reactions in cell respiration (see chapter 3). Mitochondria are different from the other organelles in that they are **semiautonomous**; i.e., they contain their own DNA (which is circular) and ribosomes, which enable them to produce some of their own proteins and to self-replicate by **binary fission.** Mitochondria are believed by many to have been early prokaryotic cells that evolved a symbiotic relationship with the ancestors of eukaryotic cells.

TEACHER TIP

FUN FACT: Mitochondria are only inherited from the mother. That means if a woman has a genetic defect in one of her mitochondrial genes, she will pass it on to all of her children; conversely, a man cannot pass it on to *any* of his children.

J. CELL WALL

Many eukaryotic cells such as plant cells and fungi are surrounded by a tough outer cell wall that protects the cell from external stimuli and desiccation. Animal cells are **not** surrounded by a cell wall.

K. CENTRIOLES

Centrioles are a specialized type of microtubule (see below) involved in spindle organization during cell division and are **not** bound by a membrane. Animal cells usually have a pair of centrioles that are oriented at right angles to each other and lie in a region called the **centrosome.** Plant cells do **not** contain centrioles.

L. CYTOSKELETON

The cytoskeleton gives the cell mechanical support, maintains its shape, and functions in cell motility. It is composed of microtubules, microfilaments, and intermediate filaments.

Microtubules are hollow rods made up of polymerized **tubulins** that radiate throughout the cell and provide it with support. Microtubules provide a framework for organelle movement within the cell. Centrioles, which direct the separation of chromosomes during cell division, are composed of microtubules (see chapter 4). **Cilia** and flagella are specialized arrangements of microtubules that extend from certain cells and are involved in cell motility.

Microfilaments are solid rods of **actin,** involved in cell movement as well as support. Muscle contraction, for example, is based on the interaction of actin with **myosin** in muscle cells (see chapter 6). Microfilaments move materials across the plasma membrane, for instance, in the contraction phase of cell division, and in amoeboid movement.

Intermediate filaments are a collection of fibers involved in maintenance of cytoskeletal integrity. Their diameters fall between those of microtubules and microfilaments.

MCAT FAVORITE

Gradients rule! Be on the lookout throughout biology for examples in which gradients drive physiological function:

- Oxygen-carbon dioxide exchange in tissues and lungs
- Urine formation in the kidneys
- Depolarization of neurons and conduction of the action potential
- Proton gradient in mitochondria
- Exchange of materials between the maternal and fetal blood across the placenta

MOVEMENT ACROSS THE CELL MEMBRANE

Substances can move into and out of cells in various ways. Some methods occur passively, without energy, while others are active and require energy expenditure (ATP).

A. SIMPLE DIFFUSION

Simple diffusion is the net movement of dissolved particles down their concentration gradients—from a region of higher concentration to a region of lower concentration. This is a passive process (see Figure 1.5). **Osmosis** is the simple diffusion of water from a region of lower solute concentration to a region of higher solute concentration. If a membrane is impermeable to a particular solute, then water will flow across the membrane until the differences in the solute concentrations have been equilibrated. Differences in the concentration of substances to which the membrane is impermeable affect the direction of osmosis. When the cytoplasm of the cell has a lower solute concentration than the extracellular medium, the medium is said to be **hypertonic** to the cell and water will flow out, causing the cell to shrink. When the cytoplasm of a cell has a higher solute concentration than the extracellular medium, the medium is said to be **hypotonic** to the cell and water will flow in, causing the cell to swell; if too much water flows in, the cell may **lyse.** When the solute concentrations inside and outside the cell are equal, the cell and the medium are said to be **isotonic,** and there is no net flow of water in either direction (see Figure 1.6).

TEACHER TIP

Movement across membranes is an MCAT favorite. With these questions, always consider the gradient in question. Where would the molecules LIKE to move and where are you TRYING to move them?

TEACHER TIP

Hyper- and hypotonicity are commonly tested using an RBC and the Na/K ATPase, which can control the volume of a RBC placed in a stressful environment.

B. FACILITATED DIFFUSION

Facilitated diffusion (passive transport) is the net movement of dissolved particles down their concentration gradient with the help of carrier molecules. This process, like simple diffusion, does not require energy (see Figure 1.5).

C. ACTIVE TRANSPORT

Active transport is the net movement of dissolved particles against their concentration gradient with the help of transport proteins. Unlike diffusion, active transport requires energy (see Figure 1.5). Active transport is required to maintain membrane potentials in specialized cells such as neurons (see chapter 12).

BRIDGE

Diffusion is the biological version of a ball rolling down a hill—down its potential energy gradient. Active transport is the biological equivalent of pushing a ball up a hill; energy, in the form of ATP, must be expended and work is performed.

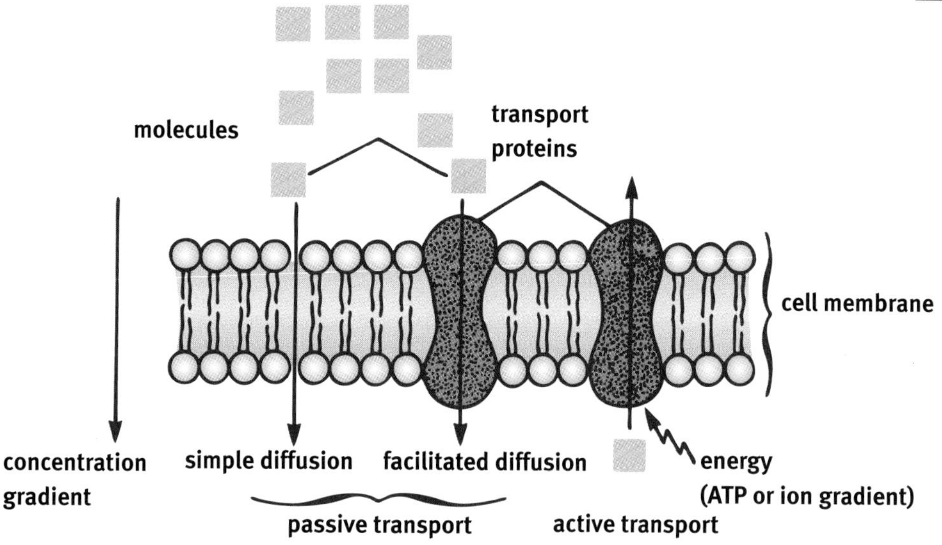

Figure 1.5. Movement Across Memberances

EXCLUSIVE

Notice how the "O" in Hyp-o-tonic looks like a swollen cell.

H_2O H_2O H_2O

isotonic solution	hypotonic solution	hypertonic solution

Figure 1.6. Osmosis

MCAT SYNOPSIS

Types of transport:

Passive diffusion
- Down gradient
- No carrier
- No energy required

Facilitated diffusion
- Down gradient
- Carrier
- No energy required

Active transport
- Against gradient
- Carrier
- Energy required

D. ENDOCYTOSIS

Endocytosis is a process in which the cell membrane invaginates, forming a vesicle that contains extracellular medium (see Figure 1.7). Pinocytosis is the ingestion of fluids or small particles, and **phagocytosis** is the engulfing of large particles. Particles may first bind to receptors on the cell membrane before being engulfed.

E. EXOCYTOSIS

In exocytosis, a vesicle within the cell fuses with the cell membrane and releases its contents to the outside. Fusion of the vesicle with the cell membrane can play an important role in cell growth and intercellular signalling (see Figure 1.7). Note that in both endocytosis and exocytosis, the material never actually crosses through the cell membrane.

Table 1.1: Movement Across the Cell Membrane

	Diffusion	Osmosis	Facilitated Transport	Active Transport
Concentration Gradient	High ⟶ Low	High ⟶ Low	High ⟶ Low	Low ⟶ High
Membrane Protein Required	No	No	Yes	Yes
Energy Required	NO—this is a PASSIVE process	NO—this is a PASSIVE process	NO—this is a PASSIVE process	YES—this is a ACTIVE process. Requires ATP
Type of Molecule/s Transported	Small nonpolar (O_2, CO_2, etc . . .)	H_2O	Large nonpolar (e.g. glucose)	Polar molecules or ions (e.g. Na^+, Cl^-, K^+, etc . . .)

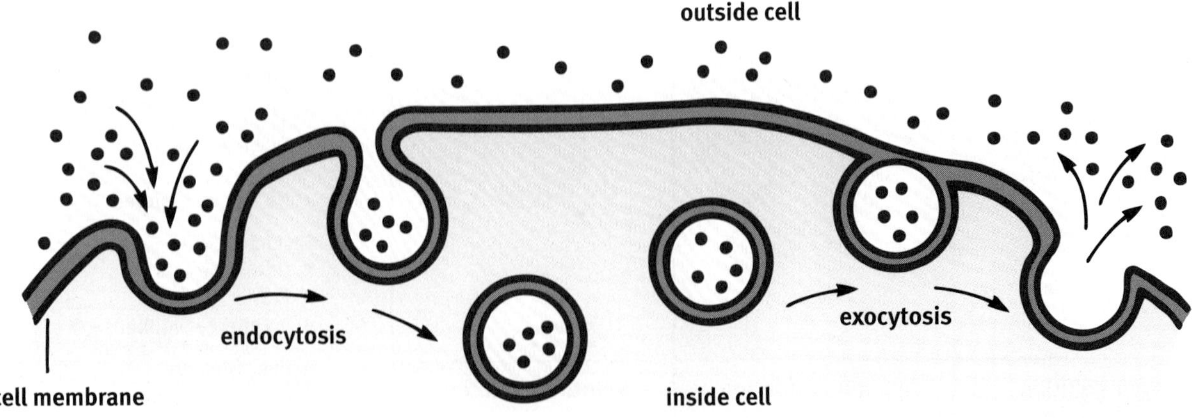

Figure 1.7. Endocytosis and Exocytosis

TISSUES

Tissues are groups of morphologically and functionally related cells. The four basic types of tissue found in the body are **epithelial, connective, nervous,** and **muscle.**

A. EPITHELIAL TISSUE

Epithelial tissue covers the surfaces of the body and lines the cavities, protecting them against injury, invasion, and desiccation. Epithelium is also involved in absorption, secretion, and sensation.

B. CONNECTIVE TISSUE

Connective tissue is involved in body support and other functions. Specialized connective tissues include bone, cartilage, tendons, ligaments, adipose tissue, and blood.

C. NERVOUS TISSUE

Nervous tissue is composed of specialized cells called neurons that are involved in the perception, processing, and storage of information concerning the internal and external environments (see chapter 12).

D. MUSCLE TISSUE

Muscle tissue has a great contractile capability and is involved in body movement. The three types of vertebrate muscle tissue are **skeletal** muscle, **cardiac** muscle, and **smooth** muscle (see chapter 6).

VIRUSES

Viruses are unique acellular structures composed of nucleic acid enclosed by a protein coat. Viruses range in size from 20–300 mm. In contrast, prokaryotes are 1–10 mm and eukaryotic cells are 10–100 mm. The nucleic acid can be either linear or circular, and has been found in four varieties: single-stranded DNA, double-stranded DNA, single-stranded RNA, and double-stranded RNA. The protein coat, or **capsid,** is composed of many protein subunits and may be enclosed by a membranous envelope.

TEACHER TIP

KEY POINT: Exo– and endocytosis allow the cell to "compartmentalize" certain functions, creating specific environments favorable to reactions such as digestion.

CLINICAL CORRELATE

Diseases caused solely by viruses include the common cold, measles, mumps, chicken pox, croup, polio, influenza, hepatitis, and AIDS. Fighting viruses with drugs is trickier than fighting bacteria because the viruses actually live inside host cells, and viruses don't have any organelles of their own. To date, the few antiviral medications that exist work by interfering with enzymatic reactions involved in viral replication. More success in combating viruses has been achieved through vaccination. Of the diseases listed above, vaccines currently exist for measles, mumps, chicken pox, polio, influenza, and hepatitis.

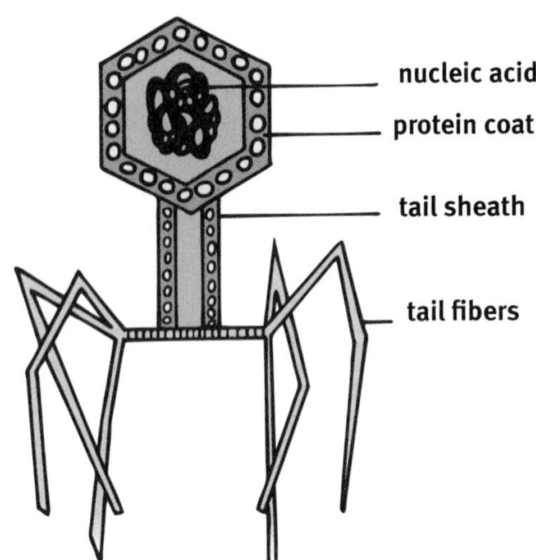

Figure 1.8. Bacteriophage

TEACHER TIP

Viruses evade the immune system in a very different way than bacteria. Most bacteria never enter a cell, whereas viruses MUST do so in order to replicate. This has immune system implications that will be discussed later.

Viruses are **obligate intracellular parasites**; i.e., they can express their genes and reproduce only within a living host cell, because they lack the structures necessary for independent activity and reproduction. A virus attaches itself to a host cell and injects its nucleic acid, taking control of protein synthesis within the cell. The viral genome replicates itself many times, produces new protein coats, and assembles new **virions** that leave the host cell in search of new hosts. Viruses that exclusively infect bacteria are called **bacteriophages.** The bacteriophage injects its nucleic acid into a bacterial cell; the phage capsid does not enter the cell (see chapter 14).

PRACTICE QUESTIONS

1. A new laboratory has just finished constructing an autoradiography developing room. It wishes to test the equipment with a control experiment. If radiolabeled antibodies against estrogen receptors are added to an antibody-permeable common eukaryotic cell line, where should the fluorescence appear on autoradiography?

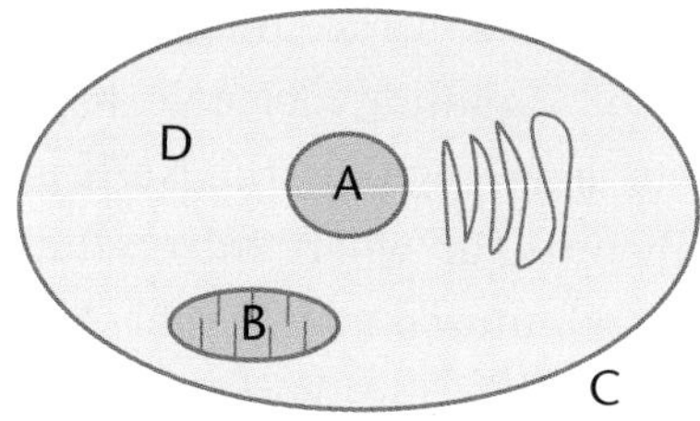

A. A—nucleus
B. B—mitochondrion
C. C—cell membrane
D. D—cytoplasm

2. A cancer researcher has developed a new radioactive antibody to identify the organizational structure of eukaryotic microtubules more precisely during the cell cycle. What other cellular structures might this antibody label?

A. Flagella of spermatozoa
B. Actin filaments of muscle cells
C. Prokaryotic cilia
D. Nuclear pores

3. A patient is brought to the ER after an occupational exposure to toxic compound X, a substance which is metabolized by the liver. A biopsy of the liver would likely show which of the following?

A. Hypochromic rough endoplasmic reticulum
B. Hyperplasia with nuclear irregularities
C. Proliferation of the smooth endoplasmic reticulum
D. Cell wall breakdown with early stages of cell death

4. The drug colchicine blocks microtubule polymerization without destruction of the tubulin monomers. Its ability to interfere with cellular motility, specifically that of pro-inflammatory immune cells, makes colchicine useful in the treatment of gout. Which of the following is a possible mechanism of action of colchicine?

A. Stabilization of centrioles
B. Binding the tubulin polymerization site
C. Hydrolase activity at the tubulin polymerization site
D. Increasing tubulin production

5. An investigator hypothesizes that a trial cancer drug interferes with protein folding after protein synthesis. In order to test its effects, a radiolabeled version of Drug A was added to a culture of cells. Of the following cellular locations, which would likely be identified upon autoradiography?

A. Nucleus and endoplasmic reticulum
B. Endoplasmic reticulum
C. Cytoplasm and endoplasmic reticulum
D. Nucleus and Golgi apparatus

6. Lactose intolerance results in diarrhea caused from an influx of lactose due to the absence of certain brush border enzymes that break down lactose. On the other hand, secretory diarrhea can be caused by pathogens (i.e., cholera), which pump chloride ions (Cl^-) into the gastrointestinal lumen. Which of the following statements is true about these processes?

   I. Lactose is osmotically active, creating a diffusion gradient into the lumen.
   II. The movement of chloride ions in secretory diarrhea creates a hypotonic lumen.
   III. Lactose can be absorbed in the absence of brush border enzymes.

   A. I
   B. I and II
   C. I and III
   D. I, II, and III

7. Antidiuretic hormone (ADH, aka vasopressin) increases the permeability of the collecting ducts of the nephron to water. Which of the following statements is correct about the ensuing process?

   A. Water channels allow water to move down its gradient and into the nephron, diluting the urine.
   B. Water channels actively pump water against its gradient out of the nephron, concentrating the urine.
   C. Water channels allow electrolytes and water to move down their gradient and out of the nephron, without changing the tonicity of the urine.
   D. Water channels allow water to move down its gradient and out of the nephron, concentrating the urine.

8. Which of the following statements about membrane carrier proteins is true?

   A. Carrier proteins transport molecules against their diffusion gradient.
   B. Small nonpolar molecules often require carrier proteins to cross the cell membrane.
   C. Carrier proteins allow large polar molecules to cross the cell membrane.
   D. Carrier protein transport is required for steroid transport into the cell.

9. Increases in the intracellular levels of cyclic-AMP, a cell-signaling molecule, have been shown to down-regulate the Na/K pump. An experiment is run where intracellular electrolytes are monitored while cyclic-AMP is depleted from cells and then replenished. Which of the following accurately depicts the levels of *intracellular* electrolytes during this experiment in response to cAMP replenishing?

   A. Increase in $[Na^+]$ and decrease in $[K^+]$
   B. Increase in $[Na^+]$ and increase in $[K^+]$
   C. Decrease in $[Na^+]$ and decrease in $[K^+]$
   D. Decrease in $[Na^+]$ and increase in $[K^+]$

10. An antiport is a type of membrane protein that is involved in *secondary active transport*, where the movement of one molecule *against* its diffusion gradient is coupled to the movement of another molecule *down* its diffusion gradient.

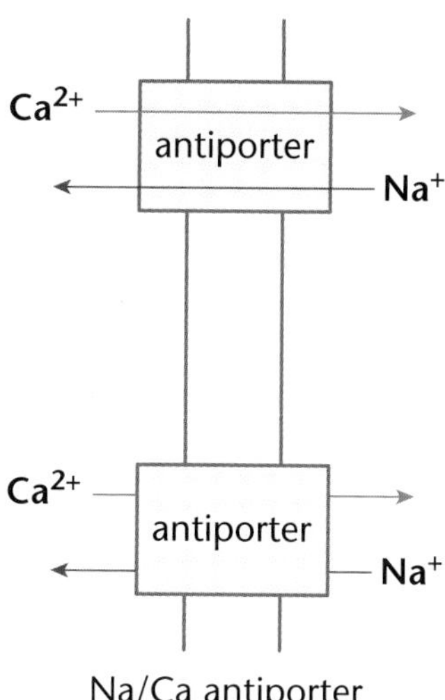

Na/Ca antiporter

Given the information provided, which of the following statements is true?

A. Secondary active transport differs from active transport in that it requires ATP.
B. In the Na/Ca^{2+} antiporter, calcium moves from an area of low concentration to high concentration, and sodium moves from an area of low concentration to high concentration.
C. The Na/K pump is an antiporter.
D. Antiporters take advantage of the diffusion gradient of one molecule in order to transport another molecule.

11. Scientists discover a new disease that causes a defect in all connective tissues. Which of the following would likely be unaffected by this disease?

A. Tendons
B. Epidermis
C. Bone
D. Blood

12. Lysozyme is a free enzyme found in solution and secretions such as teardrops and mucus. It is also believed to be present in storage vesicles within immune cells. Which of the following is a probable mechanism explaining the presence of lysozyme in both secretions and immune cells?

A. Lysozyme is manufactured in immune cells and then released into body fluids via exocytosis.
B. Lysozyme is manufactured in the extracellular space and is engulfed by immune cells via phagocytosis.
C. Lysozyme is manufactured in immune cells and then released into body fluids via endocytosis.
D. Lysozyme is manufactured in all cells and is permanently sequestered in storage vesicles.

13. ATP-binding cassette (ABC) transporters are a large family of transmembrane proteins that transport a wide variety of products across the cell membrane. They have been shown to play an important role in some forms of drug resistance, where they transport large drug molecules against their diffusion gradient out of tumor cells. Which of the following likely describes the type of movement facilitated by ABC transporters?

A. Simple diffusion
B. Facilitated diffusion
C. Exocytosis
D. Active transport

14. With the discovery of deep sea hydrothermal vents in the 20th century, hundreds of new species were cataloged. If a team of scientists wanted to quickly identify a unicellular organism from a hydrothermal vent as either a prokaryote or eukaryote, what characteristics would be important to look for via light microscopy?

I. Cell wall
II. Nucleus
III. Ribosomal subunit sizes

A. I
B. I and II
C. II and III
D. I, II and III

15. In the search for a vaccine against the human immunodeficiency virus (HIV), researchers were faced with a major problem: Certain HIV envelope proteins that are heavily glycosylated interfere with their detection by the immune system. The organelle within the host cell that is primarily responsible for glycosylation of proteins is also responsible for

A. storage of glycogen.
B. aerobic respiration.
C. production of secretory vesicles.
D. protein synthesis.

CHAPTER 2

ENZYMES

Enzymes are protein catalysts that accelerate reactions, such as those in metabolic pathways, by reducing the initial energy **(activation energy)** necessary for them to proceed. The enzyme does not change the equilibrium point of a reaction; it changes only the rate at which it is attained. During the course of reactions, the enzymes themselves are neither consumed nor changed. Most enzyme reactions are reversible; the product synthesized by an enzyme can also be decomposed by the same enzyme. Figure 2.1 compares an uncatalyzed reaction with an enzymatically catalyzed reaction. The activation energy of the catalyzed reaction is lower, yet the overall **change in free energy** (ΔG) of the two reactions remains the same.

TEACHER TIP

Enzymes are the most common place to see an overlap between the BS and PS sections of the MCAT. Be sure to know what each part of these types of curves means in both thermodynamic terms and biological ones.

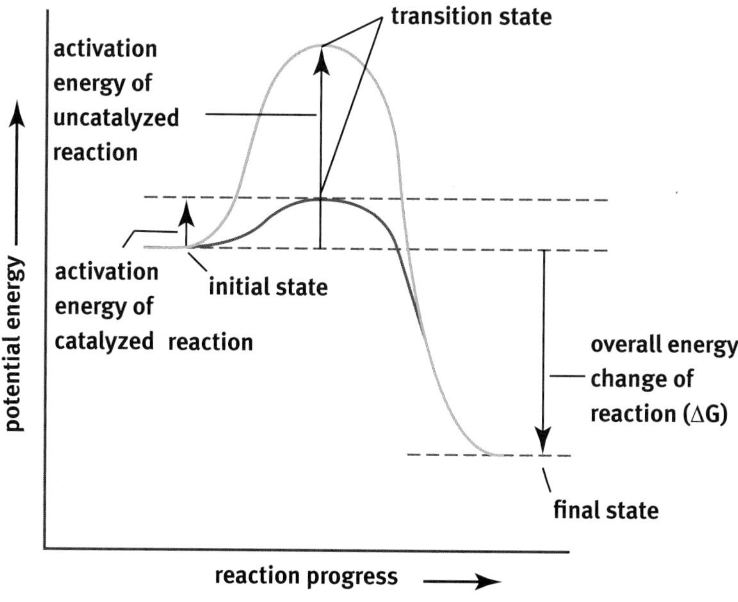

Figure 2.1. Reaction Coordinate

IN A NUTSHELL

Enzymes:

- Lower activation energy of a reaction
- Increase the rate of the reaction
- Do not affect the overall ΔG of the reaction
- Are not changed or consumed in the course of the reaction

TEACHER TIP

Enzymes very often break down or create molecules (H_2O_2, OCl^-) that would be very damaging to the cell if they were released into the cytoplasm. Recall from the last chapter how cells deal with these reactive species, which are necessary for certain reactions.

ENZYME SPECIFICITY

Enzymes are very selective; they may catalyze only one reaction or one specific class of closely related reactions. Urease, for example, selectively catalyzes the breakdown of urea. (Note that the suffix *ase* generally denotes an enzyme.) Chymotrypsin, on the other hand, selectively catalyzes the hydrolysis of specific types of peptide bonds, enabling it to catalyze the hydrolysis of more than one type of peptide (see chapter 7).

The molecule upon which an enzyme acts is called the **substrate.** There is an area on each enzyme to which the substrate bonds to form an **enzyme-substrate complex.** This area, the **active site,** has a three-dimensional shape into which the substrate fits and is held at a particular orientation. There are two models describing the formation of an enzyme-substrate complex: the **lock and key theory** and the **induced fit hypothesis.**

A. THE LOCK AND KEY THEORY

This theory holds that the spatial structure of an enzyme's active site (lock) is exactly complementary to the spatial structure of its substrate (key). Their 3-D configurations are such that the active site and the substrate fit together, forming an enzyme-substrate complex.

B. THE INDUCED FIT HYPOTHESIS

The induced fit hypothesis describes the active site of an enzyme as having some flexibility of shape. When the appropriate substrate comes in contact with the active site, the conformation of the active site changes such that it surrounds the substrate, creating a close fit (see Figure 2.2). A substrate of the wrong shape will not induce a conformational change in the enzyme's active site, thereby preventing the formation of an enzyme-substrate complex.

Studies suggest that the induced fit hypothesis is more plausible than the lock and key theory, and induced fit is currently more widely accepted.

Table 2.1. Activation Energy

1. LOWER the ACTIVATION ENERGY
2. INCREASE the RATE OF THE REACTION
3. DO NOT alter the equilibrium constant
4. ARE NOT CHANGED OR CONSUMED in the reaction (This means that they will appear in both the reactants and products.)
5. Enzymes are pH and temperature sensitive, with optimal activity at specific pH ranges and temperatures
6. DO NOT affect the overall ΔG of the reaction
7. Are SPECIFIC for a particular REACTION or CLASS of REACTIONS

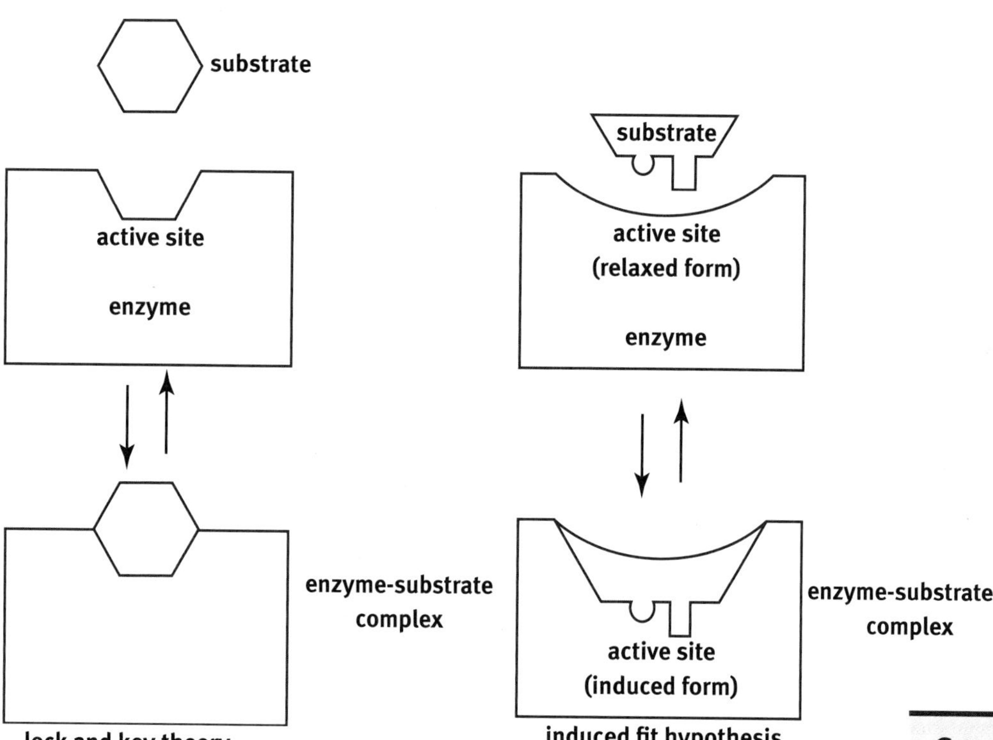

Figure 2.2. Models for Enzyme-Substrate Interactions

CLINICAL CORRELATE

Deficiencies in vitamin cofactors can result in devastating disease. Thiamin is an important cofactor for several enzymes involved in cellular metabolism and nerve conduction. Thiamin deficiency, often seen in alcoholics, results in a disease known as Wernicke-Korsokoff syndrome. In this disorder, patients suffer from a variety of neurological deficits, including delirium, balance problems, and in severe cases, the inability to form new memories.

COFACTORS

Many enzymes require the incorporation of a nonprotein molecule to become catalytically active. These molecules, called **cofactors,** can aid in binding the substrate to the enzyme or in stabilizing the enzyme in an active conformation. An enzyme devoid of its necessary cofactor is called an **apoenzyme** and is catalytically inactive, while an enzyme containing its cofactor is called a **holoenzyme.** Cofactors can be bound to their enzymes by weak noncovalent interactions or by strong covalent bonds. Tightly bound cofactors are called **prosthetic groups.**

TEACHER TIP

Vitamins come in 2 major classes: fat and water soluble. This is important to consider in digestive diseases, where different parts of the GI tract may be affected by different disease processes. Loss of parts of the GI tract may cause various vitamin deficiencies.

Two important types of cofactors are metal cations (e.g., Zn^{2+}, Fe^{2+}) and small organic groups (e.g., biotin). These latter organic cofactors are called **coenzymes.** Most coenzymes cannot be synthesized by the body and are obtained from the diet as vitamin derivatives. Lack of a particular vitamin can impair the action of its corresponding enzyme and lead to disease.

ENZYME KINETICS

The rate of an enzyme-catalyzed reaction is related to a number of factors, including the concentrations of both the enzyme and the substrate, and environmental variables such as temperature and pH.

A. EFFECTS OF CONCENTRATION

The concentrations of substrate [S] and enzyme [E] during the course of a reaction greatly affect the reaction rate. When the concentration of the substrate is low compared to that of the enzyme, many of the active sites are unoccupied and the reaction rate is low. Initial increases in the substrate concentration (at constant enzyme concentration) lead to proportional increases in the rate of the reaction because unoccupied active sites on the enzyme readily bind to the additional substrate. However, once most of the active sites are occupied, the reaction rate levels off, regardless of further increases in substrate concentration. At high concentrations of substrate, the reaction rate approaches its **maximal velocity, V_{max}**. At this point, increases in substrate concentration will no longer increase reaction rate (see Figure 2.3.)

TEACHER TIP

MM kinetics may not be your favorite topic to learn but *know these kinetics thoroughly*. They are one of the most commonly appearing MCAT topics.

According to the Michaelis-Menten model proposed in 1913, an enzyme-substrate complex, ES, is formed at rate k_1 from enzyme E and substrate S. The ES complex can either dissociate into E and S at rate k_2, or form product P at rate k_3. The relationship between the three rates is defined by the **Michaelis constant, K_m**, as $\frac{(k_2 + k_3)}{k_1}$, or the ratio of the breakdown of the ES complex to its formation.

$$E + S \underset{k_2}{\overset{k_1}{\rightleftharpoons}} ES_{\frac{1}{2}} \xrightarrow{k_3} E + P$$

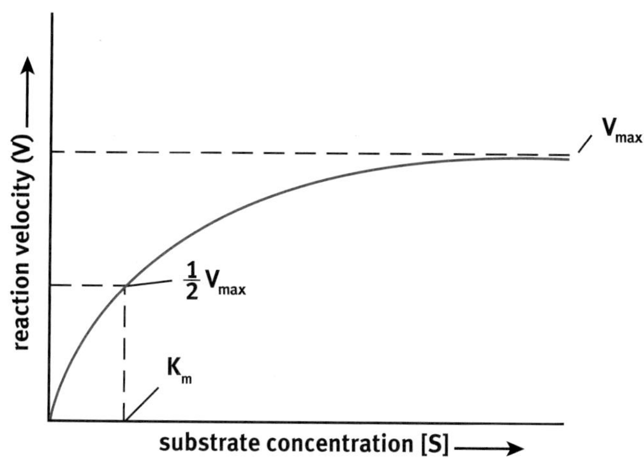

Figure 2.3. Michaelis-Menten Model

MCAT SYNOPSIS

You can assess an enzyme's affinity for a substrate by noting the K_m. A low K_m reflects a high affinity for the substrate (low [S] required for 50 percent enzyme saturation). Conversely, a high K_m reflects a low affinity of the enzyme for the substrate.

When the reaction rate is equal to ½ V_{max}, K_m = [S] and can be understood as the point at which half of the enzyme's active sites are filled (see Figure 2.3). When [S] is less than K_m, changes in substrate concentration greatly affect the reaction rate. In contrast, at high concentrations of substrate, [S] is larger than K_m, and V approaches V_{max}.

B. EFFECTS OF TEMPERATURE

Rates of enzyme-catalyzed reactions tend to double for every 10°C increase in temperature until their optimal temperature is reached. For most enzymes operating in the human body, the optimal temperature is 37°C. At higher temperatures, enzymes become denatured: their 3-D structure is destroyed and the enzyme becomes nonfunctional. Enzymes that are partially denatured can sometimes regain their activity upon being cooled (see Figure 2.4).

TEACHER TIP

Consider how the human body uses this. What part of the human body might require enzymes that work at a lower temperature? The answer will appear in a few chapters!

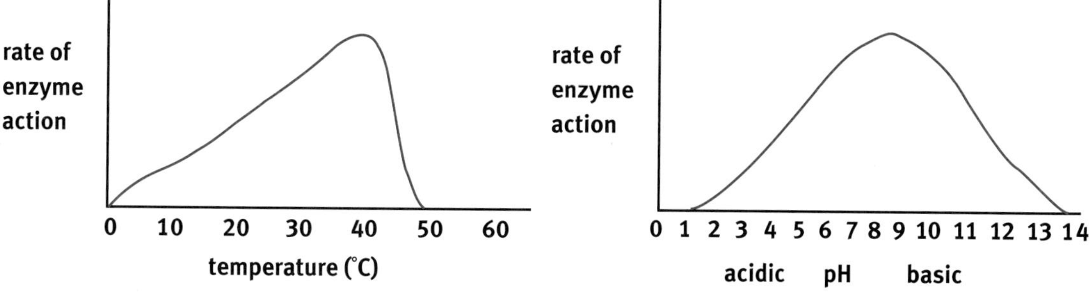

Figure 2.4. Effects of Temperature and pH on Enzyme Activity

C. EFFECTS OF pH

For each enzyme there is also an optimal pH above and below which enzymatic activity declines. Maximal activity of many human enzymes occurs around pH 7.4 (7.35–7.45), which is the pH of most body fluids and tissues. Plueral fluid is an exception and has a standard pH closer to 7.6. The other exceptions include pepsin, which works best in the highly acidic conditions of the stomach (pH = 2), and pancreatic enzymes, which work optimally in the alkaline conditions of the small intestine (pH = 8.5).

REGULATION OF ENZYMATIC ACTIVITY

TEACHER TIP

Consider that digestive enzymes chew up fats, proteins, and carbohydrates—the very same compounds that your body is made of. How do these enzymes know to digest your food but not your body? Very simply, THEY DON'T!! Instead, we regulate their activity in a coordinated manner.

The regulation of enzymatic activity is accomplished in a number of ways, most notably through allosteric effects and inhibitory interactions.

A. ALLOSTERIC EFFECTS

An **allosteric enzyme** has at least one active or catalytic site and at least one separate regulatory site. Often, these enzymes possess a quarternary structure. An allosteric enzyme oscillates between two configurations—an active state capable of catalyzing a reaction, and an inactive state that cannot. An interaction between an allosteric enzyme and a **regulator** (a molecule other than the substrate that binds to the enzyme) can stabilize either configuration, depending on the type of regulator involved. There are two types of regulators—**allosteric inhibitors** and **allosteric activators.** An inhibitor prevents an enzyme from binding to its substrate by stabilizing the inactive conformation, whereas an activator stabilizes the active configuration, promoting the formation of enzyme-substrate complexes.

TEACHER TIP

This cooperative binding of Hb results in a characteristic sigmoidal binding curve, which is an MCAT favorite.

Another allosteric effect involves increased affinity of an enzyme for its substrate. Sometimes the binding of a regulator at the allosteric site, or the binding of substrate at one of the enzyme's active sites, may stimulate the other active sites on the enzyme to bind more efficiently by increasing their affinity for the substrate. This type of cooperation is not unique to allosteric enzymes. Hemoglobin is composed of four subunits, each with its own oxygen-binding site; the binding of oxygen at one subunit increases the affinity for oxygen at the remaining three active sites (see chapter 9).

B. INHIBITION

An enzyme's activity may be regulated by one of the products of the reactions it catalyzes, or by a substance that binds to the enzyme and inhibits it from binding substrate. These interferences with enzymatic activity

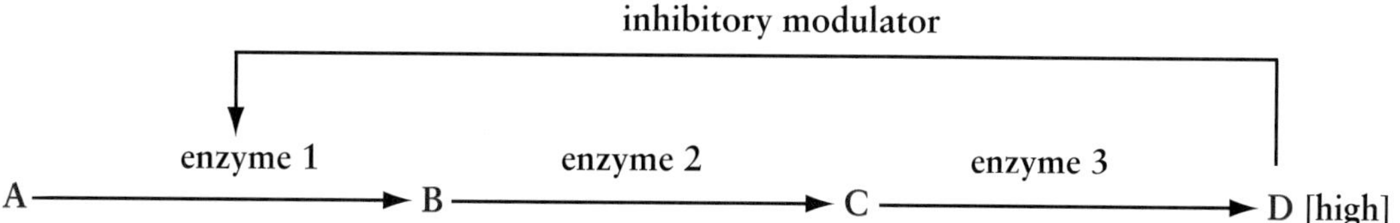

Figure 2.5. Negative Feedback

can be categorized as **feedback inhibition, competitive inhibition,** and **noncompetitive inhibition.**

1. Feedback Inhibition

Many biological reactions are regulated by feedback inhibition mechanisms, in which the end product of a sequence of enzymatic reactions becomes an allosteric modulator (in this case, an inhibitor) of one of the preceding enzymes in the sequence. In the reaction sequence shown, (Figure 2.5), product D is an inhibitory modulator for enzyme 1. Thus, when the concentration of D reaches some critical level, virtually all enzyme 1 molecules are inhibited and production of B (and thus of C and D) is halted. The process is sometimes reversible and can be instantaneous; as D levels decrease, enzyme 1 inhibition decreases, and A is again converted to B. This feedback process allows organisms to avoid overproduction of metabolites. (For an additional discussion of feedback inhibition see chapter 11.)

TEACHER TIP

This process is widely used in all biological organisms. Its opposite (feed-forward activation) is rarely used, though we will see a special example with estrogen and the menstrual cycle when we study reproduction.

2. Competitive Inhibitors

Competitive inhibitors compete with the substrate directly by binding to the active site of the enzyme. The active site of an enzyme is specific for a particular substrate or class of substrates. However, it is possible for molecules that are structurally similar to the substrate to bind to the active site of the enzyme. If this similar molecule is present in a concentration comparable to the concentration of the substrate, it will compete with the substrate for bonding sites on the enzyme and it will interfere with enzyme activity. This is known as competitive inhibition because the enzyme is inhibited by the inactive substrate, or competitor, so called because it *competes* with the substrate for the active site. Competitive inhibition is reversible with increased concentrations of substrate.

TEACHER TIP

Inhibition is commonly tested in an experimental passage. If you add more substrate and inhibition decreases (i.e., enzymatic activity goes back up), you know you are dealing with competitive inhibition. If inhibition remains the same (i.e., no change in enzymatic activity), you're dealing with noncompetitive inhibition.

3. Noncompetitive Inhibitors

A noncompetitive inhibitor is a substance that forms strong covalent bonds with an enzyme and consequently may not be displaced by the addition of excess substrate. Therefore, noncompetitive inhibition is irreversible. A noncompetitive inhibitor may be bonded at, near, or

CLINICAL CORRELATE

The concept of competitive inhibition has relevance in the clinical setting. For example, methanol (wood alcohol), if ingested, is enzymatically converted to toxic metabolites that can cause blindness and even death. Administration of intravenous ethanol is the treatment of choice for a patient suffering from methanol poisoning. Ethanol works by competing with methanol for the active sites of the enzymes involved.

remote from the active site. This is an example of allosteric inhibition. Noncompetitive inhibition can be overcome by increasing the concentration of the enzyme.

INACTIVE ENZYMES

A **zymogen** is an enzyme that is secreted in an inactive form. The zymogen is cleaved under certain physiological conditions to the active form of the enzyme. Important examples of zymogens include pepsinogen, trypsinogen, and chymotrypsinogen, which are cleaved in the digestive tract to yield the active enzymes pepsin, trypsin, and chymotrypsin, respectively (see chapter 7).

PRACTICE QUESTIONS

1. Which of the following best represents the amount of energy conserved through using an enzyme for the reaction depicted in the following graph?

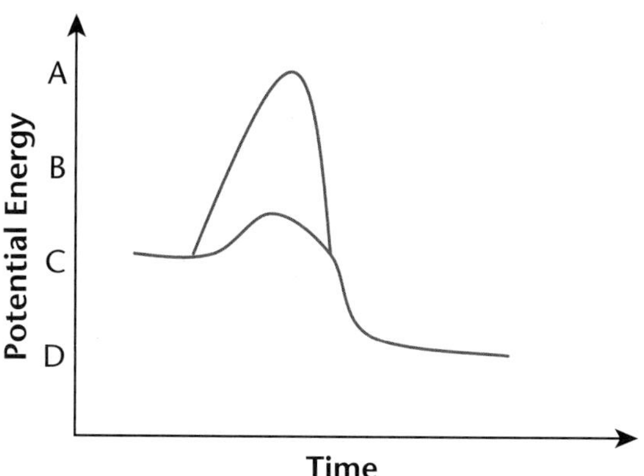

A. A – B
B. A + B
C. B – C
D. B + D

2. In the equation below, substrate C is an allosteric inhibitor to enzyme 1. Which of the following is another mechanism caused by substrate C?

A ⟶ enzyme 1 ⟶ B ⟶ enzyme 2 ⟶ C

A. Competitive inhibition
B. Irreversible inhibition
C. Feedback enhancement
D. Negative feedback

3. Which of the following would initiate a competitive inhibition of the production of substrate C in the metabolic pathway shown below?

A ⟶ enzyme 1 ⟶ B ⟶ enzyme 2 ⟶ C
⟶ enzyme 3 ⟶ D

A. Allosteric inhibition of enzyme 1
B. Allosteric inhibition of enzyme 3
C. Substrate D fits into the active site of enzyme 3
D. Substrate D fits into the active site of enzyme 1

4. When lactase hydrolyzes milk sugars, which of the following occurs?

A. Lactase retains its structure after the reaction.
B. Lactose retains its structure after the reaction.
C. Lactase increases the activation energy of the reaction.
D. Lactose decreases the activation energy of the reaction.

5. In a chemical reaction that they mediate, what are enzymes' function?

A. Change the potential energy level of the reaction
B. Change the potential energy levels of the products
C. Change the activation energy of the reaction
D. Change the enzyme energy levels of the reaction

6. Bonding between atoms within an enzyme such as trypsin is best described as

A. peptide.
B. saccharide.
C. ionic.
D. Van der Waals.

7. Which organelle is likely to contain extra protection, such as a double membrane?

A. Golgi body
B. Endoplasmic reticulum
C. Lysosome
D. Ribosome

8. Lipase does all of the following EXCEPT

A. break down lipids.
B. speed up the rate of fatty acid production.
C. slow down the rate of glycerol production.
D. increase its rate of activity with higher lipid concentrations.

9. In the graph below, which of the following best describes the chemical activity depicted by region "X" ?

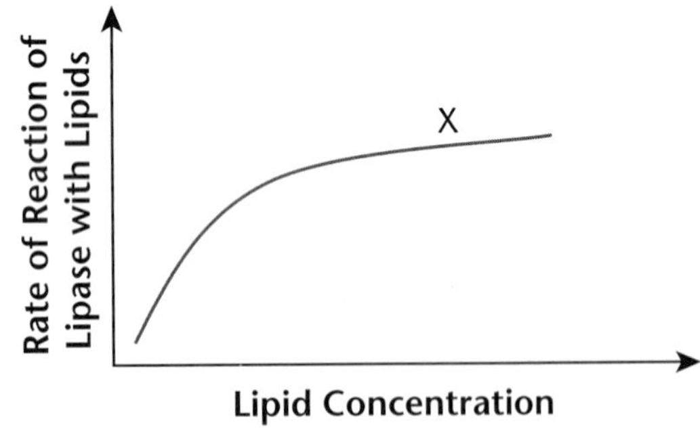

A. Active sites on lipase enzymes are all occupied by lipids.
B. Lipase concentration decreases with the rate of the reaction.
C. Lipid concentration increases with the rate of the reaction.
D. Active sites on lipid molecules are all occupied by lipase.

10. Which of the following is true of the amino acids of an active site found in a hemoglobin molecule?

A. They are all found on the primary protein chains.
B. They are all found on the secondary protein chains.
C. They are found on different tertiary chains.
D. They are found within the carboxylic acid groups on the chains.

11. In any enzyme-mediated chemical reaction, which of the following applies?

A. It is always endergonic.
B. It is always exergonic.
C. The overall energy change of the reaction is the same as the uncatalyzed version.
D. The overall energy change of the reaction is never the same as the uncatalyzed version.

12. An allosteric interaction with enzyme "X" will always

A. inhibit the activity of enzyme "X."
B. enhance the activity of enzyme "X."
C. block the substrate from the active site.
D. change the shape of enzyme "X."

CHAPTER 3

CELLULAR METABOLISM

Cellular metabolism is the sum total of all chemical reactions that take place in a cell. These reactions can be generally categorized as either **anabolic** or **catabolic.** Anabolic processes are energy-requiring, involving the biosynthesis of complex organic compounds from simpler molecules. Catabolic processes release energy as they break down complex organic compounds into smaller molecules. The metabolic reactions of cells are coupled so that energy released from catabolic reactions can be harnessed to fuel anabolic reactions.

TRANSFER OF ENERGY

A. THE FLOW OF ENERGY

The ultimate energy source for living organisms is the sun. **Autotrophic** organisms, such as green plants, convert sunlight into **bond energy** stored in the bonds of organic compounds (chiefly glucose) in the anabolic process of **photosynthesis.** Autotrophs do not need an exogenous supply of organic compounds. **Heterotrophic** organisms obtain their energy catabolically, via the breakdown of organic nutrients that must be ingested. Figure 3.1 is an energy flow diagram for biological systems; note that some energy is dissipated as heat at every stage.

TEACHER TIP

Link to Physics: Remember that no machine—even a biological one—is perfectly efficient. Primarily, this energy will be lost in the form of heat.

Glucose plays an essential role in the energetics of cell metabolism. The production of glucose ($C_6H_{12}O_6$) by autotrophs involves the breaking of C–O and O–H bonds in CO_2 and H_2O, and the forming of C–H, C–O, C–C, and O–H bonds in glucose. The net reaction of photosynthesis:

$$6CO_2 + 6H_2O + \text{Energy} \longrightarrow \underset{\text{glucose}}{C_6H_{12}O_6} + 6O_2$$

Heterotrophic organisms metabolize glucose and other organic molecules to release the stored bond energies. The net reaction of glucose catabolism, which is essentially the reversal of photosynthesis, is:

$$\underset{\text{glucose}}{C_6H_{12}O_6} + 6O_2 \longrightarrow 6CO_2 + 6H_2O + \text{Energy}$$

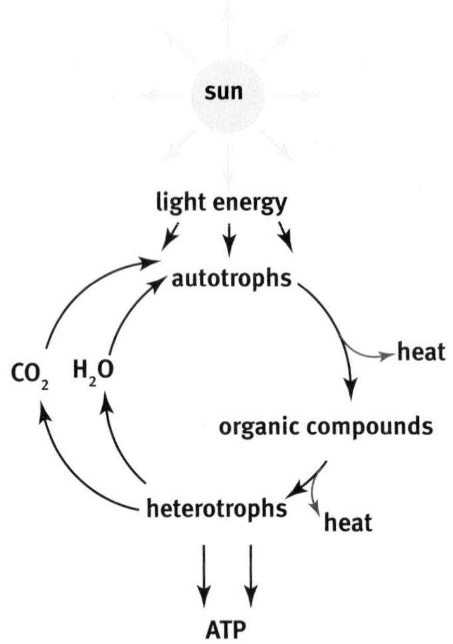

sun
light energy
autotrophs
heat
CO_2 H_2O
organic compounds
heterotrophs
heat
ATP

Figure 3.1. Energy Flow in Biological Systems

B. ENERGY CARRIERS

During metabolism, the cell uses various molecular carriers, such as **ATP** and the coenzymes **NAD⁺, NADP⁺,** and **FAD,** to shuttle energy between reactions.

1. ATP

ATP, or **adenosine triphosphate,** is the cell's main energy currency. Through its formation and degradation, cells have a quick way of releasing and storing energy. ATP is synthesized during glucose catabolism. ATP is composed of the nitrogenous base adenine, the sugar ribose, and three weakly linked phosphate groups. The energy of ATP is stored in the covalent bonds attaching these phosphate groups, often referred to as high-energy bonds.

Hydrolysis of ATP to **ADP (adenosine diphosphate)** and **P_i (inorganic phosphate)** releases stored bond energy that the cell can use

TEACHER TIP

Why are these bonds high energy? Because the large number of negative charges in close proximity requires a good deal of energy to keep coupled.

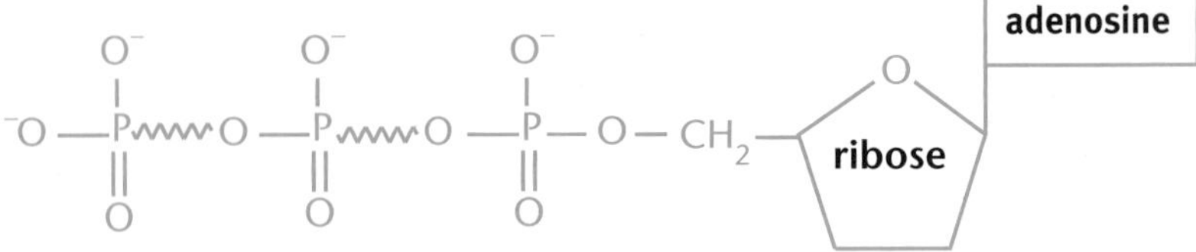

Figure 3.2. ATP

in metabolic processes. Approximately 7 kcal of energy are released per mole of ATP. This provides energy for **endergonic** (endothermic) reactions such as muscle contraction, motility, and the active transport of substances across plasma membranes. ATP may also be hydrolyzed into **AMP (adenosine monophosphate)** and **PP_i (pyrophosphate)**:

$$ATP \longrightarrow ADP + P_i + 7 \text{ kcal/mole}$$

$$ATP \longrightarrow AMP + PP_i + 7 \text{ kcal/mole}$$

Alternatively, ADP and P_i combine to form ATP; in this way the cell regenerates its ATP supply. This process requires energy (supplied by the degradation of glucose):

$$ADP + P_i + 7 \text{ kcal/mole} \longrightarrow ATP$$

2. NAD$^+$, NADP$^+$, and FAD

A second mechanism by which the cell stores chemical energy is in the form of **high potential electrons.** Electrons are transferred as **hydride ions (H:$^-$)** or as pairs of hydrogen atoms. During glucose oxidation, hydrogen atoms are removed. Most of these are accepted by the carrier coenzymes **NAD$^+$ (nicotinamide adenine dinucleotide), FAD (flavin adenine dinucleotide),** and **NADP$^+$ (nicotinamide adenine dinucleotide phosphate).** These molecules transport the high-energy electrons of the hydrogen atoms to a series of carrier molecules on the inner mitochondrical membrane that are collectively known as the **electron transport chain.**

Oxidation refers to the loss of an electron. NAD$^+$, NADP$^+$, and FAD are referred to as oxidizing agents because they cause other molecules to lose electrons and undergo oxidation. In the process, they themselves undergo **reduction**; that is, they gain electrons. For example, when NAD$^+$ accepts electrons in the form of a hydride ion it is reduced to **NADH,** while the donating molecule is oxidized. Likewise, when FAD accepts electrons in the form of hydrogen atoms, it is reduced to **$FADH_2$.** In their reduced forms, NADH, NADPH, and $FADH_2$ all behave as reducing agents. NADH transfers its electrons to another electron acceptor (e.g., the first carrier of the electron transport chain), thereby reducing it, and in the process NADH is oxidized back to NAD$^+$. NADPH is found in plant, not animal, cells. Thus, these coenzymes temporarily store and release energy in the form of electrons through their successive oxidations and reductions.

MCAT SYNOPSIS

In general, NAD$^+$, NADP$^+$, and FAD are all *reduced* during catabolic processes; their reduced forms (NADH, NADPH, and $FADH_2$) are *oxidized* during anabolic processes

TEACHER TIP

Link to Gen. Chem.: Hydride ions are one of the strongest reducing agents that you'll see on the exam. Remember lithium aluminum hydride and sodium borohydride.

MCAT SYNOPSIS

Animal cells store energy in high potential electrons in NADH and $FADH_2$.

TEACHER TIP

These redox reactions do not themselves produce usable energy. Rather they create high energy elections that can then be passed to a final acceptor (oxygen). That, in turn, is coupled to ATP generation.

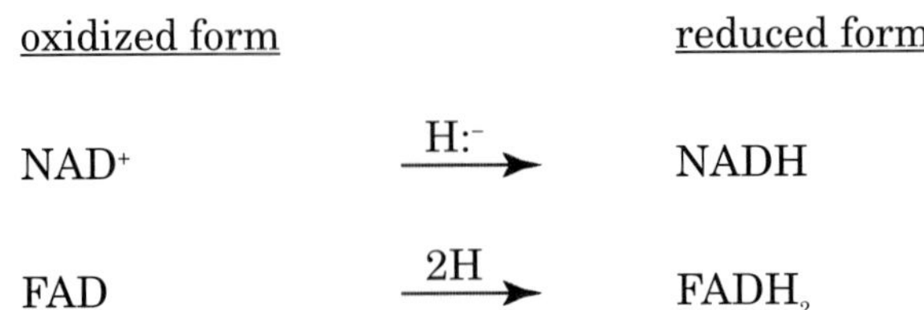

Figure 3.3. Reduction of NAD^+ and FAD

GLUCOSE CATABOLISM

The degradative oxidation of glucose occurs in two stages, **glycolysis** and **cellular respiration.**

A. GLYCOLYSIS

The first stage of glucose catabolism is glycolysis. Glycolysis is a series of reactions that lead to the oxidative breakdown of glucose into two molecules of **pyruvate** (the ionized form of pyruvic acid), the production of ATP, and the reduction of NAD^+ into NADH. All of these reactions occur in the cytoplasm and are mediated by specific enzymes. The glycolytic pathway is outlined below in Figure 3.4.

TEST TIP

You do *not* need to memorize the individual reactions of glycolysis for the MCAT. You will need to memorize them in medical school.

TEACHER TIP

You *do* need to know the net input and output of these reactions. Also, know that this reaction is ANAEROBIC. It can occur in the absence of oxygen.

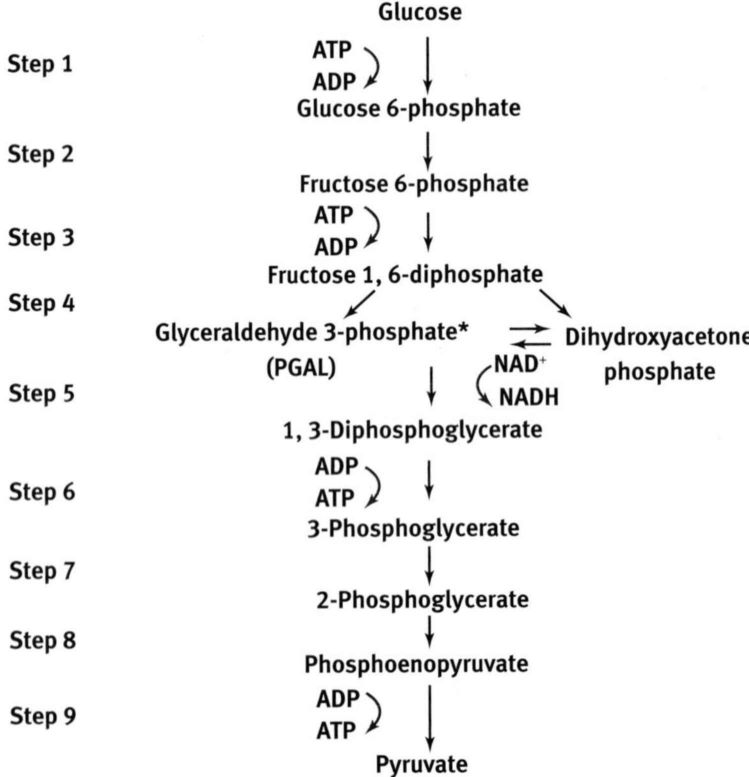

Figure 3.4. Glycolysis

1. Glycolytic Pathway

Note that at step 4, fructose 1, 6-diphosphate is split into 2 three-carbon molecules: **dihydroxyacetone phosphate** and **glyceraldehyde 3-phosphate (PGAL).** Dihydroxyacetone phosphate is isomerized into PGAL so that it can be used in subsequent reactions. Thus, 2 molecules of PGAL are formed per molecule of glucose, and all of the subsequent steps occur twice for each glucose molecule.

From 1 molecule of glucose (a six-carbon molecule), 2 molecules of pyruvate (a three-carbon molecule) are obtained. During this sequence of reactions, 2 ATP are used (in steps 1 and 3) and 4 ATP are generated (two in step 6, and two in step 9). Thus, there is a net production of 2 ATP per glucose molecule. This type of phosphorylation is called **substrate level phosphorylation,** because ATP synthesis is directly coupled with the degradation of glucose without the participation of an intermediate molecule such as NAD^+. One NADH is produced per PGAL, for a total of 2 NADH per glucose.

TEACHER TIP

Know these numbers; they are commonly tested.

The net reaction for glycolysis is:

$$\text{Glucose} + 2\text{ADP} + 2\text{P}_i + 2\text{NAD}^+ \longrightarrow$$
$$2\text{Pyruvate} + 2\text{ATP} + 2\text{NADH} + 2\text{H}^+ + 2\text{H}_2\text{O}$$

This series of reactions occurs in both prokaryotic and eukaryotic cells. However, at this stage, much of the initial energy stored in the glucose molecule has not been released and is still present in the chemical bonds of pyruvate. Depending on the capabilities of the organism, pyruvate degradation can proceed in one of two directions. Under **anaerobic** conditions (in the absence of oxygen), pyruvate is reduced during the process of fermentation. Under **aerobic** conditions (in the presence of oxygen), pyruvate is further oxidized during cell respiration in the mitochondria.

TEACHER TIP

Know the difference between *total* and *net output*. Glycolysis results in an output of 4 ATP but the net output is 2 ATP, as 2 ATP are required to drive the process.

B. CELLULAR RESPIRATION—ANAEROBIC

Cellular respiration can be described as aerobic or anaerobic.

2. Fermentation

NAD^+ must be regenerated for glycolysis to continue in the absence of O_2. This is accomplished by reducing pyruvate into **ethanol** or **lactic acid.** Fermentation refers to all of the reactions involved in this process—glycolysis and the additional steps leading to the formation of ethanol or lactic acid. Fermentation produces only 2 ATP per glucose molecule.

BRIDGE

The conversion of acetaldehyde to ethanol is a typical reduction reaction of an aldehyde to an alcohol.

a. Alcohol fermentation

Alcohol fermentation commonly occurs only in yeast and some bacteria. The pyruvate produced in glycolysis is decarboxylated to become acetaldehyde, which is then reduced by the NADH generated in step 5 of glycolysis to yield ethanol.

In this way, NAD^+ is regenerated and glycolysis can continue.

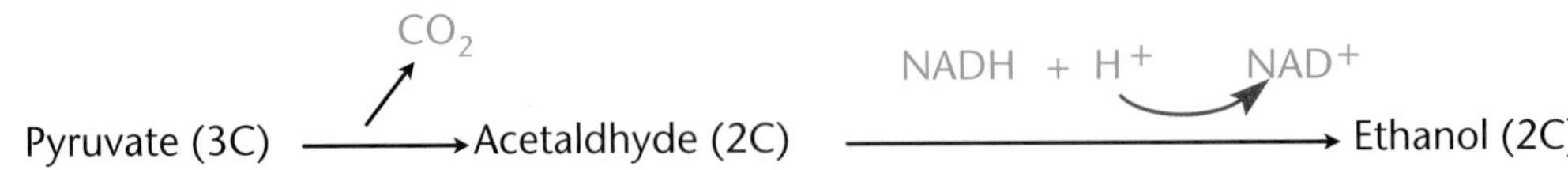

TEACHER TIP

This regeneration of usable intermediates from lactic acid once oxygen has been restored is known as the Cori cycle and it occurs in the liver.

b. Lactic acid fermentation

Lactic acid fermentation occurs in certain fungi and bacteria and in human muscle cells during strenuous activity. When the oxygen supply to muscle cells lags behind the rate of glucose catabolism, the pyruvate generated is reduced to lactic acid. As in alcohol fermentation, the NAD^+ used in step 5 of glycolysis is regenerated when pyruvate is reduced. In humans, lactic acid may accumulate in the muscles during exercise, causing a decrease in blood pH that leads to muscle fatigue. Once the oxygen supply has been replenished, the lactic acid is oxidized back to pyruvate and enters cellular respiration. The amount of oxygen needed for this conversion is known as **oxygen debt.**

$$\text{Pyruvate (3C)} \xrightarrow{\text{NADH} + H^+ \;\to\; NAD^+} \text{Lactic acid (3C)}$$

TEACHER TIP

KEY POINT: Remember that glucose has six carbons. None of these are lost during glycolysis. All are passed though to pyruvate decarboxylation and the TCA cycle where they are lost in the form of CO_2.

C. CELLULAR RESPIRATION—ANAEROBIC

Cellular respiration is the most efficient catabolic pathway used by organisms to harvest the energy stored in glucose. Whereas glycolysis yields only 2 ATP per molecule of glucose, cellular respiration can yield 36–38 ATP. Cellular respiration is an aerobic process; oxygen acts as the final acceptor of electrons that are passed from carrier to carrier during the final stage of glucose oxidation. The metabolic reactions of cell respiration occur in the eukaryotic mitochondrion and are catalyzed by reaction-specific enzymes. Cellular respiration can be divided into three stages: **pyruvate decarboxylation,** the **citric acid cycle,** and the **electron transport chain.**

1. Pyruvate Decarboxylation

The pyruvate formed during glycolysis is transported from the cytoplasm into the mitochondrial matrix where it is decarboxylated; i.e., it loses a CO_2, and the acetyl group that remains is transferred to **coenzyme A** to form **acetyl CoA.** In the process, NAD^+ is reduced to NADH.

$$\text{Pyruvate (3 C)} + \text{Coenzyme A} \xrightarrow{NAD^+ \;\rightarrow\; NADH + H^+} \text{Acetyl CoA (2C)}$$

2. Citric Acid Cycle

The citric acid cycle is also known as the **Krebs cycle** or the **tricarboxylic acid cycle (TCA cycle).** The cycle begins when the two-carbon acetyl group from acetyl CoA combines with **oxaloacetate,** a four-carbon molecule, to form the six-carbon **citrate.** Through a complicated series of reactions, 2 CO_2 are released, and oxaloacetate is regenerated for use in another turn of the cycle (Figure 3.5).

For each turn of the citric acid cycle 1 ATP is produced by substrate level phosphorylation via a GTP intermediate. In addition, electrons

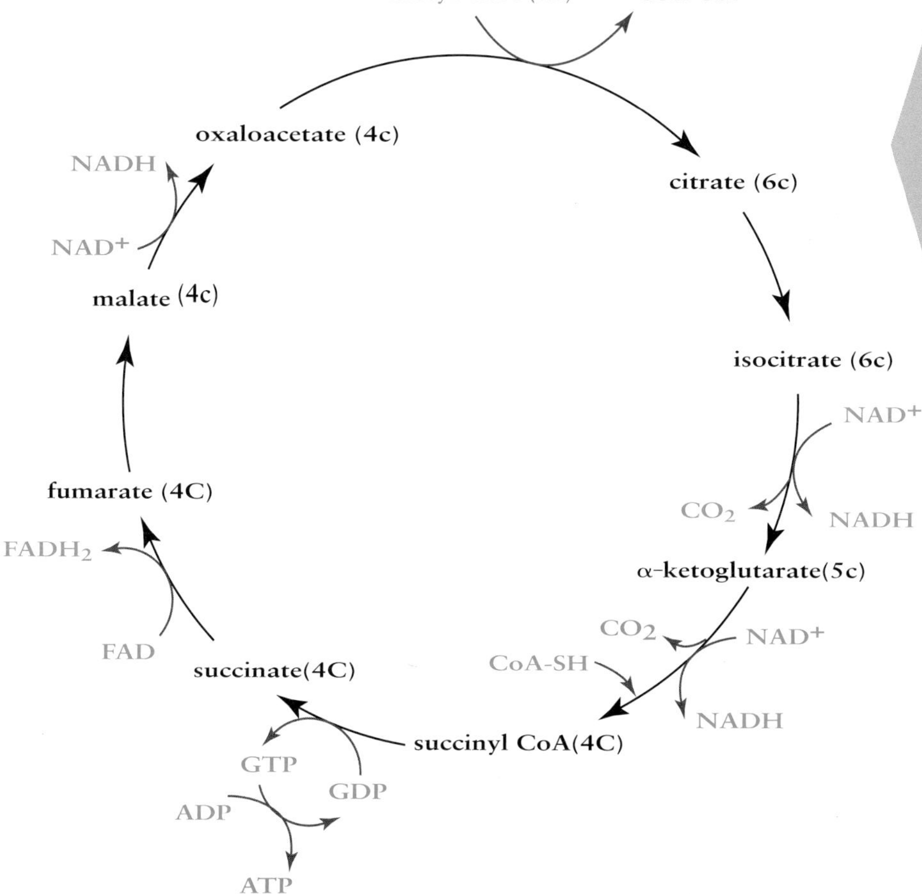

Figure 3.5. Citric Acid Cycle

TEACHER TIP

You do *not* need to know the eight intermediates of the TCA cycle. You should know that the major purpose of this cycle is to generate high-energy intermediates that can be used to make ATP. Note that some ATP is generated from GTP directly. This is known as substrate level phosphorylation.

are transferred to NAD^+ and FAD, generating NADH and $FADH_2$, respectively. These coenzymes then transport the electrons to the electron transport chain, where more ATP is produced via **oxidative phosphorylation.** Studying the cycle, we can do some bookkeeping; keep in mind that for each molecule of glucose, 2 pyruvates are decarboxylated and channeled into the citric acid cycle.

$$2 \times 3 \text{ NADH} \longrightarrow 6 \text{ NADH}$$
$$2 \times 1 \text{ FADH}_2 \longrightarrow 2 \text{ FADH}_2$$
$$2 \times 1 \text{ GTP (ATP)} \longrightarrow 2 \text{ ATP}$$

The net reaction of the citric acid cycle per glucose molecule is:

$$2\text{Acetyl CoA} + 6\text{NAD}^+ + 2\text{FAD} + 2\text{ATP} + 2\text{P}_i + 4\text{H}_2\text{O} \longrightarrow 4\text{CO}_2 + 6\text{NADH} + 2\text{FADH}_2 + 2\text{ATP} + 4\text{H}^+ + 2\text{CoA}$$

MCAT SYNOPSIS

Energy checkpoint:

2ATP	(from glycolysis)
2NADH	(from glycolysis)
2NADH	(from decarboxylation of pyruvate)
6NADH	(TCA cycle)
$2FADH_2$	(TCA cycle)
2ATP	(TCA cycle)

3. Electron Transport Chain

a. Electron transfer

The electron transport chain **(ETC)** is a complex carrier mechanism located on the inside of the inner mitochondrial membrane. During oxidative phosphorylation, ATP is produced when high energy potential electrons are transferred from NADH and $FADH_2$ to oxygen by a series of carrier molecules located in the inner mitochondrial membrane. As the electrons are transferred from carrier to carrier, free energy is released, which is then used to form ATP. Most of the molecules of the ETC are **cytochromes,** electron carriers that resemble hemoglobin in the structure of their active site. The functional unit contains a central iron atom, which is capable of undergoing a reversible redox reaction; that is, it can be alternatively reduced and oxidized.

FMN (flavin mononucleotide) is the first molecule of the ETC. It is reduced when it accepts electrons from NADH, thereby oxidizing NADH to NAD^+. Sequential redox reactions continue to occur as the electrons are transferred from one carrier to the next; each carrier is reduced as it accepts an electron and is then oxidized when it passes it on to the next carrier.

The last carrier of the ETC, **cytochrome a_3,** passes its electron to the final electron acceptor, O_2. In addition to the electrons, O_2 picks up a pair of hydrogen ions from the surrounding medium, forming water.

$$2\text{H}^+ + 2\text{e}^- + \frac{1}{2}\text{O}_2 \longrightarrow \text{H}_2\text{O}$$

TEACHER TIP

KEY POINT: Oxygen is the final electron acceptor in the ETC and the result is the formation of a water molecule.

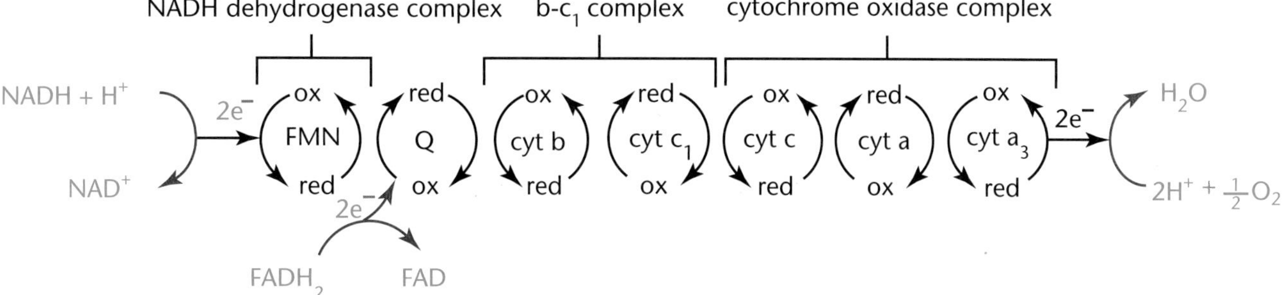

Figure 3.6. Electron Transport Chain

Without oxygen, the ETC becomes backlogged with electrons. As a result, NAD^+ cannot be regenerated and glycolysis cannot continue unless lactic acid fermentation occurs. Likewise, ATP synthesis comes to a halt if respiratory poisons such as **cyanide** or **dinitrophenol** enter the cell. Cyanide blocks the transfer of electrons from cytochrome a_3 to O_2. Dinitrophenol uncouples the electron transport chain from the proton gradient established across the inner mitochondrial membrane.

MCAT SYNOPSIS

Everything the human body does to deliver inhaled oxygen to tissues (discussed in later chapters) comes down to the role oxygen plays as the final electron acceptor in the electron transport chain. Without oxygen, ATP production is not adequate to sustain human life. Similarly, the CO_2 generated in the citric acid cycle (see Figure 3.5) is the same carbon dioxide we exhale.

b. ATP generation and the proton pump

The electron carriers are categorized into three large protein complexes: **NADH dehydrogenase,** the **b-c_1 complex,** and **cytochrome oxidase.** There are energy losses as the electrons are transferred from one complex to the next; this energy is then used to synthesize 1 ATP per complex. Thus, an electron passing through the entire ETC supplies enough energy to generate 3 ATP. NADH delivers its electrons to NADH dehydrogenase complex, so that for each NADH, 3 ATP are produced. However, $FADH_2$ bypasses the NADH dehydrogenase complex and delivers its electrons directly to **carrier Q (ubiquinone),** which lies between the NADH dehydrogenase and b-c_1 complexes. Therefore, for each $FADH_2$, there are only two energy drops, and only 2 ATP are produced.

MCAT SYNOPSIS

1 NADH ⟶ 3 ATP

1 $FADH_2$ ⟶ 2 ATP

The operating mechanism in this type of ATP production involves coupling the oxidation of NADH to the phosphorylation of ADP. The coupling agent for these two processes is a **proton gradient** across the inner mitochondrial membrane, maintained by the ETC. As NADH passes its electrons to the ETC, free hydrogen ions (H^+) are released and accumulate in the mitochondrial matrix. The ETC pumps these ions out of the matrix, across the inner mitochondrial membrane, and into the intermembrane space at each of the

TEACHER TIP

Large multicellular organisms absolutely must have the ability to generate ATP via oxidative phosphorylation. Glycolysis alone is insufficient for these organisms to maintain life.

three protein complexes. The continuous translocation of H^+ creates a positively charged acidic environment in the intermembrane space. This electrochemical gradient generates a **proton-motive force,** which drives H^+ back across the inner membrane and into the matrix. However, to pass through the membrane (which is impermeable to ions), the H^+ must flow through specialized channels provided by enzyme complexes called **ATP synthetases.** As the H^+ pass through the ATP synthetases, enough energy is released to allow for the phosphorylation of ADP to ATP. The coupling of the oxidation of NADH with the phosphorylation of ADP is called **oxidative phosphorylation.**

MCAT SYNOPSIS

Event	Location
Glycolysis	Cytoplasm
Fermentation	Cytoplasm
Pyruvate to Acetyl CoA	Mitochondrial matrix
TCA cycle	Mitochondrial matrix
Electron transport chain	Inner mitochondrial membrane

C. REVIEW OF GLUCOSE CATABOLISM

It is important to understand how all of the events described above are interrelated. Figure 3.7 is a eukaryotic cell with a mitochondrion magnified for detail.

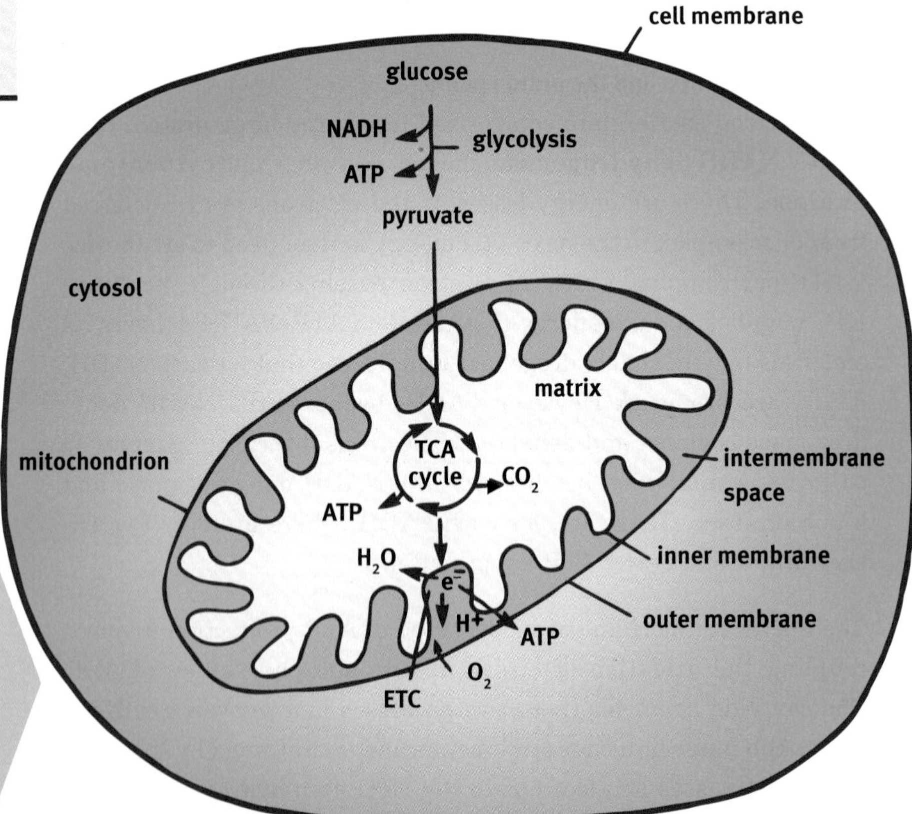

Figure 3.7. Schematic of Glucose Catabolism

TEACHER TIP

KEY POINT: The cell compartmentalizes the glycolytic pathway in a different location from pyruvate decarboxylation and the TCA cycle and ETC. Know where these processes occur—they are a perennial MCAT favorite.

To calculate the net amount of ATP produced per molecule of glucose we need to tally the number of ATP produced by substrate level phosphorylation and the number of ATP produced by oxidative phosphorylation.

1. Substrate Level Phosphorylation

Degradation of 1 glucose molecule yields a net of 2 ATP from glycolysis and 1 ATP for each turn of the citric acid cycle. Thus, a total of 4 ATP are produced by substrate level phosphorylation.

TEACHER TIP

This ATP is actually made in the form of GTP, which is energetically equivalent.

2. Oxidative Phosphorylation

Two pyruvate decarboxylations yield 1 NADH each for a total of 2 NADH. Each turn of the citric acid cycle yields 3 NADH and 1 $FADH_2$, for a total of 6 NADH and 2 $FADH_2$ per glucose molecule. Each $FADH_2$ generates 2 ATP, as previously discussed. Each NADH generates 3 ATP except for the 2 NADH that were reduced during glycolysis; these NADH cannot cross the inner mitochondrial membrane and must transfer their electrons to an intermediate carrier molecule, which delivers the electrons to the second carrier protein complex, Q. Therefore, these NADH generate only 2 ATP per glucose. So the 2 NADH of glycolysis yield 4 ATP, the other 8 NADH yield 24 ATP, and the 2 $FADH_2$ produce 4 ATP, for a total of 32 ATP by oxidative phosphorylation.

MCAT SYNOPSIS

In an ANAEROBIC environment, eukaryotic cells can generate only 2 net ATP; in an AEROBIC environment, these cells can generate a net of 36 ATP!

The total amount of ATP produced during eukaryotic glucose catabolism is therefore 4 via substrate level phosphorylation plus 32 via oxidative phosphorylation, for a total of 36 ATP. (For prokaryotes the yield is 38 ATP, because the 2 NADH of glycolysis don't have any mitochondrial membranes to cross and therefore don't lose energy.) See Table 3.1 for a summary of eukaryotic ATP production.

Table 3.1. Eukaryotic ATP Production per Glucose Molecule

Glycolysis		
2 ATP invested (steps 1 and 3)	−2	ATP
4 ATP generated (steps 6 and 9)	+4	ATP (substrate)
2 NADH × 2 ATP/NADH (step 5)	+4	ATP (oxidative)
Pyruvate Decarboxylation		
2 NADH × 3 ATP/NADH	+ 6	ATP (oxidative)
Citric Acid Cycle		
6 NADH × 3 ATP/NADH	+18	ATP (oxidative)
2 $FADH_2$ × 2 ATP/$FADH_2$	+ 4	ATP (oxidative)
2 GTP × 1 ATP/GTP	+ 2	ATP (substrate)
Total	**+136**	**ATP**

TEACHER TIP

The body's ability to use a variety of energy sources is the basis for different fad diets. Regardless of the intake, though, the same three types of intermediate molecules (carbohydrates, proteins, and fats) are used to run the body.

ALTERNATE ENERGY SOURCES

When glucose supplies run low, the body uses other energy sources. These sources are used by the body in the following preferential order: other carbohydrates, fats, and proteins. These substances are first converted to either glucose or glucose intermediates, which can then be degraded in the glycolytic pathway and TCA cycle.

A. CARBOHYDRATES

Disaccharides are hydrolyzed into monosaccharides, most of which can be converted into glucose or glycolytic intermediates. Glycogen stored in the liver can be converted, when needed, into glucose 6-phosphate, a glycolytic intermediate.

B. FATS

Fat molecules are stored in adipose tissue in the form of triglyceride. When needed, they are hydrolyzed by lipases to fatty acids and glycerol, and are carried by the blood to other tissues for oxidation. Glycerol can be converted into PGAL, a glycolytic intermediate. A fatty acid must first be "activated" in the cytoplasm; this process requires 2 ATP. Once activated, the fatty acid is transported into the mitochondrion and taken through a series of **beta-oxidation cycles** that convert it into two-carbon fragments, which are then converted into acetyl CoA. Acetyl CoA then enters the TCA cycle. With each round of β-oxidation of a saturated fatty acid, 1 NADH and 1 $FADH_2$ are generated.

CLINICAL CORRELATE

Diabetic ketoacidosis (DKA) occurs when diabetics (primarily insulin dependent) fail to take their insulin. The blood glucose levels accumulate and the cells are, ironically, starved for glucose because there is no insulin. As a result, their bodies resort to the breakdown of fats, which produces β-ketoacids, eventually resulting in a coma, as they build up in the bloodstream.

Of all the high-energy compounds used in cellular respiration, fats yield the greatest number of ATP per gram. This makes them extremely efficient energy storage molecules. Thus, while the amount of glycogen stored in humans is enough to meet the short-term energy needs of about a day, the stored fat reserves can meet the long-term energy needs for about a month.

C. PROTEINS

The body degrades amino acids (the building blocks of proteins) only when there is not enough carbohydrate available. Most amino acids undergo a **transamination** reaction in which they lose an amino group to form an α-keto acid. The carbon atoms of most amino acids are converted into acetyl CoA, pyruvate, or one of the intermediates of the citric acid cycle. These intermediates enter their respective metabolic pathways, allowing cells to produce fatty acids, glucose, or energy in the form of ATP.

METABOLIC MAP

Below is a diagram illustrating the relationship between fats, protein, and carbohydrate catabolism. Note where the products of fats and protein catabolism feed into the reactions of carbohydrate catabolism.

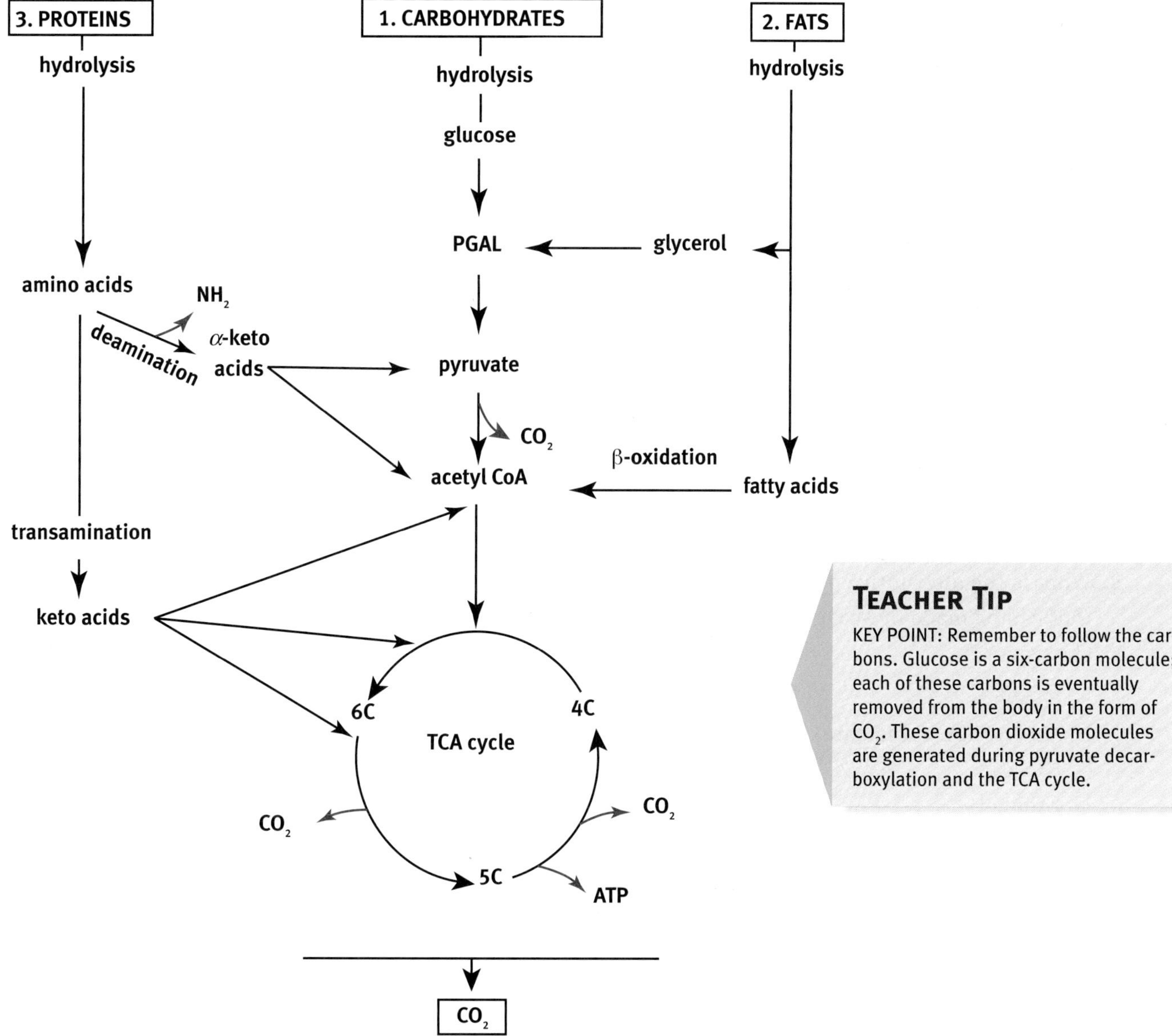

Figure 3.8. Nutrient Metabolism

TEACHER TIP

KEY POINT: Remember to follow the carbons. Glucose is a six-carbon molecule; each of these carbons is eventually removed from the body in the form of CO_2. These carbon dioxide molecules are generated during pyruvate decarboxylation and the TCA cycle.

PRACTICE QUESTIONS

1. Red blood cells (RBC) metabolize glucose anaerobically due to the absence of mitochondria. Which process is of primary importance to provide energy for RBCs?

   A. Electron transport chain
   B. Oxidative phosphorylation
   C. Citric acid (Krebs) cycle
   D. Glycolysis

2. Which part of the process of catabolism of glucose can be referred to as respiratory and accounts for the greatest portion of oxygen use by the body, producing the highest amount of ATP?

   A. Pyruvate decarboxylation
   B. Electron transport chain
   C. Glycolysis
   D. Citric acid (Krebs) cycle

3. What is the alternative product to lactic acid that can be made by yeast in the absence of oxygen?

   A. Pyruvate
   B. Acetyl CoA and lactate
   C. Glucose
   D. Ethanol

4. A researcher is staining cells with a fluorescent marker, which binds to the enzyme pyruvate dehydrogenase to experimentally verify its location. This enzyme catalyzes the reaction shown below. Theoretically, the fluorescence is expected at which location?

   Alcohol Dehydrogenase

   Ethanol ⟶ Acetaldehyde

   A. Cytoplasm
   B. Inner membrane of mitochondria
   C. Matrix of mitochondria
   D. Rough endoplasmic reticulum

5. β-ketoacids detected in a patient's urine signal the catabolism of

   A. fats.
   B. proteins.
   C. carbohydrates.
   D. nucleic acids.

6. ATP consists of the base adenine, ribose, and three phosphates. It is structurally similar to which of the following?

   A. Phospholipid
   B. Amino acid
   C. Nucleic acid
   D. Monosaccharide

7. In the process of breaking down amino acids, which of the following groups must be detached before the amino acid can enter the citric acid cycle?

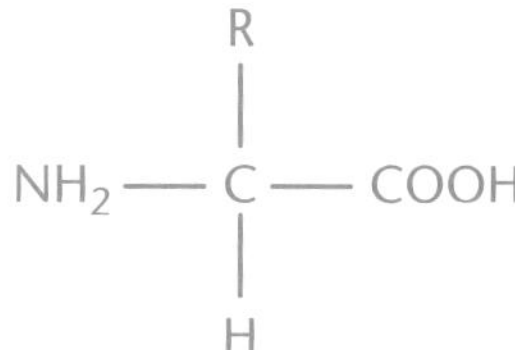

A. R-radical group of amino acid
B. COOH-carboxylic group of amino acid
C. H-proton of amino acid
D. NH_2^- amino group

8. For which of the following situations is anaerobic glycolysis of primary importance?

I. Oxygen supply is limited to the tissue.
II. Glucose supply is limited.
III. Tissues have few or no mitochondria.

A. I, II and III
B. I and III
C. I only
D. I and II

9. As lactic acid accumulates in the skeletal muscle during intense exercise, all of the following must be taking place EXCEPT

A. oxidative phosphorylation.
B. pyruvate conversion to lactate.
C. intracellular pH decreas.
D. anaerobic glycolysis.

10. Lipitor, one of the "statin" medications, competitively inhibits one of the rate-limiting steps in cholesterol synthesis. It can be inferred that

A. Lipitor binds at a site different from where the substrate binds.
B. Lipitor binds to the active site of the enzyme.
C. Lipitor binds to cholesterol.
D. None of the above

11. Phosporylation of glucose to glucose 6-phosphate is catalyzed by the enzyme hexokinase. As glucose 6-phosphate accumulates, it inhibits hexokinase activity. This is an example of what kind of activity?

A. Hormonal regulation
B. Negative feedback
C. Positive feedback loop
D. Parasympathetic regulation

12. How many lactate molecules are generated for each glucose molecule entering anaerobic glycolysis?

A. 3
B. 1
C. 4
D. 2

13. What molecule enters the tricarboxylic acid cycle in a cell?

A. Glucose
B. Acetyl CoA
C. NAD^+
D. Malate

14. What high-energy molecule is responsible for the production of most ATP as it passes its electrons along the electron transport chain?

A. $FADH^2$
B. NADH
C. GTP
D. Cytochrome a

15. According to the table below, one molecule of Acetyl CoA produces:

High-Energy Molecules Produced	ATP Conversion
3NADH	NADH ⟶ 3ATP
$FADH_2$	$FADH_2$ ⟶ 2ATP
GTP	GTP ⟶ ATP

What is the total amount of ATP yielded by the catabolism of one glucose molecule via the Krebs cycle?

A. 6 ATP
B. 12 ATP
C. 24 ATP
D. 36 ATP

16. In which part of glucose catabolism is CO_2 produced?

A. Tricarboxylic acid cycle
B. Electron transport chain
C. Phosphorylation
D. Glycolysis

CHAPTER 4

REPRODUCTION

Reproduction is the process by which an organism perpetuates itself and its species, ensuring the precise duplication of genetic material and its representation in successive generations. Reproduction can be divided into three topics: **cell division, asexual reproduction,** and **sexual reproduction.**

CELL DIVISION

Cell division is the process by which a cell doubles its organelles and cytoplasm, replicates its DNA, and then divides in two. For unicellular organisms, cell division is a means of reproduction, while for multicellular organisms it is a method of growth, development, and replacement of worn-out cells. Prokaryotes and eukaryotes differ in their means of cell division.

Prokaryotes divide by a process called **binary fission** (a type of asexual reproduction). The single DNA molecule attaches to the plasma membrane during replication and duplicates, while the cell continues to grow in size. The cell membrane pinches inward, splitting the cell into two equal halves, with each daughter cell receiving a complete copy of the original chromosome.

Eukaryotic cell division is more complicated than binary fission because cells must duplicate and equally distribute chromosomes, organelles, and cytoplasm to both daughter cells. Eukaryotic **somatic,** or **autosomal,** cells contain the diploid number of chromosomes characteristic of its species, which is designated as **2N (N** is the number of chromosomes found in a **haploid** cell, or **gamete).** The diploid number for humans is 46, and the haploid number is 23; 23 chromosomes are inherited from each parent.

> **TEACHER TIP**
>
> KEY POINT: In autosomal cells, division results in two identical (genetically) daughter cells. In germ line cells, the daughters are NOT equivalent.

The life cycle of a eukaryotic cell can be broken down into four distinct stages collectively known as the **cell cycle.**

A. THE CELL CYCLE

The four stages of the cell cycle are designated as **G_1, S, G_2,** and **M.** The first three stages of the cell cycle are **interphase** stages, that is, they occur between cell divisions. The fourth stage, **mitosis,** includes the actual cell division.

TEACHER TIP

Some cells never divide again once they are mature. This group includes neurons and muscle cells. They exist in an offshoot of G_1 called G_0, which is maintenance phase.

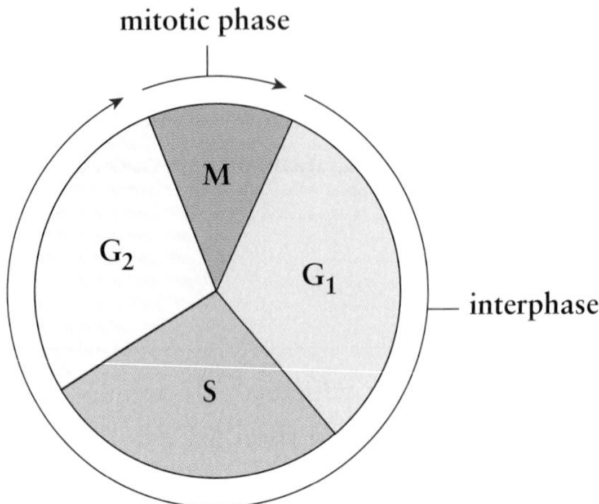

Figure 4.1. The Cell Cycle

1. Interphase

This is by far the longest part of the cell cycle. A cell normally spends at least 90 percent of the cycle in interphase.

a. G1 stage (presynthetic gap)

This stage is one of intense biochemical activity and growth. The cell doubles in size and new organelles such as mitochondria, ribosomes, endoplasmic reticulum, and centrioles are produced. A typical cell proceeds through the G_1 stage, passing a **restriction point,** after which it is committed to continue through the rest of the cell cycle and divide. However, some cells, including specialized skeletal muscle cells and nerve cells, never pass this point, instead entering a nondividing phase sometimes referred to as **G_0.**

b. S stage (synthesis)

In the synthetic stage each chromosome is replicated so that during division, a complete copy of the genome can be distributed to both daughter cells. After replication, the chromosomes, consist of two identical **sister chromatids** held together at a central region called the **centromere.** The ends of the chromosome are called the **telomeres.** Note that after DNA replication, the cell still contains the diploid number (2N) of chromosomes, but because each chromosome now consists of two chromatids, cells entering G_2 actually contain twice as much DNA as cells in G_1.

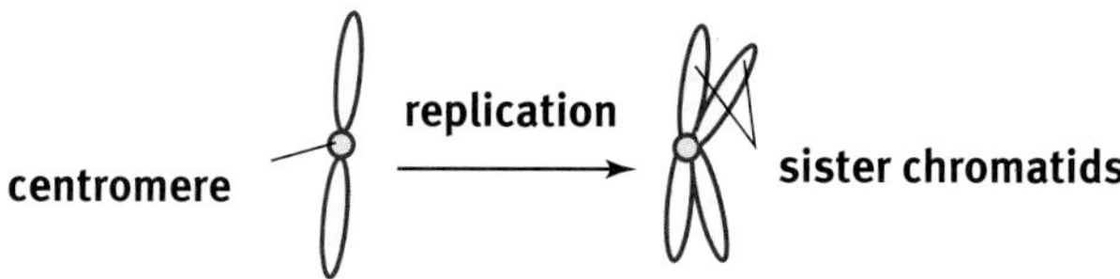

Figure 4.2. Chromosome Replication

MCAT SYNOPSIS

Each chromatid is a complete, double-stranded molecule of DNA. Sister chromatids are identical copies of each other. The term "chromosome" may be used to refer to either the single chromatid or the pair of chromatids attached at the centromere.

c. G_2 stage (postsynthetic gap)

The cell continues to grow in size, while assembly of new organelles and other cell structures continues.

2. M Stage (Mitotic Stage)

This stage consists of mitosis and **cytokinesis**. Mitosis is the division and distribution of the cell's DNA to its two daughter cells such that each cell receives a complete copy of the original genome. Cytokinesis refers to the division of cytoplasm that follows.

a. Mitosis

During interphase, the nucleus is membrane-bound and clearly visible, and one or more nucleoli may be observed. Individual chromosomes are not visible under a light microscope because they are active and uncoiled. The DNA appears granular and is called **chromatin.** As mitosis begins, the chromosomes coil up, condense, and become visible under high-power microscopy. This coiling facilitates their movement during the later stages of mitosis.

TEACHER TIP

Know the difference between chromosomes and chromatids. An autosomal cell never has more than the 2N (46 in human) number of chromosomes except in disease conditions. It will have 92 chromatids, however, right before mitosis.

Chromosome movement is dependent on certain cytoplasmic organelles. The centrioles, which are typically found in pairs, are cylindrical organelles located outside of the interphase nucleus in an area referred to as the **centrosome.** During the first stage of mitosis, the centrioles, which have already replicated, migrate to opposite poles of the cell, and a system of **spindle fibers** composed of microtubules and associated proteins appears near each pair of centrioles. The spindle fibers radiate outward from the centrioles, forming structures called **asters.** The asters extend toward the center of the nucleus, forming the **spindle apparatus.** The movement of chromosomes toward opposite poles of the cell during the later stages of mitosis is caused by the shortening of the spindle apparatus.

Although mitosis is a continuous process, four stages are discernible: **prophase, metaphase, anaphase,** and **telophase.**

TEACHER TIP

Failure in mitosis or its regulation often results in an unequal distribution of genetic material to the daughter cells. Most of the time, the cell will undergo cell death if this occurs. However, this sort of unregulated cell division without regard to the genomic stability is a hallmark of cancer.

- **Prophase**
  The chromosomes condense, the centriole pairs separate and move toward opposite poles of the cell, and the spindle apparatus forms between them. The nuclear membrane dissolves, allowing spindle fibers to enter the nucleus, while the nucleoli become less distinct or disappear. **Kinetochores,** with attached **kinetochore fibers,** appear at the chromosome centromere.

- **Metaphase**
  The centriole pairs are now at opposite poles of the cell. The kinetochore fibers interact with the fibers of the spindle apparatus to align the chromosomes at the **metaphase plate** (equatorial plate), which is equidistant to the two poles of the spindle fibers.

EXCLUSIVE

Mitosis = PMAT

Prophase:	chromosomes condense; spindles form
Metaphase:	chromosomes align
Anaphase:	sister chromatids separate
Telophase:	new nuclear membranes form

- **Anaphase**
  The centromeres now split, so that each chromatid has its own distinct centromere, thus allowing the sister chromatids to separate. The telomeres are the last part of the chromatids to separate. The sister chromatids are pulled toward the opposite poles of the cell by the shortening of the kinetochore fibers.

- **Telophase**
  The spindle apparatus disappears. A nuclear membrane forms around each set of chromosomes and the nucleoli reappear. The chromosomes uncoil, resuming their interphase form. Each of the two new nuclei has received a complete copy of the genome identical to the original genome and to each other. Cytokinesis occurs.

See Figure 4.3 for a summary of mitosis.

b. Cytokinesis

Near the end of telophase, the cytoplasm divides into two daughter cells, each with a complete nucleus and its own set of organelles. In animal cells, a cleavage furrow forms; the cell membrane indents along the equator of the cell and finally pinches through the cell, separating the two nuclei.

The life cycle of a cell is not an arbitrary series of events; cell division is a specified sequence of events dictated by the nucleus. For example, a typical somatic cell is programmed to divide between 20 and 50 times and then die. As mentioned earlier, some cells, such as

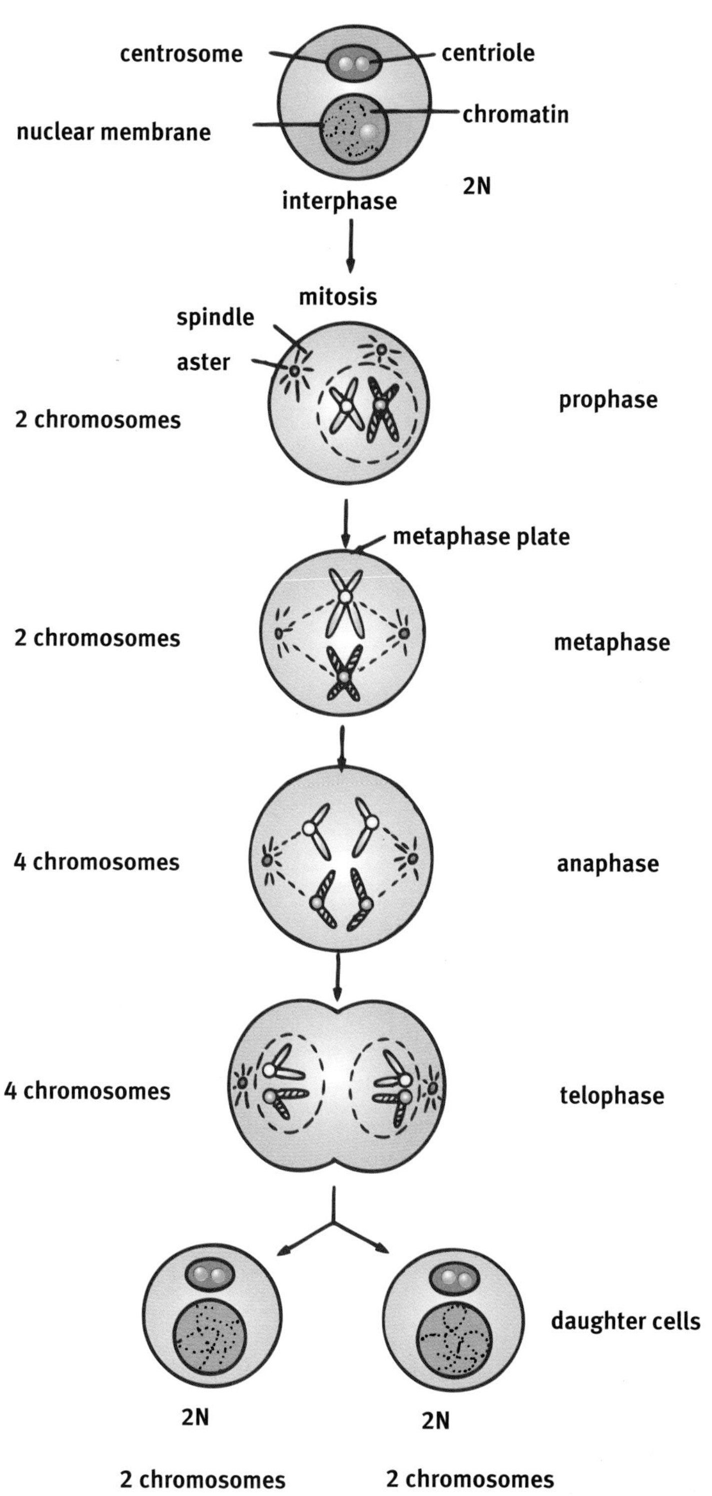

Figure 4.3. Mitosis

MCAT SYNOPSIS

Mitosis
1) Somatic cells
2) Diploid → Diploid
2N → 2N
3) 2 Daughter cells

CLINICAL CORRELATE

Cancer cells are cells in which mitosis has gone wild. The challenge of cancer therapy (chemotherapy) is to kill cancer cells without destroying the body's normal cells. Because cancer cells typically divide faster than normal cells, most chemotherapeutic agents work by targeting rapidly dividing cells. They do so by a variety of mechanisms such as inhibiting DNA synthesis or affecting spindle formation or function.

TEACHER TIP

KEY POINT: The MCAT loves to test the differences between mitosis and meiosis. Be sure to note that the diploid number is maintained throughout mitosis, whereas the process of meiosis results in haploid cells.

muscle and nerve cells, never divide at all. Cancer cells can divide indefinitely; they do not respond to the control mechanisms that normally regulate cell division.

Teacher Tip

Asexual reproduction doesn't allow for as much genetic diversity to be generated—one of the major benefits of sexual reproduction.

ASEXUAL REPRODUCTION

Asexual reproduction is the production of offspring without fertilization. New organisms are formed by division of a single parent cell. Offspring are essentially genetic carbon copies of their parent cells. Thus, except for random mutations, the offspring are genetically identical to the parent cells. The different types of asexual reproduction are **binary fission, budding, regeneration,** and **parthenogenesis.**

A. BINARY FISSION

Binary fission is a simple form of asexual reproduction seen in prokaryotes. The circular chromosome replicates and a new plasma membrane and cell wall grow inward along the midline of the cell, dividing it into two equally sized cells, each containing a duplicate of the parent chromosome. A very similar process occurs in some primitive eukaryotic cells.

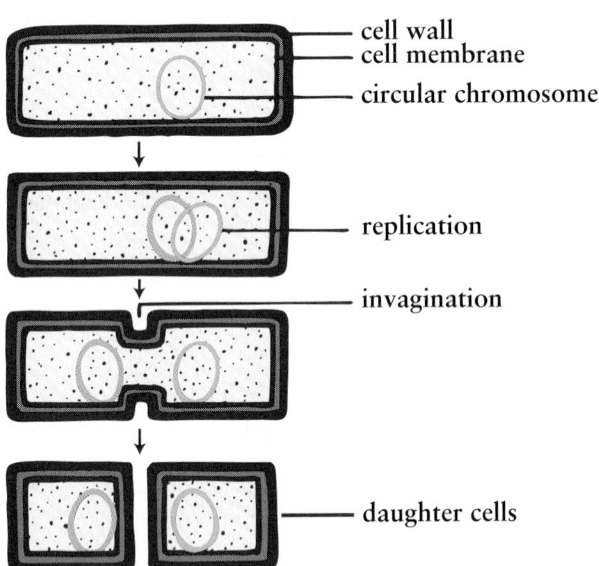

Figure 4.4. Binary Fission

B. BUDDING

Budding is the replication of the nucleus followed by unequal cytokinesis. The cell membrane pinches inward to form a new cell that is smaller in size but genetically identical to the parent cell and which subsequently grows to adult size. The new cell may separate immediately from the parent or it may remain attached to it, develop as an outgrowth, and separate at a later stage. Budding occurs in hydra and yeast.

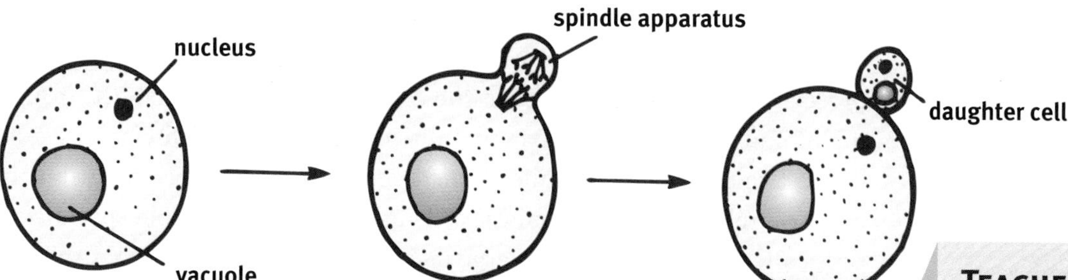

Figure 4.5. Budding

TEACHER TIP

Binary fission results in two cells of equal size, whereas budding results in cells of unequal size. Both cases, however, give rise to genetically identical cells.

C. REGENERATION

Regeneration is the regrowth of a lost or injured body part. Replacement of cells occurs by mitosis. Some lower animals such as hydra and starfish have extensive regenerative capabilities. If a starfish loses an arm, it can regenerate a new one; the severed arm may even be able to regenerate an entire body, as long as the arm contains a piece of an area called the central disk. Salamanders and tadpoles can generate new limbs. The extent of regeneration depends on the nerve damage to the severed body part. In adult birds and mammals, regeneration is usually limited to the healing of tissues, although some internal organs, such as the liver, have considerable regenerative capabilities as long as part of the organ remains viable.

TEACHER TIP

In fact, liver transplants can now be done from living donors. Only part of the liver is removed and transplanted. The donor's liver will enlarge in both the donor and recipient until it reaches the appropriate size.

D. PARTHENOGENESIS

Parthenogenesis is the development of an unfertilized egg into an adult organism. This process occurs naturally in certain lower organisms. For example, in most species of bees and ants, the males develop from unfertilized eggs, and several species of all-female, parthenogenetic salamander exist. The eggs of some higher organisms can be induced to develop parthenogenetically (although the process does not occur naturally), with the resulting embryos surviving for variable lengths of time. Frog eggs have been induced to develop into tadpoles, and unfertilized rabbit eggs have been stimulated to develop into adult rabbits. Because the organism develops from a haploid cell, all of its cells will be haploid.

SEXUAL REPRODUCTION

Sexual reproduction differs from asexual reproduction in that there are two parents involved, and the end result is genetically unique offspring. Sexual reproduction occurs via the fusion of two gametes—specialized sex cells produced by each parent. **Meiosis** is the process whereby these

TEACHER TIP

Unlike asexual reproduction, the offspring will be genetically unique from either of the parents—who are also genetically unique from one another.

sex cells are produced. Meiosis is similar to mitosis in that a cell duplicates its chromosomes before undergoing the process. However, mitosis preserves the diploid number of the cell, while meiosis halves it, resulting in haploid cells. Furthermore, mitosis comprises one division resulting in two diploid cells, while meiosis comprises two divisions resulting in four haploid gametes. Somatic cells undergo mitosis, while specialized cells called **gametocytes** undergo meiosis. During fertilization, two haploid gametes fuse, restoring the diploid number.

MCAT FAVORITE

Remember that MITOSIS occurs in all of the cells of the body that divide. MEIOSIS occurs only in the sex cells (a.k.a., "germ cells" or gametocytes) found in the reproductive system (the testes and ovaries).

A. MEIOSIS

As in mitosis, the gametocyte's chromosomes are replicated during the S phase of the cell cycle and the centrioles replicate at some point during interphase. The first round of division (meiosis I) produces two intermediate daughter cells. The second round of division (meiosis II), similar to mitosis, involves the separation of the sister chromatids, resulting in four genetically distinct haploid gametes. Each meiotic division has the same four stages as mitosis.

1. Meiosis I

a. Prophase I

The chromatin condenses into chromosomes, the spindle apparatus forms, and the nucleoli and nuclear membrane disappear. **Homologous chromosomes** (chromosomes that code for the same traits, one inherited from each parent), come together and intertwine in a process called **synapsis.** Because at this stage each chromosome consists of two sister chromatids, each synaptic pair of homologous chromosomes contains four chromatids and is, therefore, often called a **tetrad.** Sometimes chromatids of homologous chromosomes break at corresponding points and exchange equivalent pieces of DNA; this process is called **crossing over.** Note that crossing over occurs between homologous chromosomes and not between sister chromatids of the same chromosome. (The latter are identical, so crossing over would not produce any change.) Those chromatids involved are left with an altered but structurally complete set of genes. The chromosomes remain joined at points called **chiasmata** where the crossing over occurred. Such **genetic recombination** can "unlink" **linked genes** (see chapter 13), thereby increasing the variety of genetic combinations that can be produced via gametogenesis. Recombination among chromosomes results in increased genetic diversity within a species. Note that sister chromatids are no longer identical after recombination has occurred (see Figure 4.6).

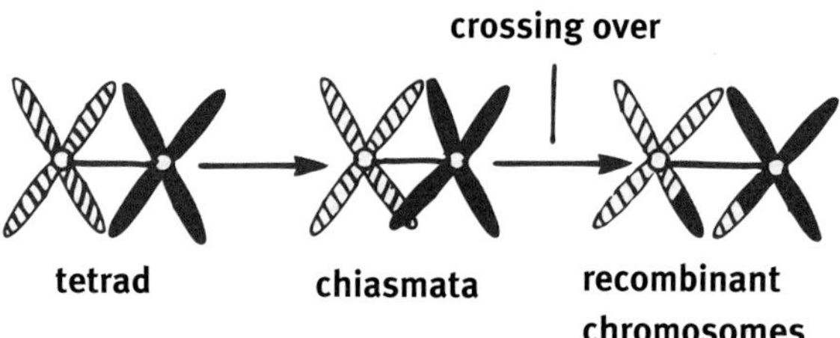

Figure 4.6. Synapsis

MCAT SYNOPSIS

Meiosis = PMAT × 2

PMAT
↓
PMAT

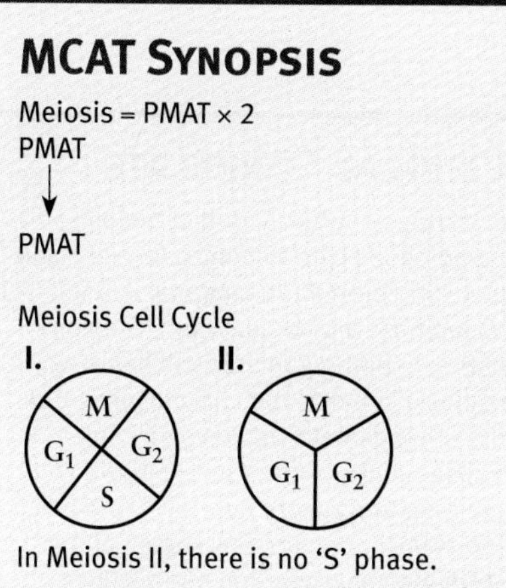

In Meiosis II, there is no 'S' phase.

TEACHER TIP

It is critical to understand how meiosis I differs from mitosis. The chromosome number is halved (reductional division) in meiosis I. The daughter cells have the haploid number of chromosomes (23 in humans). Meiosis II is similar to mitosis in that sister chromatids are separated from one another.

b. Metaphase I

Homologous pairs (tetrads) align at the equatorial plane, and each pair attaches to a separate spindle fiber by its kinetochore.

c. Anaphase I

The homologous pairs separate and are pulled to opposite poles of the cell. This process is called **disjunction,** and it accounts for a fundamental **Mendelian law** (see chapter 13). During disjunction, each chromosome of paternal origin separates (or disjoins) from its homologue of maternal origin, and either chromosome can end up in either daughter cell. Thus, the distribution of homologous chromosomes to the two intermediate daughter cells is random with respect to parental origin. Each daughter cell will have a unique pool of **alleles** (genes coding for alternative forms of a given trait; e.g., yellow flowers or purple flowers) from a random mixture of maternal and paternal origin.

d. Telophase I

A nuclear membrane forms around each new nucleus. At this point each chromosome still consists of sister chromatids joined at the centromere. The cell divides (by cytokinesis) into two daughter cells, each of which receives a nucleus containing the haploid number of chromosomes. Between cell divisions there may be a short rest period, or **interkinesis,** during which the chromosomes partially uncoil.

2. Meiosis II

This second division is very similar to mitosis, except that meiosis II is not preceded by chromosomal replication.

a. Prophase II

The centrioles migrate to opposite poles and the spindle apparatus forms.

Clinical Correlate

If, during anaphase I or II of meiosis, homologous chromosomes (anaphase I) or sister chromatids (anaphase II) fail to separate (nondisjunction), then one of the resulting gametes will have two copies of a particular chromosome and the other gamete will have no copies. Subsequently, during fertilization, the resulting zygote may have one too many or one too few copies of the chromosome. Note that nondisjunction can affect both the autosomal chromosomes (e.g., trisomy 21; Down's syndrome) and the sex chromosomes (Klinefelter's; Turner's).

MCAT Synopsis

1) Sex cells
2) Diploid ⟶ Haploid
   2N ⟶ 1N
3) 4 daughter cells in males (except in females; there is only 1 daughter cell)

Teacher Tip

In females, the other cells generated contain genetic material but they are incapable of undergoing fertilization and creating a zygote.

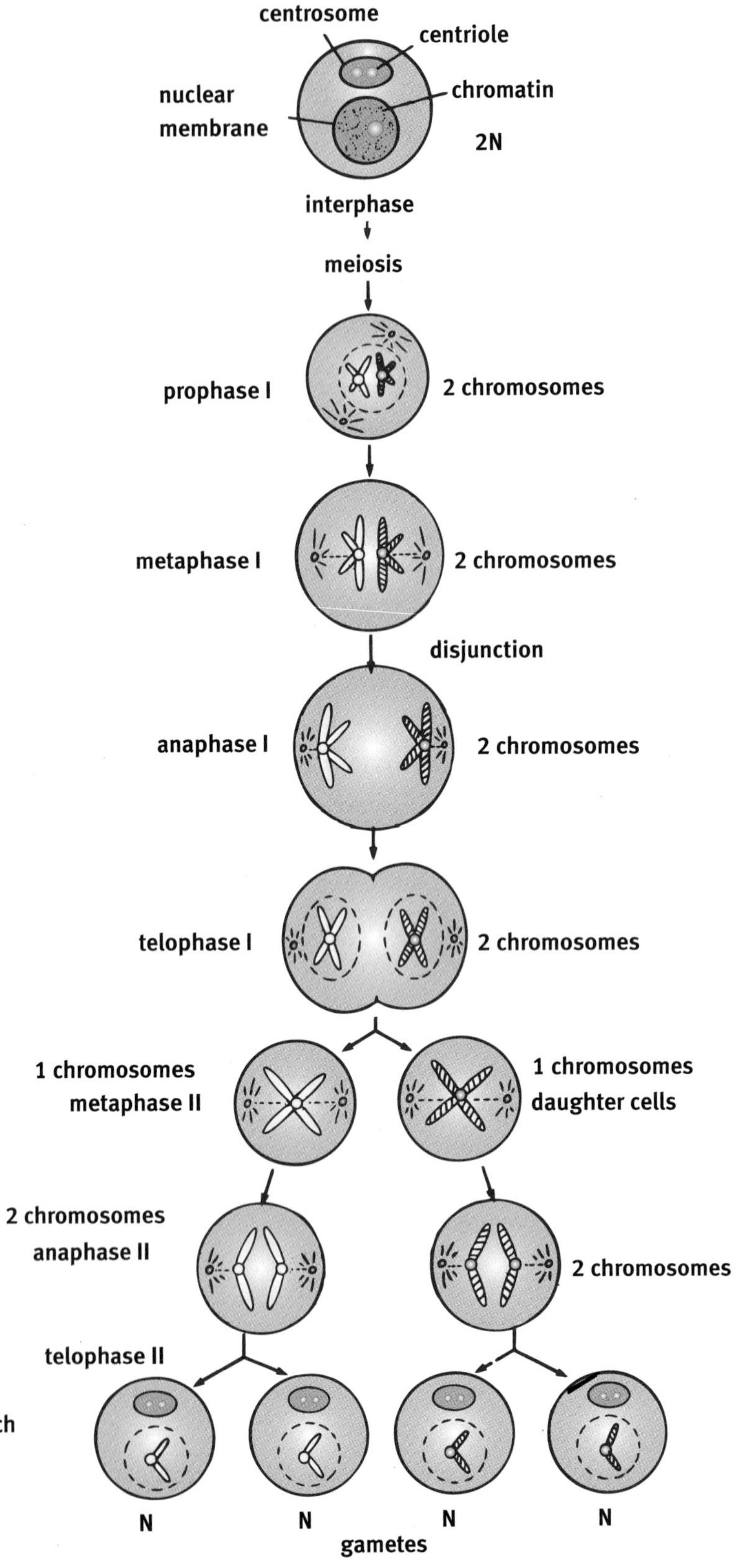

Figure 4.7. Meiosis

b. Metaphase II

The chromosomes line up along the equatorial plane. The centromeres divide, separating the chromosomes into pairs of sister chromatids.

c. Anaphase II

The sister chromatids are pulled to opposite poles by the spindle fibers.

d. Telophase II

A nuclear membrane forms around each new (haploid) nucleus. Cytokinesis follows and two daughter cells are formed. Thus, by the completion of meiosis II, four haploid daughter cells are produced per gametocyte. (In women, only one of these becomes a functional gamete.)

The random distribution of chromosomes in meiosis, coupled with crossing over in prophase I, enables an individual to produce gametes with many different genetic combinations. Thus, as opposed to asexual reproduction, which produces identical offspring, sexual reproduction produces genetic variability in offspring. The possibility of so many different genetic combinations is believed to increase the capability of a species to evolve and adapt to a changing environment.

> **MCAT SYNOPSIS**
>
> | Mitosis | Meiosis |
> |---|---|
> | 2N ⟶ 2N | 2N ⟶ N |
> | Occurs in all dividing cells | Occurs in sex cells only |
> | Homologous chromosomes don't pair up | Homologous chromosomes pair up at metaphase plate forming tetrads |
> | No crossing over | Crossing over can occur |

B. HUMAN SEXUAL REPRODUCTION

Human reproduction is a highly complex process involving not only sexual intercourse between male and female but also interactions between the reproductive and endocrine systems within the body. Children are the product of fertilization—the fusion of **sperm** and **egg** (the gametes) in the female reproductive tract. The gametes are produced in the primary reproductive organs, or **gonads.**

> **MCAT SYNOPSIS**
>
> To remember the pathway of sperm, think SEVEN UP.
>
> Seminiferous tubules
> Epididymus
> Vas deferens
> Ejaculatory duct
> (Nothing)
> Urethra
> Penis

1. Male Reproductive Anatomy

The male gonads, called the **testes,** contain two functional components: the **seminiferous tubules** and the **interstitial cells (cells of Leydig).** Sperm are produced in the highly coiled seminiferous tubules, where they are nourished by **Sertoli cells.** The interstitial cells, located between the seminiferous tubules, secrete **testosterone** and other **androgens** (male sex hormones) (see chapter 11). The testes are located in an external pouch called the **scrotum,** which maintains testes temperature 2–4°C lower than body temperature, a condition essential for sperm survival. Sperm pass from the seminiferous tubules into the coiled tubules of the **epididymis.** Here they acquire

> **TEACHER TIP**
>
> Common MCAT topic: Enzymes have a temperature range in which they maximally work. Consider what this means in terms of enzymes, which work in the testes.

motility, mature, and are stored until **ejaculation.** During ejaculation they travel through the **vas deferens** to the ejaculatory duct and then to the **urethra.** The urethra passes through the **penis** and opens to the outside at its tip. In males, the urethra is a common passageway for both the reproductive and excretory systems.

CLINICAL CORRELATE

In older males, the prostate often enlarges. Because it surrounds the urethra, this commonly results in urinary frequency and urgency.

Sperm is mixed with **seminal fluid** as it moves along the reproductive tract; seminal fluid is produced by three glands: the **seminal vesicles,** the **prostate gland,** and the **bulbourethral glands.** The paired seminal vesicles secrete a fructose-rich fluid that serves as an energy source for the highly active sperm. The prostate gland releases an alkaline milky fluid that protects the sperm from the acidic environment of the female reproductive tract. Finally, the bulbourethral glands secrete a small amount of viscous fluid prior to ejaculation; the function of this secretion is not known. Seminal fluid aids in sperm transport by lubricating the passageways through which the sperm will travel. Sperm plus seminal fluid is known as **semen.**

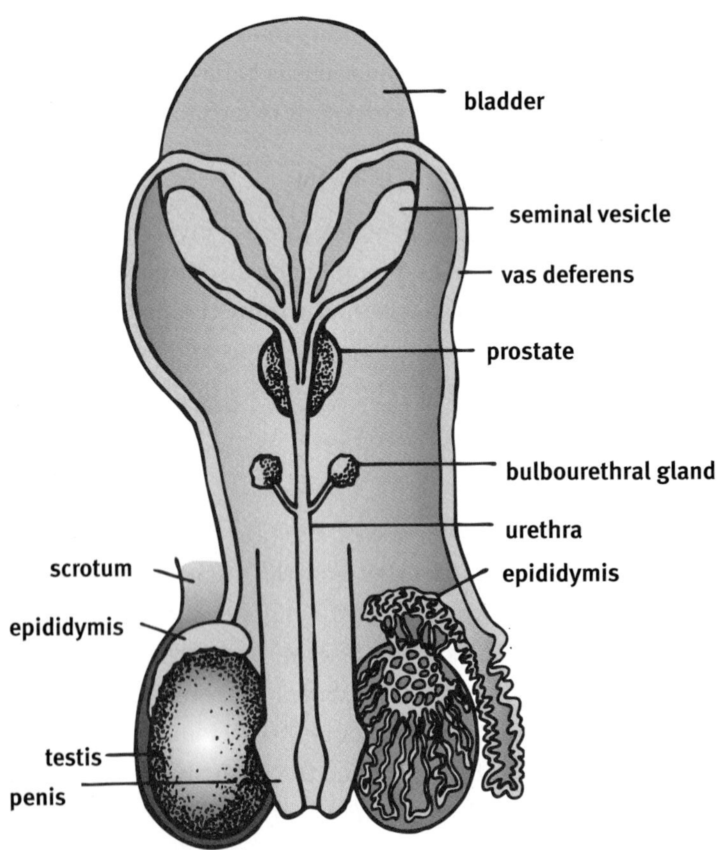

Figure 4.8. Male Reproductive Tract

2. Spermatogenesis

Spermatogenesis, or sperm production, occurs in the seminiferous tubules. Diploid cells called **spermatogonia** differentiate into diploid cells called **primary spermatocytes,** which undergo the first meiotic division to yield two haploid **secondary spermatocytes** of equal size; the second meiotic division produces four haploid **spermatids** of equal size. Following meiosis, the spermatids undergo a series of changes leading to the production of mature sperm, or **spermatozoa,** which are specialized for transporting the sperm nucleus to the egg, or **ovum.** The mature sperm is an elongated cell with a head, neck, body, and tail. The head consists almost entirely of the nucleus. The tail (flagellum) propels the sperm, while mitochondria in the neck and body provide energy for locomotion. A caplike structure called the **acrosome,** derived from the Golgi apparatus, develops over the anterior half of the head. The acrosome contains enzymes needed to penetrate the tough outer covering of the ovum. After a male has reached sexual maturity, approximately three million primary spermatocytes begin to undergo spermatogenesis per day, the maturation process taking a total of 65–75 days.

MCAT SYNOPSIS

spermatogonia (2N)
↓
1° spermatocytes (2N)
↓ meiosis I
2° spermatocytes (N)
↓ meiosis II
spermatids (N)
↓
spermatozoa (N)

TEACHER TIP

Spermatogenesis in males is a 1:4 division whereas in females it is 1:1.

3. Female Reproductive Anatomy

The female gonads, called the **ovaries,** produce eggs **(ova),** and secrete the hormones estrogen and progesterone (see chapter 11). The ovaries are found in the abdominal cavity, below the digestive system. The ovaries consist of thousands of **follicles**; a follicle is a multilayered sac of cells that contains, nourishes, and protects an immature ovum. It is actually the follicle cells that produce estrogen. Once a month, an immature ovum is released from the ovary into the abdominal cavity and drawn into the nearby **fallopian tube.** The inner surface of the fallopian tube is lined with cilia that create currents that move the ovum into and along the tube. Each fallopian tube opens into the upper end of a muscular chamber called the **uterus,** which is the site of fetal development. The lower, narrow end of the uterus is called the **cervix.** The cervix connects with the **vaginal canal,** which is the site of sperm deposition during intercourse and is also the passageway through which a baby is expelled during childbirth. The external female genitalia is referred to as the **vulva.** Note that in the mammalian (placental) female, the reproductive and excretory systems are distinct from one another; i.e., the urethra and the vagina are not connected.

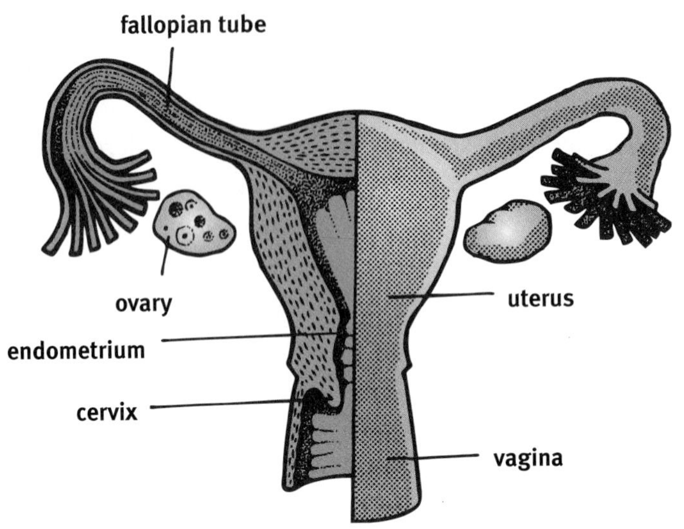

Figure 4.9. Female Reproductive Tract

4. Oogenesis

Oogenesis, which is the production of female gametes, occurs in the ovarian follicles. At birth, all of the immature ova, known as **primary oocytes,** that a female will produce during her lifetime are already in her ovaries. Primary oocytes are diploid cells that form by mitosis in the ovary. After menarche (the first time a female gets her period), one primary oocyte per month completes meiosis I, yielding two daughter cells of unequal size—a **secondary oocyte** and a small cell known as a **polar body.** The secondary oocyte is expelled from the follicle during ovulation. Meiosis II does not occur until fertilization. The oocyte cell membrane is surrounded by two layers of cells; the inner layer is the **zona pellucida,** the outer layer is the **corona radiata.** Meiosis II is triggered when these layers are penetrated by a sperm cell, yielding two haploid cells—a mature ovum and another polar body. (The first polar body may also undergo meiosis II; eventually, the polar bodies die.) The mature ovum is a large cell containing a lot of cytoplasm, RNA, organelles, and nutrients needed by a developing embryo.

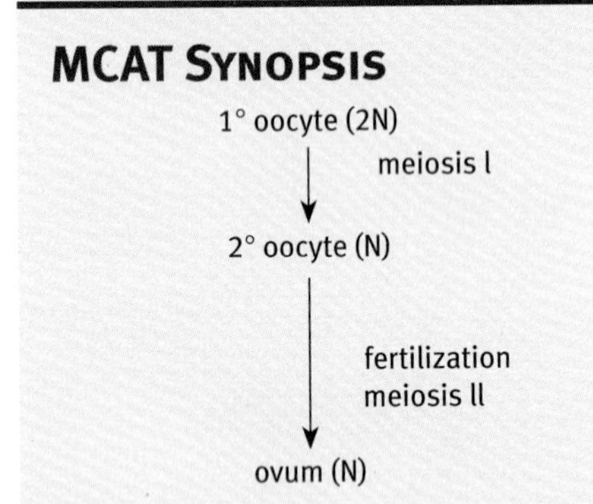

TEACHER TIP

Sometimes the egg will implant in the fallopian tube instead of the uterus. This condition is known as an *ectopic pregnancy* and is a medical emergency due to the risk of rupture and hemorrhage as the zygote enlarges.

Women ovulate approximately once every four weeks (except during pregnancy and, usually, lactation) until menopause, which typically occurs between the ages of 45 and 50. During menopause, the ovaries become less sensitive to the hormones that stimulate follicle development (FSH and LH), and eventually they atrophy. The remaining follicles disappear, estrogen and progesterone levels greatly decline, and ovulation stops. The profound changes in hormone levels are often accompanied by physiological and psychological changes that persist until a new balance is reached.

5. Fertilization

An egg can be fertilized during the 12–24 hours following ovulation. Fertilization occurs in the lateral, widest portion of the fallopian tube. Sperm must travel through the vaginal canal, cervix, uterus, and into the fallopian tubes to reach the ovum. Sperm remain viable and capable of fertilization for one to two days following intercourse.

The first barrier that the sperm must penetrate is the corona radiata. Enzymes secreted by the sperm aid in penetration of the corona radiata. The acrosome is responsible for penetrating the zona pellucida; it releases enzymes that digest this layer, thereby allowing the sperm to come into direct contact with the ovum cell membrane. Once in contact with the membrane, the sperm forms a tubelike structure called the **acrosomal process,** which extends to the cell membrane and penetrates it, fusing the sperm cell membrane with that of the ovum. The sperm nucleus now enters the ovum's cytoplasm. It is at this stage of fertilization that the ovum completes meiosis II.

The acrosomal reaction triggers a **cortical reaction** in the ovum, causing calcium ions to be released into the cytoplasm; this, in turn, initiates a series of reactions that result in the formation of the **fertilization membrane.** The fertilization membrane is a hard layer that surrounds the ovum cell membrane and prevents multiple fertilizations. The release of Ca^{2+} also stimulates metabolic changes within the ovum, greatly increasing its metabolic rate. This is followed by the fusion of the sperm nucleus with the ovum nucleus to form a diploid zygote. The first mitotic division of the zygote soon follows (see chapter 5).

6. Multiple Births

a. Monozygotic (identical) twins

Monozygotic twins result when a single zygote splits into two embryos. If the splitting occurs at the two-cell stage of development, the embryos will have separate chorions and separate placentas; if it occurs at the blastula stage, then the embryos will have only one chorionic sac and will therefore share a placenta and possibly an amnion (see chapter 5). Occasionally the division is incomplete, resulting in the birth of "Siamese" twins, which are attached at some point on the body, often sharing limbs and/or organs. Monozygotic twins are genetically identical, because they develop from the same

TEACHER TIP

Identical twins are commonly used to study the interaction between genes and the environment. Because they have the same genetic complement, they can be studied to see how much of an effect the environment has in contributing to a certain condition (e.g., schizophrenia).

zygote. Monozygotic twins are therefore of the same sex, blood type, and so on.

b. Dizygotic (fraternal) twins

Dizygotic twins result when two ova are released in one ovarian cycle and are fertilized by two different sperm. The two embryos implant in the uterine wall individually, and each develops its own placenta, amnion, and chorion (although the placentas may fuse if the embryos implant very close to each other). Fraternal twins share no more characteristics than any other siblings, because they develop from two distinct zygotes.

PRACTICE QUESTIONS

1. How many chromatids does a eukaryotic somatic cell inherit from each parent?

   A. N
   B. 2N
   C. 4N
   D. ½N

2. Cytokinesis is the process by which a cell's cytoplasm splits into two equal parts to form two daughter cells. Disproportionate splitting of the cytoplasm is a natural phenomenon of

   A. binary fission, the asexual reproduction seen in prokaryotes.
   B. parthogenesis.
   C. nothing; unequal cytokinesis never occurs.
   D. the reproductive cycle of yeast.

3. At what point does crossing over between sister chromatids occur?

   A. During prophase of meiosis
   B. During prophase of mitosis
   C. During anaphase II of meiosis
   D. It does not occur in meiosis

4. In order to amplify the DNA sequence indicated below, which of the following primers would you use?

   5' GGCTAAGATCTGAATTTTCCAAG ...

   TTGGGCAATAATAATGTAGCGCCTT 3'

   A. Primer 1:
   5' GGCTAAGATCTGAATTTTCCAAG 3'
   Primer 2:
   5' AAGGCGCTACATTATTATTGCCCAA 3'
   B. Primer 1:
   5' GAACCTTTTAAGTCTAGAATCGG
   Primer 2:
   5' AACCCGTTATTATTACATCGCGGAA 3'
   C. Primer 1:
   5' CCGATTCTAGACTTAAAAGGTTC 3'
   Primer 2:
   5' TTCCGCGATGTAATAATAACGGGTT 3'
   D. Primer 1:
   5' GAACCTTTTAAGTCTAGAATCGG 3'
   Primer 2:
   5' TTCCGCGATGTAATAATAACGGGTT 3'

5. The following sequence of genetic code is taken from the middle of a protein. Referring to the genetic code table provided below, what is the amino acid sequence for the protein produced by the following gene? Assume that the coding frame starts at the first nucleotide.

5' TCTAGCCTGAACTAATGC 3'
3' AGATCGGACTTGATTACG 5'

ISOLEUCINE	ATT, ATC, ATA
LEUCINE	CTT, CTC, CTA, CTG, TTA, TTG
VALINE	GTT, GTC, GTA, GTG
PHENYLALANINE	TTT, TTC
METHIONINE	ATG
CYSTEINE	TGT, TGC
ALANINE	GCT, GCC, GCA, GCG
GLYCINE	GGT, GGC, GGA, GGG
PROLINE	CCT, CCC, CCA, CCG
THREONINE	ACT, ACC, ACA, ACG
SERINE	TCT, TCC, TCA, TCG, AGT, AGC
TYROSINE	TAT, TAC
TRYPTOPHAN	TGG
GLUTAMINE	CAA, CAG
ASPARAGINE	AAT, AAC
HISTIDINE	CAT, CAC
GLUTAMIC ACID	GAA, GAG
ASPARTIC ACID	GAT, GAC
LYSINE	AAA, AAG
ARGININE	CGT, CGC, CGA, CGG, AGA, AGG
STOP CODONS	TAA, TAG, TGA

A. Amino—Ala Leu Val Gln Ala Ser—Carboxy
B. Carboxy—Ala Leu Val Gln Ala Ser—Amino
C. Amino—Ser Ser Leu Asp Leu Cys—Carboxy
D. Amino—Arg Ser Asp Leu Iso Thr—Carboxy

6. Polymorphism refers to an instance in nature in which two or more distinct phenotypes exist in a species. A polymorphic Simple Sequence Repeat (SSR) marker from four individuals is amplified via PCR. The products yield the following gel:

A B C D

Which of the following statements is not possible?

A. Individuals B and C are the parents of individuals A and D.
B. Individuals A and D are the parents of individuals B and C.
C. Individuals A and B are the parents of individuals C and D.
D. Individuals A and C are related.

7. The process by which DNA replicates is considered "semiconservative." Semiconservative refers to the fact that

A. if radiolabeled DNA of bacterial strain A is introduced to a culture of unlabeled bacteria strain B, descendants of the strain will have more DNA contributed from A than from B.
B. in DNA replication, one strand of the newly synthesized DNA will be a complement of the original parental strand, and one strand will be an exact replica of the original parental strand.
C. in DNA replication, half of each strand of newly synthesized DNA is a complement of the original parental strand, but half of each strand of newly synthesized DNA is an exact replica of the original parental strand.
D. DNA strands are antiparallel and the two strands of the replicated DNA are complements of one another.

8. Which of the following graphs accurately represents LH levels during the female menstrual cycle?

A.
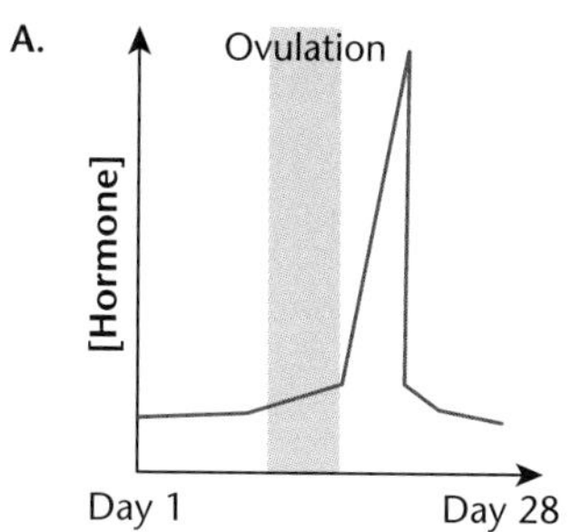

B.
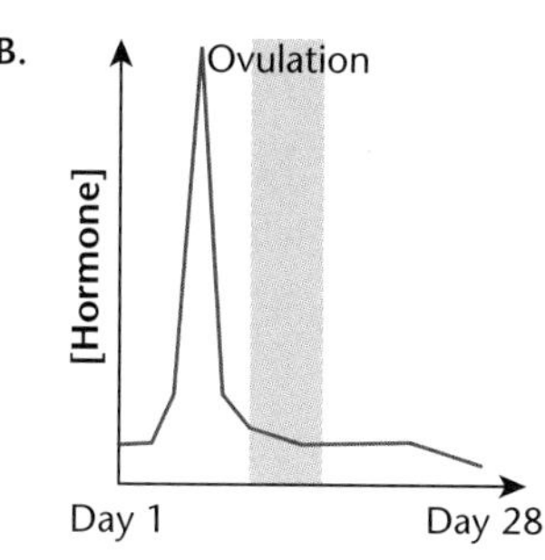

C.
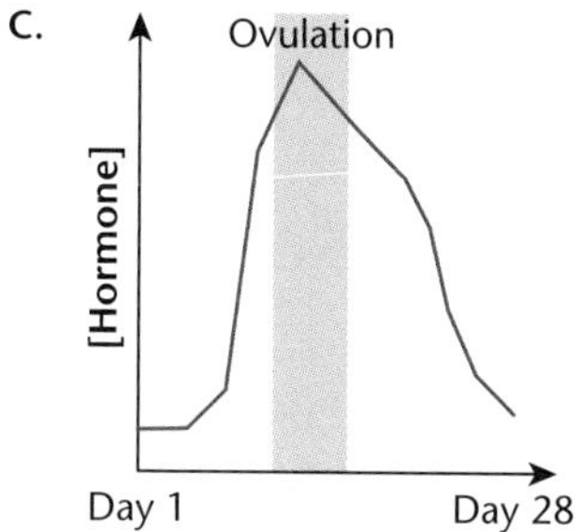

D.
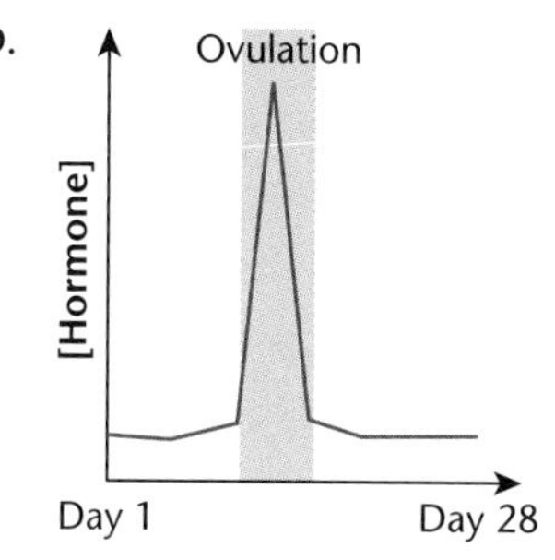

9. DHT or dihydroxytestosterone is a hormone secreted by the embryonic testes, which stimulates the development of male external genitalia. If compound A breaks down DHT, what would be the primary effect of introducing high levels of compound A to an embryo in the early stages of development?

A. The embryo would develop into a fetus lacking external genitalia.
B. The embryo would develop into a fetus with female external genitalia.
C. The embryo would be unable to complete development into a fetus.
D. The embryo would develop into a fetus with both female and male external genitalia.

10. Mullerian-inhibiting substance is secreted by embryonic Sertoli cells. Based on this fact, which of the following statements must be false?

A. Mullerian ducts develop into male sex accessory ducts.
B. Mullerian ducts develop into female sex accessory ducts.
C. Female sex accessory ducts are the default condition.
D. Wolffian ducts develop into male sex accesory ducts.

11. Spermatogenesis and spermiogenesis are the two processes by which immature male germ cells—also known as spermatogonium—produce sperm.

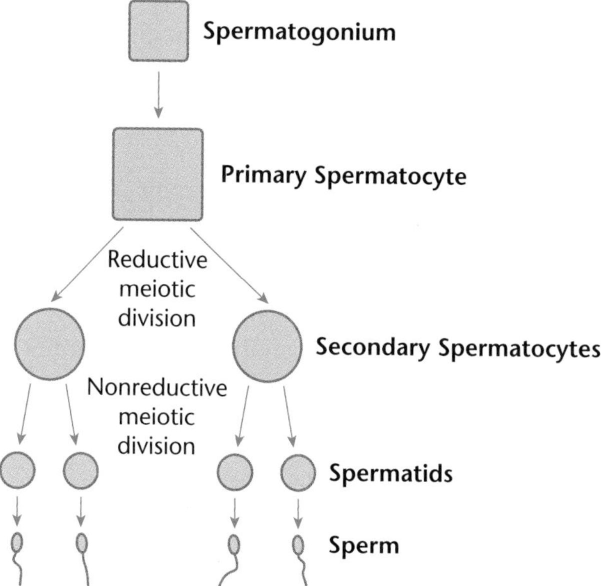

If four male germ cells undergo spermatogenesis and spermiogenesis, what will they produce?

A. 8 (2N) sperm
B. 8 (N) sperm
C. 16 (N) sperm
D. 16 (½N) sperm

12. Down syndrome, also known as trisomy 21, results from a chromosomal abnormality wherein all cells have an extra copy of the 21st chromosome. Mosaic Down syndrome is a specific case in which some, but not all, cells have an extra copy of the 21st chromosome. Which of the following could possibly cause full Down syndrome, where all cells are affected?

A. Disruption of anaphase in mitosis
B. Disruption of telophase in mitosis
C. Disruption of anaphase II in meiosis
D. Duplication event involving chromosome 21

13. In which of the following situations would male infertility be readily apparent without additional testing?

A. Blockage of the seminiferous tubules
B. Blockage of the bulbourethral gland
C. Blockage of the urethra
D. Blockage of the vas deferens

14. Though fraternal twins share their mother's womb and are born only seconds apart, they are no more genetically similar to one another than normal, non-twin siblings. Which of the following is a reasonable explanation for fraternal twins?

A. A zygote splits into two embryos at the two-cell stage of development.
B. A zygote splits into two embryos at the blastula stage of development.
C. Two ova are released in one ovarian cycle and are fertilized by two different sperm.
D. Two ova are released in one ovarian cycle and are fertilized by the same sperm.

15. Mary had an infection which caused large amounts of scarring, blocking her fallopian tubes. Which of the following statements is true?

A. Ovulation will occur less frequently.
B. Urination will become impossible.
C. Fertilization will be less likely.
D. Menstruation will become impossible.

16. In what location are male sperm stored?

A. Vas deferens
B. Seminiferous tubules
C. Sertoli cells
D. Epididymis

17. Your friend gives you one brown and one black guinea pig for your birthday. You know that in this particular species of guinea pig, coat color is controlled by one gene. You also know that this gene has one dominant allele and one recessive allele. After mating the two guinea pigs, you find that you have two black and two brown offspring. What can you conclude?

A. One guinea pig is homozygous and one is heterozygous.
B. Both guinea pigs are homozygous.
C. Both guinea pigs are heterozygous.
D. It is impossible to determine from the information given if any of the above are true.

18. Estradiol and estrogen can bind to the same steroid receptors. However, when estradiol and estrogen are present in equal concentrations, a larger proportion of the estradiol is found bound to the receptors. Which of the following would increase the amount of estrogen bound to the receptors?

A. Introducing an estrogen analog
B. Introducing an estradiol analog
C. Increasing the concentration of estradiol
D. Increasing the concentration of estrogen

FETAL CIRCULATION

KEY CONCEPTS

Fetal circulation

Fetal structures

Fetal lungs are supplied with only enough blood to nourish the lung tissue itself because fetal lungs do not function prior to birth. Obstruction of which fetal structure would cause an increase in blood supply to fetal lungs?

1) Identify the unique structures involved in fetal circulation.

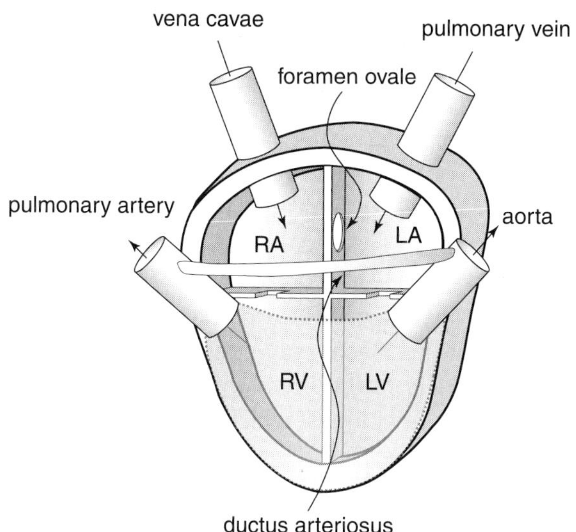

Fetal circulation differs from adult circulation in several important ways. The major difference is that in fetal circulation, blood is oxygenated in the placenta because, as the question states, fetal lungs are nonfunctional before birth. The fetal circulatory route contains three shunts that divert blood flow away from the developing fetal liver and lungs. The umbilical vein carries oxygenated blood from the placenta to the fetus. The blood bypasses the fetal liver by way of a shunt called the ductus venosus, before converging with the inferior vena cava. The inferior and superior vena cavae return deoxygenated blood to the right atrium. Because the oxygenated blood from the umbilical vein mixes with the deoxygenated blood of the vena cavae, the blood entering the right atrium is only partially oxygenated. Most of this blood bypasses the pulmonary circulation and enters the left atrium directly from the right atrium by way of the foramen ovale, a shunt that diverts blood away from the right ventricle and pulmonary artery. The remaining blood in the right atrium empties into the right ventricle and is pumped to the lungs via the pulmonary artery. Most of this blood is shunted directly from the pulmonary artery to the aorta via the ductus arteriosus, diverting even more blood away from the fetal lungs.

TAKEAWAYS

Understand the differences in fetal circulation and adult circulation and be able to apply that knowledge to situations in which the normal flow of blood is altered.

2) Examine the normal flow of blood to fetal lungs.

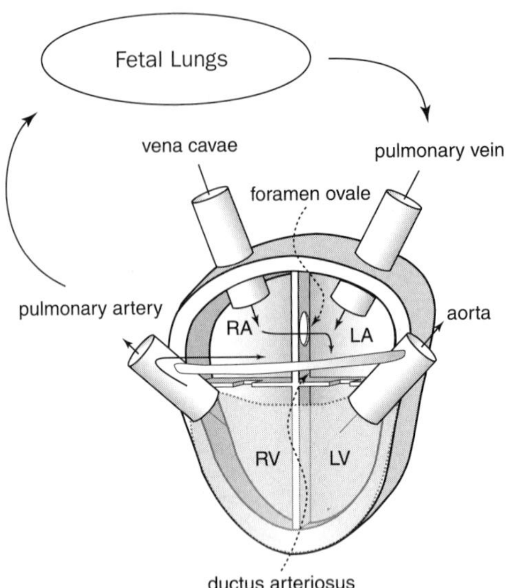

In the fetus, the pulmonary arteries carry oxygenated blood to the lungs, though this blood is by no means saturated with oxygen. The blood that is delivered to the lungs is further deoxygenated there because the blood unloads its oxygen to the fetal lungs, which need it for proper development. Remember, gas exchange does not occur in the fetal lungs—it occurs in the placenta. The deoxygenated blood then returns to the left atrium via pulmonary veins. Despite the fact that this blood mixes with the partially oxygenated blood that crossed over from the right atrium (via the foramen ovale) before being pumped into the systemic circulation by the left ventricle, the blood delivered via the aorta has an even lower partial pressure of oxygen than the blood that was delivered to the lungs. Deoxygenated blood is returned to the placenta via the umbilical arteries.

THINGS TO WATCH OUT FOR

Remember that the umbilical vein in the fetus carries oxygenated blood.

---

3) Determine which structure is most critical in bypassing fetal lungs.

The ductus arteriosus and foramen ovale shunt blood from the pulmonary arteries to the systemic circulation, bypassing the lungs. Obstruction of either structure would cause an increase in blood supply to the fetal lungs because all of the blood pumped into the pulmonary arteries by the right ventricle would then have to flow through the lungs—there would be no place else for it to go.

Remember: *There are three important shunts that divert blood flow in the fetus: the ductus venosus, the foramen ovale, and the ductus arteriosus.*

SIMILAR QUESTIONS

1) What symptoms might a baby have if the ductus arteriosus fails to close at birth?
2) What symptoms might a baby have if the foramen ovale fails to close at birth?
3) At birth, there is a reversal in the pressure gradient between the atria. What is responsible for this reversal?

CHAPTER 5

EMBRYOLOGY

Embryology is the study of the development of a unicellular zygote into a complete multicellular organism. In the course of nine months, a unicellular human zygote undergoes cell division, cellular differentiation, and morphogenesis in preparation for life outside the uterus. Much of what is known about mammalian development stems from the study of less complex organisms such as sea urchins and frogs.

EARLY DEVELOPMENTAL STAGES

A. CLEAVAGE

Early embryonic development is characterized by a series of rapid mitotic divisions known as **cleavage.** These divisions lead to an increase in cell number without a corresponding growth in cell protoplasm, i.e., the total volume of cytoplasm remains constant. Thus, cleavage results in progressively smaller cells, with an increasing ratio of nuclear-to-cytoplasmic material. Cleavage also increases the surface-to-volume ratio of each cell, thereby improving gas and nutrient exchange. An **indeterminate cleavage** is one that results in cells that maintain the ability to develop into a complete organism. Identical twins are the result of an indeterminate cleavage (see chapter 4). A **determinate cleavage** results in cells whose future **differentiation** pathways are determined at an early developmental stage. Differentiation is the specialization of cells that occurs during development.

The first complete cleavage of the zygote occurs approximately 32 hours after fertilization. The second cleavage occurs after 60 hours, and the third cleavage after approximately 72 hours, at which point the eight-celled embryo reaches the uterus. As cell division continues, a solid ball of embryonic cells, known as the **morula,** is formed. **Blastulation** begins when the morula develops a fluid-filled cavity called the **blastocoel,** which by the fourth day becomes a hollow sphere of cells called the **blastula.** The mammalian blastula is called a **blastocyst** (see Figure 5.1) and consists of two cell groups: the **inner cell mass,** which protrudes

TEACHER TIP

FUN FACT: Morula is a Latin word meaning *mulberry*, which is what the developing ball of cells looks like at this early point in time.

into the blastocoel, and the **trophoblast,** which surrounds the blastocoel and later gives rise to the chorion.

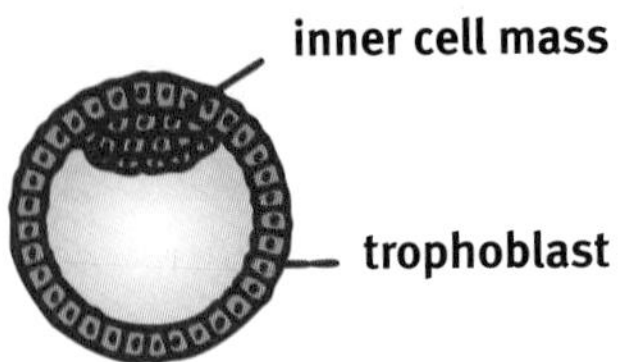

Figure 5.1. Mammalian Blastocyst

Clinical Correlate

Sometimes the blastula implants itself outside of the uterus, a situation referred to as an ectopic pregnancy. Ectopic pregnancies occur most often in the fallopian tube (over 95 percent). The embryo usually aborts spontaneously. The tube may rupture, and a considerable amount of hemorrhaging may occur.

B. IMPLANTATION

The embryo implants in the uterine wall during blastulation, approximately five to eight days after fertilization. The uterus is prepared for implantation by the hormone progesterone (see chapter 11), which causes glandular proliferation in the **endometrium**—the mucosal lining of the uterus. The embryonic cells secrete proteolytic enzymes that enable the embryo to digest tissue and implant itself in the endometrium. Eventually, maternal and fetal blood exchange materials at this site, later to be the location of the placenta.

C. GASTRULATION

Teacher Tip

These three layers are what organs arise from; they are a perennial MCAT favorite—especially for discrete questions. Knowing them is an easy way to get points.

Once implanted, cell migrations transform the single cell layer of the blastula into a three-layered structure called a **gastrula.** In the sea urchin, gastrulation begins with the appearance of a small invagination on the surface of the blastula. An inpocketing forms as cells continue to move toward the invagination, eventually eliminating the blastocoel. The result is a two-layered cup, with a differentiation between an outer cellular layer—the **ectoderm,** and an inner cellular layer—the **endoderm.** The newly formed cavity of the two-layered gastrula is called the **archenteron,** and later develops into the gut. The opening of the archenteron is called the **blastopore.** (In organisms classified as **deuterostomes,** such as humans, the blastopore is the site of the future anus, whereas in organisms classified as **protostomes,** the blastopore is the site of the future mouth.) Proliferation and migration of cells into the space between the ectoderm and the endoderm gives rise to a third cell layer, called the **mesoderm.** These three **primary germ layers** are responsible for the differential development of the tissues, organs, and systems of the body at later stages of growth.

- **Ectoderm**—integument (including the epidermis, hair, nails, and epithelium of the nose, mouth, and anal canal), the lens of the eye, and the nervous system.

- **Endoderm**—epithelial linings of the digestive and respiratory tracts (including the lungs), and parts of the liver, pancreas, thyroid, and bladder.
- **Mesoderm**—musculoskeletal system, circulatory system, excretory system, gonads, connective tissue throughout the body, and portions of digestive and respiratory organs.

TEACHER TIP

KEY POINT: The MCAT commonly tests the adrenal glands in the context of germ layers. The adrenal cortex is derived from the mesoderm, *but* the adrenal medulla is derived from the ectoderm because it contains some nervous tissue.

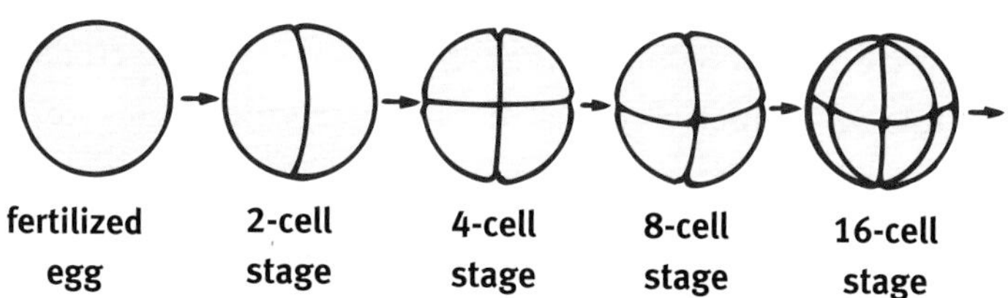

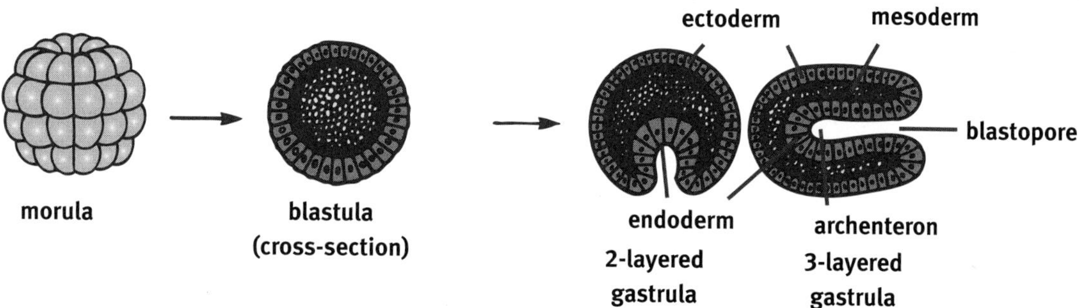

Figure 5.2. Amphibian Cleavage and Gastrulation

Despite the fact that all embryonic cells are derived from a single zygote and therefore have the same DNA, cells and tissues differentiate to perform unique and specialized functions. Most of this differentiation is accomplished through selective transcription of the genome. As the embryo develops, different tissue types express different genes. Most of the genetic information within any given cell is never expressed.

Induction is the influence of a specific group of cells (sometimes known as the **organizer**) on the differentiation of another group of cells. Induction is most often mediated by chemical substances **(inducers)** passed from the organizer to adjacent cells. In development of the eyes, lateral outpocketings from the brain (optic vesicles) grow out and touch the overlying ectoderm. The optic vesicle induces the ectoderm to thicken and form the lens placode. The lens placode then induces the optic vesicle to flatten and invaginate inward, forming the optic cup. The optic cup then induces the lens placode to invaginate and form the cornea and lens. Experiments with frog embryos show that if this ectoderm is transplanted to the trunk (after the optic vesicles have grown out), a lens will develop in the trunk. If, however, the ectoderm is transplanted before the outgrowth of the optic vesicles, it will not form a lens.

D. NEURULATION

By the end of gastrulation, regions of the germ layers begin to develop into a rudimentary nervous system; this process is known as **neurulation.** A rod of mesodermal cells, called the **notochord,** develops along the long-itudinal axis just under the dorsal layer of ectoderm. The notochord has an inductive effect on the overlying ectoderm, causing it to bend inward and form a groove along the dorsal surface of the embryo. The dorsal ectoderm folds on either side of the groove; these **neural folds** grow upward and finally fuse, forming a closed tube. This is the **neural tube,** which gives rise to the brain and spinal cord **(central nervous system).** Once the neural tube is formed, it detaches from the surface ectoderm. The cells at the tip of each neural fold are called the **neural crest** cells. These cells migrate laterally and give rise to many components of the **peripheral nervous system,** including the sensory ganglia, autonomic ganglia, adrenal medulla, and Schwann cells (see chapter 12).

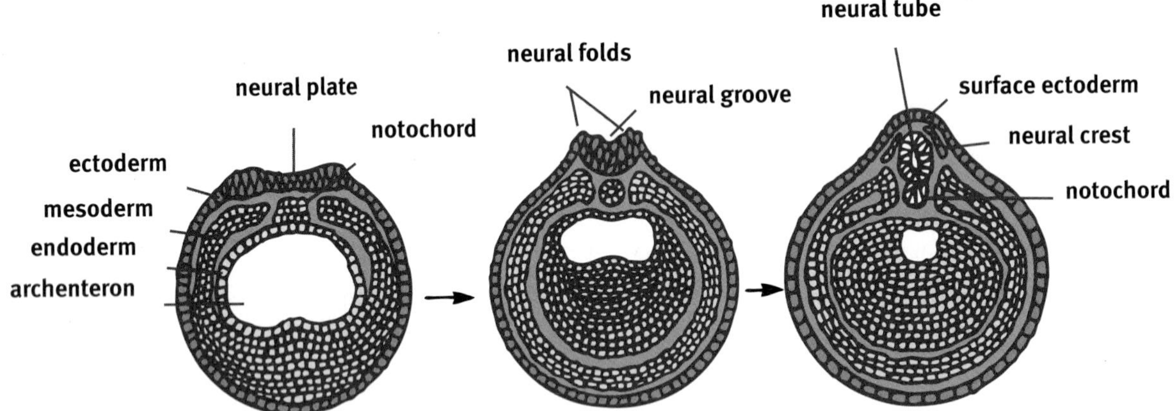

Figure 5.3. Neurulation

FETAL RESPIRATION

The growing **fetus** (the embryo is referred to as a fetus after eight weeks of **gestation**) receives oxygen directly from its mother through a specialized circulatory system. This system not only supplies oxygen and nutrients to the fetus, but removes carbon dioxide and metabolic wastes as well. The two components of this system are the **placenta** and the **umbilical cord,** which both develop in the first few weeks following fertilization.

TEACHER TIP

KEY POINT: Though the fetus gets its nutrients and oxygen from the mother, there is no actual mixing of the blood supplies. Instead, the placenta allows for the close proximity of the fetal and maternal blood stream so that diffusion can occur.

TEACHER TIP

The fetal blood supply is opposite in terms of oxygenation. The umbilical artery carries DEOXYGENATED blood and the umbilical vein carries OXYGENATED blood.

The placenta and the umbilical cord are outgrowths of the four extra-embryonic membranes formed during development: the **amnion, chorion, allantois,** and **yolk sac.** The amnion is a thin, tough membrane containing a watery fluid called **amniotic fluid.** Amniotic fluid acts as a shock absorber of external and localized pressure from uterine contractions during **labor.** Placenta formation begins with the chorion, a membrane that completely surrounds the amnion. About two weeks after fertilization the chorion extends villi into the uterine wall. These **chorionic villi** become closely associated with endometrial cells, developing into the spongy tissue of the placenta. A third membrane, the allantois, develops as an outpocketing of the gut. The blood vessels of the allantoic wall enlarge and become the **umbilical vessels,** which will connect the fetus to the developing placenta. The yolk sac, the site of early development of blood vessels, becomes associated with the umbilical vessels. At some point the allantois and yolk sac are enveloped by the amnion, forming the primitive **umbilical cord,** which is the initial connection between the fetus and the placenta. The mature umbilical cord consists of the umbilical vessels, which developed from the allantoic vessels, surrounded by a jellylike matrix. As the embryo grows, it remains attached to the placenta by the umbilical cord, which permits it to float freely in the amniotic fluid.

The placenta is the site of nutrition, respiration, and waste disposal for the fetus. Water, glucose, amino acids, vitamins, and inorganic salts diffuse across maternal capillaries into fetal blood. **Fetal hemoglobin (Hb-F)** has a greater affinity for oxygen than does adult hemoglobin **(Hb-A)**; consequently, oxygen preferentially diffuses into fetal blood. Concurrently, metabolic wastes and carbon dioxide diffuse in the opposite direction—from fetal blood into maternal blood. Note that the circulatory systems of the mother and the fetus are not directly connected, so maternal and fetal blood do not mix. As can be seen in Figure 5.5, all exchange of material between maternal and fetal blood vessels occurs in the placenta via diffusion.

MCAT SYNOPSIS

Remember, gas exchange in the fetus occurs across the placenta. Fetal lungs do not become functional until birth.

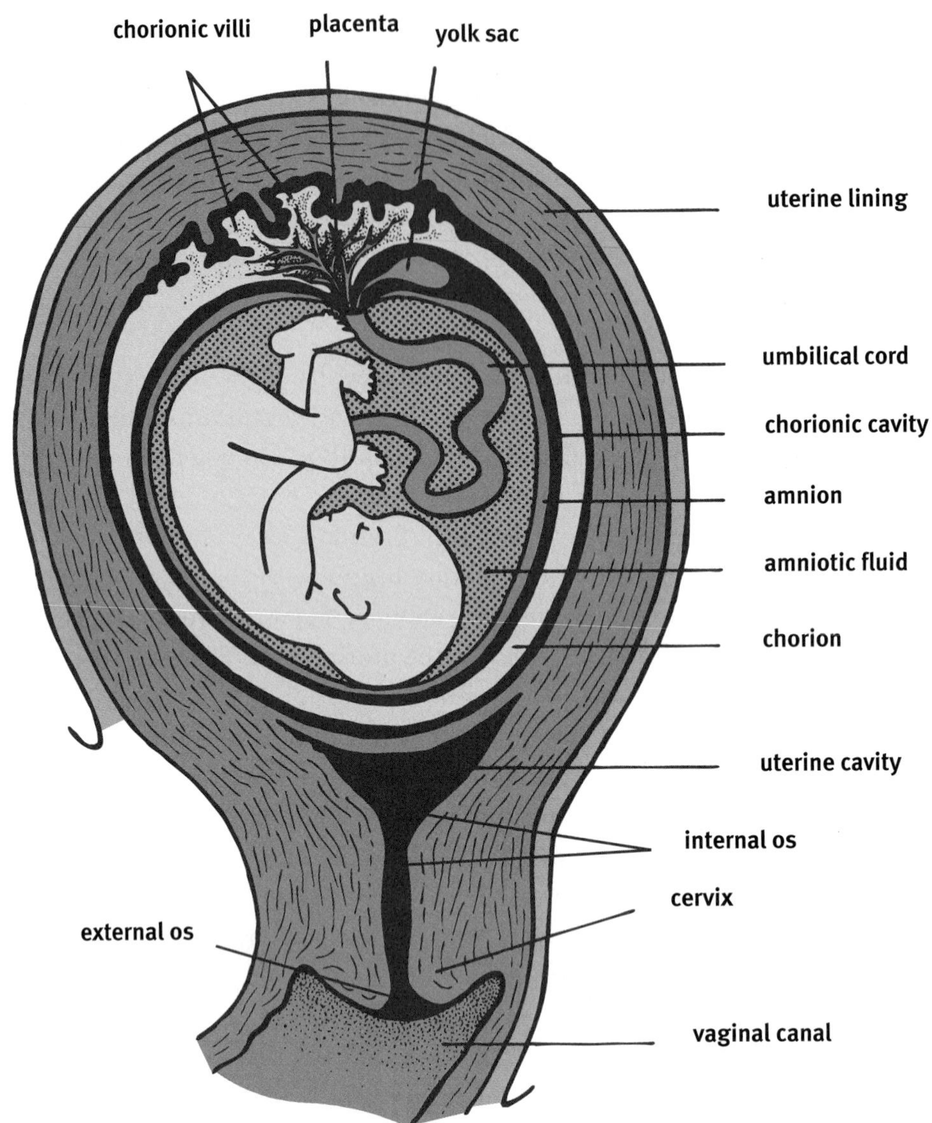

Figure 5.4. Human Fetus

TEACHER TIP

Consider what the fetal Hb curve would look like compared to adult Hb. In order for fetal Hb to "steal" the oxygen from the maternal/adult Hb, it must have a higher affinity, so the curve is shifted to the left.

In addition to nutritive and respiratory functions, the placenta offers the fetus some immunological protection by preventing the diffusion of foreign matter (e.g., bacteria) into fetal blood. However, the placenta is permeable to viruses, alcohol, and many drugs and toxins, all of which can adversely affect fetal development. The placenta also functions as an endocrine gland, producing the hormones progesterone, estrogen, and human chorionic gonadotropin (HCG)—all of which are essential for maintaining a pregnancy (see chapter 11). The presence of HCG in urine is the simplest test for pregnancy.

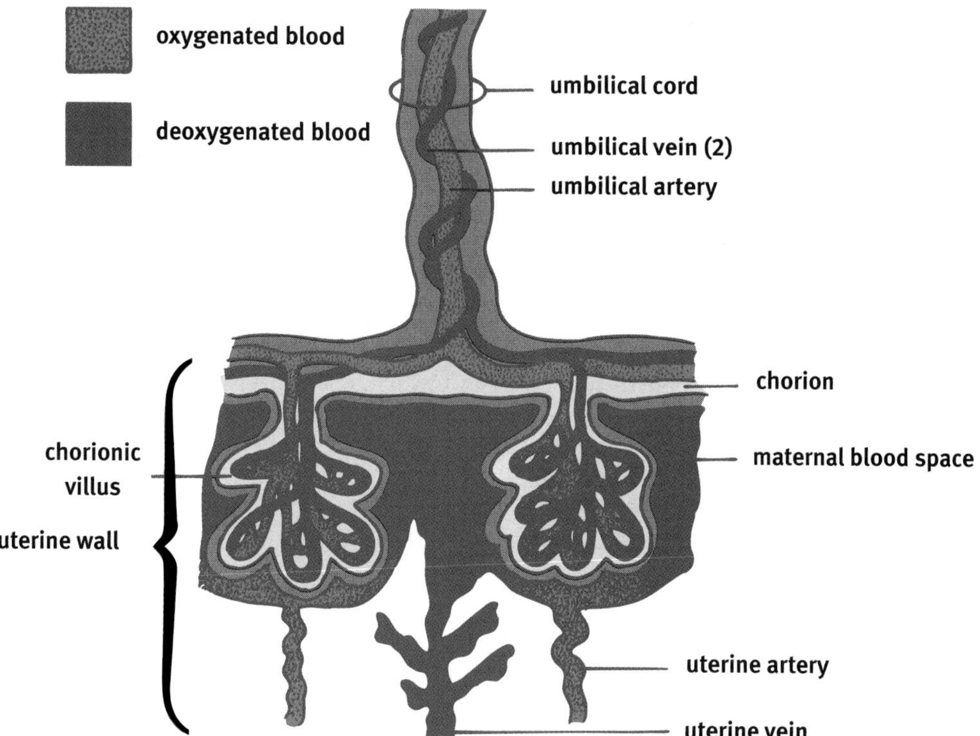

Figure 5.5. Placenta

FETAL CIRCULATION

Fetal circulation differs from adult circulation in several important ways. The major difference is that in fetal circulation, blood is oxygenated in the placenta (because fetal lungs are nonfunctional prior to birth), while in adult circulation, blood is oxygenated in the lungs. In addition, the fetal circulatory route contains three shunts that divert blood flow away from the developing fetal liver and lungs. The **umbilical vein** carries oxygenated blood from the placenta to the fetus. The blood bypasses the fetal liver by way of a shunt called the **ductus venosus,** before converging with the inferior vena cava. The inferior and superior venae cavae return deoxygenated blood to the right atrium. Because the oxygenated blood from the umbilical vein mixes with the deoxygenated blood of the venae cavae, the blood entering the right atrium is only partially oxygenated. Most of this blood bypasses the pulmonary circulation and enters the left atrium directly from the right atrium by way of the **foramen ovale,** a shunt that diverts blood away from the pulmonary arteries. The remaining blood in the right atrium empties into the right ventricle and is pumped into the pulmonary artery. Most of this blood is shunted directly from the pulmonary artery to the aorta via the **ductus arteriosus,** diverting

MCAT SYNOPSIS

A small amount of blood must reach the pulmonary circulation in order to nourish the developing fetal lungs.

TEACHER TIP

These three bypasses are all closed in the adult. If they remain patent (open), they can lead to severe hemodynamic problems.

even more blood away from the lungs. This means that in the fetus, the pulmonary arteries carry partially oxygenated blood to the lungs. The blood that does reach the lungs is further deoxygenated as the blood unloads its oxygen to the developing lungs. Remember, gas exchange does not occur in the fetal lungs—it occurs in the placenta. The deoxygenated blood then returns to the left atrium via the pulmonary veins. Despite the fact that this blood mixes with the partially oxygenated blood that crossed over from the right atrium (via the foramen ovale) before being pumped into the systemic circulation by the left ventricle, the blood delivered via the aorta has an even lower partial pressure of oxygen than the blood that was delivered to the lungs. This deoxygenated blood is returned to the placenta via the **umbilical arteries.**

In contrast, in adult circulation, deoxygenated blood enters the right atrium, the right ventricle pumps this blood to the lungs via the pulmonary arteries (those same arteries that carried partially oxygenated blood in the fetus), and gas exchange occurs in the lungs. Oxygenated blood is returned to the left atrium via the pulmonary veins (those same veins that carried deoxygenated blood in the fetus), and the left ventricle pumps the blood into circulation via the aorta. (For a more complete discussion of adult circulation, see chapter 9.)

MCAT Synopsis

Fetal circulation can be considered the opposite of adult circulation.

Umbilical vein = oxygenated blood

Umbilical arteries = deoxygenated blood

Three shunts shift fetal blood from the right-sided circulation to the left-sided circulation:

1) Ductus venosus (shunts blood from the fetal liver)
2) Ductus arteriorsus (shunts blood from the lungs)
3) Foramen ovale (shunts blood from the lungs)

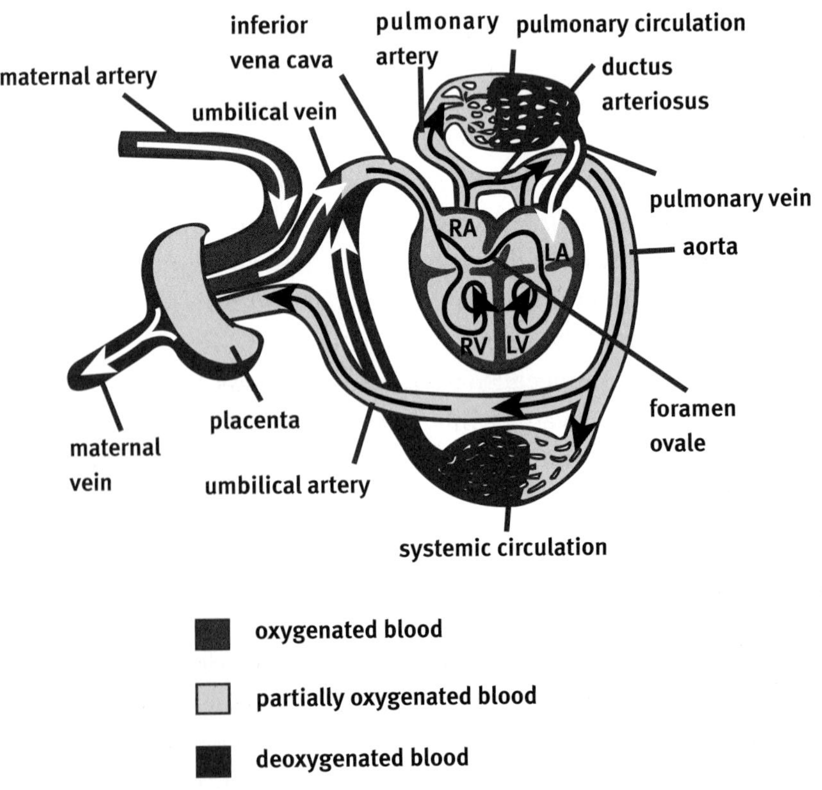

Figure 5.6. Fetal Circulation

After birth, a number of changes occur in the circulatory system as the fetus adjusts to breathing on its own. The lungs expand with air and rhythmic breathing begins. Resistance in the pulmonary blood vessels decreases, causing an increase in blood flow through the lungs. When umbilical blood flow stops, blood pressure in the inferior vena cava decreases, causing a decrease in pressure in the right atrium. In contrast, left atrial pressure increases due to increased blood flow from the lungs. Increased left atrial pressure coupled with decreased right atrial pressure causes the foramen ovale to close. In addition, the ductus arteriosus constricts and later closes permanently. The ductus venosus degenerates over a period of time, completely closing in most infants three months after birth. The infant begins to produce adult hemoglobin, and by the end of the first year of life little fetal hemoglobin can be detected in the blood.

TEACHER TIP

Understanding why blood flows from the right atrium to the left in the fetus may seem more like a physics concept—and it is. But it is commonly tested in the Biology section as well. This is a common MCAT trend—topics which are applicable to both the Physics section and the Biology section.

GESTATION

Human pregnancy, or gestation, is approximately nine months (266 days), and can be subdivided into three **trimesters.** The primary developments that occur during each trimester are described below.

A. FIRST TRIMESTER

During the first weeks, the major organs begin to develop. The heart begins to beat at approximately 22 days, and soon afterward, the eyes, gonads, limbs, and liver start to form. By five weeks the embryo is 10 mm in length; by six weeks the embryo has grown to 15 mm. The cartilaginous skeleton begins to turn into bone by the seventh week (see chapter 6). By the end of eight weeks, most of the organs have formed, the brain is fairly developed, and the embryo is referred to as a fetus. At the end of the third month, the fetus is about 9 cm long.

B. SECOND TRIMESTER

During the second trimester, the fetus does a tremendous amount of growing. It begins to move around in the amniotic fluid, its face appears human, and its toes and fingers elongate. By the end of the sixth month, the fetus is 30–36 cm long.

TEACHER TIP

Advances in medicine have allowed babies to be born as early as 24 weeks, which is far short of a normal 39. Though these children may live, there are often severe consequences given that fetal development isn't complete at 24 weeks. These problems are most apparent in the respiratory system where the amount of surfactant is insufficient.

C. THIRD TRIMESTER

The seventh and eighth months are characterized by continued rapid growth and further brain development. During the ninth month, antibodies are transported by highly selective active transport from the mother to the fetus for protection against foreign matter. The growth rate slows and the fetus becomes less active, as it has less room to move about.

BIRTH

Childbirth is accomplished by labor, a series of strong uterine contractions. Labor can be divided into three distinct stages. In the first stage, the cervix thins out and dilates, and the amniotic sac ruptures, releasing its fluids. During this time contractions are relatively mild. The second stage is characterized by rapid contractions, resulting in the birth of the baby, followed by the cutting of the umbilical cord. During the final stage, the uterus contracts, expelling the placenta and the umbilical cord.

PRACTICE QUESTIONS

1. During meiosis, haploid cells are created from diploid parent cells. The process occurs only in sexual reproduction, and it involves two complete division cycles. At what stage of mitotic division do the recently condensed chromosomes align in the equatorial region of the cell, in preparation for separation?

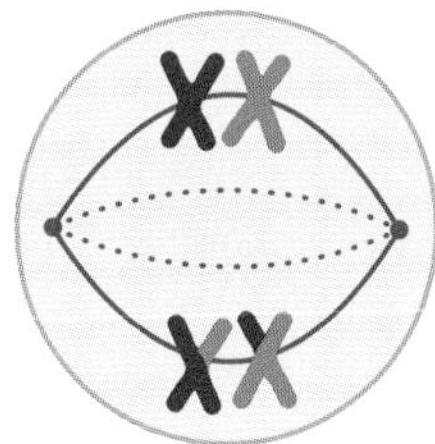

   A. Anaphase
   B. Telophase
   C. Metaphase
   D. Prophase

2. At what stage does dormancy occur in primary oocytes?

   A. Metaphase I
   B. Prophase II
   C. Metaphase II
   D. Prophase I

3. What is the origin of mitochondrial DNA?

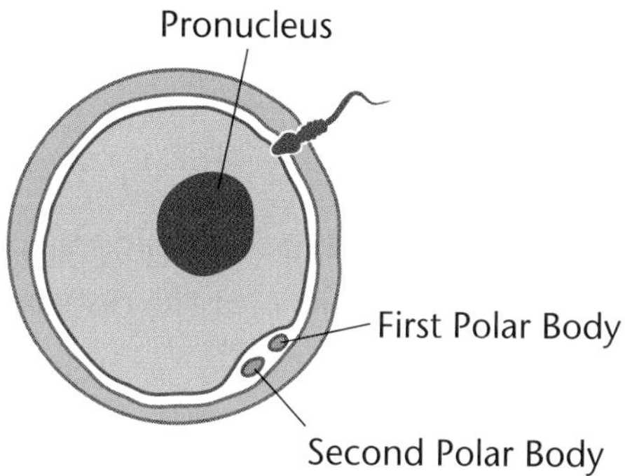

   A. Equal paternal and maternal DNA
   B. Random combination of paternal and maternal DNA
   C. Paternal only
   D. Maternal only

4. Gonadotropin-releasing hormone (GnRH) is synthesized by hypothalamic neurosecretory cells, which in turn stimulates the release of two ovarian stimulating hormones, follicle-stimulating hormone (FSH) and lutenizing hormone (LH). FSH and LH are produced by which of the following?

   A. Ovaries
   B. Adrenal gland
   C. Anterior pituitary
   D. Posterior pituitary

5. Which of the following cells is capable of prolonged dormancy?

   A. First polar body
   B. Primary oocyte
   C. Second polar body
   D. Secondary oocyte

6. The process by which one of the two copies of X-chromosomes in mammalian females becomes inactivated is called

A. attenuation.
B. attrition.
C. lyonization.
D. hybridization.

7. At approximately what week of development does the placenta take over the responsibility of producing progesterone?

A. Week 2
B. Week 4
C. Week 6
D. Week 8

8. You are scheduled to assist in a delivery today and the chief resident wants to find out if you understand the different types of twins. You mention dizygotic and you're asked to clarify what that means. You say that dizygotic twins are

A. the fertilization of one secondary oocyte by one sperm.
B. twins genetically identical.
C. one blastocyst that split.
D. twins not genetically identical.

9. Which pharyngeal arch exists only transiently during embryonic development?

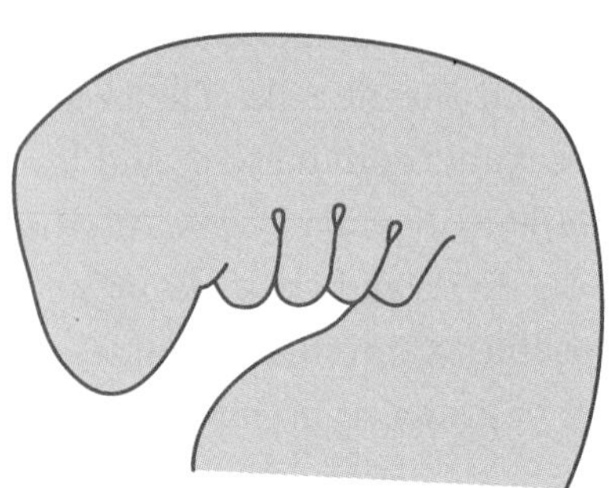

A. III
B. IV
C. V
D. VI

10. The three germ layers will give rise to all the tissues and organs of the body. The mesoderm layer will eventually develop which of the following?

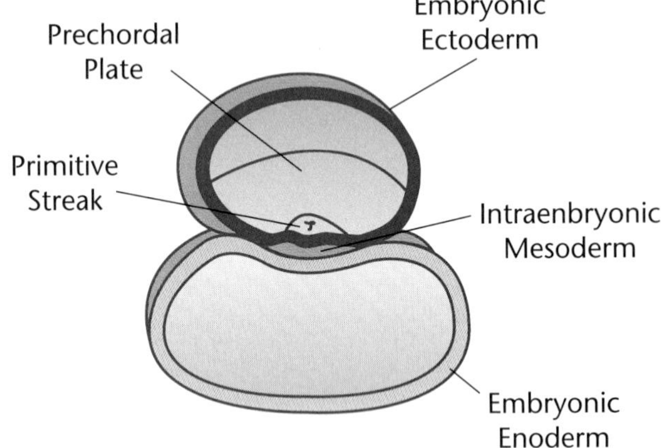

A. Central nervous system
B. Pituitary gland
C. Heart
D. Thyroid and parathyroid glands

11. In fetal circulation, through which shunt does the majority of oxygenated-enriched blood reach the systemic circulation?

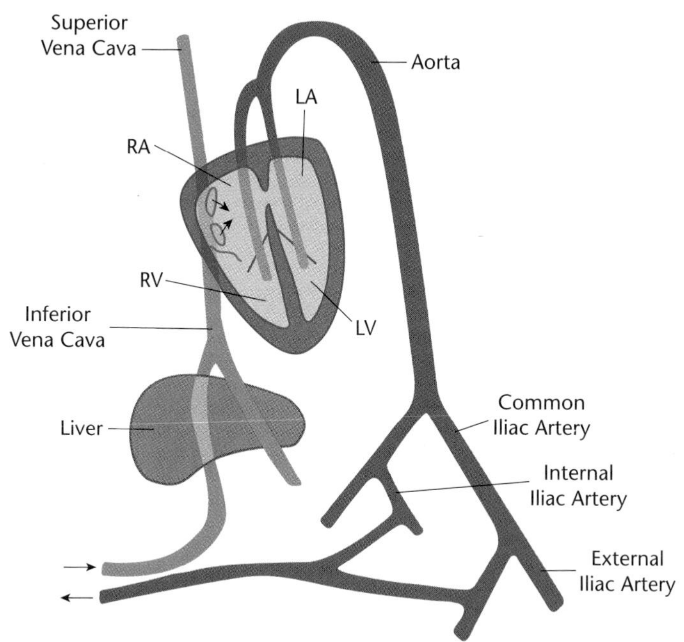

A. Ductus arteriosus
B. Ductus venosus
C. Foramen ovale
D. Umbilical arteries

12. One of the first signs of gastrulation is the formation of the

A. notochord.
B. tertiary chorionic villi.
C. primitive streak.
D. neural tube.

13. Somites are derived from which intraembryonic mesoderm layer?

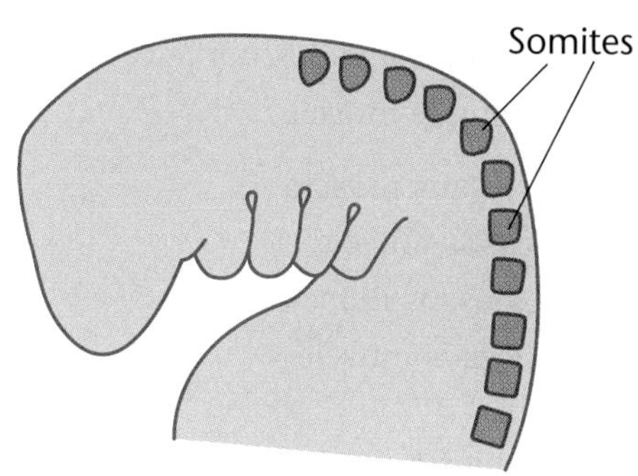

A. Paraxial mesoderm
B. Lateral mesoderm
C. Intraembryonic somatic mesoderm
D. Intraembryonic visceral mesoderm

14. Intraembryonic coelom divides the lateral mesoderm into two distinctive layers, the intraembryonic somatic mesoderm and intra embryonic visceral mesoderm. By the fourth week of development, the intraembryonic coelom becomes the

A. kidneys and gonads.
B. body cavities.
C. cartilage and bone.
D. nucleus pulposus.

15. During embryological development, which organ system is the first to reach a functional state?

A. Nervous system
B. Cardiovascular system
C. Respiratory system
D. Skeletal system

16. All the extrinsic muscles of the tongue are supplied by the hypoglossal nerve (CN XII) except one, which is supplied by the pharyngeal branch of the vagus nerve (CN X). Which extrinsic tongue muscle is it?

A. Genioglossus muscle
B. Hyoglossus muscle
C. Palatoglossus muscle
D. Styloglossus muscle

17. Which of the following is the correct order of hematopoiesis by embryonic organs?

A. Liver, thymus, spleen, bone marrow
B. Liver, spleen, thymus, bone marrow
C. Thymus, liver, spleen, bone marrow
D. Thymus, spleen, liver, bone marrow

18. By what week of development can phenotypic sexual differentiation first be recognized?

A. Week 1
B. Week 6
C. Week 7
D. Week 12

CHAPTER 6

MUSCULOSKELETAL SYSTEM

The musculoskeletal system forms the basic internal framework of the vertebrate body. Muscles and bones work in close coordination to produce voluntary movement. In addition, bone and muscle perform a number of other independent functions.

SKELETAL SYSTEM

The skeleton functions primarily as the physical support of an organism. In contrast to the external skeleton **(exoskeleton)** of arthropods, vertebrates have an internal skeleton, or **endoskeleton.** The mammalian skeleton is divided into the **axial** and **appendicular** skeletons. The axial skeleton is the basic framework of the body, consisting of the skull, the vertebral column, and the rib cage. The appendicular skeleton consists of the limb bones and the pelvic and pectoral girdles. In addition to providing the lever upon which skeletal muscles act during locomotion, the skeleton surrounds and protects delicate organs such as the brain and the spinal cord. Furthermore, skeletal bone marrow houses much of the body's blood-forming elements.

Teacher Tip

FUN FACT: An adult human has 206 bones. Over 100 of these are in the feet and hands.

The two major components of the skeleton are **cartilage** and **bone.**

CARTILAGE

Cartilage is a type of connective tissue that is softer and more flexible than bone. It is made of a firm but elastic matrix called **chondrin,** which is secreted by specialized cells called **chondrocytes.** Cartilage is the principal component of embryonic skeletons in higher animals. During mammalian development, however, much of it hardens and calcifies into bone. Cartilage is retained in adults in places where firmness and flexibility are needed. For example, in humans, the external ear, the nose, the walls of the larynx and trachea, and the skeletal joints contain cartilage. Most cartilage is avascular (i.e., contains no blood or lymph vessels) and is devoid of nerves; it receives nourishment from capillaries located in nearby connective tissue and bone via diffusion through the surrounding fluid.

Teacher Tip

Cartilage continues to grow throughout life. This is why the noses and ears of many older individuals seem larger than the other features on the face.

BONE

Bone is a specialized type of mineralized connective tissue that has the ability to withstand physical stress. Ideally designed for body support, bone tissue is hard and strong, while at the same time, somewhat elastic and lightweight.

A. MACROSCOPIC BONE STRUCTURE

There are two basic types of bone: **compact bone** and **spongy bone.** Compact bone is dense bone that does not appear to have any cavities when observed with the naked eye. Spongy bone, also called **cancellous bone,** is much less dense, and consists of an interconnecting lattice of bony spicules (trabeculae); the cavities in between the spicules are filled with **yellow** and/or **red bone marrow.** Yellow marrow is inactive and infiltrated by adipose tissue; red marrow is involved in blood cell formation (see chapter 9).

Teacher Tip

The epiphyseal plates seal as a result of the effects of sex hormones (testosterone in males and estrogen in females). Thus, growth continues through puberty until around the age of 25, when the process is complete, Most of the growth, however, is done between the onset of puberty and the age of 18.

The bones of the appendages, the **long bones,** are characterized by a cylindrical shaft called a **diaphysis** and dilated ends called **epiphyses.** The diaphysis is primarily compact bone surrounding a cavity containing bone marrow. The epiphyses are spongy bone surrounded by a thin layer of compact bone. The **epiphyseal plate** is a disk of cartilaginous cells separating the diaphysis from the epiphysis and is the site of longitudinal growth. A fibrous sheath called the **periosteum** surrounds the long bone and is the site of attachment to muscle tissue. Some periosteum cells differentiate into bone-forming cells.

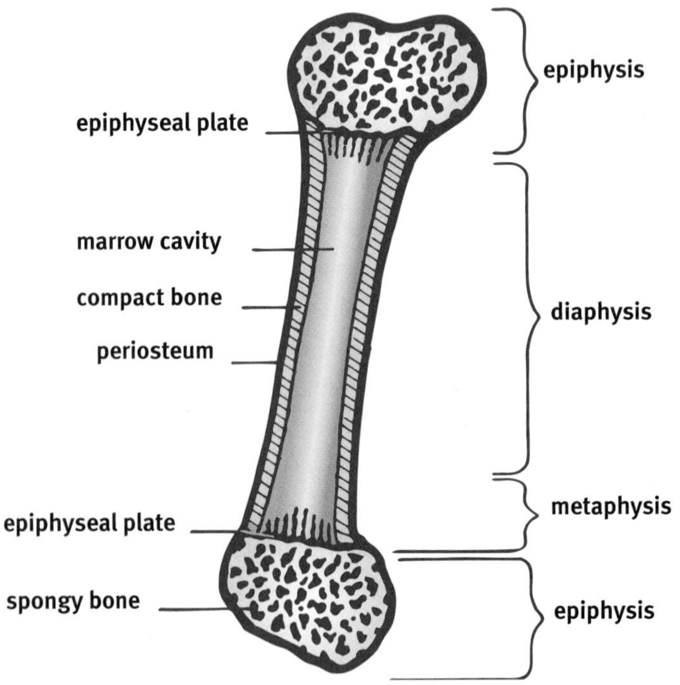

Figure 6.1. Long Bone

B. MICROSCOPIC BONE STRUCTURE

Compact bone is a dense, hardened **bone matrix,** which contains both organic and inorganic components. The organic components include proteins (principally collagen fibers and glycoproteins), while the inorganic components include calcium, phosphate, and hydroxide (which combine and harden to form **hydroxyapatite crystals**), as well as sodium, potassium, and magnesium ions. The association of hydroxyapatite crystals with collagen fibers gives bone its characteristic strength.

The bony matrix is deposited in structural units called **osteons (Haversian systems).** Each osteon consists of a central microscopic channel called a **Haversian canal,** surrounded by a number of concentric circles of bony matrix called **lamellae.** There are blood vessels, nerve fibers, and lymph in the Haversian canals, vascularizing and innervating bone tissue. Interspersed within the matrix are spaces called **lacunae,** which house mature bone cells called **osteocytes.** Osteocytes are involved in bone maintenance. Radiating from each lacuna are a number of minute canals called **canaliculi.** The canaliculi interconnect with each other and with the Haversian canals, allowing for exchange of nutrients and wastes (see Figure 6.2).

MCAT SYNOPSIS

Don't forget that bone is much more dynamic than you might think. Bone is both vascular and innervated. The bone's blood supply can become infected after an injury (a disease known as osteomyelitis) and if you break a bone, it will hurt (a lot). In addition, remember that bone is in a dynamic equilibrium between being broken down (by osteoCLASTS) and being built up (by osteoBLASTS.) This is known as bone remodeling.

TEACHER TIP

We know from our MCAT synopsis that bone growth is dynamic. The benefit of this is it allows for remodeling as different stresses in the environment impinge on the body.

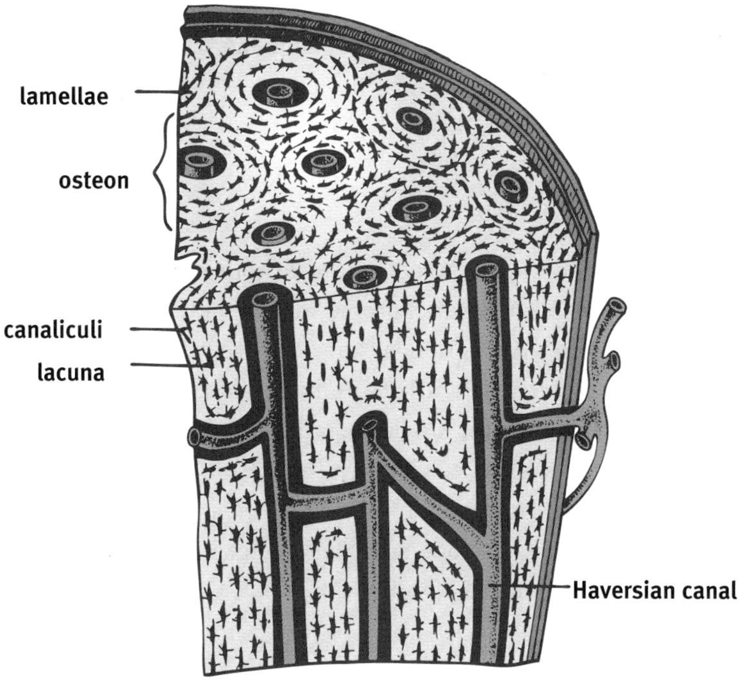

Figure 6.2. Microscopic Bone Structure

Two other types of cells found in bone tissue are **osteoblasts** and **osteoclasts.** Osteoblasts synthesize and secrete the organic constituents of the bone matrix; once they have become surrounded by their matrix, they mature into osteocytes. Osteoclasts are large, multinucleated cells involved in **bone resorption.**

Clinical Correlate

Osteoporosis is the most common bone disease in the United States. Affecting primarily post-menopausal women, osteoporosis causes hundreds of thousands of hip fractures annually. Osteoporosis is caused by loss of bone mass; it is thought to be the result of increased osteoclast resorption and some concomitant slowing of bone formation. It is believed that estrogen helps prevent osteoporosis by inhibiting osteoclast activity.

C. BONE FORMATION (OSSIFICATION)

Bone formation occurs by either **endochondral ossification** or by **intramembranous ossification.** In endochondral ossification, existing cartilage is replaced by bone. Long bones arise primarily through endochondral ossification. In intramembranous ossification, **mesenchymal** (embryonic, undifferentiated) connective tissue is transformed into, and replaced by, bone.

D. BONE REMODELING

Bone matrix is dynamic; i.e., it is continuously and simultaneously degraded and reformed. During **bone reformation,** inorganic ions (e.g., calcium and phosphate) are absorbed from the blood for use in bone formation; in the process of **bone resorption** (degradation), these ions are released into the blood. These two processes are collectively known as **bone remodeling.** Vitamin D and hormones such as parathyroid hormone and calcitonin are all involved in the regulation of bone remodeling (see chapter 11). Bone use and stress during exercise are also factors in bone remodeling.

JOINTS

Joints are connective tissue structures that join bones together. Bones that do not move relative to each other, such as skull bones, are held in place by **immovable joints.** Bones that do move relative to one another are held together by **movable joints** and are additionally supported and strengthened by **ligaments.** Movable joints consist of a **synovial capsule,** which encloses a **joint cavity (articular cavity).** Movement is facilitated by **synovial fluid,** which lubricates the joint, and by **articular cartilage** on the opposing bone surfaces, which is smooth and reduces tension during movement (see Figure 6.3).

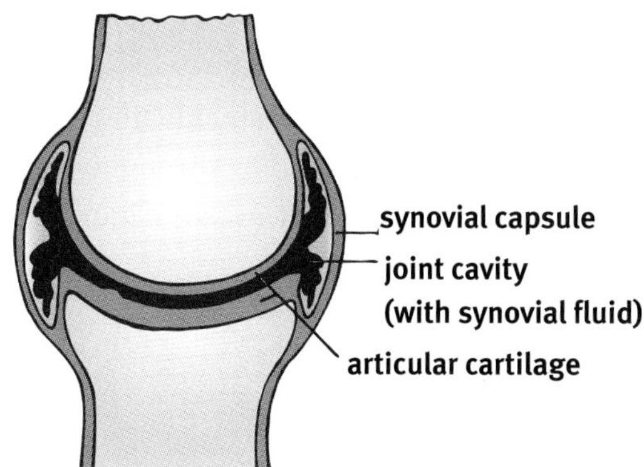

Figure 6.3. Movable Joint

> **TEACHER TIP**
>
> The degeneration of joint cartilage results in one of the most common medical conditions in this country: arthritis. Bones come in direct contact with one another due to cartilage loss, causing pain and stiffness.

MUSCULAR SYSTEM

Muscle tissue consists of bundles of specialized contractile fibers held together by connective tissue. There are three morphologically and functionally distinct types of muscle in mammals: **skeletal muscle, smooth muscle,** and **cardiac muscle.**

Table 6.1. Skeletal Muscle

Smooth Muscle	Cardiac Muscle	Skeletal Muscle
• Nonstriated	• Striated	• Striated
• 1 nucleus per cell	• 1–2 nuclei per cell	• Multinucleated cells
• Involuntary/Autonomic nervous system	• Involuntary/Autonomic nervous system	• Voluntary/Somatic nervous system
• Smooth continuous contractions	• Strong forceful contractions	• Strong forceful contractions

> **TEACHER TIP**
>
> KEY POINT: Cardiac muscle is a hybrid of skeletal and smooth muscle.

SKELETAL MUSCLE

Skeletal muscle is responsible for voluntary movements and is innervated by the **somatic nervous system** (see chapter 12). A muscle is a bundle of parallel fibers. Each fiber is a multinucleated cell created by the fusion of several mononucleate embryonic cells. The nuclei are usually found at the periphery of the cell. Embedded in the fibers are filaments called **myofibrils,** which are further divided into contractile units called **sarcomeres.** The myofibrils are enveloped by a modified endoplasmic reticulum that stores calcium ions and is called the **sarcoplasmic reticulum.** The cytoplasm of a muscle fiber is called **sarcoplasm,** and the cell membrane

> **TEACHER TIP**
>
> DON'T PANIC: Sarcoplasmic reticulum is just a fancy name for the endoplasmic reticulum in muscle cells.

is called the **sarcolemma.** The sarcolemma is capable of propagating an action potential (see chapter 12), and is connected to a system of **transverse tubules (T system)** oriented perpendicularly to the myofibrils. The T system provides channels for ion flow throughout the muscle fibers, and can also propagate an action potential (see Figure 6.4).

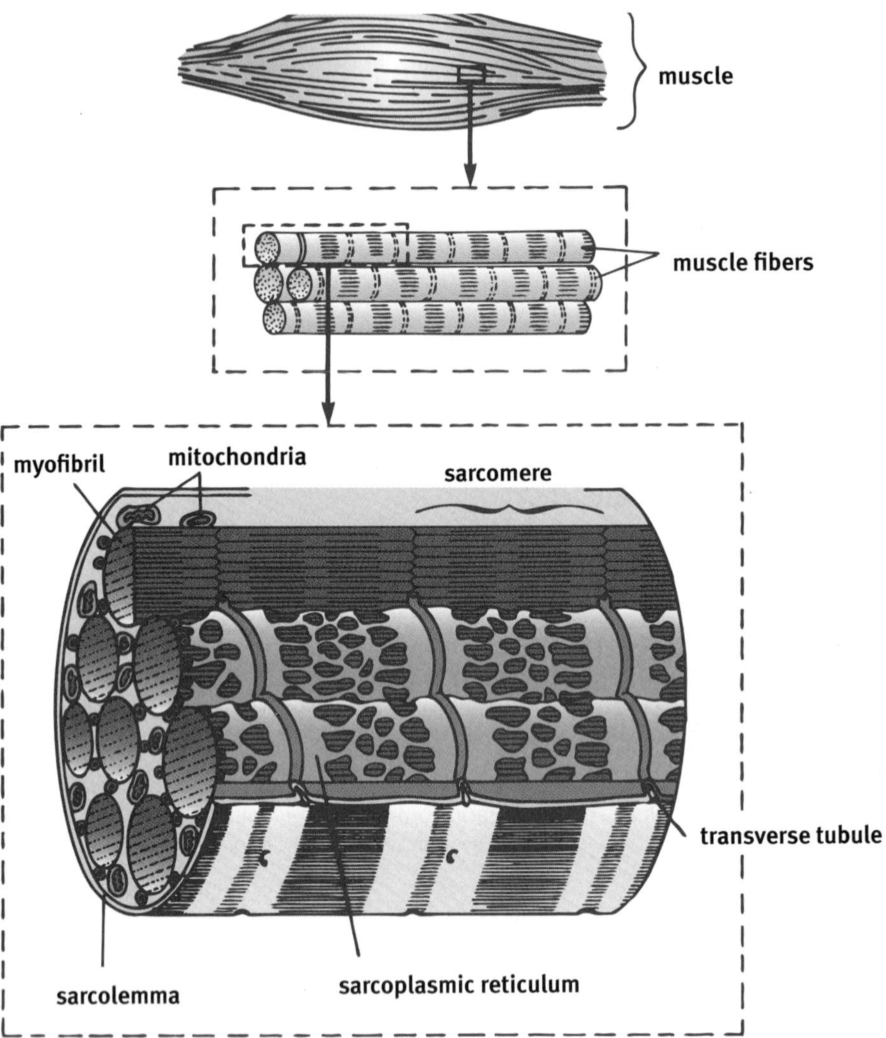

Figure 6.4. Skeletal Muscle

Teacher Tip

The MCAT requires you to be able to apply what you have learned. Think about what types of muscles would be red versus white. When would you want to be able to use fast or slow twitch fibers?

Skeletal muscle has striations of light and dark bands, and is therefore also referred to as **striated** muscle. Skeletal muscle fibers can be characterized as either red or white. **Red fibers** (slow-twitch fibers) have a high **myoglobin** content (a protein resembling hemoglobin) and many mitochondria. They derive their energy primarily from aerobic respiration and are capable of sustained and vigorous activity. **White fibers** (fast-twitch fibers) are anaerobic and therefore contain less myoglobin and fewer mitochondria than red fibers. White fibers have a greater rate of contraction than red fibers; however, white fibers fatigue more easily.

THE SARCOMERE

A. STRUCTURE

The sarcomere is composed of **thin** and **thick filaments.** The thin filaments are chains of globular **actin** molecules associated with two other proteins, **troponin** and **tropomyosin.** The thick filaments are composed of organized bundles of **myosin** molecules; each myosin molecule has a head region and a tail region.

MCAT Synopsis

H-Band = Myosin only
I-Band = Actin only
A-Band = Entire myosin fiber

Electron microscopy reveals that the sarcomere is organized as follows: **Z lines** define the boundaries of a single sarcomere and anchor the thin filaments. The **M line** runs down the center of the sarcomere. The **I band** is the region containing thin filaments only. The **H zone** is the region containing thick filaments only. The **A band** spans the entire length of the thick filaments and any overlapping portions of the thin filaments. Note that during contraction, the A band is not reduced in size, while the H zone and I band are.

Teacher Tip

Z lines, I band, and H zone all get smaller or closer together during contraction because they are defined relative to one another. The A band remains constant because it is defined as the total length of the thick fibers, regardless of state of contraction.

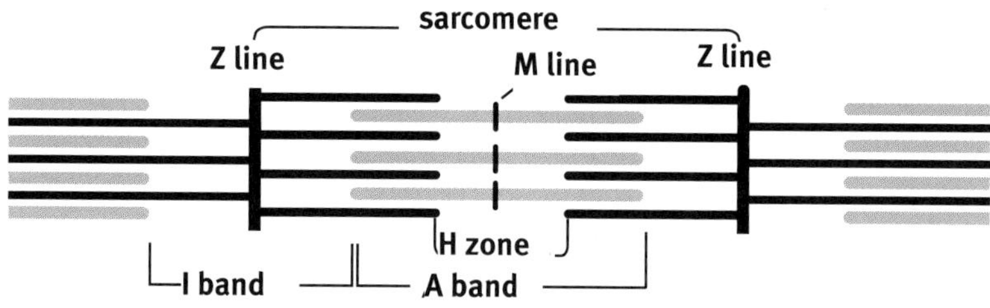

Figure 6.5. Sarcomere

B. CONTRACTION

1. Initiation

Muscle contraction is stimulated by a message from the somatic nervous system sent via a **motor neuron.** The link between the **nerve terminal (synaptic bouton)** and the sarcolemma of the muscle fiber is called the **neuromuscular junction.** The space between the two is known as the **synapse,** or **synaptic cleft.** Depolarization of the motor neuron results in the release of **neurotransmitters** (e.g., acetylcholine) from the nerve terminal. The neurotransmitter diffuses across the synaptic cleft and binds to special receptor sites on the sarcolemma. If enough of these receptors are stimulated, the permeability of the sarcolemma is altered and an **action potential** is generated (see chapter 12). The action

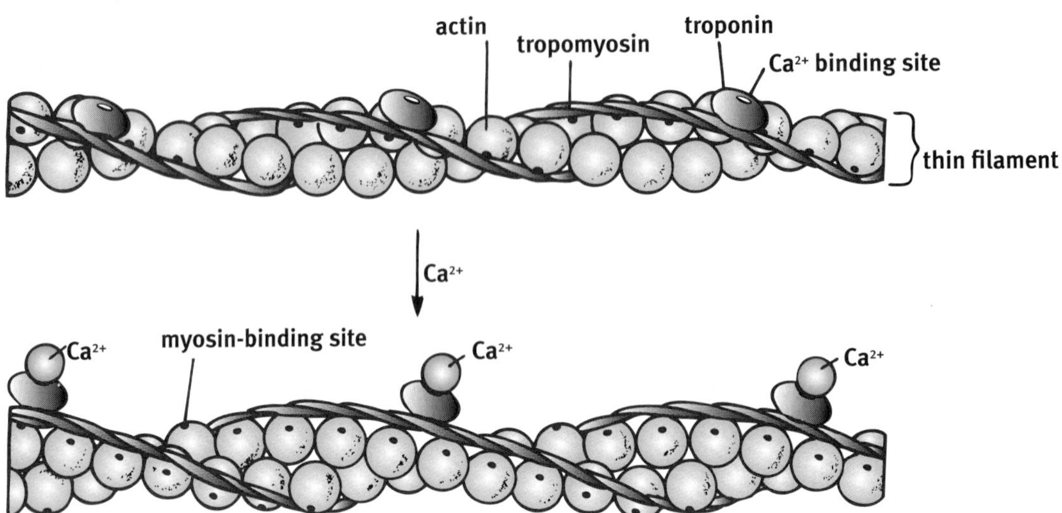

Figure 6.6. Thin Filament

potential then quickly spreads through the transverse tubules to sequentially contract the entire muscle with spontaneous synchronization.

2. Shortening of the Sarcomere

Once an action potential is generated, it is conducted along the sarcolemma and the T system, and into the interior of the muscle fiber. This causes the sarcoplasmic reticulum to release Ca^{2+} into the sarcoplasm. The Ca^{2+} binds to the troponin molecules, causing the tropomyosin strands to shift, thereby exposing the **myosin-binding sites** on the actin filaments (see Figure 6.6).

The free globular heads of the myosin molecules move toward and then bind to the exposed binding sites on the actin molecules, forming actin-myosin cross-bridges. In creating these cross-bridges, the myosin pulls on the actin molecules, drawing the thin filaments toward the center of the H zone and shortening the sarcomere (see Figure 6.7). ATPase activity in the myosin head provides the energy for the powerstroke that results in the dissociation of the myosin head from the actin. (An ATPase is an enzyme that hydrolyzes ATP.) The myosin returns to its original position and is now free to bind to another actin molecule and repeat the process, thus further pulling the thin filaments towards the center of the H zone.

MCAT FAVORITE

When the muscle contracts—the H and I bands are eliminated.

MCAT SYNOPSIS

Think of tropomyosin as the chaperone responsible for protecting actin's binding sites from the advances of the myosin head. In the presence of Ca^{2+}, troponin changes its conformation and moves tropomyosin away from its guard position, thereby allowing myosin to bind to actin and the action to begin.

3. Relaxation

When the sarcolemmic receptors are no longer stimulated, the Ca^{2+} is pumped back into the sarcoplasmic reticulum. The products of ATP hydrolysis are released from the myosin head, a new ATP binds to the

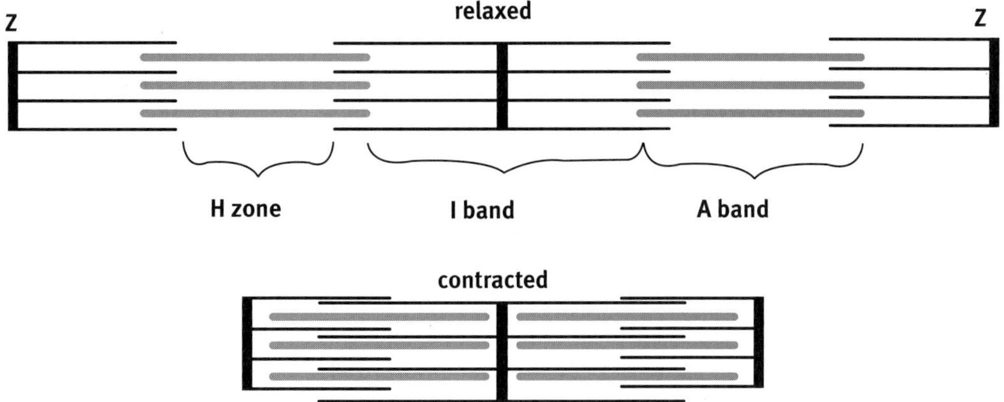

Figure 6.7. Contraction

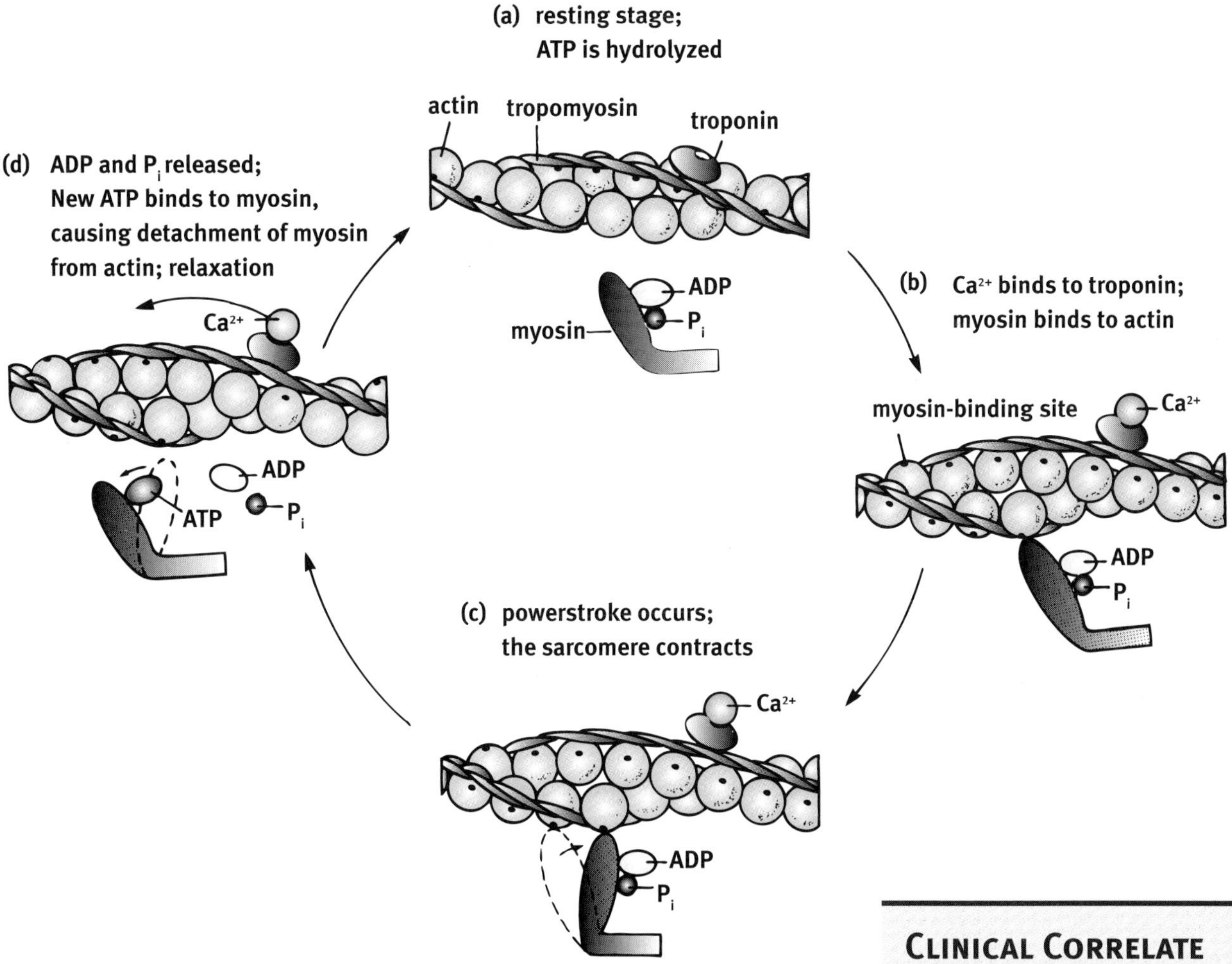

Figure 6.8. ATPase Activity

Clinical Correlate

Rigor mortis is the "stiffening" of muscles after death. This results from the lack of ATP to relax the muscle.

head, resulting in the dissociation of the myosin from the thin filament, and the sarcomere returns to its original width.

TEACHER TIP

THINK: Why do muscle fibers contract in an all-or-none fashion? Because they are innervated by neurons whose basic signal is an action potential, which is an all-or-none phenomenon.

C. STIMULUS AND MUSCLE RESPONSE

1. Stimulus Intensity

Individual muscle fibers generally exhibit an **all-or-none response**; only a stimulus above a minimal value called the **threshold value** can elicit contraction. The strength of the contraction of a single muscle fiber cannot be increased, regardless of the strength of the stimulus. Whole muscle, on the other hand, does not exhibit an all-or-none response. Although there is a minimal threshold value needed to elicit a muscle contraction, the strength of the contraction can increase as stimulus strength is increased by involving more fibers. A maximal response is reached when all of the fibers have reached the threshold value and the muscle contracts as a whole.

Tonus refers to the continual low-grade contractions of muscle, which are essential for both voluntary and involuntary muscle contraction. Even at rest, muscles are in a continuous state of tonus.

2. Simple Twitch

A simple twitch is the response of a single muscle fiber to a brief stimulus at or above the threshold stimulus and consists of a **latent period,** a **contraction period,** and a **relaxation period.** The latent period is the time between stimulation and the onset of contraction. During this time lag, the action potential spreads along the sarcolemma and Ca^{2+} ions are released. Following the contraction period, there is a brief relaxation period in which the muscle is unresponsive to a stimulus; this period is known as the **absolute refractory period.** This is followed by a **relative refractory period,** during which a greater-than-normal stimulus is needed to elicit a contraction (see Figure 6.9).

3. Summation and Tetanus

When the fibers of a muscle are exposed to very frequent stimuli, the muscle cannot fully relax. The contractions begin to combine, becoming stronger and more prolonged. This is known as **frequency summation.** The contractions become continuous when the stimuli are so frequent that the muscle cannot relax. This type of contraction is known as **tetanus** and is stronger than a simple twitch of a single fiber. If tetanization is prolonged, the muscle will begin to fatigue (see Figure 6.9).

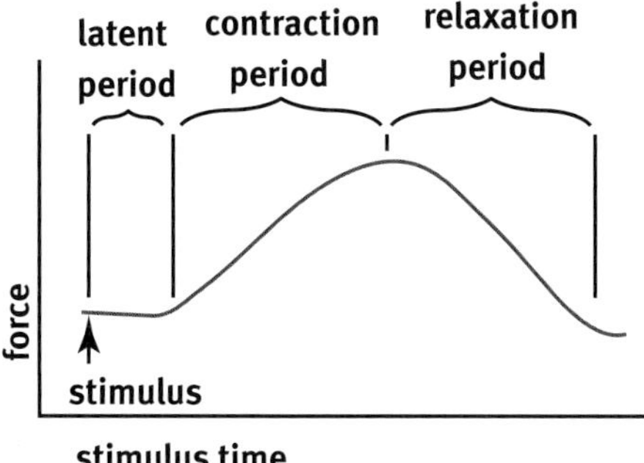

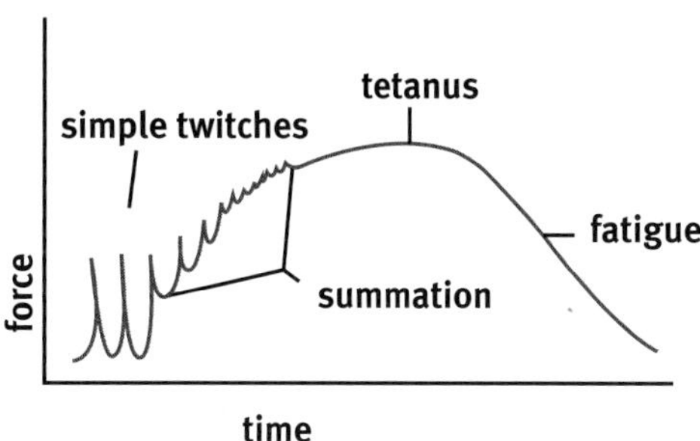

Figure 6.9. Simple Twitch and Summation/Tetanus

SMOOTH MUSCLE

Smooth muscle is responsible for involuntary actions and is innervated by the **autonomic nervous system** (see chapter 12). Smooth muscle is found in the digestive tract, bladder, uterus, and blood vessel walls, among other places. Smooth muscle cells possess one centrally located nucleus. While smooth muscle cells also contain actin and myosin filaments, these filaments lack the organization of skeletal sarcomeres; consequently, smooth muscles lack the striations of skeletal muscle.

As in skeletal muscle, smooth muscle contractions result from the sliding of actin and myosin over one another and are regulated by an influx of calcium ions. However, smooth muscle contractions are slower and are capable of being sustained longer than skeletal muscle contractions. Smooth muscle typically has both inhibitory and excitatory synapses that regulate contraction via the nervous system. Smooth muscle also has the property of reflexively contracting without nervous stimulation; this is called **myogenic** activity.

MCAT Synopsis

Skeletal Muscle
- Striated
- Voluntary
- Somatic innervation
- Many nuclei per cell
- Ca^{2+} required for contraction

Cardiac Muscle
- Striated
- Involuntary
- Autonomic innervation
- One to two nuclei per cell
- Ca^{2+} required for contraction

Smooth Muscle
- Nonstriated
- Involuntary
- Autonomic innervation
- One nucleus per cell
- Ca^{2+} required for contraction

CARDIAC MUSCLE

The muscle tissue of the heart is composed of cardiac muscle fibers. These fibers possess characteristics of both skeletal and smooth muscle fibers. As in skeletal muscle, actin and myosin filaments are arranged in sarcomeres, giving cardiac muscle a striated appearance. However, cardiac muscle cells generally have only one or two centrally located nuclei. Cardiac muscle is innervated by the autonomic nervous system, which serves only to modulate its inherent beat, because cardiac muscle, like smooth muscle, is myogenic (see chapter 9).

Teacher Tip

The MCAT loves to test the fact that smooth muscle exhibits myogenic activity. Striated muscle requires descending input from the nervous system. Smooth muscle, however, will contract even without this input. Of course, the nervous system can regulate smooth muscle as well.

ENERGY RESERVES

A. CREATINE PHOSPHATE

High-energy compounds, such as fatty acids, glycogen, and glucose, can be degraded in muscle cells to produce ATP. In addition, energy can be temporarily stored in a high-energy compound called **creatine phosphate.** During resting periods, creatine phosphate is produced via a reaction that transfers a high-energy phosphate group from ATP to creatine. During exercise, the reaction proceeds in reverse, resynthesizing ATP from creatine phosphate and ADP, thus replenishing the ATP supply without the need for additional oxygen.

FLASHBACK

Remember, in the absence of oxygen, pyruvate is reduced to lactic acid in the cytoplasm, and the TCA cycle and electron transport chain do not come into play. Lactic acid build-up is responsible for the "feel the burn" stage of vigorous exercise. See chapter 3.

$$\text{creatine} + \text{ATP} \rightleftharpoons \text{creatine phosphate} + \text{ADP}$$

B. MYOGLOBIN

Myoglobin is a hemoglobin-like protein found in muscle tissue. Myoglobin has a high O_2 affinity; it binds to O_2 from the bloodstream and holds onto it. During strenuous exercise, when muscle cells rapidly run out of available O_2, myoglobin releases its O_2. In this way, myoglobin acts as an additional oxygen reserve for active muscle. However, during strenuous exercise, the oxygen supply to muscles may be insufficient to meet its energy demands, despite the extra O_2 supplied by myoglobin. During this period the muscle obtains additional energy via anaerobic respiration, resulting in the build-up of lactic acid (see chapter 3).

TEACHER TIP

This acid can be converted back into energy-producing intermediates once sufficient levels of oxygen become available. This process occurs in the liver and is known as the Cori cycle.

CONNECTIVE TISSUE

The major function of connective tissue is to bind and support other tissue. Connective tissue is a sparsely scattered population of cells contained in an amorphous ground substance which may be liquid, jelly-like, or solid. **Loose connective tissue** is found throughout the body. It binds epithelium to underlying tissues and is the packing material that holds organs in place. It contains proteinaceous fibers of three types: **collagenous fibers,** which are composed of collagen and have great tensile strength; **elastic fibers,** which are composed of elastin and endow connective tissue with resilience; and **reticular fibers,** which are branched, tightly woven fibers that join connective tissue to adjoining tissue. There are two major cell types in loose connective tissue: **fibroblasts,** which secrete substances that are components of extracellular fibers, and **macrophages,** which engulf bacteria and dead cells via phagocytosis.

Dense connective tissue is connective tissue with a very high proportion of collagenous fibers. The fibers are organized into parallel bundles that give the fibers great tensile strength. Dense connective tissue forms **tendons,** which attach muscle to bone, and **ligaments,** which hold bones together at the joints.

MUSCLE-BONE INTERACTIONS

Locomotion is dependent on interactions between the skeletal and muscular systems. If a given muscle (including associated joints) is attached to two bones, contraction of the muscle will cause only one of the two bones to move. The end of the muscle attached to the stationary bone is called the **origin**; in limb muscles it corresponds to the **proximal end.** The end of the muscle attached to the bone that moves during contraction is called the **insertion**; in limb muscles, the insertion corresponds to the **distal end.**

Often muscles work in antagonistic pairs; one relaxes while the other contracts. Such is the case in the arm, where the biceps and triceps work antagonistically. When you move your hand toward your shoulder, the biceps contract and the triceps relax; when you move your hand down again, the biceps relax and the triceps contract (see Figure 6.10). There are also **synergistic muscles,** which assist the principal muscles during movement.

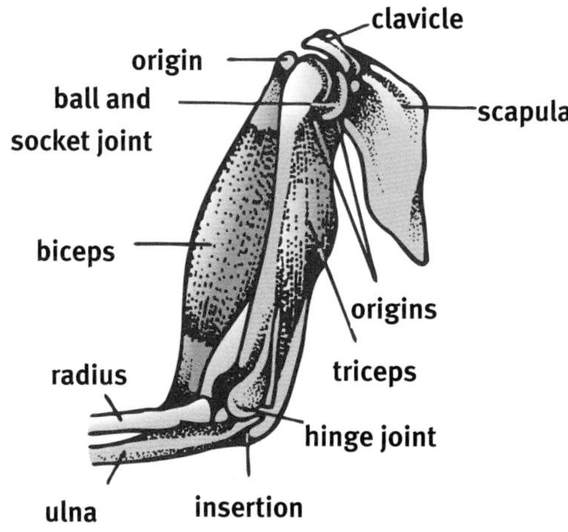

Figure 6.10. Muscles of the Upper Arm

A **flexor** muscle will contract to decrease the angle of a joint, whereas an **extensor muscle** will contract to straighten the joint. An **abductor** moves a part of the body away from the body's midline; an **adductor** moves a part of the body toward the midline.

PRACTICE QUESTIONS

1. Cartilage and bone have various differences. Which of the following scenarios would be expected given the known differences?

   A. Bone fractures heal more quickly than ruptured tendons.
   B. Bone fractures heal more slowly than ruptured tendons.
   C. Bone fractures bleed less than ruptured tendons.
   D. Bone fractures heal at the same rate as ruptured tendons.

2. Which cell layer gives rise to the skeletal system?

   A. Ectoderm
   B. Mesoderm
   C. Endoderm
   D. Epithelial cell layer

3. Which of the following is the most important element involved in muscle contraction?

   A. Iron
   B. Magnesium
   C. Phosphate
   D. Calcium

4. The bone marrow serves several functions. Which of the following cell types is derived from the bone marrow?

   A. Lymphocyte
   B. Epithelial
   C. Neuron
   D. Keratinocyte

5. A long-distance runner has exhausted the stores of glycogen in her liver, and the stores in the muscle are running low. She is forced to rely on anaerobic metabolism at the end of her workout. How many ATPs will she produce in this anaerobic state, compared to an aerobic state?

   A. 2 versus 38
   B. 36 versus 38
   C. 15 versus 38
   D. 1 versus 38

6. A patient with elevated parathyroid hormone may be expected to show signs of which of the following?

   A. Rheumatoid arthritis
   B. Osteoporosis
   C. Migraine
   D. Ankle sprain

7. In death, the production of ATP ceases. Which of the following findings will be present in this state?

   A. Muscles will be stiff and rigid.
   B. Muscles will be relaxed but not contracted.
   C. Muscles will be contracted but not relaxed.
   D. Muscles will be completely flaccid and able to be relaxed and contracted.

8. Storage of calcium and phosphate in the bones requires absorption of calcium from the intestinal track and by the kidneys from blood filtrate. Vitamin D plays an important role in this process of absorption; it is ingested and is also made in the skin. What two organs are responsible for activating vitamin D once it is present in the body?

A. Brain and lungs
B. Lungs and intestine
C. Kidney and liver
D. Liver and lungs

9. The musculoskeletal system depends upon input from the nervous system to drive its activities. Smooth muscle is innervated by which of the following systems?

A. Autonomic nervous system
B. Somatic nervous system
C. Parasympathetic but not sympathetic nervous system
D. Sympathetic but not parasympathetic nervous system

10. Weight lifting causes skeletal muscles to increase in size. By what process does this primarily occur?

A. Hypertension
B. Hyperplasia
C. Hypertrophy
D. Hyperextension

11. In the figure below, which band of the sarcomere does not change length during muscle contraction?

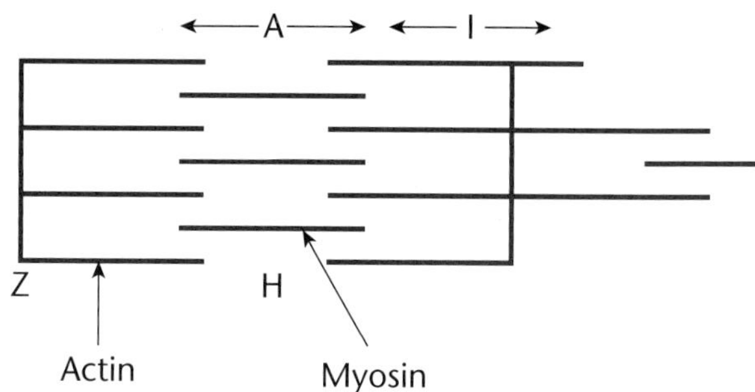

A. Z
B. I
C. H
D. A

12. Excitatory estrogen receptors have been recently found on osteoblasts. During menopause, there is a sharp decrease in the amount of estrogen production. Which of the following can be expected?

A. Decrease in the ratio of osteoclast/osteoblast activity
B. Increase in the ratio of osteoclast/osteoblast activity
C. Increase in the ratio of osteoblast/osteoclast activity
D. No change in the ratio of osteoblast/osteoclast activity

13. A patient has recently been diagnosed with primary hyperparathyroidism. The physician sends his blood to the lab for routine electrolyte testing. Which of the following lab findings is consistent with primary hyperparathyroidism?

A. Elevated serum calcium and low parathyroid hormone level
B. Elevated serum calcium and elevated parathyroid hormone level
C. Low serum calcium and low parathyroid hormone level
D. Low serum calcium and elevated parathyroid hormone level

CHAPTER 7

DIGESTION

Digestion consists of the degradation of large molecules into smaller molecules that can be absorbed into the bloodstream and used directly by cells. **Intracellular digestion** occurs within the cell, usually in membrane-bound vesicles. **Extracellular digestion** refers to a digestive process that occurs outside of the cell, within a lumen or tract. Mammals have a one-way digestive tract known as the **alimentary canal**. Mammalian digestive tracts tend to be complex and are organized into regions specialized for the digestion and absorption of specific nutrients.

Teacher Tip

The individual molecules that the body can absorb will be discussed in detail later. The big-picture concept to keep in mind is that all foods are broken down into simple sugars, amino acids and peptides, and fats.

The human digestive tract begins with the **oral cavity** and continues with the **pharynx,** the **esophagus,** the **stomach,** the **small intestine,** and the **large intestine** (see Figure 7.1). Accessory organs, such as the **salivary glands,** the **pancreas,** the **liver,** and the **gall bladder,** also play essential roles in the digestive process.

Most body surfaces (e.g., the skin and lungs, and the linings of the nose, mouth, esophagus, stomach, and intestines) are covered or lined by continuous sheets of epithelial cells. Epithelial cells are joined tightly together, facilitating their ability to act as a barrier against mechanical injury, invading organisms, and fluid loss. The free surface of epithelium is exposed to air or liquid and may be ciliated. The inner surface is attached to underlying connective tissue by a **basement membrane.**

THE ORAL CAVITY

The oral cavity (the mouth) is where mechanical and chemical digestion of food begins. Mechanical digestion is the breakdown of large food particles into smaller particles through the biting and chewing action of teeth (mastication). While mechanical digestion does not lead to changes in the molecular composition of food, the total surface area of the food is increased, allowing for faster and more efficient enzymatic action. **Chemical digestion** refers to the enzymatic breakdown of macromolecules into smaller molecules and begins in the mouth when the salivary glands secrete saliva. Saliva lubricates food to facilitate swallowing and

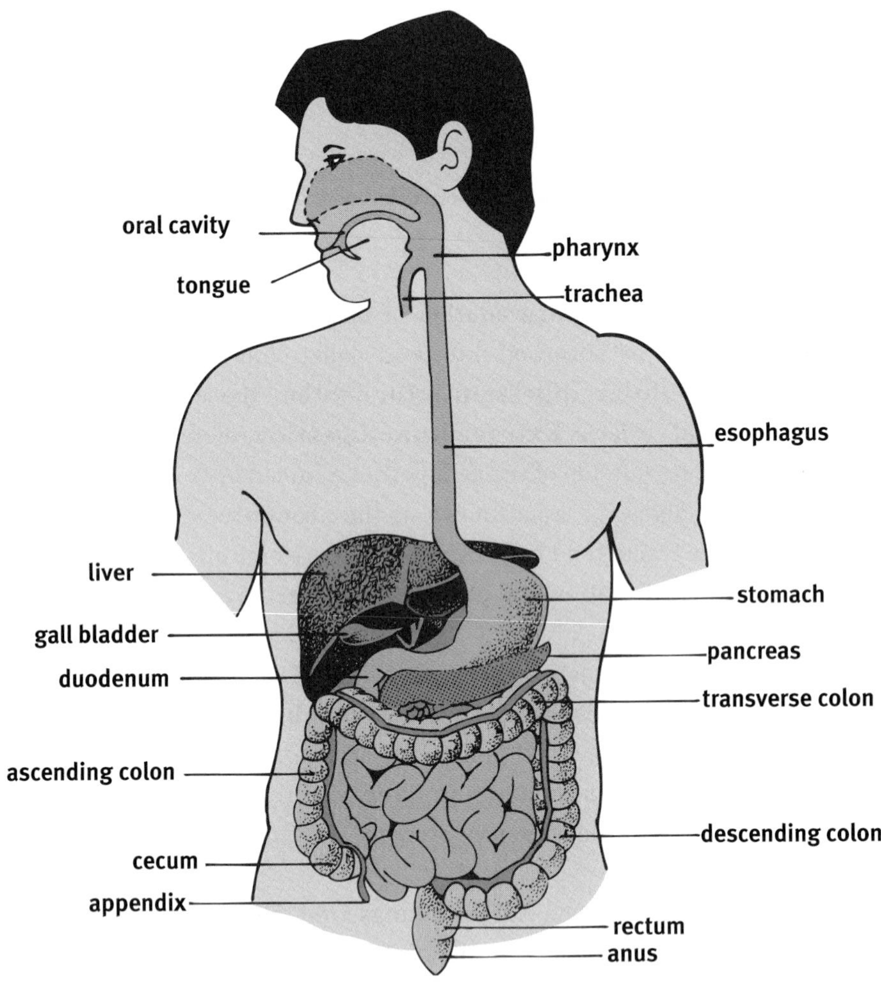

Figure 7.1. Human Digestive Tract

MCAT Synopsis

If you chew on a plain cracker long enough without swallowing, you'll start to taste sugar. This is the result of salivary amylase breaking down complex carbohydrates into simple sugars. Feel free to try this at home.

Teacher Tip

Salivary amylase is actually redundant in terms of carbohydrate digestion. Pancreatic amylase is capable of carrying out the same function.

provides a solvent for food particles. Saliva is secreted in response to a nervous reflex triggered by the presence of food in the oral cavity. Saliva contains the enzyme salivary amylase (ptyalin), which hydrolyzes starch into simple sugars. However, since food does not remain in the mouth for long, only a small portion of starch is hydrolyzed there. The muscular tongue, containing the taste buds, manipulates the food, rolls it into a ball called a bolus, and pushes the bolus into the pharynx.

THE PHARYNX

The pharynx is the cavity that leads food from the mouth into the esophagus. The pharynx also functions in respiration as the passageway through which air enters the trachea. During swallowing, the opening of the trachea is covered by a flap called the **epiglottis,** thereby preventing food particles from being aspirated into the lungs.

THE ESOPHAGUS

The esophagus is the muscular tube leading from the pharynx to the stomach. Food is moved down the esophagus by rhythmic waves of involuntary muscular contractions called **peristalsis.** When a wave of peristalsis spreads down the esophagus, a specialized ring of muscle in the lower esophagus opens, allowing food to enter the stomach. Following the peristaltic wave, this muscle, called the **lower esophageal sphincter** or **cardiac sphincter,** returns to its normal closed state, thus preventing the regurgitation of stomach contents into the esophagus.

MCAT SYNOPSIS

The initial contraction of the upper esophagus is voluntary; however, once irritated, the involuntary peristalsis proceeds. This is why we can cough up food when it "feels" like we are about to choke.

TEACHER TIP

Weakness in the lower esophageal sphincter can lead to classical "heartburn" after eating.

THE STOMACH

The stomach, a large, muscular organ located in the upper abdomen, stores and partially digests food. The walls of the stomach are lined by the thick gastric mucosa, which contains the **gastric glands** and **pyloric glands.** The gastric glands are stimulated by nervous impulses from the brain, which responds to the sight, taste, and/or smell of food. The gastric glands are composed of three types of secretory cells: **mucous cells, chief cells,** and **parietal cells.** Mucous cells secrete mucus, which protects the stomach lining from the harshly acidic juices (pH = 2) present in the stomach. **Gastric juice** is composed of the secretions of the chief cells and the parietal cells. Chief cells secrete **pepsinogen,** the zymogen of the protein-hydrolyzing enzyme **pepsin.** The chief cells also secrete intrinsic factor, which plays a role in the absorption of vitamin B^{12}. Parietal cells secrete **hydrochloric acid (HCl).** HCl kills bacteria, dissolves the intercellular "glue" holding food tissues together, and facilitates the conversion of pepsinogen to pepsin. Pepsin hydrolyzes specific peptide bonds to yield polypeptide fragments. The pyloric glands secrete the hormone **gastrin** in response to the presence of certain substances in food. Gastrin stimulates the gastric glands to secrete more HCl and also stimulates muscular contractions of the stomach, which churn food. This churning produces an acidic, semifluid mixture of partially digested food known as **chyme.**

At the junction of the stomach and the small intestine is the muscular **pyloric sphincter,** which regulates the passage of chyme from the stomach into the small intestine via alternating contractions and relaxations. Although nutrient absorption occurs in the small intestine, alcohol and certain drugs (e.g., aspirin) can be directly absorbed into the systemic circulation through capillaries in the stomach wall.

CLINICAL CORRELATE

Zollinger-Ellison syndrome is a rare disease resulting from a gastrin-secreting tumor (gastrinoma). Typically, the tumor is found in the pancreas. As you would expect, the excess gastrin stimulates an increase in HCl production in the stomach. Not surprisingly, the most notable feature of ZE is the presence of severe, intractable ulcer disease.

THE SMALL INTESTINE

Chemical digestion is completed in the small intestine. The small intestine is divided into three sections: the **duodenum,** the **jejunum,** and the **ileum.** In order to maximize the surface area available for digestion and absorption, the intestine is extremely long (greater than six meters in length) and highly coiled. In addition, numerous fingerlike projections called **villi** extend out of the intestinal submucosa, and tiny cytoplasmic projections called **microvilli** project from the surface of the individual cells lining the villi (see Figure 7.2). The total surface area of the small intestine is approximately 300 m^2.

CLINICAL CORRELATE

Severe narrowing of the pyloric sphincter can result in a condition known as pyloric stenosis. Most commonly seen in infants, the hallmark symptom of pyloric stenosis is projectile vomiting. In addition, a mass can often be palpated in the belly and peristaltic waves may be visible across the baby's abdomen. Pyloric stenosis can be surgically corrected.

A. DIGESTIVE FUNCTIONS

Most digestion in the small intestine occurs in the duodenum, where the secretions of the intestinal glands, pancreas, liver, and gall bladder mix together with the acidic chyme entering from the stomach. The presence of chyme triggers hormonal release, which in turn stimulates and regulates the secretions of the small intestine and its accessory organs.

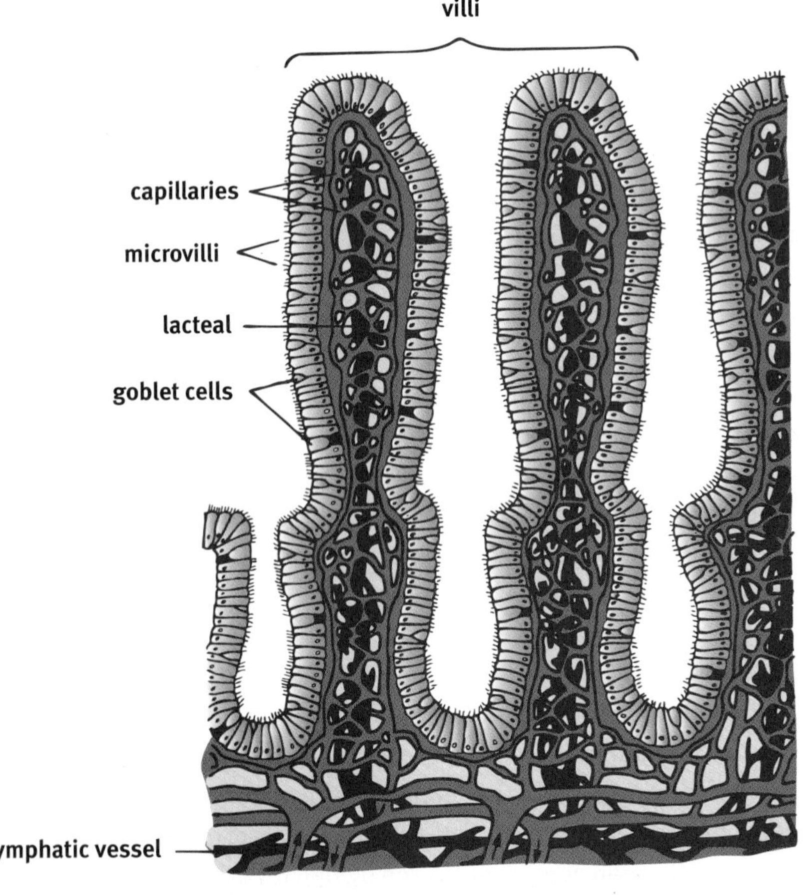

Figure 7.2. Intestinal Villi

The intestinal mucosa secretes enzymes that hydrolyze carbohydrates into monosaccharides, such as **maltase, lactase,** and **sucrase,** and **peptidases,** which hydrolyze dipeptides and oligo peptides. The hormone **secretin** is released by the duodenum in response to the acidity of chyme, stimulating the pancreas to secrete **pancreatic juice.** The enzymes of the small intestine function optimally at a slightly basic pH and are denatured by acid; pancreatic juice is an alkaline fluid (due to a high concentration of bicarbonate) that helps neutralize the acidity of chyme and contains enzymes that digest carbohydrates, proteins, and lipids. **Trypsinogen** is a proteolytic zymogen secreted by the pancreas and is converted to its active form, **trypsin,** by an enzyme called **enterokinase** (secreted by the intestinal glands). Trypsin then converts another pancreatic zymogen, **chymotrypsinogen,** to its active form, **chymotrypsin.** Each of these enzymes cleaves specific peptide bonds within proteins, producing polypeptide fragments. The pancreas also secretes **carboxypeptidase** (also secreted as a zymogen and activated by trypsin). Proteolytic enzymes in the pancreatic juice break down proteins into dipeptides and oligopeptides. Then, similar to the hydrolysis of carbohydrates, the intestinal mucosa breaks these compounds into amino acids by secreting amino peptidase.

TEACHER TIP

These enzymes are key to proper digestion. Only simple sugars (monosaccharides) can be absorbed by the gut. Without these enzymes, the sugars will either pass through the body unchanged or be digested by bacteria in the colon.

CLINICAL CORRELATE

Lactose intolerance results from the absence of lactase. Hence, lactose passes to the colon undigested. This results in the symptoms experienced by those with this deficiency.

TEACHER TIP

Having trouble keeping the sections of the small intestine in order? Just think of the stock market. The major index—Dow Jones Industrials—is in the same order as the small intestine—duodenum, jejunum, ileum.

The hormone **CCK (cholecystokinin)** is secreted into the bloodstream by the duodenum in response to the presence of chyme. CCK stimulates the secretion of pancreatic enzymes and the release of **bile.** Bile is an alkaline fluid synthesized and secreted by the liver, stored and concentrated in the gall bladder, and released into the duodenum. Bile is composed of bile salts, bile pigments, and cholesterol. Bile salts are molecules with a water-soluble region on one end and a fat-soluble region on the other. This structure, similar to that of detergents, allows bile salts to emulsify, i.e. dissolve, fat globules and to surround and maintain these particles in finely dispersed complexes called **micelles,** which are soluble in aqueous media. This process is called the **emulsification** of fat and exposes more of the lipids' surface area to the actions of **lipases,** which hydrolyze molecules of fat into glycerol and fatty acids. The amount of bile released is proportional to the amount of fat ingested. If the chyme is particularly fatty, the duodenum releases the hormone **enterogastrone,** which inhibits stomach peristalsis, thus slowing down the release of chyme into the small intestine (fats take a longer time to digest than the other macromolecules).

MCAT SYNOPSIS

We've now reviewed two important "good" functions of cholesterol: contributor to the fluidity of cell membranes (chapter 1) and key component of bile. More to come . . .

In addition to hormonal regulation, the digestive processes are also stimulated by the **parasympathetic nervous system** and inhibited by the **sympathetic nervous system** (See chapter 12).

B. ABSORPTIVE FUNCTIONS

The majority of nutrient absorption occurs across the walls of the jejunum and the ileum (a small amount of absorption occurs in the duodenum). Monosaccharides are absorbed via active transport and facilitated diffusion into the epithelial cells lining the villi; amino acids are absorbed into the epithelium via active transport. Monosaccharides, amino acids, and small fatty acids diffuse directly into the intestinal capillaries and enter portal circulation via the **hepatic portal vein.** Larger fatty acids, glycerol, and cholesterol diffuse into the mucosal cells; the fatty acids and glycerol recombine to form triglycerides, which, along with phosphoglycerides and cholesterol, are packaged into protein-coated droplets called **chylomicrons.** The chylomicrons are secreted into tiny lymph vessels within the villi called **lacteals,** which lead into the lymphatic system; the lymphatic system converges with venous blood at the thoracic duct located in the neck. The chylomicrons are processed in the bloodstream and delivered to the liver. They are repackaged there and released into the bloodstream as LDLs, VLDLs, and HDLs (lipoproteins or proteins complexed with lipids).

Vitamins and minerals are also absorbed in the small intestine. The fat-soluble vitamins (A, D, E, and K) are absorbed along with fats, and most water-soluble vitamins (e.g., the vitamin B complexes and vitamin C) are absorbed via simple diffusion into the circulatory system. Approximately seven liters of fluid enter the small intestine every day; the majority of it is absorbed through the walls of the small intestine.

THE LARGE INTESTINE

TEACHER TIP

KEY POINT: Although the large intestine reabsorbs massive amounts of water, it is the kidneys that actually regulate total body water. More on this process later.

The large intestine is approximately 1.5 m long and consists of six parts: the **cecum,** the **ascending colon, transverse colon, descending colon, sismoid colon,** and the **rectum.** The cecum is a blind outpocketing at the junction of the small and large intestines. At the tip of the cecum is a small, fingerlike projection called the **appendix.** The appendix is a **vestigial structure** (see chapter 15) containing lymphoid tissue that is often surgically removed if it becomes infected. The colon functions in the absorption of salts and the absorption of any water not already absorbed by the small intestine. If digested matter moves through the colon too quickly, too little water is absorbed, causing diarrhea and dehydration. Alternatively, if movement through the bowels is too slow, too much water is absorbed, causing constipation. The rectum stores **feces,** which consist of bacteria (particularly **E. coli**), water, undigested food, and unabsorbed

Table 7.1. Digestive Enzymes

Nutrient	Enzyme	Site of Production	Site of Function	Function
Carbohydrates	Salivary amylase (Ptyalin)	Salivary glands	Mouth	Hydrolyzes starch to maltose
	Pancreatic amylase	Pancreas	Small intestine	Hydrolyzes starch to maltose
	Maltase	Intestinal glands	Small intestine	Hydrolyzes maltose to two glucose molecules
	Sucrase	Intestinal glands	Small intestine	Hydrolyzes sucrose to glucose and fructose
	Lactase	Intestinal glands	Small intestine	Hydrolyzes lactose to glucose and galactose
Proteins	Pepsin (secreted as pepsinogen)	Gastric glands	Stomach	Hydrolyzes specific peptide bonds
	Trypsin (secreted as trypsinogen)	Pancreas	Small intestine	Hydrolyzes specific peptide bonds Converts chymotrypsinogen to chymotry
	Chymotrypsin (secreted as chymotrypsinogen)	Pancreas	Small intestine	Hydrolyzes specific peptide bonds
	Carboxy-peptidase	Pancreas	Small intestine	Hydrolyzes terminal peptide bond at carboxyl end
	Aminopeptidase	Intestinal glands	Small intestine	Hydrolyzes terminal peptide bond at amino end
	Dipeptidases	Intestinal glands	Small intestine	Hydrolyzes pairs of amino acids
	Enterokinase	Intestinal glands	Small intestine	Converts trypsinogen to trypsin
Lipids	Bile*	Liver	Small intestine	Emulsifies fat
	Lipase	Pancreas	Small intestine	Hydrolyzes lipids

*Note that bile is NOT an enzyme.

digestive secretions (e.g., enzymes and bile). The **anus** is the opening through which wastes are eliminated and is separated from the rectum by two sphincters that regulate elimination.

ACCESSORY ORGANS

A. LIVER

The liver has many functions such as storage of glycogen, gluconeogenesis, conversion of ammonia to urea, lipid metabolism, synthesis of the majority of proteins in the human blood stream, detoxification of drugs and their metabolites in the blood stream, and production and secretion of bile into the gastrointestinal tract to emulsify fats.

TEACHER TIP

Though the gallbladder stores bile, it isn't completely necessary for life. High fat diets commonly result in formation of stones or sludge within the gall-bladder or cystic duct. If this blockage cannot be cleared, the gallbladder may have to be removed. This is known as a cholecystectomy.

B. GALLBLADDER

The gall bladder is primarily responsible for the storage and secretion of excess bile.

C. PANCREAS

The pancreas has both exocrine and endocrine function. The endocrine function of the pancreas arises from its production of insulin and glucagons, and somatostatin primarily relates to glucose metabolism. In contrast, the exocrine function of the pancreas refers to its secretions of bicarbonate and digestive enzymes such as trypsin, chymotrypsin, enterokinase, amylase, and lipase into the small intestine for digestion.

TEACHER TIP

Many of the digestive enzymes could be fairly damaging to the body. Thus, they are often secreted as inactive precursors (zymogens).

SUMMARY OF DIGESTION

Digestion begins in different parts of the digestive tract for each of the three classes of macromolecules. Carbohydrate digestion begins in the mouth; protein digestion begins in the stomach; and lipid digestion begins in the small intestine. Table 7.1 is a summary of the digestive enzymes.

PRACTICE QUESTIONS

1. The digestive system has two main functions: breaking down large food molecules into small molecules and absorption of these small molecules, minerals, and water into the body. There are four major activities of the gastrointestinal tract which will accomplish these two main functions. Which of the following is not one of the activities?

   A. Propulsion
   B. Secretion
   C. Opsonization
   D. Digestion

2. What is the correct linear arrangement of the gastrointestinal tract?

   A. Mouth, trachea, stomach, duodenum, anus
   B. Mouth, trachea, jejunum, large intestine, anus
   C. Mouth, esophagus, jejunum, duodenum, anus
   D. Mouth, esophagus, duodenum, ileum, anus

3. The autonomic nervous system of the gastrointestinal tract has both extrinsic and intrinsic components. The extrinsic system is comprised of the sympathetic and parasympathetic innervations, while the intrinsic system is comprised of the enteric nervous system. The parasympathetic nervous system of the gastrointestinal tract is supplied by both the vagus nerve (CN X) and the pelvic nerve. Which portion of the gastrointestinal tract is not supplied by the vagus nerve?

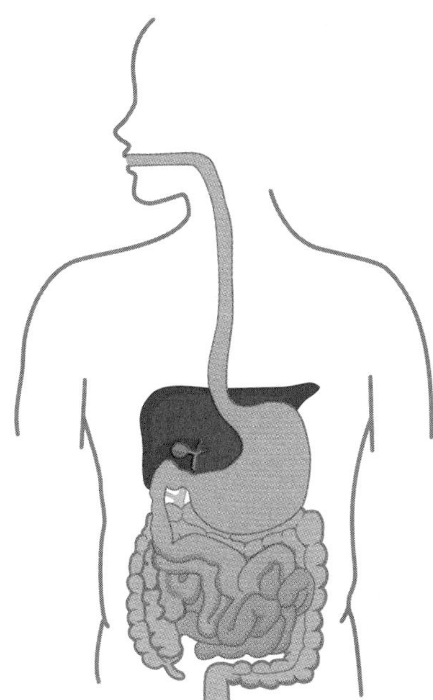

   A. Transverse colon
   B. Stomach wall
   C. Small intestine
   D. Ascending colon

4. Which subdivision of the gastrointestinal wall contains the main blood vessels of the gastrointestinal tract?

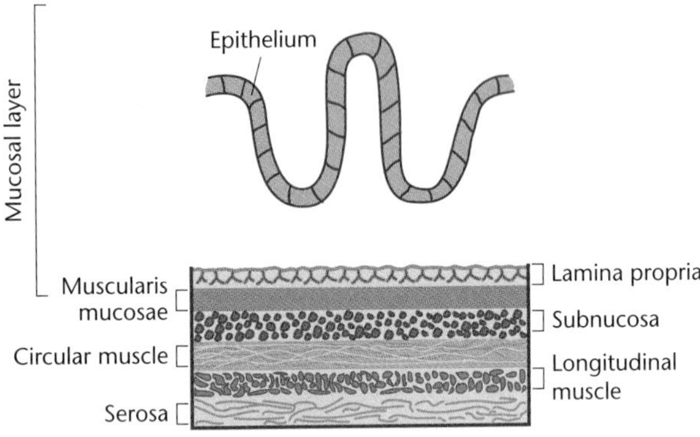

A. Mucosal layer
B. Muscularis mucosae
C. Lamina propria
D. Submucosal layer

5. An apparently healthy newborn develops excessive vomiting and abdominal distension a few hours after birth. The vomitus contains bile. Radiographic examination shows a gas-filled stomach and dilated, gas-filled small bowel loops, but no air is present in the large intestine. A diagnosis of a congenital obstruction of the small bowel is made. Where is the obstruction most likely to be located?

A. Jejunum
B. Duodenum
C. Ileum
D. Appendix

6. Which of the following is not a function of cholecystokinin (CCK)?

A. Stimulation of gallbladder contraction
B. Inhibition of H^+ secretion
C. Secretion of pancreatic HCO_3^-
D. Inhibition of gastric emptying

7. Chief cells located in the stomach secrete inactive pepsinogen. Which of the following is required to start the conversion process of pepsinogen into its active form, pepsin?

A. HCO_3^-
B. H_2CO_3
C. HCl
D. $CaCl_2$

8. Hirschsprung's disease, or congenital aganglionic megacolon, is a disease in which a portion of the colon lacks ganglion cells in the myenteric plexus. What is a likely symptom of this disease?

A. Diarrhea
B. Weight loss due to malabsorption
C. Constipation
D. Dehydration

9. During embryonic development, structures within the abdomen undergo numerous rotations before attaining their final abdominal position. With the stomach as the central point, a structure that is attached posterior to the stomach would find itself where in relation to the stomach after the final rotation?

A. Posterior to the stomach
B. Right of the stomach
C. Anterior to the stomach
D. Inferior to the stomach

10. What process is required to convert primary bile acids into secondary bile acids?

A. Conjugation
B. Dehydroxylation
C. Dehydration
D. Methylation

11. Which amino acid is used to conjugate secondary bile acids, thereby forming bile salts?

A. Arginine
B. Carnitine
C. Glycine
D. Phenylalanine

12. Which of the following is not a function of bile acid?

A. Cholesterol elimination
B. Cholesterol solubilization
C. Absorption of vitamins B_1, B_2, B_6, B_{12}, and C
D. Lipid emulsification

13. Saliva is secreted from acinar cells within the salivary glands. It is then modified by ductal cells within the glands, causing the once isotonic solution to become hypotonic. Acinar cells also secrete other products into saliva, such as enzymes required for initial digestion of lipids and starch. What enzyme found in saliva is also secreted by the pancreas?

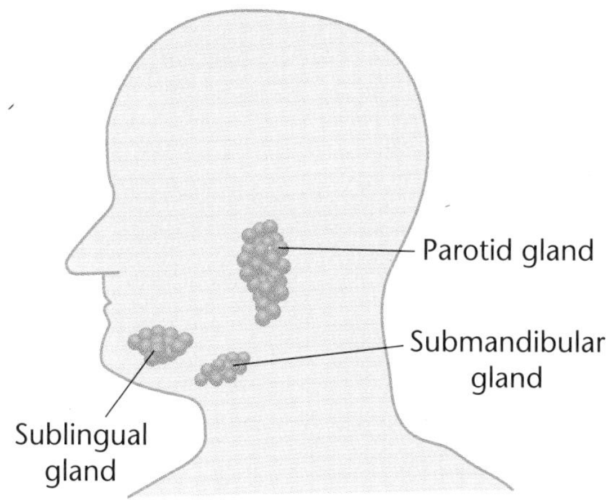

A. Pepsin
B. Chymotrypsin
C. Amylase
D. Trypsin

14. The pancreas contains groups of hormone-producing cells known as islets of Langerhans. Some of these cells produce insulin, while others produce glucagon. There is a third cluster of cells which have the ability to inhibit the secretion of both insulin and glucagon. This paracrine hormone is known as:

A. aldosterone.
B. somatostatin.
C. vasopressin.
D. cholecystokinin.

15. Cholecystokin (CCK) is secreted into the duodenum in response to the presence of fat and protein in the intestine. CCK inhibits further gastric emptying, while enhancing the digestive process within the duodenum. Other digestive products are secreted into the intestine due to CCK EXCEPT

A. pancreatic lipase.
B. hepatic bile.
C. somatostatin.
D. chymotrypsin.

16. Starch is a polysaccharide carbohydrate composed of numerous glucose monosaccharides joined together by glycosidic bonds. In which part of the digestive tract does the digestion of starch begin?

A. Stomach
B. Duodenum
C. Mouth
D. Jejunum

17. Where does final disaccharide digestion and absorption take place?

A. Stomach
B. Jejunum
C. Mouth
D. Sigmoid colon

18. The abdominal aorta is the largest artery in the abdominal cavity. Three major branches of the abdominal aorta are considered to be the main sources of blood to the abdomen and abdominal organs. Which one of these branches is not a major blood source to the abdomen?

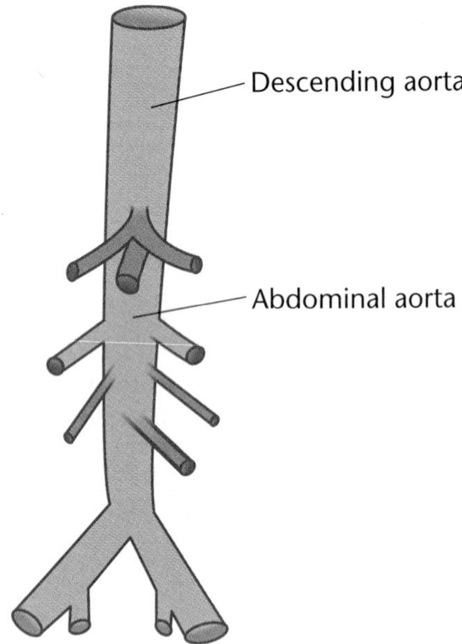

A. Superior mesenteric artery
B. Inferior mesenteric artery
C. Common iliac
D. Celiac trunk

DIGESTIVE SYSTEM

In the gastric phase of digestion, food in the stomach, particularly the presence of amino acids and peptides, causes G cells to secrete gastrin, which in turn stimulates parietal cells. Gastrin secretion is normally inhibited once acidic chyme, with a pH less than 3, reaches the duodenum. What physiological condition would be the result of a gastrin-secreting tumor?

1) Determine the role of gastrin in the stomach.

According to the question stem, gastrin stimulates parietal cells when food is present in the stomach. Parietal cells secrete HCl, and therefore gastrin is a physiological agonist of HCl secretion. Once the chyme reaches a certain acidity (pH < 3) and moves into the small intestine, gastrin secretion is inhibited and therefore HCl secretion is decreased.

---

2) Determine the role of HCl in the stomach.

In the stomach, HCl is necessary for the proper function of pepsin because the proper pH for pepsin is between 1 and 3.

---

3) Examine what occurs when acidic chyme reaches the small intestine.

Once the chyme moves into the small intestine, the pH needs to be increased in order to reach the optimal pH (≈ 8) for pancreatic proteases and lipases. Therefore, gastrin release is inhibited and the pancreas is stimulated to secrete bicarbonate in order to neutralize the acid. The pancreas also releases hydrolytic enzymes such as amylase, trypsinogen, chymotrypsinogen, and pancreatic lipases.

---

4) Examine the effect of a gastrin-secreting tumor.

A gastrin-secreting tumor will secrete gastrin at all times and will not be inhibited by normal feedback mechanisms such as the presence of chyme in the small intestine. This gastrin will continually stimulate parietal cells to produce HCl. This excess of acid will move with the chyme into the small intestine. Normal amounts of bicarbonate will be released; however, this is not enough to neutralize such an excess of HCl effectively.

---

5) Determine the effects of an acidic environment in the small intestine.

Pancreatic juices require a less acidic environment than do stomach enzymes. If the environment in the small intestine is too acidic, then pancreatic secretions will be unable to function normally. While proteins and carbohydrates are partially digested before they reach the small intestine, fats do not begin digestion until they reach the duodenum. If pancreatic lipases are unable to

KEY CONCEPTS

Digestive enzymes

Pancreatic enzymes

Pancreas

Duodenum

Gastric acid

TAKEAWAYS

Having a good understanding of the normal digestive system provides a strong basis for evaluating the effects of abnormalities that may occur within the system.

THINGS TO WATCH OUT FOR

An acidic duodenal pH will affect the functioning ability of all of the pancreatic enzymes, but protein absorption can still occur because proteins are digested in the stomach. Carbohydrate digestion does not rely on pancreatic secretions. Absorption can still occur because carbohydrates begin digestion in the mouth and continue to be broken down by maltase and sucrase in the intestinal brush border.

function due to an excessively acidic environment, they will not be able to digest lipids. This hypersecretion of gastrin will lower the pH of the duodenum so that pancreatic lipases are inactivated. This will result in the malabsorption of lipids, also known as steatorrhea.

Remember: *The pH levels of the stomach and the small intestine affect the ability of enzymes to function properly.*

SIMILAR QUESTIONS

1) A patient with a peptic ulcer takes a large overdose of antacid. This would affect the activity of what enzyme?
2) Pancreatic ductal cells secrete bicarbonate, which is moved into the intestinal lumen. What would be the physiological results if these ductal cells were destroyed by an autoimmune disorder?
3) Pancreatitis is a disease that prevents the pancreas from being able to produce adequate amounts of lipase enzymes. What will be the physiological results of this disease?

OSMOSIS

The sodium potassium pump is an ATPase that pumps 3 Na^+ out of the cell and 2 K^+ into the cell for each ATP hydrolyzed. Cells can use the pump to help maintain cell volume. What would most likely happen to the rate of ATP consumption if a cell were moved to a hypertonic environment?

KEY CONCEPTS

Hypertonic solution

Hypotonic solution

Sodium potassium pump

1) Determine the relationship between two solutions to predict the flow of water.

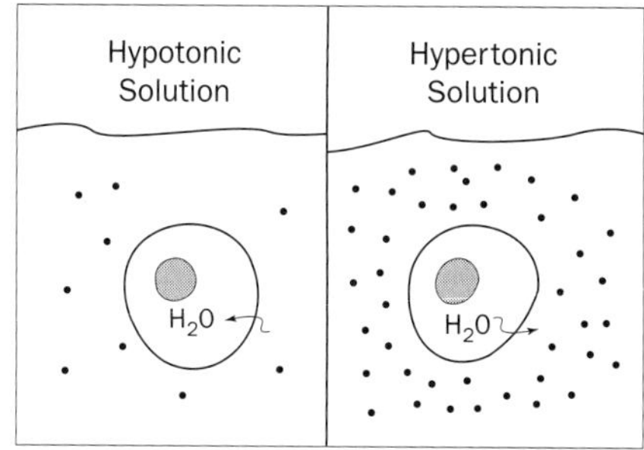

A hypertonic environment means that the environment is more concentrated than the cell is. Note that you can similarly express this condition by stating that the cell is hypotonic to the environment. A hypotonic solution is one that is less concentrated than the solution to which it is being compared.

The cell is being moved into a hypertonic environment, which means that the environment is more concentrated with solutes than the interior of the cell. Thus, we can predict that water will flow out of the cell.

TAKEAWAYS

Questions that involve osmosis are usually combined with other biology topics (particularly kidney function) to create a multistep solution. The key is to have a solid understanding of what hypertonic and hypotonic mean, and how the terms can be used interchangeably to describe the same state.

---

2) Given the flow of water, determine how the biological function in question will be affected.

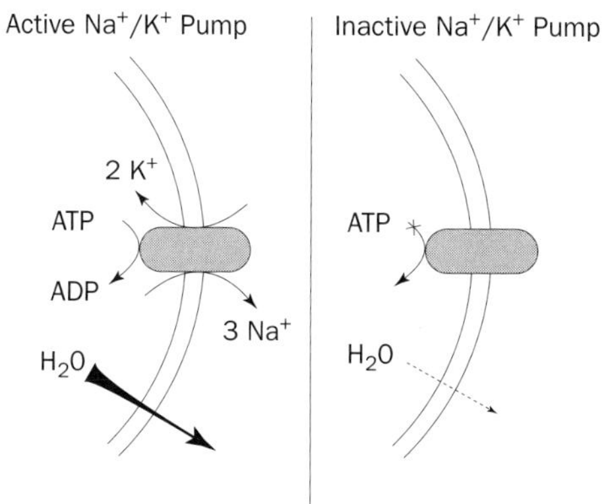

Water will flow out of the cell, thus decreasing cell volume. To counter this effect, ATP consumption will decrease to maintain cell volume.

THINGS TO WATCH OUT FOR

Some students presume that the scenario presented will eventually return to equilibrium and may actually predict that ATP consumption will decrease and then increase. However, the question stem does not speak of a return to equilibrium. Be wary of trying to read too much into the question.

The sodium potassium pump moves in two potassium ions as it moves out three sodium ions. The net effect is to decrease cell solute concentration as the cell loses one ion per each pump. The pump is dependent upon ATP consumption; therefore, relative to its current rate of ATP consumption, an increase in consumption will decrease cell volume whereas a decrease in consumption will increase cell volume.

SIMILAR QUESTIONS

1) Antidiuretic hormone (ADH) directly increases the ability of the blood to reabsorb water from the nephron. If an individual's blood becomes hypotonic with respect to the filtrate, would ADH secretion increase or decrease?
2) The reabsorption of water from the filtrate increases as the concentration of the interstitial fluid increases. Using the terms "hypertonic" and "hypo-osmotic," describe the relationship between the interstitial fluid and the filtrate as well as the relationship between the filtrate and the interstitial fluid.
3) Alcohol and caffeine block the activity of ADH, a hormone that increases the ability of the blood to reabsorb water from the filtrate. An individual drinks a large coffee in the morning, and when he goes to the restroom finds that his urine is nearly colorless. Was the urine produced hypotonic, isotonic, or hypertonic to the blood?

CHAPTER 8

RESPIRATION

Respiration is a broad term referring to the exchange of gases between an organism and its external environment, the transport of these gases within the organism, and the diffusion of gases into and out of cells. (Cellular respiration, discussed in chapter 3, refers to the role that these gases play in generating energy at the cellular level.) Aerobic organisms exchange CO_2 generated during cellular respiration for O_2 obtained from the external environment. Higher vertebrates have developed respiratory systems whereby gas exchange occurs at a single **respiratory surface,** the **lungs.**

ANATOMY

In the human respiratory system, air enters the lungs after traveling through a series of respiratory airways, as outlined in Figure 8.1. Air enters the respiratory tract through the **external nares** (nostrils) and then travels through the nasal cavities, where it is filtered by mucous and nasal hairs. It then passes through the pharynx and into a second chamber called the **larynx.** Ingested food also passes through the pharynx en route to the esophagus. To ensure that food does not accidentally enter the larynx and induce choking, a piece of tissue called the epiglottis covers the glottis (the opening to the larynx) during swallowing, thereby channeling food into the esophagus (see chapter 7). Air passes from the larynx into the cartilaginous **trachea,** which divides into two bronchi, one entering the right lung, the other entering the left. Both the trachea and bronchi are lined by ciliated epithelial cells, which filter and trap particles inhaled along with the air. The bronchi repeatedly branch into smaller bronchi, the terminal branches of which are called **bronchioles.** Each bronchiole is surrounded by clusters of small air sacs called **alveoli.** Gas exchange between the lungs and the circulatory system occurs across the very thin walls of the alveoli. Each alveolus is coated with a thin layer of liquid containing **surfactant** and is surrounded by an extensive network of capillaries. Surfactant lowers the surface tension of the alveoli and facilitates gas exchange across the membranes. Three hundred million alveoli provide approximately 100 m^2 of moist respiratory surface for gas exchange.

TEACHER TIP

The mouth and nose serve several important purposes in breathing. They allow for dirt and particulate matter to be removed from the air, and they warm and humidify the air before it reaches the lungs.

Following gas exchange, air rushes back through the respiratory pathway and is exhaled.

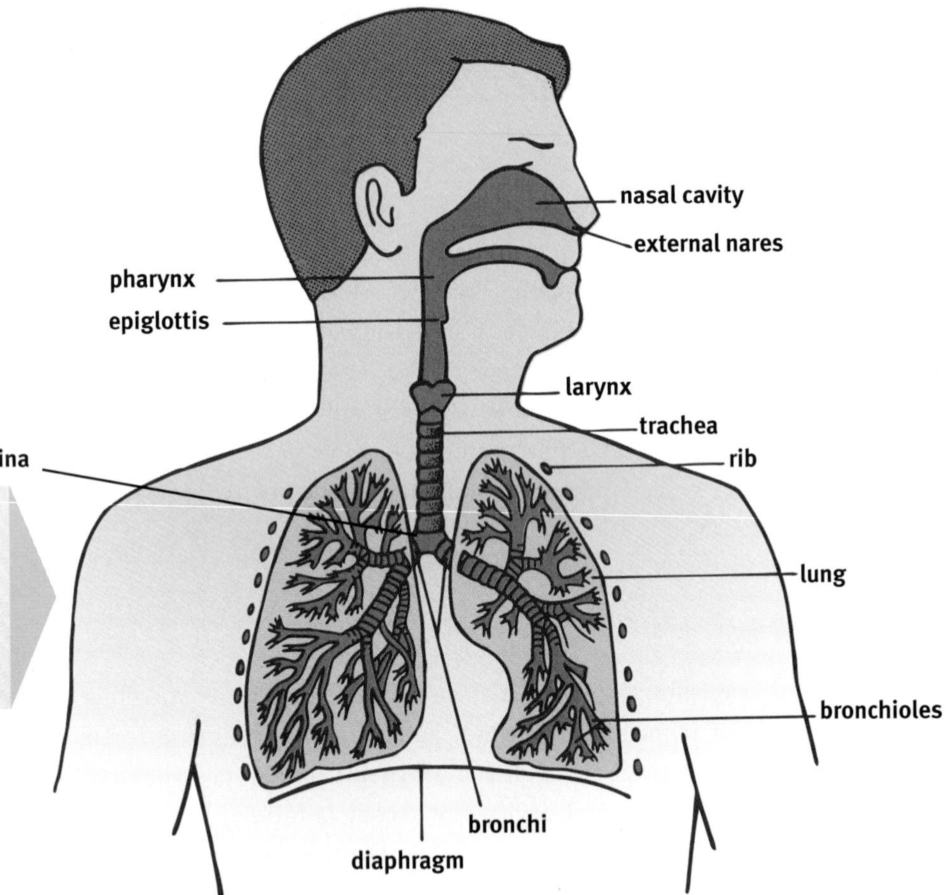

Figure 8.1. Respiratory System

TEACHER TIP

Note that the left lung has a small cut out which makes it slightly smaller than the right lung. Why might this be? It's due to the position of the heart in the thoracic cavity.

VENTILATION

Ventilation of the lungs (breathing) is the process by which air is inhaled and exhaled. The purpose of ventilation is to take in oxygen from the atmosphere and eliminate carbon dioxide from the body. The ventilating mechanism is dependent upon pressure changes in the **thoracic cavity,** the body cavity that contains the heart and lungs. The thoracic cavity is separated from the abdominal cavity by a muscle known as the **diaphragm** and is bounded on the sides by the chest wall. The lungs are surrounded by membranes called the **visceral pleura** and the **parietal pleura.** The space between the two pleura, the **intrapleural space,** contains a thin layer of fluid (see Figure 8.2). The pressure differential between the intrapleural space and the lungs (which is essentially atmospheric pressure) prevents the lungs from collapsing.

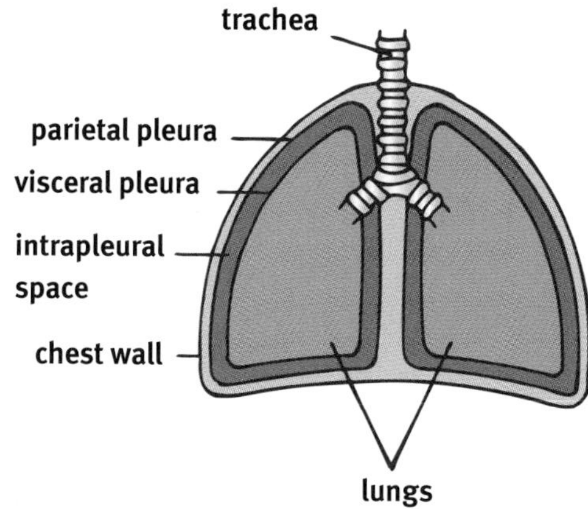

Figure 8.2. Thoracic Cavity (neutral position)

CLINICAL CORRELATE

Pneumothorax is a common result of a penetrating injury trauma to the chest. In this condition, air enters the intrapleural space, thereby increasing the intrapleural pressure and collapsing the lung. A pneumothorax is treated by inserting a needle and withdrawing air from the intrapleural space

A. STAGES OF VENTILATION

1. Inhalation

During inhalation, the diaphragm contracts and flattens, and the **external intercostal muscles** contract, pushing the rib cage and chest wall up and out. This causes the thoracic cavity to increase in volume. This volume increase, in turn, reduces the intrapleural pressure, causing the lungs to expand and fill with air. This is referred to as **negative-pressure breathing** because air is drawn in by a vacuum.

BRIDGE

Remember, Boyle's law says that the pressure and volume of gases are inversely related. This is the principle underlying negative-pressure breathing.

2. Exhalation

Exhalation is generally a passive process. The lungs and chest wall are highly elastic and tend to recoil to their original positions following inhalation. The diaphragm and external intercostal muscles relax and the chest wall pushes inward. The consequent decrease in thoracic cavity volume causes the air pressure in the intrapleural space to increase. This causes the lungs to deflate, forcing air out of the alveoli. During forced exhalation, the **internal intercostal muscles** contract, pulling the rib cage down. Surfactant reduces the high surface tension of the fluid lining the alveoli, preventing alveolar collapse during exhalation.

TEACHER TIP

KEY POINT: Inhalation and exhalation are different processes in terms of energy expenditure. Muscle contraction is required to create the negative pressure in the thoracic cavity that makes air rush in during inspiration. Expiration during calm states is entirely due to elastic recoil of the lungs and musculature. Of course, during more active states, the muscles can be used to force air out and speed the process of ventilation.

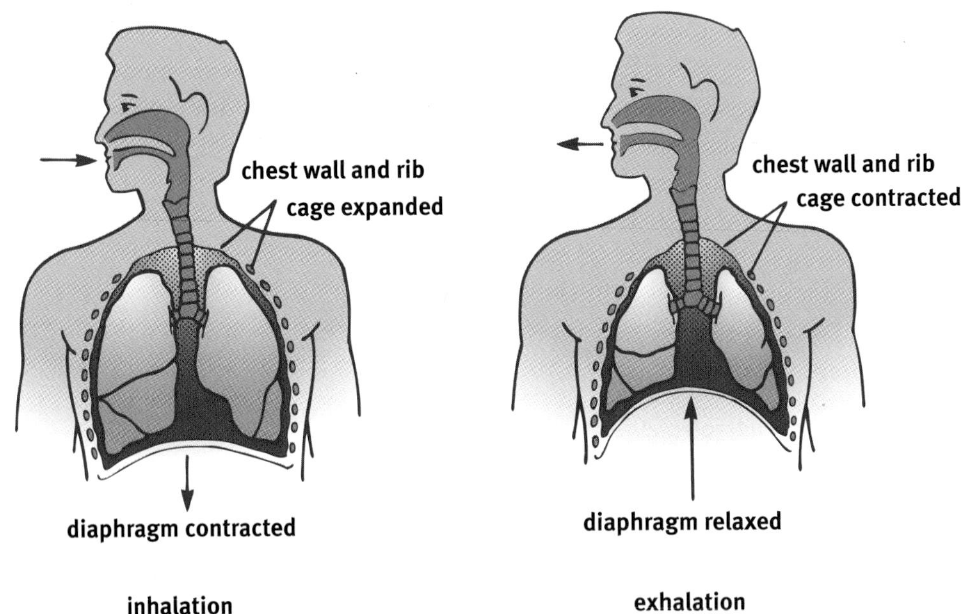

Figure 8.3. Ventilation

> **TEACHER TIP**
>
> Although we breathe oxygen in order to stay alive, it is primarily a response to rising CO_2 that drives ventilation. It is not until oxygen falls to a very low level that a lack of oxygen will drive the ventilatory response.

B. CONTROL OF VENTILATION

Ventilation is regulated by neurons (referred to as **respiratory centers**) located in the **medulla oblongata,** whose rhythmic discharges stimulate the intercostal muscles and/or the diaphragm to contract. These neural signals can be modified by **chemoreceptors** (e.g., in the aorta), which respond to changes in the pH and the partial pressure of CO_2 in the blood. For example, when the partial pressure of CO_2 rises, the medulla oblongata stimulates an increase in the rate of ventilation.

To a limited extent, ventilation can be consciously controlled by the cerebrum. However, if a person tries to hold his breath indefinitely, the high concentration of CO_2 in the blood will stimulate the medulla oblongata to "override" this conscious attempt and stimulate inhalation. Hyperventilation (deep, rapid breathing) lowers the partial pressure of CO_2 in the blood below normal; chemoreceptors sense this and send signals to the respiratory center, which temporarily inhibits breathing.

LUNG CAPACITIES AND VOLUMES

An instrument called a **spirometer** measures the amount of air normally present in the respiratory system and the rate at which ventilation occurs. The maximum amount of air that can be forcibly inhaled and exhaled from the lungs is called the **vital capacity.** The amount of air normally inhaled and exhaled with each breath is called the **tidal volume.** The residual volume is the air that always remains in the lungs, preventing the alveoli from collapsing. The **expiratory reserve volume** is the volume of air that can still be forcibly exhaled following a normal exhalation (see Figure 8.4). **Total lung capacity** is equal to the vital capacity plus the residual volume.

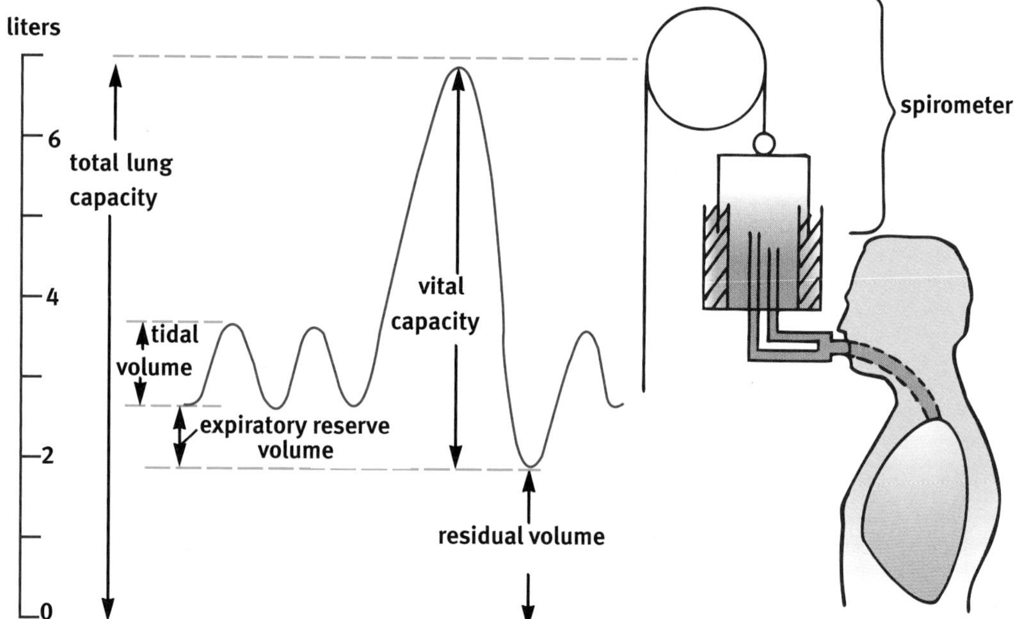

Figure 8.4. Spirometer

TEACHER TIP

KEY POINT: A certain volume of air, called residual volume, can *never* be removed from the lungs during normal breathing processes.

GAS EXCHANGE

A dense network of minute blood vessels called the pulmonary capillaries surrounds the alveoli. Gas exchange occurs by diffusion across these capillary walls and those of the alveoli; gases move from regions of higher partial pressure to regions of lower partial pressure. Blood enters the pulmonary capillaries in a deoxygenated state and thus has a lower partial pressure of O_2 than does the inhaled air in the alveoli. Hence, O_2 diffuses down its gradient into the capillaries where it binds with hemoglobin and returns to the heart via the pulmonary veins. In contrast, the partial pressure of CO_2 in the capillaries is greater than that of the inhaled alveolar air; thus CO_2 diffuses from the capillaries into the alveoli, where it is subsequently released into the external environment during exhalation (see Figure 8.5).

MCAT SYNOPSIS

O_2 in the alveoli flows down its partial pressure gradient from the alveoli into the pulmonary capillaries where it can bind to hemoglobin for transport. Meanwhile, CO_2 flows down its partial pressure gradient from the capillaries into the alveoli for expiration.

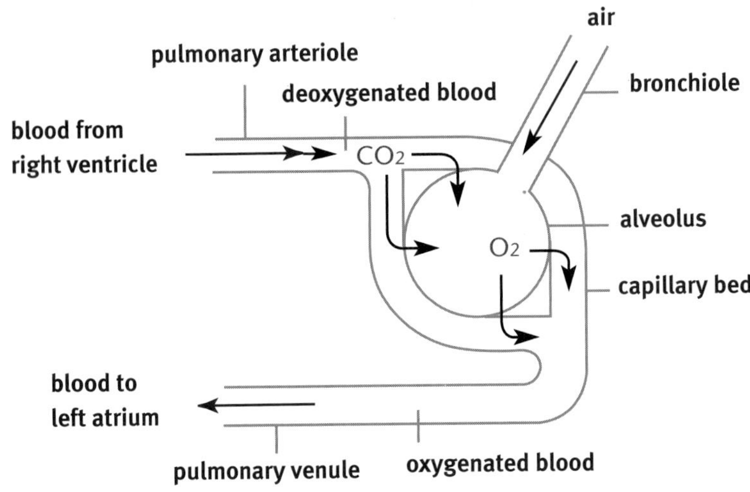

Figure 8.5. Gas Exchange

TEACHER TIP

Another of the MCAT's favorite topics is how altitude will affect both ventilation and the Hb binding curves. Be sure to learn these points for Test Day success.

At high altitudes, the partial pressure of O_2 in the atmosphere declines, making it more difficult to get sufficient oxygen to diffuse into the capillaries. The body can compensate for these conditions in a variety of ways, such as by increasing the rate of ventilation (hyperventilation) and by increasing the production of red blood cells to carry more oxygen (polycythemia). In addition, the affinity of hemoglobin for oxygen decreases to facilitate unloading of oxygen in tissues, and there is greater vascularization of the peripheral tissues.

PRACTICE QUESTIONS

1. The uncoupling agent 2, 4-dinitrophenol dissociates the proton gradient from the electron transport chain. Administration of 2, 4-dinitrophenol would have which of the following effects?

A. Increase in NADH concentrations within the mitochondria

B. Increase followed by a decrease in NADH concentrations

C. Decrease in NADH concentrations within the mitochondria

D. Decrease followed by an abrupt increase in NADH concentrations

2. A man breathes 12 times per minute with a tidal volume of 500 ml and an inspiratory reserve volume of 300 ml. His son breathes 8 times per minute with a tidal volume of 300 ml and an inspiratory reserve volume of 600 ml. Who has greater total minute ventilation?

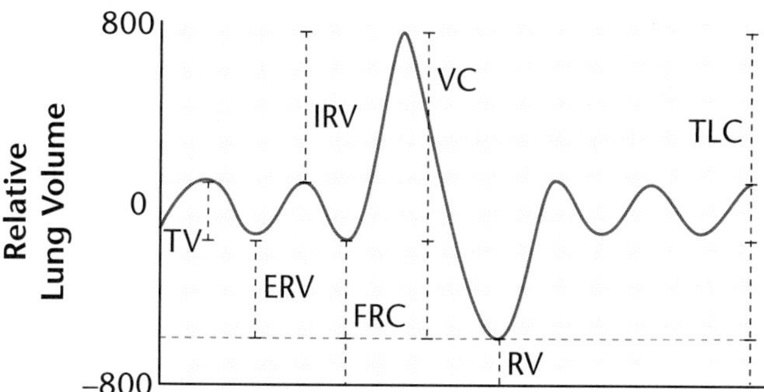

A. Man

B. Son

C. Total ventilations are equal

D. Cannot calculate minute ventilation from this data

3. Death from muscular dystrophy is often due to poor ventilation. What anatomical defect is responsible for this failure to ventilate?

A. Damaged cardiac muscle

B. Inadequate intercostal muscle function

C. Narrowed trachea

D. Poorly compliant lung tissue

4. A scientist is interested in creating an artificial surfactant to decrease surface tension on the alveoli of the lung. It is believed that this surfactant will decrease the electric recoil of the lungs. Surfactant A is made with 80 percent lipid, 10 percent water, and 10 percent protein. Surfactant B is made of 65 percent lipids and 35 percent water. Surface tension for sample A is 37 dynes/cm, while surface tension for sample B is 52 dynes/cm. What most likely accounts for the difference?

A. Greater degree of hydrophobicity in sample A due to the presence of more lipid

B. Greater degree of hydrophobicity in sample B

C. Presence of protein in sample A

D. Rate of respiration of subjects

5. When traveling to higher altitudes, the respiratory system adapts to maintain adequate oxygenation, i.e., minute ventilation (the product of respiratory rate and tidal volume). Comparing the respirations of a person at 7,000 feet to that of a person at sea level will reveal

A. a lower respiratory rate at 7,000 feet as compared to sea level.

B. a higher respiratory rate at 7,000 feet as compared to sea level.

C. a higher respiratory rate at 3,000 feet as compared to sea level.

D. the same respiratory rate at both altitudes.

6. Minute ventilation is the product of the respiratory rate and the tidal volume (volume in each breath of inspired air). How will increased minute ventilation impact the pH of arterial blood?

A. Increases pH
B. Decreases pH
C. There will be no change in pH
D. An initial increase, followed by sharp decrease

7. In the figure below, what line represents the oxygen dissociation curve during exercise?

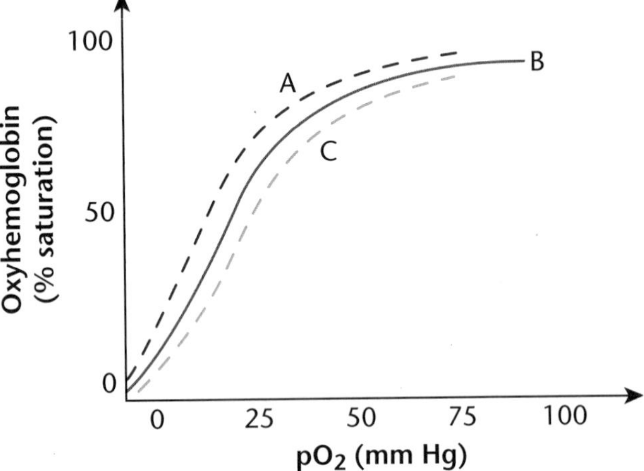

A. A
B. B
C. C
D. D

8. Pulmonary fibrosis is a disease process that results in replacement of the lung parenchyma (alveoli), which is normally very compliant, with fibrous scar tissue that is dense and cartilaginous. There is no known cure. As patients with pulmonary fibrosis progress, which of the following would be expected observations?

A. Increased lung volume with hyperoxygenation
B. Decreased lung volume with hyperoxygenation
C. Increased lung volume with hypoxia
D. Decreased lung volume with hypoxia

9. What element is crucial to proper functioning of hemoglobin?

A. Copper
B. Iron
C. Manganese
D. Selenium

10. Where is the respiratory drive centered?

A. Forebrain
B. Midbrain
C. Brainstem
D. Cerebellum

11. Under normal conditions, air is driven into the respiratory system via

A. positive airway pressure.
B. negative intrapleural pressure.
C. positive intrapleural pressure.
D. functional reserve capacity.

12. Via what route is unoxygenated blood driven from the right ventricle of the heart to the lung for oxygenation?

A. Pulmonary arteries
B. Pulmonary veins
C. Aorta
D. Foramen ovale

13. CO_2 is transported in the blood via all the following forms, EXCEPT

A. acetyl CoA.
B. dissolved in plasma.
C. carbamino compounds.
D. bicarbonate.

14. Blood in the pulmonary veins is rich in which of the following?

A. Oxyhemoglobin
B. Lactic acid
C. Chyme
D. Hemoglobin

KEY CONCEPTS

Respiratory system

Alveoli

Oxygen exchange

Physiological dead space

Anatomical dead space

Alveolar dead space

TAKEAWAYS

The respiratory system is intimately linked to the circulatory system. Oxygen is delivered to tissues, and CO_2 is removed from tissues and ultimately removed from the lungs through capillaries.

THINGS TO WATCH OUT FOR

Under resting conditions, alveolar oxygen equilibrates with the arterial blood of the pulmonary capillary. This is considered a perfusion-limited exchange. Under conditions of exercise, the partial pressures of oxygen do not equilibrate along the length of the pulmonary capillary and the partial pressure gradient is maintained.

RESPIRATORY SYSTEM

The volume of the lungs that does not participate in gas exchange is considered physiological dead space. There are two types of dead space that are seen at rest: anatomical and alveolar. Anatomical dead space is in the conducting areas, such as the mouth and trachea, where oxygen enters the respiratory system but does not contact alveoli. Alveolar dead space is the area in the alveoli that does contact air but lacks sufficient circulation to participate in gas exchange. How can physiological dead space be reduced?

1) Examine each type of dead space separately

Anatomical dead space refers to the air that remains in the mouth and trachea with every breath. Because the size and length of the mouth and trachea are set and relatively unchangeable, it is unlikely that physiological dead space can be decreased through the anatomical dead space.

Alveolar dead space involves alveoli that contact air but do not participate in gas exchange. Because the alveoli are normal, they are capable of participating in gas exchange under the right conditions; therefore, alveolar dead space can be reduced.

---

2) Review the method of gas exchange at the tissues and in the lungs.

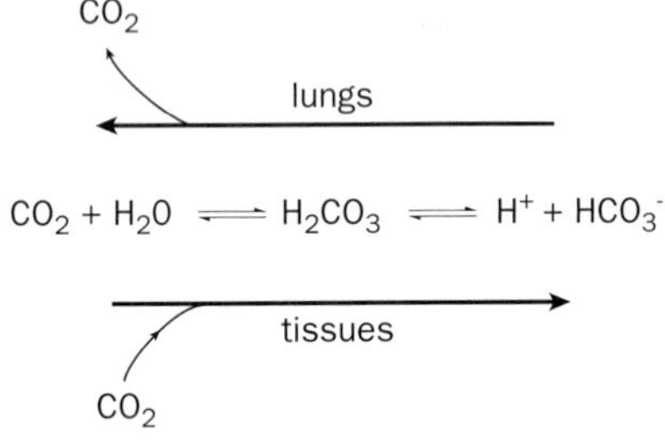

In the normal lung, O_2 will diffuse from alveolar air into the pulmonary capillary. When the partial pressures of O_2 in alveolar air and capillary blood equilibrate, the diffusion stops. Normally this occurs before the blood in the pulmonary capillary passes out of the lungs and is considered perfusion-limited gas exchange. This O_2 is bound to hemoglobin and is taken and released to the tissues. CO_2 is produced by the tissues and diffuses into capillary blood, where it is carried to the lungs as HCO_3^-. At the lungs, the reaction is reversed and CO_2 is exhaled.

---

3) Determine why some alveoli do not participate in gas exchange.
There is not sufficient blood flow through the capillaries of these "dead space" alveoli to induce them to participate in gas exchange. There must be blood flow in order for gas exchange to occur.

---

4) Determine how to increase blood flow through the lungs.
If pulmonary blood flow were increased, then more alveoli would be perfused with blood and would therefore participate in gas exchange. Increasing pulmonary blood flow would require increasing the output of the right ventricle. Cardiac output increases during exercise because there is an increased heart rate and increased venous return due to skeletal muscle activity. Therefore, exercise would increase the amount of pulmonary blood flow. This increased flow of blood through the lungs would recruit more alveoli for gas exchange and therefore reduce alveolar and physiological dead space.

Remember: *Gas exchange occurs between alveolar air and the pulmonary capillaries. In order to increase the number of alveoli being used for gas exchange, the amount of pulmonary blood available for gas exchange must also be increased.*

SIMILAR QUESTIONS

1) What is the result if blood flow to the left lung is completely blocked by a pulmonary embolism?
2) If an area of the lung is not ventilated due to an obstruction, what is the partial pressure of oxygen (Po_2) of the pulmonary capillary in that area?
3) At what point will the diffusion of air from the alveoli to the capillary stop?

CHAPTER 9

CIRCULATION

Higher organisms rely on a complex **cardiovascular system** to transport respiratory gases, nutrients, and wastes to and from cells. A secondary circulatory system, the **lymphatic system,** collects excess body fluids and returns them to the cardiovascular circulation.

THE CARDIOVASCULAR SYSTEM

The human cardiovascular system is composed of a muscular four-chambered **heart,** a network of **blood vessels,** and the **blood** itself. The right side of the heart pumps deoxygenated blood into the lungs via the pulmonary arteries. Oxygenated blood returns from the lungs to the left side of the heart via the pulmonary veins. It is then pumped into the **aorta,** which branches into a series of arteries. The arteries branch into arterioles, and then into microscopic capillaries. Exchange of gases, nutrients, and cellular waste products occurs via diffusion across capillary walls. The capillaries then converge into venules, and eventually into veins, leading deoxygenated blood back toward the right side of the heart. Blood returning from the lower body and extremities enters the heart via the **inferior vena cava,** while deoxygenated blood from the upper head and neck region flows through the **jugular vein** and into the **superior vena cava,** which also leads into the right atrium of the heart. The blood then flows to the right ventricle through the tricuspid valve. From the right ventricle, the blood goes to the pulmonary artery and is pumped to the lungs to be oxygenated (see chapter 8). The blood then returns from the lungs to the left atrium via the pulmonary veins. The left atrium then pumps the blood to the left ventricle through the mitral valve. Finally, the blood enters systemic circulation as it enters the aorta from the left ventricle. Oxygenated blood is supplied to heart muscle by the **coronary arteries.** The first branches off the aorta; **the coronary veins** and **coronary sinus** return deoxygenated blood to the right side of the heart.

Teacher Tip

Link to Physics: The heart and blood vessels are analogous to a pair of pumps that are linked in series. The right heart is a low-pressure system that sends blood to the lungs, whereas the left heart is a high pressure system that sends blood to the body.

In systemic circulation there are three special circulatory routes, referred to as **portal systems,** in which blood travels through *two* capillary beds before returning to the heart. There is a portal system in the liver (hepatic portal circulation), in the kidneys (see chapter 10), and in the brain (hypophyseal portal circulation; see chapter 11).

A. THE HEART

The heart is the driving force of the circulatory system. The right and left halves can be viewed as two separate pumps: The right side of the heart pumps deoxygenated blood into pulmonary circulation (toward the lungs), while the left side pumps oxygenated blood into systemic circulation (throughout the body). The two upper chambers are called **atria** and the two lower chambers are called ventricles. The atria are thin-walled, while the **ventricles** are extremely muscular. The left ventricle is more muscular than the right ventricle because it is responsible for generating the force that propels systemic circulation and because it pumps against a higher resistance.

TEACHER TIP

Because the right heart only pumps to the lungs, which are quite close, it can operate at lower pressures; consequently the right heart is not as muscled as the left. The left heart, responsible for the body, is more well-developed and can pump more strongly to move blood through the vasculature.

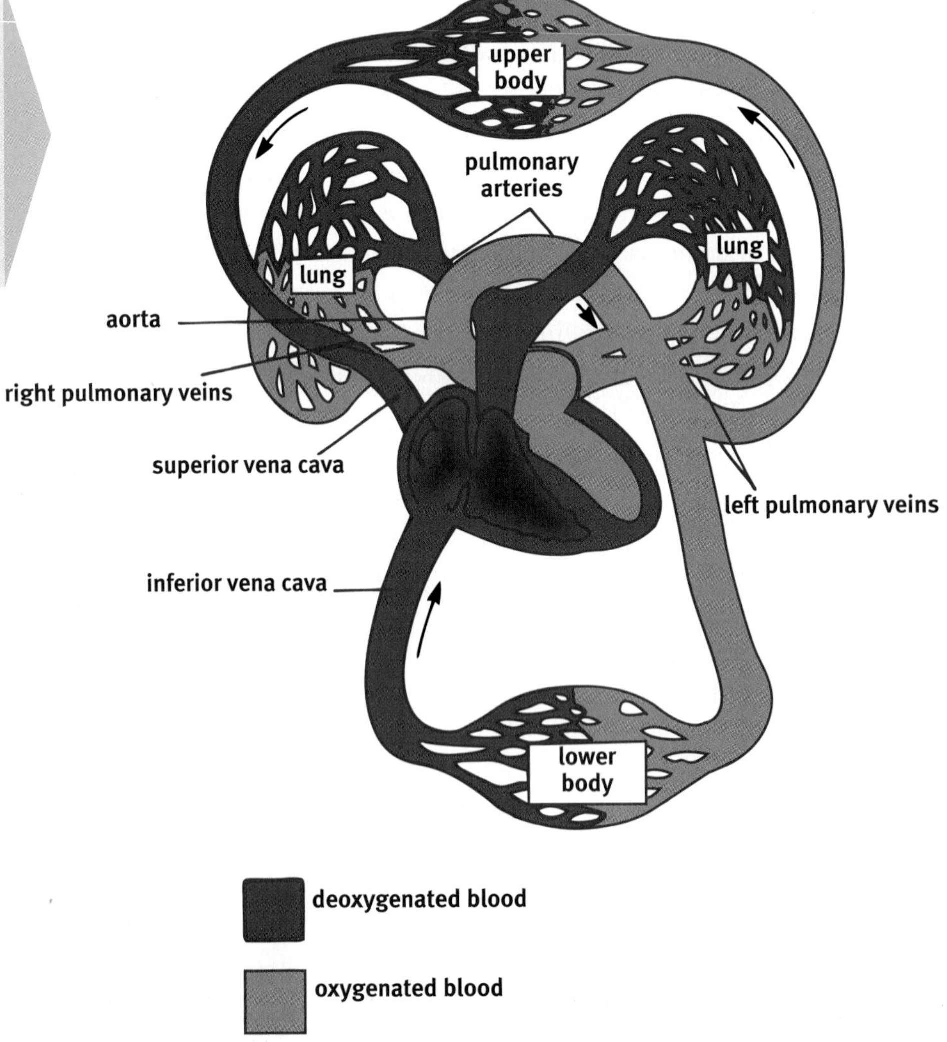

Figure 9.1. Circulation

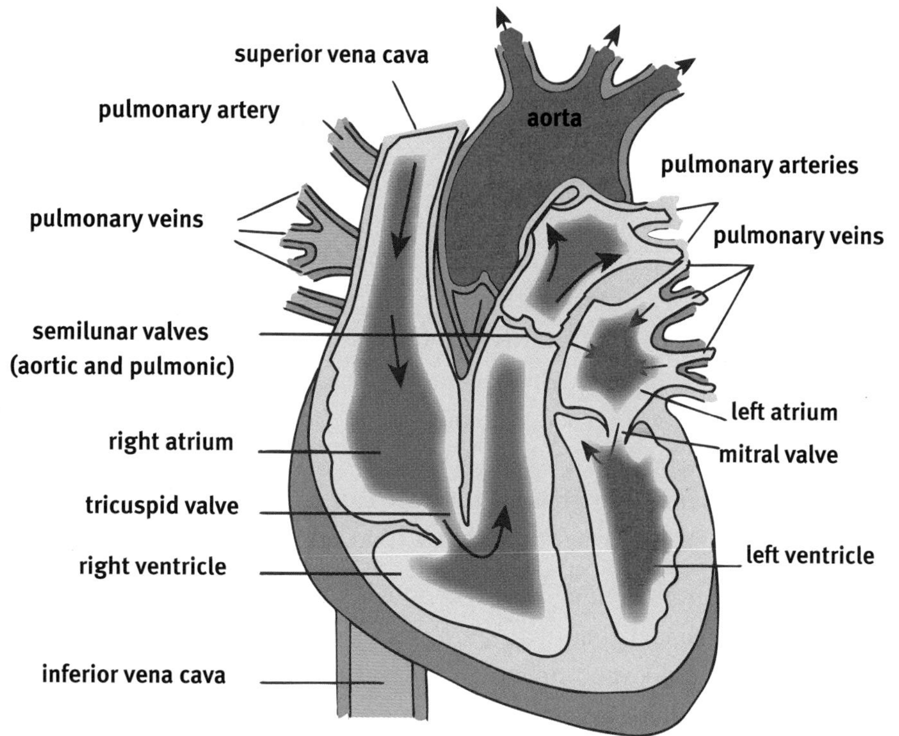

Figure 9.2. Human Heart

MCAT SYNOPSIS

Blood Flow

Superior and inferior vena cavae
↓
Right atrium
↓
Right ventricle
↓
Pulmonary artery
↓
Lungs
↓
Pulmonary veins
↓
Left atrium
↓
Left ventricle
↓
Aorta

1. Valves

The **atrioventricular valves,** located between the atria and ventricles on both sides of the heart, prevent backflow of blood into the atria. The valve on the right side of the heart has three cusps and is called the **tricuspid valve.** The valve on the left side of the heart has two cusps and is called the **mitral valve.** The **semilunar valves** have three cusps and are located between the left ventricle and the aorta (the aortic valve) and between the right ventricle and the pulmonary artery (the pulmonic valve).

CLINICAL CORRELATE

The "lub dubs" you hear when you listen to someone's heart with a stethoscope are referred to as the heart sounds. The first heart sound, S1, is produced when the two atrioventricular valves close at the start of systole. (Those valves must close so that the blood flows out of the heart instead of back up into the atria). The second heart sound, S2, is produced when the two semilunar valves close at the conclusion of systole. (If they didn't close at that point, blood would flow back into the ventricles.)

2. Contraction

a. Phases

The heart's pumping cycle is divided into two alternating phases, **systole** and **diastole,** which together make up the **heartbeat.** Systole is the period during which the ventricles contract. Diastole is the period of cardiac muscle relaxation during which blood drains into all four chambers. **Cardiac output** is defined as the total volume of blood the left ventricle pumps out per minute. Cardiac output = **heart rate** (number of heartbeats per minute) × **stroke volume** (volume of blood pumped out of the left ventricle per contraction).

TEACHER TIP

There is a limit to how fast the heart can beat. Because the heart fills with blood when it isn't contracting (diastole), the faster the heart beats, the less time there is for blood to enter the heart. Thus, as the heart beats faster, there are diminishing returns in terms of the amount of blood supplied to the body.

b. Mechanism and control

Cardiac muscle (see chapter 6) contracts rhythmically without stimulation from the nervous system, producing impulses that spread through its internal conducting system. An ordinary cardiac contraction originates in, and is regulated by, the **sinoatrial (SA) node** (the **pacemaker**), a small mass of specialized tissue located in the wall of the right atrium. The SA node spreads impulses through both atria, stimulating them to contract simultaneously. The impulse arrives at the **atrioventricular (AV) node,** which conducts slowly, allowing enough time for atrial contraction and for the ventricles to fill with blood. The impulse is then carried by the **bundle of His (AV bundle),** which branches into the right and left bundle branches and through the **Purkinje fibers** in the walls of both ventricles, generating a strong contraction.

The **autonomic nervous system** (see chapter 12) modifies the rate of heart contraction. The parasympathetic system innervates the heart via the **vagus nerve** and causes a decrease in the heart rate. The sympathetic system innervates the heart via the cervical and upper thoracic ganglia and causes an increase in the heart rate. The adrenal medulla exerts hormonal control via epinephrine (adrenaline) secretion, which causes an increase in heart rate (see chapter 11).

Clinical Correlate

The heart's electrical impulses can be detected on the body's surface by placing electrodes on the skin on opposite sides of the heart. A recording of these currents is called an electrocardiogram (a.k.a., ECG or EKG). Electrocardiograms are incredibly powerful tools for assessing the status of a patient's heart. A normal EKG is shown below.

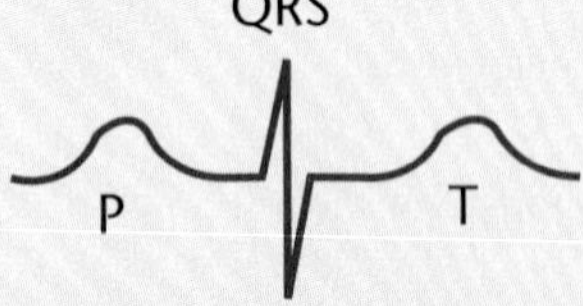

Because depolarization will precede cardiac muscle contraction, the electrical spokes of the EKG occur just before a cardiac contractile event. The P wave occurs immediately before the atria contract and the QRS complex occurs just before the ventricles contract. The T wave represents ventricular repolarization.

Teacher Tip

Cardiac muscle is a hybrid of smooth muscle and striated muscle. It can beat without descending input due to the presence of the SA node, AV node, and Purkinje; however, much like we saw earlier with smooth muscle, this rate can be affected by the descending input.

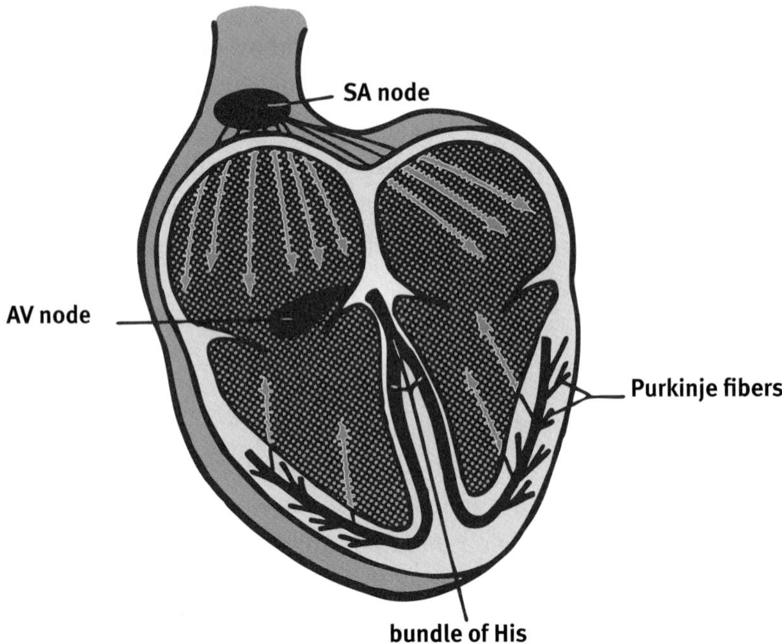

Figure 9.3. Contraction

B. BLOOD VESSELS

The three types of blood vessels are arteries, veins, and capillaries. **Arteries** are thickly-walled, muscular, elastic vessels that transport oxygenated blood away from the heart—except for the pulmonary arteries, which transport deoxygenated blood from the heart to the lungs. **Veins** are relatively thinly walled, inelastic vessels that conduct deoxygenated blood towards the heart—except for the pulmonary veins, which carry oxygenated blood from the lungs to the heart. Much of the blood flow in veins depends on their compression by skeletal muscles during movement, rather than on the pumping of the heart. Venous circulation is often at odds with gravity; thus larger veins, especially those in the legs, have valves that prevent backflow. **Capillaries** have very thin walls composed of a single layer of endothelial cells across which respiratory gases, nutrients, enzymes, hormones, and wastes can readily diffuse. Capillaries have the smallest diameter of all three types of vessels; red blood cells must often travel through them single file.

TEACHER TIP

When the valves break down in larger veins, the blood begins to pool rather than return to the heart. This is commonly seen in many individuals as varicose veins.

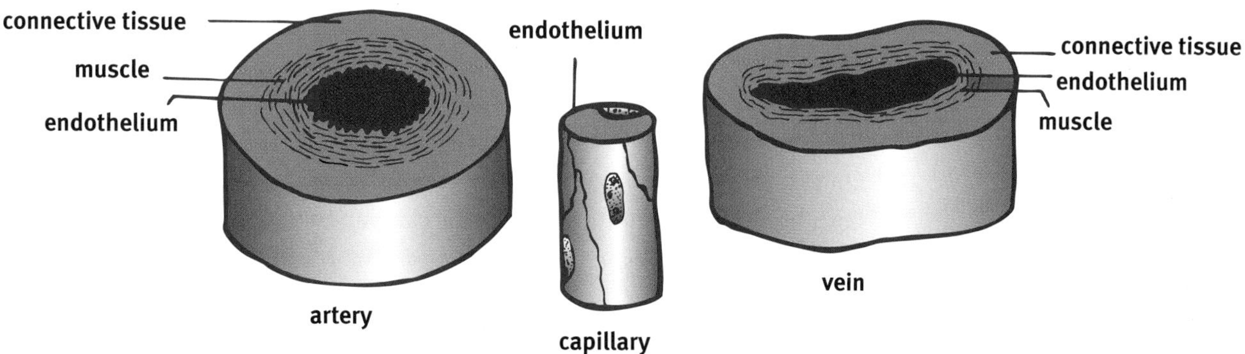

Figure 9.4. Blood Vessels

C. BLOOD PRESSURE

Blood pressure is the force per area that blood exerts on the walls of the blood vessels. Blood pressure is measured by an instrument called a **sphygmomanometer** (a.k.a., "blood pressure cuff") and is expressed as systolic pressure/diastolic pressure. As blood flows through the circulatory system from artery to capillary, blood pressure gradually drops, due to friction between blood and the walls of the vessels, and to the increase in cross-sectional area afforded by the numerous capillary beds (see Figure 9.5).

BRIDGE

In Physics pressure is defined as force/area. This holds true for blood pressure as well.

TEACHER TIP

KEY POINT: The major drop in blood pressure occurs across the arterioles. This is necessary because the veins, especially the capillaries, are thin-walled and would not be able to deal with the pressure levels seen in the arterial side of the vasculature.

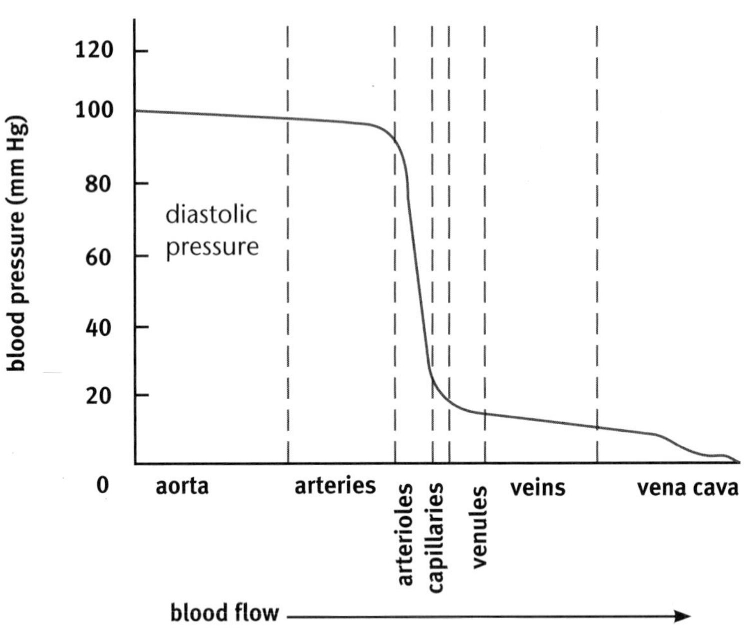

Figure 9.5. Blood Pressure

BLOOD

CLINICAL CORRELATE

Thallasemia is a condition where either the β-chain or α-chain is misconfigured. This results in anemia when only 1 chain β is affected. However, if both of the β- or α-chains are affected, the patient often dies in childhood or before birth.

A. COMPOSITION

On the average, the human body contains 4–6 liters of blood. Blood has both liquid (55 percent) and cellular components (45 percent; formed elements). **Plasma** is the liquid portion of the blood. It is an aqueous mixture of nutrients, salts, respiratory gases, wastes, hormones, and blood proteins (e.g., immunoglobulins, albumin, and fibrinogen). The cellular components of the blood are **erythrocytes, leukocytes,** and **platelets.**

1. Erythrocytes (red blood cells)

Erythrocytes are the oxygen-carrying components of blood. An erythrocyte contains approximately 250 million molecules of **hemoglobin,** each of which can bind up to four molecules of oxygen. Adult hemoglobin consists of 2β chains and 2α chains. Erythrocytes have a distinct biconcave, disklike shape, which gives them both increased surface area for gas exchange and greater flexibility for movement through those tiny capillaries. Erythrocytes are formed from stem cells in the bone marrow, where they lose their nuclei, mitochondria, and membranous organelles. Because erythrocytes lack mitochondria, they are anaerobic and obtain their ATP via glycolysis alone. Once mature, erythrocytes circulate in the blood for about 120 days, after which they are phagocytized by special cells in the spleen and liver. There are about 5 million erythrocytes per one mm^3 of blood.

2. Leukocytes (white blood cells)

Leukocytes arise from stem cells in the marrow of long bones. Leukocytes are larger than erythrocytes and have protective functions. The number of leukocytes in the blood varies widely; there are normally 5,000–10,000 leukocytes per one mm^3 of blood, but this number substantially increases when the body is battling an infection. There are three types of leukocytes: **granular leukocytes, lymphocytes,** and **monocytes.**

Granular leukocytes are nonspecific and attack general invading pathogens, such as bacteria or parasites. Granular leukocytes **(neutrophils, basophils,** and **eosinophils)** play key roles in inflammation, allergic reactions, pus formation, and the destruction of invading bacteria and parasites. Neutrophiles predominantly fight bacterial infections, where eosmophiles are associated with parasitic infections. Basophiles are responsible for allergies and allergic reactions through the release of histamine.

Lymphocytes play an important role in the **immune response**; they are produced in the lymph nodes, tonsils, spleen, appendix, thymus, and bone marrow and are involved in the production of **antibodies.** As a result, lymphocytes are involved in the specific immune response against a specific invading pathogen. For example, if you have antibodies against influenza virus, you can still be infected with another strain. The two types of lymphocytes are **B lymphocytes** and **T lymphocytes.** Monocytes are involved in the nonspecific immune response. They phagocytize foreign matter and organisms such as bacteria. Some monocytes migrate from the blood to tissue, where they mature into stationary cells called **macrophages.** Macrophages have greater phagocytic capability than monocytes.

> **TEACHER TIP**
>
> HIV causes a loss of a certain subset of T cells known as helper T cells (CD4+). While this alone is not particularly detrimental to the organism, a loss of these cells prevents activation of other lymphocytes and generation of an immune response. This is why people infected with HIV are more susceptible to disease.

3. Platelets

Platelets are cell fragments approximately 2–3 μm in diameter and are also formed in the bone marrow. Platelets lack nuclei and function in clot formation. There are about 250,000–500,000 platelets per one mm^3 of blood.

> **CLINICAL CORRELATE**
>
> Anasarca is a condition of generalized edema in the tissues. It is caused by very low albumin concentration in the blood, i.e. low osmotic pressure in the capillary at the venule end.

B. BLOOD ANTIGENS

Erythrocytes have characteristic cell-surface proteins **(antigens).** Antigens are macromolecules that are foreign to the host organism and trigger an immune response. The two major groups of red blood cell antigens are the **ABO group** and the **Rh factor.**

1. ABO Group

There are four ABO blood groups, **A, B, AB,** and **O**; see Table 9.1.

Teacher Tip

You are almost guaranteed to see at least one question on blood groups. It is critical that you learn how the system works (A/B codominant).

Table 9.1

Blood Type	Antigen in Red Blood Cell	Antibodies Produced
A	A	anti-B
B	B	anti-A
AB (universal recipient)	A and B	none
O (universal donor)	none	anti-A and anti-B

Clinical Correlate

When an Rh^- woman delivers an Rh^+ fetus, she stands a good chance of being exposed to the baby's Rh^+ blood cells. This may lead to the development of antibodies against the Rh antigen, which can cause problems (erythroblastosis fetalis) with future Rh^+ pregnancies. This problem can be avoided in most cases by giving the mother Rh immune globulin (RhoGAM) immediately after delivery. Administration of immune globulin (which is a type of passive immunization) will suppress the development of active immunity on the mother's part, preventing the production of antibodies to the Rh antigen.

It is extremely important during blood transfusions that donor and recipient blood types be appropriately matched. The aim is to avoid transfusion of red blood cells that will be clumped ("rejected") by antibodies (proteins in the immune system that bind specifically to antigens) present in the recipient's plasma. The rule of blood matching is as follows: If the donor's antigens are already in the recipient's blood, no clumping occurs. Type AB blood is termed the **"universal recipient,"** as it has neither anti-A nor anti-B antibodies. Type O blood is considered to be the **"universal donor"**; it will not elicit a response from the recipient's immune system because it does not possess any surface antigens (see chapter 13 for further discussion of ABO blood groups).

2. Rh Factor

The Rh factor is another antigen that may be present on the surface of red blood cells. Individuals may be Rh^+, possessing the Rh antigen, or Rh^-, lacking the Rh antigen. Consideration of the Rh factor is particularly important during pregnancy. An Rh^- woman can be sensitized by an Rh^+ fetus if fetal red blood cells (which will have the Rh factor) enter maternal circulation during birth. If this woman subsequently carries another Rh^+ fetus, the anti-Rh antibodies she produced when sensitized by the first birth may cross the placenta and destroy fetal red blood cells. This results in severe anemia for the fetus, known as **erythroblastosis fetalis.** Erythroblastosis is not caused by ABO blood-type mismatches between mother and fetus, because anti-A and anti-B antibodies cannot cross the placenta.

FUNCTIONS OF THE CIRCULATORY SYSTEM

Blood transports nutrients and O_2 to tissue, and wastes and CO_2 from tissue. Platelets are involved in injury repair. Leukocytes are the main component of the immune system.

A. TRANSPORT OF GASES

Erythrocytes transport O_2 throughout the circulatory system. Actually, it is the hemoglobin molecules in erythrocytes that bind to O_2. A hemoglobin molecule is composed of four polypeptide chains, each containing a prosthetic heme group. Each heme group is capable of binding to one molecule of oxygen. Thus, each hemoglobin molecule is capable of binding to four molecules of O_2. The binding of O_2 at the first heme group induces a conformational change that facilitates the binding of O_2 at the other three heme groups. Similarly, the unloading of O_2 at one heme group facilitates the unloading of O_2 at the other three heme groups. This cooperation between the heme groups is an allosteric effect (see chapter 2); this is reflected in hemoglobin's S-shaped **dissociation curve** (see Figure 9.6).

TEACHER TIP

Hemoglobin has four subunits (i.e., quaternary structure). This is what allows it to shift when oxygen binds and gives the classic sigmoidal binding curve. Myoglobin is a single subunit (i.e., no quaternary structure). Its curve is not sigmoidal. This is a concept commonly tested on the MCAT.

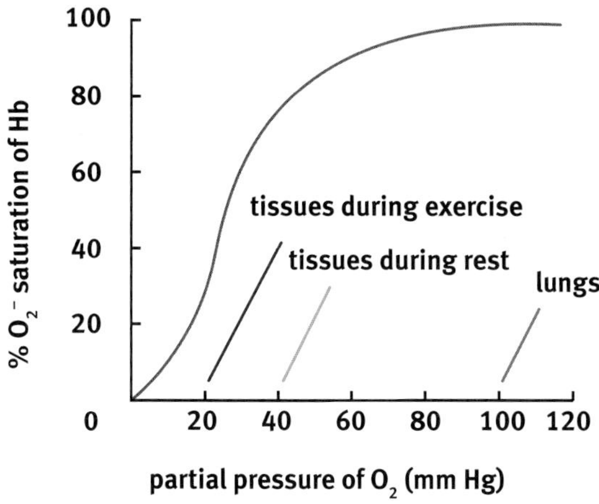

Figure 9.6. Hemoglobin Dissociation Curve

Hemoglobin also binds to CO_2. Carbon dioxide diffuses from tissue into erythrocytes, where it combines with H_2O to form carbonic acid (H_2CO_3). Carbonic acid then dissociates into a bicarbonate ion (HCO_3^-) and a hydrogen ion (H^+). The H^+ binds to the hemoglobin molecule, while HCO_3^- diffuses into the plasma. There is an allosteric relationship between the concentrations of CO_2, H^+, and O_2, known as the **Bohr effect.** According to the Bohr effect, increasing concentrations of H^+ (a decrease in pH) and CO_2 (an increase in HCO_3^-) in the blood decrease hemoglobin's O_2 affinity.

MCAT Synopsis

Only a small percentage of carbon dioxide is actually bound directly to hemoglobin to form carboxyhemoglobin; most of the CO_2 is dissolved in plasma and lives as HCO_3^-.

Thus, the presence of high concentrations of H^+ and CO_2 in metabolically active tissue, such as muscle, enhances the release of O_2 to this tissue. Conversely, a high concentration of O_2, as in the alveolar capillaries, promotes O_2 uptake and CO_2 release from hemoglobin. In the lungs, HCO_3^- and H^+ reassociate to form CO_2 and H_2O, which are expelled during exhalation (see chapter 8). Both formation and dissociation of carbonic acid are catalyzed by the enzyme **carbonic anhydrase.**

$$CO_2 + H_2O \xrightleftharpoons{\text{carbonic anhydrase}} H_2CO_3 \rightleftharpoons H^+ + HCO_3^-$$

B. TRANSPORT OF NUTRIENTS AND WASTES

MCAT Synopsis

Think of it this way—hydrostatic pressure pushes fluid out of vessels while osmotic pressure pulls fluid back into the vessels. Hydrostatic pressure is dependent on the blood pressure driven by the heart; osmotic pressure is dependent on the number of particles dissolved in the plasma.

Amino acids and simple sugars are absorbed into the bloodstream at the intestinal capillaries and transported to the liver via the hepatic portal vein. After processing, they are transported throughout the body. Fats enter the lymphatic system through lymph capillaries in the small intestine and drain into the bloodstream at the large veins of the neck, thereby bypassing the liver. Throughout the body, metabolic waste products (e.g., water, urea, and carbon dioxide) diffuse into capillaries from surrounding cells; these wastes are then delivered to the appropriate excretory organs (see chapter 10).

The exchange of materials is greatly influenced by the balance between the **hydrostatic pressure** and the **osmotic pressure** of the blood and tissue fluids. The hydrostatic pressure at the arteriole end of the capillaries is greater than the hydrostatic pressure of the surrounding tissue fluids (interstitial fluid). This causes fluid to move out of the capillaries at the arteriole end. However, because blood has a higher solute concentration than the tissue fluid, osmotic pressure causes fluid to move back into the capillaries at the venule end. Proteins, such as albumin, are primarily responsible for the majority of this osmotic pressure.

Clinical Correlate

Anasarca is a condition of generalized edema in the tissues. It is caused by very low albumin concentration in the blood, i.e., low osmotic pressure in the capillary at the venule end.

As shown in Figure 9.7, the hydrostatic pressure at the arteriole end of the capillary bed is approximately 36 mm Hg, while the opposing osmotic pressure is approximately 25 mm Hg. This 11 mm Hg difference favors the hydrostatic pressure, and so there is a net flow of fluid out of the capillaries. At the venule end of the capillary bed, the osmotic pressure across the wall is greater than the hydrostatic pressure, which has dropped to 15 mm Hg. This difference tends to draw fluid into the capillaries. Hence, most of the fluid is forced out of the capillaries at the arteriole

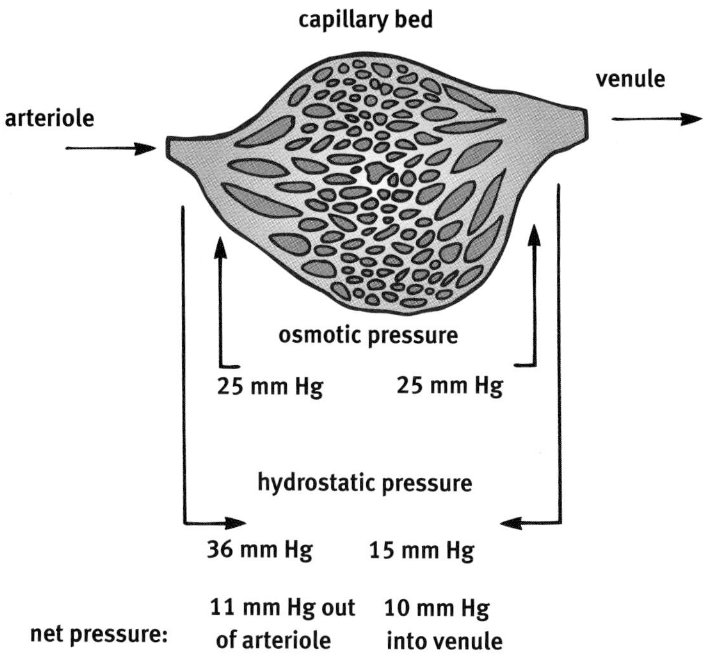

Figure 9.7. Net Fluid Flow at Capillary Bed

> **TEACHER TIP**
> Note how much lower the pressure is here than in the arteries (normal 120/80). Recall that this pressure drop occurs across the arterioles and is necessary because the capillaries cannot handle higher pressure. They are only a single cell thick so that gas exchange can occur.

end and is reabsorbed by the capillaries at the venule end. The remaining fluid is transported back into the blood via the lymphatic system.

C. CLOTTING

When platelets come into contact with the exposed collagen of a damaged vessel, they release a chemical that causes neighboring platelets to adhere to one another, forming a platelet plug. Subsequently, both the platelets and the damaged tissue release the clotting factor **thromboplastin.** Thromboplastin, with the aid of its cofactors calcium and vitamin K, converts the inactive plasma protein **prothrombin** to its active form, **thrombin.** Thrombin then converts **fibrinogen** (another plasma protein) into **fibrin.** Threads of fibrin coat the damaged area and trap blood cells to form a **clot.** Clots prevent extensive blood loss while the damaged vessel heals itself. People suffering from the genetic disease **hemophilia** lack one of the agents involved in clot formation and bleed excessively, even from minor cuts and bruises (see chapter 13).

D. IMMUNOLOGICAL REACTIONS

The body has the ability to distinguish between "self" and "nonself," and to "remember" nonself entities (antigens) that it has previously encountered. These defense mechanisms are an integral part of the **immune system.** The immune system is composed of two **specific defense mechanisms**: **humoral immunity,** which involves the production of antibodies; and

> **TEACHER TIP**
> In some individuals this ability to distinguish between self and nonself is lost, resulting in a class of diseases known as auto-immune diseases. Type I diabetes is a result of auto-immunity to the beta cells of the pancreas and is an MCAT favorite.

cell-mediated immunity, which involves cells that combat fungal and viral infection. Lymphocytes are responsible for both of these immune mechanisms. The body also has a number of nonspecific defense mechanisms.

1. Humoral Immunity

One of the body's defense mechanisms is the production of antibodies. Humoral immunity is responsible for the proliferation of antibodies following exposure to antigens. Antibodies, also called **immunoglobulins** (Igs), are complex proteins that recognize and bind to specific antigens and trigger the immune system to remove them. Antibodies either attract other cells (such as leukocytes) to phagocytize the antigen, or cause the antigens to clump together (agglutinate) and form large insoluble complexes, facilitating their removal by phagocytic cells. An antibody molecule consists of four polypeptide chains—two identical **heavy chains** and two identical **light chains**—held together by disulfide linkages and noncovalent bonds. Certain regions on the chains (called **variable regions**) serve as antigen-binding sites; these sites are structured so as to bind to one specific antigen. The remaining part of the chains (the **constant regions**) aid in the process by which foreign antigens are destroyed (see Figure 9.8). There are five types of constant regions—M, A, D, G, and E—defining five classes of immunoglobulins: **IgM, IgA, IgD, IgG,** and **IgE.**

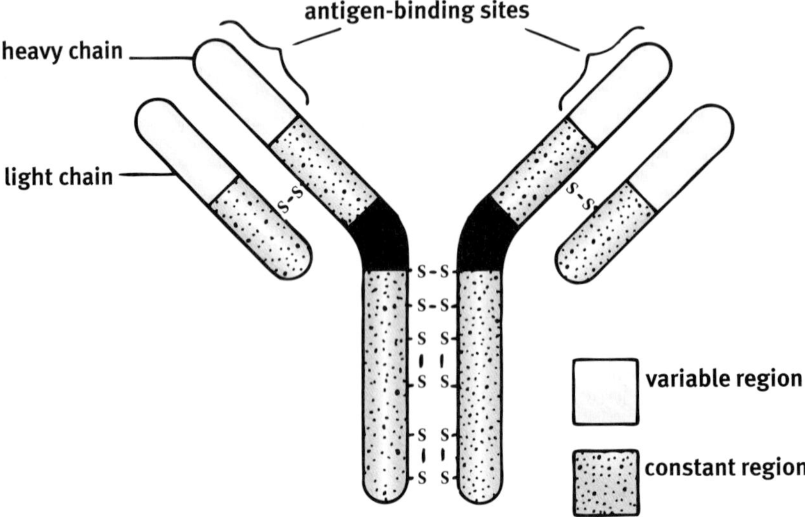

Figure 9.8. Antibody Structure

The lymphocytes involved in the humoral response are the B lymphocytes, or **B cells,** which originate in the bone marrow and differentiate in the spleen, lymph nodes, and other lymphatic organs. When exposed to a specific antigen, B lymphocytes specific for that antigen proliferate. Some of the daughter cells become **memory cells,** and others become **plasma cells (effector cells)**; this is known as the **primary response.** Plasma cells produce and release antibodies specific for the antigen. It generally takes 7–10 days for the plasma cells to generate a sufficient amount of antibody. Memory cells "remember" the antigen and are long-lived in the bloodstream, sometimes remaining there permanently. Memory cells are able to elicit a more immediate response upon subsequent exposure to the same antigen; this is referred to as the **secondary response.**

Active immunity refers to the production of antibodies during an immune response. Active immunity can be conferred by vaccination; an individual is injected with a weakened, inactive, or related form of a particular antigen, that stimulates the immune system to produce specific antibodies against it. Active immunity may require weeks to build up. **Passive immunity** involves the transfer of antibodies produced by another individual or organism. Passive immunity is acquired either passively or by injection. For example, during pregnancy, some maternal antibodies cross the placenta and enter fetal circulation, conferring passive immunity upon the fetus. Although passive immunity is acquired immediately, it is very short-lived, lasting only as long as the antibodies circulate in the blood system.

TEACHER TIP

Sometimes the organisms that cause diseases are so similar in structure that the immune system can be fooled—even for our benefit. When Edward Jenner was trying to find a treatment for smallpox, he inoculated his son with infectious particles from a different but related disease, cowpox. While the child contracted cowpox, he became immunized to smallpox due to the similarity of the two diseases!

2. Cell-Mediated Immunity

The lymphocytes involved in cell-mediated immunity are T lymphocytes, or **T cells,** which develop in bone marrow and mature and proliferate in the thymus. T cells act primarily against the body's own cells that are infected by a fungus or virus. T cells differentiate into effector cells: **cytotoxic T cells** destroy antigens directly; **helper T cells** activate other B and T cells, as well as nonlymphocyte cells such as macrophages, through the secretion of **lymphokines** (e.g., interleukins); **suppressor T cells** regulate other B and T cells to decrease their activity against antigens. Some T cells differentiate into memory cells. These events constitute the primary components of a cell-mediated response. During a secondary response, these memory cells proliferate vigorously and produce a large number of cytotoxic T cells to combat the invader.

TEACHER TIP

Recall that viruses must be inside of cells in order to replicate, thus they can often evade the immune system. One way that the immune system deals with this problem is by using cytotoxic T cells to kill virally infected cells.

T cells play important roles in allergic reactions and in the rejection of organ transplants. Sometimes pollen or certain foods can act as antigens, stimulating the release of substances (e.g., **histamine**) responsible for allergic symptoms, such as hives and mucous membrane inflammation. Cell-mediated immunity plays an important role in transplant rejection; i.e., tissue from a donor is recognized by the recipient as foreign because the recipient's body does not recognize the antigens on the transplanted cells, and in response, cytotoxic T cells are sent out to destroy the foreign cells. In certain diseases, the body mistakenly identifies its own cells as foreign and elicits an **autoimmune** response, destroying its own cells.

3. Nonspecific Defense Mechanisms

The body employs a number of nonspecific defenses against foreign material: 1) Skin is a physical barrier against bacterial invasion. In addition, pores on the skin's surface secrete sweat, which contains an enzyme that attacks bacterial cell walls. 2) Passages (e.g., the respiratory tract) are lined with ciliated mucous-coated epithelia, which filter and trap foreign particles. 3) Macrophages engulf and destroy foreign particles. 4) The **inflammatory response** is initiated by the body in response to physical damage: injured cells release histamine, which causes blood vessels to dilate, thereby increasing blood flow to the damaged region. Granulocytes attracted to the injury site phagocytize antigenic material. An inflammatory response is often accompanied by a fever. 5) Proteins called **interferons** are produced by cells under viral attack. Interferons diffuse to other cells, where they help prevent the spread of the virus.

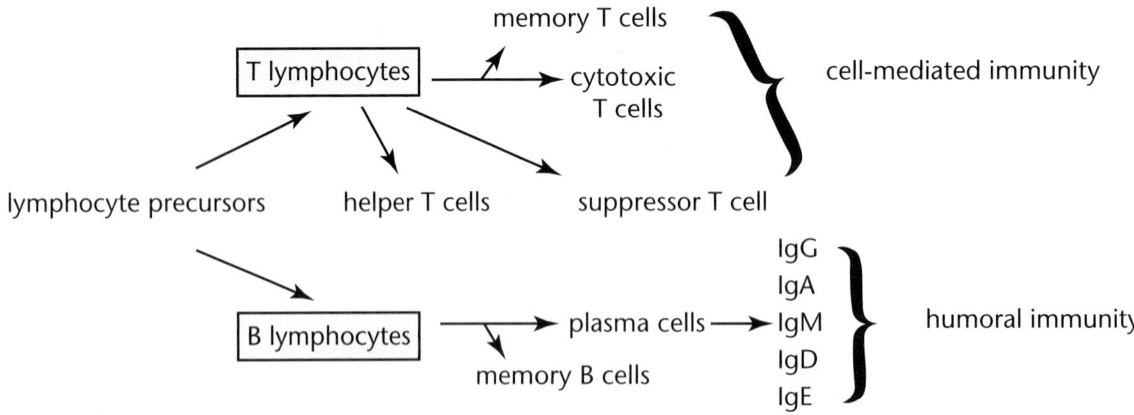

Figure 9.9. Lymphocyte Differentiation

THE LYMPHATIC SYSTEM

The lymphatic system is a secondary circulatory system distinct from cardiovascular circulation. Its vessels transport excess interstitial fluid, called **lymph,** to the cardiovascular system, thereby keeping fluid levels in the body constant. **Lymph capillaries** (lacteals) collect fats by absorbing chylomicrons in the small intestine and transporting them to cardiovascular circulation (see chapter 7). Lymph capillaries are closed at one end and lead into other lymph vessels that have valves to prevent the backflow of lymph. These lymph vessels then converge in the region of the upper chest and neck, where they drain into the large veins of the cardiovascular system. Lymph flow is regulated by contraction of neighboring skeletal muscles and rhythmic contractions of the lymphatic vessels themselves. **Lymph nodes** are swellings along lymph vessels containing phagocytic cells (leukocytes) that filter the lymph, removing and destroying foreign particles.

TEACHER TIP

Flashback to Digestion: Recall that unlike carbohydrates and proteins (amino acids), fat molecules are taken up by the lymphatics and dumped directly into the circulation. Thus, they (unlike carbohydrates and proteins) are not seen by the liver before entering the circulation.

PRACTICE QUESTIONS

1. At any given time, there is more blood in the venous system than the arterial system. Which of the following features of a vein allows this?

A. Relative lack of smooth muscle in the wall
B. Presence of valves
C. Proximity of veins to lymphatic vessels
D. Thin endothelial lining

2. Which of the following is the body's primary mechanism for buffering the blood?

A. Fluid intake
B. Absorption of nutrients in the gastrointestinal system
C. Carbon dioxide produced from metabolism
D. Reabsorption in the kidney

3. A deficiency of eosinophils would predispose the body to which of the following?

A. Giardia
B. Sickle cell disease
C. Hepatitis B
D. Influenza

4. Allergic reactions are mediated by which of the following?

A. Granules in basophils
B. Nucleus of eosinophils
C. IgG of red blood cells
D. Granules in neutrophils

5. Systolic blood pressure is the pressure at which

A. the aortic valve is open.
B. the mitral valve is open.
C. the pulmonic valve is closed.
D. venous valves are closed.

6. Diastolic blood pressure is measured when

A. right ventricular pressure is equal to left ventricular pressure.
B. arterial pressure equals venous pressure.
C. ventricular pressure is less than atrial pressure.
D. pulmonic artery pressure is equal to aortic pressure.

7. Which of the following correctly demonstrates the relationship between the parasympathetic nervous system and heart rate at rest?

A. Administration of intravenous epinephrine increases heart rate.
B. Blocking the sympathetic nervous system at rest does not alter the heart rate.
C. Blocking acetylcholine receptors at rest does not alter the heart rate.
D. Administration of intravenous acetylcholine increases the heart rate.

8. Following are the sample lab results from Rh testing in a family:

	Rh Factor
Mother	Negative
Father	Positive
1st Child	Positive

It is not known whether the mother received immunoglobulins against Rh factor (antigen D) in her first pregnancy. Based on the data above, if the mother is six months pregnant with a second child by the same father, which of the following is most likely?

A. Red blood cells of the first child are circulating within the mother.
B. The father's Rh factor protects the fetus against auto-immune attack.
C. The mother's immune system may be generating antibodies against Rh.
D. Administration of Rh immune globin at this point would provide protection to the fetus.

9. Which of the following conveys the most strength to a clot?

A. Thrombin
B. Fibrinogen
C. Platelets
D. Fibrin

10. The porto-hepatic system lies in series with the upper and lower body with respect to the heart as diagramed below.

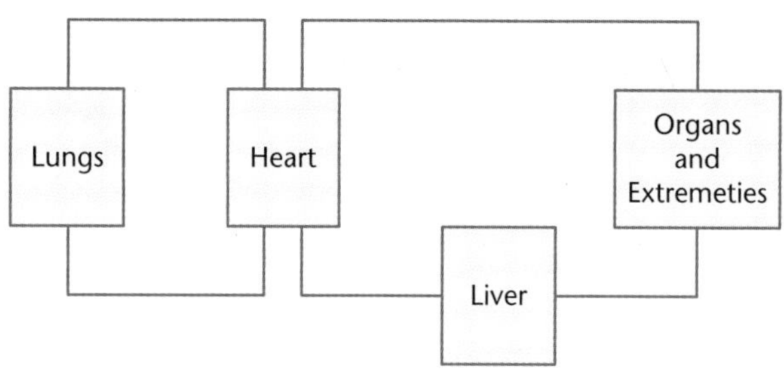

Placement of the porto-hepatic system in series serves which of the following functions?

A. Oxygenates liver tissue
B. Enhances absorption of water
C. Increases venous return to the heart
D. Filters deoxygenated blood

11. What is the half-life of epinephrine given the graph of epinephrine clearance below?

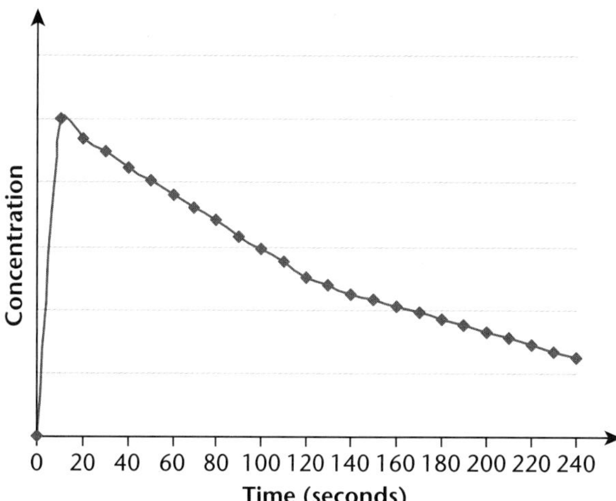

A. 60 seconds
B. 90 seconds
C. 120 seconds
D. 180 seconds

12. Which of the following is described in the graph of antibody producton below?

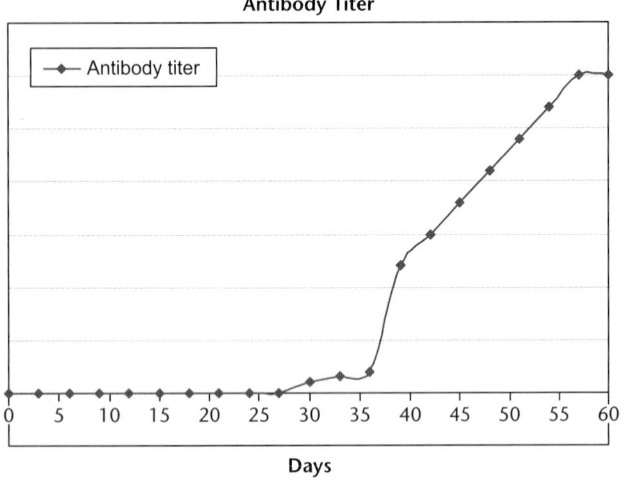

A. Passive immunization
B. Exposure to a new antigen
C. Exposure to a previously recognized antigen
D. Lymphocytopenia

13. Put the following in chronological order.

1. Rearrangement of heavy and light chains
2. First exposure to antigen
3. Proliferation of B cells into memory and plasma cells
4. Binding of antibody to antigen
5. Phagocytosis

A. 2, 3, 1, 4, 5
B. 2, 1, 4, 3, 5
C. 2, 3, 4, 1, 5
D. 4, 2, 3, 1, 5

14. Pus is primarily composed of phagocytosed bacterial remnants. Which of the following would you expect to find in a microscopic sample of pus?

A. Red blood cells, white blood cells, and platelets
B. Granulocytes, monocytes, and macrophages
C. Eosinophils, basophils, and neutrophils
D. Collagen, white blood cells, and calcium

15. An acute, uncompensated drop in stroke volume would preferentially spare which of the following body parts?

A. Left-upper extremity
B. Right-upper extremity
C. Brain
D. Heart

CIRCULATION

Increased O_2 consumption in the left ventricle coupled with left ventricular hypertrophy and a heart murmur is most likely the result of what condition, and what symptoms would be seen in a patient with this condition?

1) Examine the reasons for increased O_2 consumption in the heart.

O_2 consumption in the heart increases when there is increased afterload (or increased aortic pressure), increased heart rate, increased contractility, and/or increased size of the heart.

---

2) Examine the reasons for left ventricular hypertrophy.

Left ventricular hypertrophy is the abnormal enlargement of the muscle of the left ventricle. This thickening occurs when the left ventricle has to work harder to generate enough force to overcome greater pressure as it is pumping (greater afterload).

---

3) Review the flow of blood through the heart.

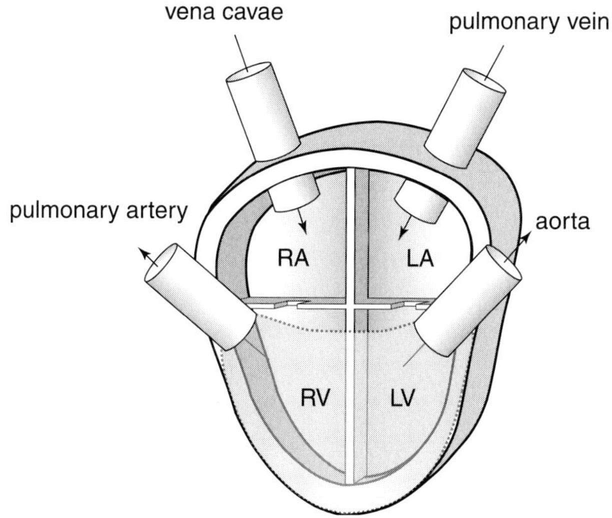

Blood travels into the right atrium through the vena cava. It moves through the tricuspid valve into the right ventricle and is then passed into the pulmonary artery, which carries it to the lungs. After leaving the lungs, blood travels through the pulmonary vein to the left atrium, then through the mitral valve into the left ventricle. The left ventricle pumps blood through the aortic valve into the aorta.

KEY CONCEPTS

Circulation

Cardiac circulation

Cardiac oxygen consumption

Blood volume

TAKEAWAYS

It's important to be able to integrate knowledge from different areas, in this case O_2 consumption, blood flow, and the pathway of the heart, when examining a question.

SIMILAR QUESTIONS

1) Where would a patient diagnosed with stenosis of the mitral valve experience the greatest increase in blood pressure?
2) If a tracer substance were injected into a patient's superior vena cava, which structure would it reach last before leaving the heart?
3) The decrease in the number of pulmonary capillaries due to the loss of functional lung tissue will most likely result in a pressure overload. Where will this overload occur?

4) Determine the cause of the heart murmur.

Heart murmurs result from turbulent blood flow through the heart, particularly through the valves. Deformities of a valve will cause blood flow through the valve to become turbulent and create a heart murmur.

---

5) Determine the cause of the left ventricular hypertrophy and the increased O_2 consumption.

The left ventricle thickens and uses more oxygen because it cannot easily pump the blood through the aortic valve into the aorta. Stenosis is a condition in which the leaves of a heart valve adhere to each other, decreasing the volume of blood flow through the valve. Therefore, a stenotic aortic valve would make pumping blood through the aortic valve more difficult and lead to increased O_2 consumption and left ventricular hypertrophy.

---

6) Determine the effects of decreased blood flow due to aortic stenosis.

If less blood can be pumped from the left ventricle into the aorta, the ability to supply the body with blood will be reduced. This can cause blood to back up into the lungs and cause shortness of breath, especially with activity, as well as chest pain. Also, because less blood will be going out to the body, weakness can result; further, because less blood will be going to the brain, fainting is also a symptom of aortic stenosis.

Remember: *Knowing the pathway that blood takes through the heart is essential!*

NORMAL OXYGEN DISSOCIATION CURVE

How does the oxygen dissociation curve of arterial blood differ from the curve for venous blood, and what accounts for this difference?

1) Review the normal oxygen dissociation curve.

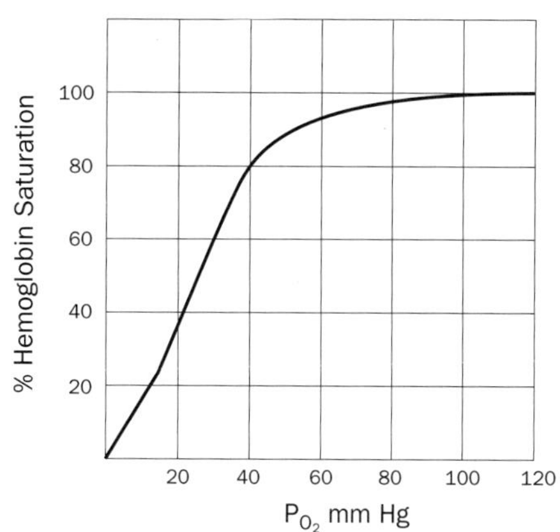

The oxygen dissociation curve shows the percent saturation of hemoglobin as a function of the partial pressure of O_2 (Po_2). At Po_2 = 100 mm Hg, hemoglobin saturation is 100 percent, which means that four oxygen molecules are bound to the hemoglobin. At Po_2 = 40 mm Hg, hemoglobin is 80 percent saturated and at Po_2 = 25 mm Hg, hemoglobin is 50% saturated with oxygen molecules. The cooperative binding of O_2, meaning the binding of the first O_2 molecule, facilitates the binding of the next and results in a sigmoidal, or S-shaped, curve.

---

2) Examine how arterial blood differs from venous blood.

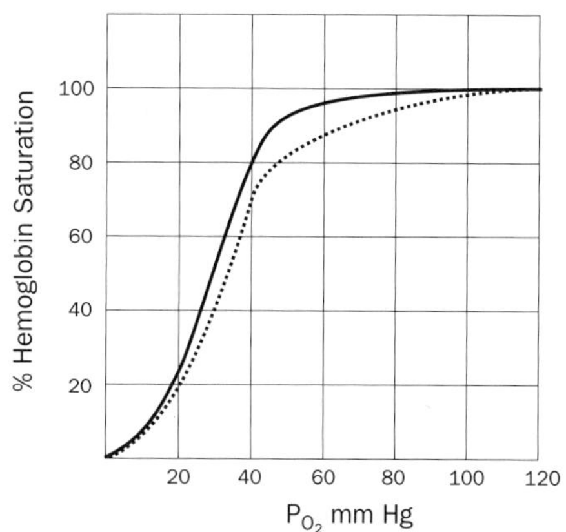

After blood passes through the lungs and into the arteries, the hemoglobin is 100 percent saturated with oxygen. The tissues of the body produce CO_2 as waste. The increase in CO_2 at the tissues decreases the pH of the tissues.

KEY CONCEPTS

Oxygen dissociation curve

Arterial blood saturation

Venous blood saturation

Right/left shift

Bohr effect

TAKEAWAYS

It is important to understand how to read the oxygen dissociation curve and how changes in the curve equate to changes in the affinity of hemoglobin for oxygen. Increases in Pco_2, decreases in pH, and increases in temperature shift the curve to the right. The opposite of those, a decrease in Pco_2, an increase in pH, or a decrease in temperature shift the curve to the left.

THINGS TO WATCH OUT FOR

Right shifts of the curve are more common, but don't forget the factors that shift the curve to the left.

SIMILAR QUESTIONS

1) How is the P_{50} of venous blood different from that of arterial blood?
2) How will the fetal oxygen dissociation curve differ from that of an adult?
3) How will arterial Po_2 be affected by living at a high altitude?

Increases in CO_2 or decreases in pH decrease the affinity of hemoglobin for oxygen and cause the curve to shift slightly to the right, increasing the Po_2 and facilitating the unloading of O_2 at the tissues. The tissues keep Po_2 low by consuming O_2 for aerobic metabolism, so that the O_2 diffusion gradient is maintained. In arterial blood, the hemoglobin saturation at 40 mm Hg is 80 percent, but in venous blood the Hb saturation at 40 mm Hg is 75 percent. Therefore, about 5 percent more oxygen is released. This right shift of the curve is known as the Bohr effect. An increase in temperature also causes a right shift.

At the lungs, alveolar gas has a Po_2 of 100 mm Hg. O_2 diffuses from the alveolar air into the capillaries. O_2 is bound very tightly to hemoglobin because at a Po_2 of 100 mm Hg, hemoglobin has a very high affinity for O_2. This maintains the partial pressure gradients and facilitates the diffusion of oxygen into the blood.

ABNORMAL OXYGEN DISSOCIATION CURVE

Carbon monoxide (CO) binding to hemoglobin occurs in competition with oxygen (O_2) to hemoglobin binding; hemoglobin's affinity for CO is over 200 times its affinity for O_2. However, the binding of CO at one site increases the affinity for O_2 at the remaining sites. Draw the oxygen dissociation curve for CO poisoning, measuring hemoglobin oxygen content (in units of mL O_2/dL) on the vertical axis.

KEY CONCEPTS

Oxygen dissociation curve

Carbon monoxide

Hemoglobin

Left shift

1) Visualize the normal oxygen dissociation curve.

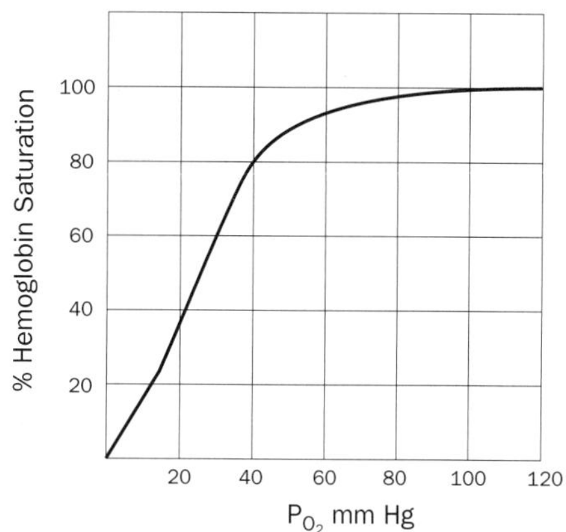

The oxygen dissociation curve shows the percent saturation of hemoglobin as a function of the partial pressure of O_2 (Po_2). At Po_2 = 100 mm Hg, hemoglobin saturation is 100 percent, which means that four oxygen molecules are bound to the hemoglobin. At Po_2 = 40 mm Hg, hemoglobin is 80 percent saturated and at Po_2 = 25 mm Hg, hemoglobin is 50 percent saturated with oxygen molecules. The cooperative binding of O_2, meaning the binding of the first O_2 molecule, facilitates the binding of the next and results in a sigmoidal, or S-shaped, curve.

TAKEAWAYS

Be familiar with the concepts of Po_2 and Pco_2, what factors change their values, and how they are represented graphically.

---

2) Examine the effect that CO binding has on O_2 binding.

The question stem states that CO competes with O_2 when binding hemoglobin. Because hemoglobin affinity is 200 times greater for CO than for O_2, hemoglobin will preferentially bind CO first on a hemoglobin molecule. This will decrease the amount of O_2 that can bind to hemoglobin and therefore decrease the amount of O_2 that is in the blood.

Things to Watch Out For

Right shifts in the dissociation curve (Bohr effect) are more commonly seen, but be prepared for the factors that can cause the curve to shift to the left.

Similar Questions

1) How will exercise affect the oxygen dissociation curve?
2) What type of physical reaction would high Pco_2 cause?
3) What would the oxygen dissociation curve look like in a patient with metabolic alkalosis?

3) Determine the effect that CO binding will have on the oxygen dissociation curve.

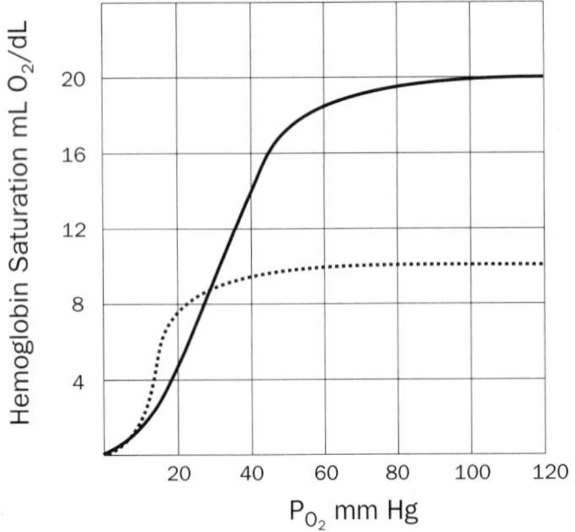

The question stem also states that the binding of CO increases hemoglobin affinity for O_2 at the remaining sites. Any physiological factor (i.e., decreased Pco_2, increased pH, or decreased temperature) that increases the affinity of hemoglobin for oxygen has the effect of shifting the curve to the left. Any physiological factor (i.e., increased Pco_2, decreased pH, or increased temperature) that decreases the affinity of hemoglobin for oxygen has the effect of shifting the curve to the right. The right shift is known as the Bohr effect. However, in this case the affinity of hemoglobin for oxygen is increased and there will be a left shift in the oxygen dissociation curve. It is this left shift that makes CO poisoning so deadly; with CO bound to hemoglobin, the O_2 molecules are bound so tightly that they cannot be off-loaded at the tissues and thus asphyxia occurs.

Remember: *The oxygen dissociation curve can be shifted to the left or to the right based on physiological conditions.*

LYMPHATIC SYSTEM

Approximately 20 L/day of fluid filters across capillaries. Reabsorption across capillaries is approximately 16 L/day, and therefore the excess fluid must be returned to circulation by the lymphatic system. Lymphatic vessels are attached to the underlying connective tissue by fine filaments. What purpose do these filaments serve?

KEY CONCEPTS

Lymphatic system

Lymphatic vessels

Blood vessels

1) Examine the structure of lymph vessels.

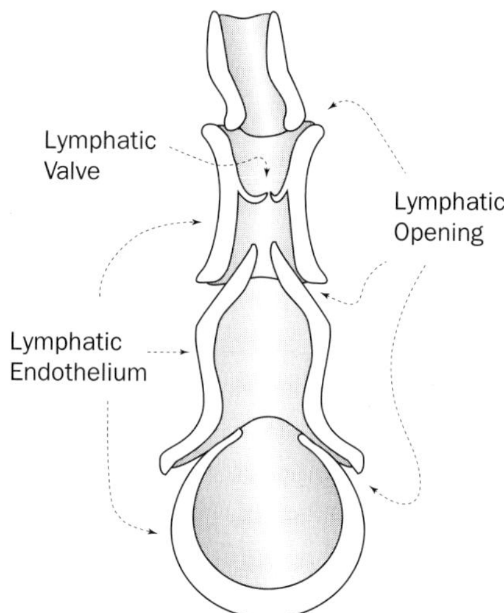

Lymphatic vessels have very thin walls that do not contain the smooth muscle that is found in arteries. Lymph vessels contain valves that ensure the unidirectional flow of lymph through the vessels. Filtrate from blood vessels, including cells and protein that have moved into the interstitial fluid compartment, is picked up by the lymphatic vessels. Lymphatic vessels called lacteals absorb fats from the gastrointestinal tract. The filtrate is moved through the system of lymphatic vessels, passing through lymph nodes where foreign particles are destroyed and removed. It rejoins blood circulation at the thoracic duct and superior vena cava.

TAKEAWAYS

The lymphatic system plays a very important role in returning fluid, cells, and proteins back to the blood stream, but it relies on the movement of skeletal muscles in order to accomplish this role.

---

2) Determine how interstitial fluid moves through lymph vessels.
Because lymphatic vessels do not have smooth muscle in their walls, they must rely on outside forces to move the lymph fluid through the vessels. The movement of skeletal muscles around the lymphatic vessels aids in moving lymph along, and their one-way valves prevent backflow of this fluid.

THINGS TO WATCH OUT FOR

Although the lymphatic system has some similarities with the circulatory system, lymphatic vessels are closed-ended, they do not connect in a complete circuit, and they are unidirectional.

SIMILAR QUESTIONS

1) If a patient's lymphatic channels have been obstructed by the spread of malignant tumors, what will result?
2) What physiological conditions can contribute to excess fluid in the interstitial space?
3) How does the lymphatic system return interstitial proteins to the blood?

3) Determine how interstitial fluid enters lymphatic vessels.

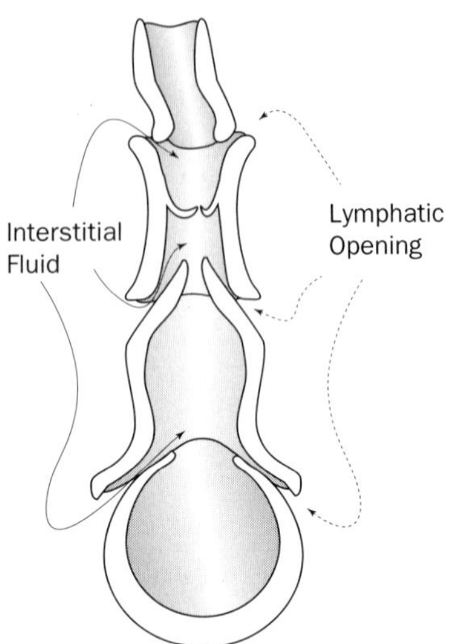

Capillaries have tight junctions between their endothelial cells. These tight junctions prevent unregulated passage of solutes in and out of the capillary lumen. Lymphatic vessels do not possess these tight junctions but rather have openings through which the interstitial fluid, complete with cells and proteins, can pass into the vessel. Because the lymph vessels are attached by fine filaments to their underlying connective tissue, skeletal muscle contraction will pull on these filaments and distort the lymphatic vessel. This distortion causes spaces to open between the endothelial cells of the vessel and allows the interstitial fluid to enter.

Remember: *Lymphatic vessels differ from blood vessels in that they lack smooth muscle around the vessel and lack tight junctions between endothelial cells.*

CHAPTER 10

HOMEOSTASIS

Homeostasis is the process by which a stable internal environment within an organism is maintained. Some important homeostatic mechanisms include the maintenance of a water and solute balance **(osmoregulation),** the removal of metabolic waste products **(excretion),** the regulation of blood glucose levels, and the maintenance of a constant internal body temperature **(thermoregulation).** In mammals, the primary homeostatic organs are the **kidneys,** the **liver,** the **large intestine,** and the **skin.**

> **TEACHER TIP**
>
> KEY POINT: Maintenance of an internal environment wouldn't be that hard if the external environment weren't changing. However, in the real world it is; thus, homeostasis becomes an absolutely critical adaptation to life.

THE KIDNEYS: OSMOREGULATION

The kidneys regulate the concentration of salt and water in the blood through the formation and excretion of urine. The kidneys are bean-shaped and are located behind the stomach and liver. Each kidney is composed of approximately one million units called **nephrons.**

A. STRUCTURE

The kidney is divided into three regions: the **cortex,** the **medulla,** and the **pelvis.** Blood enters the kidney through the **renal artery,** which divides into many **afferent arterioles** that run through the medulla and into the cortex (see Figure 10.1). Each afferent arteriole branches into a convoluted network of capillaries called a **glomerulus** (see Figure 10.2). Rather than converging directly into a vein, the capillaries converge into an **efferent arteriole,** which divides into a fine capillary network known as the **vasa recta.** The vasa recta enmeshes the nephron tubule and then converges into the **renal vein.** This arrangement of tandem capillary beds is a portal system (see chapter 9).

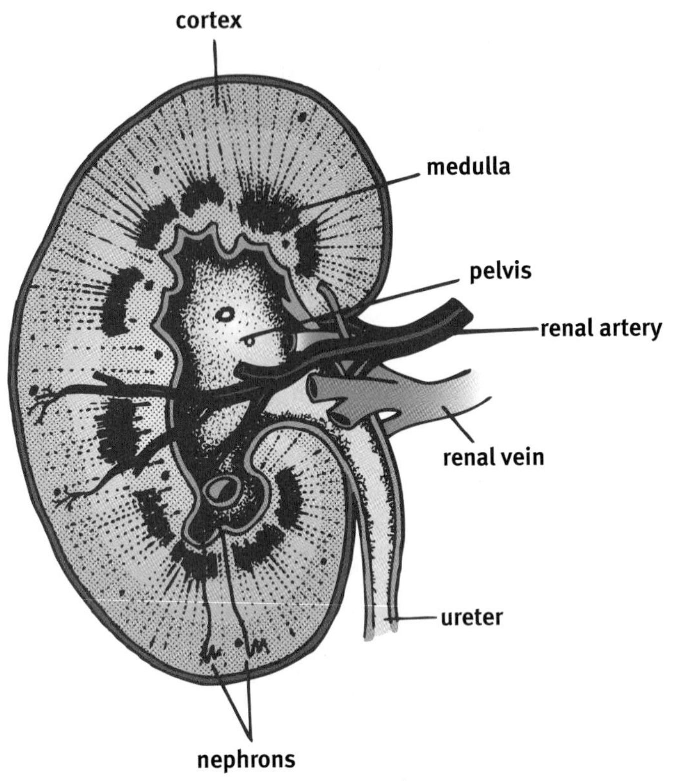

Figure 10.1. Kidney

TEACHER TIP

It is the kidneys, not the large intestine, that are primarily responsible for water balance in living organisms. As well, the kidney is the only place in the body where there are two arterioles in series. This system allows for a relatively high pressure to be created across the glomerulus, something critical for the filtration process.

A nephron consists of a bulb called **Bowman's capsule,** which embraces a glomerulus and leads into a long coiled tubule that is divided into five units: the **proximal convoluted tubule,** the **descending limb** of the **loop of Henle,** the **ascending limb** of the **loop of Henle,** the **distal convoluted tubule,** and the **collecting duct.** The nephron is positioned such that the loop of Henle runs through the medulla, while the convoluted tubules and Bowman's capsule are in the cortex (see Figure 10.2).

B. FUNCTION

1. Overview

Filtration, secretion, and **reabsorption** are the three processes that regulate salt and water balance in the blood.

MCAT SYNOPSIS

Imagine that the glomerulus is like a sieve or collander. Small molecules dissolved in the fluid will pass through the glomerulus (e.g., glucose that is later reabsorbed), while large molecules such as proteins and blood cells will not. If blood cells or protein are found in the urine, this indicates a problem at the level of the glomerulus.

a. Filtration

Blood pressure forces 20 percent of the blood plasma entering the glomerulus into the surrounding Bowman's capsule. The fluid and small solutes entering the nephron are called the **filtrate.** The filtrate is isotonic with blood plasma. Molecules too large to filter through the glomerulus, such as blood cells and albumin, remain in the circulatory system.

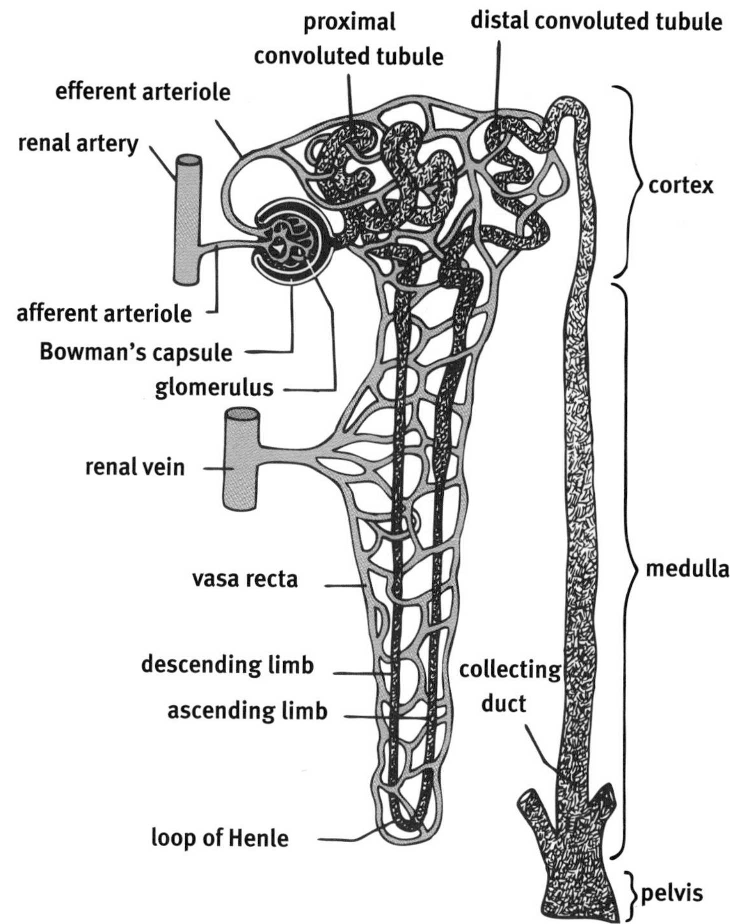

Figure 10.2. Nephron

b. Secretion

The nephron secretes substances such as acids, bases, and ions from the interstitial fluid into the filtrate by both passive and active transport. Secretion maintains blood pH, potassium concentration in the blood, and nitrogenous waste concentration in the filtrate.

c. Reabsorption

Essential substances (glucose, salts, and amino acids) and water are reabsorbed from the filtrate and returned to the blood. This results in the formation of concentrated urine, which is hypertonic to the blood.

2. Nephron Function

Through the selective permeability of its walls and the maintenance of an osmolarity gradient, the nephron reabsorbs nutrients, salts, and water from the filtrate and returns them to the body, thus maintaining the bloodstream's solute concentration.

TEACHER TIP

The kidneys are without a doubt the MCAT's favorite organ systems. Take time to understand the intricacies of the major processes that the kidney undertakes.

CLINICAL CORRELATE

In certain conditions (e.g., congestive heart failure), the body tends to accumulate excess water in the form of fluid in the lungs or in peripheral tissues. The judicious use of a diuretic drug can help the body get rid of excess fluids. Diuretics typically inhibit the reabsorption of sodium in one or more regions of the nephron, thereby increasing sodium excretion. The increased sodium excretion, in turn, results in an increased excretion of water, thereby relieving the body of some of its excess fluid.

a. Selective permeability

The walls of the proximal tubule and the descending limb of the loop of Henle are permeable to water. The walls of the lower ascending limb are permeable only to salt. In the presence of ADH, the walls of the collecting duct are permeable to water and urea but only slightly permeable to salt.

> **TEACHER TIP**
>
> Flashback to Chapter 1: The entire system under which the kidney operates is membrane transport. Both active and passive transport are used, and the extent to which they are used depends on the specific section of the nephron in question. The key point is that membrane permeability is absolutely necessary for the kidneys to work.

b. Osmolarity gradient

The selective permeability of the tubules establishes an **osmolarity gradient** in the surrounding interstitial fluid. By exiting and then reentering at different segments of the nephron, solutes create an osmolarity gradient, with tissue osmolarity increasing from cortex to inner medulla. The solutes that contribute to the maintenance of the gradient are urea and salt (Na^+ and Cl^-). Urea diffuses out of the collecting duct; it eventually reenters the nephron by diffusing into the ascending limb. Salt is cycled between the two limbs of the loop of Henle. Na^+ and Cl^- diffuse out of the lower half of the ascending limb, while the upper half actively pumps out Na^+ (Cl^- passively follows). This combination of passive diffusion and active transport of solutes maximizes water conservation and the excretion of urine hypertonic to the blood (see Figure 10.3).

> **TEACHER TIP**
>
> KEY POINT: Water is not reabsorbed by itself. In fact, it is not usually pumped at all. The kidney moves ions (primarily Na and Cl) to create gradients that water will follow.

c. Flow of filtrate

Filtrate enters Bowman's capsule and flows into the proximal convoluted tubule, where virtually all glucose, amino acids, and other important organic molecules are reabsorbed via active transport. In addition, 60–70 percent of the Na^+ in the filtrate is reabsorbed (by both active and passive mechanisms); water and Cl^- passively follow. The filtrate then flows down the descending limb into the renal medulla, where there is an increasing ionic concentration in the interstitial fluid, causing more water to diffuse out of the nephron. The filtrate flows through the ascending limb, which is impermeable to water, and then into the distal convoluted tubule. The filtrate continues through the collecting duct, where water reabsorption is under hormonal (ADH) control. The remaining filtrate, urine, is hypertonic to the blood and highly concentrated in urea and other solutes.

> **MCAT SYNOPSIS**
>
> The kidneys function to eliminate wastes (urea, H+) generated by metabolic activity, while reabsorbing various important substances (glucose, amino acids, sodium) for re-use by the body. Generation of a solute concentration gradient from cortex to medulla allows a considerable amount of water to be reabsorbed. Excretion of a concentrated urine serves to limit water losses from the body and helps preserve blood volume.

C. HORMONAL REGULATION

Hormonal regulation plays a key role in urine formation. Two hormones that regulate water reabsorption are **aldosterone** and **ADH.**

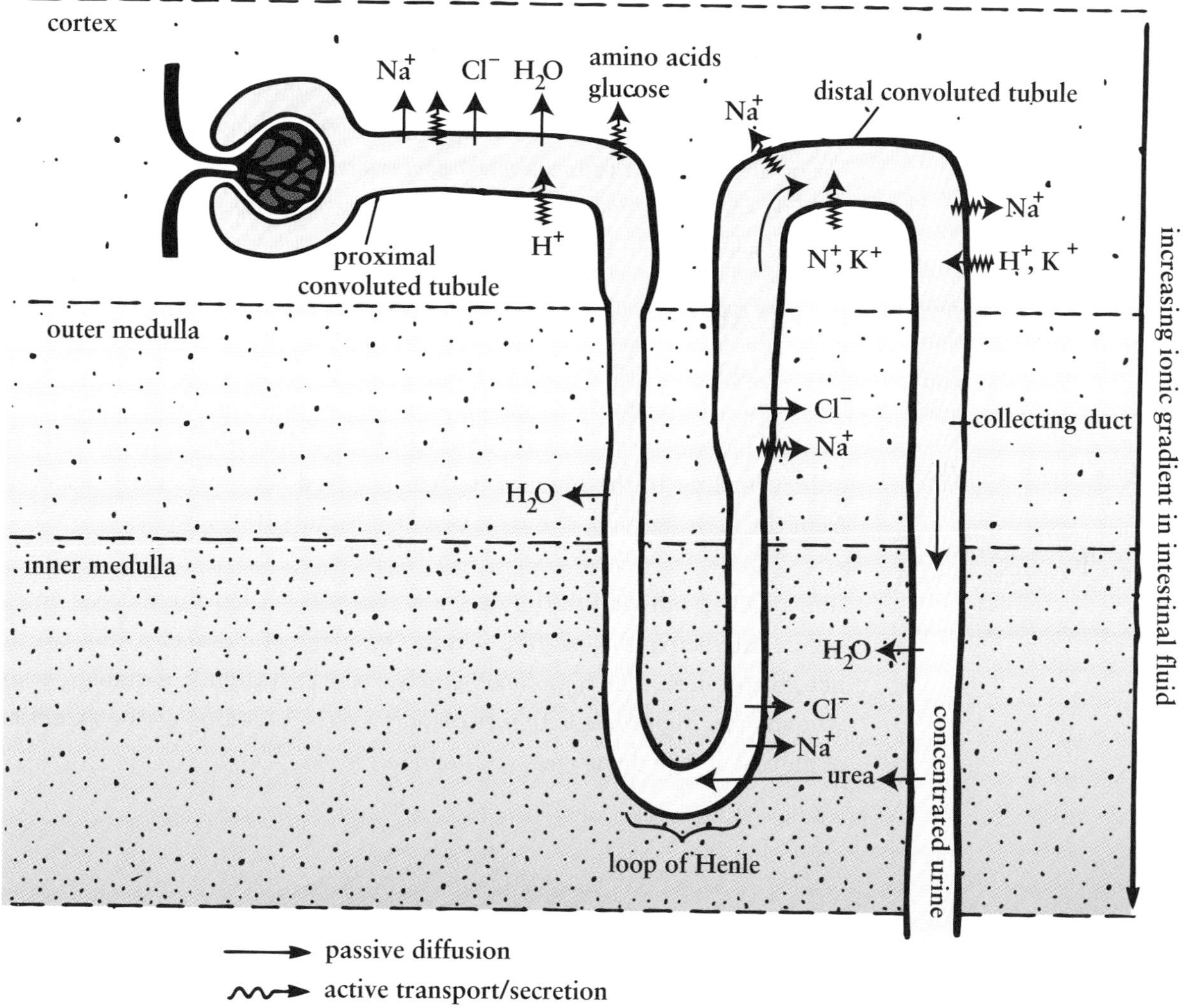

Figure 10.3. Selective Permeability and Osmolarity Gradient in the Nephron

1. Aldosterone

Aldosterone, which is produced by the adrenal cortex, stimulates both the reabsorption of Na^+ from the collecting duct and the secretion of K^+. Reabsorption of Na^+ increases water reabsorption, leading to a rise in blood volume, and hence a rise in blood pressure. In a person suffering from **Addison's disease,** aldosterone is produced insufficiently or not at all. This causes overexcretion of urine with a high Na^+ concentration, which causes a considerable drop in blood pressure. Aldosterone secretion is regulated by the **renin-angiotensin system** (see chapter 11).

TEACHER TIP

It is critical to know how aldosterone and ADH exert their effects. Aldosterone directly increases sodium reabsorption and water follows. ADH makes the CCD more leaky (permeable) to water such that it will reenter the interstitium. The ultimate effect is similar but the mechanism in which they work is slightly different.

2. ADH (Antidiuretic Hormone)

ADH, also known as **vasopressin,** is formed in the hypothalamus and stored in the posterior pituitary. As an "antidiuretic," it causes increased water reabsorption. It acts directly on the collecting duct, increasing its permeability to water. The amount of ADH produced is dependent on plasma osmolarity. A high solute concentration in the blood causes increased ADH secretion, while a low solute concentration in the blood reduces ADH secretion. Alcohol and caffeine inhibit ADH secretion, causing excess excretion of dilute urine and dehydration (see chapter 11).

MCAT SYNOPSIS

While aldosterone and ADH ultimately do the same thing (increase water reabsorption in the kidney), they have different mechanisms of action: ADH directly increases water reabsorption from the nephron's collecting duct, while aldosterone indirectly increases water reabsorption by increasing sodium reabsorption from the collecting duct.

D. EXCRETION

By the time filtrate exits the nephron, most of the water has been reabsorbed. The remaining fluid, composed of urea, uric acid, and other wastes, leaves the collecting tubule and exits the kidney via the **ureter,** a duct leading to the bladder. Urine is stored there until it is excreted from the body through the **urethra** (see Figure 10.4).

In a healthy individual, the nephron reabsorbs all of the glucose entering it, producing glucose-free urine. The urine of a diabetic, however, is not glucose-free. The high blood glucose concentration in a diabetic overwhelms the nephron's active transport system, leading to the excretion of glucose in the urine (see chapter 11).

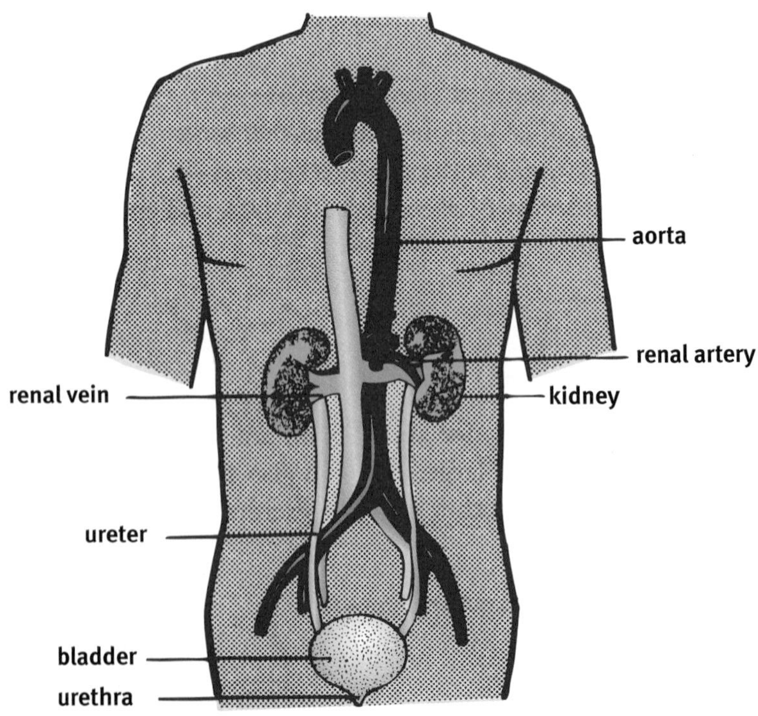

Figure 10.4. Human Excretory System

THE LIVER

The liver helps regulate blood glucose levels and produces urea. Glucose and other monosaccharides absorbed during digestion are delivered to the liver via the **hepatic portal vein** (see chapter 7). Glucose-rich blood is processed by the liver, which converts excess glucose to glycogen for storage. If the blood has a low glucose concentration, the liver converts glycogen into glucose and releases it into the blood, restoring blood glucose levels to normal. In addition, the liver synthesizes glucose from noncarbohydrate precursors via the process of **gluconeogenesis.** Glycogen metabolism is under both hormonal and nervous control (see chapter 11).

The liver is also responsible for the processing of nitrogenous wastes. Excess amino acids are absorbed in the small intestine and transported to the liver via the hepatic portal vein. There the amino acids undergo a process called **deamination,** in which the amino group is removed from the amino acid and converted into ammonia, a highly toxic compound. In a complex biochemical process, the liver combines ammonia with carbon dioxide to form urea, a relatively nontoxic compound, which is released into the blood and eventually excreted by the kidneys.

TEACHER TIP

KEY POINT: Recall that when we discussed cells, compartmentalization was a key way in which cells were able to carry out fairly dangerous reactions without damaging themselves. Here again in the liver, we see the compartmentalization of a damaging molecule (ammonia) and its conversion to a nontoxic intermediate (urea) which can be excreted.

The liver is also responsible for:

- Detoxification of toxins
- Storage of iron and vitamin B_{12}
- Destruction of old erythrocytes
- Synthesis of bile
- Synthesis of various blood proteins
- Defense against various antigens
- Beta-oxidation of fatty acids to ketones
- Interconversion of carbohydrates, fats, and amino acids

THE LARGE INTESTINE

The large intestine absorbs water and sodium not previously absorbed in the small intestine (see chapter 7). However, the large intestine also functions as an excretory organ for excess salts. Excess calcium, iron, and other salts are excreted into the colon and then eliminated with the feces.

THE SKIN: OSMOREGULATION AND THERMOREGULATION

A. STRUCTURE

The skin is the largest organ of the body, comprising an average of 16 percent of total body weight. The two major layers of the skin are the **epidermis** and the **dermis,** beneath which lies subcutaneous tissues, sometimes called the **hypodermis.**

The epidermis is the outermost epithelial layer and is composed of five cellular layers: the **stratum basalis (or stratum germinativum),** the **stratum spinosum,** the **stratum granulosum,** the **stratum lucidum,** and the **stratum corneum.** The deepest layer, the stratum basalis, continuously proliferates, pushing older epidermal cells outward. As the older cells reach the outermost layer (stratum corneum), they die, lose their nuclei, and transform into squames (scales) of keratin. The keratinized cells of the stratum corneum are tightly packed, serving as a protective barrier against microbial attack. Hair projects above the surface of the epithelium; sweat pores open to the surface.

The dermis can be subdivided into a layer of loose connective tissue known as the **papillary layer** and a layer of dense connective tissue known as the **reticular layer.** Within the dermis are the sweat glands, the sense organs, blood vessels, and the bulbs of hair follicles.

The **hypodermis,** composed of loose connective tissue, is abundant in fat cells and binds the outer skin layers to the body (see Figure 10.5).

B. FUNCTION

TEACHER TIP

The skin is also involved in the production of vitamin D via the effect sunlight has on it. Recall that vitamin D is critical in bone maintenance.

The skin protects the body from microbial invasion and from environmental stresses, such as dry weather and wind. Specialized epidermal cells called **melanocytes** synthesize the pigment **melanin,** which protects the body from ultraviolet light. The skin is a receptor of stimuli, such as pressure and temperature. The skin is also an excretory organ (removing excess water and salts from the body) and a thermoregulatory organ (helping control both the conservation and release of heat).

Sweat glands secrete a mixture of water, dissolved salts, and urea via sweat pores. As sweat evaporates, the skin is cooled. Thus, sweating has both an excretory and a thermoregulatory function. Sweating is under nervous control.

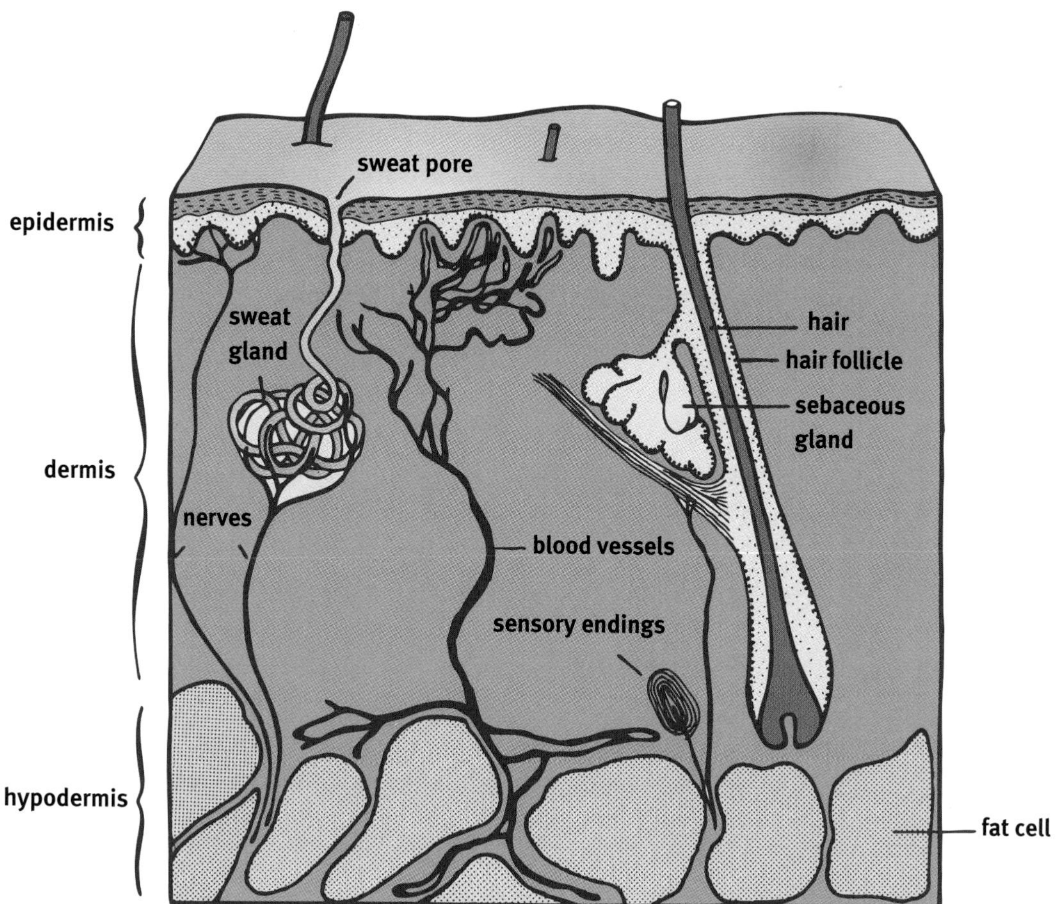

Figure 10.5. Human Skin

Subcutaneous fat in the hypodermis insulates the body. Hair entraps and retains warm air at the skin's surface. Hormones such as epinephrine can increase the metabolic rate, thereby increasing heat production. In addition, muscles can generate heat by contracting rapidly (shivering). Heat loss can be inhibited through the constriction of blood vessels in the dermis. Likewise, dilation of these same blood vessels dissipates heat.

Alternative mechanisms are used by some mammals to regulate their body temperature. For example, **panting** is a cooling mechanism that evaporates water from the respiratory passages. Most mammals have a layer of fur; fur traps and conserves heat. Some mammals exhibit varying states of **torpor** in the winter months in order to conserve energy; their metabolism, heart rate, and respiration rate greatly decrease during these months. **Hibernation** is a type of torpor during which the animal remains dormant over a period of weeks or months with body temperature maintained below normal. Animals with a constant body temperature are referred to as **homeotherms (endotherms).**

MCAT Synopsis

While this chapter focuses on the homeostatic roles played by the kidney, liver, and skin, you should be aware that homeostasis is not limited to those organs; all the organs of the body are involved in one way or another in preserving physiologic equilibrium.

Teacher Tip

Homeostasis is largely maintained automatically. This is partially done through local, organ-level effects, but the master control for homeostatic mechanisms is via the endocrine system: the topic of our next chapter and a common MCAT topic.

THYROID GLAND: THERMOREGULATION

The basal metabolic rate of the human body contributes a great deal to the warmth or coolness of the body. The thyroid hormones, primarily thyroxine, control the basal metabolic rate (see chapter 11). When there is overproduction of these hormones (hyperthyroidism), the person will feel excessively warm. When there is a decrease in the level of these hormones (hypothyroidism), the person will feel cold.

PRACTICE QUESTIONS

1. Which of the following is a normal finding in the filtrate when the glomerulus is functioning properly?

   A. Erythrocytes are in the filtrate.
   B. Albumin (69 kD) is in the filtrate.
   C. Glucose is in the filtrate.
   D. Large (larger than 69 kD) proteins are in the filtrate.

2. An increase in aldosterone will NOT cause

   A. reabsorption of Na^+ from collecting duct.
   B. an increase in blood pressure.
   C. urine with a high concentration of Na^+.
   D. urine with a low concentration of Na^+.

3. Which of the following would most likely happen after ingesting a large quantity of water quickly?

   A. Vasopressin secretion is stimulated.
   B. Vasopressin secretion is inhibited.
   C. Aldosterone production is stimulated.
   D. There is increased reabsorption of water from the collecting duct.

4. Which of the following properly traces the order of the structural pathway that filtrate follows in a nephron?

   A. Bowman's capsule, proximal convoluted tubule, loop of Henle, collecting duct
   B. Glomerulus, proximal convoluted tubule, loop of Henle, distal convoluted tubule
   C. Glomerulus, collecting duct, proximal convoluted tubule, distal convoluted tubule
   D. Bowman's capsule, distal convoluted tubule, loop of Henle, collecting duct

5. Which of the following is NOT a function of the liver?

   A. Production of bile from cholesterol
   B. Production of essential amino acids via interconversion from other amino acids
   C. Storage of vitamins and iron
   D. Production of energy by metabolizing fat

6. Which of the following is NOT a function of the epidermis?

   A. Sweat production
   B. Protection against harmful bacteria
   C. Protection against excess water loss
   D. Protection against ultraviolet radiation

7. Which of the following organs is NOT responsible for thermoregulation?

   A. Thyroid gland
   B. Skin
   C. Kidneys
   D. All of the above are responsible for thermoregulation.

8. Where in the nephron is glucose normally reabsorbed?

   A. Bowman's capsule
   B. Proximal convoluted tubule
   C. Loop of Henle
   D. Distal convoluted tubule

9. Assuming that vasopressin release is completely blocked, which of the following will occur after aldosterone release?

   A. Slight increase or no change in blood pressure due to osmoregulation of the kidneys
   B. Decrease in urine volume
   C. Decrease in Na^+ reabsorption
   D. Decrease in K^+ secretion

10. Which of the following situations would NOT result in a higher perceived temperature?

A. A patient who just finished exercising
B. Hyperthyroidism
C. Vascular disease, which results in constriction of blood vessels in the dermis
D. Overactive sweat glands

11. A patient's urine is sweet-smelling, and she has been diagnosed as diabetic. What is the most likely reason glucose appears in her urine?

A. Glucose reabsorption in the proximal convoluted tubule has stopped occurring.
B. Glucose reabsorption in the distal convoluted tubule is not occurring.
C. There is an increased secretion of glucose across the distal convoluted tubule.
D. There is an oversaturation of glucose such that glucose transporters in the proximal tubule are overwhelmed.

12. The image below illustrates the reaction of glycogenolysis, the formation of glucose from the breakdown of glycogen. Which of the following statements is true about this process?

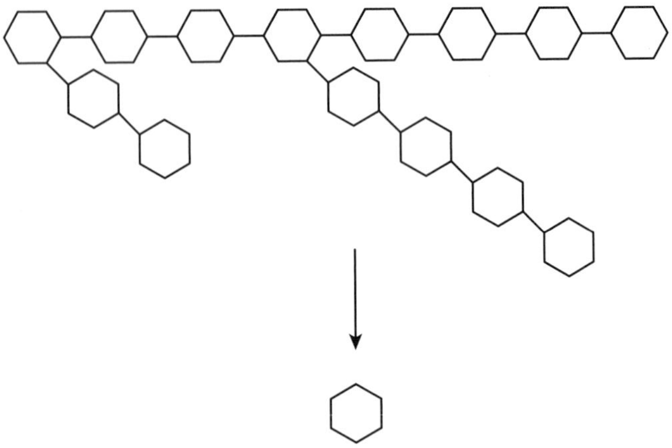

A. This process is impaired in those with impaired kidney function.
B. The reaction is stimulated by high glucose levels in the body.
C. The reaction may result in an increased production of fat.
D. The reaction is solely under hormonal control.

13. The image below illustrates the transport of glucose and sodium from the lumen of a nephron tubule to the renal interstitium. Which of the following is true about the glucose transport depicted here?

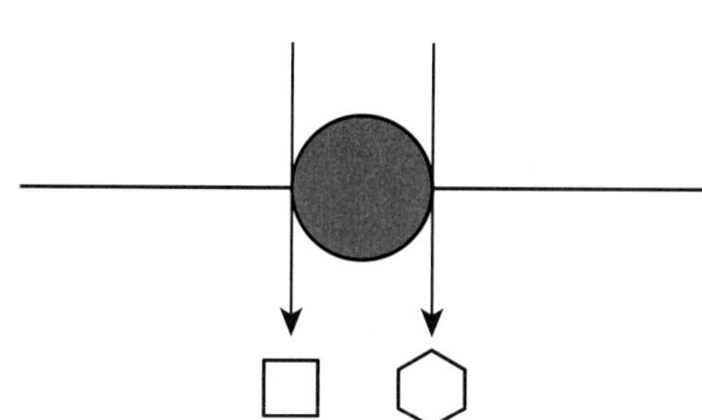

A. This transport occurs at the distal convoluted tubule of the nephron.
B. The Na^+/Glucose transporter is malfunctioning in the nephrons of all diabetic patients.
C. This transport occurs at the collecting duct of the nephron.
D. This is active transport.

14. In which section of the nephron is water NOT reabsorbed?

A. Proximal convoluted tubule
B. Descending loop of Henle
C. Ascending loop of Henle
D. Collecting duct

KEY CONCEPTS

Starling forces

Capillary filtration

Plasma proteins

Glomerular capillaries

TAKEAWAYS

As blood flows through a capillary, fluid that is lost at the arterial end is reabsorbed at the venule end when normal blood proteins are present. Changes in Starling forces alter the conditions where capillaries are present. An increase in capillary hydrostatic pressure or an increase in interstitial oncotic pressure will lead to capillary filtration. An increase in capillary oncotic pressure or interstitial hydrostatic pressure will oppose capillary filtration.

THINGS TO WATCH OUT FOR

Remember that proteins act as a solute, and water will flow to the areas of higher solute concentration.

STARLING FORCES

A patient with kidney disease has extensive damage to the glomerular capillaries. These capillaries have become permeable to plasma proteins. What other symptoms will this patient have as a result of this kidney damage?

1) Determine the effect of glomerular capillaries that are permeable to proteins.

Glomerular capillaries do not normally allow the passage of plasma proteins or red blood cells. If the capillaries are damaged so that plasma proteins enter the renal tubule, these proteins will be lost because they cannot be reabsorbed along the tubule.

---

2) Examine the forces at work on capillaries.

The relationship of the different forces at work in the capillaries is explained by Starling forces as follows. Capillary hydrostatic pressure (P_c) is blood pressure, and it is the major force in capillary filtration. Osmotic pressure is the major force that keeps fluid from leaving the capillaries and is considered the oncotic pressure (π_c) of the plasma proteins. The interstitial fluid also has hydrostatic pressure (P_i), which opposes filtration out of the capillary. The proteins of the interstitial fluid exert oncotic pressure (π_i) and tend to favor filtration out of the capillary. To recap in simpler terms, the blood pressure in the capillary tries to force fluid out the capillary, whereas the pressure of the fluid in the interstitial space tries to hold the fluid in the capillary. The proteins in the interstitial space try to "suck" fluid out of the capillary, whereas the proteins in the blood try to hold the fluid in the capillary.

When blood enters the arterial end of a capillary, the P_c pressure acts to force fluids to leave the capillary and enter the interstitial space. This loss of fluid along the capillary increases the concentration of the solute, or proteins, in the blood. This increase in oncotic pressure "pulls" fluid back into the capillary at the venous end. Any fluid that is not returned to the capillary is generally picked up by the lymphatic system.

---

3) Determine the effect when proteins are lost from the blood.

The loss of plasma proteins will cause a drop in oncotic pressure in the blood. As a result, water that leaves the arteriole end of the capillary will not be reabsorbed at the venule end. Fluid in large quantities cannot be picked up by the lymphatic system, so this fluid will remain in the interstitial space and back up in the extremities, a condition known as edema. The failure of fluid to be reabsorbed from the interstitial space also leads to a large drop in blood volume and therefore blood pressure.

SIMILAR QUESTIONS

1) What factors increase the loss of fluid to the interstitial space at the arterial end of a capillary?
2) What physiological conditions can increase capillary oncotic pressure?
3) What symptoms will patients with inadequate lymphatic function have?

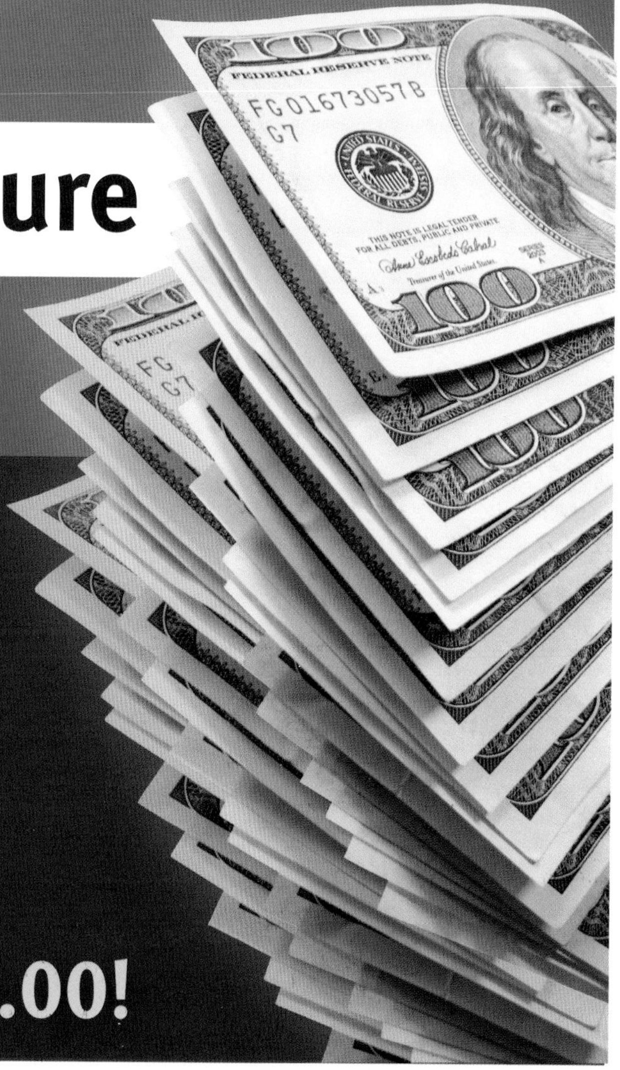

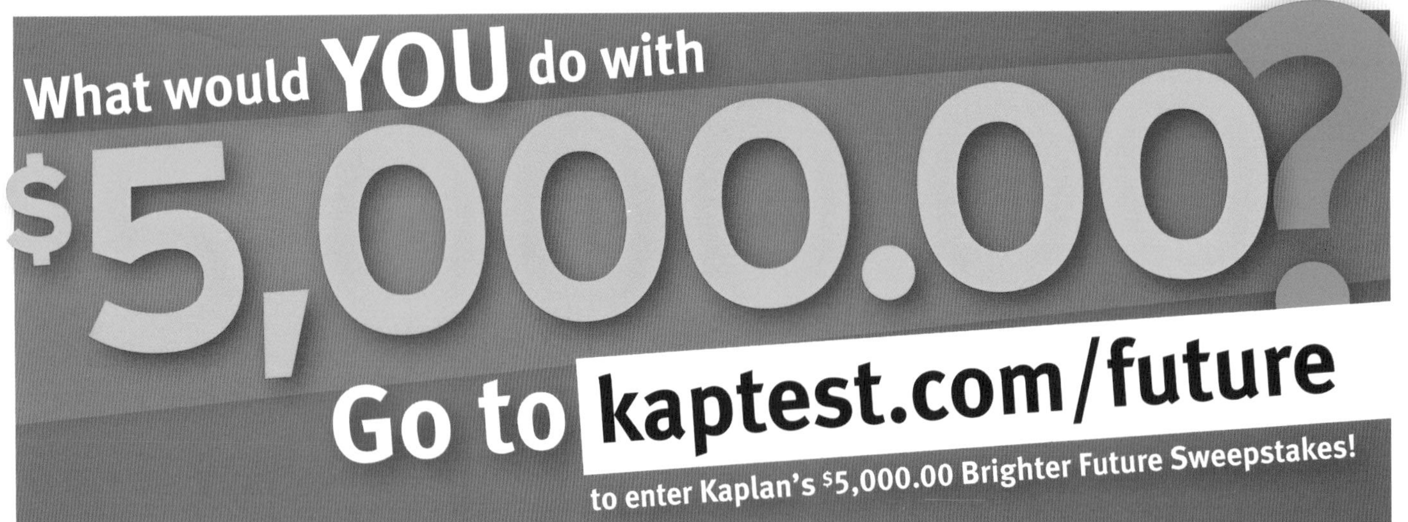
What would YOU do with
$5,000.00?
Go to kaptest.com/future
to enter Kaplan's $5,000.00 Brighter Future Sweepstakes!

Kaplan $5,000 Brighter Future Sweepstakes 2009 Complete and Official Rules

1. NO PURCHASE IS NECESSARY TO ENTER OR WIN. A PURCHASE WILL NOT INCREASE YOUR CHANCES OF WINNING.
2. PROMOTION PERIOD. The "Kaplan $5,000 Brighter Future Sweepstakes" ("Sweepstakes") commences at 6:59 A.M. EST on April 1, 2009 and ends at 11:59 P.M. EST on March 31, 2010. Entry forms can be found online at kaptest.com/brighterfuturesweeps. All online entries must be received by March 31, 2010 at 11:59 P.M. EST.
3. ELIGIBILITY. This Sweepstakes is open to legal residents of the 50 United States and the District of Columbia and Canada (excluding the Province of Quebec) who are sixteen (16) years of age or older as of April 1, 2009. Officers, directors, representatives and employees of Kaplan (from here on called "Sponsor"), its parent, affiliates or subsidiaries, or their respective advertising, promotion, publicity, production, and judging agencies and their immediate families and household members are not eligible to enter.
4. TO ENTER. To enter simply go to kaptest.com/brighterfuturesweeps and fill-out the online entry form between April 1, 2009 and March 31, 2010. As part of your entry, you will be asked to provide your first and last name, email address, permanent address and phone number, parent or legal guardian name if under eighteen (18), and the name of your undergraduate school.

LIMIT ONE ENTRY PER PERSON AND EMAIL ADDRESS. Multiple entries will be disqualified. Entries are void if they contain typographical, printing or other errors. Entries generated by a script, macro or other automated means are void. Entries that are mutilated, altered, incomplete, mechanically reproduced, tampered with, illegible, inaccurate, forged, irregular in any way, or otherwise not in compliance with these Official Rules are also void. All entries become the property of the Sponsor and will not be returned to the entrant. Sponsor and those working on its behalf will not be responsible for lost, late, misdirected or damaged mail or email or for Internet, network, computer hardware and software, phone or other technical errors, malfunctions and delays that may occur. Entries will be deemed to have been submitted by the authorized account holder of the email account from which the entry is made. The authorized account holder is the natural person to whom an email address is assigned by an Internet access provider, online service provider or other organization (e.g. business, educational institution, etc.) responsible for assigning email addresses for the domain associated with the submitted email address. By entering or accepting a prize in this Sweepstakes, entrants agree to be bound by the decisions of the judges, the Sponsor and these Official Rules and to comply with all applicable federal, state and local laws and regulations. Odds of winning depend on the number of eligible entries received.
5. WINNER SELECTION. Two (2) winners will be selected for the First Prize; two (2) winners for the Second Prize, five (5) winners for the Third Prize, five (5) winners for Fourth Prize, five (5) winners for the Fifth Prize, and 25 winners for the Sixth Prize from all eligible entries received in a random drawing to be held on or about May 11, 2010. The drawing will be conducted by an independent judge whose decisions shall be final and binding in all regards. Participants need not be present to win. Please note that if the entrant selected as the winner resides in Canada, he/she will have to correctly answer a timed, test-prep question in order to be confirmed as the winner and claim the prize.
6. WINNER NOTIFICATION AND VALIDATION. Winners of the drawing will be notified by mail within 10 days after the drawing. An Affidavit of Eligibility and Compliance with these Official Rules and a Liability and (unless prohibited) Publicity Release must be executed and returned by the potential winner within twenty-one (21) days after prize notification is sent. If the winner is under eighteen (18) years of age, the prize will be awarded to the winner's parent or legal guardian who will be required to execute an affidavit. Failure of the potential winner to complete, sign and return any requested documents within such period or the return of any prize notification or prize as undeliverable may result in disqualification and selection of an alternate winner in Sponsor's sole discretion. You are not a winner unless your submissions are validated.

In the event that a winner chooses not to accept his or her prize, does not respond to winner notification within the time period noted on the notification or does not return a completed Affidavit of Eligibility and Compliance with these Official Rules and a Liability and (unless prohibited) Publicity Release within twenty-one (21) days after prize notification is sent, the prize may be forfeited and an alternate winner selected in Sponsor's sole discretion.
7. PRIZES.
- First Prize: Two (2) winners will be selected to win $5,000.00 USD.
- Second Prize: Two (2) winners will be selected to win $1,000.00 USD.
- Third Prize: Five (5) winners will be selected to win their choice of a Free Kaplan SAT, ACT, GMAT, GRE, LSAT, MCAT, DAT, OAT, or PCAT Classroom Course (retail value up to $1,899).
- Fourth Prize: Five (5) winners will be selected to win their choice of Ten (10) Free Hours of GMAT, GRE, LSAT, MCAT, DAT, OAT, PCAT Private Tutoring (retail value of $1,500), or Ten (10) Free Hours of SAT, ACT, PSAT Premier Tutoring (retail value of $2,000).
- Fifth Prize: Five (5) winners will be selected to win their choice of Three (3) Free Hours of Admissions Consulting for Precollege (retail value of $450) or three (3) Free Hours of Business School, Law School, Grad School or Med School Admissions Consulting (retail value of $729).
- Sixth Prize: Twenty-five (25) winners will be selected to win $100.00 USD.

For winners of the Third and Fourth Prizes, the winner must redeem the course at Kaplan locations in the US offering them and have completed the program before December 31, 2012.

Prizes are not transferable. No substitution of prizes for cash or other goods and services is permitted, except Sponsor reserves the right in its sole discretion to substitute any prize with a prize of comparable value. Any applicable taxes or fees are the winner's sole responsibility. All prizes must be redeemed within 21 days of notice of award and course prizes used by December 31, 2012.
8. GENERAL CONDITIONS. By entering the Sweepstakes or accepting the Sweepstakes prize, winner accepts all the conditions, restrictions, requirements and/or regulations required by the Sponsor in connection with the Sweepstakes. Unless otherwise prohibited by law, acceptance of a prize constitutes permission to use winner's name, picture, likeness, address (city and state) and biographical information for advertising and publicity purposes for this and/or similar promotions, without prior approval or compensation. Acceptance of a prize constitutes a waiver of any claim to royalties, rights or remuneration for said use. Winner agrees to release and hold harmless the Sponsor, its parent, affiliates and subsidiaries, and each of their respective directors, officers, employees, agents, and successors from any and all claims, damages, injury, death, loss or other liability that may arise from winner's participation in the Sweepstakes or the awarding, acceptance, possession, use or misuse of the prize. Sponsor reserves the right in its sole discretion to modify or cancel all or any portions of the Sweepstakes because of technical errors or malfunctions, viruses, hackers, or for other reasons beyond Sponsor's control that impair or corrupt the Sweepstakes in any manner. In such event, Sponsor shall award prizes at random from among the eligible entries received up to the time of the impairment or corruption. Sponsor also reserves the right in its sole discretion to disqualify any entrant who fails to comply with these Official Rules, who attempts to enter the Sweepstakes in any manner or through any means other than as described in these Official Rules, or who attempts to disrupt the Sweepstakes or the kaptest.com website or to circumvent any of these Official Rules.
9. WINNERS' LIST. Starting August 15, 2010, a winners' list may be obtained by sending a self-addressed, stamped envelope to: "$5,000 Kaplan Brighter Future Sweepstakes" Winners' List, Kaplan Test Prep and Admissions Marketing Department, 1440 Broadway, 8th Floor New York, NY 10018. All winners' list requests must be received by December 1, 2010.
10. USE OF ENTRANT AND WINNER INFORMATION. The information that you provide in connection with the Sweepstakes may be used for Sponsor's and select Corporate Partners' purposes to send you information about Sponsor's and its Corporate Partners' products and services. If you would like your name removed from Sponsor's mailing list or if you do not wish to receive information from Sponsor or its Corporate Partners, write to:

Direct Marketing Department
Attn: Kaplan Brighter Future Sweepstakes Opt Out
1440 Broadway
8th Floor
New York NY 10018

11. SPONSOR. The Sponsor of this Sweepstakes is: Kaplan Test Prep and Admissions and Kaplan Publishing, 1440 Broadway, 8th Floor New York, NY 10018.
12. THIS SWEEPSTAKES IS VOID WHERE PROHIBITED, TAXED OR OTHERWISE RESTRICTED BY LAW.

CHAPTER 11

ENDOCRINE SYSTEM

The endocrine system acts as a means of internal communication, coordinating the activities of the organ systems. **Endocrine glands** (see Figure 11.1) synthesize and secrete chemical substances called **hormones** directly into the circulatory system. (In contrast, **exocrine glands,** such as the gall bladder, secrete substances that are transported by ducts.) Hormones regulate the function of **target organs** or tissues.

Teacher Tip

KEY POINT: Unlike the other organ systems we have discussed thus far, the basis of the endocrine system is ACTION AT A DISTANCE. Each organ has a local effect that is then passed though the bloodstream to affect the entire organism.

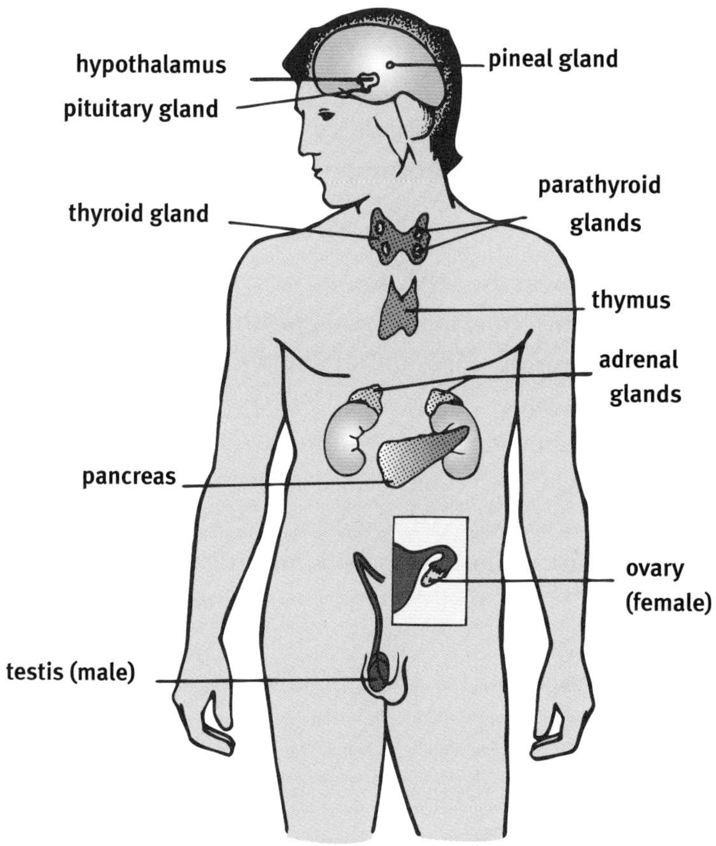

hypothalamus
pituitary gland
pineal gland
thyroid gland
parathyroid glands
thymus
adrenal glands
pancreas
ovary (female)
testis (male)

Figure 11.1. Human Endocrine System

ENDOCRINE GLANDS

Glands that synthesize and/or secrete hormones include the **pituitary, hypothalamus, thyroid, parathyroids, adrenals, pancreas, testes, ovaries, pineal, kidneys, gastrointestinal glands, heart,** and **thymus.** Some hormones regulate a single type of cell or organ, while others have more widespread actions. The specificity of hormonal action is determined by the presence of specific receptors on or in the target cells.

TEACHER TIP

While it seems like the pituitary has all the power, the anterior pituitary is being controlled by the hypothalamus directly above it. This makes the hypothalamus the "master control gland."

A. PITUITARY GLAND

The pituitary **(hypophysis)** is a small, trilobed gland lying at the base of the brain. The two main lobes, **anterior** and **posterior,** are functionally distinct. (In humans, the third lobe, the intermediate lobe, is rudimentary.)

1. Anterior Pituitary

The anterior pituitary synthesizes both direct hormones, which directly stimulate their target organs, and tropic hormones, which stimulate other endocrine glands to release hormones. The hormonal secretions of the anterior pituitary are regulated by hypothalamic secretions called **releasing/inhibiting hormones** or factors.

TEACHER TIP

Flashback to enzymes: remember that enzymes were often regulated via feedback inhibition. The endocrine system is exactly the same. As levels of the final effector molecule rise, the feedback to the hypothalamus and pituitary decrease their actions.

a. Direct hormones

- **Growth hormone (GH, somatotropin)**

  GH promotes bone and muscle growth, inhibits the uptake of glucose by certain cells, and stimulates the breakdown of **fatty acid,** thus conserving glucose. GH secretion is stimulated by the hypothalamic releasing hormone **GHRH** and inhibited by somatostatin. Secretion is also under neural and metabolic control. In children, a GH deficiency can lead to stunted growth **(dwarfism),** while overproduction of GH results in **gigantism.** Overproduction of GH in adults causes **acromegaly,** a disorder characterized by a disproportionate overgrowth of bone, localized especially in the skull, jaw, feet, and hands.

- **Prolactin**

  Prolactin stimulates milk production and secretion in female **mammary glands.**

b. Tropic hormones

- **Adrenocorticotropic hormone (ACTH)**

  ACTH stimulates the adrenal cortex to synthesize and secrete glucocorticoids and is regulated by the releasing hormone **corticotropin releasing factor (CRF).**

- **Thyroid-stimulating hormone (TSH)**
  TSH stimulates the thyroid gland to absorb iodine and then synthesize and release thyroid hormone. TSH is regulated by the releasing hormone **TRH.**

- **Luteinizing hormone (LH)**
  In females, LH stimulates ovulation and formation of the corpus luteum. In males, LH stimulates the interstitial cells of the testes to synthesize **testosterone.** LH is regulated by **estrogen, progesterone,** and **gonadotropin releasing hormone (GnRH).**

- **Follicle-stimulating hormone (FSH)**
  In females, FSH causes maturation of ovarian follicles; in males, FSH stimulates maturation of the seminiferous tubules and sperm production. FSH is regulated by estrogen and by GnRH.

EXCLUSIVE

To remember the six hormones of the anterior pituitary, think FLAT PiG:

FSH
LH
ACTH
TSH
Prolactin
i(gnore)
GH

2. Posterior Pituitary

The posterior pituitary does not synthesize hormones; it stores and releases the hormones **oxytocin** and **ADH,** which are produced by the neurosecretory cells of the hypothalamus. Hormone secretion is stimulated by action potentials descending from the hypothalamus.

TEACHER TIP

The posterior pituitary is controlled differently than the anterior. The posterior pituitary serves simply as a jumping off point for the hormones ADH and oxytocin (made in the hypothalamus) and does not make any hormones of its own.

a. Oxytocin

Oxytocin, which is secreted during childbirth, increases the strength and frequency of uterine muscle contractions. Oxytocin secretion is also induced by suckling; oxytocin stimulates milk secretion in the mammary glands.

b. Antidiuretic hormone (ADH, vasopressin)

ADH increases the permeability of the nephron's collecting duct to water, thereby promoting water reabsorption and increasing blood volume (see chapter 10). ADH is secreted when plasma osmolarity increases, as sensed by **osmoreceptors** in the hypothalamus, or when blood volume decreases, as sensed by **baroreceptors** in the circulatory system.

B. HYPOTHALAMUS

The hypothalamus is part of the forebrain and is located directly above the pituitary gland. The hypothalamus receives neural transmissions from other parts of the brain and from peripheral nerves that trigger specific responses from its neurosecretory cells. The neurosecretory cells regulate pituitary gland secretions via negative feedback mechanisms and through the actions of inhibiting and releasing hormones.

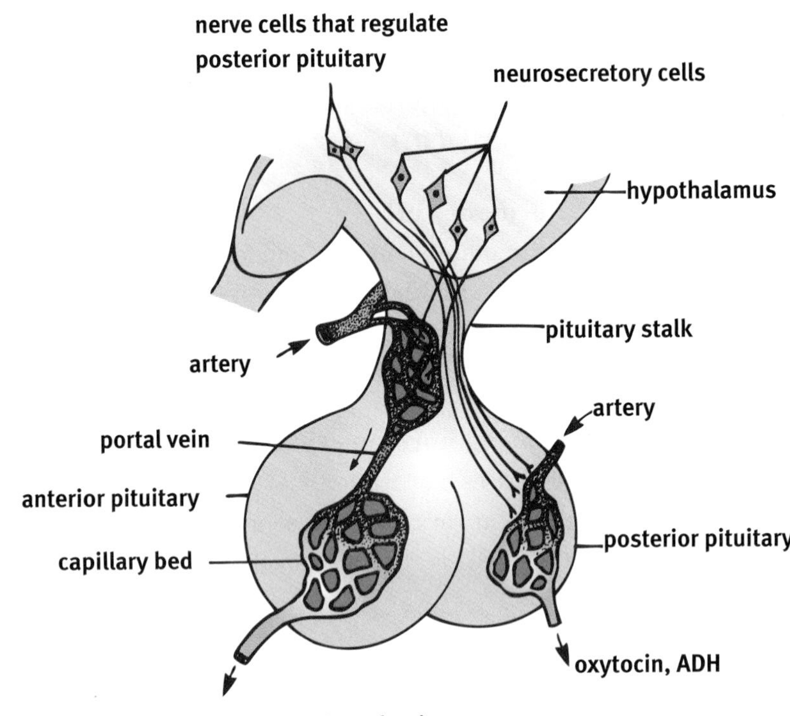

Figure 11.2. Hypothalamus and Pituitary Gland

1. Interactions with Anterior Pituitary

Hypothalamic releasing hormones are hormones that stimulate or inhibit the secretions of the anterior pituitary. For example, GnRH stimulates the anterior pituitary to secrete FSH and LH. Releasing hormones are secreted into the **hypothalamic–hypophyseal portal system** (see Figure 11.2). In this circulatory pathway, blood from the capillary bed in the hypothalamus flows through a portal vein into the anterior pituitary, where it diverges into a second capillary network. In this way, releasing hormones can immediately reach the anterior pituitary.

TEACHER TIP

While most of the hormones in the anterior pituitary require a factor from the hypothalamus to be released (e.g., GnRH for FSH and LH), prolactin is actually the opposite. As long as the hypothalamus secretes prolactin inhibitory factor (PIF, dopamine), no prolactin will be released. It is the *absence* of PIF that allows for prolactin release. This fact is worth knowing for Test Day.

Oversecretion of hormones is potentially harmful to an organism and so a preventive mechanism, called **negative feedback,** has evolved (see chapter 2). A high hormone level inhibits further production of that hormone. For example, when plasma levels of adrenal cortical hormones reach a critical level, the hormones themselves exert an inhibitory effect on the pituitary and on the hypothalamus, inhibiting CRF and ACTH release. In the absence of CRF, the anterior pituitary stops ACTH secretion, and the adrenal cortex stops secreting adrenal cortical hormones. When adrenal hormone levels are too low, the hypothalamus is stimulated to release CRF. This stimulates the anterior pituitary to secrete

ACTH, which, in turn, stimulates the adrenal cortex to release adrenal cortical hormones (see Figure 11.3).

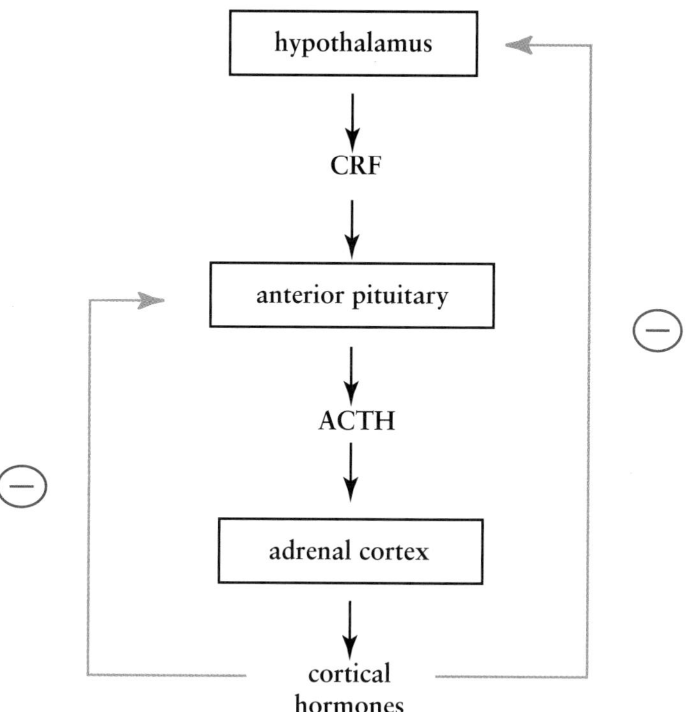

Figure 11.3. Negative Feedback Mechanism

2. Interactions with Posterior Pituitary

Neurosecretory cells in the hypothalamus synthesize both oxytocin and ADH and transport them via their axons into the posterior pituitary for storage and secretion.

C. THYROID GLAND

The thyroid gland is a bilobed structure located on the ventral surface of the trachea. It produces and secretes **thyroxine, triiodothyronine (the thyroid hormones),** and **calcitonin.**

1. Thyroid Hormones (Thyroxine and Triiodothyronine)

Thyroxine (**T_4**) and triiodothyronine (**T_3**) are derived from the iodination of the amino acid tyrosine. Thyroid hormones are necessary for growth and neurological development in children. They increase the rate of cellular respiration and the rate of protein and fatty acid synthesis and degradation in many tissues. High plasma levels of thyroid hormones inhibit TRH and TSH secretion, thereby returning plasma levels to normal.

TEACHER TIP

Iodine is absolutely required for the thyroid to carry out its function. In the Western world, shortage of iodine is very rare, as most salt is now iodized.

MCAT SYNOPSIS

PTH increases Ca^{2+}
CalciTONIN decreases Ca^{2+}
(CalciTONIN tones down Ca^{2+})

If you remember this simple principle, you'll be able to PREDICT their respective effects on bone, intestinal absorption of calcium and urinary excretion/reabsorption of calcium. You don't need to memorize anything, just THINK.

Inflammation of the thyroid or iodine deficiency causes **hypothyroidism,** in which thyroid hormones are undersecreted or not secreted at all. Common symptoms of hypothyroidism include a slowed heart rate and respiratory rate, fatigue, cold intolerance, and weight gain. Hypothyroidism in newborn infants, called **cretinism,** is characterized by mental retardation and short stature. In **hyperthyroidism,** the thyroid is overstimulated, resulting in the oversecretion of thyroid hormones. Symptoms often include increased metabolic rate, feelings of excessive warmth, profuse sweating, palpitations, weight loss, and protruding eyes. In both disorders, the thyroid often enlarges, forming a bulge in the neck called a **goiter.**

2. Calcitonin

Calcitonin decreases plasma Ca^{2+} concentration by inhibiting the release of Ca^{2+} from bone. Calcitonin secretion is regulated by plasma Ca^{2+} levels.

TEACHER TIP

Just like insulin and glucagon, which are secreted from the pancreas, PTH and calcitonin are antagonistic to one another. Think of them in pairs. Their primary function is to regulate calcium levels in the blood.

D. PARATHYROID GLANDS

The parathyroid glands are four small pea-shaped structures embedded in the posterior surface of the thyroid. These glands synthesize and secrete **parathyroid hormone (PTH),** which, together with calcitonin and vitamin D, regulates plasma Ca^{2+} concentration. In turn, the plasma Ca^{2+} concentration regulates PTH secretion by means of a negative feedback mechanism. PTH raises the Ca^{2+} concentration in the blood by stimulating Ca^{2+} release from bone and decreasing Ca^{2+} excretion in the kidneys. In addition, PTH converts vitamin D into its active form, which stimulates intestinal calcium absorption.

E. ADRENAL GLANDS

The adrenal glands are situated on top of the kidneys and consist of the **adrenal cortex** and the **adrenal medulla.**

1. Adrenal Cortex

In response to stress, ACTH stimulates the adrenal cortex to synthesize and secrete the steroid hormones, which are collectively known as **corticosteroids.** The corticosteroids, derived from cholesterol, include **glucocorticoids, mineralocorticoids,** and **cortical sex hormones.**

MCAT SYNOPSIS

Yet another "good" function of cholesterol: key precursor for steroid hormones.

a. Glucocorticoids

Glucocorticoids, such as **cortisol** and **cortisone,** are involved in glucose regulation and protein metabolism. Glucocorticoids raise blood glucose levels by promoting gluconeogenesis and decrease protein synthesis. They also reduce the body's immunological and inflammatory responses. Cortisol secretion is governed by a negative feedback mechanism.

b. Mineralocorticoids

Mineralocorticoids, particularly **aldosterone,** regulate plasma levels of sodium and potassium and, consequently, the total extracellular water volume. Aldosterone causes active reabsorption of sodium and passive reabsorption of water in the nephron (see chapter 10). This results in a rise in both blood volume and blood pressure. Aldosterone also stimulates the secretion of potassium ion and hydrogen ion into the nephron and their subsequent excretion in urine.

TEACHER TIP

Too much volume in the vasculature results in high blood pressure (hypertension). One way to relieve this is to decrease the volume of fluid by preventing the kidneys from reabsorbing as much fluid. Certain drugs known as ACE-inhibitors do this by preventing the conversion of angiotensin I to angiotensin II. This prevents aldosterone from being released and salt and water are not reabsorbed, thereby decreasing fluid volume.

Aldosterone secretion is regulated by the **renin-angiotensin** system. When blood volume falls, the juxtaglomerular cells of the kidney produce **renin**—an enzyme that converts the plasma protein **angiotensinogen** to **angiotensin I.** Angiotensin I is converted to **angiotensin II,** which stimulates the adrenal cortex to secrete aldosterone. Aldosterone helps to restore blood volume by increasing sodium reabsorption at the kidney, leading to an increase in water reabsorption. This removes the initial stimulus for renin production.

c. Cortical sex hormones

The adrenal cortex secretes small quantities of **androgens** (male sex hormones) in both males and females. Because, in males, most of the androgens are produced by the testes, the physiologic effect of the adrenal androgens is quite small. In females, however, overproduction of the adrenal androgens may have masculinizing effects, such as excessive facial hair.

2. Adrenal Medulla

The secretory cells of the adrenal medulla can be viewed as specialized sympathetic nerve cells that secrete hormones into the circulatory system. The adrenal medulla produces **epinephrine (adrenaline)** and **norepinephrine (noradrenaline),** both of which belong to a class of amino acid-derived compounds called **catecholamines.** Epinephrine increases the conversion of glycogen to glucose in liver and muscle tissue, causing a rise in blood glucose levels and an increase in the basal metabolic rate. Both epinephrine and norepinephrine increase the rate and strength of the heartbeat and dilate and constrict blood vessels in such a way as to increase the blood supply to skeletal muscle,

FLASHBACK

The secretions of the exocrine pancreas (see chapter 7) are components of the pancreatic juice that enters into the duodenum:

- Amylase (carbohydrate digestion)
- Lipase (lipid digestion)
- Trypsin, chymotrypsin and carboxypeptidase (protein digestion)

the heart, and the brain, while decreasing the blood supply to the kidneys, skin, and digestive tract. These effects are known as the **"fight or flight response,"** and are elicited by sympathetic nervous stimulation in response to stress. Both of these hormones are also neurotransmitters (see chapter 12).

F. PANCREAS

The pancreas is both an exocrine organ and an endocrine organ. The exocrine function is performed by the cells that secrete digestive enzymes into the small intestine via a series of ducts. The endocrine function is performed by small glandular structures called the **islets of Langerhans,** which are composed of **alpha, beta,** and **delta cells.** Alpha cells produce and secrete **glucagon**; beta cells produce and secrete **insulin**; delta cells produce and secrete **somatostatin.**

MCAT SYNOPSIS

Insulin decreases plasma glucose. Glucagon increases plasma glucose.

Don't forget that growth hormone, the glucocorticoids, and epinephrine are also capable of increasing plasma glucose.

1. Glucagon

Glucagon stimulates protein and fat degradation, the conversion of glycogen to glucose, and gluconeogenesis, all of which serve to increase blood glucose levels. Glucagon secretion is stimulated by a decrease in blood glucose and by gastrointestinal hormones (e.g., CCK and gastrin) and is inhibited by high plasma glucose levels. Glucagon's actions are largely antagonistic to those of insulin.

TEACHER TIP

There are two types of diabetes. One is due to auto-immune destruction of the beta cells of the pancreas (type I) while the other is due to the body resisting the effects of insulin (type II).

2. Insulin

Insulin is a protein hormone secreted in response to a high blood glucose concentration. It stimulates the uptake of glucose by muscle and adipose cells and the storage of glucose as glycogen in muscle and liver cells, thus lowering blood glucose levels (see Figure 11.4). It also stimulates the synthesis of fats from glucose and the uptake of amino acids. Insulin's actions are antagonistic to those of glucagon and the glucocorticoids. Insulin secretion is regulated by blood glucose levels. Overproduction of insulin causes **hypoglycemia** (low blood glucose levels). Underproduction of insulin, or an insensitivity to insulin, leads to **diabetes mellitus,** which is characterized by **hyperglycemia** (high blood glucose levels). High blood glucose levels lead to excretion of glucose and water loss. In addition, diabetes is associated with weakness and fatigue, and may lead to **ketoacidosis,** which is a dangerous lowering of blood pH due to excess keto acids and fatty acids in the plasma.

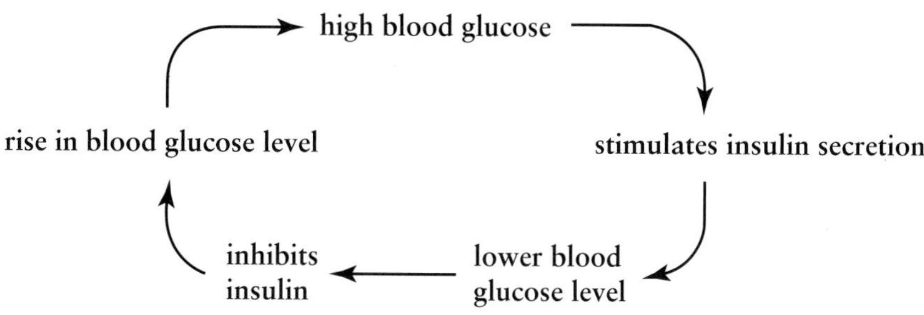

Figure 11.4. Regulation of Insulin Secretion

NOTE

Somatostatin is always inhibitory, regardless of where it acts.

3. Somatostatin

Pancreatic somatostatin secretion is increased by high blood glucose or high amino acid levels, leading to both decreased insulin and glucagon secretion. Somatostatin is also regulated by CCK and GH levels.

G. TESTES

The interstitial cells of the testes produce and secrete androgens, e.g., testosterone (see chapter 4). Testosterone induces embryonic sexual differentiation and male sexual development at puberty and maintains secondary sex characteristics. Testosterone secretion is controlled by a negative feedback mechanism involving FSH and LH. Insensitivity to testosterone results in a syndrome called **testicular feminization,** in which a genetic male (XY) has female secondary sexual characteristics.

H. OVARIES

The ovaries synthesize and secrete estrogens and progesterone. The secretion of both estrogens and progesterone is regulated by LH and FSH, which, in turn, are regulated by GnRH.

1. Hormones

a. Estrogens

Estrogens are steroid hormones necessary for normal female maturation. They stimulate the development of the female reproductive tract and contribute to the development of secondary sexual characteristics and sex drive. Estrogens are also responsible for the thickening of the **endometrium** (uterine wall). Estrogens are secreted by the ovarian follicles and the **corpus luteum.**

TEACHER TIP

The MCAT likes to test your ability to identify FSH, LH, estrogen, and progesterone throughout the menstrual cycle. Be sure to know when each peaks.

b. Progesterone

Progesterone is a steroid hormone secreted by the corpus luteum during the luteal phase of the menstrual cycle. Progesterone stimulates the development and maintenance of the endometrial walls in preparation for implantation.

2. The Menstrual Cycle

The hormonal secretions of the ovaries, the hypothalamus, and the pituitary play important roles in the female reproductive cycle. From **puberty** through **menopause,** interactions between these hormones result in a monthly cyclical pattern known as the **menstrual cycle.** The menstrual cycle may be divided into the **follicular phase, ovulation,** the **luteal phase,** and **menstruation** (see Figure 11.5).

a. Follicular phase

The follicular phase begins with the cessation of the **menstrual flow** from the previous cycle. During this phase, FSH and LH act together to promote the development of several ovarian follicles, which grow and begin secreting estrogen. Rising levels of estrogen in the latter half of this phase stimulate GnRH secretion, which in turn further stimulates LH secretion.

> **MCAT SYNOPSIS**
>
> - Follicles mature during the follicular phase (FSH, LH).
> - The LH surge at midcycle triggers ovulation.
> - A ruptured follicle becomes corpus luteum and secretes estrogen and progesterone to build up uterine lining in preparation for implantation; LH and FSH inhibited.
> - If fertilization doesn't occur, corpus luteum atrophies, progesterone and estrogen levels decrease, menses occurs, and LH and FSH levels begin to rise again.

b. Ovulation

Midway through the cycle **ovulation** occurs—a mature ovarian follicle bursts and releases an **ovum.** Ovulation is caused by a surge in LH which is preceded by and, in part, caused by a peak in estrogen levels.

c. Luteal phase

Following ovulation, LH induces the ruptured follicle to develop into the corpus luteum, which secretes estrogen and progesterone. Progesterone causes the glands of the endometrium to mature and produce secretions that prepare it for the implantation of an embryo. Progesterone and estrogen are essential for the maintenance of the endometrium. Progesterone and estrogen together inhibit secretion of GnRH, thereby inhibiting LH and FSH secretion. This prevents the maturation of additional follicles during the remainder of the cycle.

d. Menstruation

If the ovum is not fertilized, the corpus luteum atrophies. The resulting drop in progesterone and estrogen levels causes the endometrium (with its superficial blood vessels) to slough off, giving rise to the menstrual flow **(menses).** Progesterone and estrogen levels decline and GnRH is no longer inhibited. GnRH restimulates LH and FSH secretion, and so the cycle begins anew. However, if the ovum is fertilized, menstruation ceases for the duration of the pregnancy.

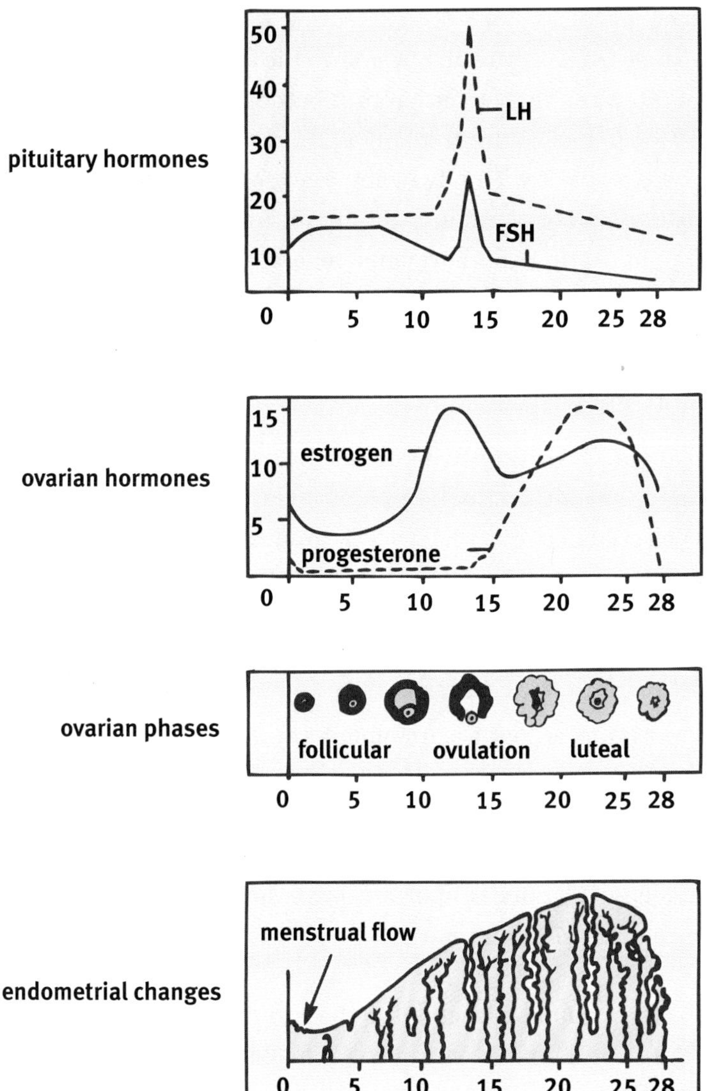

Figure 11.5. The Menstrual Cycle

CLINICAL CORRELATE

Oral contraceptive pills (OCPs) are simply estrogen and progesterone preparations. They block conception by inhibiting LH and FSH release (negative feedback), thereby inhibiting ovulation.

TEACHER TIP

Flashback to embryology: Recall that a woman is born with all of her eggs frozen in meiosis I. No new eggs are generated during a woman's lifetime. Following menarche and until puberty, one egg per month will complete meiosis I and begin meiosis II. This egg will be ovulated and, if fertilized, will rapidly complete meiosis II before combining with the sperm's genetic material to create a zygote.

3. Pregnancy

During the first trimester of pregnancy, the corpus luteum is preserved by **human chorionic gonadotropin (HCG),** a hormone produced by the blastocyst and the developing placenta. Hence, progesterone and estrogen secretion by the corpus luteum is maintained during the first trimester. During the second trimester, HCG levels decline, but progesterone and estrogen levels rise, since they are now secreted by the placenta itself. High levels of progesterone and estrogen inhibit GnRH secretion, thus preventing FSH and LH secretion and the onset of a new menstrual cycle.

CLINICAL CORRELATE

Urine pregnancy tests, including the home variety, are designed to test for the presence of HCG in the urine. HCG can be detected in the urine one to two weeks after conception.

4. Menopause

Menopause is the period in a woman's life (usually between the ages of 45 and 55) when menstruation first becomes irregular and eventually stops. Menopause is the result of a progressive decline in the functioning of the ovaries with advancing age; some follicles fail to rupture, ovulation does not occur, and less estrogen is produced by the ovaries, thereby disrupting the hormonal regulation of other glands. Women undergoing menopause may experience symptoms such as bloating, hot flashes, and headaches.

I. PINEAL GLAND

The pineal gland is a tiny structure at the base of the brain that secretes the hormone **melatonin.** The role of melatonin in humans is unclear, but it is believed to play a role in the regulation of **circadian rhythms**—physiological cycles lasting 24 hours. Melatonin secretion is regulated by light and dark cycles in the environment.

J. OTHER ENDOCRINE ORGANS

Glandular tissue is found throughout the mucosa of the stomach and intestines. The primary stimulus for gastrointestinal hormone release is the presence of food in the gut, though neural input and exposure to other hormones also affect their release. Over 20 gastrointestinal peptides have been isolated; important examples are gastrin, secretin, and CCK (see chapter 7).

Clinical Correlate

Patients with chronic kidney disease can become anemic due to impaired erythropoietin production, causing inadequate red cell production from the bone marrow. Recently, genetically engineered erythropoietin has been employed to stimulate the bone marrow to produce more red blood cells in such patients.

Although the primary function of the kidneys is urine formation (see chapter 10), special cells within the kidneys have important endocrine functions. **Renin,** an enzyme secreted by the kidney, is involved in the regulation of aldosterone secretion. **Erythropoietin** is secreted by the kidney in response to decreased renal oxygen levels and stimulates bone marrow to produce red blood cells.

It has also been discovered that the heart and brain are endocrine organs; they release **atrial natriuretic hormone (ANH) and brain natriuretic peptide (BNP),** respectively. ANH and BNP are involved in the regulation of salt and water balance.

The thymus gland is located in the front neck region and secretes hormones such as **thymosin** during childhood. Thymosin stimulates T lymphocyte development and differentiation (see chapter 9). The thymus atrophies by adulthood, after the immune system has fully developed. See Table 11.1 for a listing of the principal hormones.

Table 11.1. Principal Hormones in Humans

Hormone	Source	Action
Growth hormone	Anterior pituitary	Stimulates bone and muscle growth
Prolactin	Anterior pituitary	Stimulates milk production and secretion
Adrenocorticotropic hormone (ACTH)	Anterior pituitary	Stimulates the adrenal cortex to synthesize and secrete glucocorticoids
Thyroid-stimulating hormone (TSH)	Anterior pituitary	Stimulates the thyroid to produce thyroid hormones
Luteinizing hormone (LH)	Anterior pituitary	Stimulates ovulation in females; testosterone synthesis in males
Follicle-stimulating hormone (FSH)	Anterior pituitary	Stimulates follicle maturation in females; spermatogenesis in males
Oxytocin	Hypothalamus; stored in posterior pituitary	Stimulates uterine contractions during labor, and milk secretion during lactation
Vasopressin (ADH)	Hypothalamus; stored in posterior pituitary	Stimulates water reabsorption in kidneys
Thyroid hormone	Thyroid	Stimulates metabolic activity
Calcitonin	Thyroid	Decreases the blood calcium level
Parathyroid hormone	Parathyroid	Increases the blood calcium level
Glucocorticoids	Adrenal cortex	Increase blood glucose level and decreases protein synthesis
Mineralocorticoids	Adrenal cortex	Increase water reabsorption in the kidneys
Epinephrine and Norepinephrine	Adrenal medulla	Increase blood glucose level and heart rate
Glucagon	Pancreas	Stimulates conversion of glycogen to glucose in the liver; increases blood glucose
Insulin	Pancreas	Lowers blood glucose and increases storage of glycogen
Somatostatin	Pancreas	Suppresses secretion of glucagon and insulin
Testosterone	Testis	Maintains male secondary sexual characteristics
Estrogen	Ovary/placenta	Maintains female secondary sexual characteristics
Progesterone	Ovary/placenta	Promotes growth/maintenance of endometrium
Melatonin	Pineal	Unclear in humans
Atrial natriuretic hormone	Heart	Involved in osmoregulation
Thymosin	Thymus	Stimulates T lymphocyte development

MECHANISMS OF HORMONE ACTION

Hormones are classified on the basis of their chemical structure into three major groups: **peptide hormones, steroid hormones,** and **amino acid-derived hormones.** There are two ways in which hormones affect the activities of their target cells: via extracellular receptors or intracellular receptors.

A. PEPTIDES: SECONDARY MESSENGER

Peptide hormones range from simple short peptides (amino acid chains) such as ADH, to complex polypeptides such as insulin. Synthesis of peptide hormones begins with the synthesis of a large polypeptide (see chapter 14). The polypeptide is then cleaved into smaller protein units and transported to the Golgi apparatus, where it is further modified into the active hormone. The hormone is packaged into secretory vesicles and stored until it is released by the cell via exocytosis.

MCAT Synopsis

Peptide hormones:

- Surface receptors
- Generally act as first messengers

Steroid hormones:

- Intracellular receptors
- Hormone/receptor binding to DNA promotes transcription of specific genes

Peptide hormones act as **first messengers.** Their binding to specific receptors on the surface of their target cells triggers a series of enzymatic reactions within each cell, the first of which may be the conversion of ATP to **cyclic adenosine monophosphate (cAMP)**; this reaction is catalyzed by the membrane-bound enzyme **adenylate cyclase.** Cyclic AMP acts as a **second messenger,** relaying messages from the extracellular peptide hormone to cytoplasmic enzymes and initiating a series of successive reactions in the cell. This is an example of a **cascade effect**; with each step, the hormone's effects are amplified. Cyclic AMP activity is inactivated by the cytoplasmic enzyme **phosphodiesterase.**

B. STEROIDS: PRIMARY MESSENGER

Teacher Tip

Flashback to the cell: Membrane trafficking is an MCAT favorite. The differences in the precursor molecules for steroid and peptide hormones governs their ability to cross membranes, which in turn controls where their receptors exist, which in turn affects what type of effects they will have on the cell.

Steroid hormones, such as estrogen and aldosterone, belong to a class of lipid-derived molecules with a characteristic ring structure. They are produced by the testes, ovaries, placenta, and adrenal cortex. In the synthesis of steroid molecules, precursors already present in the cell (such as cholesterol) undergo enzymatic reactions that convert them into active hormones. Steroid hormones pass through the cell membrane with ease because they are lipid-soluble. Steroid hormones are not stored, but are secreted at a rate determined by their rate of synthesis.

Steroid hormones enter their target cells directly and bind to specific receptor proteins in the cytoplasm. This receptor-hormone complex enters the nucleus and directly activates the expression of specific genes by binding to receptors on the chromatin. This induces a change in mRNA transcription and protein synthesis.

C. AMINO ACID DERIVATIVES

Amino acid derivatives are hormones composed of one or two modified amino acids. They are synthesized in the cytoplasm of glandular cells. Some are further modified and stored in granules until the cell is stimulated to release them, while others are initially synthesized as component parts of larger molecules and stored.

Some amino acid–derived hormones, such as epinephrine, activate their target cells as peptide hormones do; i.e., via second messengers. Others, such as thyroxine, act in the same manner as steroid hormones, entering the nucleus of their target cells and regulating gene expression.

PRACTICE QUESTIONS

Questions 1 and 2 refer to the paragraph below.

Antidiuretic hormone (ADH) is a peptide hormone produced in the hypothalamus and released by the posterior pituitary in response to an increase in serum osmolarity. Diabetes insipidus is a disease characterized by a physical or functional lack of antidiuretic hormone and production of dilute urine.

1. One would expect which of the following derangements in a patient with diabetes insipidus?

A. Increase in urine osmolarity
B. Decrease in serum osmolarity
C. Increase in serum glucose
D. Decrease in urine osmolarity

2. Given the symptoms of diabetes insipidus, one would expect ADH to act on

A. Na/K/Cl channels in the Loop of Henle.
B. NaCl channels in the distal collecting tubule.
C. H_2O channels in the distal collecting tubule and collecting duct.
D. Na/H channels in the proximal tubule.

3. Which of the following hormonal abnormalities most likely accounts for an elevated heart rate?

A. Elevated estrogen
B. Elevated growth hormone
C. Decreased aldosterone
D. Increased T_3

4. Thyroid hormone exerts its effects by

A. direct elevation of cyclic AMP.
B. direct augmentation of gene transcription.
C. indirect elevation of cyclic AMP.
D. indirect depression of phosphodiesterase.

5. Exogenous administration of T_4 is as efficacious as T_3 in treating hypothyroidism because of

A. adequate iodine intake.
B. adequate levels of deiodinase.
C. adequate levels of thyroperoxidase.
D. circulating levels of thyroglobulin.

6. Which of the following observations would be expected in the thyroid gland if serum calcium levels were to rise?

A. Increased activation of the second messenger pathway leading to an increase in calcitonin secretion
B. Decreased activation of the second messenger pathway leading to a decrease in calcitonin secretion
C. Reduced calcium influx into the cell leading stimulation of calcitonin release
D. Decreased transmembrane potentials across C cells of the thyroid leading to stimulation of calcitonin release

	1	A
X	2	B
	3	A
X	4	A
X	5	A
X	6	D
	7	C
X	8	B
	9	A
	10	B
	11	A
	12	B
	13	B
	14	D
X	15	B
X	16	A
	17	A
X	18	D
	19	D
	20	D
	21	A
	22	D
	23	A
	24	D
	25	B
	26	B
	27	D
	28	C
X	29	B
X	30	A
	31	D
X	32	D

X	33	C
	34	B
	35	A
	36	A
X	37	A
X	38	C
X	39	C
X	40	B
	41	C
X	42	B
	43	B
X	44	D
X	45	C
X	46	D
X	47	B
	48	B
X	49	D
	50	A
X	51	D
X	52	C

80 - 55 = 25

80 / 25 = 3

7. $GLUT_4$ is the main transporter of glucose into cells following the administration of insulin. Given that $GLUT_4$ is thought to be a glucose/sodium symporter, which of the following changes in extracellular concentrations would you expect after the administration of insulin and glucose?

	Sodium	Potassium	Glucose
A.	Increase	Increase	Increase
B.	Increase	Increase	Decrease
C.	Increase	Decrease	Increase
D.	Decrease	Increase	Increase
E.	Decrease	Decrease	Increase

8. The secretory endometrium is maintained by the change of hormone levels in which of the following patterns?

	Estrogen	Progesterone	FSH
A.	Decrease	No change	No change
B.	No change	Decrease	No change
C.	No change	No change	Increase
D.	Increase	Increase	No change
E.	Increase	Increase	Decrease

9. Administration of steroids exacerbates hyperglycemia secondary to type II diabetes by which of the following mechanisms?

A. Inhibition of white blood cell migration to the source of injury
B. Induction of pancreatic beta cell destruction
C. Induction of lipolysis and glycogenolysis in the liver
D. Augmentation of muscle mass leading to increased demand for glucose

10. Stimulation of glucose metabolism is a direct effect of which of the following hormones?

	Thyroid Hormone	Growth Hormone	Estrogen
A.	+	–	–
B.	–	+	–
C.	–	–	+
D.	+	+	–
E.	+	+	+

11. Radioactive iodine (I_{131}) would be likely to destroy cells in which of the following organs?

A. Kidney
B. Lung
C. Thyroid
D. Liver

12. Whereas norepinephrine is synthesized in many parts of the body to mediate the fight-or-flight response in animals, it is made into epinephrine in the

A. hypothalamus.
B. anterior pituitary.
C. posterior pituitary.
D. adrenal medulla.

13. Menstruation generally does not occur once a pregnancy has been established because of the inhibitory effects of

A. testosterone secretion from the placenta.
B. estrogen and progesterone secretion from the corpus luteum.
C. beta-HCG secretion from the corpus luteum.
D. estrogen secretion from the uterine lining.

14. Drugs with dopaminergic antagonist activity are commonly used to treat the symptoms of many psychotic diseases. Which of the following side effects is most commonly seen with use of these drugs?

    A. Parkinsonism
    B. Impaired lactogenesis
    C. Uterine contractions
    D. Increased blood pressure

15. Primary aldosteronism, a condition in which unusually high levels of aldosterone are produced from the adrenal cortex, would likely cause which of the following electrolyte abnormalities?

    A. Low sodium (hyponatremia)
    B. Low potassium (hypokalemia)
    C. Low blood pressure (hypotension)
    D. High levels of angiotensin II

16. The following lab results reflect which of the following conditions?

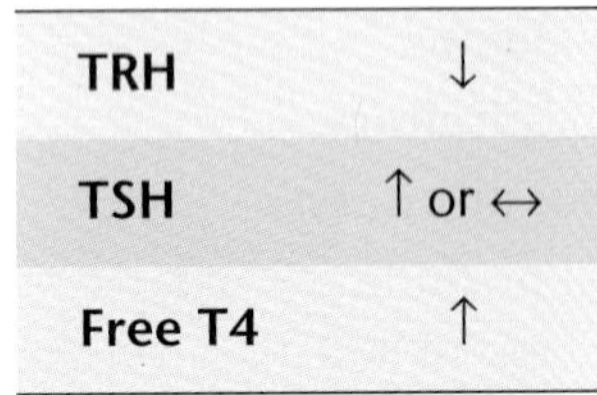

TRH	↓
TSH	↑ or ↔
Free T4	↑

    A. Primary hyperthyroidism
    B. Secondary hyperthyroidism
    C. Tertiary hyperthyroidism
    D. Primary hypothyroidism

17. Prepubertal exposure to estrogen would cause which of the following?

    A. Early onset of regular menses
    B. Axillary hair eruption
    C. Breast development
    D. Uterine contraction

18. Administration of progesterone daily prevents pregnancy primarily by which of the following mechanisms?

    A. Thickening the endometrial lining
    B. Inhibiting cholesterol synthesis in the ovary
    C. Contracting the uterus to prevent implantation
    D. Impairing sperm motility through the uterus and fallopian tubes

19. PTH secretion causes a rise in serum calcium by which of the following mechanisms?

    A. Increased cardiac muscle activity
    B. Release of protein bound calcium in the blood
    C. Release of stored calcium from GI mucosal cells
    D. Increased osteoclastic activity in the bone

MENSTRUAL CYCLE

During the follicular phase of the menstrual cycle, a dominant follicle is produced that secretes estrogen. If this follicle produces normal amounts of estrogen during the early days of its maturity but declines in estrogen production by day 10 of the menstrual cycle, what would be the result?

1) Visualize the menstrual cycle, focusing on the follicular phase.

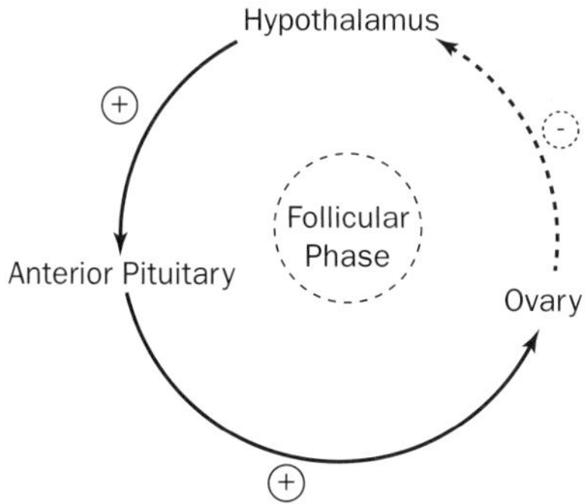

In the follicular phase, the hypothalamus secretes GnRH, which acts on the anterior pituitary to promote the release of FSH. FSH acts on the ovary and promotes the development of several ovarian follicles. The mature follicle begins secreting estrogen.

---

2) Determine the normal role of estrogen up until day 10.

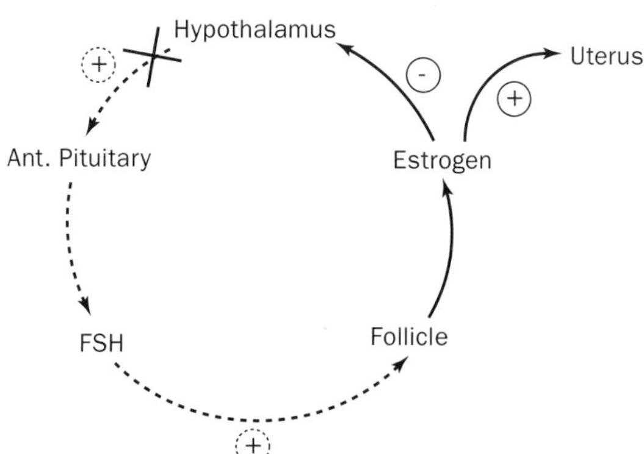

Estrogen has both positive and negative feedback effects in the menstrual cycle. Early in the follicular phase, the estrogen acts on the uterus, causing vascularization of the uterine wall. It also acts in a negative feedback loop to

KEY CONCEPTS

Menstrual cycle

FSH

LH

Estrogen

Progesterone

Positive/negative feedback

TAKEAWAYS

It is important to have a good understanding of the normal way that systems such as the menstrual cycle function. Using that knowledge, different variables, such as disease or dysfunction, can be applied to the system and the results of that dysfunction can be found in a methodical way.

inhibit the release of FSH from the anterior pituitary in order to prevent the development of multiple eggs. Because the question stem states that early levels of estrogen are normal, vascularization of the uterus and inhibition of FSH will both occur normally.

---

3) Determine the normal role of estrogen after day 10.

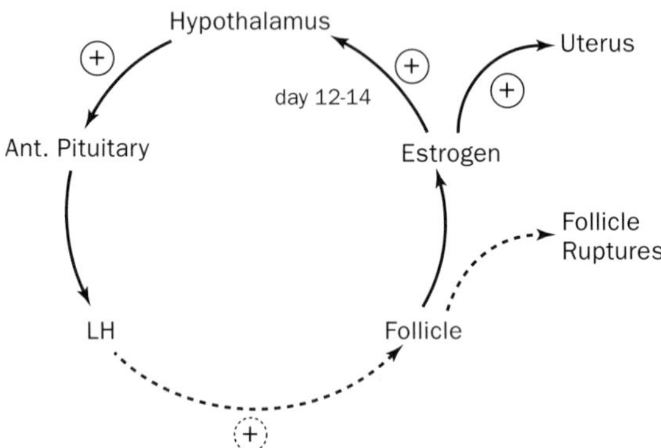

The question also states that estrogen levels decline after day 10. Now focus on the role of estrogen after day 10. Estrogen levels increase rapidly around day 12 of the cycle, and this burst of estrogen has a positive feedback effect on the secretion of FSH and LH. This results in the LH surge. The LH surge is responsible for ovulation, or the release of an egg.

---

4) Examine the consequence a decrease in estrogen after day 10.

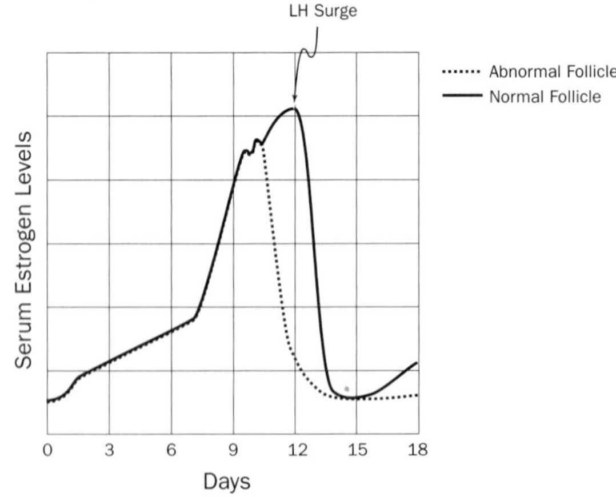

Therefore, if estrogen levels decrease after day 10 rather than increase as they normally should, then there will be no ovulation.

THINGS TO WATCH OUT FOR

Estrogen has both negative and positive feedback effects on FSH and LH at different times in the menstrual cycle. Remember that estrogen levels fall dramatically after the LH surge but rise again during the luteal phase. During this phase, however, both estrogen and progesterone are now produced by the corpus luteum, and both have a negative feedback effect.

SIMILAR QUESTIONS

1) At what point in the follicular phase is FSH inhibited?
2) What are the actions of estrogen in the follicular phase of the menstrual cycle?
3) How can ovulation during the menstrual cycle be prevented?

CHAPTER 12

NERVOUS SYSTEM

The nervous system enables organisms to receive and respond to **stimuli** from their external and internal environments. **Neurons** are the functional units of the nervous system. A neuron converts stimuli into electrochemical signals that are conducted through the nervous system.

NEURONS

A. STRUCTURE

The neuron is an elongated cell consisting of **dendrites,** a **cell body,** and an **axon.** Dendrites are cytoplasmic extensions that receive information and transmit it toward the cell body. The cell body **(soma)** contains the nucleus and controls the metabolic activity of the neuron. The **axon hillock** connects the cell body to the axon (nerve fiber), which is a long cellular process that transmits impulses away from the cell body. Most mammalian axons are ensheathed by an insulating substance known as **myelin,** which allows axons to conduct impulses faster. Myelin is produced by cells known as **glial cells.** (**Oligodendrocytes** produce myelin in the central nervous system, and **Schwann cells** produce myelin in the peripheral nervous system.) The gaps between segments of myelin are called **nodes of Ranvier.** Ultimately, the axons end as swellings known as **synaptic terminals** (sometimes also called synaptic boutons or knobs) (see Figure 12.1). Neurotransmitters are released from these terminals into the **synapse** (or **synaptic cleft**), which is the gap between the axon terminals of one cell and the dendrites of the next cell.

TEACHER TIP

There are many types of neurons in the body. They don't all have the same structure or even a complete set of axons and dendrites, though they do all have the ability to signal chemically following electrical excitation.

B. FUNCTION

Neurons are specialized to receive signals from sensory receptors or from other neurons in the body and transfer this information along the length of the axon. Impulses, known as **action potentials,** travel the length of the axon and invade the nerve terminal, thereby causing the release of neurotransmitter into the synapse. When a neuron is at rest, the potential difference between the extracellular space and the intracellular space is called the **resting potential.**

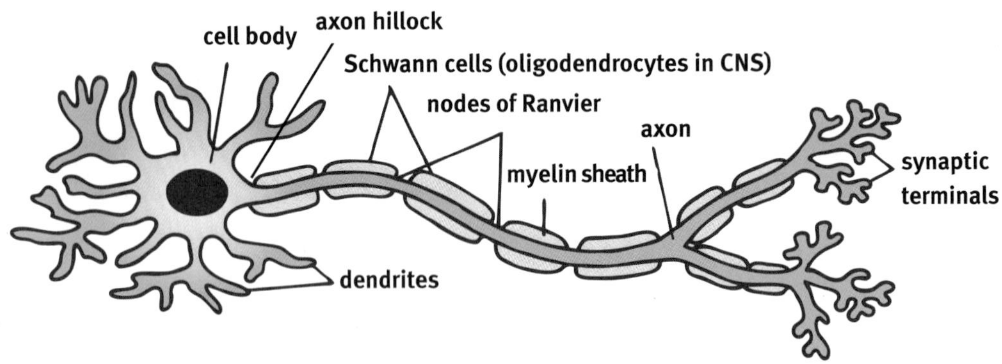

Figure 12.1. Peripheral Nerve

Teacher Tip

Flashback: Remember that the Na/K ATPase isn't only present in neurons. We saw it earlier in RBC as a way to control cell tonicity. The Na/K ATPase is able to make both on osmotic and electrogenic contribution to the cell.

1. Resting Potential

Even at rest, a neuron is polarized. This potential difference is the result of an unequal distribution of ions between the inside and outside of the cell. A typical resting membrane potential is –70 millivolts (mV), which means that the inside of the neuron is more negative than the outside. This difference is due to selective ionic permeability of the neuronal cell membrane and is maintained by the **Na^+/K^+ pump** (also called the Na^+/K^+ ATPase).

The concentration of K^+ is higher inside the neuron than outside; the concentration of Na^+ is higher outside than inside. Additionally, negatively charged proteins are trapped inside of the cell. The resting potential is created because the neuron is selectively permeable to K^+, so K^+ diffuses down its concentration gradient, leaving a net negative charge inside. (Neurons do not allow much Na^+ to enter the cell under resting conditions, so the cell remains polarized.)

Because the transmission of action potentials leads to the disruption of the ionic gradients (see next section), the gradients must be restored by the Na^+/K^+ pump. This pump, using ATP energy, transports 3 Na^+ out for every 2 K^+ it transports into the cell (see Figure 12.2).

MCAT Synopsis

Na^+ wants to go into the cell because it is more negative inside (electrical gradient) and because there is less Na^+ inside (chemical gradient).

2. Action Potential

The nerve cell body receives both excitatory and inhibitory impulses from other cells. If the cell becomes sufficiently excited or **depolarized** (i.e., the inside of the cell becomes less negative), an action potential is generated. The minimum **threshold membrane potential** (usually around –50 mV) is the level at which an action potential is initiated.

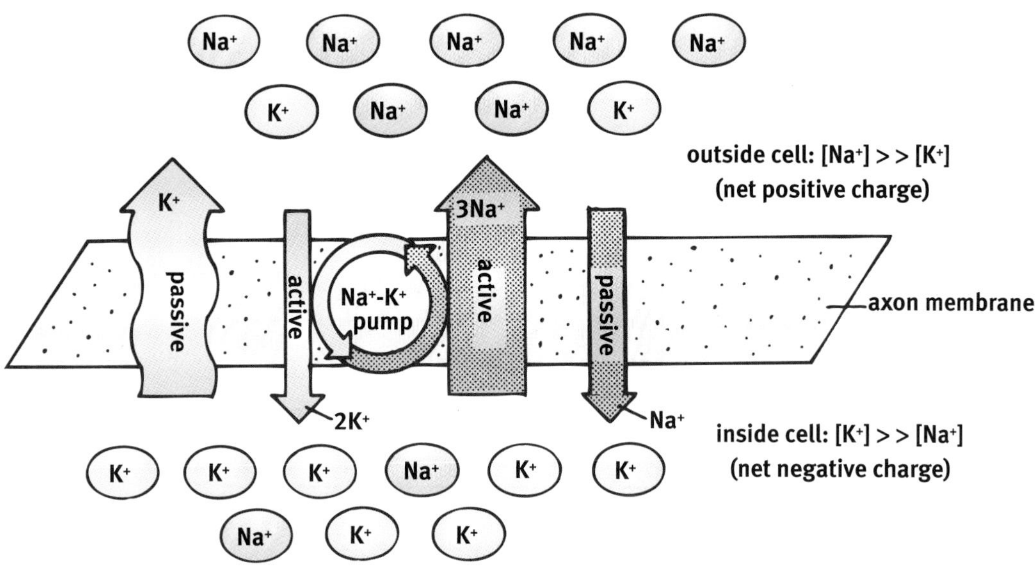

Figure 12.2. Resting Potential of a Neuron

Ion channels located in the nerve cell membrane open in response to these changes in voltage and are therefore called **voltage-gated ion channels.** An action potential begins when **voltage-gated Na^+ channels** open in response to depolarization, allowing Na^+ to rush down its **electrochemical gradient** into the cell, causing a rapid depolarization of that segment of the cell. The voltage-gated Na^+ channels then close, and **voltage-gated K^+ channels** open, allowing K^+ to rush out down its electrochemical gradient. This returns the cell to a more negative potential, a process known as **repolarization.** In fact, the neuron may shoot past the resting potential and become even more negative inside than normal; this is called **hyperpolarization** (see Figure 12.3). Immediately following an action potential, it may be very difficult or impossible to initiate another action potential; this period of time is called the **refractory period.**

TEACHER TIP

Flashback to the musculoskeletal system: As we saw in muscles, each fiber twitches in an all-or-nothing fashion. We see now (and remember) that this is due to how they are innervated. Because each muscle fiber has only one neuron innervating it, when the neuron fires, the muscle contracts. Because neurons fire in an all-or-nothing fashion, so too must the muscle fiber.

The action potential is often described as an **all-or-none response.** This means that whenever the threshold membrane potential is reached, an action potential with a consistent size and duration is produced. Neuronal information is coded by the frequency and number of action potentials rather than the size of the action potential. (In other words, the harder you hit your thumb with a hammer, the more action potentials will travel up your pain fibers, but the size and duration of each individual action potential will remain the same.)

CLINICAL CORRELATE

Local anesthetics work by blocking the voltage-gated Na^+ channels. These drugs work particularly well on sensory neurons, and therefore block the transmission of pain. They work so well on pain neurons because these neurons have small axonal diameters and have little or no myelin. This makes it easier to prevent action potential propagation.

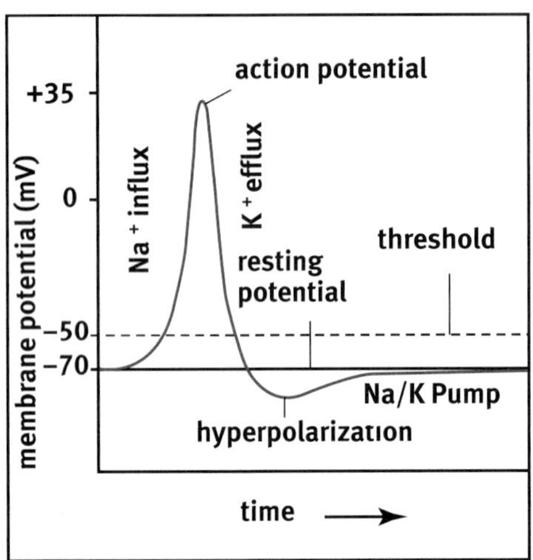

Figure 12.3. Action Potential

TEACHER TIP

This insulation by myelin is extremely effective. A human spinal cord is about the thickness of a finger. Without the insulation, the cord would have to be almost as big as a telephone pole in order to prevent signal loss.

3. Impulse Propagation

If there is an adequate stimulus, the action potential will first be initiated at the axon hillock. Na^+ rushes into the neuron and diffuses to adjacent parts of the axon, causing nearby voltage-gated Na^+ channels to open. This occurs as previous segments are repolarizing. This chain of events (depolarization followed by a subsequent repolarization) continues along the length of the axon (see Figure 12.4). Although axons can theoretically propagate action potentials bidirectionally, information transfer will occur only in one direction: from dendrite to synaptic terminal. (This is because synapses operate only in one direction and because refractory periods make the backward travel of action potentials impossible.) Different axons can propagate action potentials at different speeds. The greater the diameter of the axon and the more heavily it is myelinated, the faster the impulses will travel. Myelin increases the conduction velocity by insulating segments of the axon, so that the membrane is permeable to ions only in the nodes of Ranvier. In this way, the action potential "jumps" from node to node; this process is called **saltatory conduction.**

SYNAPSE

The synapse is the gap between the axon terminal of one neuron (called the **presynaptic neuron** because it is before the synapse) and the dendrites of another neuron **(postsynaptic neuron).** Neurons may also communicate with postsynaptic cells other than neurons, such as cells in muscles or glands; these are called **effector cells.** The vast majority of synapses in the human are **chemical synapses.** In chemical synapses,

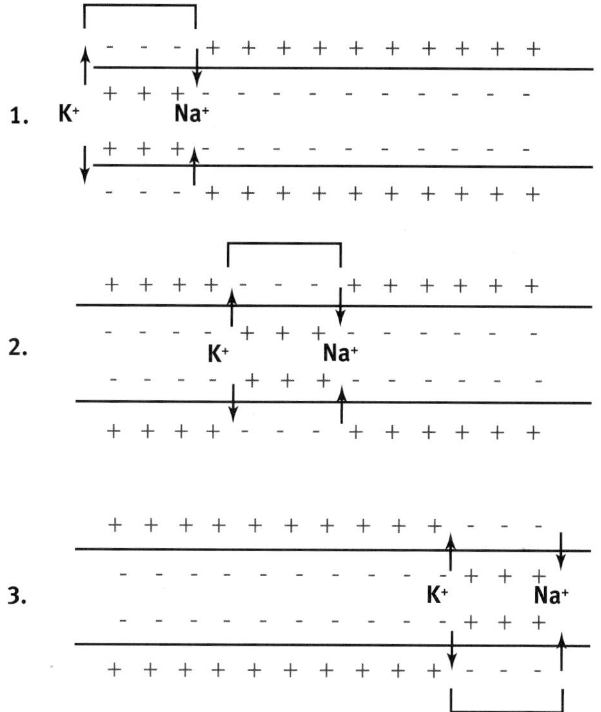

Figure 12.4. Propagation of an Action Potential

the nerve terminal contains thousands of membrane-bound vesicles full of chemical messengers known as **neurotransmitters.** When the action potential arrives at the nerve terminal and depolarizes it, the synaptic vesicles fuse with the presynaptic membrane and release neurotransmitter into the synapse via a calcium-dependent process of exocytosis. The neurotransmitter diffuses across the synapse and acts on receptor proteins embedded in the postsynaptic membrane (see Figure 12.5). Depending on the nature of the receptor, the neurotransmitter may have an excitatory or an inhibitory effect on the postsynaptic cell. Neurotransmitter is removed from the synapse in a variety of ways: it may be taken back up into the nerve terminal (via a protein known as an **uptake carrier**) where it may be reused or degraded; it may be degraded by enzymes located in the synapse (e.g., **acetylcholinesterase** inactivates the neurotransmitter acetylcholine); it may simply diffuse out of the synapse.

CLINICAL CORRELATE

Many common drugs (either in clinical use or street drugs) modify processes that occur in the synapse. For instance, cocaine acts by blocking neuronal uptake carriers, thus prolonging the action of neurotransmitters in the synapse by preventing neurotransmitter re-entry into the nerve terminal. There are clinically useful drugs (e.g., drugs used to treat glaucoma) that inhibit acetylcholinesterase, thereby elevating synaptic levels of acetylcholine. Nerve gases are extremely potent acetylcholinesterase inhibitors which have been used in war and in recent terrorist activities. Nerve gas causes rapid death by preventing the action of skeletal muscle (most importantly, the diaphragm)—leading to respiratory arrest.

TEACHER TIP

KEY POINT: It is critical to understand the difference between electrical and chemical transmission and that neurons use both. Within a neuron, electricity is used to pass messages in an all-or-nothing fashion. Between neurons, chemical molecules are used to pass messages in a modulated manner that is dependent on how much neurotransmitter is released.

ORGANIZATION OF THE VERTEBRATE NERVOUS SYSTEM

There are many different kinds of neurons in the vertebrate nervous system. Neurons that carry information about the external or internal environment to the brain or spinal cord are called **afferent neurons.**

MCAT SYNOPSIS

Afferent neurons are sensory neurons and efferent neurons are motor neurons.

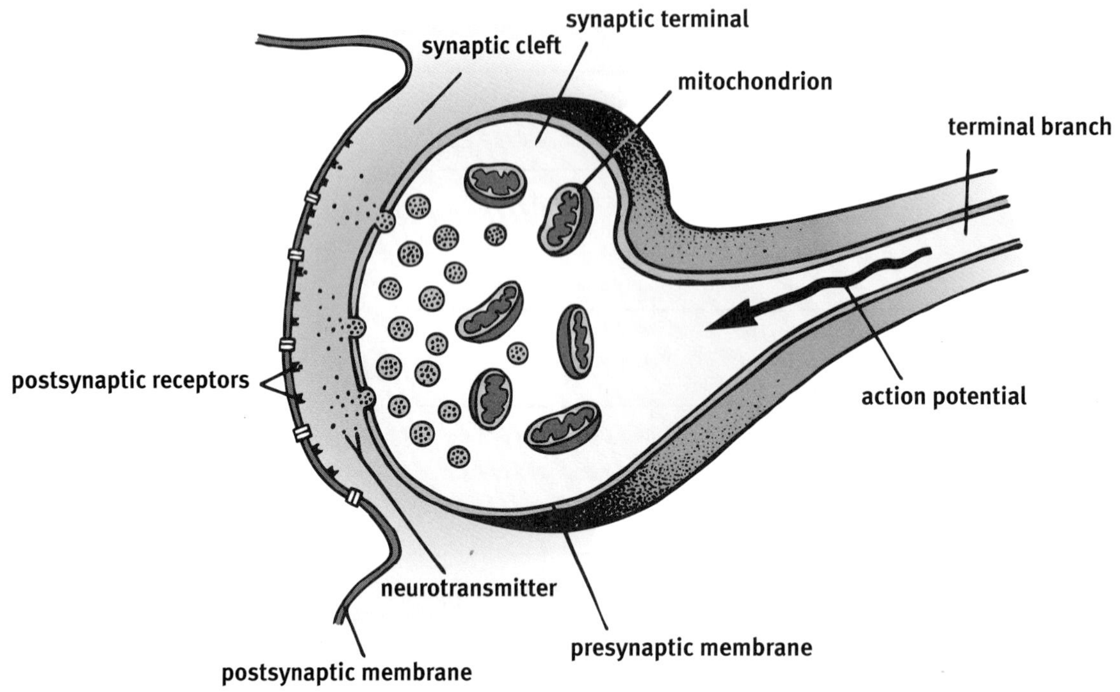

Figure 12.5. The Synapse

Neurons that carry commands from the brain or spinal cord to various parts of the body (e.g., muscles or glands) are called **efferent neurons.** Some neurons **(interneurons)** participate only in local circuits; their cell bodies and their nerve terminals are in the same location.

TEACHER TIP

While it may seem complex to separate the nervous system into these two divisions, it is actually quite simple. The CNS is the brain and spinal cord. Everything else falls under the purview of the PNS.

Nerves are essentially bundles of axons covered with connective tissue. A nerve may carry only sensory fibers (a **sensory nerve**), only motor fibers (a **motor nerve**), or a mixture of the two (a **mixed nerve**). Neuronal cell bodies often cluster together; such clusters are called **ganglia** in the periphery; in the central nervous system, they are called **nuclei.** The nervous system itself is divided into two major systems, the **central nervous system** and the **peripheral nervous system** (see Figure 12.6).

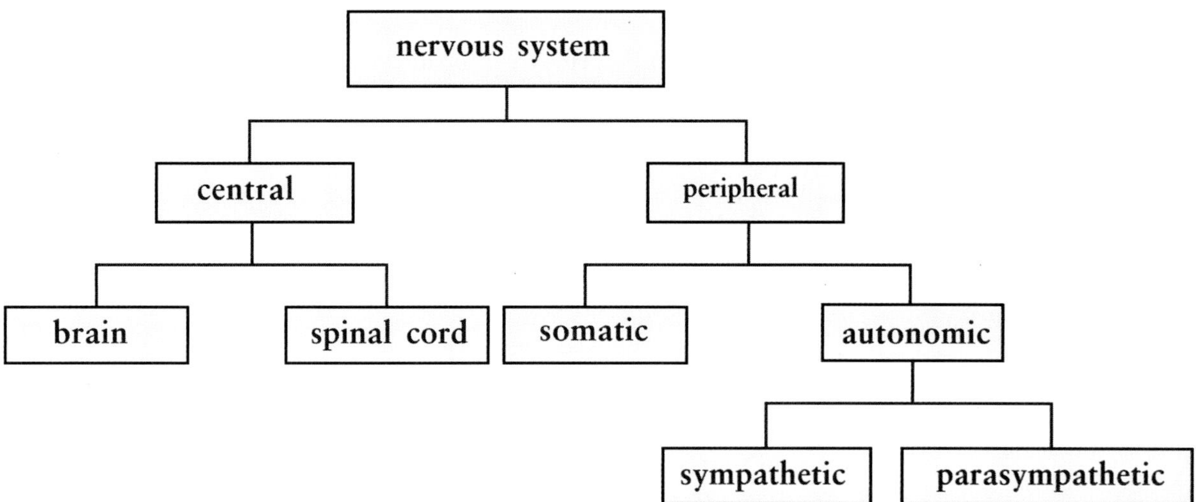

Figure 12.6. Organization of the Vertebrate Nervous System

A. CENTRAL NERVOUS SYSTEM

The central nervous system (CNS) consists of the **brain** and the **spinal cord.**

1. Brain

The brain is a jellylike mass of neurons that resides in the skull. Its functions include interpreting sensory information, forming motor plans, and cognitive function (thinking). The brain consists of **gray matter** (cell bodies) and **white matter** (myelinated axons). The brain can be divided into the **forebrain, midbrain,** and **hindbrain.**

> **TEACHER TIP**
>
> As much as the digestive system has infoldings to increase the effective surface area, so too does the brain. The increased folds (gyri) in the human cerebral cortex allow for higher-level cognitive functions to be carried out.

a. Forebrain

The forebrain consists of the **telencephalon** and the **diencephalon.** The telencephalon consists of right and left hemispheres; each hemisphere can be divided into four different lobes: **frontal, parietal, temporal,** and **occipital.** A major component of the telencephalon is the **cerebral cortex,** which is the highly convoluted gray matter that can be seen on the surface of the brain. The cortex processes and integrates sensory input and motor responses and is important for memory and creative thought. Right and left cerebral cortices communicate with each other through the **corpus callosum.**

The diencephalon contains the **thalamus** and **hypothalamus.** The thalamus is a relay and integration center for the spinal cord and cerebral cortex. The hypothalamus controls visceral functions such as hunger, thirst, sex drive, water balance, blood pressure, and temperature regulation. It also plays an important role in the control of the endocrine system (see chapter 11).

Clinical Correlate

Have you ever wondered why a person staggers when he or she gets very drunk? It is because alcohol has profound effects on the cerebellum.

Teacher Tip

The brainstem is the most primitive part of the brain conserved from the most simple of organisms. It drives the basic functions from breathing to the heart beating. Recall that the respiratory system can be driven by chemoreceptors in the brainstem that are sensitive to CO_2 levels.

b. Midbrain

The midbrain is a relay center for visual and auditory impulses. It also plays an important role in motor control.

c. Hindbrain

The hindbrain is the posterior part of the brain and consists of the **cerebellum,** the **pons,** and the **medulla.** The cerebellum helps to modulate motor impulses initiated by the motor cortex and is important in the maintenance of balance, hand-eye coordination, and the timing of rapid movements. One function of the pons is to act as a relay center to allow the cortex to communicate with the cerebellum. The medulla (also called the medulla oblongata) controls many vital functions such as breathing, heart rate, and gastrointestinal activity. Together, the midbrain, pons, and medulla constitute the **brainstem.**

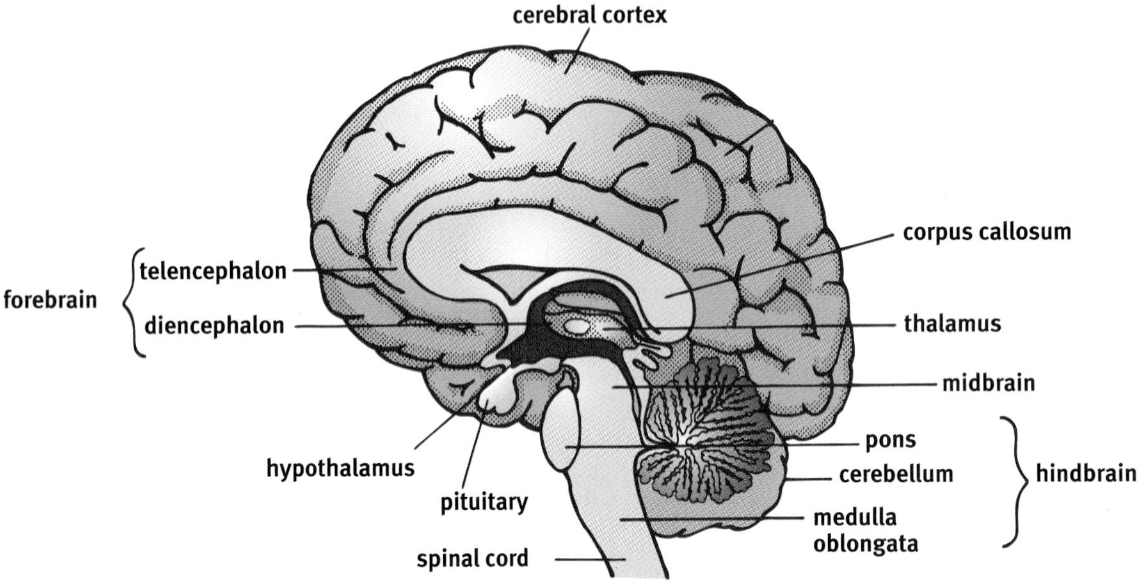

Figure 12.7. Human Brain

2. Spinal Cord

The spinal cord is an elongated structure, continuous with the brainstem, that extends down the dorsal side of vertebrates. Nearly all nerves that innervate the viscera or muscles below the head pass through the spinal cord, and nearly all sensory information from below the head passes through the spinal cord on the way to the brain. The spinal cord can also integrate simple motor responses (e.g., reflexes) by itself. A cross-section of the spinal cord reveals an outer white matter area containing motor and sensory axons and an inner gray matter area containing nerve cell bodies. Sensory information enters the spinal cord dorsally; the cell bodies of these sensory neurons are located in the **dorsal root ganglia.** All motor information exits the spinal cord ventrally. Nerve branches entering and leaving the cord are called **roots** (see Figure 12.8). The spinal cord is divided into four regions (going in order from the brainstem to the tail): **cervical, thoracic, lumbar,** and **sacral.**

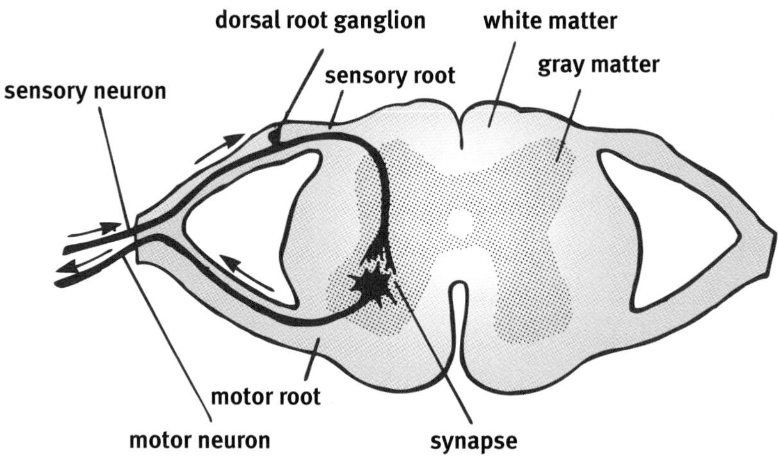

Figure 12.8. Spinal Cord

CLINICAL CORRELATE

The injury that the late actor Christopher Reeve sustained was so devastating because he damaged his spinal cord at the high cervical levels. Most of his spinal cord was essentially disconnected from his brain so the communication between his body and his brain was severely compromised, producing a state of paralysis and a lack of sensation below the neck.

B. PERIPHERAL NERVOUS SYSTEM

The peripheral nervous system (PNS) consists of 12 pairs of cranial nerves, which primarily innervate the head and shoulders, and 31 pairs of spinal nerves, which innervate the rest of the body. Cranial nerves exit from the brainstem and spinal nerves exit from the spinal cord. The PNS has two primary divisions: the somatic and the autonomic nervous systems, each of which has both motor and sensory components.

1. Somatic Nervous System

The somatic nervous system (SNS) innervates skeletal muscles and is responsible for voluntary movement. Motor neurons release the neurotransmitter acetylcholine (ACh) onto ACh receptors located on skeletal muscle. This causes depolarization of the skeletal muscle, leading to muscle contraction. In addition to voluntary movement, the somatic nervous system is also important for reflex action. There are both **monosynaptic** and **polysynaptic** reflexes.

CLINICAL CORRELATE

There is an autoimmune disorder called myasthenia gravis, in which the body mounts an immune response against the acetylcholine receptors on the skeletal muscle. People with this disorder can become quite weak and fatigued. Patients are affected to varying degrees: you may not be able to observe much of a problem or the patient may be confined to a wheelchair.

TEACHER TIP

Consider the purpose of this system: While a knee-jerk reflex can certainly be amusing to watch, there is a deeper reason. The stretch on the patellar tendon makes the body think that the muscle may be getting overstretched. In response, contraction occurs.

- Monosynaptic reflex pathways have only one synapse between the sensory neuron and the motor neuron. The classic example is the **knee-jerk reflex.** When the tendon covering the patella (kneecap) is hit, stretch receptors sense this and action potentials are sent up the sensory neuron and into the spinal cord. The sensory neuron synapses with a motor neuron in the spinal cord, which in turn, stimulates the quadriceps muscle to contract, causing the lower leg to kick forward (see Figures 12.8 and 12.9).

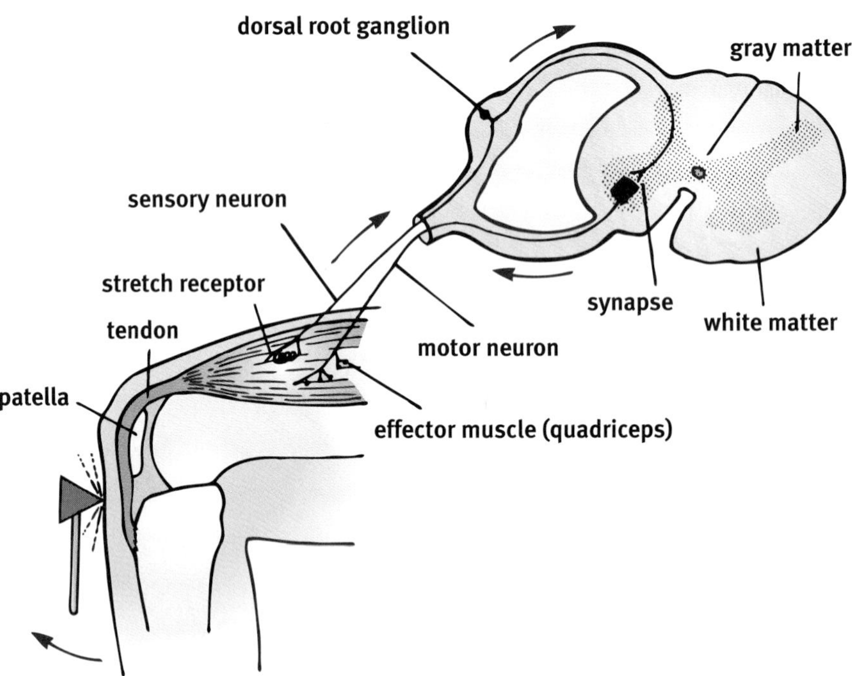

Figure 12.9. Reflex Arc for Knee-Jerk

MCAT SYNOPSIS

Reflexes occur at the level of the spinal cord, and do not require the participation of the brain. There are two advantages to this. First, the brain has enough to do and doesn't necessarily want to get involved in everything. Second, reflexes are often designed to be fast responses. For instance, if you put your hand on the stove, you probably don't want to analyze the pain before you remove your hand from the flames.

- In polysynaptic reflexes, sensory neurons synapse with more than one neuron. A classic example of this is the **withdrawal reflex.** When a person steps on a nail, the injured leg withdraws in pain, while the other leg extends to retain balance.

TEACHER TIP

Many students have trouble with the autonomic nervous system. It does control many functions within the body but think simply and in big-picture terms. Autonomic means AUTOMATIC. If it is a body function that you don't have to think about, it probably has at least some autonomic input. From there you simply need to decide whether it is sympathetic (flight or fight) or parasympathetic (rest and digest).

2. Autonomic Nervous System

The autonomic nervous system **(ANS)** is sometimes also called the involuntary nervous system because it regulates the body's internal environment without the aid of conscious control. Whereas the somatic nervous system innervates skeletal muscle, the ANS innervates cardiac and smooth muscle. Smooth muscle is located in areas such as blood vessels, the digestive tract, the bladder, and bronchi, so it isn't surprising that the ANS is important in blood pressure control, gastrointestinal motility, excretory processes, respiration, and reproductive processes. ANS pathways are characterized by a two-neuron system. The first neuron (preganglionic neuron) has a cell body located within the CNS and its axon synapses in peripheral ganglia. The second neuron (postganglionic neuron) has its cell body in the ganglia and then synapses on cardiac or smooth muscle. The ANS is comprised of two subdivisions, the **sympathetic** and the **parasympathetic nervous systems,** which generally act in opposition to one another.

a. Sympathetic nervous system

The sympathetic division is responsible for the "flight or fight" responses that ready the body for action. It basically does everything you would want it to do in an emergency situation. It increases blood pressure and heart rate; it increases blood flow to skeletal muscles and it decreases gut motility. The preganglionic neurons emerge from the thoracic and lumbar regions of the spinal cord and use acetylcholine as their neurotransmitter; the postganglionic neurons typically release norepinephrine. The action of preganglionic sympathetic neurons also causes the adrenal medulla to release adrenaline (epinephrine) into the bloodstream.

b. Parasympathetic nervous system

The parasympathetic division acts to conserve energy and restore the body to resting activity levels following exertion ("rest and digest"). It acts to lower heart rate and to increase gut motility. One very important parasympathetic nerve that innervates many of the thoracic and abdominal viscera is called the **vagus nerve.** Parasympathetic neurons originate in the brainstem (cranial nerves) and the sacral part of the spinal cord. Both the preganglionic and postganglionic neurons release acetycholine.

MCAT Synopsis

The first neuron in the autonomic nervous system is called the preganglionic neuron and the second is the postganglionic neuron.

MCAT Synopsis

To help you remember the effects of the sympathetic nervous system ("fight or flight"), imagine that you are being chased by a bear. What would you expect or want to happen?

- Increased heart rate and breathing rate
- Blood directed away from skin and toward big muscles (want blood flow to muscle to facilitate running away)
- Decreased digestion
- Pupil dilation

SPECIAL SENSES

The body has three types of sensory receptors to monitor its internal and external environment: **interoceptors, proprioceptors,** and **exteroceptors.** Interoceptors monitor aspects of the internal environment such as blood pressure, the partial pressure of CO_2 in the blood, and blood pH. Proprioceptors transmit information regarding the position of the body in space. These receptors are located in muscles and tendons to tell the brain where the limbs are in space and are also located in the inner ear to tell the brain where the head is in space. Exteroceptors sense things in the external environment such as light, sound, taste, pain, touch, and temperature.

Teacher Tip

KEY POINT: Be sure to know which neurotransmitters are released pre- and postsynaptically at sympathetic and parasympathetic neurons. This is a classic case for an MCAT discrete question.

TEACHER TIP

Color blindness is a result of lacking one, two, or three of these sets of cones. Total color blindness is most commonly due to a complete lack of cones.

BRIDGE

The lens in the eye is a converging (convex) lens. A convex lens with a smaller radius of curvature (i.e., thicker) has more refractive power and a shorter focal length (good for near vision). A lens with a larger radius of curvature (i.e., flatter) has less refractive power and a longer focal length (good for far vision). A convex lens forms an inverted and reversed image on the focal plane (i.e., the retina); it is up to the brain to sort that out.

1. The Eye

The eye detects light energy (as photons) and transmits information about intensity, color, and shape to the brain. The eyeball is covered by a thick, opaque layer known as the **sclera,** which is also known as the white of the eye. Beneath the sclera is the **choroid** layer, which helps to supply the retina with blood. The innermost layer of the eye is the **retina,** which contains the photoreceptors that sense the light. The transparent **cornea** at the front of the eye bends and focuses light rays. The rays then travel through an opening called the **pupil,** whose diameter is controlled by the pigmented, muscular **iris.** The iris responds to the intensity of light in the surroundings (light makes the pupil constrict). The light continues through the lens, which is suspended behind the pupil. The lens, the shape of which is controlled by the **ciliary muscles,** focuses the image onto the retina. In the retina are photoreceptors that **transduce** light into action potentials. There are two main types of photoreceptors: **cones** and **rods.** Cones respond to high-intensity illumination and are sensitive to color, while rods detect low-intensity illumination and are important in night vision. The cones and rods contain various pigments that absorb specific wavelengths of light. The cones contain three different pigments that absorb red, green, and blue wavelengths; the rod pigment, **rhodopsin,** absorbs one wavelength. The photoreceptor cells synapse onto **bipolar cells,** which in turn synapse onto **ganglion cells.** Axons of the ganglion cells bundle to form the right and left **optic nerves,** which conduct visual information to the brain. The point at which the optic nerve exits the eye is called the **blind spot** because photoreceptors are not present there. There is also a small area of the retina called the **fovea,** which is densely packed with cones and is important for high acuity vision (see Figure 12.10).

The eye also has its own circulation system. Near the base of the iris, the eye secretes aqueous humor, which travels to the anterior chamber of the eye from which it exits and eventually joins venous blood.

2. The Ear

The ear transduces sound energy (pressure waves) into impulses perceived by the brain as sound. The ear is also responsible for maintaining equilibrium (balance) in the body.

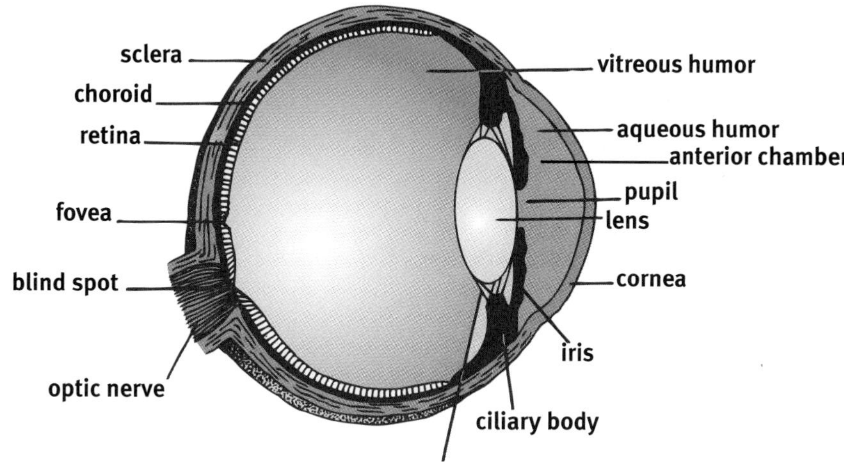

Figure 12.10. Human Eye

CLINICAL CORRELATE

Some people develop a plumbing problem in the eye and cannot adequately drain aqueous humor. This disease is called glaucoma. Because of the draining problem, pressure builds in the anterior chamber and is transmitted to the vitreous humor, leading to increased pressure on the optic nerve. If the pressure is not relieved, this condition can permanently damage the optic nerve and lead to blindness.

Sound waves pass through three regions as they enter the ear. First, they enter the **outer ear,** which consists of the **auricle** (pinna) and the **auditory canal.** At the end of the auditory canal is the **tympanic membrane (eardrum)** of the **middle ear,** which vibrates at the same frequency as the incoming sound. Next, the three bones, or **ossicles (malleus, incus,** and **stapes),** amplify the stimulus and transmit it through the **oval window,** which leads to the fluid-filled **inner ear.** The inner ear consists of the **cochlea** and the **semicircular canals.** The cochlea contains the **organ of Corti,** which has specialized sensory cells called hair cells. Vibration of the ossicles exerts pressure on the fluid in the cochlea, stimulating the hair cells to transduce the pressure into action potentials, which travel via the **auditory (cochlear) nerve** to the brain for processing (see Figure 12.11).

TEACHER TIP

KEY POINT: This is another classic place where the MCAT may test some of your physics knowledge in the BS section. The basis of hearing is sound waves so don't be surprised if you get a question about longitudinal waveforms.

The three semicircular canals are each perpendicular to the other two and filled with a fluid called **endolymph**. At the base of each canal is a chamber with sensory hair cells; rotation of the head displaces endolymph in one of the canals, putting pressure on the hair cells in it. This changes the nature of impulses sent by the vestibular nerve to the brain. The brain interprets this information to determine the position of the head.

3. The Chemical Senses

The chemical senses are taste and smell. These senses transduce chemical changes in the environment, specifically in the mouth and nose, into **gustatory** and **olfactory** sensory impulses, which are interpreted by the nervous system.

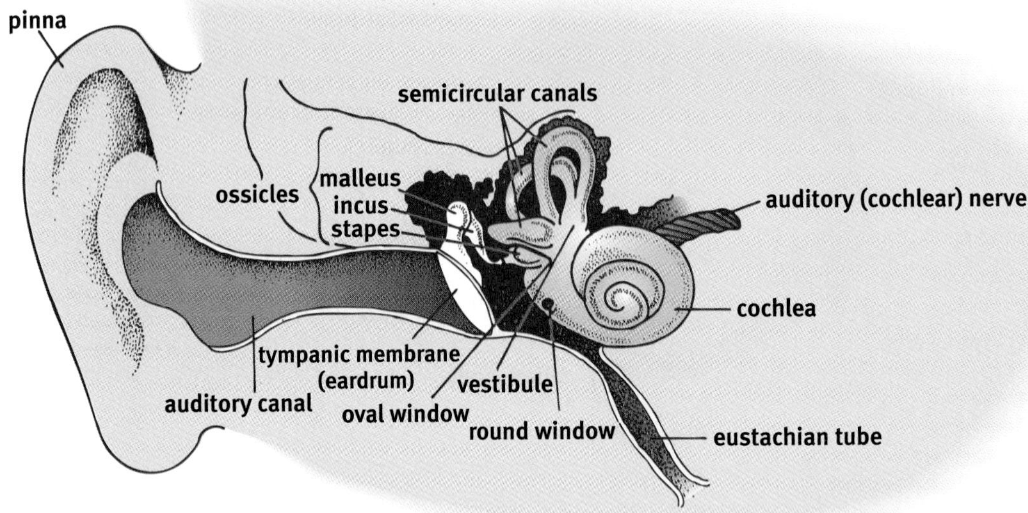

Figure 12.11. Human Ear

a. Taste

Taste receptors, or **taste buds,** are located on the tongue, the soft palate, and the epiglottis. Taste buds are composed of approximately 40 epithelial cells. The outer surface of a taste bud contains a **taste pore,** from which microvilli, or **taste hairs,** protrude. The receptor surfaces for taste are on the taste hairs. Interwoven around the taste buds is a network of nerve fibers that are stimulated by the taste buds. These neurons transmit gustatory information to the brainstem via three cranial nerves. There are four kinds of taste sensations: sour, salty, sweet, and bitter. Although most taste buds will respond to all four stimuli, they respond preferentially; i.e., at a lower threshold, to one or two of them.

b. Smell

Olfactory receptors are found in the olfactory membrane, which lies in the upper part of the nostrils over a total area of about 5 cm^2. The receptors are specialized neurons from which **olfactory hairs,** or **cilia,** project. These cilia form a dense mat in the nasal mucosa. When odorous substances enter the nasal cavity, they bind to receptors in the cilia, depolarizing the olfactory receptors. Axons from the olfactory receptors join to form the **olfactory nerves.** The olfactory nerves project directly to the **olfactory bulbs** in the base of the brain.

TEACHER TIP

Have you ever gone into a room with a very strong smell, which, after a while was hardly noticeable? Olfactory receptors can be overpowered and after constant stimulation, will desensitize to a given stimulus. This desensitization is a hallmark of much of the nervous system.

PRACTICE QUESTIONS

1. Myelin sheaths do NOT serve which of the following functions?

   A. Saltatory conduction
   B. Protection of axons
   C. Prevention of leakage of current
   D. Increase in speed of signal transmission

2. The Nernst equation shown below determines the membrane potential of a neuron for only one ion. “Out” denotes the extracellular concentration whereas “in” denotes in the intracellular concentration. Assuming sodium ions are the major determinant of resting potential (E) and that (RT)/F > 0, which of the following about resting potential is true?

$$E = \frac{RT}{F} \ln \frac{[Na^+]_{out}}{[Na^+]_{in}}$$

   A. E > 0
   B. E < 0
   C. E = 0
   D. E is indeterminable.

3. A postsynaptic potential stimulates the cell body of a neuron directly. The potential is strong enough to overcome threshold and cause action potential propagation at the axon hillock of a postsynaptic neuron. Which of the following is the main reason why the postsynaptic potential does not progress back down from the cell body toward the dendrites?

   A. The membrane of the neuron does not have a requisite amount of ion channels.
   B. No myelin sheath is around the neuron.
   C. The above statement is not true. The postsynaptic potential does in fact progress down toward the dendrites.
   D. None of the above is true.

4. During a flight-or-fight response, which of the following is NOT expected to occur?

   A. Inhibition of sexual arousal
   B. Acetylcholine release at synaptic clefts
   C. Pupil constriction
   D. Increase in heart rate

5. In a sympathetic response, which of the following is activated?

   A. Gastrointestinal activity
   B. Redirection of blood from digestive tract to muscles
   C. Cardiac contractility decreases
   D. Constriction of blood circulation in muscles

6. Which of the following statements of the parasympathetic nervous system is true?

   I. It is subject to control by the brain stem.
   II. Signals are transmitted mainly by interneurons
   III. It causes a decrease in heart rate.

   A. I
   B. II
   C. III
   D. I and III

7. The following is a graph of an action potential. At the top of the peak at 20 ms, which of the following best characterizes what is occurring?

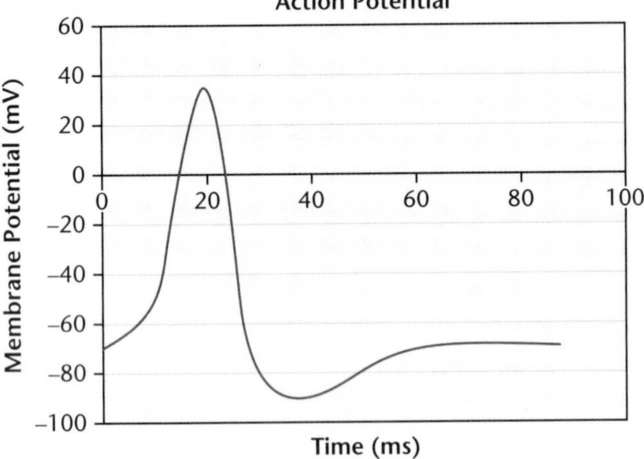

A. Some sodium channels have inactivated and some potassium channels have begun to open.
B. All sodium channels are open and all potassium channels are closed.
C. Sodium channels are beginning to open and some potassium channels have inactivated.
D. Both sodium and potassium channels are closed.

8. The following is a diagram of a rod cell. When there is an absence of light, the sodium channels of the rod cell are open. When there is light detected by the pigments found in the top section of the diagram, the sodium channels close. Which of the following is NOT a reasonable conclusion based on this information?

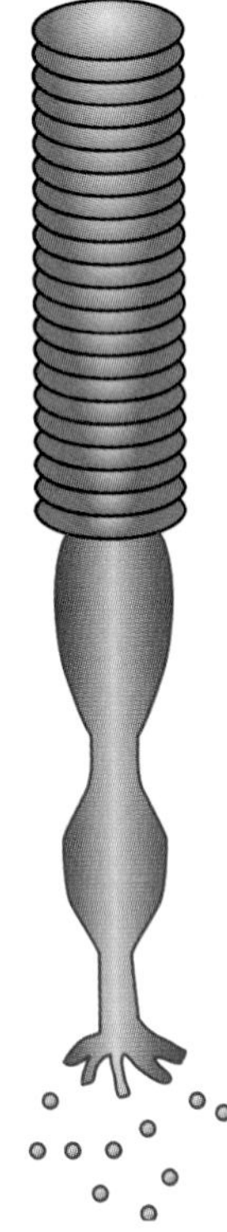

A. Depolarization of the cell occurs when the external environment is dark.
B. The neurotransmitter (shown at the bottom of the diagram) released by this cell transmits a signal that there is light detected by the pigments of the rod cell.
C. The diagram shown depicts a situation when the external environment is dark.
D. Hyperpolarization, not depolarization, signals when the external environment is lit.

9. The following is a picture of a typical nerve synapse. Which of the following is true without being readily observed in the diagram?

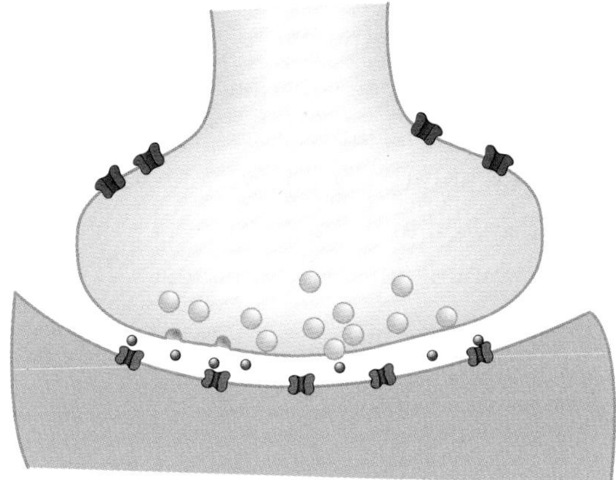

A. Vesicles contain neurotransmitters, which do not determine whether there is an excitatory or inhibitory response.
B. Voltage-gated calcium channels are independent of the formation of neurotransmitter-containing vesicles.
C. The degree of postsynaptic response is independent of the amount of neurotransmitter release into the synapse.
D. None of the above

10. Which of the following gives eyes their color (blue, green, brown, or red)?

A. Cornea
B. Pupil
C. Iris
D. Lens

11. A patient has suffered physical trauma to her right eye and has found that her vision is impaired mainly in the center of her field of view. She has great deficit in reading and color recognition in that eye. What is the most likely area of the injury to the right eye?

A. Any part of the retina
B. Optic nerve
C. Fovea
D. Blind spot

12. The following is a graph of a cardiac action potential. Skeletal muscle action potentials, by contrast, have a more gradual increase in potential and decrease more drastically without a pronounced plateau. Which of the following is true of cardiac muscle action potentials?

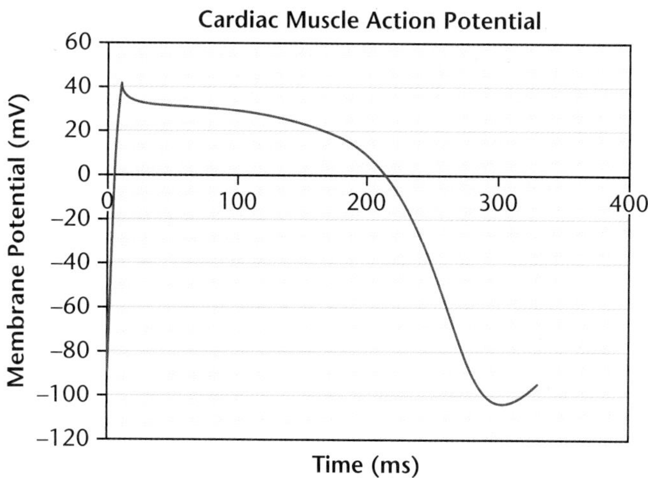

A. Sodium channels and potassium channels open faster in cardiac muscle than they do in skeletal muscle.
B. Sodium channels open faster in cardiac muscle but potassium channels open more slowly.
C. Sodium channels and potassium channels open more slowly in cardiac muscle.
D. Sodium channels open more slowly in cardiac muscle but potassium channels open faster.

13. Multiple sclerosis is a disease where the central nervous system is sporadically demyelinated and is believed to be autoimmune in nature. Which of the following is the most likely immunological target?

A. Schwann cells
B. Astrocytes
C. Lymphocytes
D. Leukocytes

14. A clinical researcher discovers a developmental defect in the retina. Based on experimental data, it seems that the disorders stem from a mutation that affects fetal development in the first trimester. Which of the following is the most likely fetal site affected?

A. Endoderm
B. Mesoderm
C. Ectoderm
D. Neuroblastula

15. Tetrapropylammonium ion (TPA) is a known inhibitor of the Na^+/K^+ pump. When administered to motor neurons, there will be a(n)

A. inability to contract muscles immediately on administration.
B. initial ability to contract but inability to contract subsequently.
C. initial ability to contract followed by quick relaxation and spasms.
D. continuous muscular spasms.

ACTION POTENTIAL

A nerve action potential is depicted below. If, during the action potential, a stimulus were to be applied as indicated by the arrow, what would result?

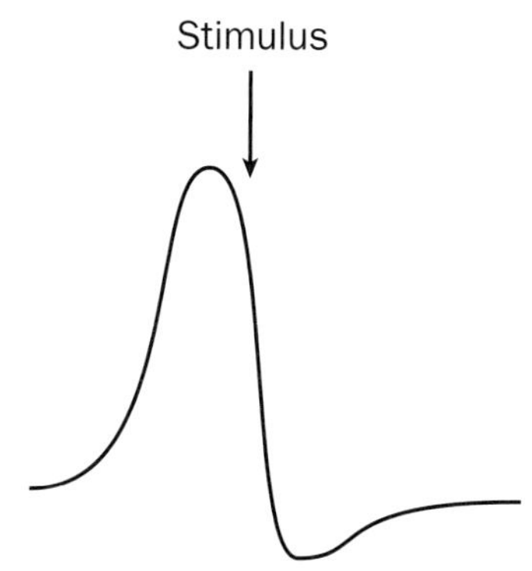

KEY CONCEPTS

Action potentials

Depolarization

Refractory periods

1) Visualize the graph of the action potential.

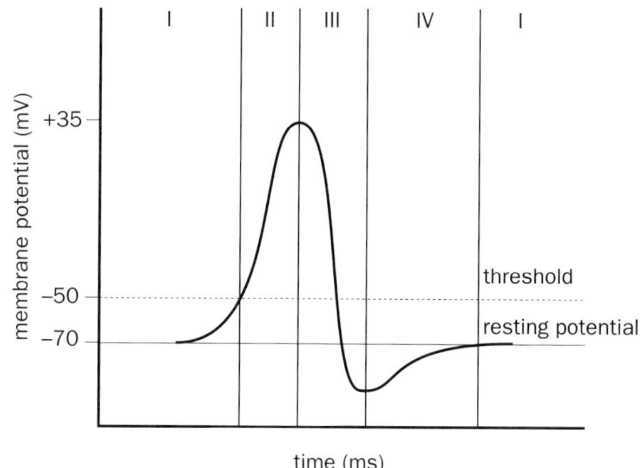

TAKEAWAYS

It is important to understand each stage of the action potential, including which gates are open or closed and which ions are flowing.

Region I—The cell is at rest and all gates are closed.

Region II—Depolarization: sodium gates are open and sodium flows into the cell, moving the membrane towards the sodium equilibrium potential.

Region III—Repolarization: sodium gates close and potassium gates open, moving the cell closer to the potassium equilibrium potential.

Region IV—Hyperpolarization: all gates are closed and the cell is ready to undergo another action potential, but the distance to the threshold is farther so it is harder to stimulate the cell. This is known as the relative refractory period.

SIMILAR QUESTIONS

1) At what point in the action potential is sodium closest to its electrochemical equilibrium?
2) What forces can increase the speed of an action potential?
3) How can an action potential be inhibited?

2) Review the characteristics of the action potential.
Action potentials propagate by the spread of currents to adjacent membranes; they are considered "all or nothing" because once threshold is reached, an action potential will continue. During an action potential (regions II and III) no other action potential can be elicited, no matter how large the stimulus. This is known as the absolute refractory period.

---

3) Evaluate the region in which the new stimulus is being applied.
The new stimulus being applied to the action potential occurs during repolarization. This is also during the absolute refractory period, a time during which no new action potentials can be elicited. Therefore, the new stimulus will not produce a new action potential.

Remember: *Action potentials are all or nothing. Once one begins it will continue, and a new action potential cannot be stimulated until after the absolute refractory period.*

CHAPTER 13

GENETICS

Genetics is the study of how traits are inherited from one generation to the next. The basic unit of heredity is the **gene.** Genes are composed of DNA and are located on chromosomes. When a gene exists in more than one form, the alternate forms are called **alleles.** The genetic makeup of an individual is the individual's **genotype**; the physical manifestation of the genetic makeup is the individual's **phenotype.** Some phenotypes correspond to a single genotype, while other phenotypes correspond to several different genotypes.

TEACHER TIP

Know the difference between genotype and phenotype. If you are given the genotype of an organism, you should be able to predict the phenotype. However, if you are given the phenotype, you cannot always predict the genotype because dominant and recessive alleles are present.

MENDELIAN GENETICS

In the 1860s, Gregor Mendel developed the basic principles of genetics through his experiments with the garden pea. Mendel studied the inheritance of individual pea traits by performing genetic crosses: He took **true-breeding** individuals (which, if self-crossed, produce progeny only with the parental phenotype) with different traits, mated them, and statistically analyzed the inheritance of the traits in the progeny.

A. MENDEL'S FIRST LAW: LAW OF SEGREGATION

Mendel postulated four principles of inheritance:

- Genes exist in alternate forms (now referred to as alleles).
- An organism has two alleles for each inherited trait, one inherited from each parent.
- The two alleles segregate during meiosis, resulting in gametes that carry only one allele for any given inherited trait.
- If two alleles in an individual organism are different, only one will be fully expressed and the other will be silent. The expressed allele is said to be **dominant,** the silent allele, **recessive.** In genetics problems, dominant alleles are typically assigned capital letters, and recessive alleles are assigned lower case letters. Organisms that contain two copies of the same allele are **homozygous** for that trait; organisms that carry two different alleles are **heterozygous.**

1. Monohybrid Cross

The principles of Mendelian inheritance can be illustrated in a cross between two true-breeding pea plants, one with purple flowers and the other with white flowers. Since only one trait is being studied in this particular mating, it is referred to as a **monohybrid cross.** The individuals being crossed are the **Parental** or **P generation**; the progeny generations are the **Filial** or **F generations,** with each generation numbered sequentially (e.g., F_1, F_2, etc.).

The purple flower parent has the genotype PP (i.e., it has two P alleles) and is homozygous dominant. The white flower parent has the genotype pp and is homozygous recessive. When these individuals are crossed, they produce F_1 plants that are 100 percent heterozygous (genotype = Pp). Because purple is dominant to white, all the F_1 progeny have the purple flower phenotype.

2. Punnett Square

One way of predicting the genotypes expected from a cross is by drawing a **Punnett square** diagram. The parental genotypes are arranged around a grid, as shown in Figure 13.1. Because the genotype of each progeny will be the sum of the alleles donated by the parental gametes, their genotypes can be determined by looking at the intersections on the grid. A Punnett square indicates all the potential progeny genotypes, and the relative frequencies of the different genotypes and phenotypes can be easily calculated (see Figure 13.1).

TEACHER TIP

Being able to create and read Punnett squares is one of the most valuable skills on the MCAT. One passage will likely be devoted to genetics and will require that you draw and analyze at least one Punnett square.

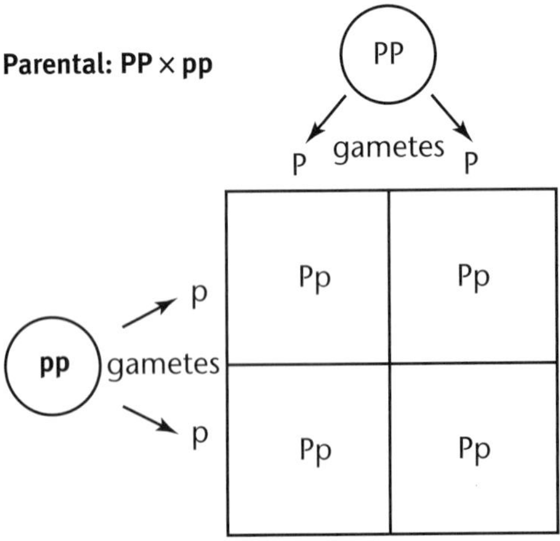

Figure 13.1. Monohybrid Cross

When the F_1 generation from our monohybrid cross is **self-crossed,** i.e., Pp × Pp, the F_2 progeny are more genotypically and phenotypically diverse than their parents. Because the F_1 plants are heterozygous, they will donate a P allele to half of their descendants and a p allele to the other half. One-fourth of the F_2 plants will have the genotype PP; 50 percent will have the genotype Pp; and 25 percent will have the genotype pp. Because the homozygous dominant and heterozygous genotypes both produce the dominant phenotype, purple flowers, 75 percent of the F_2 plants will have purple flowers, and 25 percent will have white flowers (see Figure 13.2).

This is a standard pattern of Mendelian inheritance. Its hallmarks are the disappearance of the silent (recessive) phenotype in the F_1 generation and its subsequent reappearance in 25 percent of the individuals in the F_2 generation.

TEACHER TIP

This common pattern of inheritance for a cross (disappearance of the silent allele in the F_1 with its reappearance in F_2) is worth memorizing. You should also learn the distribution for a dihybrid cross.

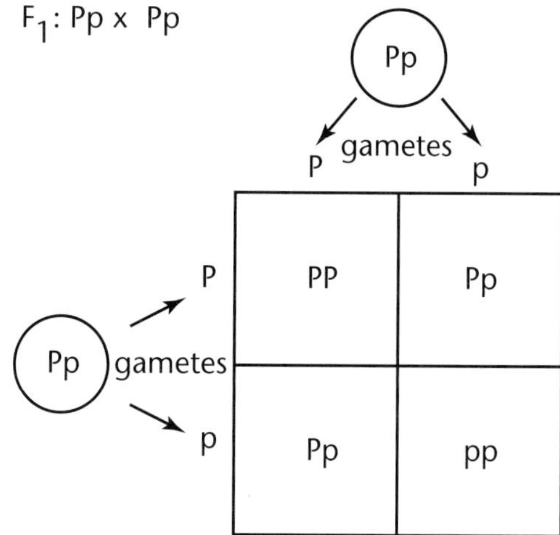

F_2 genotypes: 1:2:1; 1PP: 2Pp:1pp

F_2 phenotypes: 3:1; 3 purple:1 white

Figure 13.2. Self-Cross of F_1 Generation

3. Testcross

Only with a recessive phenotype can genotype be predicted with 100 percent accuracy. If the dominant phenotype is expressed, the genotype can be either homozygous dominant or heterozygous. Thus, homozygous recessive organisms always breed true. This fact can be used to determine the unknown genotype of an organism with a dominant phenotype. In a procedure known as a **testcross** or **backcross,** an organism with a dominant phenotype of unknown genotype (Ax) is crossed with a phenotypically recessive organism (genotype aa). Because

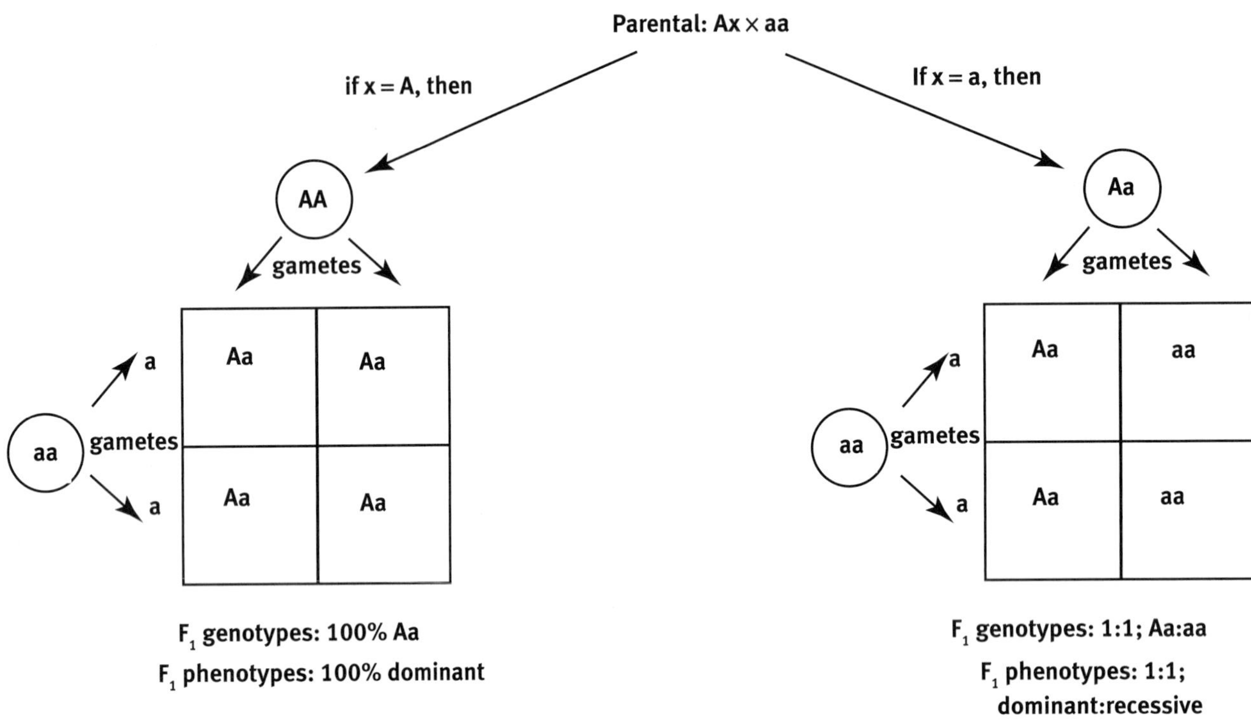

Figure 13.3. Testcross

Teacher Tip

Can you think of why we wouldn't use a homozygous DOMINANT organism for the testcross? Because then we wouldn't be able to tell the genotype of the test animal. Phenotypically, all of the animals would be the same because they would have at least one dominant allele from the homozygous dominant organism. Using the recessive organism allows us to work backward and determine genotype from phenotype (which usually isn't possible).

the recessive parent is homozygous, it can donate only the recessive allele, a, to the progeny. If the dominant parent's genotype is AA, all of its gametes will carry an A, and thus all of the progeny will have genotype Aa. If the dominant parent's genotype is Aa, half of the progeny will be Aa and express the dominant phenotype, and half will be aa and express the recessive phenotype. In a testcross, the appearance of the recessive phenotype in the progeny indicates that the phenotypically dominant parent is genotypically heterozygous (see Figure 13.3).

B. MENDEL'S SECOND LAW: LAW OF INDEPENDENT ASSORTMENT

1. Dihybrid Cross

The principles of the monohybrid cross can be extended to a dihybrid cross in which the parents differ in two traits, as long as each trait assorts independently; i.e., the alleles of unlinked genes assort independently during meiosis. This is known as Mendel's **law of independent assortment.**

In the following example, a purple-flowered tall pea plant is crossed with a white-flowered dwarf pea plant; both plants are doubly homozygous (tall is dominant to dwarf, T = tall allele, t = dwarf allele;

purple is dominant to white, P = purple allele, p = white allele). The purple parent's genotype is TTPP, and it thus produces only TP gametes; the white parent's genotype is ttpp and produces only tp gametes. The F_1 progeny will all have the genotype TtPp and will be phenotypically dominant for both traits.

When the F_1 generation is self-crossed (TtPp × TtPp), it produces four different phenotypes: tall purple, tall white, dwarf purple, and dwarf white, in the ratio 9:3:3:1, respectively. This is the typical pattern for Mendelian inheritance in a dihybrid cross between heterozygotes with independently assorting traits (see Figure 13.4).

MCAT SYNOPSIS

Note that each trait assorts individually in a 3:1 ratio, as in a monohybrid cross. There are nine purple tall and three purple dwarf, for a total of 12 purple; and there are three white tall and one white dwarf, for a total of four white. Hence, the purple:white ratio is 12:4 = 3:1. Likewise, the tall:dwarf ratio is 3:1.

TEACHER TIP

KEY POINT: Much as we learned the common 3:1 distribution for a monohybrid cross, this 9:3:3:1 distribution is worth learning for dihybrid crosses.

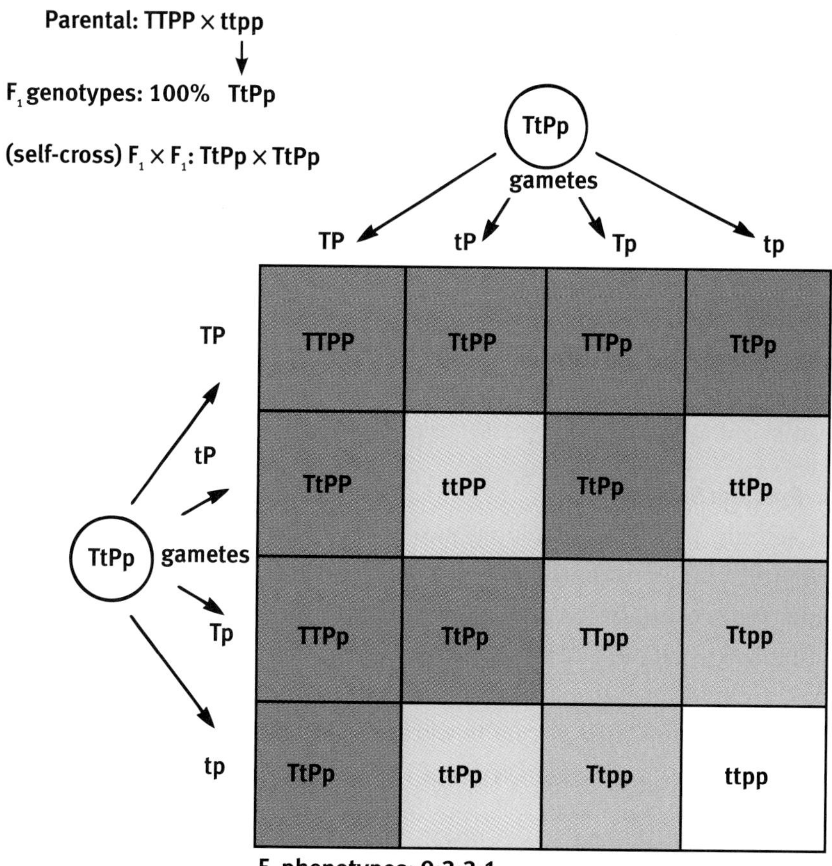

Figure 13.4. Dihybrid Cross

2. Statistical Calculations

Each F_1 parent in the dihybrid cross can produce four possible gametes: TP, Tp, tP, and tp. The probability of a particular genotype appearing in the F_2 progeny can be determined by calculating the number

TEACHER TIP

Don't fret over memorizing these numbers. Simply keep in mind that for most questions you'll be asked with multiple genes, assortment of them is mutually independent (i.e., inheritance of one gene does not affect the other). From there, the fractions are usually pretty easy to work out.

of different gamete combinations that will produce this genotype. For example, the genotype TTPP can be produced in only one way, by the fusion of two TP gametes. Because 1/4 of each parent's gametes will be TP, 1/4 of the other parent's gametes will also be TP, 1/4 × 1/4 or 1/16 of the total progeny will be TTPP. In statistical terms, the probability that one parent will donate a particular gamete (1/4 in this case) is independent of the probability that the other parent will donate a particular gamete (also 1/4). Consequently, the probability of producing a genotype that requires the occurrence of both these independent events is equal to the *product* of the individual probabilities that these events will occur (1/16).

In contrast, the genotype TtPp can be produced by four different gamete combinations, TP + tp; Tp + tP; tP + Tp; and tp + TP. The probability of any one of these combinations is 1/4 × 1/4 or 1/16 (e.g.,1/4 of one parent's gametes will be TP, and 1/4 of the other parent's gametes will be TP; the probability of these gametes fusing is the product of the individual probabilities). Because there are four ways to produce a TtPp genotype, the frequency of the TtPp genotype in the F_2 generation is 1/16 + 1/16 + 1/16 + 1/16 = 4/16 = 1/4. In statistical terms, the probability of producing a genotype that can be the result of more than one event is equal to the *sum* of the individual probabilities that these events will occur. (Note that statistical calculations are most accurate with a large sample size.)

3. Problem Solving

In solving problems involving two independently assorted traits, it generally helps to consider each trait individually. For example, consider the cross between a purple tall plant of unknown genotype and a white tall plant, also of unknown genotype. The F_1 generation consists of 62 tall plants with purple flowers, 59 tall plants with white flowers, 20 dwarf plants with purple flowers, and 21 dwarf plants with white flowers. What are the genotypes of the parental generation?

Because both parents are tall, but the F_1 generation contains dwarf plants, both parents must be heterozygous for tallness and hence of genotype Tt. If so, then tall plants should outnumber dwarf plants in the F_1 generation by a ratio of 3 to 1. In fact, the ratio of tall plants (62 + 59 = 121) to dwarf plants (20 + 21 = 41) is 121:41 or approximately 3:1.

In addition, one parent is white; it must therefore be homozygous pp. But Because the F_1 generation contained white-flowered plants, the purple parent must also have the allele for white flowers. If we now look at the segregation of purple and white alone, we find that the ratio of purple (62 + 20 = 82) to white (59 + 21 = 80) is almost 1:1. This is the ratio expected in a cross between a heterozygous dominant individual (Pp) and a homozygous recessive (pp). Thus, the genotype of the purple tall parent must be TtPp, and the genotype of the white tall parent must be Ttpp.

THE CHROMOSOMAL THEORY OF INHERITANCE

The principles of Mendelian genetics reflect the linear arrangement of genes on chromosomes. **Diploid** species have chromosome pairs **(homologues).** In diploids, the alleles for a given trait are segregated; one allele is located on one chromosome, and the other allele is found on its homologue.

A. SEGREGATION AND INDEPENDENT ASSORTMENT

Mendelian segregation and independent assortment are the consequences of chromosomal behavior during meiosis. Prior to meiosis, each chromosome is replicated, but the daughter copy remains attached to the parental chromosome via the centromere, forming sister chromatids. The sister chromatids pair with their homologues and align at the equatorial plate during metaphase I. During the first meiotic division, the homologous pairs separate, and following cytokinesis, the number of chromosomes per cell is reduced from 2N to N. This is the step in meiosis during which segregation and independent assortment occur. In the second meiotic division, the sister chromatids separate. Each gamete receives the haploid (N) complement of chromosomes; i.e., one sister chromatid from every homologous pair. The fusion of two gametes during fertilization restores the diploid number, 2N.

FLASHBACK

Now may be an opportune time to review meiosis. See chapter 4.

TEACHER TIP

What is the value of segregation and independent assortment? It allows for greater genetic diversity in the offspring.

B. NONINDEPENDENT ASSORTMENT: GENETIC LINKAGE

Not all traits assort independently in a dihybrid cross. In the sweet pea plant, the allele for purple-colored pollen (A) is dominant to the allele for red pollen (a); the allele for long pollen (B) is dominant to the allele for round pollen (b). In a cross between two purple long dihybrids (AaBb × AaBb), if the two traits assort independently, then the expected phenotypic ratio is 9 purple long:3 purple round:3 red long:1 red round. The purple long F_1 progeny have the **parental phenotype**, purple long; the other phenotypes are **recombinant phenotypes**, Because they recombine the parental traits. However, in this dihybrid cross, the F_1 genotypic ratio is 4 AABB:8 AaBb:4 aabb, or 1:2:1. The F_1 phenotypic ratio

TEACHER TIP

KEY POINT: The 3:1 and 9:3:3:1 distribution we learned for monohybrid and dihybrid crosses, respectively, only works if the genes are inherited independently (i.e., not linked). If they are linked, then the numbers aren't valid. Don't worry about this too much, though. It's far more likely you'll be asked IF genes are linked than if you can calculate the exact statistical numbers.

is 12 purple long:4 red round, or 3:1; the parental phenotype is overly represented in the progeny. In fact, the segregation pattern for these two traits in a dihybrid cross is like that of a single trait in a monohybrid cross. This is because genes A and B are **linked**; they are located on the same chromosome and are usually inherited together. This means that the parent AaBb does not produce four different types of gametes (AB, Ab, aB, ab). Instead, only two different gametes are produced; in this case, AB and ab. (If the two types of gametes were Ab and aB, then the genotypic ratio would have been 1 AAbb:2 AaBb:1 aaBB.)

Genetic linkage is a direct result of the organization of genes along chromosomes: linked genes are located on the same chromosome. Recall that during meiosis I, homologous chromosomes segregate into different cells. If two genes are located on the same chromosome, they tend to segregate together. The degree of genetic linkage can be tight and complete, with no recombinant phenotypes. Linkage can also be weak, as when the number of recombinants in the F_1 progeny approaches the number expected from independent assortment. Tightly linked genes recombine at a frequency close to 0 percent; weakly linked genes recombine at frequencies approaching 50 percent.

C. RECOMBINATION FREQUENCIES: GENETIC MAPPING

Linked genes can recombine at frequencies between 0 and 50 percent to produce recombinants. The recombinant chromosomes arise through the physical exchange of DNA between homologous chromosomes paired during meiosis. This process is called **crossing over** or **genetic recombination** (see chapter 4). Crossing over can unlink linked genes (see Figure 13.5).

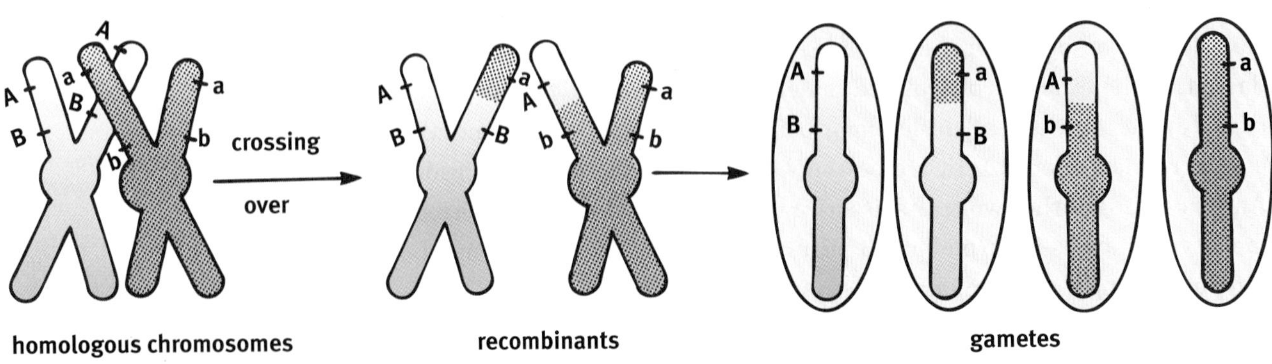

Figure 13.5. Crossing Over

The degree of genetic linkage is a measure of how far apart two genes are on the same chromosome. The probability of a crossover and exchange occurring between two points is generally directly proportional to the distance between the points. For example, pairs of genes that are far apart from each other on a chromosome have a higher probability of being separated during crossing over than pairs of genes that are located close to each other. Thus, the frequency of genetic recombination between two genes is related to the distance between them.

TEACHER TIP

KEY POINT: Crossing over allows for increased genetic diversity and hopefully greater reproductive fitness of the offspring. While this is a simple point and has been repeated many times already, it should indicate to you how important a concept it will be on the MCAT.

Recombination frequencies can be used to construct a **genetic map.** One **map unit** is defined as a 1 percent **recombinant frequency.** Recombination frequencies are roughly additive. If genes are found on a map in the order XYZ, then the recombination frequency between X and Y plus the recombination frequency between Y and Z will be roughly equal to the recombination frequency between X and Z. Likewise, if you are given the recombinant frequencies for X and Y, X and Z, and Y and Z (which can be determined by dividing the number of recombinant offspring by the total number of offspring), then you can determine the relative positions of these genes on the chromosome. In Figure 13.6, we are given that X and Y have a recombination frequency of 8 percent; i.e., they are 8 map units apart. If X and Z recombine 12 percent of the time, then they are 12 map units apart. Depending on where you draw Z in relation to X on your map, Y and Z are either 20 map units apart, or 4 map units apart. Since we are also given that Y and Z recombine with a frequency of 4 percent, the genes are in the order XYZ (or ZYX) on the chromosome.

FLASHBACK

Recall in chapter 4 that crossing over occurs when the homologous chromosomes pair up into tetrads during prophase I.

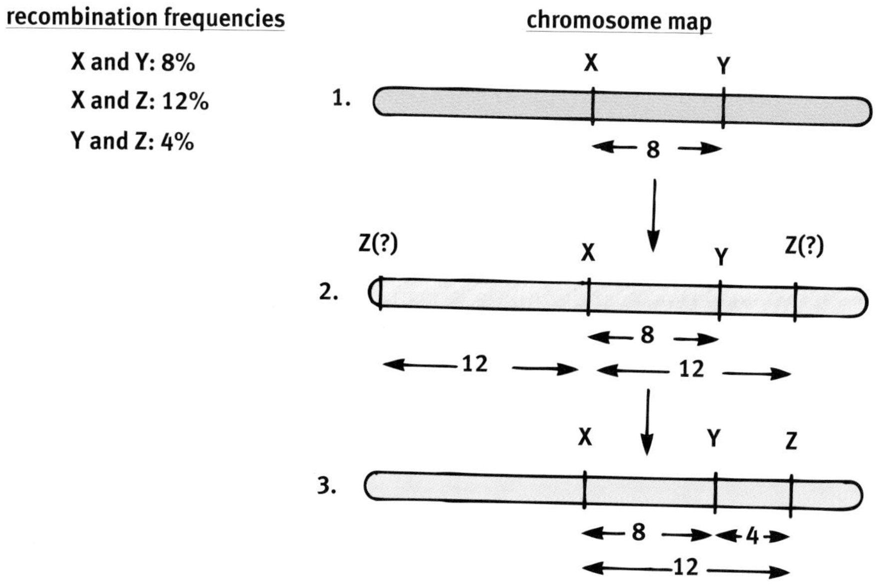

Figure 13.6. Chromosome Mapping

VARIATIONS ON MENDELIAN GENETICS

In real life, inheritance patterns are often more complicated than Mendel would have hoped. One major source of complication is in the relationship between phenotype and genotype. In theory, 100 percent of individuals with the recessive phenotype have a homozygous recessive genotype, and 100 percent of individuals with the dominant phenotype have either homozygous or heterozygous genotypes. Such clean concordance between genotype and phenotype is not always the case.

A. INCOMPLETE DOMINANCE

Some progeny phenotypes are apparently blends of the parental phenotypes. The classic example is flower color in snapdragons: homozygous dominant red snapdragons when crossed with homozygous recessive white snapdragons produce 100 percent pink progeny in the F_1 generation. When F_1 progeny are self-crossed, they produce red, pink, and white progeny in the ratio of 1:2:1, respectively (see Figure 13.7). The pink color is the result of the combined effects of the red and white genes in heterozygotes. An allele is **incompletely dominant** if the phenotype of the heterozygote is an intermediate of the phenotypes of the homozygotes.

TEACHER TIP

This 1:2:1 distribution is distinct from the 3:1 we saw with classic monohybrid crosses.

B. CODOMINANCE

Codominance occurs when multiple alleles exist for a given gene and more than one of them is dominant. Each dominant allele is fully dominant when combined with a recessive allele, but when two dominant alleles are present, the phenotype is the result of the expression of both dominant alleles simultaneously.

The classic example of codominance and multiple alleles is the inheritance of ABO blood groups in humans. Blood type is determined by three different alleles, I^A, I^B, and i. Only two alleles are present in any single individual, but the population contains all three alleles. I^A and I^B are both dominant to i. Individuals who are homozygous I^A or heterozygous I^Ai have blood type A; individuals who are homozygous I^B or heterozygous I^Bi have blood type B; and individuals who are homozygous ii have blood type O. However, I^A and I^B are codominant; individuals who are heterozygous I^AI^B have a distinct blood type, AB, which combines characteristics of both the A and B blood groups.

FLASHBACK

Remember: Type A individuals carry the A antigen on their RBCs and have circulating anti-B antibodies. Type B folks carry the B antigen and have circulating anti-A antibodies. Type O individuals have neither antigen and both antibodies. Type ABs have both antigens but neither antibodies. See chapter 9.

C. PENETRANCE AND EXPRESSIVITY

A dominant allele is not necessarily expressed to the same degree in all individuals who carry it; phenotype is a combination of genetics and

snapdragons

R = allele for red flowers

r = allele for white flowers

Parental: RR × rr (red × white)

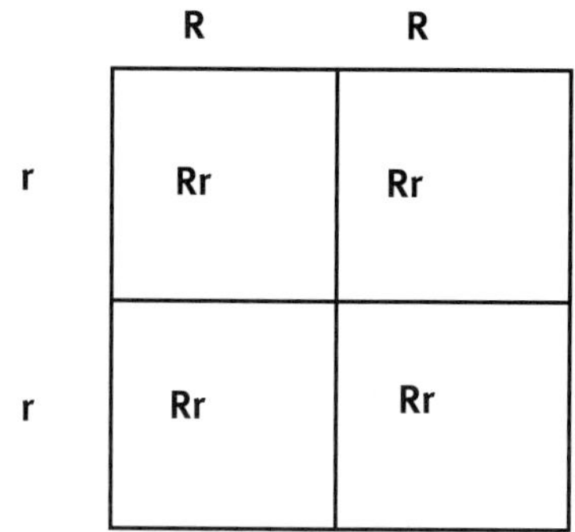

F_1 genotypic ratio: 100% Rr

F_1 phenotypic ratio: 100% pink

F_1: Rr × Rr (pink × pink)

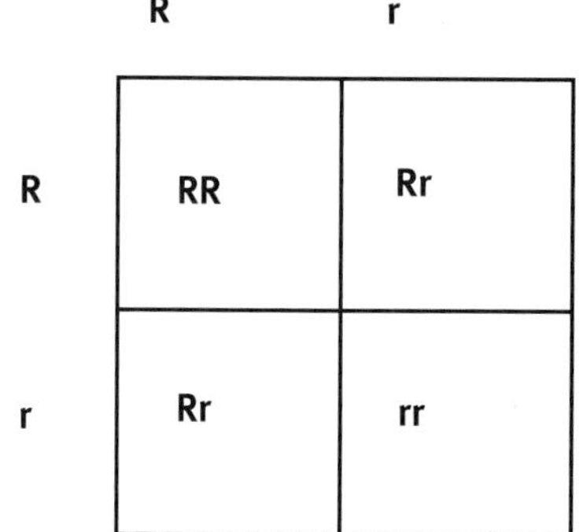

F_1 genotypic ratio: 1RR:2Rr:1rr

F_2 phenotypic ratio: 1 red:2 pink:1 white

Figure 13.7. Incomplete Dominance

environment. The **penetrance** of a genotype is the percentage of individuals in the population carrying the allele who actually express the phenotype associated with it. The **expressivity** of a genotype is the degree to which the phenotype associated with the genotype is expressed in individuals who carry the allele. Both penetrance and expressivity can be affected by environment; e.g., in the fruitfly *Drosophila melanogaster,* the dominant gene curly (C^Y) gives rise to adult flies with abnormal wings that curl up if the pupae are kept at 25°C, but remain uncurled if the pupae are kept at 19°C. At 25°C, C^Y is 100 percent penetrant, whereas at 19°C, C^Y is 0 percent penetrant. The expressivity is the degree of curliness of the wings.

D. INHERITED DISORDERS

1. Recessive

Recessively inherited disorders are caused by recessive alleles that are inherited as simple recessive traits. Individuals homozygous for the recessive allele exhibit the disorder, while heterozygotes are **carriers** of the disorder, and are capable of passing the allele on to their offspring. Individuals afflicted with such disorders are usually the result of a mating between two carriers. As in a typical dominant/recessive monohybrid cross, one-fourth of the offspring of such a mating are predicted to have the disorder. The disorders can be mild, like albinism, a lack of skin pigmentation; or **lethal,** like Tay-Sachs disease, which results from a malfunctioning enzyme that causes lipids to accumulate in the brain, causing death in early childhood. Since these alleles are recessive and do not typically affect carriers, the allele remains in the gene pool, "hidden" in carriers who are not selected against by natural selection. Most lethal genes are **early acting,** i.e., they program an early death for homozygotes, typically during embryonic development. Sometimes, lethal genes impart an advantage to heterozygous individuals, as in the case of sickle-cell anemia. Heterozygous individuals are resistant to malaria, while homozygous individuals have abnormal hemoglobin, which causes the painful and often fatal anemia.

TEACHER TIP

Keep this early-versus late-acting idea in mind. You may be asked if a condition is likely to be recessive or dominant based on a phenotypic model.

2. Dominant

Lethal alleles can also be dominant. These are **late-acting** genes; the classic example is the gene for Huntington's chorea in humans. Huntington's chorea is 100 percent penetrant and fully dominant; all individuals carrying the allele succumb to the disease. Since the Huntington's chorea gene isn't expressed until middle age, most of its victims have already had children by the time of diagnosis; assuming the other parent is normal, 50 percent of the children are predicted to inherit the Huntington's chorea gene.

E. SEX DETERMINATION

Different species vary in their systems of sex determination. In sexually differentiated species, most chromosomes exist as pairs of homologues called **autosomes** but sex is determined by a pair of **sex chromosomes.** All humans have 22 pairs of autosomes; additionally, females have a pair of homologous **X chromosomes,** and males have a pair of heterologous chromosomes, an **X** and a **Y** chromosome. The sex chromosomes pair during meiosis and segregate during the first meiotic division. Because females can produce only gametes containing the X chromosome, the

MCAT SYNOPSIS

The odds of a child being a boy or a girl are 50 percent. That means that regardless of how many sons or daughters a couple might have, the odds of having a boy or girl the next time around remains 50 percent. Each fertilization is an independent event!

gender of a zygote is determined by the genetic contribution of the male gamete. If the sperm carries a Y chromosome, the zygote will be male; if it carries an X chromosome, the zygote will be female. For every mating there is a 50 percent chance that the zygote will be male and a 50 percent chance that it will be female.

TEACHER TIP

The male completely determines the sex of the child. This has certain implications for sex-linked diseases. Because they are usually on the X-chromosome, a male can never pass a sex-linked disease onto his sons.

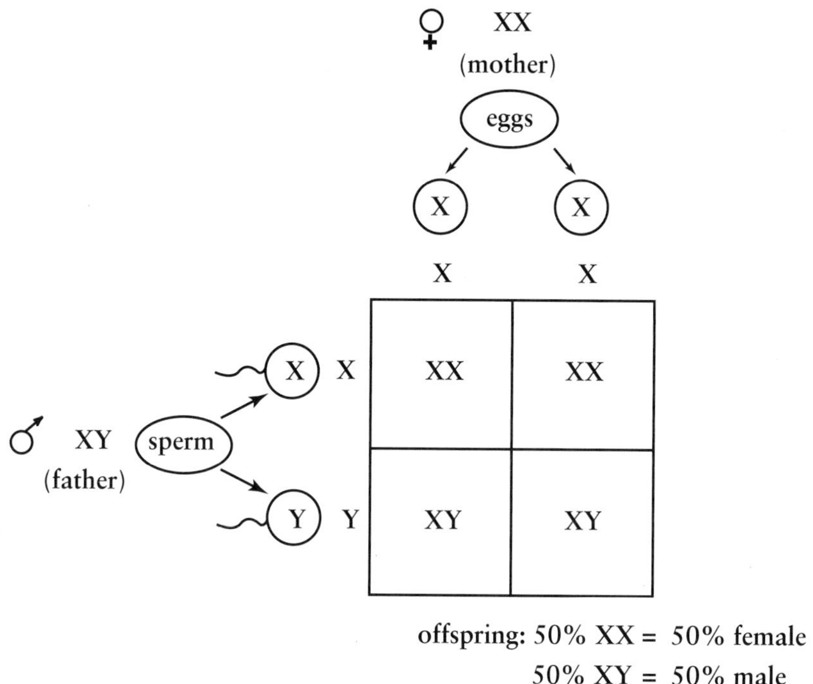

Figure 13.8. Sex Determination in Humans

Genes that are located on the X or Y chromosome are called **sex-linked.** In humans, most sex-linked genes are located on the X chromosome, though some Y-linked traits have been found (e.g., hair on the outer ears).

F. SEX LINKAGE

In humans, females have two X chromosomes, and males have only one. As a result, recessive genes that are carried on the X chromosome will produce the recessive phenotypes whenever they occur in males, since no dominant allele is present to mask them. The recessive phenotype will thus be much more frequently found in males. Examples of sex-linked recessives in humans are the genes for hemophilia and for color blindness.

TEACHER TIP

KEY POINT: Although females have 2 X-chromosomes, one of these is inactivated in each cell early during development.

The pattern of inheritance for a sex-linked recessive is somewhat complicated. Because the gene is carried on the X chromosome, and males pass the X chromosome only to their daughters, affected males *cannot* pass

a. Cross between a carrier female (X^hX) and a normal male (XY):

	X^h	X
X	X^hX	XX
Y	X^hY	XY

offspring
25% X^hX = 25% carrier female
25% XX = 25% normal female
25% X^hY = 25% hemophiliac male
25% XY = 25% normal male

b. Cross between a carrier female (X^hX) and a hemophiliac male (X^hY)

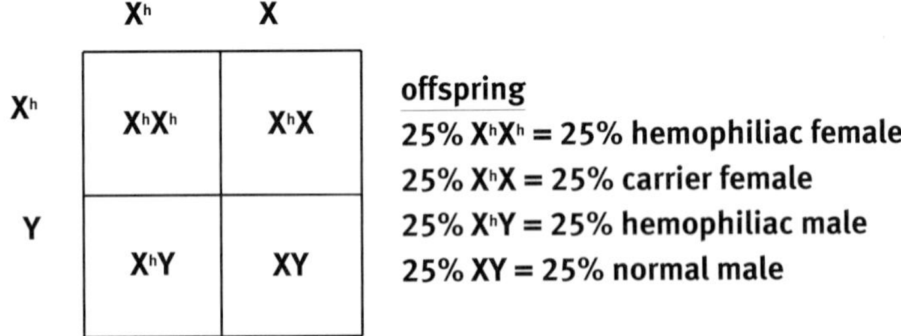

	X^h	X
X^h	X^hX^h	X^hX
Y	X^hY	XY

offspring
25% X^hX^h = 25% hemophiliac female
25% X^hX = 25% carrier female
25% X^hY = 25% hemophiliac male
25% XY = 25% normal male

Figure 13.9. Inheritance of Hemophilia Gene

the trait to their male offspring. Affected males will pass the gene to *all* of their daughters. However, unless the daughter also receives the gene from her mother, she will be a phenotypically normal carrier of the trait. Because all of the daughter's male children will receive their only X chromosome from her, half of her sons will receive the recessive sex-linked allele (see Figure 13.9). Thus, sex-linked recessives generally affect only males; they cannot be passed from father to son, but can be passed from father to grandson via a daughter who is a carrier, thereby skipping a generation.

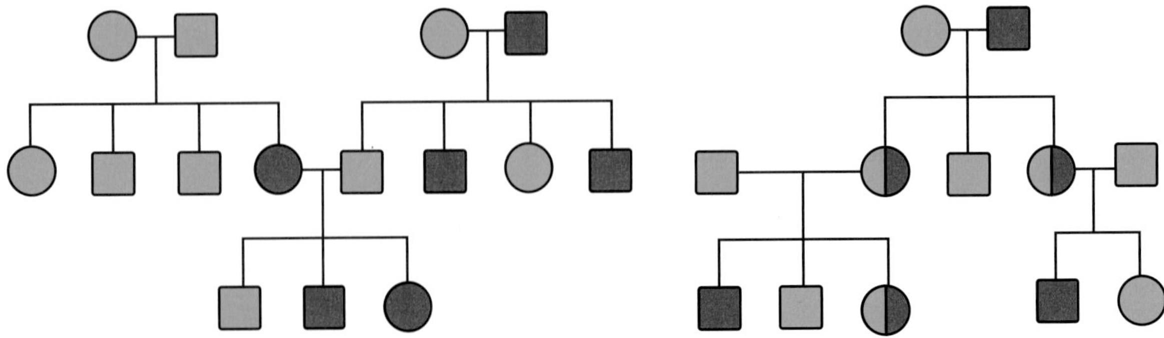

Figure 13.10a. Autosomal Recessive

Figure 13.10b. Sex-linked Recessive

PEDIGREE ANALYSIS

Ethical constraints forbid geneticists from performing testcrosses on human populations. Instead, they must rely on examining matings that have already occurred. A **pedigree** is a family tree depicting the inheritance of a particular genetic trait over several generations. By convention, males are indicated by squares and females by circles. Matings are indicated by horizontal lines, and descendants are listed below. Individuals affected by the trait are generally shaded, and unaffected individuals are unshaded. When carriers of sex-linked traits have been identified (typically, female heterozygotes), they are usually half shaded in family trees.

A human pedigree for a recessive autosomal trait, such as albinism, is shown in Figure 13.10a (an affected child born to parents that are normal) and, for a sex-linked trait, such as hemophilia, in Figure 13.10b (the key here is more affected males than females). In analyzing pedigrees, look for individuals with the recessive phenotype. Such individuals have only one possible genotype: homozygous recessive. Matings between them and the dominant phenotype behave as testcrosses; the ratio of phenotypes among the offspring allows deduction of the dominant genotype.

MCAT FAVORITE

When analyzing a pedigree, look for the recessive phenotype (you'll know the genotype) and work from there. If only males are affected, suspect sex linkage.

TEACHER TIP

Pedigrees are probably the most common type of informational passage seen on the MCAT. Because there are only seven passages, you can't guarantee that an entire one will be about pedigrees, but you will have at least a discrete question.

CHROMOSOMAL ABERRATIONS

Chromosome number and structure can be altered by abnormal cell division during meiosis or by mutagenic agents.

A. NONDISJUNCTION

Nondisjunction is either the failure of homologous chromosomes to separate properly during meiosis I, or the failure of sister chromatids to separate properly during meiosis II (usually in a secondary spermatocyte or secondary oocyte). In the case of a secondary spermatocyte, it results in one gamete with two copies of the chromosome (polyploid), two normal haploid gametes, and one gamete with no copies of the chromosome (aneuploid). The resulting zygote may have either three copies of that chromosome, called **trisomy** (somatic cells will have **2N + 1** chromosomes) or a single copy of that chromosome, called **monosomy** (somatic cells will have **2N – 1** chromosomes). A classic case of trisomy is the birth defect **Down's syndrome,** which is caused by trisomy of **chromosome 21.** Victims of Down's syndrome are of short stature, have characteristic facial features, and are mentally retarded. They are also usually sexually underdeveloped and have shorter-than-normal lifespans.

CLINICAL CORRELATE

Chronic Myeloid Leukemia (CML) is associated with a specific chromosomal abnormality called the Philadelphia chromosome. The Philadelphia chromosome represents a reciprocal translocation from chromosome 22 to chromosome 9. The presence of the Philadelphia chromosome is a reliable marker for CML.

TEACHER TIP

The human body deals with extra sex chromosomes better than it does with extra autosomal chromosomes. In fact, the only autosomal aberration compatible with long-term life is trisomy-21.

Most monosomies and trisomies are lethal, causing the embryo to spontaneously abort early in the pregnancy.

Nondisjunction of the sex chromosomes may also occur, resulting in individuals with extra or missing copies of the X and/or Y chromosomes. **XXY** individuals are afflicted with **Klinefelter's syndrome**; they are sterile males with abnormally small testes. **XO** females have only one sex chromosome and suffer from **Turner's syndrome**; they fail to develop secondary sexual characteristics and are sterile and of short stature. **XXX** females are referred to as **metafemales** and are usually mentally retarded and sometimes infertile. **XYY** males are normal males, though they tend to be taller than average and, according to some studies, may be more violent.

B. CHROMOSOMAL BREAKAGE

Chromosomal breakage may occur spontaneously or be induced by environmental factors, such as mutagenic agents and X rays. The chromosome that loses a fragment is said to have a deficiency. The fragment may join with its homologous chromosome, resulting in a **duplication,** or it may join with a nonhomologous chromosome, an event termed a **translocation.** The fragment may also rejoin its original chromosome but in the reverse position; this is known as an **inversion.** For example, Down's syndrome can also be caused by the translocation of a chromosome 21 fragment.

PRACTICE QUESTIONS

1. A 46-year-old man had a brother who died at the age of three from infantile Tay-Sachs disease, which is always fatal by age six. What is the probability that this man is a carrier of a disease gene?

   A. 100%
   B. 25%
   C. 50%
   D. Cannot be determined from the information given

2. During which phase of the meiotic division is crossing-over expected to occur?

   A. Anaphase I
   B. Prophase I
   C. Anaphase II
   D. Telophase I

3. A scientist interested in preparing a genetic map would expect a higher probability of a crossing-over to occur when

   A. the genes are located farther apart on the chromosome.
   B. there are fewer genes on the chromosome.
   C. there are more genes on the chromosome.
   D. the genes are located close to each other on the chromosome.

4. A mother with blood type I (O) has two children, one with blood type II (A) and another from the same father with blood type III (B). It can be concluded that the father's blood type is

   A. type III (B).
   B. type II (A).
   C. type IV (AB).
   D. Cannot be determined without further information

5. The ABO blood system is encoded by a single gene located on chromosome 9. How many primary alleles does this gene have?

   A. 1
   B. 2
   C. 3
   D. 4

6. Before the blood type system was discovered, the fatal transfusion of blood type III (B) to an individual with blood type II (A) would result in an agglutination (clumping) reaction between

   A. anti-A antibodies of the receiver and antigens A of the donor's blood.
   B. anti-A and anti-B antibodies of the donor's blood with antigens A of the receiver.
   C. anti-B antibodies of the donor's blood with antigens B of the receiver.
   D. anti-B antibodies of the receiver with antigens B of the donor's blood.

7. A couple has two sons. What is the probability that their next child is a boy?

   A. 50%
   B. 25%
   C. 12.5%
   D. 6.25%

8. A customer is interested in buying a purebred dog (homozygous dominant) in which black coat color is dominant. To make sure that the black dog he is offered is a purebred and not a heterozygote, which of the following would be the best mating to test the genotype?

A. Mating with a purebred (homozygous dominant)
B. Mating with a heterozygous dog
C. Mating with a homozygous recessive dog
D. Either A or B

9. Albinism is an autosomal recessive disease that disrupts the metabolic pathway normally leading to the production of the pigment melanin. If a man and a woman who are both carriers of a disease allele have a child, what is the probability of a phenotypically healthy child

A. 100%
B. 75%
C. 50%
D. 25%

10. Retinoblastoma, a disorder causing a malignant eye tumor, is an autosomal dominant disease with about 90 percent penetrance. This most likely means

A. 90 percent of people carrying the disease allele develop the disease.
B. 90 percent of people carrying the disease allele don't develop the disease.
C. 10 percent of people carrying the disease allele develop the disease.
D. 90 percent of people homozygous for the disease allele develop the disease.

11. Marfan syndrome is an autosomal dominant disorder affecting the cardiovascular system, the skeleton and the eye. This is an example of

A. full penetrance.
B. codominance.
C. imprinting.
D. pleiotropy.

12. Down syndrome is caused by trisomy 21. This is most likely the result of which of the following?

A. Nondisjunction
B. Insertion
C. Deletion
D. Inversion

13. A man who has phenylketonuria, an autosomal recessive disorder, marries a woman who is a carrier of the recessive allele of this gene. They have four sons. What is the probability that all children are affected?

A. $\frac{1}{2}$
B. $\frac{1}{4}$
C. $\frac{1}{8}$
D. $\frac{1}{16}$

14. Duchenne muscular dystrophy is a recessive X-linked disorder. If both sons in a family are affected, it can be inferred that the mother's genotype is which of the following?

I. Homozygous recessive
II. Homozygous dominant
III. Heterozygous

A. Only I
B. II or III
C. I or III
D. I, II, or III

15. From the pedigree of family X shown below, what is the most likely mode of inheritance?

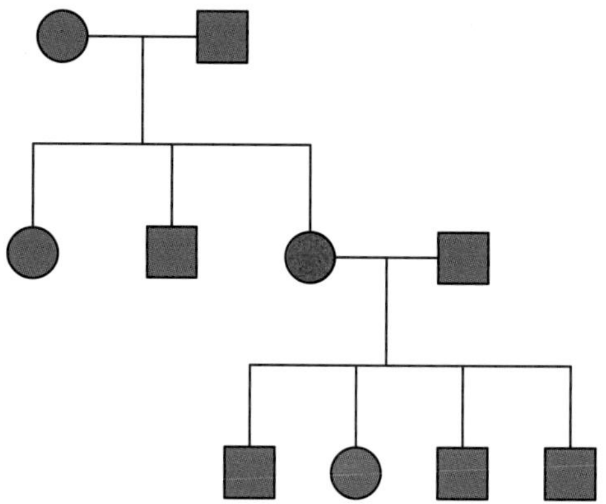

A. X-linked recessive
B. Autosomal recessive
C. Autosomal dominant
D. Mitochondrial inheritance

16. The pedigree below is for adult polycystic kidney disease, an autosomal dominant disorder. What is the risk that the offspring in generation III will develop the disorder?

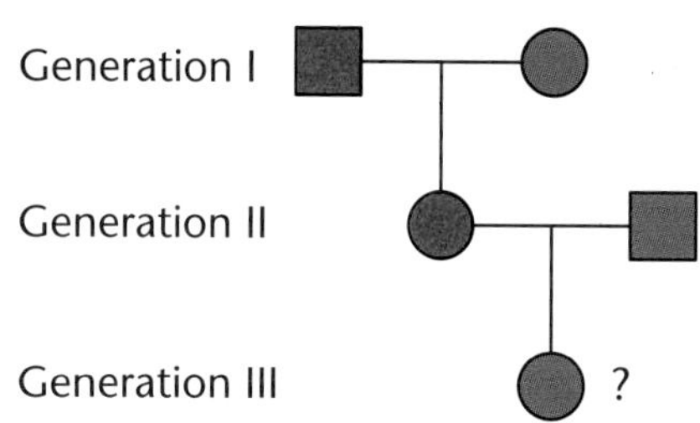

A. 100%
B. 75%
C. 50%
D. Cannot be determined without further information

17. The pedigree below is for Leber's hereditary optic neuropathy. This disorder has a mitochondrial mode of inheritance. All offspring of affected females have the disorder. This is most likely due to which of the following?

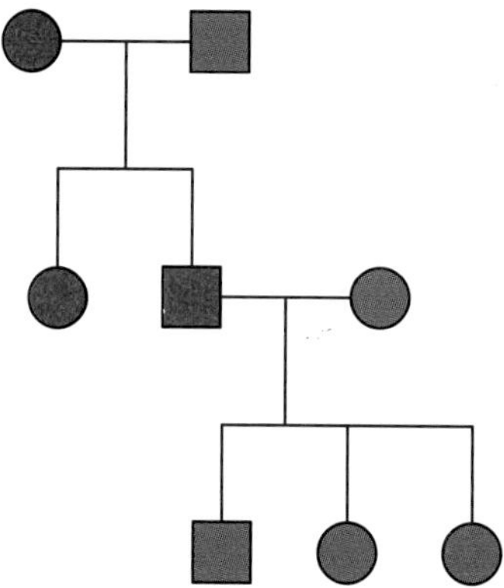

I. Males don't pass mitochondria to offspring.
II. The condition is X-linked.
III. Mitochondria are located in the cytoplasm.

A. I only
B. I and II
C. I and III
D. I, II, and III

18. Based on the pedigree below, which of the following can be concluded?

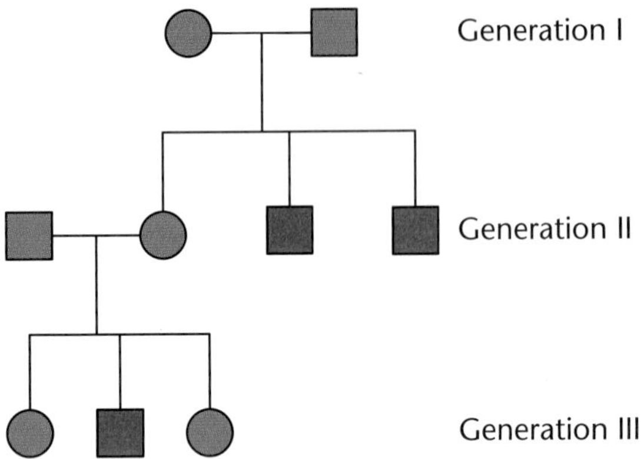

A. The disorder is X-linked dominant.
B. The father in generation II is a carrier of the disease.
C. This is an autosomal recessive disorder.
D. The mother in generation I is a carrier of the disease.

19. Having an extra chromosome 18, as shown on the drawing, leads to Edwards syndrome and is an example of

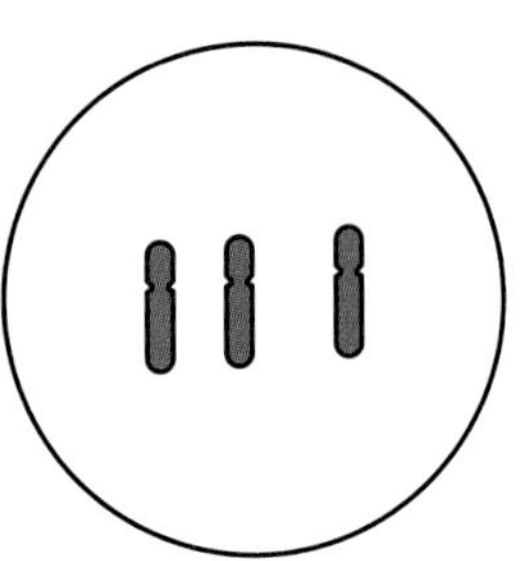

A. polyploidy.
B. triploidy.
C. monosomy.
D. aneuploidy.

20. A genetic disorder affects 1 in 10,000 members of the population. Determine the frequency of the normal allele of the gene in this population.

A. 0.01
B. 9999
C. 0.99
D. 0.0001

CLASSICAL GENETICS—PROBABILITY & PENETRANCE

Dystonia is a syndrome of involuntary spasms and sustained contractions of the muscles. One form of the disease is childhood dystonia, in which dystonia begins in the leg or foot and eventually spreads to involve the entire body. If one parent has this type of dystonia, while the other parent has no alleles for the disease, a child of those parents has a 50 percent chance of having the genotype for the disease. Given that the gene's penetrance is 40 percent, if a man with the disease (his mother was homozygous recessive) and a woman with no alleles for the disease have two children, what is the probability that both children will be healthy?

KEY CONCEPTS

Penetrance

Genotype

Phenotype

Probability

1) Identify the inheritance pattern.
No generation is skipped, and gender does not matter; thus, dystonia is an autosomal, dominant trait.

Whether it is presented in a pedigree diagram or indirectly given in the question stem, the inheritance pattern should be identified quickly. In the question stem above, we are told that if just one parent has the disease, there is at least a 50 percent chance she will pass it on to a child; thus, the trait must be dominant. The probabilities cited in the question stem are independent of the gender of the parent or the child; thus, sex-linked inheritance is ruled out.

---

2) Identify the relevant genotypes to set up the Punnet square.
Because the man is afflicted with the disease, and we have determined that the disease is autosomal dominant, he must be homozygous (DD) for the trait or heterozygous (Dd). Because his mother was homozygous recessive (dd), he must be heterozygous for the disease, as he received one recessive allele from his mother. The woman has no alleles for the disease and thus must be homozygous recessive (dd).

	D	**d**
d	Dd	dd
d	Dd	dd

The relevant genotypes may vary depending on the question. In this question, the relevant genotypes are those of the parents because we are interested in the probability of conceiving a healthy child.

TAKEAWAYS

After identifying the pattern of inheritance for the gene and the genotypes of the parental generation, set up the Punnet square to aid in the calculations of the probability questions posed. Unless otherwise stated, it is safe to assume that the penetrance of a gene in a given question is 100 percent.

---

3) Use the Punnet square to calculate the probability for each event.
The probability that the couple will bear two healthy children is $(80\%)^2 = 64\%$.

There is a 50 percent chance that a child will be homozygous recessive (healthy) and a 50 percent chance that the child will inherit the genotype for the disease. However, because penetrance is only 40 percent, there is only a 20 percent ($50\% \times 40\%$) chance of the child actually expressing the disease. Therefore, there is an 80 percent chance that the child will be healthy.

Recall that penetrance is the dependence of an organism's phenotype on the genotype. One hundred percent penetrance signifies no environmental effects, whereas 0 percent penetrance signifies no genetic influence of a particular gene on a physical trait. Here, we have 40 percent penetrance, which means that only 40 percent of the heterozygotes will actually suffer from childhood dystonia.

Remember: *To find the probabilities of both events occurring, multiply the probabilities of each event.*

THINGS TO WATCH OUT FOR

Beware of tricky probability questions. One typical trap was on your diagnostic: a disease is expressed in individuals who are homozygous recessive for the gene. Given parents who are both heterozygotes, what is the probability that a healthy child will be homozygous dominant? The Punnet square indicates 25 percent, but the trick is that we know the child is healthy; thus, there are only three possible outcomes—not four. Therefore, the probability is ⅓ instead of ¼.

SIMILAR QUESTIONS

1) The phenotype of an individual is known, but her genotype is not. Given a pedigree, could you determine the probability that she is homozygous dominant for this trait?
2) If normal parents have a colorblind son, what is the probabllity that he inherited the gene for colorblindness from his mother? What is the probability that he inherited the gene from his father?
3) A woman with blood genotype B marries a man with blood genotype A. What is the chance that their first child will have blood type B? What is the chance that their first and second children will have blood type B?

CHAPTER 14

MOLECULAR GENETICS

Genes are composed of **DNA (deoxyribonucleic acid),** which contains information coded in the sequence of its base pairs, providing the cell with a blueprint for protein synthesis. Furthermore, DNA has the ability to self-replicate, which is crucial for cell division, and hence for organismal reproduction. DNA is the basis of heredity; self-replication ensures that its coded sequence will be passed on to successive generations. This is the central dogma of molecular genetics and it is summarized in Figure 14.1.

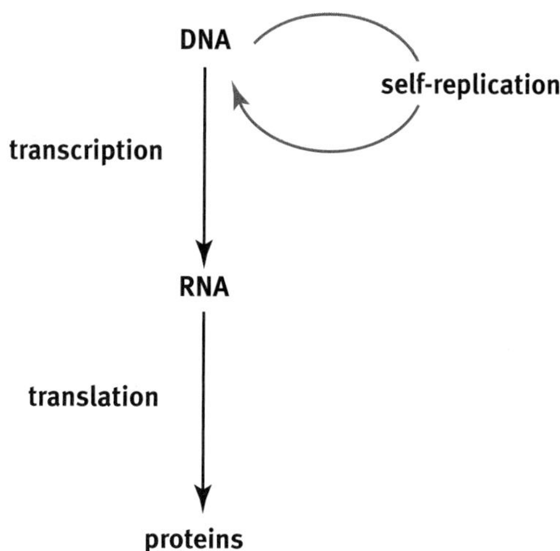

Figure 14.1. Central Dogma of Molecular Genetics

TEACHER TIP

The MCAT has become increasingly focused on molecular genetics, of which this theory forms the core. Also important to know is that some viruses (retroviruses, including HIV) use RNA as their genetic material, which is then turned back into DNA in a process called reverse transcription.

DNA

A. STRUCTURE

The basic unit of DNA is the **nucleotide,** which is composed of **deoxyribose** (a sugar) bonded to both a **phosphate group** and a **nitrogenous base.** There are two types of bases: the double-ringed **purines** and the single-ringed **pyrimidines.** The purines in DNA are **adenine (A)** and **guanine (G),** and the pyrimidines are **cytosine (C)** and **thymine (T)** (see Figure 14.2).

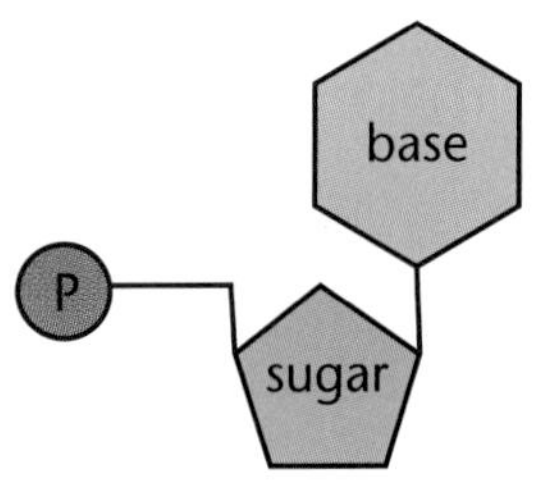

Figure 14.2. Nucleotide

Nucleotides bond together to form polynucleotides. The 3′ hydroxyl group of the sugar on one nucleotide is joined to the 5′ hydroxyl group of the adjacent sugar by a phosphodiester bond. The phosphate and sugar form a chain with the bases arranged as side groups off the chain.

MCAT Synopsis

Due to complementary base pairing in DNA, the amount of A will equal the amount of T and G will equal C. Also, because G is triple bonded to C, the higher the G/C content of DNA, the more tightly bound the two strands will be.

A DNA molecule is a **double-stranded helix** with the sugar-phosphate chains on the outside of the helix and the bases on the inside. T always forms **two** hydrogen bonds with A; G always forms **three** hydrogen bonds with C. This **base-pairing** forms "rungs" on the interior of the double helix that link the two polynucleotide chains together (see Figure 14.3).

Teacher Tip

If A-T forms two hydrogen bonds and C-G forms three, what does this mean about the relative stability of DNA strands that are A/T-rich versus those that are C/G-rich? Because H-bonds are INTER-molecular interactions, you can use heat to melt the two strands of DNA apart. This is the basis of the polymerase chain reaction. This A/T versus C/G ratio tells us how high the temperature needs to be, with more C/G requiring a higher temperature.

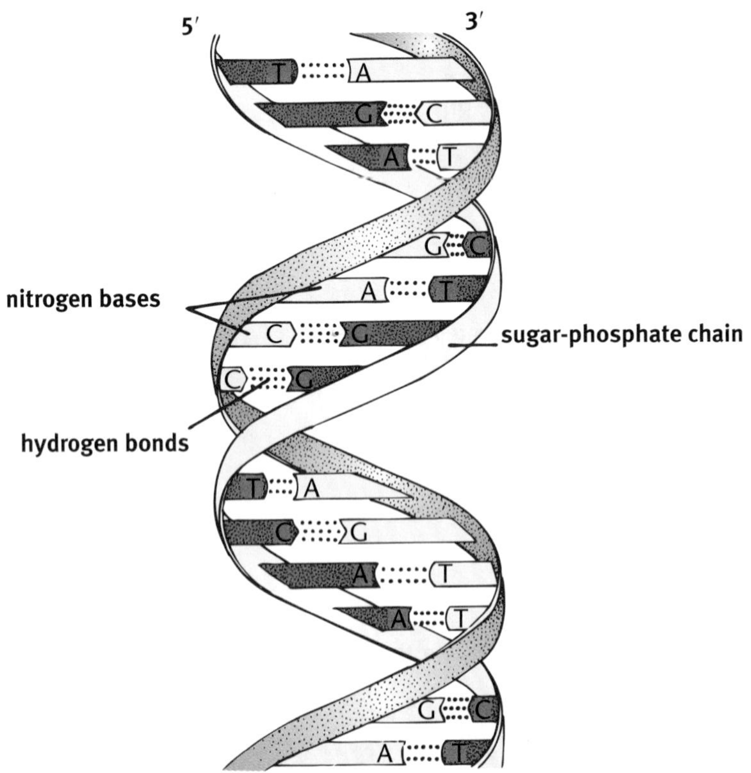

Figure 14.3. DNA Molecule

The strands are positioned **antiparallel** to each other, i.e., one strand has a **5′ → 3′ polarity,** and its complementary strand has a **3′ → 5′ polarity.** The 5′ end is designated as the end with a free hydroxyl group (or phosphate group) bonded to the 5′ carbon of the terminal sugar; the 3′ end is designated as the one with a free hydroxyl group attached to the 3′ carbon of the terminal sugar. This is known as the **Watson-Crick** model of DNA (see Figure 14.4).

MCAT Synopsis

1) Watson-Crick double helix
2) Antiparallel
3) 5′ → 3′ polarity
4) Adenine bonds to thymine with 2-hydrogen bonds
5) Cytosine bonds to guanine with 3-hydrogen bonds

5′end

5′ → 3′

3′end

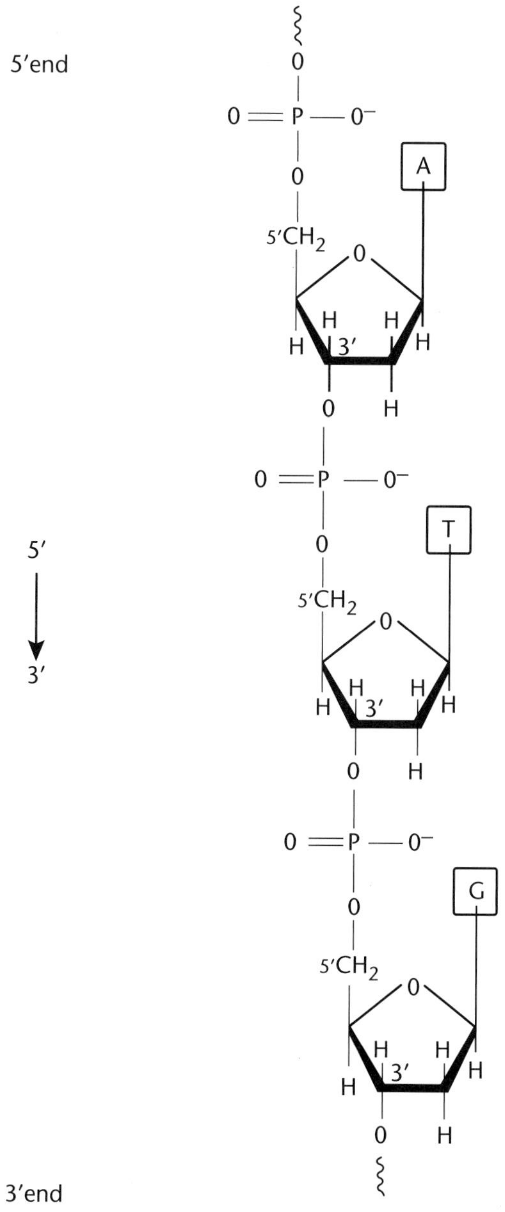

Figure 14.4. Single-Stranded DNA

Teacher Tip

One of the most common MCAT topics is the 5′ → 3′ nature of DNA. This may be in the form of a discrete or passage-based question. It may be on transcription, translation, or general base pairing. The bottom line is that DNA and RNA work in a 5′ → 3′ direction.

B. DNA REPLICATION (EUKARYOTIC)

Teacher Tip

Previous MCAT administrations have asked how you can tell the new strand from the old immediately following replication. The answer is methylation. As DNA ages, methyl groups may be added to it for a variety of reasons. When the new complimentary strand is synthesized, these methyl groups aren't immediately present, so you can tell the old strand from the new simply by looking for methylation!

1. Semiconservative Replication

During replication, the helix unwinds and each strand acts as a template for complementary base-pairing in the synthesis of two new daughter helices. Each new daughter helix contains an intact strand from the parent helix and a newly synthesized strand; thus DNA replication is **semiconservative.** The daughter DNA helices are identical in composition to each other and to the parent DNA (see Figure 14.5).

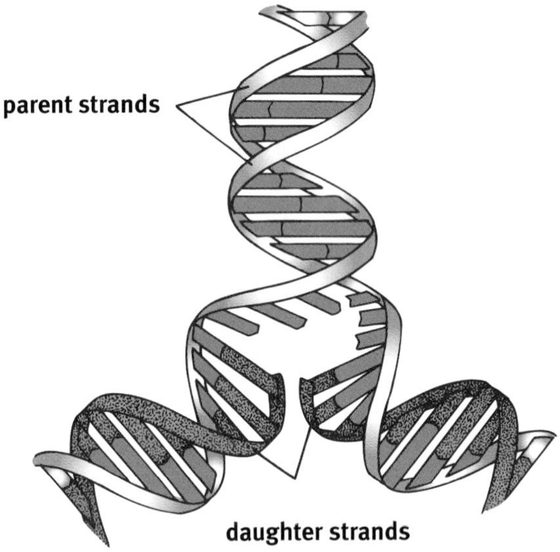

Figure 14.5. Semiconservative Replication

2. Origin of Replication

As the helix unwinds, both strands are simultaneously copied with the aid of more than a dozen enzymes, at the rate of about 50 nucleotide additions per second (in mammals). Replication begins at specific sites along the DNA called **origins of replication** and proceeds in both directions simultaneously. As replication proceeds in a given direction, a **replication fork** forms (see Figure 14.6).

Teacher Tip

Bacteria have topoisomerases as well. Some of our antibiotics poison these as their mechanism of actions. Because the topoisomerases of bacteria are somewhat different from ours, the human isn't hurt. We also use topoisomerase poisons in cancer treatment. In that case, we want to stop cell division so we prevent DNA replication (requied for cell division) by keeping it from unwinding.

3. Unwinding and Initiation

The enzyme **helicase** unwinds the helix, while **single-strand binding** protein (SSB) binds to the single strands and stabilizes them, preventing them from recoiling and reforming a double helix. **DNA gyrase** is a type of *topoisomerase* that enhances the action of helicase by the introduction of negative supercoils into the DNA molecule.

A **primer** chain, usually several nucleotides long and composed of RNA, is necessary for the initiation of DNA synthesis. An RNA polymerase, **primase,** synthesizes the primer, which binds to a segment of DNA to

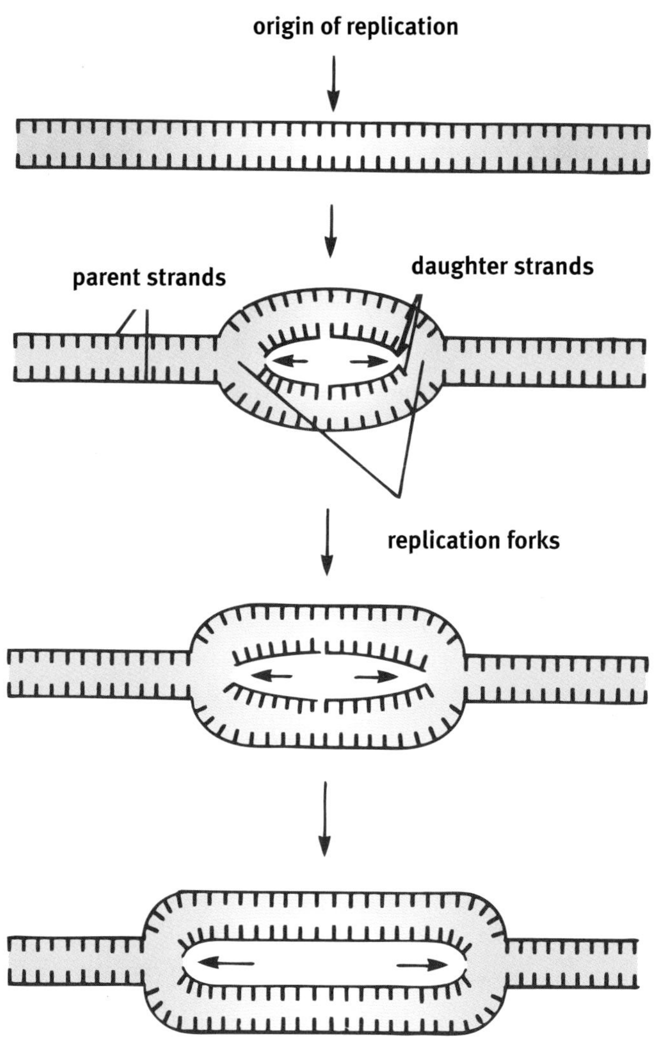

Figure 14.6. Origin of Replication

TEACHER TIP

There are approximately three billion base pairs in the human genome. This complete genome is present in every single one of your autosomal cells. In order for DNA replication to proceed at a rapid enough rate, there are thousands and thousands of origins of replication in the genome.

which it is complementary and serves as the site for nucleotide addition. The first nucleotide binds to the 3′ end of the primer chain.

4. Synthesis

DNA synthesis proceeds in the 5′ → 3′ direction and is catalyzed by a group of enzymes collectively known as **DNA polymerases.** The double-stranded DNA ahead of the DNA polymerase is unwound by a helicase, and SSB again keeps the unwound DNA in a single-stranded form so that both strands can serve as templates. DNA gyrase concurrently introduces negative supercoils to relieve the tension created during unwinding. As the helix unwinds, free nucleotides (attached to pyrophosphate groups [PPi]) are aligned opposite the parent strands. The nucleotides form phosphodiester linkages, releasing the pyrophosphate, and the bases form H-bonds with their complements.

TEACHER TIP

Replication is subject to the 5′ → 3′ rule. This means that one strand—the lagging—is synthesized DISCONTINUOUSLY. Prior MCAT administrations have ask which strand is more likely to be subject to errors. Not surprisingly, it is the lagging strand, as the replication machinery has to hop on and off more often.

One daughter strand is the **leading strand** and the other daughter strand is the **lagging strand.** The leading strand is continuously synthesized by DNA polymerase in the 5′ → 3′ direction. The lagging strand is synthesized discontinuously in the 5′ → 3′ direction (since DNA polymerase synthesizes only in that direction) as a series of short segments known as **Okazaki fragments**; however, overall growth of the lagging strand occurs in the 3′ → 5′ direction (see Figure 14.7). The lagging strand loops through DNA polymerase in the same direction as the leading strand. The looped segment of the lagging strand is primed with RNA, and DNA polymerase adds a short sequence of nucleotides (approximately 1,000). The lagging strand is released and a new loop is formed. Primase again synthesizes a short stretch of primer to initiate the formation of another Okazaki fragment. The RNA primers are removed and replaced by DNA. The gaps between the Okazaki fragments are also filled in with DNA. Finally, the fragments are covalently linked by the enzyme **DNA ligase** (see Figure 14.7).

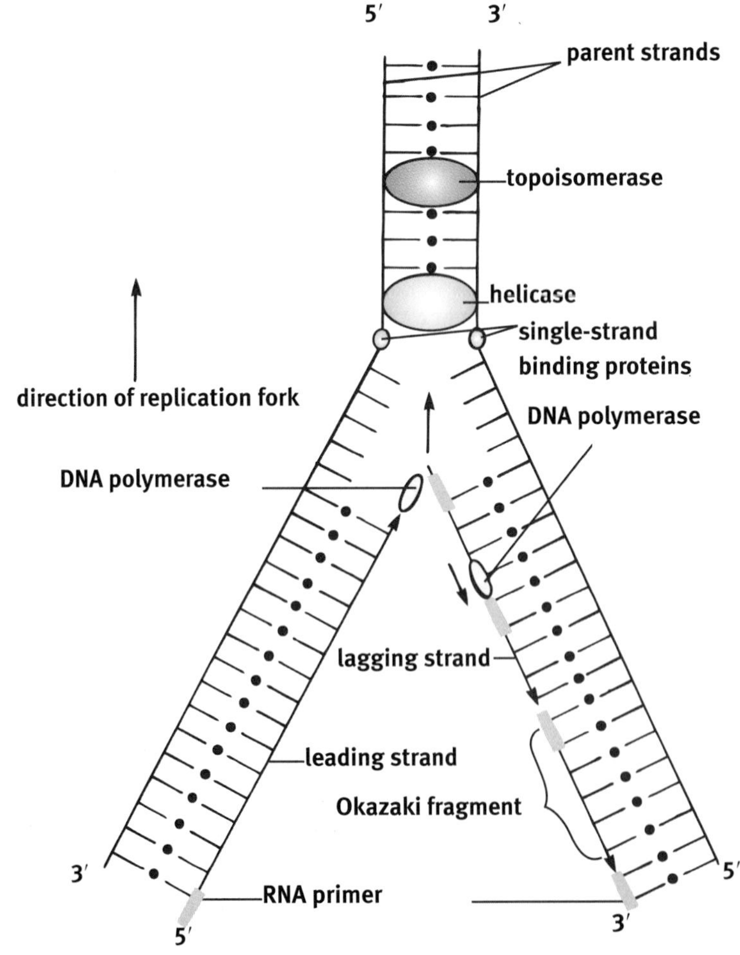

Figure 14.7. DNA Replication

RNA

RNA, ribonucleic acid, is a polynucleotide structurally similar to DNA except that its sugar is ribose, it contains uracil (U) instead of thymine, and it is usually **single-stranded.** RNA can be found in both the nucleus and the cytoplasm. There are several types of RNA, all of which are involved in some aspect of protein synthesis: **mRNA, tRNA, rRNA,** and **hnRNA.**

A. MESSENGER RNA (mRNA)

mRNA carries the complement of a DNA sequence and transports it from the nucleus to the ribosomes, where protein synthesis occurs. mRNA is **monocistronic**; i.e., one mRNA strand codes for one polypeptide.

B. TRANSFER RNA (tRNA)

tRNA is found in the cytoplasm and aids in the translation of mRNA's nucleotide code into a sequence of amino acids. tRNA brings amino acids to the ribosomes during protein synthesis. There is at least one type of tRNA for each amino acid, and approximately 40 known types of tRNA.

C. RIBOSOMAL RNA (rRNA)

rRNA is a structural component of ribosomes and is the most abundant of all RNA types. rRNA is synthesized in the nucleolus.

D. HETEROGENEOUS NUCLEAR RNA (hnRNA)

hnRNA is a large ribonucleoprotein complex that is the precursor of mRNA.

MCAT SYNOPSIS

DNA:

- Double-stranded
- Sugar = deoxyribose
- Base pariing: A/T, G/C
- Found in nucleus only

RNA:

- Single-stranded
- Sugar = ribose
- Base pairing: A/U, G/C
- Found in nucleus and cytoplasm

TEACHER TIP

mRNA is the messenger. The DNA codes for proteins but can't carry out any of the enzymatic reactions itself. Proteins can carry out the reactions but need to know how to build themselves in order to do the right chemistry. mRNA takes the work orders from the DNA to the ribosomes to create the proteins, which allow for reactions necessary for life to occur.

PROTEIN SYNTHESIS (EUKARYOTIC)

A. TRANSCRIPTION

Transcription is the process whereby information coded in the base sequence of DNA is transcribed into a strand of mRNA. The strand of mRNA is synthesized from a DNA template in a process similar to DNA replication. The DNA helix unwinds at the point of transcription, and synthesis occurs in the $5' \rightarrow 3'$ direction, using only one DNA strand (the **antisense strand**) as a template. The base-pairing rules are the same as for DNA, with U replacing T (G bonds with C; A bonds with U). mRNA is synthesized by the enzyme **RNA polymerase,** which must bind to sites on the DNA called **promoters** to begin RNA synthesis. Synthesis continues until the polymerase encounters a **termination sequence,** which signals RNA polymerase to stop transcription, thus allowing the DNA helix to reform. The mRNA strand is then processed and leaves the nucleus through nuclear pores.

KAPLAN EXCLUSIVE

INtrons are cut **OUT!**
Exons are **ex**pressed.

B. POST-TRANSCRIPTIONAL RNA PROCESSING

Most eukaryotic DNA does not code for proteins; noncoding or "garbage" sequences are found between coding sequences. A typical gene consists of several coding sequences, **exons,** interrupted by noncoding sequences, **introns.** The RNA initially transcribed is a precursor molecule, hnRNA, which contains both introns and exons. During hnRNA processing, the introns are cleaved and removed, while the exons are spliced to form a mRNA molecule coding for a single polypeptide. Processing occurs within the nucleus, and is also necessary for tRNA and rRNA production (see Figure 14.8).

Teacher Tip

You might be asked what is necessary for a piece of RNA to become a message. The RNA that is synthesized from the DNA must be processed in three ways: 1) a 5′ guanosyl cap must be added; 2) a poly-A tail must be added; and 3) introns must be removed. Failure to complete these steps will result in degradation of the pre-mRNA.

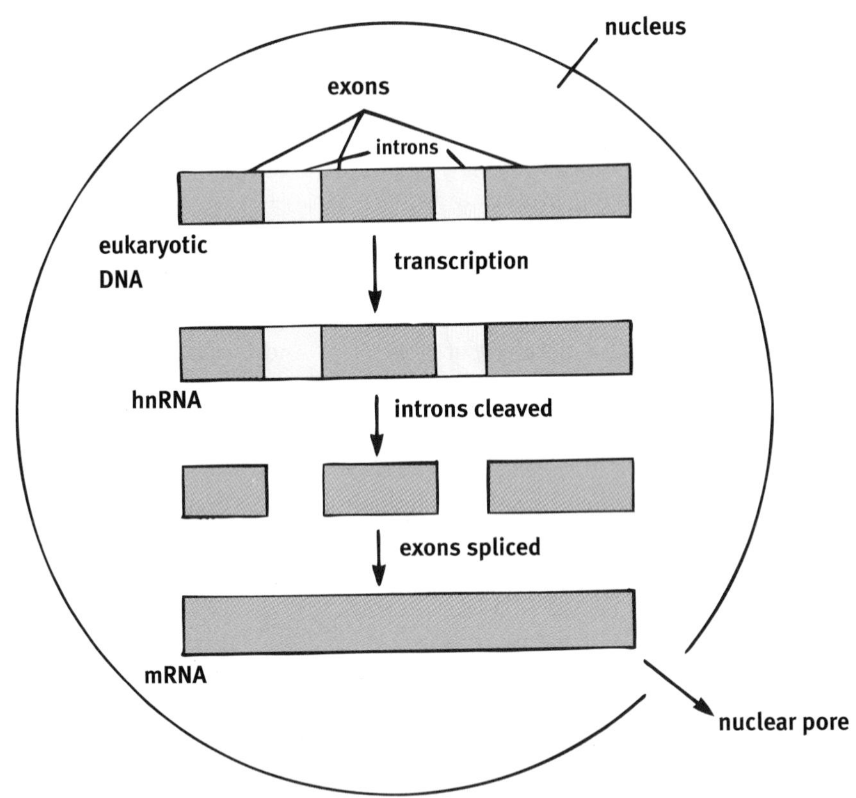

Figure 14.8. mRNA Processing

C. THE GENETIC CODE

The language of DNA consists of four "letters": A, T, C, and G. The language of proteins consists of 20 "words": the 20 amino acids. The DNA language must be translated by mRNA in such a way as to produce the 20 words in the amino acid language; hence, the **triplet code.** (A 2-letter [doublet] code would not suffice; with only four letters in the DNA alphabet, there would be only $4^2 = 16$ words possible—not enough to code for all 20 amino acids.) The base sequence of mRNA is translated as a series of triplets, otherwise known as **codons.** A sequence of three consecutive bases codes for a particular amino acid; e.g., the codon GGC specifies glycine, and the codon GUG specifies valine. The genetic code is universal for almost all organisms. (The exceptions are found in single-celled eukaryotes called ciliated protozoa, in mycoplasma, and in the mitochondria of several species.)

MCAT SYNOPSIS

Each codon represents only one amino acid, but most amino acids are represented by more than one codon.

Given that there are 4^3, or 64, different codons possible based on the triplet code, and there are only 20 amino acids that need to be coded, the code must contain synonyms. Most amino acids have more than one codon specifying them. This property is referred to as the **degeneracy** or **redundancy** of the genetic code (see Table 14.1).

TEACHER TIP

The genetic code is mostly degenerate for commonly used amino acids. AA like glycine and proline, which are necessary to make collagen, are completely redundant at the third position, whereas those AA used less commonly may have only one or two coding sequences.

Table 14.1. The Genetic Code

First Base (5′)	Second Base: U		Second Base: C		Second Base: A		Second Base: G		Third Base (3′)
U	UUU	Phe	UCU	Ser	UAU	Tyr	UGU	Cys	U
U	UUC	Phe	UCC	Ser	UAC	Tyr	UGC	Cys	C
U	UUA	Leu	UCA	Ser	UAA	***Stop***	UGA	***Stop***	A
U	UUG	Leu	UCG	Ser	UAG	***Stop***	UGG	Trp	G
C	CUU	Leu	CCU	Pro	CAU	His	CGU	Arg	U
C	CUC	Leu	CCC	Pro	CAC	His	CGC	Arg	C
C	CUA	Leu	CCA	Pro	CAA	Gln	CGA	Arg	A
C	CUG	Leu	CCG	Pro	CAG	Gln	CGG	Arg	G
A	AUU	Ile	ACU	Thr	AAU	Asn	AGU	Ser	U
A	AUC	Ile	ACC	Thr	AAC	Asn	AGC	Ser	C
A	AUA	Ile	ACA	Thr	AAA	Lys	AGA	Arg	A
A	AUG	Start or Met	ACG	Thr	AAG	Lys	AGG	Arg	G
G	GUU	Val	GGU	Ala	GAU	Asp	GGU	Gly	U
G	GUC	Val	GGC	Ala	GAC	Asp	GGC	Gly	C
G	GUA	Val	GGA	Ala	GAA	Glu	GGA	Gly	A
G	GUG	Val	GGG	Ala	GAG	Glu	GGG	Gly	G

D. TRANSLATION

Translation is the process whereby mRNA codons are translated into a sequence of amino acids. Translation occurs in the cytoplasm and involves tRNA, ribosomes, mRNA, amino acids, enzymes, and other proteins.

1. tRNA

tRNA brings amino acids to the ribosomes in the correct sequence for polypeptide synthesis; tRNA "recognizes" both the amino acid and the mRNA codon. This dual function is reflected in its three-dimensional structure: one end contains a three-nucleotide sequence, the **anticodon,** which is complementary to one of the mRNA codons; the other end is the site of amino acid attachment and consists of a CCA sequence for all tRNA. Each amino acid has its own **aminoacyl-tRNA synthetase,** which has an active site that binds to both the amino acid and its corresponding tRNA, catalyzing their attachment to form an **aminoacyl-tRNA complex.** (This is an energy-requiring process.)

FLASHBACK

You can think of DNA as being responsible for genotype and protein as being responsible for phenotype. See chapter 13.

TEACHER TIP

The catalyzation reaction requires energy. Although the most common energy currency of the cell is ATP, this process actually uses energy generated from GTP (a similar molecule). While this seems like a minor point, it is one of those exceptions often tested on the exam.

2. Ribosomes

Ribosomes are composed of two subunits (consisting of proteins and rRNA), one large and one small, that bind together only during protein synthesis. Ribosomes have three binding sites: one for mRNA, and two for tRNA: the **P site** (peptidyl-tRNA binding site) and the **A site** (aminoacyl-tRNA complex binding site). The P site binds to the tRNA attached to the growing polypeptide chain, while the A site binds to the incoming aminoacyl-tRNA complex.

3. Polypeptide Synthesis

Polypeptide synthesis can be divided into three distinct stages: **initiation, elongation,** and **termination.** All three stages are energy-requiring and are mediated by enzymes.

MCAT SYNOPSIS

DNA → DNA = replication (new DNA synthesized in 5′ → 3′ direction)

DNA → RNA = transcription (new RNA synthesized in 5′ → 3′ direction)

RNA → protein = translation (mRNA read in 5′ → 3′ direction)

a. Initiation

Synthesis begins when the small ribosomal subunit binds to the mRNA near its 5′ end in the presence of proteins called **initiation factors.** The ribosome scans the mRNA until it binds to a start codon (AUG). The initiator aminoacyl-tRNA complex, **methionine-tRNA** (with the anticodon 3′-UAC-5′), base pairs with the start codon. The large ribosomal unit then binds to the small one, creating a complete ribosome with the met-tRNA complex sitting in the P site.

b. Elongation

Hydrogen bonds form between the mRNA codon in the A site and its complementary anticodon on the incoming aminoacyl-tRNA complex. The enzyme **peptidyl transferase** catalyzes the formation of a peptide bond between the amino acid attached to the tRNA in the A site and the met attached to the tRNA in the P site. Following peptide bond formation, a ribosome carries uncharged tRNA in the P site and peptidyl-tRNA in the A site. The cycle is completed by **translocation,** in which the ribosome advances three nucleotides along the mRNA in the 5′ → 3′ direction. In a concurrent action, the uncharged tRNA from the P site is expelled and the peptidyl-tRNA from the A site moves into the P site. The ribosome then has an empty A site ready for entry of the aminoacyl-tRNA corresponding to the next codon (see Figure 14.9).

TEACHER TIP

AUG is both the start codon and the only codon for methionine. The first AUG that the ribosome encounters will not only start polypeptide synthesis but will also put a methionine in that postion. Thus, all polypeptide chains start with methionine, though it is commonly removed during post-translation modifications. Further AUG sequences in the mRNA simply add another methionine to the chain.

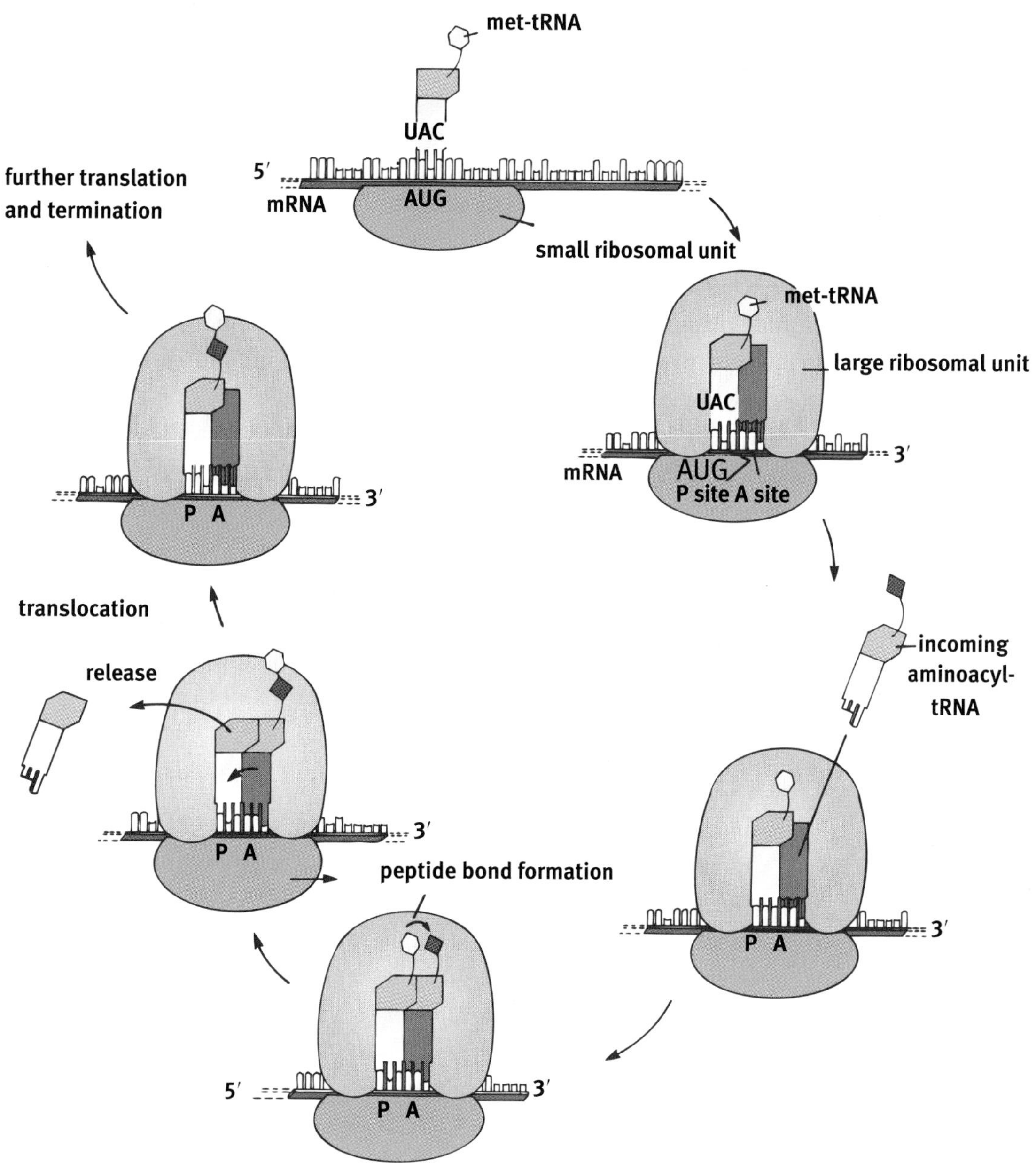

Figure 14.9. Initiation and Elongation

c. Termination

Polypeptide synthesis terminates when one of three special mRNA **termination codons** (UAA, UAG, or UGA) arrives in the A site. These codons signal the ribosome to terminate translation; they do not code for amino acids. Instead of another aminoacyl-tRNA complex coming into the A site and binding to the codon, a protein called **release factor** binds to the termination codon, causing a water molecule to be added to the polypeptide chain. This reaction

> **MCAT Favorite**
>
> Point mutations do not result in a change of the length of the genome or gene, even if it is a nonsense mutation and results in a truncated protein. This is because point mutations are always substitutions.

precipitates the release of the polypeptide chain from the tRNA and the ribosome itself; the ribosome then dissociates into its two subunits. Frequently, many ribosomes simultaneously translate a single mRNA molecule, forming a structure known as a **polyribosome.**

TEACHER TIP

PTM are a great way for a peptide to know where it is targeted. Cells have many different compartmentalized structures and functions to carry out. PTM often are the way in which proteins are correctly sorted within the cell.

E. POST-TRANSLATIONAL MODIFICATIONS

During and after its release, the polypeptide assumes the characteristic conformation determined by the primary sequence of amino acids. Disulfide bonds can form within or between polypeptide chains. There are often other post-translational modifications made to the polypeptide before it becomes a functional protein. For example, there might be cleavages and/or additions at the terminal ends of the chain; certain amino acids within the chain might be phosphorylated, carboxylated, methylated, or glycosylated.

MCAT SYNOPSIS

A nonsense mutation is a mutation that produces a premature termination of the polypeptide chain by changing one of the codons to a stop codon. Nonsense mutation can have disastrous effects. Thalassemia is a genetic disease in which erythrocytes are produced with little or no functional hemoglobin leading to severe anemia. Thalassemia can be caused by a variety of different mutations: point mutations can change a codon into a stop codon; frame-shift mutations (insertions and deletions) can introduce a stop codon in the altered reading frame.

F. MUTATIONS

A mutation is a change in the base sequence of DNA that may be inherited by offspring. The common types of mutations are **base-pair substitutions, base-pair insertions,** and **base-pair deletions.**

1. Types of Mutations

a. Point mutations

A point mutation occurs when a single nucleotide base is substituted by another. If the substitution occurs in a noncoding region, or if the substitution is transcribed into a codon that codes for the same amino acid, there will be no change in the amino acid sequence (a "silent" mutation). If the substitution changes the sequence, the result can range from insignificant to lethal, depending on the effect the substitution has on the protein. Sickle-cell anemia most commonly results from a single base-pair substitution; sickle-cell hemoglobin has a valine (codon GUG) where normal hemoglobin has a glutamic acid (codon GAG).

TEACHER TIP

Recall from the previous page that silent mutations result from the degeneracy of the genetic code. It makes sense that those amino acids that are used most commonly are redundant. That way, if the third position gets changed, no effect will be seen in the organism.

b. Frame shift mutations

Base-pair insertions and deletions involve the addition or loss of nucleotides, respectively. Such mutations usually have more serious effects on the coded protein, because nucleotides are read as a series of triplets. The addition or loss of a nucleotide(s) (except in multiples of three) will change the **reading frame** of the mRNA and is known as a **frameshift mutation.** The protein, if synthesized at all, will most likely be nonfunctional.

2. Mutagenesis

Mutagenesis is the creation of mutations; it can be caused by internal genetic "mistakes" or by external cancer-causing agents called **mutagens.** Internal mistakes can occur during DNA replication, resulting in gene mutations and dysfunctional proteins. Physical mutagens, such as X rays and ultraviolet radiation, and chemical mutagens, such as base analogs, all result in mutations. Furthermore, DNA itself can act as a mutagen; mobile pieces of DNA called **transposons** can insert themselves in genes and cause mutation.

> **MCAT FAVORITE**
>
> Remember, a mutation will only be inherited if it occurs in the germ (sex) cell line. Mutations limited to somatic cells will not be passed on to the next generation. They may, however, play an important role in the development of tumors.

VIRAL GENETICS

The viral genome contains anywhere from several to several hundred genes and has either double-stranded **or** single-stranded DNA **or** RNA. Viruses are highly specific with respect to host selection and can be generally grouped into plant viruses, animal viruses, and bacteriophages (DNA viruses that infect bacteria).

A. INFECTION OF HOST CELL

A virus can only infect a host cell that has a surface receptor for the virus' capsid (protein coat). Viruses enter their host cells by a variety of mechanisms. Some viruses introduce only their nucleic acid into the host cell's cytoplasm, while others enter the host cell entirely (their nucleic acid is liberated from its capsid intracellularly).

B. GENOME REPLICATION AND TRANSCRIPTION

1. DNA-Containing Viruses

Viral DNA is replicated and viral mRNA is transcribed inside the host cell's nucleus (or nuclear region), using the host's DNA polymerases, RNA polymerases, and nucleotide pool. A few DNA viruses replicate and transcribe in the cytoplasm; these viruses must bring their own DNA and RNA polymerases with them.

2. RNA-Containing Viruses

Viral RNA is replicated and is transcribed in the host cell's cytoplasm. An enzyme called **RNA replicase** transcribes new RNA from an RNA template. Some viruses bring RNA replicase with them into the host; otherwise a portion of viral RNA functions as mRNA, which is translated to RNA replicase immediately after entering the host cell. **Retroviruses** are a special group of RNA viruses that use their genome as a template for DNA synthesis rather than for RNA synthesis.

CLINICAL CORRELATE

HIV, the virus that causes AIDS, is a retrovirus.

DNA is synthesized by the enzyme **reverse transcriptase.** The retroviral DNA becomes integrated into the host DNA. When viral DNA becomes integrated into host DNA it is called a **provirus** (animal viruses) or **prophage** (bacteriophages). The proviral DNA is later transcribed into mRNA that is needed for prophage assembly.

TEACHER TIP

For our purposes, viruses are not considered alive. They have genetic material and are capable of using that material to make proteins and other viruses, but only when they are with a cell whose machinery they can use. Viruses cannot make more of themselves without a host to do it in.

C. TRANSLATION AND PROGENY ASSEMBLY

The mRNA transcribed from viral nucleic acid is translated into the polypeptide chains that compose the viral protein coats with the aid of the host cell's tRNA, amino acids, ribosomes, and enzymes. Viral progeny self-assemble; the protein-nucleic acid configuration forms either spontaneously or with the aid of viral enzymes. A single virus is capable of producing hundreds of progeny.

D. PROGENY RELEASE

Once assembled, viral progeny may be released either by lysis of the host cell or by **extrusion,** a process similar to budding. In extrusion, the progeny are enclosed in vesicles derived from the host cell membrane; this permits viral replication without killing the host cell. The process of viral replication and extrusion in animal viruses is called a **productive cycle** (see Figure 14.10).

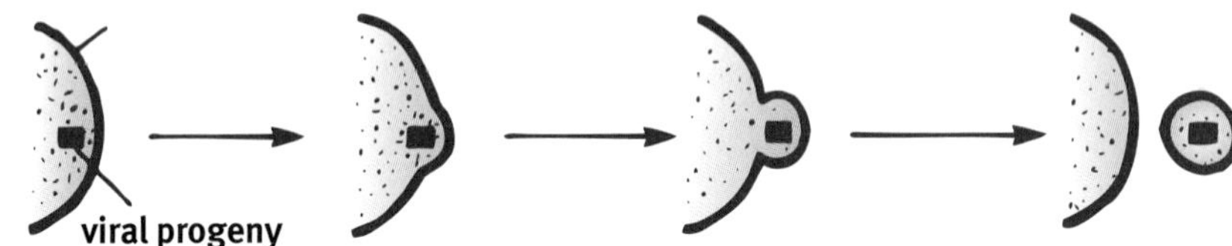

Figure 14.10. Extrusion

TEACHER TIP

Link to immunology: Think about how your body or a bacteria has to respond to a viral threat. Viruses are INSIDE of the cells. They have to be in order to use the cellular machinery. When your body fights bacteria, they are (usually) outside of the cells so different mechanisms can be used. In order to kill a virus, the infected cell is often killed in the process. This is fine in the case of cells, which are replaced over time (like those lining your throat), but what about neurons which don't regrow? Your body cannot kill these so it uses different mechanisms to keep the virus in check. Bottom line: Viruses create a whole host of problems as a result of their unique position status as being alive or not.

E. BACTERIOPHAGE

A bacteriophage infects its host bacterium by attaching to it, boring a hole through the bacterial cell wall, and injecting its DNA, while its protein coat remains attached to the cell wall. Once inside its host, the bacteriophage enters either a **lytic cycle** or a **lysogenic cycle.**

1. Lytic Cycle

The phage DNA takes control of the bacterium's genetic machinery and manufactures numerous progeny. The bacterial cell then bursts (lyses), releasing new virions, each capable of infecting other bacteria. Bacteriophages that replicate by the lytic cycle, killing their host cells, are called **virulent.**

2. Lysogenic Cycle

If the bacteriophage does not lyse its host cell, it becomes integrated into the bacterial genome in a harmless form (prophage or probacteriophage), lying dormant for one or more generations. The virus may stay integrated indefinitely, replicating along with the bacterial genome. However, either spontaneously or as a result of environmental circumstances (e.g., radiation, ultraviolet light, or chemicals), the prophage can reemerge and enter a lytic cycle (see Figure 14.11). Bacteria containing prophages are normally resistant to further infection ("superinfection") by similar phages.

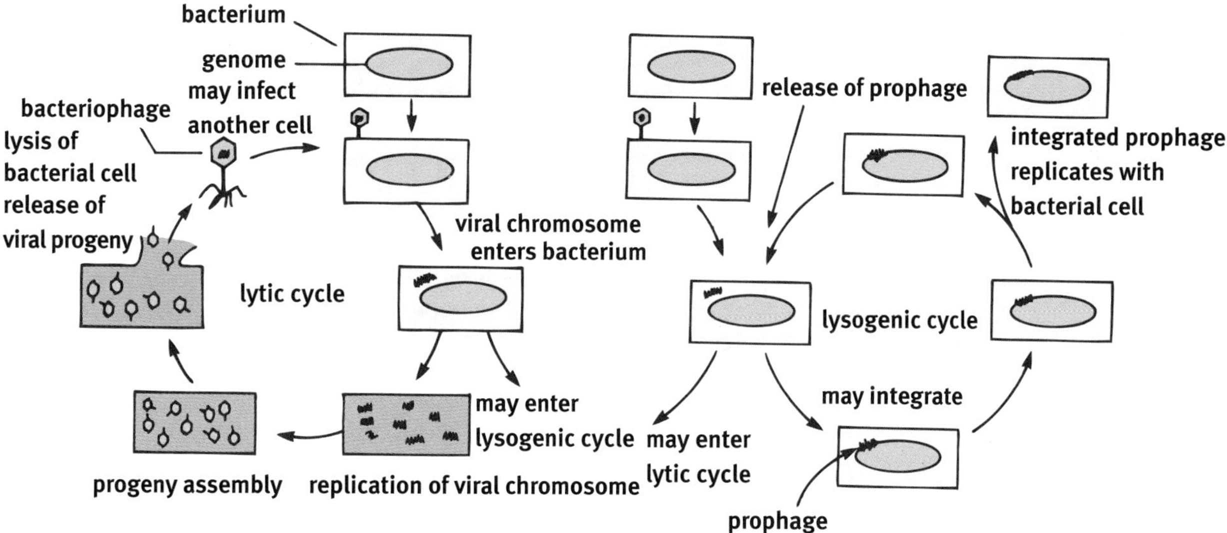

Figure 14.11. Bacteriophage Life Cycle

BACTERIAL GENETICS

A. BACTERIAL GENOME

The bacterial genome consists of a single circular chromosome located in the nucleoid region of the cell (see chapter 1). Many bacteria also contain smaller circular rings of DNA called **plasmids,** which contain accessory genes. **Episomes** are plasmids that are capable of integration into the bacterial genome. Because the bacterial chromosome is not separated from the cytoplasm by a nuclear membrane, transcription and translation occur almost simultaneously. As soon as a small portion of newly synthesized mRNA separates from its DNA template, translation begins. A strand of prokaryotic mRNA may be **polycistronic,** i.e., coding for more than one polypeptide (usually a group of related proteins).

B. REPLICATION

Replication of the bacterial chromosome begins at a unique origin of replication and proceeds in both directions simultaneously. DNA is synthesized in the 5′ → 3′ direction. Replication occurs at the rate of approximately 500 nucleotide additions per second.

TEACHER TIP

While bacteria are simple, failure to evolve their genome will result in negative selection or lack of a selection. These mechanisms allow for evolution to occur. Keep in mind that evolution occurs in response to a selection pressure. Most bacteria used to be susceptible to antibiotics such as penicillin. Overuse of these drugs, however, has led to a selective pressure for bacteria to develop resistance to penicillin and other antibiotics. These resistances may then be passed on via these mechanisms to other bacteria.

C. GENETIC VARIANCE

Bacterial cells reproduce by binary fission and proliferate very rapidly under favorable conditions. Although binary fission is an asexual process, bacteria have three mechanisms for increasing the genetic variance of a population: **transformation, conjugation,** and **transduction.**

1. Transformation

Transformation is the process by which a foreign chromosome fragment (plasmid) is incorporated into the bacterial chromosome via recombination, creating new inheritable genetic combinations.

2. Conjugation

Conjugation can be described as sexual mating in bacteria; it is the transfer of genetic material between two bacteria that are temporarily joined. A cytoplasmic **conjugation bridge** is formed between the two cells and genetic material is transferred from the **donor male (+) type** to the **recipient female (–) type.** The bridge is formed from appendages called **sex pili,** which are found on the donor male. Only bacteria containing plasmids called **sex factors** are capable of forming pili and conjugating. The best studied sex factor is the **F factor** in *Escherichia coli*. Bacteria possessing this plasmid are termed **F^+ cells,** those without it are called **F^- cells.** During conjugation between an F^+ and an F^- cell, the F^+ cell replicates its F factor and donates the copy to the recipient, converting it to an F^+ cell (see Figure 14.12). Plasmids that do not induce pili formation may transfer into the recipient cell along with the sex factor.

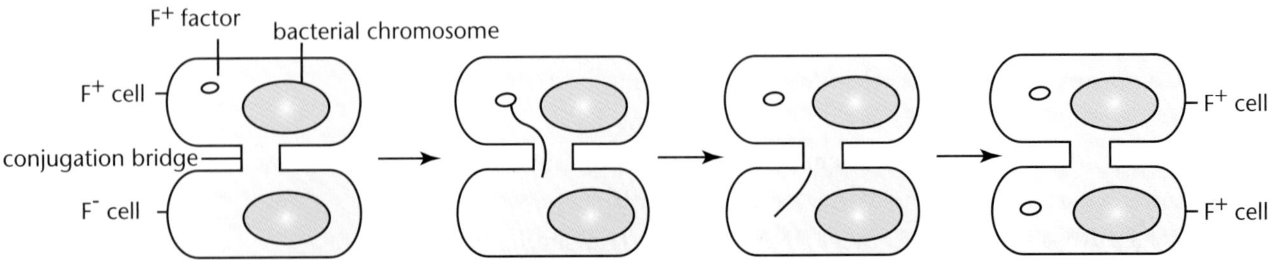

Figure 14.12. Conjugation

Sometimes the sex factor becomes integrated into the bacterial genome. During conjugation the entire bacterial chromosome replicates and begins to move from the donor cell into the recipient cell. The conjugation bridge usually breaks before the entire chromosome is transferred, but the bacterial genes that enter the recipient cell can easily recombine with the bacterial genes already present to form novel genetic combinations. These bacteria are called **Hfr cells,** meaning that they have a high frequency of recombination.

3. Transduction

Transduction is when fragments of the bacterial chromosome accidentally become packaged into viral progeny produced during a viral infection. These virions may infect other bacteria and introduce new genetic arrangements through recombination with the new host cell's DNA (see Figure 14.13). This process is similar to conjugation and may reflect an evolutionary relationship between viruses and plasmids.

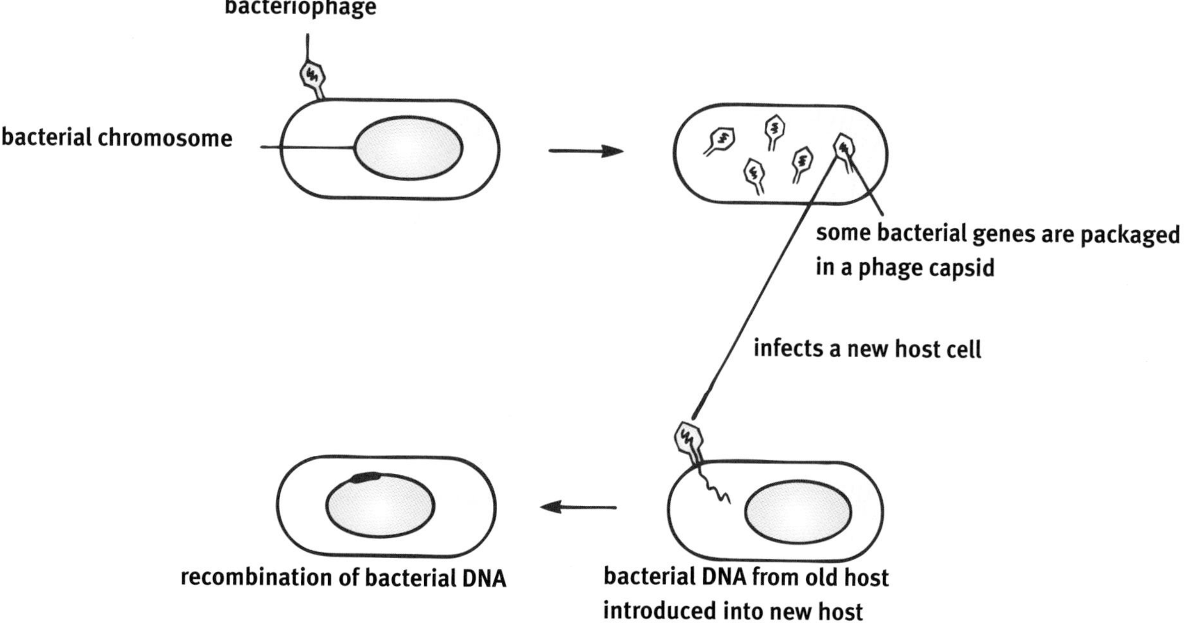

Figure 14.13. Transduction

D. GENE REGULATION

The regulation of gene expression (transcription) enables prokaryotes to control their metabolism. Regulation of transcription is based on the accessibility of RNA polymerase to the genes being transcribed and is directed by an **operon,** which consists of **structural genes,** an **operator gene,** and a **promoter gene.** Structural genes contain sequences

TEACHER TIP

Although bacteria are much simpler and their genomes are quite different (smaller, circular, no introns), they are still subject to levels of control. Gene regulation is critical to all organisms' survival; cancer (simply defined as unregulated cell division), for instance, is due to a loss of genetic regulation of cell division.

of DNA that code for proteins. The operator gene is the sequence of nontranscribable DNA that is the repressor binding site. The promoter gene is the noncoding sequence of DNA that serves as the initial binding site for RNA polymerase. There is also a **regulator gene,** which codes for the synthesis of a repressor molecule that binds to the operator and blocks RNA polymerase from transcribing the structural genes.

Regulation may be via **inducible systems** or **repressible systems.** Inducible systems are those that require the presence of a substance, called an **inducer,** for transcription to occur. Repressible systems are in a constant state of transcription unless a **corepressor** is present to inhibit transcription.

TEACHER TIP

What sorts of systems would you want to be inducible? Why make a system inducible at all? Recall that gene expression (from transcription to the final protein product) is energetically expensive. Any cell looks to do it at a minimum level of energy expenditure while maintaining maximal output. Inducible systems in bacteria are one way to do this—by preventing gene expression when it is unnecessary.

1. Inducible Systems

In an inducible system, the repressor binds to the operator, forming a barrier that prevents RNA polymerase from transcribing the structural genes. The repressor is active until it binds to the inducer. For transcription to occur, an inducer must bind to the repressor, forming an **inducer-repressor complex.** This complex cannot bind to the operator, thus permitting transcription. The proteins synthesized are thus said to be inducible. The structural genes typically code for an enzyme, and the inducer is usually the substrate, or a derivative of the substrate, upon which the enzyme normally acts. When the substrate (inducer) is present, enzymes are synthesized; when it is absent, enzyme synthesis is negligible. In this manner, enzymes are transcribed only when they are actually needed. An example of an inducible system is the ***lac* operon** (see Figure 14.14).

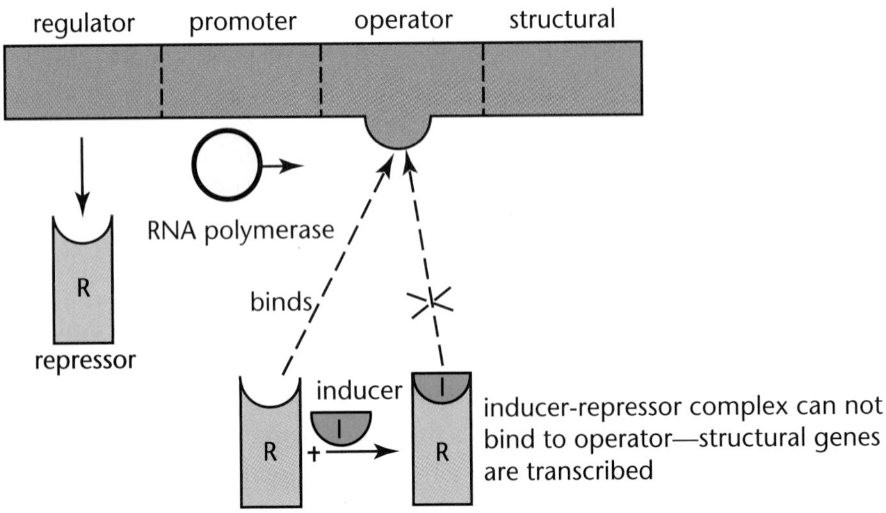

Figure 14.14. Inducible System

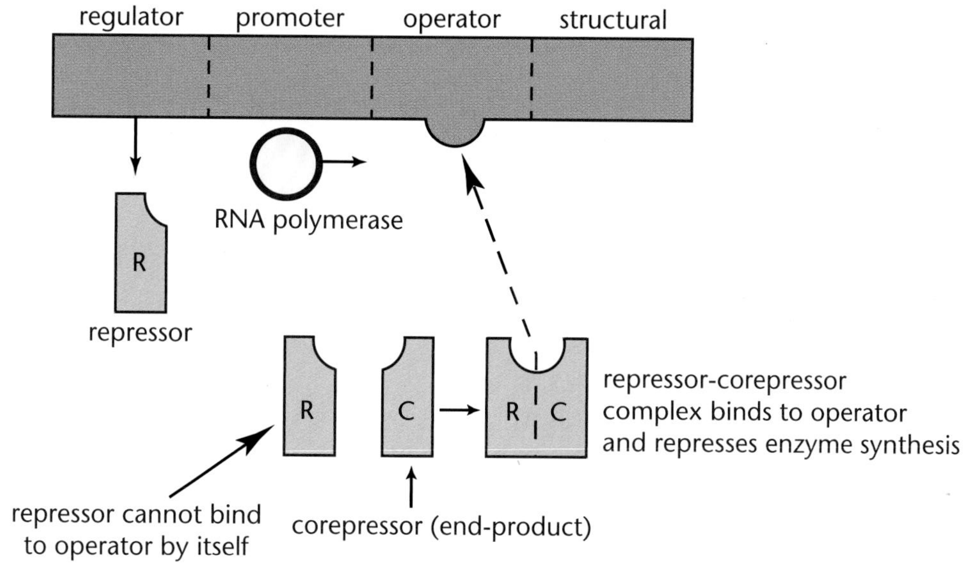

Figure 14.15. Repressible System

2. Repressible Systems

In a repressible system, the repressor is inactive until it combines with the corepressor. The repressor can bind to the operator and prevent transcription only when it has formed a **repressor-corepressor complex.** Corepressors are often the end-products of the biosynthetic pathways they control. The proteins produced (usually enzymes) are said to be repressible since they are normally being synthesized; transcription and translation occur until the corepressor is synthesized. An example of a repressible system is the ***trp* operon** (see Figure 14.15)

> **TEACHER TIP**
>
> Much as we want to be able to turn genes on as needed, we'd also like to be able to turn them off. Repressible systems allow us to do this.

PRACTICE QUESTIONS

1. In the laboratory you have made a DNA primer with the sequence 5′-AGCGCTAT-3′. Which of the following sequences will the primer most likely recognize?

A. 5′-TCGCGATA-3′
B. 5′-ATAGCGCT-3′
C. 5′-AGCGCTAT-3′
D. 5′-CGCATATG-3′

2. In the laboratory you are working on a silencing RNA project, where small strands of RNA are introduced into cells to bind DNA and activate a DNA lysis pathway. If the DNA sequence you want to recognize is 5′-TAGATCC-3′, which of the following RNA sequences would be most appropriate to use?

A. 5′-GGATCTA-3′
B. 5′-AUCUAGG-3′
C. 5′-ATCTAGG-3′
D. 5′-GGAUGUA-3′

3. A new disease is discovered. It is the result of a point mutation in the area of a gene coding for an intron interfering with post-transcriptional RNA processing. Where in the cell does this process occur?

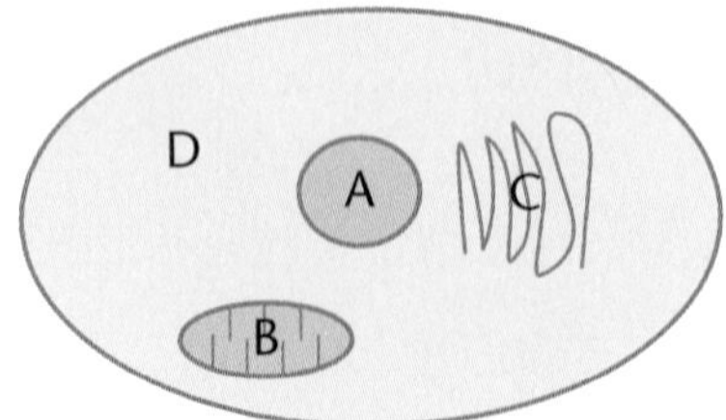

A. Nucleus
B. Mitochondria
C. Endoplasmic reticulum
D. Cytoplasm

4. Which of the following mutations can result in the introduction of a premature stop codon into a DNA sequence?

I. Point mutation
II. Frame-shift insertion
III. Frame-shift deletion

A. I
B. III
C. II and III
D. I, II, and III

5. Varicella virus, the DNA virus responsible for chicken pox, replicates in the cytoplasm of its host cell. Which of the following is most likely true about varicella virus replication?

A. It is reverse trancriptase-dependent.
B. It utilizes the host DNA polymerase.
C. It requires the encoding for DNA polymerase in its viral genome.
D. It requires co-infection with another virus to provide the necessary DNA polymerase.

6. Which of the following comparisons between eukaryotic and prokaryotic DNA polymerase enzymes is correct?

A. Eukaryotic DNA polymerases always have 3′→5′ polymerase activity.
B. Prokaryotic DNA polymerases always have 3′→5′ polymerase activity.
C. Prokaryotic DNA polymerases never have 5′→3′ polymerase activity.
D. Eukaryotic DNA polymerases never have 5′→3′ exonuclease activity.

7. Which of the following is true of eukaryotic DNA synthesis on the lagging strand of a DNA replication fork?

 I. It occurs in the 5′→3′ direction.
 II. It connects the 5′ phosphate group to the 3′ hydroxyl group.
 III. It requires a primer.

A. I and II
B. I and III
C. II and III
D. All of the above

8. Which of the following correctly depicts a eukaryotic peptide?

A. NH_3 — Met — Val — COOH

B. NH_3 — Arg — Met — COOH

C. NH_3 — Arg — Met — NH_3

D. COOH — Met — Val — NH_3

9. Which of the following statements appropriately identifies the role of the helicase and topoisomerase enzymes in DNA replication?

A. Helicase unwinds the DNA strands while topoisomerase winds them.
B. Helicase winds the DNA strands while topoisomerase unwinds them.
C. Helicase unwinds the DNA strands while topoisomerase relieves the resulting tension.
D. Topoisomerase unwinds the DNA strands while helicase relieves the resulting tension.

10. The addition of CAG repeats into the Huntingtin gene correlates with the risk of developing Huntington's disease. How would you categorize this type of mutation?

A. Nonsense
B. Insertion
C. Frame-shift
D. Silent

11. After spending a day in the sun without wearing any sun protection, Dr. X is worried about possible sun damage. What are the likely effects of his exposure?

	Epithelial Cell Damage	DNA Damage Repair	Germ Cell Mutation
A.	Yes	No	No
B.	Yes	Yes	Yes
C.	No	No	Yes
D.	Yes	Yes	No

12. The most common types of point mutations involve the substitution of a purine for a purine or a pyramidine for a pyramidine. Which of the following substitutions fits one of these patterns?

A. Adenine to thymine
B. Adenine to cytosine
C. Guanine to thymine
D. Cytosine to thymine

13. Macrolide antibiotics act by binding the large ribosomal subunit in bacteria, inhibiting ribosomal translocation. Which of the following translation steps would be directly affected by a macrolide?

A. Peptide elongation
B. Binding of the small ribosomal subunit to RNA
C. Binding of the small and large ribosomal subunits
D. Aminoacylation of the tRNA

KEY CONCEPTS

Transcription

Antisense strand

Sense strand

TAKEAWAYS

When solving any transcription problems, follow these rules:

- G pairs with C and T pairs with A.
- In RNA, T is replaced with U.
- The sense strand of the DNA = the transcribed hnRNA with U replacing T.
- The antisense strand and the sense strand are complements of each other.

THINGS TO WATCH OUT FOR

Note that the sequence described above is for problems that ask for DNA sequence from RNA sequence. In problems that ask for RNA sequence from DNA sequence, perform step 3 first, followed by step 2, and then step 1.

Be careful to maintain the correct polarity in every step of the problem. The newly synthesized strand is built in the 5′ to 3′ direction, and the reading frame is read in the 3′ to 5′ direction.

DNA TRANSCRIPTION

An RNA strand with the sequence 5′-GACTGAUCAGACTA-3′ was erroneously created when a mutant RNA polymerase substituted a thymine for the second cysteine when it encountered a GG in the reading frame of the DNA. What is the antisense strand of the DNA from which this RNA was transcribed? (Assume that "GA" is not in the antisense strand.)

1) Determine the correct primary structure of RNA.

We can substitute CC for CT in the fragment in order to produce the correct sequence of RNA: 5′-GACCGAUCAGACCA-3′.

In this case, when C precedes T, we know that it is due to the mutant polymerase. The first G in the DNA sequence GG will correctly have been transcribed as C, but the second G will have been incorrectly transcribed as T, yielding CT instead of CC.

---

2) Determine the sense strand.

We can simply replace the uracils with thymines to get the following sense strand: 5′-GACCGATCAGACCA-3′.

Transcription always proceeds in the 5′ to 3′ direction starting at the 3′ end of the anti-sense strand. The RNA corresponds to the sense strand (minus any introns that were spliced out—in this problem we will assume there were no introns).

We are working backwards, going from RNA to DNA. The RNA produced represents the sense strand with the thymines replaced by uracil.

---

3) Determine the antisense strand.

5′-GACCGATCAGACCA-3′ → sense strand
3′-CTGGCTAGTCTGGT-5′ → anti-sense strand

The antisense strand of DNA is the complement of the sense strand of DNA. We can determine the sense strand by remembering that G pairs with C, that T pairs with A, and that the antisense strand is antiparallel to the sense strand (meaning that the 3′ end of the sense strand will line up with the 5′ end of the antisense strand and vice versa).

SIMILAR QUESTIONS

1) What is the base sequence of the mRNA produced from the following sense strand of DNA: 3′-TAGGGTACGTACCTA-5′?
2) What are the possible primary structures of mRNA produced from the antisense strand 3′-GAATACCAGTAGTATTTGCCGATGACTAGTTAGCCGTTAGC-5′ after splicing by a splisosome that makes blunt end cuts between GG in the sequence 5′-CGGC-3′?

DNA REPLICATION

The following molecule of DNA is replicated using two cycles of PCR in the presence of N^{15} labeled guanine. What percentage of the DNA strands will contain the labeled guanine in both strands (sense and antisense strands)?

5′-CATACTGATCATCTAGCGTATGCGT-3′
3′-GTATGACTAGTAGATCGCATACGCA-5′

KEY CONCEPTS

Semiconservative replication

DNA

1) Determine what happens after the first round of replication.
DNA replication is semiconservative, which means that for every strand of original DNA, one new strand of DNA is synthesized as its new complement.

Our templates for this first round of replication are:

5′-CATACTGATCATCTAGCGTATGCGT-3′
3′-GTATGACTAGTAGATCGCATACGCA-5′

Neither of these original strands contains the labeled guanine. So the first round of replication gives us:

5′-CATACTGATCATCTAGCGTATGCGT-3′
3′-GTATGACTAGTAGATCGCATACGCA-5′*

and

5′-CATACTGATCATCTAGCGTATGCGT-3′*
3′-GTATGACTAGTAGATCGCATACGCA-5′

where the * marks strands containing the labeled guanine.

The original strand with the 5′ to 3′ polarity at the site of replication will be the lagging strand because nucleotides can only be added in the 5′ to 3′ direction. Primase lays down a new primer to which DNA polymerase can bind in intervals of about 500 nucleotides, so that its new complementary strand can be created in short fragments called Okazaki fragments. The primer for these Okazaki fragments is RNA and is replaced with DNA before ligase joins the short fragments together. This process eliminates the need to create the replicate strand in the 3′ to 5′ direction.

TAKEAWAYS

DNA replication is semiconservative. The newly synthesized strand of DNA will be identical to the old complementary strand, provided that there are no mutations.

---

2) Determine what happens after the second round of replication.
Our templates for the second round of replication are:

5′-CATACTGATCATCTAGCGTATGCGT-3′
3′-GTATGACTAGTAGATCGCATACGCA-5′*

and

5′-CATACTGATCATCTAGCGTATGCGT-3′
3′-GTATGACTAGTAGATCGCATACGCA-5′*

So this second round of replication gives us:

5′-CATACTGATCATCTAGCGTATGCGT-3′
3′-GTATGACTAGTAGATCGCATACGCA-5′*

and

5′-CATACTGATCATCTAGCGTATGCGT-3′*
3′-GTATGACTAGTAGATCGCATACGCA-5′*

and

5′-CATACTGATCATCTAGCGTATGCGT-3′*
3′-GTATGACTAGTAGATCGCATACGCA-5′*

and

5′-CATACTGATCATCTAGCGTATGCGT-3′ *
3′-GTATGACTAGTAGATCGCATACGCA-5′

with the asterisks again indicating strands containing labeled guanine.

In the second round of replicati on, the new strands from the first round of replication are used as templates to create newer strands.

---

3) Determine the percentage of DNA molecules that only have "new" strands.
fifty percent of the double stranded DNA molecules will have both strands with the labeled N^{15} guanine.

After two rounds of replication, the middle two double-stranded DNA molecules have both strands labeled with the N^{15} guanine, whereas the outer two double strands of DNA still maintain one original strand.

THINGS TO WATCH OUT FOR

Be careful in noting the polarity of the strands. Remember that DNA is always synthesized in the 5′ to 3′ direction.

SIMILAR QUESTIONS

1) What is the product after 5′-ACGAGCTATGCTACTATATG-3′ goes through two rounds of replication?
2) A molecule of DNA is replicated using three cycles of PCR in the presence of N^{15} labeled nuclei acids. What percentage of the newly formed DNA will contain an unlabeled strand?

CHAPTER 15

EVOLUTION

Evolution is a process of change and adaptation leading to the development of new life forms and genetic diversity.

THEORIES OF EVOLUTION

A. LAMARCK

Jean Baptiste Lamarck was an early evolution theorist. He formulated the concept of **use and disuse**: organs that are used extensively develop, while organs that are not used atrophy. Lamark theorized that newer, more complex species arise from older and simpler species through the accumulation and modification of **acquired characteristics.** Although it is now known that characteristics are inherited rather than acquired through use, Lamarck's work was the first systematic approach to understanding evolutionary processes.

PAVLOV'S DOG

If you see any hint of the buzz phrases "use and disuse" or "inheritance of acquired characteristics," think Lamarck. And don't forget—Lamarck was wrong!

B. DARWIN

Charles Darwin developed a theory of evolution in *The Origin of Species,* published in 1859. In it, Darwin outlined a number of basic agents leading to evolutionary change:

1. Organisms produce offspring, very few of which survive to reproductive maturity.
2. There are chance variations between individuals in any given population, some of which are inheritable. Variations that give the organism a slight advantage in the struggle for existence are called favorable variations.
3. Individuals who have inherited favorable variations are likely to live longer and produce more offspring than others; thus favorable variations become more common from generation to generation. This process is known as **natural selection.** Gradually, natural selection leads to variations that differentiate organisms into groups and ultimately into distinct species. **Fitness** is measured in terms of reproductive success and the relative genetic contribution of an

TEACHER TIP

Natural selection is not equivalent to evolution. It is simply a *mechanism* for evolution. Natural selection is equivalent to "survival of the fittest." Know this for the exam.

individual to the future of the population. Natural selection is the driving force of evolution.

MCAT Synopsis

Natural Selection:

- Chance variations occur thanks to mutation and recombination.
- If the variation is "selected for" by the environment, that individual will be more "fit" and more likely to survive to reproductive age.
- Survival of the fittest leads to an increase of those favorable genes in the gene pool.

C. NEO-DARWINISM (THE MODERN SYNTHESIS)

Most of Darwin's ideas persist in the current view of evolution, termed neo-Darwinism, or the modern synthesis. The science of genetics revealed that the ultimate source of hereditary variation lies in the processes of mutation and genetic recombination. Some gene combinations increase chances for survival and reproduction, while others decrease them. This leads to **differential reproduction**; i.e., individuals with favorable genes produce more offspring. As a result, after many generations, these favorable genes will have become pervasive in the **gene pool**; the gene pool consists of all of the genes in all individuals in a population at a given time.

Teacher Tip

Evolution is a theory, not a fact. The kinds of passages that are likely to include the topic of evolution are persuasive argument types. Be sure to consider how the passage information you are given would fit within a given mechanism or concept, e.g., punctuated equilibrium.

D. PUNCTUATED EQUILIBRIUM

One remarkable aspect of the fossil record is that many organisms do not demonstrate gradual changes; instead there seem to be short periods of rapid change with long static periods between them. To explain this phenomenon, Eldredge and Gould (1972) proposed the model of **punctuated** equilibrium. They contend that evolution is characterized by long periods of stasis "punctuated" by evolutionary changes occurring in spurts. This is in contrast to Darwin's model, which proposes that evolutionary changes accumulate gradually and evenly over time.

EVIDENCE OF EVOLUTION

Evidence supporting modern evolutionary theory is drawn from many disciplines, including **paleontology, biogeography, comparative anatomy, comparative embryology,** and **molecular biology.**

A. PALEONTOLOGY

Paleontology, which is the study of the fossil record, is of particular significance to the study of evolution. With the use of radioactive dating techniques, paleontologists are able to determine the age of fossils, thus allowing them to determine the chronological succession of species in the fossil record.

B. BIOGEOGRAPHY

Biogeography refers to the distribution of life forms throughout the globe. Darwin observed that many species found on one of the Galapagos Islands seemed more closely related to species inhabiting the neighboring mainland than to species inhabiting the other Galapagos Islands. The biogeography of the Galapagos suggests that species migrated from the mainland to neighboring islands, where they adapted to the different island environments in isolation from each other.

C. COMPARATIVE ANATOMY

Homologous structures are similar in structure and share a common evolutionary origin. A classic example of homologous structures is found in the forelimbs of mammals: bat wings, whale flippers, horse forelegs, and human arms are all modifications of a common anatomical theme. In contrast, **analogous structures** share a functional similarity but arose from different evolutionary origins. The wings of insects and birds are both adaptations for flight but evolved from separate lines of descent. **Vestigial structures** are remnants of organs that have lost their ancestral functions, and thus are evidence of evolutionary forces at work. Examples include vestiges of limb bones in the adult python and the appendix and vestiges of the tail bone (coccyx) in man.

D. COMPARATIVE EMBRYOLOGY

The stages of embryonic development in closely related organisms resemble each other, indicating common evolutionary origins. The earliest stages tend to be the most similar. For example, all chordates exhibit certain features as embryos, such as gills.

E. MOLECULAR BIOLOGY

Through comparative DNA studies, biologists have been able to detect similarities in the DNA composition of related species. Taxonomically close species have a greater percentage of similar DNA than taxonomically distant species.

GENETIC BASIS OF EVOLUTION

Genetic variation functions as the raw material for natural selection. Sources of genetic variation include inheritable mutations and recombination. Mutations are random changes in the nucleotide sequence of DNA. Recombination refers to novel genetic combinations resulting from sexual reproduction and crossing over.

FLASHBACK

If you didn't get it the first time out, it's time to revisit the concepts of recombination and mutation. See chapters 4 and 14.

TEACHER TIP

Hardy-Weinberg can seem like a lot of information to remember on Test Day, but it usually translates into easy points so it's worth learning. It is easy to learn the two equations, but how about those five criteria that must be met for this equilibrium to be in place? They basically state that *no evolution* is occurring.

A. THE HARDY-WEINBERG EQUILIBRIUM

Evolution can be viewed as a result of changing **gene frequencies** within a population. Gene frequency is the relative frequency of a particular allele. When the gene frequencies of a population are not changing, the gene pool is stable, and the population is not evolving. However, this is true only in ideal situations in which the following conditions are met:

1. The population is very large.
2. There are no mutations that affect the gene pool.
3. Mating between individuals in the population is random.
4. There is no net migration of individuals into or out of the population.
5. The genes in the population are all equally successful at reproducing.

Under these idealized conditions, a certain equilibrium will exist between all of the genes in a gene pool, which is described by the **Hardy-Weinberg equation.**

MCAT FAVORITE

All you need to know to solve any MCAT Hardy-Weinberg problem is the value of p (or p^2) or q (or q^2). From there, you can calculate everything else using $p + q = 1$ and $p^2 + 2pq + q^2 = 1$.

For a gene locus with only two alleles, T and t, p = the frequency of allele T and q = the frequency of allele t. By definition, for a given gene locus, p + q = 1, because the combined frequencies of the alleles must total 100 percent. Thus $(p + q)^2 = (1)^2$ and

$$\mathbf{p^2 + 2pq + q^2 = 1}$$

where p^2 = frequency of TT (dominant homozygotes)
$2pq$ = frequency of Tt (heterozygotes)
q^2 = frequency of tt (recessive homozygotes)

The Hardy-Weinberg equation may be used to determine gene frequencies in a large population in the absence of microevolutionary change (defined by the five conditions given above). For example, individuals from a non-evolving population can be randomly crossed to demonstrate that the gene frequencies remain constant from generation to generation. Assume that in the original gene pool the gene frequency of the dominant gene for tallness, T, is .80, and the gene frequency of the recessive gene for shortness, t, is .20. Thus, $p = .80$ and $q = .20$. In a cross between two heterozygotes, the resulting F1 genotype frequencies are: 64 percent TT, 16 percent + 16 percent = 32 percent Tt, and 4 percent tt (see the following Punnett square).

	$p = .80$ (T)	$q = .20$ (t)
$p = .80$ (T)	($p^2 = .64$) TT = 64%	($pq = .16$) Tt = 16%
$q = .20$ (t)	($pq = .16$) Tt = 16%	($q^2 = .04$) tt = 4%

The gene frequencies of the F_1 generation can be calculated as follows:

64% TT = 64% T allele + 0% t allele
32% Tt = 16% T allele + 16% t allele
4% tt = 0% T allele + 4% t allele

Gene frequencies = 80% T allele + 20% t allele

Thus, $p = .80$ and $q = .20$. These frequencies are the same as those in the parent generation, thus demonstrating Hardy-Weinberg equilibrium in a nonevolving population.

TEACHER TIP

Hardy-Weinberg equilibrium equations allow you to find two pieces of information: the relative frequency of genes in a population and the frequency of a given phenotype in the population. Remember, there will be twice as many genes as individuals in a population—because each individual has two autosomal copies of each gene.

B. MICROEVOLUTION

No population can be represented indefinitely by the Hardy-Weinberg equilibrium because such idealized conditions do not exist in nature. Real populations have unstable gene pools and migrating populations. The agents of microevolutionary change—**natural selection, mutation, assortive mating, genetic drift,** and **gene flow**—are all deviations from the five conditions of a Hardy-Weinberg population.

1. Natural Selection

Genotypes with favorable variations are selected through natural selection, and the frequency of favorable genes increases within the gene pool.

2. Mutation

Gene mutations change allele frequencies in a population, shifting gene equilibria.

3. Assortive Mating

If mates are not randomly chosen, but rather selected according to criteria such as phenotype and proximity, the relative genotype ratios will be affected, and will depart from the predictions of the Hardy-Weinberg equilibrium. On the average, the allele frequencies in the gene pool remain unchanged.

TEACHER TIP

These five points simply reinforce what we already learned. For Hardy-Weinberg equilibrium to exist, we need a stable (nonevolving) gene pool. These points are basically all exceptions to one of the rules for Hardy-Weinberg equilibrium to exist. For example, the equilibrium requires no migrations, but points 4 and 5 (genetic drift and gene flow) are both exceptions to this.

4. Genetic Drift

Genetic drift refers to changes in the composition of the gene pool due to chance. Genetic drift tends to be more pronounced in small populations, where it is sometimes called the **founder effect.**

5. Gene Flow

Migration of individuals between populations will result in a loss or gain of genes, and thus change the composition of a population's gene pool.

MODES OF NATURAL SELECTION

Natural selection is the only evolutionary process that assembles and maintains particular gene combinations over extended periods of time. Three different modes of natural selection are discussed below: **stabilizing selection, directional selection,** and **disruptive selection** (see Figure 15.1).

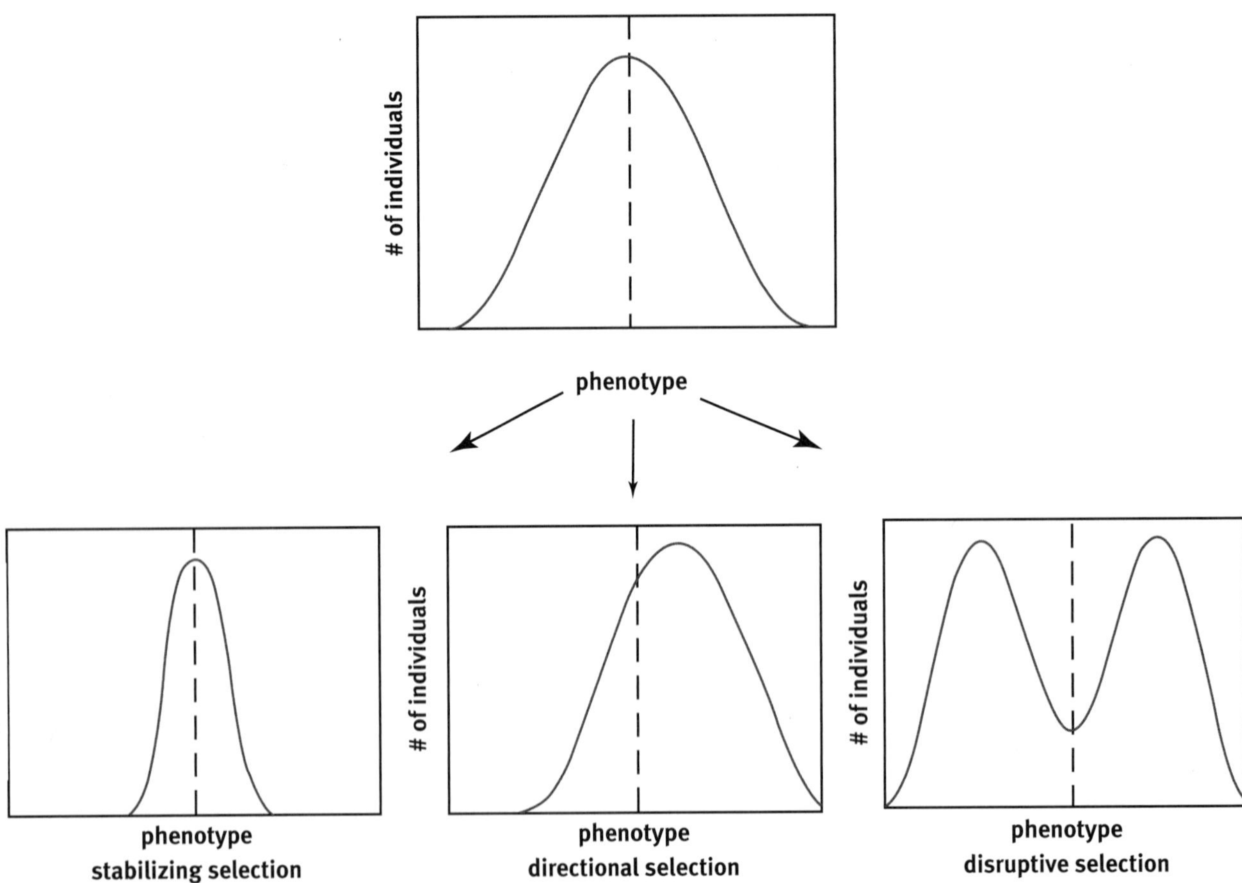

Figure 15.1. Modes of Natural Selection

A. STABILIZING SELECTION

Stabilizing selection maintains a well-adapted uniform character in a population by eliminating deviations from the norm. This process reduces the frequency of extreme phenotypes, thereby reducing variation. For example, stabilizing selection maintains human birth weights within a very narrow range.

TEACHER TIP

Again, natural selection is a theory. Each of these forms of selection would be pressured by a different environment. For the MCAT, consider why a particular situation might engender stabilizing selection rather than disruptive selection.

B. DIRECTIONAL SELECTION

Directional selection produces an adaptive change over time, with an increase in the proportion of individuals with an extreme phenotype. Directional selection occurs when organisms must adapt to a changing environment. A familiar example of directional selection is the emergence of the DDT-resistant mosquito. The introduction of DDT produced a selectional advantage for those mosquitoes possessing the mutant gene for DDT resistance. After a period of time, the population of mosquitoes all possessed the gene for DDT resistance.

C. DISRUPTIVE SELECTION

Disruptive selection favors variants of both phenotypic extremes over the intermediates, leading to the existence of two or more phenotypic forms within a population **(polymorphism).**

ALTRUISTIC BEHAVIOR

Altruistic behavior is behavior that benefits one individual at the expense of another. An example is bee societies in which worker bees are sterile but labor for the benefit of the hive. Explaining the existence of such behavior in terms of natural selection has been a challenge to Darwinian theory. **Group selection** is the now-discredited hypothesis that certain individuals in a population inherit a gene for not reproducing, thus controlling population size at an advantageous level. This hypothesis is flawed because such a gene could not be passed on by its nonreproducing carriers. However, it led to the development of **kin selection** theory, which holds that natural selection can lead to behavior that does not improve the survival of an individual but does improve the survival of his near kin. Since increasing the survival and reproductive success of near kin, who share alleles, will often increase the survival of the individual's alleles, such behavior is consistent with neo-Darwinism. Since worker bees are the genetic sisters of the queen bee, their labor ensures the survival of their own alleles. **Inclusive fitness** describes fitness as the number of an individual's alleles that are inherited by the next generation.

TEACHER TIP

Like all theories, evolution also has detractors and problems in its completeness. These challenges may seem to make the answers less clear on Test Day, but remember that the MCAT is written in a one-right/three-wrong format. If an answer isn't completely RIGHT, it is completely WRONG. Keep your basic facts in mind for Test Day success.

ADAPTIVE RADIATION

Adaptive radiation is the emergence of a number of lineages from a single ancestral species. A single species may diverge into a number of distinct species; the differences between them are those adaptive to a distinct lifestyle, or **niche.** A classic example is Darwin's finches of the Galapagos Island chain. Over a comparatively short period of time, a single species of finch underwent adaptive radiation, resulting in 13 separate species of finches, some of them on the same island. Such adaptations minimized the competition among the birds, enabling each emerging species to become firmly established in its own environmental niche.

PATTERNS OF EVOLUTION

When examining apparent similarities in form or function between two species, it is important to determine whether the similarities are the result of a close evolutionary relationship or the result of similar adaptations to similar environments. Patterns of evolution are described in terms of **convergent evolution, divergent evolution,** and **parallel evolution** (see Figure 15.2).

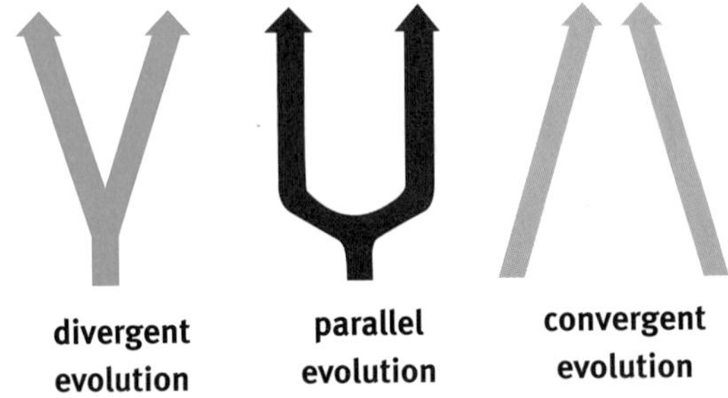

Figure 15.2. Evolutionary Patterns

A. CONVERGENT EVOLUTION

Convergent evolution refers to the independent development of similar characteristics in two or more lineages **not** sharing a recent common ancestor. For example, fish and dolphins have come to resemble one another physically, although they belong to different classes of vertebrates. They evolved certain similar features in adapting to the conditions of aquatic life.

B. DIVERGENT EVOLUTION

Divergent evolution refers to the independent development of dissimilar characteristics in two or more lineages sharing common ancestry.

For example, seals and cats are both mammals belonging to the order Carnivora, yet differ markedly in general appearance. These two species live in very different environments, and adapted to different selection pressures while evolving.

C. PARALLEL EVOLUTION

Parallel evolution refers to the process whereby related species evolve in similar ways for a long period of time in response to analogous environmental selection pressures.

TEACHER TIP

What sorts of pressures or environments might push a species to pursue divergent or convergent evolution?

ORIGIN OF LIFE

The earliest evidence of primitive prokaryotic life is found in stromatolites, which are fossilized bands of sediment that contain microorganisms approximately 3.5 billion years old. It is not clear how life on Earth originated, but a hypothesis has been developed based on a theory proposed independently by both Oparin and Haldane in the 1920s and tested for the first time in the 1950s by Stanley Miller.

A. FORMATION OF ORGANIC MOLECULES

Oparin and Haldane proposed that conditions during the early years of Earth's existence favored the abiotic synthesis of organic molecules. Carbon, hydrogen, nitrogen, and small amounts of oxygen present in the atmosphere and seas bonded together in various ways and accumulated, forming a **"primordial soup"** of organic precursor molecules. The energy for the formation of these bonds was supplied by a number of sources, including the sun, lightning, radioactive decay, and volcanic activity. Miller tested this hypothesis in a laboratory by simulating the conditions believed to have existed on primitive Earth. A mixture of gases was circulated past a source of electrical discharge (simulating lightning), and after one week, the reaction apparatus was found to contain a variety of organic compounds, including simple amino acids. During numerous modified replications of this experiment, all twenty amino acids, many lipids, and the five nitrogenous bases of DNA and RNA have all been generated. It is postulated that organic monomers were abiotically synthesized in a similar way on primitive Earth, and as they accumulated, were brought into close proximity, allowing them to react and form polymers.

TEACHER TIP

These experiments did not actually "create" life as we would understand it today from the cell theory. What they did prove was that Earth's early environment provided all the necessary reagents to create the building blocks of life (nitrogenous bases, lipids, amino acids). How these simple nonliving molecules were then able to go to the right combinations providing for life is still unclear. Knowing the extent and proof of certain theories on Test Day is critical.

B. FORMATION OF PROTOBIONTS

In laboratory experiments, abiotically produced polymers in an aqueous solution can spontaneously assemble into tiny proteinaceous droplets called **microspheres.** These microspheres have a selectively permeable membrane that separates them from their surroundings and maintains an independent internal chemical environment. Colloidal droplets called **coacervates** had been formed in Oparin's laboratory from a solution of polypeptides, nucleic acids, and polysaccharides. These coacervates are capable of carrying out enzymatic activity within their membrane if enzymes and substrate are present. Although microspheres and coacervates have some properties characteristic of life, they are not living cells. The molecular aggregates of organic polymers that are believed to have been the primitive ancestors of living cells are called **protobionts.**

C. FORMATION OF GENETIC MATERIAL

These hypothetical protobionts had the ability to grow in size and divide, but did not have a way of transmitting information to their next generation. The evolution of genetic material is difficult to map out, but it is believed that short strands of RNA were the first molecules capable of self-replication and of storing and transmitting information from one generation to the next. Experiments in the laboratory have shown that free bases can align with their complementary bases on a pre-existing short RNA sequence and bind together, creating a new short RNA chain. Natural selection may have favored RNA sequences whose three-dimensional conformations were more stable and could replicate faster. The next evolutionary step might have involved the association of specific amino acids with specific RNA bases. Thus, an RNA sequence could bring a number of amino acids together in a particular sequence and facilitate their bonding together to form a particular peptide. Natural selection could have selected for the synthesis of those peptides that enhanced the replication and/or the further activity of the RNA. Once this hereditary mechanism developed, protobionts would have been able to grow, split, and transmit important genetic information to their progeny. Self-replicating molecules eventually evolved to code for many of the molecules needed by primitive cells. Evolutionary trends led to the eventual establishment of DNA, which is a more stable molecule than RNA, as the primary warehouse of genetic information.

PRACTICE QUESTIONS

1. Lamark and Darwin are both known for their theories regarding the origin and descent of present day species. Upon which of the following statements would Darwin and Lamark have disagreed?

   A. Chronologically later organisms have a reproductive advantage over their predecessors.
   B. The evolution of new traits is fueled by chance.
   C. Present day animals are descendants of past animals.
   D. Traits become vestigial because they confer little or no reproductive advantage.

2. The fossil record of species A suggests that its evolutionary history was marked by periods of rapid change interspersed with periods of little or no change. This is an example of

   A. Eldredge and Gould's theory of punctuated equilibrium.
   B. Darwin's theory of evolution and natural selection.
   C. Lamark's theory of acquired characteristics.
   D. neo-Darwinian belief in differential reproduction.

3. Paleontologists discovered a bird fossil that stratigraphic analysis dates to around 200,000 B.C. Subsequent radioactive dating revealed that the prehistoric bird fossil contained 10 percent carbon-14. Scientists hypothesize that this fossil is related to a dinosaur fossil that contains 20 percent carbon-14. This data

   A. supports the theory that the prehistoric bird is an evolutionary descendant of the dinosaur.
   B. conflicts with the theory that the prehistoric bird is an evolutionary descendant of the dinosaur.
   C. is invalid because carbon-14 has a half-life of roughly 5,700 years, and is reliable only for dating objects up to 60,000 years old.
   D. does not support or conflict with the theory that prehistoric bird is an evolutionary descendant of the dinosaur.

4. On Tree Island off the coast of Juvialand, researchers discover a small population of swallows with brightly colored red feathers and long pointy beaks. Juvialand also has a larger population of swallows, though they have black feathers and short flat beaks. This is most likely a result of

   A. founder effect.
   B. sexual selection for red feathers over black feathers.
   C. natural selection for red feathers over black feathers,
   D. codominance between the red feather phenotype and the black feather phenotype.

5. The Bottleneck effect refers to an evolutionary event that causes a large proportion of a population to be killed off or isolated from the rest. Which of the following statements is true?

A. The Founder effect is a specific instance of the Bottleneck effect.
B. The Bottleneck effect is a specific instance of the Founder effect.
C. The Founder effect is not related to the Bottleneck effect.
D. Both the Bottleneck and Founder effects are examples of genetic drift.

6. The red bird is a descendant of the blue bird, and the orange bird is a descendant of the black bird. The blue bird and the black bird do not have a common ancestor. Which of the following statements is NOT true?

A. The blue bird's wings are analogous structures to the orange bird's wings.
B. The red bird's wings are analogous structures to the orange bird's wings.
C. The red bird's wings are analogous structures to the black bird's wings.
D. The red bird's wings are analogous structures to the blue bird's wings.

7. Given the diagram below, species Z and B are

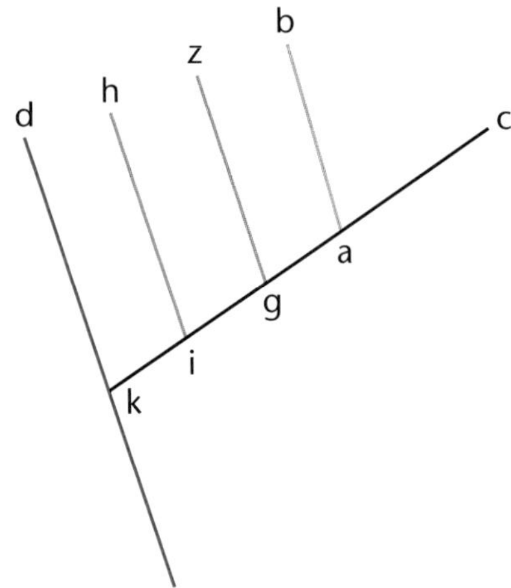

A. paraphyletic.
B. monophyletic.
C. parsimonious.
D. polyphyletic.

8. A population of gophers lives in an area with a large number of predatory squirrels. Their main means of defense is hiding in small crevices or intimidating the squirrels with their size. What evolutionary force would you expect is at play on the gophers' population?

A. Stabilizing selection
B. Directional selection
C. Disruptive selection
D. Hardy-Weinberg equilibrium

9. If p represents the frequency of allele A, and q represents the frequency of allele B in a population of hummingbirds, then assuming a state of Hardy-Weinberg equilibrium,

A. $p + q = 100$.
B. $p + q = 1$.
C. $p^2 + q^2 = 1$.
D. $p^2 + q^2 = 100$.

10. Hardy-Weinberg equilibrium refers to a population in which gene frequencies are not changing and the gene pool remains in a stable state. Which of the following conditions is necessary for this to occur?

A. Small populations, because there are fewer individuals and thus, less genetic diversity
B. Genes in a population that all confer roughly the same reproductive advantage
C. Large amount of migration between several populations, ensuring that selection remains random
D. Individuals with certain traits who mate more, thus keeping these traits in equilibrium

11. Given the following information, what do we know is true?

I. Species A and species B belong in a monophyletic group.
II. Species A and species B both have beaks.

A. Species A's beaks and species B's beaks are homologous structures.
B. Species A's beaks and species B's beaks are analogous structures.
C. Species A and species B share a common ancestor.
D. Both A and C

12. If the following conditions are true, which of the following phylogenetic trees is possible?

Condition 1: Species A, B, and E are paraphyletic.
Condition 2: Species D and C are polyphyletic.
Condition 3: Species I, E, B, Z, and A are monophyletic.

A.
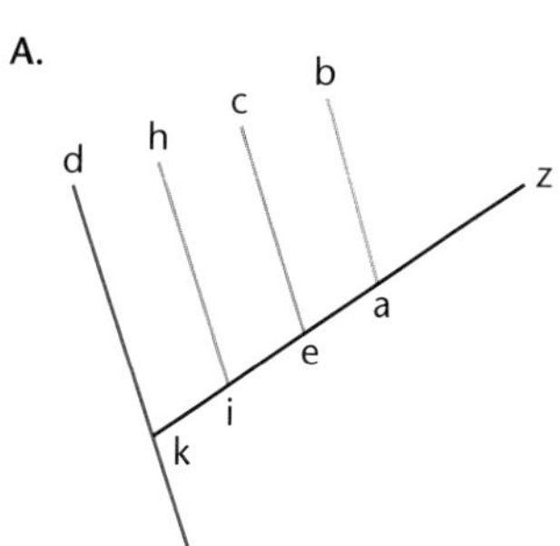

B.
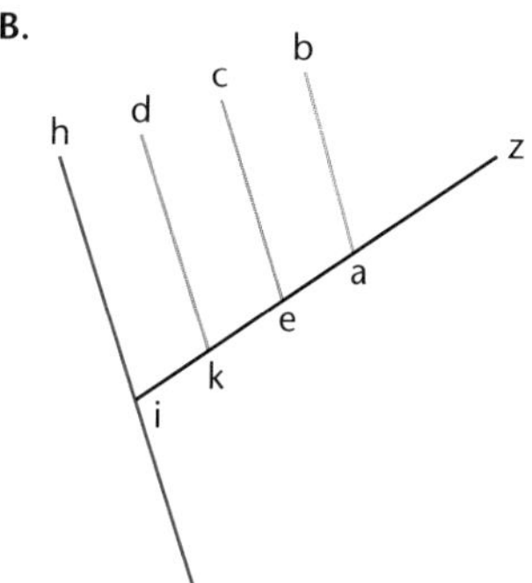

C.
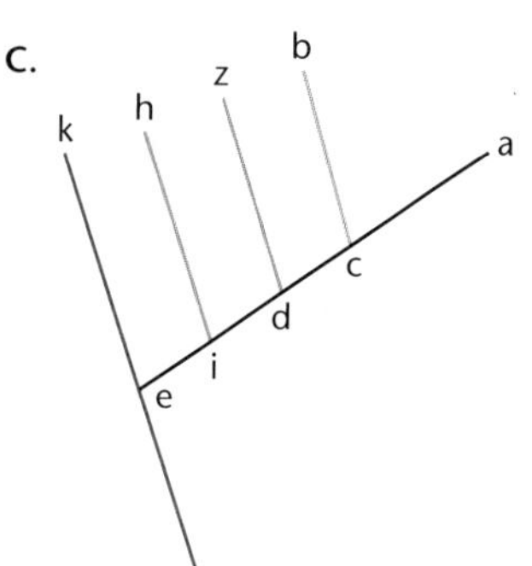

D.
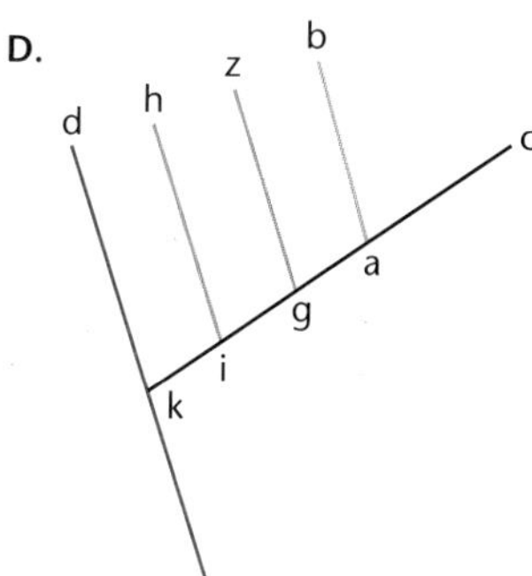

13. Given the diagram below, which of the following statements is NOT correct?

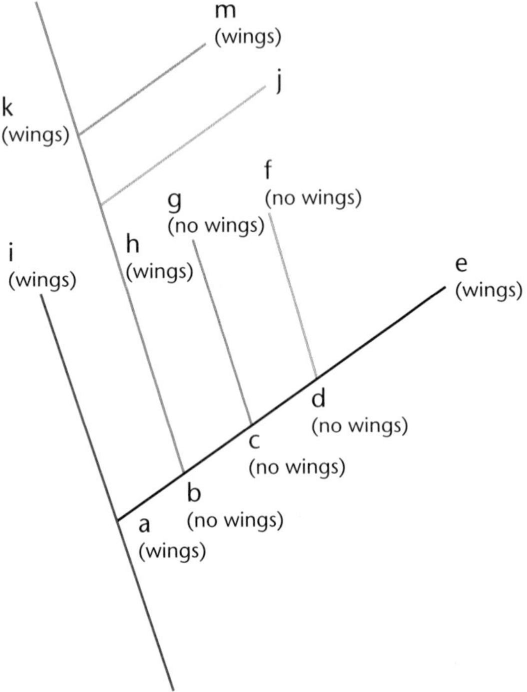

A. Species A and species M have an analogous wings trait.
B. Species A and species I have a homologous wings trait.
C. Species A and species H have a homologous wings trait.
D. Species D and species G have a homologous wings trait.

14. The founder effect is most likely a catalyst of which of the following?

A. Convergent evolution
B. Parallel evolution
C. Divergent evolution
D. Extinction

15. If a population of dogs undergoes adaptive radiation, one would expect that the environment in which the dogs lived was:

A. diverse, with a wide array of different niches.
B. homogenous, with very few different niches.
C. extremely crowded.
D. very sparsely populated.

16. Assortative mating is an evolutionary

A. phenomenon in which individuals attempt to mate with as many different genetic phenotypes as possible in order to improve genetic variation in their offspring.
B. phenomenon in which mates are not randomly chosen but rather selected according to expression of genetic phenotypes similar to their own.
C. force exerted on individuals to sacrifice personal reproductive success for the overall advantage of the group, by preventing overpopulation and overcompetition.
D. phenomenon in which individuals mate with multiple partners to maximize their chances for reproductive success.

17. A population bottleneck event is best depicted in which of the following graphs?

A.

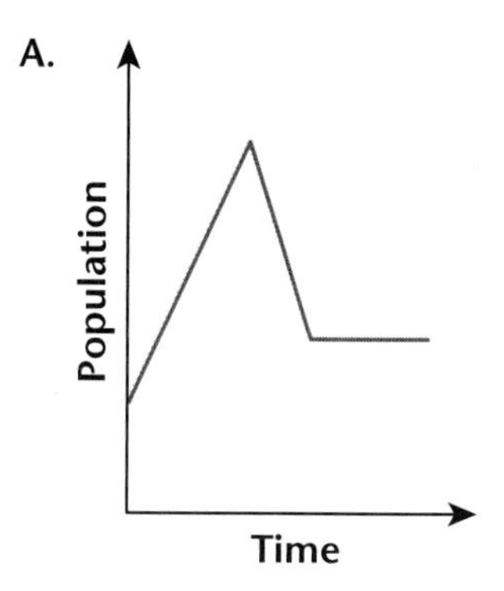

B.

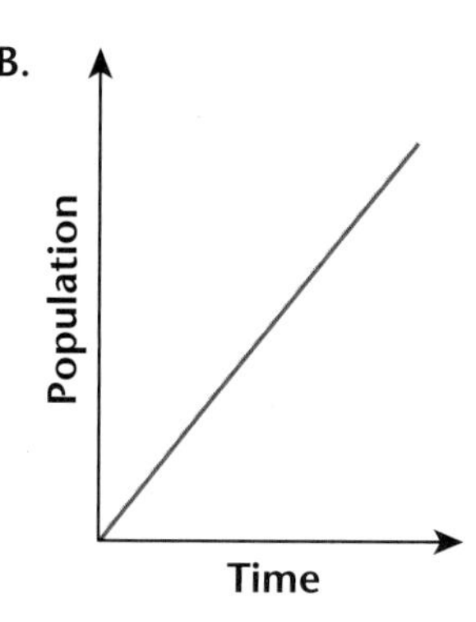

C.

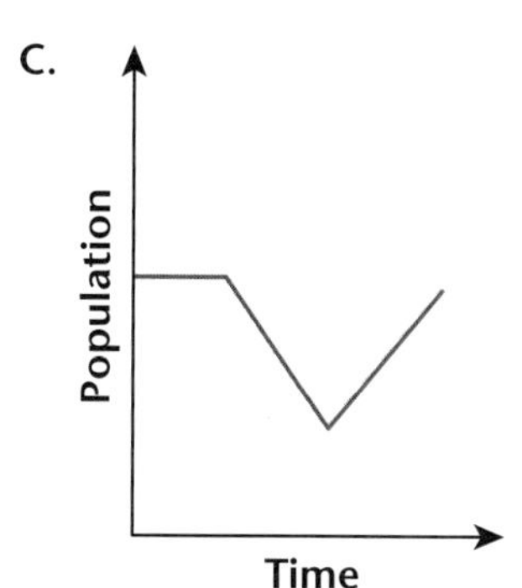

D.

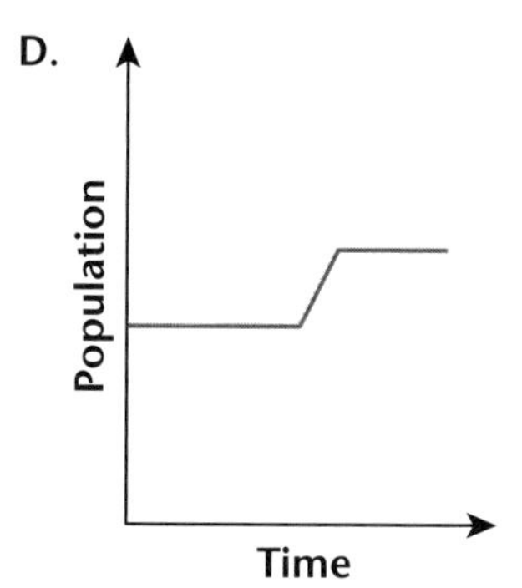

18. In honeybee populations, worker bees are born sterile and only the queen bee produces offspring. Honeybees are considered eusocial insects, a category of organisms in which not every individual reproduces. Which of the following statements is NOT true?

A. Honeybee reproduction is an instance of inclusive fitness.
B. Honeybee reproduction is an instance of altruism.
C. Honeybee reproduction is an instance of group selection.
D. Honeybee reproduction is an instance of kin selection.

19. If the frequency of allele A in a population is 80 percent and the frequency of allele B in a population is 20 percent, and that population is at Hardy-Weinberg equilibrium, what are the respective frequencies of recessive homozygotes and dominant heterozygotes in the population? Assume that allele A is dominant over allele B.

A. 4 percent recessive homozygotes, 36 percent dominant heterozygotes
B. 40 percent recessive homozygotes, 32 percent dominant heterozygotes
C. 4 percent recessive homozygotes, 32 percent dominant heterozygotes
D. 20 percent recessive homozytoes, 0 percent dominant heterozygotes

KEY CONCEPTS

Hardy-Weinberg

$p^2 + 2pq + q^2 = 1$

Gene frequency

TAKEAWAYS

Remember the Hardy-Weinberg equation for geneotypes: $p^2 + 2pq + q^2 = 1$. Note that p^2 is the homozygous dominant genotype (GG), $2pq$ is the heterozygous genotype (Gg), and q^2 is the homozygous recessive genotype (Gg).

Be sure to understand what category each percent or frequency falls under. For phenotype frequencies, consider either dominant or recessive. For genotype frequencies, consider either homozygous dominant, heterozygous, or homozygous recessive. For allele frequencies, consider dominant or recessive.

HARDY-WEINBERG

The gene for gigantism is known to be on a recessive allele. The dominant allele for the same gene codes for a normal phenotype. In North Carolina, nine people out of a sample of 10,000 were found to have gigantism phenotypes, whereas the rest had normal phenotypes. Assuming Hardy-Weinberg equilibrium, calculate the frequency of the recessive and dominant alleles as well as the number of heterozygotes in the population.

1) Solve for the frequency of the recessive allele.

gigantism = homozgygous recessive = gg = q^2

$q^2 = 9/10{,}000 = .0009$

$q = .03$

Recessive allele frequency = 3%

Refer back to the Hardy-Weinberg equation:

☞ $p^2 + 2pq + q^2 = 1$

Because gigantism will only emerge with a recessive genotype, it will be represented as gg. From the Hardy-Weinberg equation, the recessive genotype is depicted as q^2. By taking the square root of q^2 we get the frequency of the recessive gigantism allele or .03.

---

2) Solve for the frequency of the dominant allele.

$p + q = 1$

$p = 1 - q$

$1 - .03 = .97$

Dominant allele frequency = 97%

The frequency of the dominant allele plus the recessive allele equals 1. To solve for the frequency of the dominant allele, you subtract the recessive allele frequency from 1.

---

3) Solve for the heterozygous population.

$2pq$ = frequency of heterozygotes

Gg = 2 (.97) × (.03)

Gg = .058 or 6%

.058 × 10,000 = 580 people

To find the heterozygous population, we need to use the heterozygous portion of the Hardy-Weinberg equation. Plugging in $2pq$ gives us the frequency of the heterozygous genotype.

THINGS TO WATCH OUT FOR

There are five circumstances in which the Hardy-Weinberg law may fail to apply. These five are: mutation, gene migration, genetic drift, nonrandom mating, and natural selection.

SIMILAR QUESTIONS

1) Suppose a similar survey was done in New York. However, this time they found 90 people with gigantism out of a survey of 200,000 people. Calculate the same parameters with the new survey.
2) An allele x occurs with a frequency of 0.8 in a wolf pack population. Give the frequencies of the genotypes XX, Xx, and xx.
3) If the homozygous recessive frequency of a certain allele is 16 percent, determine the percentage of phonetically normal individuals.

Part II
Practice Sections

INSTRUCTIONS FOR TAKING THE PRACTICE SECTIONS

Before taking each Practice Section, find a quiet place where you can work uninterrupted. Take a maximum of 70 minutes per section (52 questions) to get accustomed to the length and scope.

Keep in mind that the actual MCAT will not feature a section made up of Biology questions alone, but rather a Biological Sciences section made up of both Biology and Organic Chemistry questions. Use the following three sections to hone your Biology skills.

Good luck!

PRACTICE SECTION 1

Time—70 minutes

QUESTIONS 1–52

Directions: Most of the questions in the following Biology Practice Section are organized into groups, with a descriptive passage preceding each group of questions. Study the passage, then select the single best answer to the question in each group. Some of the questions are not based on a descriptive passage; you must also select the best answer to these questions. In you are unsure of the best answer, eliminate the choices that you know are incorrect, then select an answer from the choices that remain.

PASSAGE I (QUESTIONS 1–7)

Certain species of hermit crabs inhabit gastropod shells for protection from predators and the environment. Studies have shown that crabs have the ability to take advantage of chemical cues emitted by gastropod flesh, not only informing them that the original shell occupant is dead, but also guiding and orienting the crab to the shell's location at a great range (Diaz et al. 1995). Factors influencing shell choice include size (Blackstone 1985), structural integrity (Rotjan et al. 2004), and material. A 1995 study by Humberto Diaz et al. showed that at closer distances, crabs also rely heavily on visual cues to locate a shell and gauge its quality. They showed specifically that crabs employ visual assessment of shell shape, in delicate combination with shell color and chemical cues, in choosing a shell. Crabs presented with a choice of silhouettes favored horizontal rectangle shapes, exhibiting distaste for vertical diamond shapes. Furthermore, crabs presented with single silhouettes had difficulty orienting to suboptimal shell shapes such as triangles, but easily oriented to optimal shell shapes, such as horizontal diamonds, (Diaz et al. 1995).

An experiment was designed by behavioral ecology students to examine the effect of color on hermit crab shell choice. They hypothesized that hermit crabs would prefer shells that offer a camouflage advantage and design an experiment to test the hypothesis that hermit crab shell choice is influenced by color.

In the first control experiment, 50 hermit crabs were presented with a choice between shells with a clear coat of paint or no paint. The shells were set on a background of natural black rocks. In the second experiment, 50 hermit crabs were presented with a choice between shells with a pink coat of paint or a clear coat of paint, set on a background of pink colored rocks. In the third experiment, 50 hermit crabs were presented with a choice between shells with a pink coat of paint and a clear coat of paint, set on a background of natural black rock.

Crabs were deshelled two hours in advance and placed in heated tanks prior to the experiment. The shells were painted immediately before use and allowed to dry for roughly 10 minutes before the experiment began.

The following morning, the shell choice of each crab was recorded. A crab was recorded as choosing a particular shell only if it was physically inside of it at the time of observation.

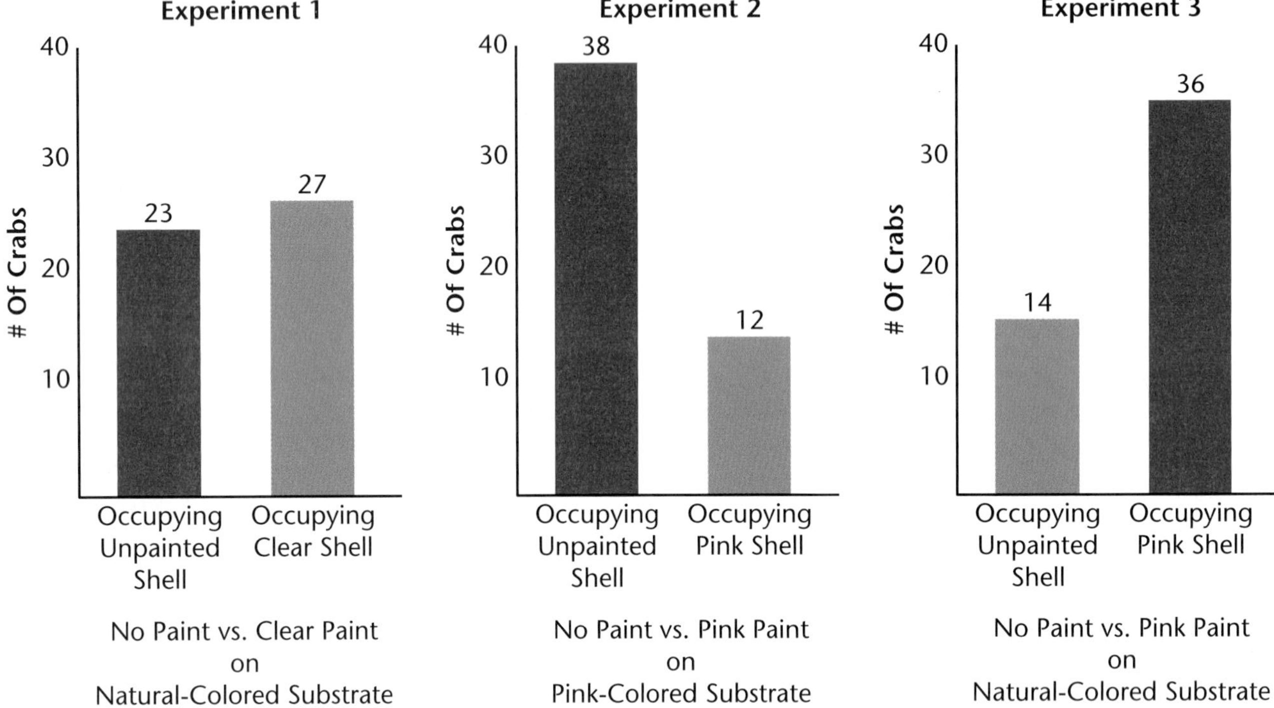

1. Which of the following would be a reasonable null hypothesis for this experiment?

A. Hermit crabs do not show preference for shells based on color.

B. Hermit crabs prefer shells most similar in color to their environment.

C. Hermit crabs prefer shells different in color to their environment.

D. Hermit crabs always prefer darker-colored shells.

2. Which of the following is not a legitimate concern over the experiment set-up?

A. Shell sizes were not identical.

B. Shells were not identical distances away from the subject crabs.

C. The black paint released olfactory signals.

D. The black paint became a dark gray after drying.

3. Based on the data, which of the following conclusions is most likely to be true?

   A. Hermit crabs show a preference for color.
   B. Hermit crabs always prefer black shells.
   C. Hermit crabs always prefer white shells.
   D. Hermit crabs prefer black shells because their natural environment is black sand.

4. Which of the following statements is least likely to explain the data?

   A. Hermit crabs communicate to one another visually.
   B. Hermit crabs' natural environment is light-colored.
   C. Hermit crabs' natural predators are all color-blind.
   D. Natural selection favors hermit crabs that stand out in their environment.

5. Based on the data, what evolutionary forces could be at play on these hermit crabs in an environment with many areas of pure pink rocks and many areas of pure black rocks?

   A. Disruptive selection
   B. Directional selection
   C. Both A and B
   D. Neither A nor B because null hypothesis is true

6. A hypothetical population of 89 black-shelled hermit crabs was discovered in the red sands of Jordan's Wadi Rum desert. Hermit crabs are not native to this region and experts believe they were introduced to the environment by South American tourists. Scientists began tracking this unique population of crabs in 1992. By 2007, only four crabs remained. These findings

   A. strongly call into question the hypothesis that shell color affects hermit crab shell choice.
   B. do not call into question the validity of the hypothesis that shell color affects hermit crab shell choice.
   C. strongly support the hypothesis that shell color affects hermit crab shell choice.
   D. are invalid because the hermit crabs are not native to Jordan.

7. The species of hermit crab used in the experiment and a second species of hermit crab are monophyletic. This second species is color-blind. Which of the following scenarios is most likely?

   A. These two species of hermit crabs do not share a common ancestor.
   B. Color-blindness is an analogous trait between the two species.
   C. This second species of hermit crab was influenced by evolutionary pressures of the founder effect.
   D. Color-blindness is a homologous trait between these two species.

PASSAGE II (QUESTIONS 8–17)

Cystic fibrosis is a serious genetic disorder causing fibrotic lesions of the pancreas, obstruction of the lungs with thick mucus, and reproductive and intestinal problems. With respiratory obstruction, some patients have mild difficulty while others experience serious problems that sharply decrease their life span. The most common form of the disease results from the loss of three nucleotides coding for the amino acid phenylalanine. The pedigree of an affected family is presented below:

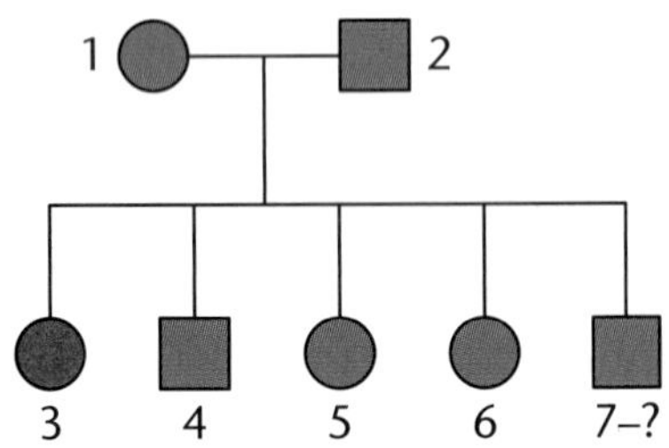

A researcher interested in identifying genotypes of each family member assayed polymorphisms revealed through the variation in length of restriction fragments containing the locus for cystic fibrosis. DNA of each family member was obtained from blood samples. Then, under specific conditions, DNA was digested by restriction enzymes, which recognize specific DNA sequences. The lengths of the DNA fragments were compared through gel electrophoresis. The fragments migrate down the gel and are separated based on their sizes. Smaller fragments move faster through the gel of specific density. The gel is shown below, with the DNA fragments moving from the top toward the bottom of the page:

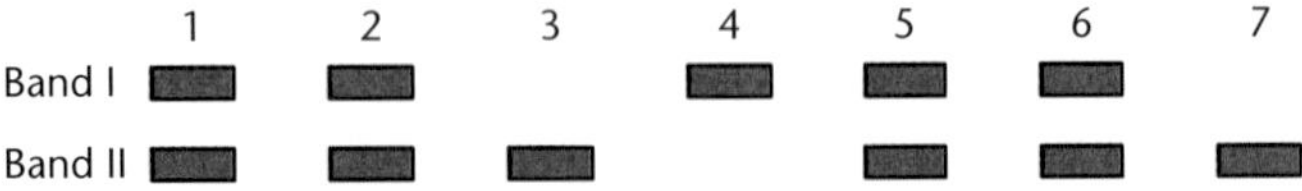

8. According to the pedigree, the disease alleles of the gene are most likely

A. codominant.
B. X-linked.
C. recessive.
D. dominant.

9. If male 7 from the pedigree marries a female carrier, the probability of their having a healthy noncarrier child is

A. 0 percent.
B. 25 percent.
C. 50 percent.
D. 75 percent.

10. According to the passage, what can be concluded about the expressivity of the disease?

A. The expressivity is homogeneous in the population.
B. Expressivity varies.
C. Expressivity approaches 90 percent.
D. There is not enough information to make a decision.

11. It can be inferred from the passage that a mutation leading to the most common form of cystic fibrosis can be classified as a (n)

A. deletion.
B. nondisjunction.
C. inversion.
D. insertion.

12. Based on the polymorphisms of DNA fragments, family member 7 is most likely

I. heterozygous.
II. homozygous recessive.
III. homozygous dominant.

A. I only
B. II only
C. I or II
D. I or III

13. Which family member is not carrying the disease allele?

A. 1
B. 4
C. 6
D. 7

14. According to the passage, when compared to the fragment with the normal allele, the speed of movement through the gel of DNA fragment containing the disease allele would be

A. slower, as the disease allele fragment is larger.
B. slower, as the disease allele fragment is shorter.
C. faster, as the disease allele fragment is larger.
D. faster, as the disease allele fragment is shorter.

15. According to its functional significance, cystic fibrosis mutation can be referred to as

A. missense.
B. nonsense.
C. silent.
D. None of the above

16. The researcher later used the restriction fragment length polymorphism method described to assay 100 members of the U.S. population for cystic fibrosis. One person had the disorder. Identify the observed frequency of the disease allele.

A. 0.01
B. 0.1
C. 1
D. 0.9

17. Family member 5 marries a carrier of the cystic fibrosis allele. On average, what proportion of their children will be affected?

A. ¼
B. ¾
C. ½
D. 0

QUESTIONS 18 THROUGH 21 ARE NOT BASED ON A DESCRIPTIVE PASSAGE.

18. Young patients after an untreated throat infection with streptococci bacteria can develop rheumatic heart disease later in life. Studies have shown that the heart disease affects primarily the mitral valve whose surface cells have proteins similar to a surface protein common to many strains of streptococcal bacteria.

Based solely on the information above, what class of disease best describes rheumatic heart disease?

A. Congenital endocrine abnormality such as type I diabetes
B. Hypersensitivity reaction such as an autoimmune disease
C. Allergic reaction such as a bee sting
D. Congenital structural abnormality of the heart such as a patent foramen ovale

19. The activation of phosphofructokinase-1 by glucagon-mediated increase in PKA activity is an example of what type of modulation of protein activity?

A. Competitive antagonism
B. Synergism
C. Noncompetitive antagonism
D. Allosteric activation

20. What is the purpose of hexokinase?

A. Phosphorylate Glucose-6-phosphate to Glucose-1, 6-bisphosphate
B. Phosphorylate Glucose-6-phosphate to Fructose-1, 6-bisphosphate
C. Isomerize Glucose-6-phosphate to Fructose-6-phosphate
D. Phosphorylate Glucose to Glucose-6-phosphate

21. Both oxalacetate and acetyl-CoA can be generated from pyruvate. Which of the following ratios, if greater than one, would favor the production of pyruvate from oxalacetate and acetyl-CoA, rather than the usual 'forward' reaction?

A. Carbon dioxide/Oxygen
B. FAD/FADH2
C. Glycogen/Glucose
D. Glucose/Fructose-1, 6-bisphosphate

PASSAGE III (QUESTIONS 22–28)

The electron transport chain (ETC) is the site of the final process in glucose catabolism where most of the ATP is produced. The ETC is comprised of a series of carrier proteins that pass electrons along the inner membrane of mitochondria. The carrier proteins are embedded in the inner membrane. Each carrier is first reduced when it accepts electrons, and then oxidized as it passes electrons along to the next carrier. In the figure below, steps 1 through 6 show ETC carriers starting with NAD^+ (nicotinamide adenine dinucleotide) and ending with molecular oxygen.

The passage of electrons along the ETC does not in itself explain ATP production. The chemiosmotic hypothesis is used to tie electron transport with phosphorylation. According to this theory, as electrons are passed from carrier to carrier in the chain, protons (H^+) are pumped across the impermeable inner mitochondrial membrane into the intermembrane space, building up the electrical and pH gradients. The energy of the gradient is responsible for ATP production. When a specific gradient is reached, accumulated protons pass through the transmembrane enzyme complex ATP-synthase from intermembrane space back into the mitochondrial matrix dissipating the gradient and making ATP.

The fact that the highly specific order of the carriers and their oxidation is tied with phosphorylation makes the final ATP synthesis fully susceptible to any interruptions along the chain. Some of the currently identified blockers and their sites of action are listed in the table below:

Inhibitors	Site blocked
Rotenone	Step 2 of ETC
Antimycin A	Step 4 of ETC
Sodium azide	Step 6 of ETC
Cyanide	Step 6 of ETC
Carbon monoxide	Step 6 of ETC
Oligomycin	Inhibits ATP synthase
2, 4-dinitrophenol	↑ Permeability of inner mitochondrial membrane

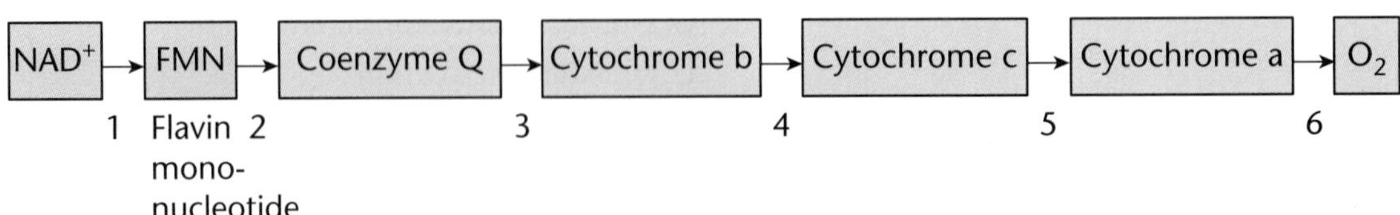

22. According to the chemiosmotic hypothesis described in the passage, the electrical and pH gradients developed across the inner mitochondrial membrane can be described as having

A. more positive charge and higher pH in the intermembrane space than in the matrix.
B. more negative charge and lower pH in the intermembrane space than in the matrix.
C. more negative charge and higher pH in the intermembrane space than in the matrix.
D. more positive charge and lower pH in the intermembrane space than in the matrix.

23. Applying the information from the previous table, in cells treated with antimycin A, all of the following can be expected EXCEPT

A. oxygen remains the final acceptor of electrons.
B. the proton gradient is decreased.
C. ATP synthesis is decreased.
D. cytochrome b is fully reduced.

24. While testing an unknown electron transport chain inhibitor, a researcher measured a high proton gradient while no ATP synthesis could be detected. Using the information in the previous table, what could be the unknown inhibitor?

A. 2,4-dinitrophenol
B. Antimycin A
C. Rotenone
D. Oligomycin

25. Application of which of the following inhibitors will prevent electrons from reaching oxygen?

I. Oligomycin
II. Rotenone and antimycin A
III. Cyanide and carbon monoxide

A. I only
B. II and III only
C. II only
D. I, II, and III

26. It can be inferred from the passage that the higher permeability of inner mitochondrial membrane due to 2,4-dinitrophenol most likely results in

A. more protons accumulated in the intermembrane space, increasing the electric gradient.
B. protons escaping the intermembrane space, decreasing the electric gradient.
C. more ATP produced by ATP synthase.
D. oxygen leaving the mitochondria.

27. It can be inferred from the passage that the mitochondrial matrix has

A. ATP synthase.
B. ADPs.
C. phosphates.
D. ADPs and phosphates.

28. A researcher is interested in isolating fully reduced cytochrome a. All of the following inhibitors can be used for this purpose EXCEPT

A. cyanide.
B. sodium azide.
C. rotenone.
D. carbon monoxide.

PASSAGE IV (QUESTIONS 29–32)

The pathophysiology of asthma involves the inflammatory cascade and constriction of bronchiole airways. Treatment of asthma requires the use of several medications in combination. Traditional treatment of asthma involves use of a beta agonist to decrease the amount of bronchiole constriction that decreases the size of the airway. Additional treatments include corticosteroids to reduce inflammation, and anticholinergic medication to decrease the amount of parasympathetic stimulation to the respiratory system. Newer medications block the leukotriene pathway that contributes to the inflammatory cascade. Other medications block IgE mediated histamine release that can trigger an asthma attack.

Many of the medications used to treat asthma are delivered directly to the lungs by inhalers. The effectiveness of the medication is directly related to the amount of medication that is present in the lung. If the inhaler is used incorrectly, more of the medication will end up in the back of the throat instead of within the lung tissue.

In any effort to determine the best inhaler for treating asthma, a scientist used three different drug delivery devices to deliver a radiolabeled bronchodilator directly to the lung. Patients were then imaged with a PET scanner to determine how much of the radiolabeled medication had been delivered directly to the lung. This technique of radiolabeling a medication for delivery is analogous to radiolabeling a monoclonal antibody that is being used for cancer treatment. The monoclonal antibody will hone to the cancer cells and block receptors crucial to the functioning of the tumor mass, while the radioactivity that is delivered will caused apoptosis and necrosis of the cancer mass. The direct use of radiolabelling, for drug delivery or treatment, has become very popular because imaging technology is sophisticated enough to detect where radioactivity is present.

The scientist delivered a set amount of radiolabeled bronchodilator to 11 asthma patients using three different inhalers. The amount of radioactivity (in Bq/unit of lung tissue) detected was as follows:

	Inhaler A	Inhaler B	Inhaler C
Subject 1	6	9	15
Subject 2	10	7	0
Subject 3	18	3	3
Subject 4	6	11	0
Subject 5	6	4	5
Subject 6	9	7	8
Subject 7	3	9	2
Subject 8	0	2	5
Subject 9	7	1	12
Subject 10	4	0	8
Subject 11	9	0	7

29. What additional variable could have affected the results?

A. Presence of pre-existing lung disease beyond asthma
B. Tidal volume
C. Sex
D. Zero order kinetics of bronchodilators

30. IgE is traditionally associated with which of the following immunocytes?

A. Neutrophil
B. Basophil
C. T-lymphocyte
D. Mast cells

31. Anticholinergic medication during an asthma attack is appropriate because

A. the parasympathetic response encourages exercise.
B. there is reduced blood flow to the lungs during exercise.
C. sympathetic drive encourages bronchodilation.
D. parasympathetic drive encourages bronchoconstriction.

32. Which inhaler, on average, was most effective in delivering bronchodilator to the lungs?

A. A
B. B
C. C
D. They were all equally effective.

QUESTIONS 33–35 ARE NOT BASED ON A DESCRIPTIVE PASSAGE.

33. Those with abetalipoproteinemia exhibit, among other things, low levels of chlyomicrons in their bloodstream. Which of the following symptoms is likely caused by this metabolic disorder?

A. Diarrhea or excessive watery stool
B. Steatorrhea or excessive fat in the stool
C. Hyperlipidemia or excessive fat in the blood stream
D. Hypertriglyceridemia or elevated levels of triglycerides in the blood stream

34. Which of the following DNA replication errors would be expected to have the LEAST severe consequence?

A. A → T
B. A → G
C. A → C
D. A → U

35. The discovery of which of the following enzymes challenged the central dogma of molecular biology and why?

A. Reverse transcriptase, because transcription was thought to be unidirectional only from DNA to RNA.
B. Reverse transcriptase, because transcription was thought to be unidirectional only from 5′ to 3′ and never 3′ to 5′.
C. Integrase, because the central dogma did not account for movement of DNA within the chromosome.
D. Integrase, because the central dogma did not account for the existence of DNA outside of the nucleus.

PASSAGE V (QUESTIONS 36–41)

Sheryl Williams, a 45-year-old real estate agent comes to your office. She is a new patient. She states up front that she's extremely busy and that she is pressed for time. Her only reason for being there is for health insurance purposes; she claims there is nothing wrong with her. With that in mind, you proceed with your history taking and physical exam. You have only just started when the patient grimaces and clutches her stomach. She asks you how much longer the exam would be.

You realize this is not typical behavior, and begin to question the patient further. She states that the pain will gradually subside within the next few hours. She says she's been having these episodes for the past few months, and thinks they must be hunger pains. Because food can worsen the pain, she has cut back on her caloric intake. As a result, she has lost weight, which she considers a good thing. You ask about other symptoms she may have, and after some consideration, she tells you that she feels bloated a lot. She mentions in passing that she has been having frequent diarrhea, and she noticed that her feces have started to look a bit oily. She wonders if she should cut back on eating fatty foods.

You sense that these are more than just hunger pains and inform Sheryl of your concerns. She agrees to further testing. You order a serum gastrin level test, secretin stimulation test, endoscopy, and abdominal CT. The test results come back indicating highly elevated serum gastrin levels. Endoscopy shows multiple small ulcers in the distal duodenum, and CT shows a small mass on the head of the pancreas.

36. The mass is determined to be a gastrinoma (a gastrin secreting tumor). The patient undergoes surgery and the tumor is removed. How does gastrin affect H^+ secretion?

A. Activates the cholecystokinin-B (CCKB) receptor
B. Activates H2 receptors
C. Activates the muscarinic (M3) receptor
D. Activates somatostatin

37. The patient noted that her feces appeared "oily." When there is fat in the stool, this condition is called steatorrhea. This could be an indication of malabsorption of dietary lipids. How does the patient's condition affect her ability to absorb lipids?

A. Inhibition of the liver to produce bile salts
B. Inactivation of pancreatic enzymes
C. Automimmune reaction to gluten
D. Facilitating intestinal colonization by flagellated bacterium

38. Which of the following substances does not stimulate H^+ secretion by gastric parietal cells?

A. GIP
B. Ach
C. Histamine
D. Gastrin

39. Gastrin is secreted from G cells located in the antrum of the stomach. One function of gastrin is to

A. promote fat digestion and absorption.
B. inhibit gastric emptying.
C. promote secretion of pancreatic and biliary HCO_3^-.
D. stimulate gastric mucosa growth.

40. The patient stated that she had been experiencing frequent diarrhea, and that the feces appeared to be oily. Why would someone with Zollinger-Ellison syndrome have frequent episodes of diarrhea?

A. Decreased ability of the large intestine to absorb water and compact feces
B. Increased parasympathetic stimulation
C. Overproduction of motilin by M cells of the small intestine in conjunction with oversecretion of gastrin by G cells
D. Malabsorption due to villi blunting

41. In Zollinger-Ellison syndrome, proper regulation over gastrin production and H^+ secretion is lost. Normally, what type of physiologic control is exhibited once the proper gastric pH is reached?

A. Baroreceptor (pressure-regulated)
B. Positive feedback control
C. Negative feedback regulated
D. Pulsatile regulation

PASSAGE VI (QUESTIONS 42–46)

Estrogen is a hormone that is very important in the female (and to a lesser extent, male) reproductive cycle and for other body structures, particularly promoting healthy bone and muscle. However, estrogen has also been implicated with many types of gynecological cancers, particularly breast cancer. Scientists have found that an ideal way to target this cancer is through targeting the enzyme-catalyzed production of estrogen. Aromatase is an enzyme in the cytochrome 450 family that catalyzes the conversion of testosterone to estrogen. This enzyme is found primarily in the brain, gonads, and adipose (fat) tissue. The first figure shows a generalized reaction coordinate under standard conditions.

Reaction Coordinate for Estrogen Production

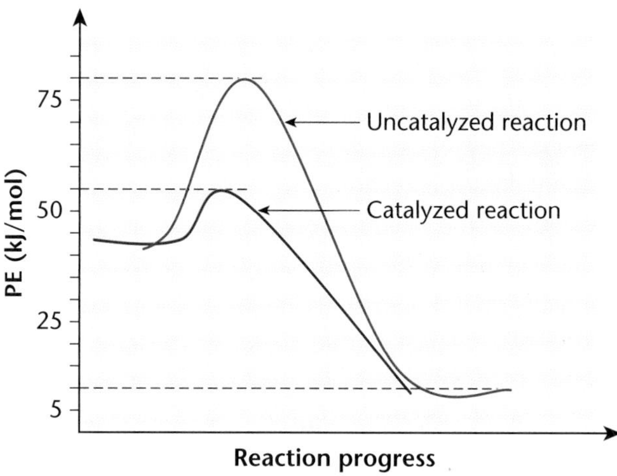

The next figure shows the Michaelis-Menten model for aromatase in the adipose (breast tissue) of a healthy woman under standard conditions.[1]

Michaelis-Menten Model of Aromatase

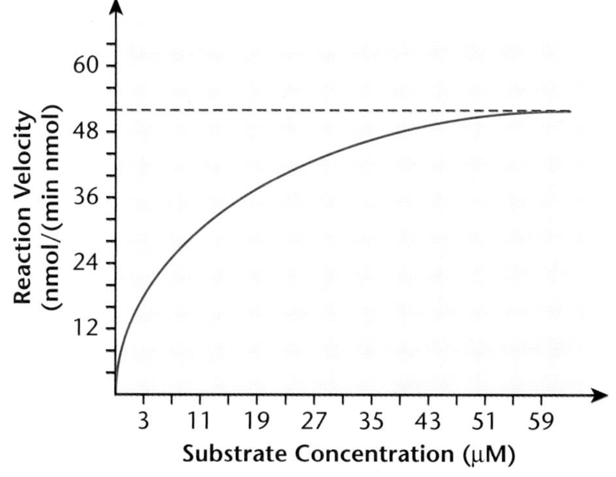

42. What is the overall change in the free energy (ΔG) of the *catalyzed* reaction?

A. 70 kJ/mol
B. 45 kJ/mol
C. 35 kJ/mol
D. 0 kJ/mol

43. By approximately what percentage does aromatase lower the activation energy of the reaction?

A. 0%
B. 33%
C. 66%
D. 100%

44. Studies have found that aromatase activity is high in obese individuals, yet in animal models, those lacking aromatase are obese. What is the best explanation for this?

A. At high concentrations of fat tissue, the aromatase reaction rate increases past the V_{max} in a nonobese individual.
B. The reaction's product serves to inhibit aromatase when it is present at high levels.
C. The enzyme requires a higher activation energy to successfully complete the reaction in the obese individual.
D. The enzyme structure changes in obese individuals, and the wrong substrate is being catalyzed by the reaction.

[1]Kagawa N., H. Hori, M.R. Waterman, and S. Yoshioka, "Characterization of Stable Human Aromatase Expressed in *E. coli*," *Steroids* 69, no. 4 (2004): 235–43.

The table below shows several types of aromatase inhibitors used in the treatment of breast cancer:[2]

Prescription Aromatase Inhibitors

Drug	Mechanism	Notes
Formestane	Suicidal	Injection only
Exemestane	Suicidal	Androgen steroid; similar affect to competitive inhibitors
Letrozole	Competitive	Approved in US
Fadrozole	Competitive	Approved in Japan only; less weight gain
Anastrozole	Competitive	Approved in US

45. What type of regulation mechanism does exemestane use?

A. Allosteric inhibition
B. Allosteric activation
C. Feedback inhibition
D. None of the above

46. 'Male menopause' is characterized by unusually low androgen levels. How can androgen levels be increased in an affected man?

A. Aromatase activation
B. Aromatase inhibition
C. Artificial injection of aromatase from female cells
D. None—aromatase has no effect in men

PASSAGE VII (QUESTIONS 47–52)

Diabetes mellitus (DM) is a metabolic disease affecting blood sugar that results from defects in insulin secretion. It is relatively common, affecting 23.6 million people in the United States, 8 percent of the U.S. population.[3] Type I, or juvenile diabetes, occurs when the body does not produce any insulin at all. Type II, often called 'adult-onset' diabetes (though children can be affected as well), occurs when the body is resistant to normal levels of insulin that are produced, and is often diagnosed in adulthood.

While diabetes does have some genetic influence, its incidence is often combined with other risk factors such as age and obesity. However, there are two rare forms of diabetes that are entirely due to genetics. Maturity-Onset Diabetes of the Young (MODY) is a monogenic form that accounts for 1–5 percent of diabetes cases in the United States. MODY is an autosomal dominant condition. There are several varieties, but each of them is due to mutations in single genes which lead to insufficient insulin production in the body. MODY is usually diagnosed when patients are in their twenties. Like Type II diabetes, MODY can be controlled without artificial insulin, and for otherwise healthy individuals, symptoms may not become apparent until later in life.

Another rare genetic form of Type II diabetes is Maternally Inherited Diabetes and Deafness (MIDD), which accounts for ~1 percent of diabetes cases. Like MODY, MIDD is usually diagnosed at a younger age than Type II diabetes, and is not associated with obesity or other typical risk factors. Unlike MODY, MIDD requires artificial insulin to control blood sugar.

The following pedigree is from an isolated rural community in the southern United States over four generations. It is unique in that the family has presented with the MODY, MIDD, and traditional forms of Type II diabetes.[4]

[2]Buzdar, A.U. "Endocrine Therapy for Breast Cancer." In *Breast Cancer*, by K.K. Hunt and J. Mendelsohn, eds. *MD Anderson Cancer Series*. Houston, TX: University of Texas Press, 2001.

[3]American Diabetes Association. Total Prevalence of Diabetes & Pre-Diabetes. http://www.diabetes.org/diabetes-statistics/prevalence.jsp

[4]Derived from C. Cervin et al., "Cosegregation of MIDD and MODY in a Pedigree: Functional and Clinical Consequences." *Diabetes* 53 (2004): 1894–1899.

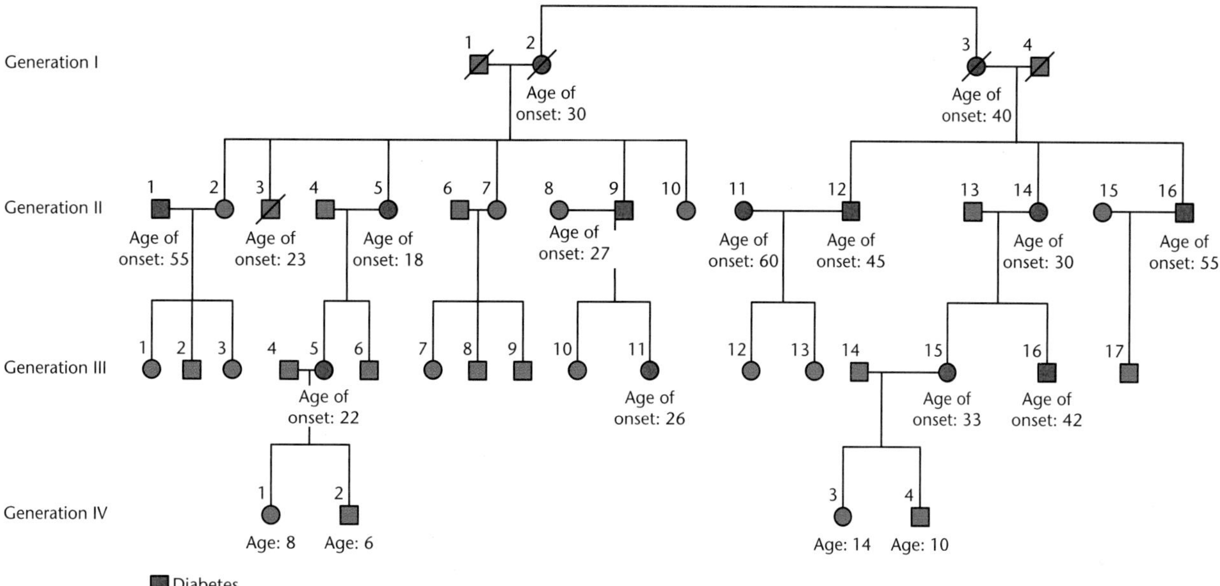

47. The two sisters in generation I of this pedigree both have diabetes. What are their genotypes? (capital letter = dominant allele, lowercase letter = recessive allele)

A. MM, MM
B. Mm, Mm
C. Mm, mm
D. None of the above

48. Based on the available information, what forms of diabetes could individual II-1 present with?

I. Type I Diabetes
II. Type II Diabetes
III. MODY
IV. MIDD

A. I or III only
B. II or IV only
C. III or IV only
D. I, II, III, or IV

49. What is the likelihood that individual IV-2 (the six-year-old boy) will develop diabetes before age 40?

A. 0%
B. 25%
C. 50%
D. 100%

50. What is the likelihood that individuals III-12 and III-13 will both develop diabetes before age 40?

A. 0%
B. 12.5%
C. 25%
D. 50%

51. If the penetrance of the MODY allele is 85 percent, what is the likelihood that all of the nondiabetic children of individuals I-1 and I-2 are heterozygous carriers?

A. 03%
B. 2.25%
C. 15%
D. 85%

52. A form of MODY, called atypical diabetes mellitus (ADM), which has been identified only in African-American and some Asian populations, is characterized by initial need for insulin that eventually gives way to Type II diabetic symptoms. If individual III-17 was to marry a heterozygote for ADM, what is the likelihood that their child would inherit a permanently insulin-dependent form of diabetes?

A. 0%
B. 25%
C. 50%
D. 100%

PRACTICE SECTION 2

Time—70 minutes

QUESTIONS 1–52

Directions: Most of the questions in the following Biology Practice Section are organized into groups, with a descriptive passage preceding each group of questions. Study the passage, then select the single best answer to the question in each group. Some of the questions are not based on a descriptive passage; you must also select the best answer to these questions. If you are unsure of the best answer, eliminate the choices that you know are incorrect, then select an answer from the choices that remain.

PASSAGE I (QUESTIONS 1–7)

Human immune deficiency virus (HIV) is responsible for over 2 million deaths annually worldwide and 40,000 thousand new infections each year in the United States. The current approach to treatment for HIV infections consists of highly active antiretroviral therapy, combination-based medical therapy. Some early therapeutics focused on the inhibition of reverse transcription and consisted of two drug classes: nucleotide/nucleoside reverse-transcriptase inhibitors (NRTIs) and nonnucleoside reverse transcriptase inhibitors (nNRTIs). NRTIs generally mimic nucleic acids and terminate chain elongation. nNRTIs generally bind to a nonactive site on reverse transcriptase to cause a conformational change that interferes with transcription.

As a student interested in the molecular genetics of infectious diseases, you decide to set up an experiment examining three antiretroviral drugs (drugs A, B, and C) that target the reverse transcriptase enzyme. You culture recombinant CD4+ T cells (one of the major targets of HIV) and infect them with HIV. You then either expose them to plain cell culture media or one of three antiretroviral drugs. After 24 hours, you process cells and measure the levels of viral RNA and reverse transcriptase activity. Your results (as compared to the control group) are shown below:

	Viral RNA Concentration	Reverse Transcriptase Activity
Drug A	↓	↔
Drug B	↓	↔
Drug C	↓	↓
Drug D	↔	↔

1. The purpose of this experiment was most likely to
   A. test the efficacy of four new antiretroviral drugs.
   B. contrast the different mechanisms of antiretroviral drugs.
   C. test a new line of recombinant T cells as models for human infection.
   D. test the reliability over time of new assays.

2. If the mechanism of drug A was related to its ability to mimic the nucleotide adenine and terminate the addition of further nucleotides to the nascent DNA strand, with which parent strand base would it pair with in reverse transcription?
   A. Thymine
   B. Guanine
   C. Uracil
   D. Cytosine

3. Given the results of the experiment, what is a possible mechanism for drug C?
   A. Binding and inhibition of viral elongation factor activity
   B. Binding and inhibition of reverse transcriptase activity
   C. Inhibition of viral entry into host cells
   D. Early DNA chain termination during reverse transcription

4. The experiment described in the passage was performed on drug D, a drug recently approved by the FDA to treat HIV. The results of the experiment show no change in viral RNA products or the reverse transcriptase activity. Which of the following best explains these results?
   A. Poor sample quality of drug D
   B. Drug D's mode of action is not related to reverse transcription
   C. Drug D is quickly metabolized to an inactive form by the host cell
   D. Drug D has no effect on the virus

5. As described in the above passage, the action of non-nucleotide reverse transcriptase inhibitors is most similar to which of the following?
   I. Competitive inhibitor
   II. Noncompetitive inhibitor
   A. I
   B. II
   C. I and II
   D. Neither I nor II

6. Based on the information in the passage, which of the following is true of nucleotide/nucleoside reverse transcriptase inhibitors?
   A. They cause early termination of translation.
   B. They are noncompetitive inhibitors of reverse transcriptase.
   C. They cannot be removed after incorporation into the virus DNA.
   D. They bind a site separate from the active enzymatic site on reverse transcriptase.

7. After cell entry and reverse transcription, HIV can become a latent provirus, inserting itself into the host genome. During this stage, where in the cell is viral DNA normally found?

A. Lysosome
B. Cytoplasm
C. Nucleus
D. Storage vesicles

PASSAGE II (QUESTIONS 8–17)

Teratology is the branch of science that focuses on the causes, mechanisms, and patterns associated with abnormal embryological development. Until the 1940s, it was believed that human embryos were protected from environmental agents such as drugs and viruses. It was thought that barriers such as the fetal membranes and the mother's abdominal and uterine walls provided sufficient protection for the developing fetus.

Then, in the 1940s, well-documented cases were being reported about certain drugs and viruses that were producing severe anatomic deformities and even fetal death. For simplicity sake, the causes of congenital anatomic anomalies are divided into genetic factors and environmental factors. But experience has shown that many of the common congenital anomalies are caused by multifactorial inheritance.

The causes of human congenital anomalies or birth defects break down into the following categories:

50–60% unknown etiology
20–25% multifactorial inheritance
7–10% environmental agents
7–8% mutant genes
6–7% chromosomal abnormalities

8. Thalidomide was popularly prescribed and ingested during the 1960s. The main targeted consumers were pregnant women suffering from morning sickness and difficulty sleeping. Because of inadequate testing, many infants were born with severe birth defects. In general, what is considered to be the most critical stage of fetal development?

A. Third trimester
B. Embryonic stage
C. Fertilization
D. Fetal stage

9. Sometimes the separation of chromosome DNA does not go accordingly, and nondisjunction occurs. This can result in gametes containing either more or less of the standard amount of genetic material. Which of the following disorders is due to nondisjunction?

A. Cystic fibrosis
B. Sickle cell disease
C. Down syndrome
D. Polycythemia vera

10. A newborn is presented to you with a huge mass located at the anal region. You recognize it as a sacrococcygeal teratoma. You know it is the persistence of the primitive streak, formed from the

A. hypoblast.
B. prochordal plate.
C. epiblast.
D. exocoelomic membrane.

11. A four year-old girl presents with five days of total blindness. There was no history of trauma, and intracranial pressure is normal. An MRI is taken and reveals a large suprasellar mass compressing upon the lateral ventricles and pituitary fossa. Urgent surgery is performed and her eyesight is eventually recovered. This tumor was most likely which of the following?

A. Medulloblastoma
B. Craniopharyngioma
C. Glioblastoma multiforme
D. Optic nerve glioma

12. Which abdominal wall defect does not involve the umbilical cord?

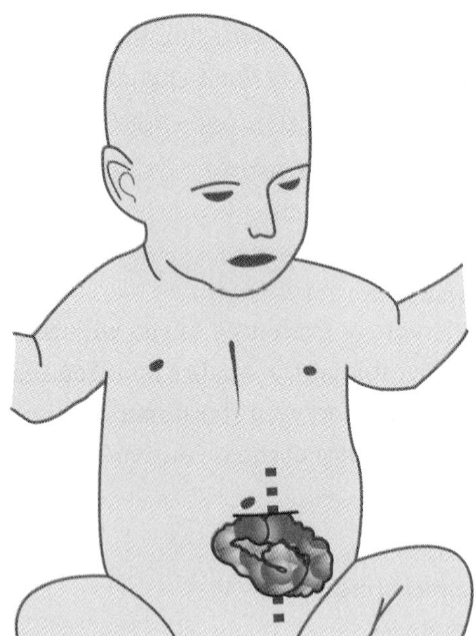

A. Myeloschisis
B. Omphalocele
C. Meckel diverticulum
D. Gastroschisis

13. A young couple comes to your office with concerns about miscarriage. They have heard stories about how a person can suddenly lose her pregnancy, and they want to know as much as they can about the subject. They mention something about extra chromosomes and want to know what that means. You explain that triploidy is which of the following?

A. 47 XXX
B. 48 XXX
C. 69 XXX
D. 92 XXXX

14. An often-seen complication of pregnancy is that of a fertilized ovum implanting itself upon tissue other than the uterine wall. There are multiple sites in which this may occur, but the most common site for an ectopic pregnancy is

A. isthmic.
B. cornual.
C. ampullary.
D. abdominal.

15. You meet with a young couple that has been trying to get pregnant for the past year without success. During your initial workup, the woman states that she has a history of PID (Pelvic Inflammatory Disorder) and wants to know if that could be the reason. What is the most common cause of PID?

A. Syphillis
B. Human papilloma virus
C. Chlamydia
D. Herpes

16. The physician is worried that the fetus may be suffering from fetal erythroblastosis, a disease caused by

A. rubella.
B. point mutation of the beta-globin chain of haemoglobin.
C. CFTR gene mutation.
D. anti-Rh antibodies.

17. The usual result of an oocyte fertilized by two sperms is

A. dizygotic twins.
B. partial mole.
C. normal pregnancy.
D. fetal gigantism.

QUESTIONS 18 THROUGH 21 ARE NOT BASED ON A DESCRIPTIVE PASSAGE.

18. Recent studies have shown that viruses can make many DNA and/or RNA transcripts from the same genomic strand of either DNA or RNA, each of which has different frames. Which of the following organisms uses a process in translation that is MOST similar to this?

A. Eukaryote
B. Prokaryote
C. Both of the above
D. Neither of the above

19. Although many classes of bacteria exhibit antibiotic resistance, researchers have noted that more classes of Gram-negative bacteria have antibiotic resistance than gram positive. What is the unique structural feature of Gram-negative bacteria which MOST LIKELY contributes to this phenomenon?

A. Capsid
B. Membrane-bound organelles
C. Inner cell wall
D. Outer cell wall

20. The lumen of the nuclear membrane is continuous with what organelle?

A. Nucleolus
B. Endoplasmic reticulum
C. Golgi apparatus
D. Ribosome

21. Which type of cell releases glucagon?

A. Beta cell
B. Alpha cell
C. Plasma cell
D. Delta cell

PASSAGE III (QUESTIONS 22–31)

The female menstrual cycle is a synchronized set of events that results in the ovulation of a solitary follicle and ensures that the uterus is prepared to receive an embryo. The cycle is controlled by gonadotropin releasing hormones (GnRH) released by the hypothalamus. The pituitary gonadotropins secrete luteinizing hormones (LH) and follicle stimulating hormones (FSH) that dictate menstruation.

The cycle is divided into three main phases. The beginning of phase 1 is typically taken to be the first day of menses. In this phase, the failure to achieve fertilization after ovulation causes the uterine lining to be discharged. Simultaneously, new tertiary follicles begin to develop. In phase 2, the follicles continue to grow. As they enlarge, they secrete increasing amounts of estradiol, which stimulates endometrial growth in preparation of implantation. Moderately high estradiol levels inhibit GnRH secretion by the hypothalamus, while very high levels of estradiol stimulate GnRH secretion. When estradiol levels reach a certain threshold, positive feedback causes LH secretion to surge. The LH surge causes meiosis to resume in the oocyte of the largest follicle, and ultimately results in ovulation at the beginning of phase 3. The corpus luteum is also formed in this phase, which secretes estradiol and progesterone. The combination of these two hormones in high concentration maintains the uterine wall, and serves as a negative feedback loop in LH production. If fertilization does not occur, the ovum begins to disintegrate, typically 24 hours after ovulation but occasionally as late as 72 hours after ovulation. In contrast, male sperm can typically survive inside a woman's reproductive tract for 72 to 96 hours.

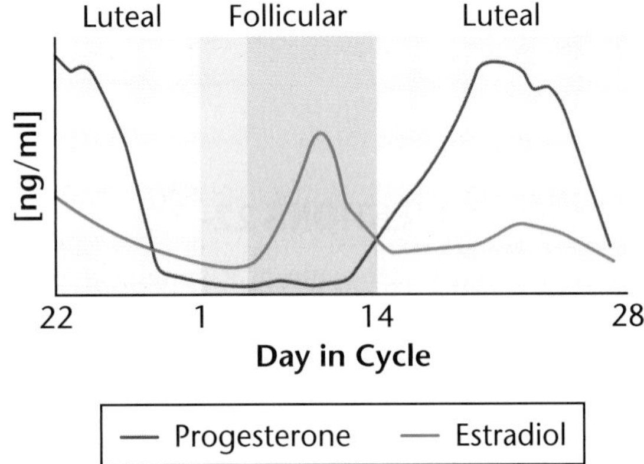

22. Which of the following is not a phase of menstruation?

A. Destructive
B. Secretory
C. Gestational
D. Proliferative

23. Below is an image of Mary's menstrual cycle. How many ova does she produce per year?

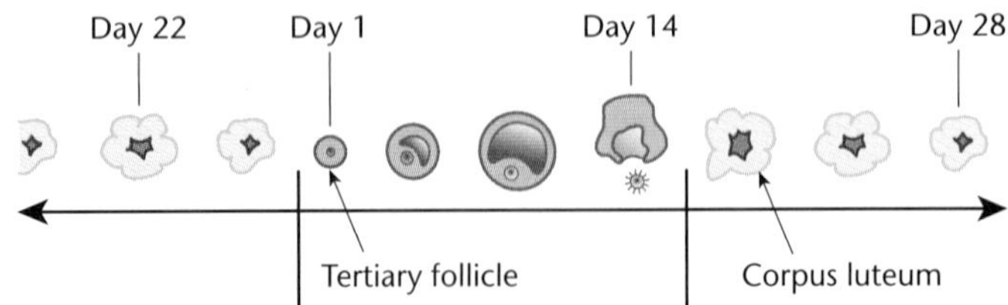

A. 11
B. 12
C. 13
D. 14

24. The corpus luteum is

A. the disintegrated ovum, when fertilization fails to occur.
B. the product of ovum and sperm fertilization.
C. the follicle before ovulation occurs.
D. the follicle following ovulation.

25. Which of the following conditions would NOT contribute to infertility?

A. Extremely low levels of body fat
B. Abnormally high levels of progesterone
C. Abnormally low levels of estrogen
D. Abnormally short luteal cycles coupled with long follicular cycles

26. The combination pill affects a woman's menstrual flow by

A. making it lighter, in that it mimics the circulating levels of progesterone and estradiol during pregnancy.
B. making it lighter, in that it mimics the surge of FSH and LH right before ovulation. This tricks your body into believing it is about to ovulate, preventing the proliferative uterine phase.
C. making it heavier, in that it mimics the circulating levels of progesterone and estradiol during pregnancy. This tricks your body into believing it is pregnant, stimulating the proliferative uterine phase.
D. making it heavier, in that it mimics the surge of FSH and LH right before ovulation. This tricks your body into believing it is about to ovulate, stimulating the proliferative uterine phase.

27. Which of the following is not contained in menstrual discharge?

A. Blood
B. Cells previously lining the vagina
C. Stratum functionalis
D. Zygote

28. At the beginning of the follicular phase, circulating estradiol levels are low. However, by midfollicular phase, estradiol has reached moderately high circulating levels. Which of the following is true of the follicular phase?

A. FSH levels are lower just before the midpoint of the follicular phase than at the beginning.
B. FSH levels are lower at the midpoint of the follicular phase than at the end.
C. FSH levels see a decline at about the midpoint of the follicular phase.
D. FSH levels are held constant throughout the menstrual cycle via a complex mechanism of positive and negative feedback loops.

29. Which of the following graphs accurately depicts the relationship between FSH and estradiol?

A.
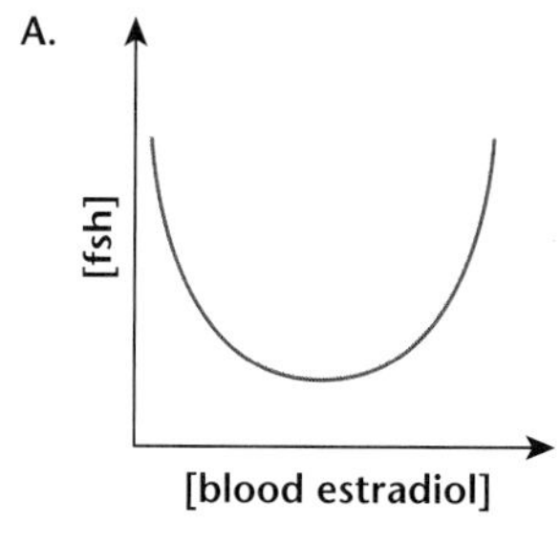

B.
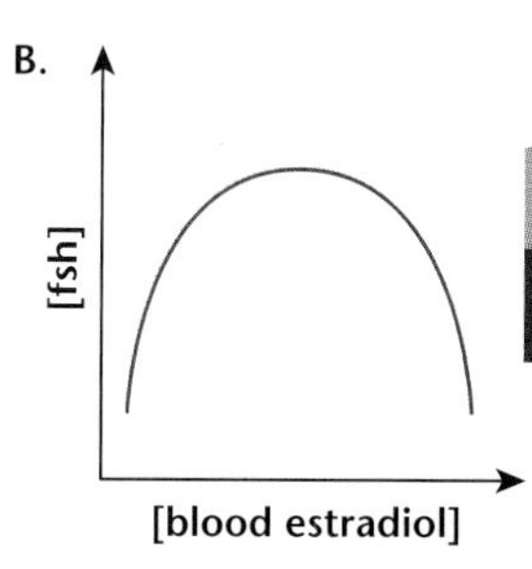

C.
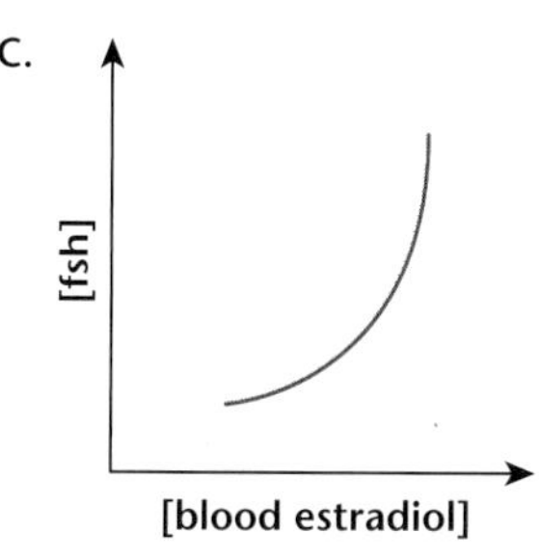

D.
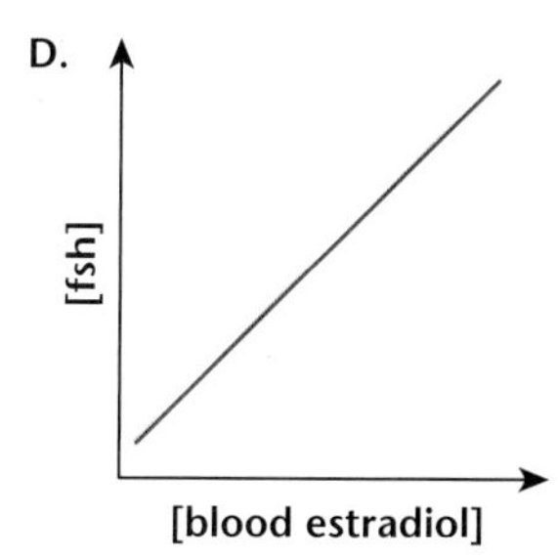

30. Studies have shown that a combination of estradiol and progesterone causes release of FSH and LH before ovulation, yet a combination of estradiol and progesterone inhibits release of FSH and LH after ovulation. Which of the following is true?

A. Very high estradiol and very high progesterone levels cause the FSH and LH surges that lead to ovulation.
B. Very high estradiol and very low progesterone levels suppress FSH and LH production after ovulation.
C. Very high estradiol and very low progesterone levels cause the FSH and LH surges that lead to ovulation. The opposite conditions contribute to FSH and LH suppression after ovulation.
D. Both A and B

31. There is a 0.3 to 0.5° Celsius rise in basal body temperature immediately after ovulation during a woman's menstrual cycle. If a couple wanted to use the basal body temperature method as a form of birth control, which of the following minimum considerations should they follow? Assume a cycle of 28 days according to the following chart.

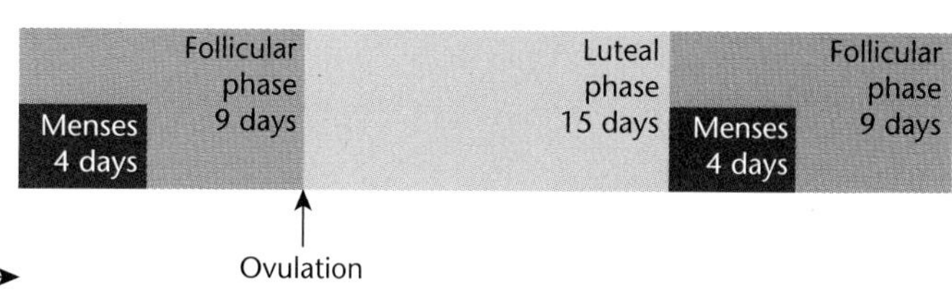

A. Limit sexual intercourse to three days after temperature rise, for 21 days.
B. Limit sexual intercourse to three days after temperature rise, for 12 days.
C. Limit sexual intercourse to 14 days after temperature rise, for 21 days.
D. Limit sexual intercourse to 14 days after temperature rise, for 12 days.

PASSAGE IV (QUESTIONS 32–38)

Mitochondrial inheritance disorders are a particular family of diseases that are inherited from mother to child. All are related to a group of underlying mutations affecting mitochondrial functioning. Because mitochondria are found in all human cells, these mitochondrial defects can affect any tissue in the body. Disease presentations include muscle weakness, strokes, epilepsy, or heart failure.

Mitochondria are the only cellular organelles, aside from the nucleus, that contain their own DNA, known as mitochondrial DNA (or mtDNA). mtDNA is inherited through the mother. Mutations in mtDNA can affect energy production within cells and therefore lead to disease. Tissues that consume the most energy are maximally affected by defective mitochondria.

As part of a laboratory experiment you isolate the mtDNA of several families who have known mitochondrial inheritance disorders. From each family you isolate gene X, a commonly mutated mitochondrial gene involved in oxidative phosphorylation. You then analyze the genes via gel electrophoresis, including a negative control of gene X from a healthy individual.

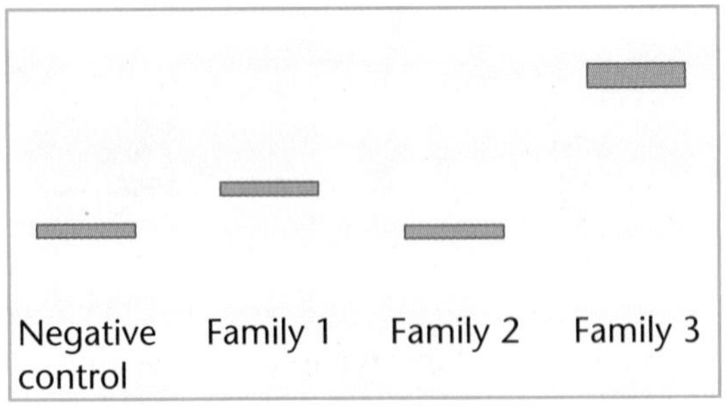

32. Given the results regarding the control gene and the gene from family 2, which of the following explains the presence of a mitochondrial inheritance disorder in family 2?

I. Mutation of another vital mitochondrial gene in family 2

II. Point mutation in gene X of family 2

III. No genetic mutations in family 2

A. I
B. II
C. III
D. I and II

33. On further investigation, it is found that gene X produces a transmembrane protein. Taking this into account, along with the information in the passage, what is the most likely location of this protein in the cell?

A. Outer mitochondrial membrane
B. Nuclear membrane
C. Inner mitochondrial membrane
D. Nonmembrane bound protein in the mitochondrial matrix

34. If we assume that a specific mitochondrial inheritance disorder affects the ability of the electron transport chain to donate electrons to oxygen, the most likely compound to increase in someone with this disorder is

A. lactic acid.
B. phospholipids.
C. alanine.
D. carbon dioxide.

35. According to the passage, mitochondrial inheritance disorders have

A. multiple genotypes and multiple phenotypes.
B. one genotype with multiple phenotypes.
C. multiple genotypes with one phenotype.
D. one genotype with one phenotype.

36. Consider a scenario where scientists have just discovered a mitochondrial inheritance disorder that does not obey the traditional maternal inheritance pattern. It is found to be due to a mutation in the nuclear DNA of the cell. Which of the following explains how a mutation in nuclear DNA could cause a disease with similar presentation to a mitochondrial inheritance disorder?

A. Mitochondrial DNA can recombine with nuclear DNA.
B. All the genes needed for mitochondrial function are located in nuclear DNA.
C. Certain nuclear DNA products are transported to the mitochondria where they play a vital role in mitochondrial function.
D. All the genes needed for mitochondrial function are located in the mitochondrial DNA.

37. The family tree below depicts the inheritance of MELAS (mitochondrial encephalomyopathy, lactic acidosis, and stroke-like episodes), a mitochondrial inheritance disorder.

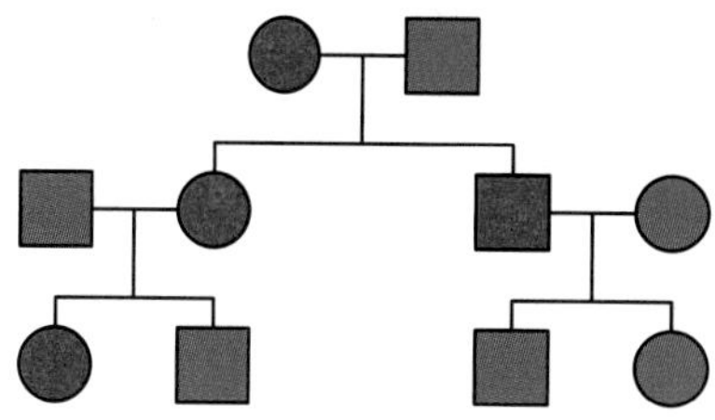

Which of the following contributes to this inheritance pattern?

I. Maternal inheritance pattern of mitochondria
II. Mitochondria possess their own separate genome
III. Sperm cell mitochondria contribute to ova during fertilization

A. I
B. II
C. I and II
D. I, II, and III

38. Which of the following statements is true of mitochondrial DNA and eukaryotic nuclear DNA?

A. Mitochondria and nuclear DNA each encode for their own ribosomes.
B. Mitochondrial DNA and nuclear DNA are always circular.
C. Mitochondrial DNA and nuclear DNA have the same pattern of inheritance.
D. Mitochondrial DNA and nuclear DNA often recombine during cell division.

QUESTIONS 39 THROUGH 41 ARE NOT BASED ON A DESCRIPTIVE PASSAGE.

39. Which of the following enzymes decomposes polysaccharides into maltose?

A. Amylase
B. Lipase
C. Trypsinogen
D. Pepsin

40. Which of the following mutations in an RNA codon would be expected to produce the least severe result?

A. AAA → AGA
B. AAA → AAG
C. AAA → GAA
D. AAA → AAT

41. What is the genetic basis for the statement, "Males drive evolution"?

A. Genes from males are dominant to those expressed by females.
B. Genes from males have been exposed to more positive selection than those of females.
C. Gametogenesis in the male produces four unique sperm cells whereas in the female it produces only one ovum.
D. Males can procreate for a longer time than females and thus a male has a larger contribution to the next generation's genes than a female.

PASSAGE V (QUESTIONS 42–48)

Epilepsy affects approximately 100 million people living in the world and afflicts all nationalities indiscriminately. Seizures are the symptoms of this disease and may vary greatly in type and degree. These seizures result from sudden excessive electrical discharges of neurons in any number of areas in the brain, manifesting in different ways such as disturbances of movement, loss of vision, loss of hearing, and abrupt changes in mood. Although epilepsy is one of the oldest conditions known to man, much is still unknown about the disorder. In the elderly, epilepsy is more likely caused by an underlying brain disease or may be the result of brain trauma. Still, there are many people, especially adolescents and infants, for whom the cause of epilepsy is unknown. In these cases the most commonly accepted theory is that there is an imbalance of neurotransmitters, which causes a lower threshold for convulsions. The following are two controversial proposed mechanisms—not mutually exclusive of each other—for how epilepsy develops from a normal, healthy brain.

The kindling model is one proposed mechanism by which epileptogenesis may occur. In the kindling model, seizures begin to occur spontaneously after repeated subconvulsive stimuli. Typically, the model is used in research to induce epilepsy in various research animals. This is done through very low, usually electrical stimulation of the brain. After a prolonged period of such stimulation, the animals would start to convulse due to voltage sensitization. This sensitization may last for as long as 12 weeks after discontinuation of stimuli.

Excitotoxicity is another proposed mechanism by which epileptogenesis may occur. The process revolves around the actions of certain endogenous excitotoxins, including glutamate, a prominent excitatory neurotransmitter. Glutamate is known to cause apoptosis when left in the synaptic cleft in elevated concentrations via overactivation of NMDA receptors. Brain trauma may actually initiate this mechanism by causing ischemia, which is defined as a restriction in blood supply to particular areas, which then through a cascade of events causes an elevated accumulation of glutamate at the synapse.

42. Based on the passage, which of the two mechanisms would be supported by a finding that carbamazepine, an anticonvulsive medication commonly used to treat epilepsy, was found to stabilize the inactivated state of the voltage-gated sodium channels responsible for action potential propagation?

A. Excitotoxicity
B. Kindling model
C. Both of the mechanisms can be supported.
D. Neither of the mechanisms can possibly be supported.

43. Which of the following accurately describes the differences between the above two models of epileptogenesis?

A. The kindling model, unlike the excitotoxicity model, concerns primarily processes at the synapse.
B. The kindling model, unlike the excitotoxicity model, does not involve the use of chemical stimulation.
C. Excitotoxicity is concerned with a possible chemical process by which epileptogenesis occurs, whereas the kindling model is mainly concerned with a possible electrical process by which epileptogenesis occurs.
D. Both models are essentially the same.

44. Assuming you accept the excitotoxicity view of epileptogenesis, which of the following methods would best treat acute seizure activity in a patient with extremely elevated concentration of glutamate?

A. Extracellular administration of an enzyme, which degrades glutamate
B. Increasing vesicle release into the synaptic clefts in the brain
C. Lowering the threshold stimulus for action potentials to occur in the brain
D. A and C

45. Glutamate is known to be the major excitatory neurotransmitter in mammals. Glutamate does NOT

A. depend on its receptors in whether it will be excitatory or inhibitory.
B. become released into the synaptic cleft by vesicles.
C. mediate epileptogenesis via its receptors.
D. All of the above

46. Based on the given information, which of the following is a plausible mechanism by which trauma to the brain results in epilepsy?

A. Ischemia depletes metabolic nutrients necessary for production of uptake carriers.
B. Trauma agitates the synaptic cleft, which increases the movement and activity of neurotransmitters.
C. Trauma causes increased action potentials.
D. A and C

47. Which of the following phenomena could plausibly explain the kindling model?

A. The phenomenon that an action potential may not occur if the threshold stimulus is reached very slowly
B. The existence of a time period after an action potential has been initiated in which no stimulus could possibly create another action potential
C. The existence of a time period after action potential initiation during which only an abnormally large stimulus could create another action potential
D. None of the above is plausible.

48. Which of the following could possibly explain an abrupt loss of balance in someone with elevated levels of glutamate in his brain?

A. Trauma to the cerebellum
B. Trauma to the thalamus
C. Trauma to the hypothalamus
D. Trauma to the brainstem

PASSAGE VI (QUESTIONS 49–52)

The human body is made up of approximately 60 percent water, with the percentage varying based on the fat content of the individual. In general, lean muscle contains about 75 percent water, while adipose tissue contains only 14 percent water. Therefore, athletes, who have very low concentrations of body fat, have particularly high water content and need to be adequately hydrated. However, for athletes in high-endurance events, such as marathon runners, excessive water concentration can actually be harmful, and sometimes fatal, as evidenced by the death of a 28-year-old female runner in the Boston Marathon in 2002 from hyponatremic encephalopathy.

Figure 1 shows sodium and potassium concentrations in a normal cell and serum. The normal sodium concentration in the blood is ~140 mEq/L.[5] Hyponatremia is a disorder caused by abnormally low sodium concentration in the blood (below 130 mEq/L) . For high-endurance athletes, sodium concentration can be rapidly diluted by drinking excess water. When this occurs in brain cells, it causes brain swelling, sometimes leading to coma or death.

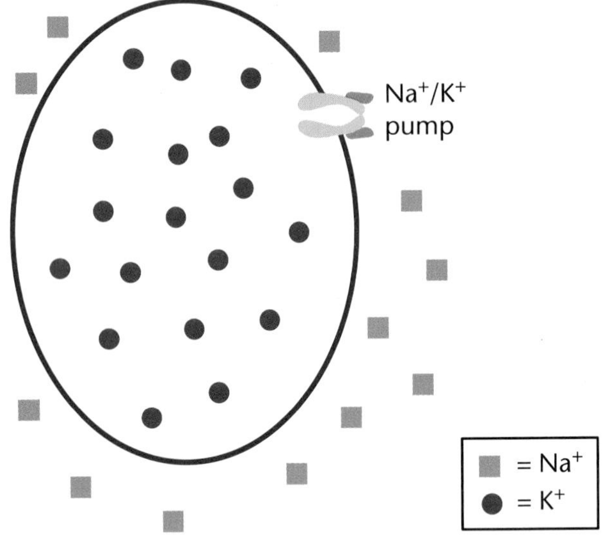

Figure 1

49. Given the information in figure 1, what is the standard H_2O concentration within and outside the cell, respectively?

A. 50%/50%
B. 60%/40%
C. 75%/25%
D. None of the above

50. What molecule is required to control the balance of sodium and water within a cell?

A. NaCl
B. Glucose
C. ATP
D. Urea

[5] http://www.ncbi.nlm.nih.gov/bookshelf/br.fcgi?book=cm&part=A5466

51. Hyponatremic encephalopathy has particularly severe consequences for women, as evidenced by the sole death in the Boston Marathon. What is the most likely explanation for this?

A. Women consume more water during strenuous exercise than men.

B. Women have a smaller brain mass than men do, so the same amount of cell deaths yields a higher proportion of lost brain capacity.

C. Sex hormones impair brain cell adaptation to excess water levels.

D. Vasopressin is present at high levels in affected women.

52. While intravenous sodium is necessary to reverse the effects of hyponatremia, doing so too rapidly can cause a serious problem in the myelin sheath. What part of the brain cell does myelin represent?

A. Nucleus

B. Cell wall

C. Cell membrane

D. Cytoplasm

PRACTICE SECTION 3

Time—70 minutes

QUESTIONS 1–52

Directions: Most of the questions in the following Biology Practice Section are organized into groups, with a descriptive passage preceding each group of questions. Study the passage, then select the single best answer to the question in each group. Some of the questions are not based on a descriptive passage; you must also select the best answer to these questions. If you are unsure of the best answer, eliminate the choices that you know are incorrect, then select an answer from the choices that remain.

PASSAGE I (QUESTIONS 1–8)

Many enzymes require certain ranges of physical conditions to be met for their proper functioning. One such enzyme, tyrosinase (also known as catechol oxidase), is responsible for coloration in the skin and hair of several animal species. There are several metabolic pathways involved in coloration that are mediated by this enzyme. For example, tyrosinase converts the amino acid tyrosine into melanin in pigment producing cells but in other cells, oxidizes catechol to become the yellow benzoquinone.

Tyrosinase is responsible for coloration in Himalayan rabbits. To understand its functioning within certain temperature ranges, an experiment was performed on the rabbits at varying temperatures. Three groups of rabbits were raised at three different temperatures. The results in the following table show the percentage of individuals of each group exhibiting a type of fur coloration:

	% Dark	% Medium	% Light
32°C Group	1	7	92
28°C Group	6	85	9
10°C Group	90	8	2

The study concluded that tyrosinase is thermoliable, meaning that it functions best at certain temperatures.

However, in humans, skin coloration, long thought to be due to tyrosinase activity, has been shown to act independent of temperature variations. While melanin synthesis pathways are mediated by tyrosinase at several stages, the extent of its role in determining skin pigmentation is unclear. Results from several studies with human epidermal cell cultures show a high correlation between melanin concentration and tyrosinase activity. This would indicate that tyrosinase levels determine skin coloration.

Other data contradict this finding. Results from several immunotitration experiments and Western immunoblots show no statistical differences between the actual numbers of tyrosinase molecules among tissue sample groups and different levels of melanin concentrations.

Thus, two alternate, opposing hypotheses are currently accepted:

- Hypothesis 1: Tyrosinase levels determine skin color because of a high correlation between the melanin concentration and tyrosinase activity.
- Hypothesis 2: Tyrosinase levels do not determine skin color because of findings from immunotitration experiments and Western immunoblots.

1. What further data would best support hypothesis 2 without refuting the results of hypothesis 1?

   A. Post-translational alterations in tyrosinase to change its activity levels differ with varying melanin levels.
   B. Genetic alterations in tyrosinase to change its activity levels differ with varying melanin levels.
   C. Tyrosinase activity varies with temperature in most animal species but not in humans.
   D. Melanin concentration and skin coloration are not positively correlated with each other.

2. From the passage, one could logically infer that the metabolic activity of tyrosinase in Himalayan rabbits is

   A. least active in cooler climates.
   B. independent of body temperature.
   C. inactive at or below cooler, arctic temperatures.
   D. more active at cooler body temperatures.

3. Based on the data presented in the passage, which region of the rabbit is likely to be dark in color at 25°C?

   A. Chest
   B. Dorsal
   C. Limb
   D. Ventral

4. Which portion of tyrosinase is most important in terms of its overall functioning?

   A. Active site
   B. Allosteric site
   C. Substrate site
   D. Enzyme-substrate complex

5. What level of structural organization of tyrosinase is first and most importantly affected by temperature changes?

   A. 0°
   B. 1°
   C. 2°
   D. 3°

[Source: Journal of Investigative Dermatology (1993) 100, 806–811; doi:10.1111/1747.ep12476630. Role of Tyrosinase as the Determinant of Pigmentation in Cultured Human Melanocytes. Ken Iozumi, George E Hoganson, Raffaele Pennella, Mark A Everett and Bryan B Fuller].

6. If a future study were conducted on chemical activity in melanin-producing cells, which finding would best support hypothesis 2 while accepting the results of hypothesis 1?

A. Gene epistasis in melanin-producing cells
B. Allosteric interactions with tyrosinase
C. Transcriptional variations within melanin producing cells
D. Elevated pH changes within cell organelles

7. Based on findings from the passage, what is true about the thermoliability of tyrosinase between 10°C and 35°C?

A. Its active site is completely denatured at 10°C.
B. Its active site is partially denatured at 10°C.
C. Its allosteric site is completely denatured at 25°C.
D. Its allosteric site is completely denatured at 35°C.

8. What other physical factors might likely determine tyrosinase activity?

A. pH
B. Pressure
C. Both of the above
D. Neither of the above

PASSAGE II (QUESTIONS 9–16)

Renal clearance (C) is given by the equation:

$$C = (U \times V)/P$$

U is the concentration of the solute in the urine, and V is the urine flow rate. P is the concentration of the solute in the blood.

The general definition for filtration fraction (FF) is defined as the percentage of blood plasma that filters through the glomerulus. Filtration fraction is given by the equation:

$$FF = GFR/RPF$$

GFR is the glomerular filtration rate and RPF is the renal plasma flow. The glomerular filtration rate is equal to the clearance of inulin, a polysaccharide that is neither secreted nor reabsorbed. RPF is approximately equal to the clearance of p-aminohippuric acid (PAH).

In standard clinical practice, plasma creatinine concentration (P_{cr}) is used to measure glomerular function. Creatinine is an inert product of creatine metabolism and is produced at a constant rate by muscle tissue. Creatinine is almost exclusively excreted by the kidney and enters the kidney via filtration through the glomerulus. The production rate of creatinine (Cr_{Prod}) is given by the equation:

$$P_{cr} \times GFR = Cr_{Prod}$$

Rearranged, the same equation gives us the plasma creatinine concentration, which is:

$$P_{cr} = Cr_{Prod}/GFR$$

Plasma Creatinine as an Index for GFR

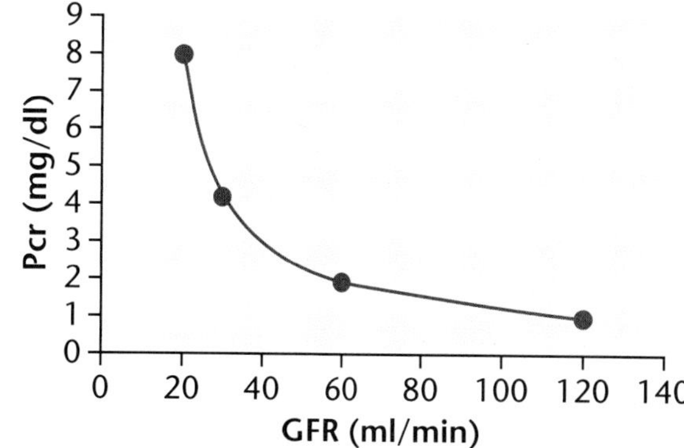

9. Which of the following cannot be true when GFR = C?

A. The solute is neither secreted nor reabsorbed.
B. The solute is inulin.
C. Glucose is reabsorbed from the proximal convoluted tubules.
D. All of the above

10. Which of the following is true when C < GFR?

A. Reabsorption of the solute has occurred
B. Secretion of the solute has occurred.
C. Both of the above
D. None of the above

11. Which of the following must be assumed when using inulin to measure glomerular filtration rate?

A. The filtered concentration of inulin is exactly the same as the plasma concentration.
B. Inulin increases the rate of filtration.
C. Inulin lowers renal plasma flow.
D. Inulin lowers renal blood flow.

12. Which of the following statements of inulin is most likely true?

A. It is bigger than an erythrocyte.
B. It is bigger than albumin.
C. It is bigger than glucose.
D. None of the above

13. No known solute is completely filtered from the blood after a single pass through the glomerular apparatus. PAH is most likely

A. bigger than an erythrocyte.
B. bigger than albumin.
C. both filtered and secreted by the kidney.
D. None of the above

14. Which of the following is true when C > GFR?

A. The solute is being secreted into the tubules of the nephron.
B. There is more filtration than clearance occurring.
C. The solute is being resabsorbed from the tubules of the nephron.
D. None of the above

15. A patient has a plasma creatinine concentration of 4 mg/dL. Her clearance of PAH is 550 mL/min. Approximately what percent of plasma is filtered by the patient's kidneys per min?

A. 5.5%
B. 7.5%
C. 10%
D. 14.5%

16. Is renal blood flow typically greater or less than the PAH clearance?

A. Greater
B. Less
C. Equal
D. Indeterminable

PASSAGE III (QUESTIONS 17–23)

Interferons are molecules produced by leukocytes and fibroblasts in response to viral infections. When a virus enters a cell and begins replication, it also stimulates transcription of antiviral genes in the infected cell, which are translated and released. These antiviral genes are responsible for the protective effect of interferons in widespread viral infections. This is thought to occur by prevention of viral RNA translation thereby blocking viral protein synthesis. A set of interferons secreted by T cells, gamma-interferons, also potentiate phagocytosis towards virally infected cells of the body.

17. The following are the results of an experiment to test interferon production in response to various pathogens.

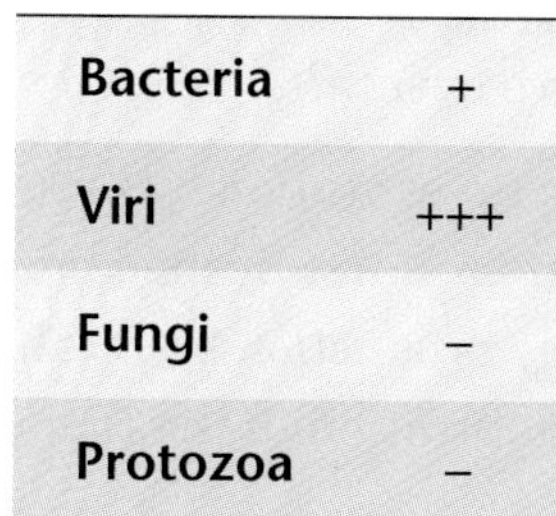

Bacteria	+
Viri	+++
Fungi	–
Protozoa	–

What is the most likely explanation for these findings?

A. Fungi and protozoa are generally extracellular pathogens.
B. Variation in the structure of bacterial cell walls.
C. Differences between prokaryotic and eukaryotic life cycles.
D. Locomotive properties of bacteria and protozoa.

18. The following are the results of an experiment where interferon was added to plates of virally infected cells two hours after initial inoculation with (high titers of a) virus. The control represents a plate of virally infected cells before and two hours after addition of culture medium. Which of the following patterns of growth would be expected in the control group, assuming the virus is cytolytic?

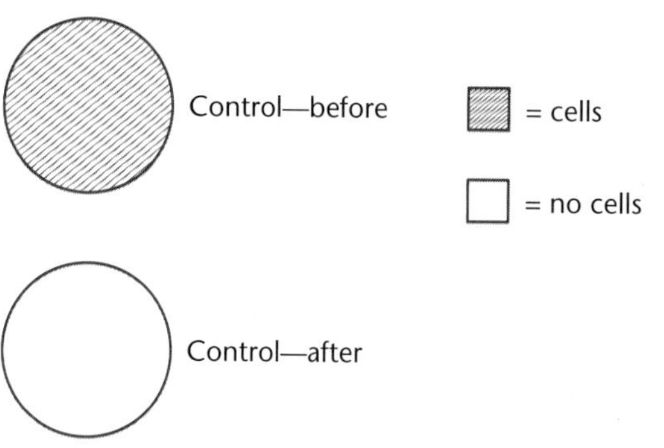

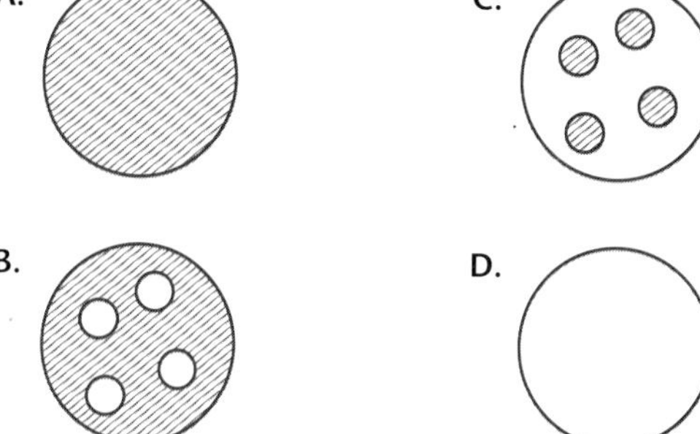

19. Which of the following findings on microscopy would provide proof that interferons inhibited viral RNA synthesis?

A. Lack of a viral envelope
B. Lack of the viral cytopathic effect
C. Lack of viral penetration into the nucleus
D. Lack of viral capsid protein

20. Gamma interferon, synthesized by T lymphocytes, stimulates the humoral immune system to fight viral infections. Which of the following findings would provide evidence that the humoral immune system has been recruited?

A. Increased phagocytosis of virally infected cells
B. Increased inflammation at the site of viral entry
C. Increased concentration of B lymphocytes at the site of viral entry
D. Increased concentration of immunoglobulins at the site of viral entry

21. Cytotoxic T cells are capable of killing virally infected cells via a number of ways. Interferon production by cytotoxic T cells leads to which of the following?

A. Involvement of immunoglobulins
B. Release of cytolytic enzymes
C. Use of intracellular machinery to break down infectious particles
D. Recruitment of macrophages to the site of infection

22. People born without a thymus would have which of the following laboratory derangements?

A. Low lymphocyte count
B. Low immunoglobulin titer
C. High immunoglobulin titer
D. High interferon concentrations

23. Certain diseases affecting tissue perfusion can have a profound effect on the efficiency of the immune system. Poor oxygen delivery would hamper which of the following immunoprotective events?

A. Antigen presentation by natural killer cells
B. Respiratory burst by macrophages
C. Antibody production by B cells
D. T cell maturation in the thymus

QUESTIONS 24 THOUGH 29 ARE NOT BASED ON A DESCRIPTIVE PASSAGE.

24. Which of the following describes the central reaction of a Western blot?

A. Insertional mutagenesis
B. Nucleotide template-directed polymerization
C. Plasmid-driven transcription
D. Nucleotide hybridization

25. Which of the following is an assumption of the Hardy-Weinberg model?

A. Mating between species occurs at a set rate.
B. Mutation occurs at a set frequency.
C. Positive selection for certain genotypes occurs but does not eliminate any genes.
D. The population being studied is large and stable.

26. Angiotensin DIRECTLY causes the release of which of the following from the adrenal cortex?

A. Renin
B. Aldosterone
C. Calcitonin
D. Thyroxine

27. Cystic fibrosis is a genetic disorder inherited through an autosomal recessive gene.

If a male heterozygous carrier and a female heterozygous carrier have a female child who is homozygous for the diseased trait, what is the chance that a second child will develop cystic fibrosis?

A. 0%
B. 12.5%
C. 25%
D. 75%

28. Given the principle of independent assortment, how many unique gametes could be produced from the genotype AaBbCc?

A. 4
B. 6
C. 8
D. 12

29. Some types of mammals have especially long loops of Henle that maintain a steep osmotic gradient. This adaptation enables the organism to

A. excrete urine that is more hypertonic.
B. excrete less sodium across the membrane.
C. produce urine that is isotonic to body fluids.
D. reabsorb more blood proteins such as albumin.

QUESTIONS 30–36 ARE NOT BASED ON A DESCRIPTIVE PASSAGE.

30. Mice are administered a drug that inhibits endocytosis. Then, they are intravenously infused with a substance that is found to accumulate rapidly inside cells. This substance is most likely a

A. steroid hormone.
B. polypeptide.
C. second messenger.
D. glucose analog.

31. The lung is a more common site for primary tuberculosis than the duodenum because

A. the mycobacterium that causes tuberculosis cannot survive in organs other than the lungs.
B. the lung has a more readily available supply of oxygen than does the alimentary canal.
C. the bile salts present in the small intestine destroy the tubercle bacilli.
D. the low pH of the digestive secretions in the stomach kills mycobacteria before they enter the duodenum.

32. An MRI scan of a child's brain reveals a tumor growing on her posterior pituitary gland. Which of the following symptoms might have predicted this finding?

A. Hypertension
B. Increased plasma calcium levels
C. Decreased plasma calcium levels
D. Precocious puberty

33. A researcher investigates the cells involved in bone formation and reabsorption. From which of the following types of cells are osteoclasts most likely to be differentiated?

A. Red blood cells
B. Fibroblasts
C. Plasma cells
D. Macrophages

34. Many runners find that smoking cigarettes decreases their speed and endurance. This finding is due to all of the following effects of nicotine EXCEPT

A. constriction of the terminal bronchioles of the lungs.
B. increase in surfactant secretion by type II alveolar epithelial cells.
C. swelling of the epithelial linings.
D. paralysis of the cilia on the surfaces of respiratory epithelial cells.

35. Which of the following structures is found in bacterial cells?

A. Ribosome
B. Mitochondrion
C. Golgi apparatus
D. Nuclear membrane

36. One type of DNA mutation that can occur as a result of environmental toxin exposure is a deletion, in which one or more nucleotides are deleted during the replication of the cell's genome. However, in mutations in which three base pairs are deleted, the mutated gene often codes for a relatively normal protein. This is likely due to

A. most DNA mutations have no effect on cellular function.
B. codons ability to expand in size to fill the gaps creates by base-pair deletions.
C. retention of the original reading frame.
D. occurrence of a back-mutation.

PASSAGE IV (QUESTIONS 37–46)

Erythropoietin (EPO) is a hormone synthesized in the kidney that is responsible for stimulating red blood cell production. Therapeutically, it is used to treat severe anemia as seen in kidney disease and cancer. However recently, it has gained notoriety as a performance-enhancing drug capable of providing the user with additional oxygen carrying capacity. Because intense aerobic training stimulates endogenous production of EPO, absolute levels are not helpful in determining whether or not an athlete has used it for doping. Current methods of detecting exogenous EPO administration extort the aberrant glycosylation of the recombinant form of EPO.

Although erythropoeisis can be stimulated by EPO, production of effective red blood cells is dependent on the availability of iron in the body. Iron is an ion integrated into the heme molecule. Formed heme molecules negatively feedback on the rate-limiting step of heme synthesis.

Endogenous EPO production is regulated by oxygen levels sensed by the kidneys. Adequate oxygen levels allow for hydroxylation and thus inactivation of hypoxia-inducible factor (HIF), a transcription factor of EPO found in kidney cells.

37. In the healthy human adult, erythropoeisis occurs in which of the following locations

I. Liver
II. Spleen
III. Skull

A. I only
B. II only
C. III only
D. I and III

38. The kidney is also involved in the processing of which of the following substances?

A. Folic acid
B. Vitamin D
C. Vitamin K
D. Riboflavin

39. Which of the following laboratory findings would you expect in a patient with chronic kidney disease who is unable to produce adequate EPO levels?

A. Larger than normal (macrocytic) red blood cells
B. Smaller than normal (microcytic) red blood cells
C. Normal sized (normocytic) red blood cells
D. Fragments of red blood cells (shistocytes)

40. Which of the following laboratory techniques would be most useful for distinguishing exogenous from endogenous EPO?

A. Northern blot
B. Peripheral smear
C. Spectrophotometry
D. Enzyme-linked immunoabsorbant assay (ELISA)

41. The following data were obtained in a mouse population exposed to varying levels of oxygen. Biologically active HIF was measured by ELISA. Red blood cell percentage by volume was measured by centrifuging a blood sample and comparing the volume of sediment to the total volume of the sample.

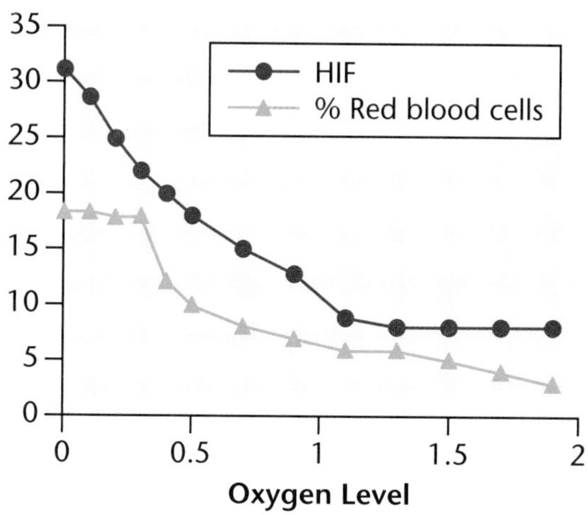

The most likely explanation for the shape of the curve at low oxygen levels in the graph above is

A. insensitivity of ELISA to high levels of HIF.
B. exhaustion of iron stores in chronic low oxygen states.
C. impairment of HIF transcription secondary to chronic low oxygen states.
D. red blood cell clumping.

42. Genetic mutations resulting in insuppressable HIF would express

A. abnormally high numbers of red blood cells.
B. abnormally low numbers of red blood cells.
C. abnormally high levels of EPO at elevated oxygen concentrations.
D. abnormally low levels of EPO at elevated oxygen concentrations.

43. Which of the following properties of the red blood cell allows it to complete its course through the circulation?

A. Lack of a nucleus
B. Lack of protein production
C. Lack of a structural protein network
D. Lack of cholesterol in the cell membrane

44. According to the passage, HIF acts at which of the following steps?

Hypoxia $\xrightarrow{A}$ EPO $\xrightarrow{B}$ Erythropoiesis $\xrightarrow{D}$ RBC

Heme precurors $\xrightarrow{C}$ Heme↑

A. Hypoxia → EPO
B. EPO → Erythropoiesis
C. Heme precursors → Heme↑
D. Erythropoiesis → RBC

45. Epinephrine works systemically to shunt blood to the skeletal muscles, brain, and heart away from nonessential organs such as the stomach, intestines, and kidneys. One would expect which of the following responses to a prolonged administration of epinephrine?

A. Increase in EPO production
B. Accelerated gastric emptying
C. Decrease in renin secretion
D. Increased endogenous catecholamine production

46. In order to bind oxygen, the iron contained in heme needs to be retained in the Fe^{2+} state. Which of the following enzymes is likely responsible for returning Fe^{3+} to its most efficient oxygen-binding state?

A. Catalase
B. Enolase
C. Reductase
D. Oxidase

PASSAGE V (QUESTIONS 47–52)

Bones break when subjected to forces greater than their mechanical strength to bear force. Whether a bone will fracture under a given load depends on both the inherent strength of the bone and the magnitude of the force. Materials, such as bone, whose mechanical properties are dependent on the loading rate of an applied force are said to be viscoelastic. The viscoelasticity of bone is important clinically because when force is applied at low speeds, bone is weak, and when force is applied at higher speeds, bone is stronger.

Fractures of bone are a common occurrence. They are important to note and treat not only because they are painful and debilitating, but also because they may reflect underlying medical disease such as an endocrine disorder or cancer.

Bone healing is divided into primary and secondary processes. Primary healing requires precise reapproximation of the fracture ends, and rarely occurs naturally. It requires rigid immobilization of the fracture and compression of the cortices of the bone together. Primary bone healing is simply the deposition of new bone across the fracture by osteoblasts. This new bone integrates into the two opposing sides through tunnels created by osteoclasts called cutting cones. There will be local bone resorption and eventual recreation of normal bone structure. In secondary bone healing the body first produces a mass of cartilage scar that is subsequently transformed to bone by matrix deposition and calcification.

In addition to serving as the framework of the body, bone is the main storage depot for calcium and phosphorus. A full 99 percent of calcium in the body is stored as hydroxyapatite in the bone. In a typical 24-hour period, 500 mg of calcium is released by the bone and 500 mg is replaced by osteoblast formation of new bone. Like calcium, phosphorus is stored in the body primarily in the bone, although nearly 100 g is present in the extracellular fluid, approximately 10 times the amount of extra-skeletal calcium. The primary circulating factors that affect calcium balance are PTH, vitamin D, calcitonin, and calcium. PTH is released by the parathyroid in response to low calcium levels and acts directly on osteoblasts, which stimulate osteoclasts to promote the release of calcium. Vitamin D must be made active by enzymatic steps in the liver and the kidney. The liver will hydroxylate vitamin D at position 25; the kidney will they add a hydroxyl group at position 24 or 1. An addition to position 24 will be an inactive form, while an addition at 1 will be an active form of vitamin D to work on calcium reabsorption in the body. Vitamin D will act at the kidney to promote reabsorption of calcium from glomerular filtrate and at the intestine to promote absorption directly from the gut.

47. Why might bone development be hampered in cloudy climates?

A. Poor development of the periosteum
B. Less sunlight to produce vitamin C from endogenous precursors
C. Barometric pressure changes increase the likelihood of a break
D. Less sunlight to produce vitamin D from endogenous precursors

48. Bone loss would result from overactivity of which of the following cells?

A. Osteoblasts
B. Osteoclasts
C. T lymphocytes
D. B lymphocytes

49. It can be inferred from the passage that the majority of bone healing occurs by

A. endochondral ossification.
B. membranous ossification.
C. primary healing.
D. secondary healing.

50. A patient who has had her thyroid removed complains of nausea, tetany, numbness, and tingling around her lips. Excess of what mineral most likely contributes to these symptoms?

A. PTH
B. Calcitonin
C. Phosphorus
D. Calcium

51. Vitamin D is stored in which of the following?

A. Interstitial fluid
B. Fat
C. Muscle
D. Liver

52. T and B cells are both developed in the bone, but T cells mature in which of the following?

A. Liver
B. Spleen
C. Thymus
D. Thyroid

Answers and Explanations

CHAPTER PRACTICE QUESTIONS

CHAPTER 1: THE CELL

1. A

Estrogen is a steroid hormone that can freely pass through the cell and nuclear membranes to bind estrogen receptors, found in the nucleus. Therefore, antibodies against estrogen receptors will be found in the nucleus. Protein hormone receptors are often found on the cell membrane, where they mediate signaling cascades within the cytoplasm when activated (C).

2. A

Microtubules are composed of tubulin and provide cellular structure and organelle movement. Eukaryotic cilia and flagella are also made up of microtubules; therefore, any antibody against microtubules will tag spermatozoa flagella in addition to cell structure elements. Actin filaments are composed on actin, a type of microfilament and other structural element within the cell. Prokaryotic cilia evolved separately from eukaryotic cilia and are not composed of microtubules.

3. C

This patient has been exposed to a toxin that is metabolized by the liver. One of the major functions of smooth endoplasmic reticulum is poison/chemical detoxification. Other functions include steroid synthesis and cellular transport packaging. Rough endoplasmic reticulum is responsible for protein synthesis (A). Hyperplasia with irregularities would signify increased cell division associated with cancer-like growth (B). While toxins may cause liver cell death, human cells do not possess cell walls (D).

4. B

Colchicine blocks polymerization of microtubules. Of the mechanisms listed, the only one which would result in blocked polymerization would be if colchicines bound the tubulin polymerization site. Stabilization of centrioles, which are made of tubulin, would enhance polymerization as taxane drugs do (A). The prompt states that colchicine acts without destroying tubulin, therefore it is unlikely that has hydrolase activity (C). Increasing tubulin production would not affect tubulin polymerization (D)

5. C

Protein folding after protein synthesis occurs in both the cytoplasm (for most soluble proteins) and the endoplasmic reticulum (for most membrane-bound and compartmentalized proteins). The nucleus and Golgi apparatus do not play a role in protein folding after synthesis (A, D)

6. A

Lactose is an osmotically active molecule that creates a diffusion gradient, drawing water into the lumen of the GI tract. As suggested by the passage, without the enzyme required to break down lactose (lactase), lactose cannot be absorbed out of the GI tract. In secretory diarrhea, the pumping of chloride ions into the GI lumen pulls sodium ions into the GI lumen as well, creating a hypertonic solution and drawing water into the GI lumen.

7. D

Antidiuretic hormone is released by the posterior pituitary when the body is dehydrated (low blood pressure/increased osmotic pressure). Its main function is to help conserve water. It does this by binding in the collecting duct of the nephron, which activates the fusion of aquaporin receptors to the cell membrane. These allow water to travel down its diffusion gradient, concentrating the urine.

8. C

Membrane carrier proteins transport molecules across cellular membranes. While small nonpolar molecules are often able to diffuse through the cellular membrane, and small polar molecules through channels, larger molecules often require carrier proteins. Steroids are able to diffuse across the membrane.

9. D

This question tests your understanding of the movement of sodium and potassium via the Na/K pump, which pumps sodium out and potassium into the cell. If cAMP were depleted, the pump would not be running, causing sodium to leak in and potassium to leak into the cell via various permeability channels. This would cause an elevated level of sodium and decreased level of potassium. Once cAMP was replenished, the Na/K pump would begin running again, pumping out sodium and pumping in potassium, reversing the previous effect.

10. D

Antiporters allow one molecular to move down its diffusion gradient in exchange for harnessing that energy to move another molecule up its diffusion gradient. Active transport such as the Na/K pump requires ATP, whereas secondary active transport does not directly require ATP (A, C). One molecule must move down the diffusion gradient in order for another molecule to move against its diffusion gradient (B)

11. B

This question is testing your knowledge of tissue types. All of the structures listed are made from connective tissues, except for epidermis, which is an example of epithelial tissue.

12. A

Enzymes are manufactured in cells (gene transcribed, translated into a protein) before being secreted into the extracellular space (in this case, the tear drops/mucus) by exocytosis (the fusing of a vesicle to the cell membrane to release its contents). Endocytosis involves cell membrane invagination to engulf extracellular medium (C).

13. D

Transport of molecules against their diffusion gradient is done by active transport. Simple diffusion is the movement of particles down their diffusion gradient (A). Facilitated diffusion is the movement of particles down their diffusion gradient with the help of carrier particles (B). Exocytosis involves the fusion of a vesicle to the cell membrane to release its contents into the extracellular space (C).

14. B

Prokaryotes have cell walls and lack nuclei. Eukaryotes have nuclei, and only fungi and plants have cell walls. Identification of the presence of a nucleus and a cell wall would be important in determining if the organism was a prokaryote or eukaryote. Ribosomal subunit size cannot be determined via light microscopy (C, D).

15. C

Glycosylation occurs in the Golgi bodies via a series of glycosylation pathways. Golgi bodies are also responsible for the production of secretory vesicles. Storage of glycogen occurs in storage vacuoles (A). Aerobic respiration occurs in the mitochondrion

(B). Protein synthesis occurs in the cytoplasm and associated with the endoplasmic reticulum (D).

CHAPTER 2: ENZYMES

1. A

(A) is correct because it represents the amount of activation energy reduced by the addition of an enzyme. The other answer choices fail to address the lowered activation energy mathematically.

2. D

(D) is correct because by limiting enzyme 1 activity, the rest of the mechanism is slowed, which is the definition of negative feedback. (A) is wrong because there is no competition for the active site with allosteric interactions. There is not enough information for (B) to be correct because we aren't given whether the inhibition is reversible or not. Generally, allosteric interactions are temporary, making this distractor wrong. (C) is wrong as it is the opposite of what is happening when the enzyme 1 is reduced in activity.

3. D

(D) is correct because it competitively reduces the rate of substrate C production. (A) and (B) fail to act competitively on the active site by definition because they are allosteric in nature. (C) is competitive but occurs after substrate C is produced in the chain, thereby not affecting the production of C but only substrate D.

4. A

(A) is correct by definition of an enzyme, whereby it remains unchanged after the reaction it catalyzes. (B) is irrelevant because it is a substrate. (C) is not true, as the enzyme would decrease the rate of a reaction; (D) is wrong because it is a substrate, which has no relevance for increasing or decreasing activation energy.

5. C

(C) is correct because, by definition, enzymes lower activation energy required for a reaction to take place. (A) and (B) are wrong because G is not altered by the enzyme. (D) is wrong because enzyme energy levels are not affected by the enzymes but by the overall kinetic energy surrounding the reaction.

6. A

(A) is correct because enzymes are proteins in nature and macromolecules, and so the other choices do not fit to bonds found in macromolecules and/or proteins in particular. (B) is a type of polysaccharide bonding, and (C) and (D) aren't found between amino acids. (D) is a possibility that may form from secondary or tertiary structures but it's not a certain choice like (A).

7. C

(C) is correct because it is the only organelle that contains hydrolytic enzymes capable of intracellular destruction if it were to leak out.

8. C

(C) is correct because glycerol is a product of lipid breakdown and it should speed up in its formation due to the enzyme lipase's activity. The other choices are all true of the enzyme's influence on a rate of a reaction.

9. A

(A) is correct because there is a limit to the amount of an enzyme's activity above a certain concentration—the enzymes' active sites are already occupied and cannot increase in their rates of processing the substrate, no matter how much more substrate is produced. The other choices make no sense as they are not addressing the slowing rate of the reaction.

10. C

(C) is correct because the quaternary structure of hemoglobin often requires the complexity of an active site to span several polypeptides. Choices A and B would produce too simplistic an active site. (D) does not make sense because relegating active site structure only to small functional groups would not befit a large macromolecule such as an enzyme.

11. C

(C) is correct because the delta G for any reaction remains unchanged. The distracter choices all point to a change in delta G making them wrong.

12. D

(D) is the only correct choice because allosteric interactions always change the shape of the enzyme. Allosteric interactions can be inhibitory or excitatory to a metabolic pathway thus making all of the distracters wrong.

CHAPTER 3: CELLULAR METABOLISM

1. D

Glycolysis is the process of primary importance in glucose catabolism in RBC as it occurs in cytoplasm. All other answer choices require mitochondria to be present.

2. B

Electron transport chain requires oxygen as a final acceptor for electrons. ETC also produces the highest amount of ATP (36 ATPs per molecule of glucose). Answer choices (A), (C), and (D) produce less ATP and don't account for the major oxygen consumption.

3. D

Pyruvate is converted to ethanol in yeast in the absence of oxygen. Other answer choices are not produced in yeast when oxygen is not present.

4. C

Conversion of pyruvate to acetyl CoA by enzyme occurs in the mitochondrial matrix before the beginning of Krebs cycle. Theoretically, the fluorescence should be expected there. Other locations are not relevant for this question.

5. A

β-ketoacids result from fat breakdown. Before fat can be converted to acetyl CoA, it goes through cycles of β-oxidation, during which β-ketoacids are produced and can be detected in the patient's urine. Other answer choices are not characterized by this product.

6. C

ATP is structurally similar to nucleic acids that also contain ribose or deoxyribose, a phosphate, and a thymine, adenine, cytosine, or a guanine base. Other answer choices have a different structure.

7. D

Before entering the citric acid cycle, amino acids need to undergo the process of transamination to detach an amino group. As a result, an α-ketoacid would be formed that then could be converted to acetyl CoA. Thus, only the amino group of the amino acid needs to be detached before the citric acid cycle can proceed, making other answer choices wrong.

8. B

Anaerobic glycolysis is of special importance when oxygen supply is limited as in the example of intense exercise and since oxygen is needed for oxidative phosphorylation choice I is correct. When tissues have few or no mitochondria, glycolysis is the main process that provides energy from glucose breakdown, as the Krebs cycle and the electron transport chain occur in the mitochondria; therefore, III is correct. Limited glucose supply does not explain the special importance of glycolysis. On the contrary, if there is less glucose present, it is even more important to break it down fully via oxidative phosphorylation to provide more energy. (A), (C), and (D) are incomplete or include wrong statements.

9. A

The question requires you to understand that the production of lactic acid involves an alternative (anaerobic) pathway to the Krebs cycle and oxidative phosphorylation (aerobic) pathway. Oxidative phosphorylation may not be happening because pyruvate is being converted to lactic acid instead of being transformed into acetyl CoA and entering the Krebs cycle (B). Production of lactic acid requires conversion of pyruvate to lactate and is the result of anaerobic glycolysis ((B) and (D) are indeed happening). As lactic acid gets accumulated, the intracellular (inside the cell) pH decreases as a general response to acid addition ((C) is occurring as well).

10. B

Competitive inhibition occurs when an inhibitor binds to an active site, preventing substrate from binding. (A) defines noncompetitive inhibition.

11. B

Negative feedback is observed when the product of the reaction inhibits further reaction as in the situation described in the question. Positive feedback (C) would further promote the reaction. There is no mention that hormones or the nervous system affect hexokinase activity, so (A) and (D) are wrong as well.

12. D

Each molecule of glucose is converted to two molecules of pyruvate during glycolysis. In anaerobic glycolysis, each molecule of pyruvate then gets transformed into a molecule of lactic acid. Thus each molecule of glucose produces two molecules of lactic acid. Other answer choices are wrong.

13. B

Acetyl CoA enters the tricarboxylic acid cycle. After glycolysis, pyruvate needs to get converted into acetyl CoA in order for the TCA cycle to proceed. In a answer (A): glucose enters glycolysis. In a answer (C): NAD^+ gets reduced during TCA cycle. In a answer (D): malate is one of the intermediate products in TCA cycle.

14. B

NADH produces about three ATPs when it passes it electrons along the electron transport chain. (A) $FADH_2$ produces two ATPs as it enters ETC further in the carrier chain. (C) GTP produces 1 ATP. (D) cytochrome a is one of the ETC carriers and is not a high-energy molecule responsible for ATP production directly.

15. C

You're asked to use the information provided to calculate the amount of ATP produced per 1 glucose molecule. First, calculate the total amount of ATP produced per 1 acetyl CoA : 3×3 (from NADH) + 2 ($FADH_2$) + 1(GTP) = 12. Then, as each glucose produces 2 Acetyl CoA, multiply the answer by 2: $2 \times 12 = 24$. The final answer is 24, (C).

16. A

CO_2 is produced during the tricarboxylic acid cycle when pyruvate molecules are modified and cleaved. Electron transport chain and phosphorylation deal with electrons and do not produce CO_2—(B) and (C) are wrong. Glycolysis breaks down glucose (6 carbons) into two 3-carbon pyruvates without releasing CO_2—(D) is wrong.

CHAPTER 4: REPRODUCTION

1. B

N represents the haploid number of an organism, or a single set of chromosomes. Eukaryotic orgaisms have haploid germ cells and diploid somatic cells. Each chromosome is made up of two sister chromatids. If a germ cell passes on N chromosomes, then it passes on 2N chromatids.

2. D

Binary fission is a process in which a cell is reproduced asexually by equal division into two parts. Parthogenesis is a form of asexual reproduction that occurs in females in which the embryo develops without fertilization by a male germ cell. Unequal cytokinesis is found in yeast reproductive cycle.

3. D

Crossing over is a form of genetic recombination in which homologous chromosomes pair up and exchange pieces of their genetic material. Crossing over occurs in prohpase I of meiosis, and is often referred to as synapsis. However, crossing over occurs between homologous chromosomes, and not between the sister chromatids of an individual chromosome. Sister chromatids are the identical pieces of DNA joined at the centromere to make up one chromosome.

4. A

DNA is amplified by a process know as PCR or the polymerase chain reaction. This process requires the use of two primers, which should bracket the region of DNA you wish to amplify. DNA polymerase is used and it synthesize new DNA in the 5′ to 3′ direction, so the primers must be complementary to the DNA regions at the 3′ to 5′ ends. Therefore, for the top strand, you need a primer complementary from the 3′ end towards the 5′ end, In answer choice (A), this is primer 2. For the bottom strand (which is not shown), you need a primer complementary from the 3′ end towards the 5′ end as well. Conveniently, the genetic code of this complementary primer would be identical to the upper strand, which is a complement of the bottom strand. In answer choice (B), this is represented by primer 1.

5. A

To complete this question, we must first determine which strand is the DNA template strand and which strand is the DNA coding strand. The DNA template strand is read 3′ to 5′ by RNA polymerase to synthesize mRNA 5′ to 3′. This mRNA therefore is identical to other DNA strand (aside from using U instead of T), also known as the coding DNA strand. mRNA is then translated 5′ to 3′ by tRNAs into amino acids.

The question states that the above genetic code is taken from the *middle* of a protein. Therefore, the mRNA must not code for any stop codons—the stop codon must be taken from outside this region. Because the mRNA is identical to the coding strand, and it is read from 5′ to 3′, the coding strand must be the strand when read from 5′ to 3′ without any stop codons. Based on this information we can determine which strand is the template strand and which strand is the coding strand.

According to the genetic code table, we see that the stop codons are TGA, TAA, TAG. We see that if the top strand is the coding strand, the mRNA would have a stop codon in it.

5′ TCU AGC CTG AAC **TAA** TGC 3′

The bottom strand does not. Therefore it must be the coding strand. Therefore the amino acid sequence that is produced must be:

5′	GCA	TTA	GTT	CAG	GCT	AGA	3′
Aminno	Ala	Leu	Val	Gln	Ala	Ser	Carboxy

6. C

Running the SSR on the gel reveals that at least four distinct phenotypes exist for this marker, which has been separated on the gel by size. Individuals A and D can be the children of B and C because the alleles they have for this marker are present in at least one of their parents, from whom they must have inherited the allele. For the same reason, individuals B and C could the children of A and D.

7. B

Semiconservative replication refers to the fact that when DNA is replicated, one strand of the newly synthesized DNA is a complement, and the other strand is identical to the original DNA. This occurs because during replication, the two strands of DNA split in two. Each strand serves as the template for creating a new complement strand. The original template and the new complement together form a new DNA helix. Conservative replication theory suggests that one of the replicated helixes is an exact math of the original DNA, while the other replicated helix is composed of strands that are both complements of the original DNA. Semiconservative replication has been proved through the use of nitrogen isotopes to track the original strands.

Semiconservative Replication Visual

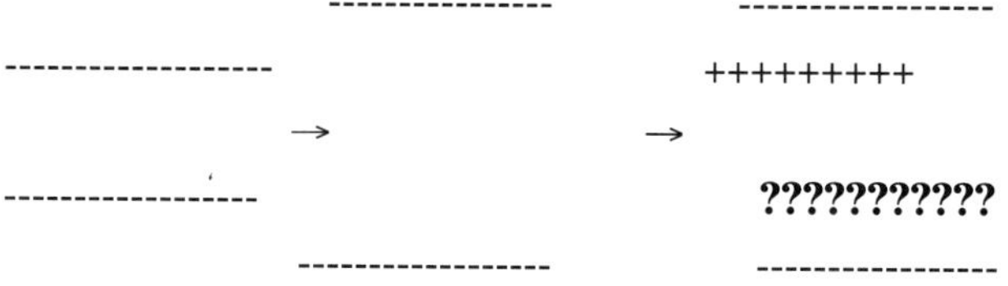

8. D

The LH surge is the catalyst for ovulation in the female menstrual cycle. It begins right at the start of ovulation and ends immediately following the start of ovulation.

9. B

This question assumes basic knowledge of embryonic development, specifically the fact that embryos develop female external genitalia as a default. In male embryos, male sex hormones turn on and turn off specific genes that cause development of male external genitalia instead. Knowing this, we can discount option (A). Without the male sexual hormones, female genitalia should develop by default. We can also discount option (C), because development would not be prevented, it would follow the default course—female development. Option (D) can also be discounted because without male sexual hormones, the genes that are required in development of male genitalia are never turned on.

10. A

Sertoli cells are found in the male reproductive system. If these cells inhibit Mullerian hormone from being release, then this hormone must not play a role in the development of the male reproductive system. Moreover, Mullerian ducts that from through the effects of Mullerian hormone must not be present in males, thus male sex accessory ducts could not develop from them. Based on the information provided, options b, c, and d are all possible. In regards to option B, if Sertoli cells must secrete Mullerian inhibiting substance, this suggests that production of Mullerian hormone and that Mullerian ducts are the default condition. For option (C), if Mullerian ducts do not develop into male sexual organs, than they likely function in the development of the female reproductive system, while Wolffian ducts likely develop into the male reproductive system.

11. C

You can see from the chart that one spermatogonium results in four sperm. This process involves one meiotic division and one nonreductive division. Therefore the ploidy of the sperm will be N.

It is important to note that spermiogenesis is not an additional step in the number of sperm produced—it is a term describing the cytoplasmic maturation that results in activation of spermatids to sperm.

12. C

Disruption of mitosis will only affect the chromosomes of the daughter cells and subsequent daughter cells of those cells. Disruption of meiosis will result in germ cells with trisomy 21 and affect all cells. A duplication even involving chromosome 21, like options (A) and (B), is isolated to one event and will not affect all cells.

13. C

If the urethra is blocked, no fluids can be secreted. This would be readily apparent. Blockage of the seminiferous tubules, bulbourethral gland, or vas deferens would cause components of seminal fluid from being secreted. However, you would be unable to detect this without testing, because the other components would still be released, and fluid would be secreted.

14. C

Options (A), (B), and (D) would all result in sibling who has a higher degree of relatedness than normal siblings, who develop from two distinct ova and two distinct sperm.

15. C

Fallopian tubes are another name for oviducts. These ducts lead from the ovaries into the uterus. Urination and menstruation would not be affected by the blockage of this pathway. Likewise, ovulation could still occur, though the produced ovum would be unable to implant into the uterus. Fertilization would be less likely because scarring will increase the difficulty of sperm reaching the egg. Male sperm swim up the uterus and through the fallopian tubes. Fertilization typically occurs in the outer ⅓ of the female fallopian tubes.

16. D

Vas deferens is the tube that carries sperm from epididymis and testes to the penis. The seminiferous tubules are tubules found in the testes that produce spermatozoa. Sertoli cells are also known as nurse cells. They are found in the seminiferous tubule walls, and aid in the development of spermatozoa. The epididymis is a tubular organ connected to the testicles. Sperm travel through them as they mature and are stored here after maturation.

17. A

Two homozygous guinea pigs would result in all offspring displaying the dominant phenotype. Two heterozygous guinea pigs would result in three offspring displaying the dominant trait and one offspring displaying the recessive trait. Only in the case of one homozygous and one heterozygous guinea pig would the offspring ratio be two dominant phenotypes to two recessive phenotypes.

18. D

An estrogen analog would compete with estrogen for the receptors. An estradiol analog would also compete with estrogen for the receptors. Increasing the concentration of estradiol would also increase competition for the estrogen receptors, especially because we know that the receptors have a greater affinity for estradiol. Thus, the answer is (D). Increasing the concentration of estrogen would help increase its ability to bind to the estrogen receptors because the ratio of estrogen to estradiol would become higher.

HIGH-YIELD SIMILAR QUESTIONS

Fetal Circulation

1. If the ductus arteriosus does not close at birth blood will continue to be shunted away from the lungs. This will lead to a decrease in oxygenated blood being sent to the body which causes

cyanosis, giving the baby a bluish appearance. The heart will increase its rate in order to pump more blood to the body and breathing rate will also increase.

2. The foramen ovale shunts some blood from the right atrium to the left atrium in order to bypass the lungs. However, blood will still move into the right ventricle and to the lungs. Therefore at rest the baby will have no symptoms since the oxygenation should be adequate. During times of strain, such as crying or feeding, the body will have higher oxygen demands and the baby will show signs of cyanosis (will turn blue).

3. Major changes occur at birth, including the closure of the umbilical vein and artery and the functioning of the lungs for gas exchange. When air fills the lungs pulmonary vascular resistance decreases dramatically. This decrease in pulmonary vascular resistance coupled with the changes in pressure due to closure of the umbilical cord raises the pressure in the left atria above the pressure in the right atria.

CHAPTER 5: EMBRYOLOGY

1. D

During prophase, chromosomes condense, nuclear envelope breaks down, and spindle formation occurs. Metaphase (C) is when the homologous pairs line up at the cell's equator. Anaphase (A) is the stage where the pairs separate and begin migrating to opposite poles of the cell. For (B), during meiosis in telophase I, microtublues are still present, and two daughter cells have been formed and are awaiting meiosis II to begin. During telophase II, microtubules of the spindle network disappear, nuclear envelopes form, and four daughter cells each with a haploid set of chromosomes are created.

2. D

Primary oocytes begin the first meiotic division before birth but enter a prolonged period of dormancy during prophase I, choice (D). This dormancy lasts until puberty, shortly before ovulation due to an LH surge. (A) Shortly before ovulation, the primary oocyte completes the first meiotic division, giving rise to a secondary oocyte and a polar body. Upon ovulation, the secondary oocyte (B) and (C) begins the second meiotic division and pauses at metaphase II.

3. D

Mitochondrial DNA in all adult cells originates from (D) maternal DNA. Once the sperm enters the cytoplasm of the oocyte, the male pronucleus is formed and the sperm tail degenerates. The sperm's mitochondrial DNA is located on the sperm's tail and therefore degenerates along with the tail.

4. C

Gonadotropin-releasing hormone (GnRH) is produced in the hypothalamus and is carried to the anterior pituitary gland by the hypophysial portal system, stimulating the release of FSH and LH. Both FSH and LH are key components in the ovarian cycle, from follicular development to ovulation and to corpus luteum formation. (A) Ovaries are important sources of estrogen and progesterone, hormones essential for the development of secondary sex characteristics and pregnancy regulation. (B) The adrenal gland is comprised of the adrenal cortex and adrenal medulla. The adrenal medulla s are the body's main source of epinephrine, norepinephrine, and dopamine. The adrenal cortex produces cortisol, aldosterone, and androgens. (D) The posterior pituitary produces oxytocin and vasopressin.

5. B

At birth, the female has about two million primary oocytes. By puberty, the number of oocytes has dropped to about 40,000. (B) Primary oocytes remain in a prolonged state of dormancy in prophase I of meiosis. Prior to ovulation, the primary oocyte completes meiosis I and a secondary oocyte is formed while the (A) first polar body is formed and degenerates. The (D) secondary oocyte remains in metaphase II of meiosis II. After ovulation and with successful fertilization, the secondary oocyte completes meiosis II to form a mature oocyte and a (C) second polar body.

6. C

Lyonization (aka X-inactivation) occurs when one of two copies of the X-chromosome in female mammals is inactivated. This is so that the female does not have twice as many X-chromosome gen products as the male (who only have one X-chromosome copy). The choice of which X-chromosome is inactivated in random. (A) Attenuation is the reduction in amplitude and intensity of a signal. (B) Attrition refers to the loss of participants such as in a study or class. (D) Hybridization in biology refers to the mating of individuals from different species or subspecies.

7. D

The corpus luteum remains functionally active through-out the first 20 weeks of pregnancy. For the first eight weeks, it is progesterone produced by the corpus luteum that maintains pregnancy. By week eight, the placenta takes over progesterone production.

8. D

Dizygotic (fraternal) twins are (D) not genetically alike. They are due to the fertilization of two separate secondary oocytes by two different sperms. Two blastocysts are implanted seperately in the uterus. Dizygotic twins have two placentas, two amniotic sacs, and two chorions. Monozygotic (identical) twins are (B) genetically identical. They are the result of (A) one secondary oocyte being fertilized by one sperm. The blastocyst was (C) split into two, and about 66 percent of the time, the twins have (E) one placenta, one chorion, and two amniotic sacs.

9. C

No human structures develop from the fifth (V) arch; it exists only transiently during embryonic development. Some notable derivatives of the other arches are:

Arch III: Glossopharyngeal nerve (CN IX); common carotid/internal carotid artery

Arch IV: Thyroid cartilage; epiglottic cartilage

Arch VI: Vagus nerve (CN X); recurrent laryngeal nerve

10. C

The cells from the three germ layers will go through countless divisions, migrations, and aggregations in order to form the various organs and tissues. The heart (C) is derived from mesoderm cells. The central nervous system and pituitary gland arise from the ectoderm, while the thyroid and parathyroid glands arise from endoderm cells.

11. D

The umbilical cord contains three major vessels, (D) two umbilical arteries and one umbilical vein. Highly oxygenated blood is delivered to the fetus via the left umbilical vein. This blood reached the inferior vena cava via the (B) ductus venosus. Passing through the inferior vena cava, blood reaches the right atrium and enters the left atrium through the (C) foramen ovale, bypassing the right ventricle. From the left atrium, blood leaves through the left ventricle, is pumped out of the aorta, and delivered throughout the body. A small amount of the blood does enter the right ventricle instead of passing through the foramen ovale, where upon this portion enters the pulmonary trunk, bypasses the fetal lungs via the (A) ductus arteriosus, and is diverted into the aortic arch.

12. C

One of the first signs of gastrulation is the formation of the primitive streak. This process leads to the formation of the three distinctive embryonic germ layers (ectoderm, mesoderm, and endoderm), with completion around day 20. The primitive streak forms a visible longitudinal axis down the midline of the embryonic disk and consists of the primitive groove, primitive knot, and primitive pit. The notochord (A) is formed of mesoderm and is located in the midline of the trilaminar embryonic disk; it is involved in the differentiation of ectoderm into neuroectoderm, (D) which later becomes the neural tube, upon which the brain and spinal cord arise. The process of formation of the tertiary chorionic villi (B) does not involve gastrulation. The chorionic villi are derived from extraembryonic mesoderm and trophoblast cells.

13. A

Somites are derived from paraxial mesoderm. Thirty-five pairs of somites are eventually formed, from which the sclerotome, myotome, and dermatome are derived. The lateral mesoderm (B) is the portion of the mesoderm on the lateral sides of the embryo, as the name states. Both the intraembryonic somatic (C) and visceral mesoderms (D) are derived from the lateral mesoderm.

14. B

By the fourth week of development, the intraembryonic coelom had been divided into three well-defined body cavities: pericardial cavity, peritoneal cavity, and two pericardioperitoneal canals. Kidneys and gonads are formed from intermediate mesoderm. Cartilage and bone are formed from sclerotome, derivatives of the paraxial mesoderm. Nucleus pulposus is formed from the notochord.

15. B

The cardiovascular system is the first organ system to reach a functional state. During the third week of development, paired endocardial heart tubes develop and fuse to form a primitive heart tube. The tube later joins with embryonic blood vessels, chorion, and umbilical vesicle to develop into the primordial cardiovascular system. At the end of the third week, the heart begins to beat and blood is circulating. Neurulation (A), the formation of the neural plate and neural tube does not begin until about 21 days into development. The respiratory system (C) does not begin development until 28 days after conception, when the larygotracheal groove starts to develop from the ventral wall of the primordial pharynx. Mesodermal cells (D) give rise to mesenchyme, from which both bone and cartilage develop. Bones appear first as mesenchymal cell condensations which form into bone models, and cartilage first appears during the fifth week of development.

16. C

All the extrinsic muscles of the tongue are supplied by the hypoglossal nerve (CN XII), except for the palatoglossus muscle (C), which is supplied from the pharyngeal branch of the vagus nerve (CN X). As for the other answer choices, most of the tongue muscles are derived from myoblasts which migrate from the occipital myotomes during fetal development. The hypoglossal nerve accompanies the myoblasts during migration and innervates the tongue muscles as they develop.

17. B

Hematopoiesis first begins around week 3 of development, within the extraembryonic visceral mesoderm surrounding the yolk sac. By week 5, certain embryonic organs take over this duty. The organ sequence is (B) liver, spleen, thymus, and bone marrow.

18. D

Upon fertilization, the genotype of the embryo (46, XX or 46, XY) is established. During weeks 1–6, the embryo is still sexually undifferentiated phenotypically. By week 7, phenotypic sexual differentiation begins. Week 12 is when the external genitalia can first be recognized.

CHAPTER 6: MUSCULOSKELETAL SYSTEM

1. A

Bone has much more innervation and capillary blood flow as compared to cartilage. Hence, they would be expected to heal faster than cartilage, i.e. ruptured tendons.

2. B

Mesoderm gives rise to the skeletal system. Mesoderm also gives rise to the musculature.

3. D

When discussing the muscle, the answer is very likely to be calcium, regardless of the question. Calcium is the most important conductor of the neuronal stimulus to the muscle. Acetylcholine diffuses across the neuromuscular junction and activates nicotinic acetylcholine receptors on the motor end plate. This causes sodium to flood the muscle fiber. The action potential spreads through the T tubule network, causing the sarcoplasmic reticulum to release calcium that binds the troponin C and initiates a muscle contraction. Iron and magnesium do not play a significant role in this process, and phosphate is not an element.

4. A

The bone marrow houses lymphocytes (T and B cells) as well as the precursors for other immunocytes, platelets, and red blood cells. The other cells are not derived from the bone marrow.

5. A

Anaerobic metabolism does not utilize oxygen to create ATP. As such, the only ATPs produced from the Krebs cycle in an anaerobic condition will be produced during glycolysis in the cytoplasm. This process yield 2 ATP. The complete cycle will result in a total of 38 ATPs being produced per unit of oxidized glucose. It is easiest to remember this by recalling that glycolysis yields 2 ATP. The game is over for the anaerobic state after this; there is no oxygen to act as the electron transport carriers, so no more ATP can be made.

6. B

Osteoporosis. Recall that PTH kicks in when calcium is low. Calcium is drawn from the bone into the blood. An inappropriate elevation in PTH will cause increased resorption of bone.

7. A

Rigor mortis is the term used to define the musculoskeletal system after someone dies. The processes of relaxation and contraction both require ATP, hence, the lack of ATP will result in rigid muscles that cannot be contracted or relaxed.

8. C

Vitamin D is ingested or developed in the skin in an inactive form. It must be hydroxylated at two positions before it becomes active in the kidney and the intestine. The kidney is responsible for hydoxylation at the 1 site, and the liver is responsible for hydroxylation at 25.

9. A

The important distinction here is 'what moves on its own, and what requires initiative to do?' Smooth muscle lines, for example, the GI tract. You don't have to think about its action—it is autonomic, or AUTOMATIC. In contrast, striated muscle required voluntary movement, and is known as somatic nervous system. The autonomic nervous system is composed of both the parasympathetic and sympathetic nervous systems; hence, answer choices (C) and (D) are wrong.

10. C

The appropriate term for the enlargement of skeletal muscles in response to exercise is hypertrophy. In this process, the number of contractile units per muscle fiber is increased, but there is not cell division. The number of cells remains the same; each cell is just larger due to the stimulus to increase the contractile force in the muscle to match the applied load. Hypertension is a term related to blood pressure and has nothing to do with muscle growth. Hyperplasia is a term meaning an increased number of cells in response to a stimulus. This is the term that will trip you up if you do not understand the fundamental basis skeletal muscle growth. Hyperextension refers to the movement of a joint beyond its normal range of motion. This can cause injury, not growth in muscle size.

11. D

This is an easy question if you understand the fundamental unit of skeletal muscle. The sarcomere is arranged between Z lines; there is no Z band. The Z line at each end is considered the boundary of an individual sarcomere. The I band is the area of sarcomere that is only thin actin monomers. The H band is the center portion of a sarcomere that is only myosin monomers. The A band is the region in which the actin and myosin fibers will overlap. When the actin and myosin engage to cause a contraction, the I and H regions shorten. The area of overlaps, the A band, will remain of the same length.

12. B

In menopause, there is a decrease of estrogen. Hence, there will be decreased stimulation of the osteoblasts. Because the osteoblasts and osteoclasts are always in constant opposition (bone remodeling theory, discuss in Kaplan Biology Homes study notes), decreaed stimulation of the osteoblasts will result in an INCREASED ration of osteoclast to osteoblast activity.

13. B

This question relies on an understanding of the feedback mechanisms of the parathyroid and the bones. In the case of bone loss, we may be suspicious of an increase in the amount of parathyroid hormone (PTH) circulating in the blood. An elevated PTH in the context of an underlying disturbance would be considered a secondary hyperparathyroidism. For example, if a patient had chronic kidney failure, they may not be absorbing calcium appropriately, and they are unable to convert vitamin D to its active form. The calcium will be low because of kidney dysfunction, and the PTH will be elevated in an effort to leech calcium from the bone to keep the serum levels normal. Primary hyperthyroidism would not be related to calcium status or loss of bone mass. Pseudo hypoparathyroidism occurs when there is a relative insensitivity of the osteoblast-osteocyte system to PTH. The PTH may be elevated, but the calcium remains low in the blood. The presence of bone loss in this patient suggests that PTH does work on the bones, in this case, to excess.

CHAPTER 7: DIGESTION

1. C

Opsonization is the coating of microbes (i.e., bacterium) with complement components, such as C3b. (A) propulsion allows for ingested food to be moved towards the rectum. (B) secretions of electrolytes and enzymes aid in (D) digestion, which allows for nutrients to reach the bloodstream.

2. D

The correct linear arrangement of the gastrointestinal tract is: (D) mouth, esophagus, stomach, duodenum, jejunum, ileum, large intestine, and anus. The trachea or windpipe is part of the respiratory system. During swallowing, the epiglottis (a lid-like flap of elastic cartilaginous tissue covered by a mucous membrane) that is attached to the root of the tongue, will prevent food from entering the trachea.

3. A

Both the vagus nerve (CN X) and the pelvic nerve are considered to be part of the parasympathetic system of the gastrointestinal tract (B), (C), and (D). The vagus nerve innervates the upper GI tract (striated muscle of the upper third of the esophagus, stomach wall, small intestine (duodenum, jejunum, ileum), and ascending colon). The pelvic nerve supplies the lower GI tract (striated muscle of the external anal canal, transverse colon, descending colon, and sigmoid colon) (A).

4. D

(A) mucosal layer is subdivided into the epithelial cells layer, lamina propria, and muscularis mucosae. The specialized epithelial cells are capable of absorption and secretion. (C) lamina propria contains some blood and lymph vessels, but it is comprised primarily of connective tissue. (B) muscularis mucosae, as the name indicates, consists of smooth muscle cells. (D) submucosal layer is considered to be the layer that contains the main blood vessels of the gastrointestinal tract.

5. C

The most frequently affected region is the ileum. The next most frequently affected region is the duodenum. The atretic ileum would probably appear as a narrow segment connecting the proximal and distal small bowel segments. Ileal atresia most likely occurred because of a prenatal interruption of the blood supply to the ileum.

6. B

Cholecystokin (CCK) is secreted by I cells, located in the mucosa of the duodenum and jejunum. Cholecystokinin is essential for fat digestion and absorption. (A) CCK stimulates gallbladder contraction, which leads to bile release into the lumen of the small intestine. Bile is required for the emulsificiation of dietary lipids. (C) CCK increases the secretion of bicarbonate from the pancreas, enhancing the effects of secretin. The process of fat digestion and absorption takes a long time in the stomach. CCK inhibits/slows down gastric emptying and increases gastric emptying time (D). Gastric inhibitory peptide (GIP) is secreted by the mucosa cells of the duodenum and jejunum. It inhibits gastric H^+ secretion (B).

7. C

When food is ingested, both gastrin and the Vagus nerve stimulates the release of pepsinogen and HCl. Pepsinogen is secreted by the chief cells of the stomach, while HCl is secreted by the stomach's parietal cells. This causes an acidic environment within the stomach, between pH 1 and 2. This causes pepsingoen to unfold and undergo an autocatalytic process, leading to active pepsin. Pepsin will then proceed with protein digestion and also convert more pepsinogen into pepsin.

8. C

The proximal, dilated megacolon has the normal number of ganglion cells, but distal to it, the section that lacks innervations is unable to relax, thereby preventing movement of intestinal contents. Constipation is a very common and typical presentation. Absorption primarily takes place in the small intestine. Only a small portion of the digestive process takes place in the large intestine (B). Instead, the large intestine primarily absorbs water and compacts feces.

9. D

During embryonic development, structures within the abdominal cavity will shift positions before reaching their final positions. During the stomach development, the stomach will undergo its first 90° rotation along the embryonic axis; therefore, posterior structures are moved to the left of the stomach. Later, a second rotation occurs—this time along the frontal plane—causing structures on the left side of the stomach to shift inferiorly. Structures that start out posterior to the stomach, then, would find their final positions to be inferior to the stomach.

10. B

In order for bile salts to be formed from cholesterol, multiple processes need to take place beforehand. Hepatocytes utilize cholesterol in order to synthesize two types of primary bile acids: cholic acid and chenodeoxycholic acid. These primary bile acids are secreted into the intestinal lumen. There, intestinal bacteria will dehydroxylate the primary bile acids, producing secondary bile acids: deoxycholic acid and lithocholic acid (B).

11. C

The liver conjugates secondary bile acids with either glycine or taurine to form bile salts. Arginine (A) is the immediate precursor of nitric oxide (NO), urea, and is necessary for the synthesis of creatine. Carnitine (B) is required for lipid transport within the cell, transporting long-chain fatty acid acyl groups into the mitochondrial matrix. Phenylalanine (D) is converted into tyrosine, which is required for the production of dopamine, norepinephrine, and epinephrine. A lack of phenylanine hydroxylase (PAH) in one's system will lead to a buildup of phenylalalanine, a genetic disorder known as phenylketonuria (PKU). If left untreated, this condition can lead to severe mental retardation and seizures.

12. C

There are four primary bile acid functions. The majority of secreted bile salts are extracted by the liver and reused (A). About 600 mg/day of bile salts are lost through fecal excretion out of the body's total bile salt pool of 2.5 g. Although the amount appears minimal, this is the only significant mechanism with which the body has to eliminate excess cholesterol. In order to prevent cholesterol from precipitating in the gallbladder, bile acids and phospholipids solubilize cholesterol in the bile (B). In order for solubilization to work, dietary lipids need to be emulsified first (D). The negatively charged bile acids surrounds the lipds, creating small lipid droplets within the intestinal lumen. The negative charges on the bile salts will repel other bile salts, tearing apart the lipid droplets. This increases the surface area, allowing for more digestive enzymes to work. Bile acids facilitate the absorption of fat-soluble vitamins (K, A, D, E)(C). Vitamins B_1, B_2, B_6, B_{12}, and C are water-soluble vitamins. These water-soluble vitamins are usually absorbed via Na^+-dependent cotransporters in the small intestine.

13. C

α-amylase found in saliva begins the process of starch and lipid digestion. Amylase is also found in pancreatic juice. Pepsinogen (A) is secreted by the chief cells of the stomach, while HCl is secreted by the stomach's parietal cells. This causes an acidic environment within the stomach, between pH 1 and 2. This causes pepsingoen to unfold and undergo an autocatalytic process, leading to active pepsin. Pepsin will then proceed with protein digestion and also convert more pepsinogen into pepsin. Trypsin (D) in produced by the pancreas, in the inactive form of trypsinogen. Trypsinogen in secreted into the small intestine and the enzyme, enteropeptidase, converts trypsingoen in the active form, trypsin. Chymotrypsin (B) is synthesized in the pancreas, in the inactive form of chymotrypsinogen. It is converted to its active form through cleavage by trypsin.

14. A

Aldosterone is produced in the adrenal cortex and increases blood volume by reabsorption of sodium in the kidneys. Somatostatin (B) is produced by the delta cells of the pancreatic islets of Langerhans. Somatostatin has the ability to inhibit insulin release from pancreatic beta cells and inhibit glucagon release from pancreatic alpha cells. Vasopressin (C) (Antidiuretic Hormone) is produced in the posterior pituitary and increases the retention of water in the kidneys. Cholecystokinin (D) is secreted into the duodenum, whose function is to stimulate the process of fat and protein digestion.

15. C

CCK stimulates the release of hepatic bile and pancreatic lipase to digest fat. CCK stimulates chymotrypsin, which is required for the digestion of protein. Somatostatin (C) is an inhibitory hormone. One of its function is the inhibition of Cholecystokinin.

16. C

The digestion of starch starts in the mouth by salivary amylase. The pancreas also produces amylase to further assist in the breakdown of starch. Protein digestion begins in the stomach (A) and continues in the small intestine. The duodenum (B) is essential in the breakdown of food. The duodenum helps regulate the rate of emptying of the stomach. The liver and gall bladder release bile, and the pancreas releases bicarbonate and digestive enzymes ie trypsin, amylase, and lipase into the duodenum to aid in food breakdown. The jejunum (D), located between the duodenum and ileum, functions mainly in absorption of digested material.

17. B

Carbohydrate digestion starts in the mouth. Final disaccharide digestion and absorption takes place in the microvilli (brush border) of the small intestine, The large intestine (colon) is primarily responsible for water reuptake.

18. C

Three major vessels supply blood to the abdomen and abdominal organs. Superior mesenteric artery (SMA) (A) supplies the distal duodenum, jejunum, ileum, and colon to the splenic flexure. Inferior mesenteric artery (IMA) (B) supplies the descending colon, sigmoid colon, and rectum. Celiac trunk (D) supplies the esophagus, stomach, proximal duodenum, liver, gallbladder, pancreas, and spleen. The answer is the common iliac, which supplies blood to the lower limbs and the pelvis, ending the abdominal aorta.

HIGH-YIELD SIMILAR QUESTIONS

Digestive System

1. A large dose of antacid would increase the pH of the stomach and therefore inactivate pepsin. The optimum pH for pepsin is between 1 and 3; pepsin is denatured and therefore inactivated at a pH greater than 5.

2. If the pancreas could not secrete bicarbonate the acidic chyme that moves into the duodenum would not be neutralized and pancreatic lipases would not be able to function. This will result in the malabsorption of lipids and steatorrhea.
3. Inadequate amounts on lipase enzymes will lead to steatorrhea. If lipids are not broken down by lipases they cannot be absorbed by the small intestine.

Osmosis

1. Decrease
2. Interstitial fluid is hypertonic to filtrate; filtrate is hypotonic/hypoosmotic to interstitial fluid
3. Hypotonic

CHAPTER 8: RESPIRATION

1. C

The electron transport chain will work fine since it is not inhibited. As a result, the NADH will transfer electrons and oxidize to NAD^+. Hence, the cell will become depleted of the NADH, but will not reap the benefits of ATP production from lack of generation of the proton gradient.

2. A

Minute ventilation is the product of tidal volume multiplied by respiratory rate. The man in this case has a minute ventilation of 6L, while the son has a minute ventilation of 2.4 L.

3. B

Inadequate intercostal muscle function will greatly compromise respiratory function. These muscles, known as accessory muscles of breathing, act to expand the chest cavity and increase the negative pressure required for respiration. Cardiac muscle is not extensive damaged in muscular dystrophy; the histology of cardiac muscle is distinct from the skeletal muscle primarily affected in muscular dystrophy. A narrowed trachea is not a hallmark of MS; the trachea is made of collagen, epithelium, and connective tissue that are not involved in the fundamental defects of skeletal muscle in muscular dystrophy. Lung tissue compliance is not a function of skeletal muscle integrity.

4. A

The surface tension is more markedly decreased with artificial surfactant A because there is a greater degree of hydrophobic molecules in the compound. These hydrophobic lipids will disrupt the loose bonds of polar molecules that are responsible for surface tension on the alveoli. The greater amount of hydrophobic molecules, the more disrupted the lattice responsible for surface tension. Sample B is less hydrophobic than A, and will integrate with the polar molecules, rather than cause a disruption of the polar lattice that promote alveolar collapse. The presence of protein in sample A does not contribute nearly as effectively to hydrophobicity as the elevated lipid in sample A. While some of the protein may be hydrophobic, much will be charged and engaged with the polar molecules. It is the increased lipid, not the presence of protein that allows A to decrease surface tension more effectively than B. The rate of respiration of subjects will have no bearing on surface tension.

5. B

At higher altitudes, there is lower oxygen concentrations, as compared to sea level. Thus, a person will feel subjectively shirt of breath and need to increase the respiratory rate to obtain more oxygen in a given amount of time.

6. B

Increased minute ventilation will result in the air in the lungs containing more carbon dioxide than they would in the case of a normal ventilation rate. As such, the carbon dioxide remaining in the lungs will diffuse into the blood and be buffered by the bicarbonate system. The result of the CO_2/H_{20} buffer will be the production of bicarbonate and hydrogen ions. Hydrogen ions will decrease the pH of the system per the equation pH = –log [H^+}.

7. C

The oxygen saturation curve is a graphical representation of the propensity of hemoglobin to 'give up' its oxygen under certain conditions. Consider what occurs during exercise. Temperature is increased in the body, oxygen is used more rapidly, and lactic acid is produced. The body becomes hot, deoxygenated, and acidic. 2, 3 DPG is produced by the red blood cells to facilitate offloading of oxygen. Delivery of oxygen to these tissues will allow the body to regain equilibrium towards homeostasis. A shift to the right off this curve signals that at identical partial pressures of oxygen, hemoglobin saturation will be lower, indicating that more oxygen is shifted off of hemoglobin and into the tissue. Under normal conditions, less than a quarter of the oxygen on hemoglobin is used by the tissues. The system is built to unload more oxygen at time of stress. You will never forget this curve shift if you just recall that exercise is the 'right' thing for the body—the curve shifts to the right. Answer (D) suggests there is no synergy, or increased uptake of oxygen at lower partial pressure, but this is not true. The relationship is not linear; it accelerates variably at different partial pressures of oxygen, as indicated by considering the answers in terms of rate of change. The sinusoidal change of correct answer (C) reflects this, while the rate of change in (D) is 0.

8. D

The replacement of the compliant lung tissue with fibrous tissue will make the lung less compliant. As a result it will "stretch" less. This will lead to low lung volumes. Destruction of the alveoli will decrease the lung's ability to effectuate gas exchange, leading to hypoxia. Patients ill then become subjectively short of breath.

9. B

Iron is the element required for proper functioning of hemoglobin. Decreased levels of iron in the blood, known as iron-deficiency anemia, will result in small red blood cells that are widely varying in their size and shape. Copper, manganese, and selenium all play important roles in the body as micronutrients, but are not important for proper functioning of hemoglobin.

10. C

The brainstem is home to the autonomic function that causes us to breath without thinking about it. The forebrain is involved with higher level thinking and executive judgment. The midbrain is responsible for sensory integration and other higher level tasks. The cerebellum is important in balance, coordination, and memory.

11. B

The most important thing to remember about respiratory mechanics is that the thoracic cavity is essentially a negative pressure system that draws air into the chest. The diaphragm plays a crucial role in this system. Upon inspiration, the diaphragm falls, increasing the size of the thoracic cavity. Recall that pressure and volume are inversely related per Charles' law. The larger the volume, the lower the pressure. The pressure in the airways becomes increasing negative relative to the ambient pressure of air outside the system. Air will be forced to fill the vacuum—in this case, the chest. This system is driven by a functioning diaphragm. Injury to neck can cause problems with respiratory because the phrenic nerve innervating the diaphragm, emerges from the spinal cord at C 3, 4, and 5. Without the phrenic nerve and a functioning diaphragm, this negative pressure system is compromised, and breathing becomes more difficult.

12. A

This question is strictly anatomy. Unoxygenated blood is sent to the lungs from the heart via the pulmonary artery. This can be tricky because it is an artery carrying deoxygenated blood, while arteries usually carry oxygenated blood. Pulmonary veins return oxygenated blood to the heart. The aorta is the major artery to the rest of the body from the left ventricle. Foramen ovale is a small hole between the atria of the heart.

13. A

Acetyl CoA is not involved in the transport of carbon dioxide in the blood. In physiologic terms, acetate is an organic molecule that is produced as the result of fatty chain oxidation. Acetyl CoA is then fed into the oxidative phosphorylation pathway and used to create ATP. (B), (C), and (D) are all used to carry carbon dioxide, with bicarb being the most heavily relied upon way of CO_2 to be transported in the blood.

14. A

Blood in the pulmonary vein is returning from the lungs, where it has been oxygenated. Oxyhemoglobin is the appropriate term for hemoglobin equipped with oxygen. Lactic acid would not be present in excess in blood in the pumolnary veins under normal conditions. Chyme is a term for food passing into the digestive system. Blood in pulmonary veins will be no more or less enriched with hemoglobin than any other blood. The key concept to remember here is that pulmonary veins equals richly oxygenated hemoglobin.

HIGH-YIELD SIMILAR QUESTIONS

Respiratory System

1. If respiration is occurring normally but there is no blood flow to the left lung then there is no gas exchange occurring in the left lung. If no oxygen is being diffused from the air into the blood and no CO_2 is being released then the Po_2 of the alveoli will equal the Po_2 of inspired air.
2. If there is an airway obstruction but blood flow to the lung is normal there is no gas exchange. The blood that flows into the lung will have the same value of Po_2 and Pco_2 as venous blood. Since no gas exchange occurs this value will remain the same for blood as it exits the lung.
3. When the Po_2 of inspired air equals the Po_2 of capillary blood then diffusion will stop.

CHAPTER 9: CIRCULATION

1. A

The relative lack of smooth muscle in the vein walls allows it to stretch in order to store a majority of the blood in the body. Valves in the veins allow for one-way flow of blood towards the heart. Both arteries and veins are close to lymphatic vessels and that has no bearing on the difference in volume. Both arteries and veins have a thin endothelial lining.

2. C

Carbon dioxide is a byproduct of metabolism in cells, which later combines with water to form bicarbonate. Food and fluid absorption of buffer are not significant sources.

3. A

Eosinophils are the body's protection against parasitic infections, such as tapeworm and the various species of malaria. Parasites, by definition, are organisms that invade and live in a host, using nutrients provided by the host and often causing damage to the host. Sickle cell anemia (B) is an inherited blood disorder. Hepatitis B (C) and influenza (D) are caused by viruses.

4. A

Allergic reactions to pollen, ragweed, pet dander, and so on. are mediated by histamine release from granules in basophils. Red blood cells and lymphocytes have nothing to do with allergic reactions. Granules of neutrophils contain enzymes aimed at damaging bacteria.

5. A

Systolic blood pressure is the pressure of blood during systole, when blood is being pumped out of the ventricles and into circulation. This would be the time at which the aortic and pulmonic valves are open, allowing blood out of the ventricles to circulate to the extremities and the lungs. The mitral valve opens during diastole to allow ventricular filling. Atrial and ventricular pressure become equal also during diastole.

6. C

Diastolic blood pressure is the pressure in the arterial system when the heart is at rest. This occurs during ventricular filling, when the ventricular pressure is less than the atrial pressure, allowing blood to fill the ventricle. Arterial pressure does not normally equal venous pressure, nor does pressure normally equalize over both sides of the heart.

7. B

The parasympathetic nervous system mediates the cardiovascular system the majority of the time because we do not often require acute augmentation of stroke volume and/or heart rate. Thus, if adrenergic input is blocked (epinephrine and norepinephrine from the sympathetic nervous system), little to no difference would be evident in our cardiovascular status. If acetylcholine receptors were blocked, the effects of the sympathetic nervous system would be amplified.

8. C

The fact that the couple's first child is Rh positive implies that during birth, the mother could potentially have been exposed to the Rh-positive blood, stimulating antibody production against Rh. Rh-immune globin administration would have no effect at this point. The red blood cells of the first child are not in the maternal circulation. The father's Rh factor will determine the Rh status of the second child. The fetus does not generate any of its own antibodies until after birth.

9. D

Insoluble fibrin conveys the most strength to a clot. Thrombin, once activated, converts fibrinogen to fibrin. Fibrin then becomes cross-linked with the help of factor XIII to assume its insoluble state.

10. D

The liver lies *in series with*, as opposed to *in parallel*, with blood coming from the upper and lower extremities after oxygen has been extracted in the capillary beds. This allows blood to be filtered for waste products before returning back to the heart to be reoxygenated.

11. C

The half-life of epinephrine is short; oftentimes, the sympathetic nervous system needs an acute augmentation of cardiac output and thus a short-lived molecule would be ideal to mediate these effects. The half-life is the amount of time required for the level of a drug to decrease by half of its original concentration. By the graph, the substance was injected at t = 10 seconds and falls to half of its original concentration approximately 120 seconds later.

12. B

The graph shows antibody levels as if the body were exposed to a new antigen. It takes time for rearrangement of heavy and light chains specific to the antigen to be formed by the B lymphocyte, and thus a lag is created between the time at which the body is exposed to an antigen and the time at which it is capable of mounting an antibody mediated defense. Passive immunization is the direct administration of preformed antibodies to a given antigen.

13. A

When an antigen is encountered, B cells are stimulated to proliferate in order to manufacture specific antibodies to the antigen. The manufacturing process requires rearrangement of the heavy and light chains so that the variable regions of the immunoglobulins bind only the antigen. Once it does, phagocytosis is triggered by the binding of the specific antibody to the antigen.

14. B

Phagocytosis plays an important role in both the non specific and humoral response to foreign pathogens. At the level of the skin, macrophages dwell in the connective tissue surrounding the organs of the body. Neutrophils are recruited to the site of entry and become part of the non specific response to invading bacteria, working in combination with monocytes and macrophages to completely decompose bacteria. The cell-mediated branch of the immune system does not result in pus formation.

15. D

The coronary arteries are the first branch off of the aorta, and would thus receive normal blood flow. Beyond the first branch, a heartbeat with a diminished stroke volume is less likely to perfuse the brain or extremities. With time, the body preferentially will protect perfusion to the brain by vasoconstricting the coronary arteries in order to improve cerebral oxygenation, but that occurs later.

HIGH-YIELD SIMILAR QUESTIONS

Circulation

1. In mitral valve stenosis the valve between the left atrium and the left ventricle narrows and restricts blood flow into the left ventricle. This increases blood pressure in the left atrium.
2. Left ventricle
3. Pulmonary arteries

Normal Oxygen Dissociation Curve

1. At P = 50 mm Hg, venous blood has about 60% hemoglobin saturation. Arterial blood, on the other hand, has greater hemoglobin saturation (approximately 90%).
2. Fetal hemoglobin has a greater affinity for O_2 than adult hemoglobin, so the curve is shifted to the left.
3. PO_2 is reduced, but over time, hemoglobin "learns" to bind oxygen at this lower pressure (shifting the curve left).

Abnormal Oxygen Dissociation Curve

1. Exercise will lead to an increase in body temperature as well as in increase in CO_2 production, and thereby a decrease in pH, by tissues. Increases in Pco_2, decreases in pH and increases in temperature all shift the oxygen dissociation curve to the right.
2. High levels of Pco_2 lead to an increase in ventilation rate in order to blow off the excess CO_2.
3. In metabolic alkalosis blood pH will be increased due to the loss of H^+ ions. Increased pH leads to a left shift in the oxygen dissociation curve.

Lymphatic System

1. If a patient's lymphatic channels are obstructed then fluid that filters into the interstitial space from capillaries cannot be returned to circulation by lymph vessels. This fluid will build up in the interstitial space and edema will result.
2. Blocked lymphatic channels, excess proteins in the interstial fluid, loss of proteins from the plasma (as can happen in kidney or liver disease)
3. Distortion of lymphatic vessels by the movement of skeletal muscles allows proteins and interstitial fluid to enter the lymphatic system. This lymph is carried through lymphatic vessels, which have valves to prevent backflow, and eventually dumped back into blood circulation at the thoracic duct or subclavian vein.

CHAPTER 10: HOMEOSTASIS

1. C

The glomerulus will allow glucose to pass through into the filtrate when functioning properly. Glucose will usually not be present in the filtrate, however, because it undergoes reabsorption in the proximal convoluted tubule, which is located adjacent to the glomerulus. (A), (B), and (D) are wrong because all three are too large to pass through the glomerulus, and only upon malfunction of the glomerulus would any of the three be present in the filtrate.

2. C

Urine will not have a high concentration of Na^+ due to reabsorption of Na^+ caused by aldosterone stimulation. (A), (B), and (D) are wrong because aldosterone stimulates reabsorption of Na^+, which increases the blood pressure and also lowers the concentration of Na^+ that will be passed in the urine.

3. B

Ingesting a large quantity of water will effect a low solute concentration in the blood. The low concentration will inhibit ADH (vasopressin) secretion such that more water will remain in the filtrate and eventually the urine. Therefore, (A) is wrong. (C) is wrong as well because an increase in water will inevitably result in a rise in blood volume, which would decrease the amount of aldosterone release from the adrenal cortex.

4. A

(B) and (C) are wrong because the glomerulus is a capillary bed and thus does not ever house the filtrate. It is across this capillary bed into the Bowman's capsule where filtrate makes its first appearance. (C) and (D) are wrong because of wrong ordering.

5. B

Although the liver will produce some amino acids by interconversion, essential amino acids cannot be synthesized by the body.

6. A

Sweat glands are in the dermis layer. The sweat pore, however, is located in the epidermis. (B) and (C) are wrong because the keratinized epidermal cells protect against harmful bacteria and excess water loss. (D) is wrong because melanocytes, which are located in the epidermis, protect against UV radiation via production of melanin.

7. C

The kidneys only regulate osmolarity of the blood and filtrate/urine. The excreted urine is no cooler or warmer than the blood in the kidneys. (A) and (B) are wrong because the thyroid gland and skin do regulate temperature. (D) is wrong because (C) is correct.

8. B

Nearly all glucose (and all other solutes) is reabsorbed from the proximal convoluted tubule. Therefore, (A), (C), and (D) are wrong.

9. A

Even though the osmolarity inside the collecting duct is smaller relative to the outside due to aldosterone release, because water will only be able to slowly passively diffuse to the outside of the duct, much more water will be staying inside the duct. Therefore, water will not be able to be reabsorbed so the blood pressure will be the same as before aldosterone release. (B) is wrong because more water will be excreted in the urine due to the blocking of vasopressin release. (C) and (D) are wrong because aldosterone will still directly cause an increase in Na^+ reabsorption and decrease in K^+ reabsorption regardless of the block on vasopressin.

10. D

A patient who has overactive sweat glands would feel cooler than normal due to more evaporation of sweat, which is mostly water. Remember, water has a relatively high heat of vaporization. (B) is wrong because hyperthyroidism would boost the basal metabolic rate of the patient, and thus, she would be warmer than normal. (A) and (C) are also wrong because both would also result in a warmer than usual patient.

11. D

In a diabetic patient, which we can assume given the patient's family history, the glucose transport across the proximal convoluted tubules cannot cope with a higher influx of glucose into the filtrate. (A) is not correct because glucose reabsorption does not stop. (B) is not correct because glucose is only reabsorbed in the proximal convoluted tubule. (C) is not correct because glucose is not secreted into the tubule.

12. C

One of the functions of the liver is the interconversion of carbohydrates and fats (as well as proteins). Higher concentrations of glucose produced from glycogenolysis may be interconverted into fat and vice-versa. (A) is wrong because the process occurs in the liver, not the kidney. (B) is wrong because low levels stimulates glycogenolysis. (D) is wrong because the reaction is also under nervous control.

13. D

This transport process requires ATP. (A) and (C) are wrong because this transport occurs at the proximal convoluted tubule. (B) is wrong because these transporters in diabetic patients are not malfunctioning, but rather the nephrons are overtaxed with a greater influx of glucose than is seen in normal patients.

14. C

Water is normally reabsorbed from the proximal convoluted tubule and descending loop of Henle. Water is also reabsorbed from the collecting duct upon vasopressin stimulation.

HIGH-YIELD SIMILAR QUESTIONS

Starling Forces

1. Factors that increase filtration out of the capillaries are: increased arterial or venous pressure (remember P_c is blood pressure), a decrease in the hydrostatic pressure of the interstitial fluid (P_i), decreased protein in the blood which lowers the π_c, or an increase in proteins in the interstitial fluid (π_i).
2. Capillary oncotic pressure will be increased by any factor that increases the protein concentration in the blood. For example, loss of fluid, as in dehydration, will increase capillary oncotic pressure.
3. Fluids and protein that are filtered from the capillary into the interstitial space are normally returned to circulation via the lymphatic system. Inadequate lymphatic function will

increase π_i which will favor filtration of fluids out of the capillaries and prevent fluid reabsorption at the venule end leading to edema.

CHAPTER 11: ENDOCRINE SYSTEM

1. D

Lack of or unresponsiveness to ADH causes an inability to concentrate urine. This would cause a dilution in urine, and a subsequent increase in serum osmolarity. An increase in serum glucose would be more evident of diabetes mellitus. Oxytocin is a hormone also released from the posterior pituitary responsible for the onset of labor as well as milk letdown.

2. C

ADH acts by concentrating urine by encouraging reabsorption of water in the distal collecting tubule and collecting duct of the nephron. Loop diuretics act upon the Na/K/Cl channels, thiazide diuretics acts upon NaCl channels and dopamine acts upon the Na/H channels of the nephron to indirectly cause water excretion.

3. D

Thyroid storm, or sudden onset hyperthyroidism, is the most common endocrine cause of an elevated heart rate. Thyroid hormone, in additional to increasing heart rate, increases the body's metabolic rate resulting in weight loss, increases the speed of nerve transmission resulting in tremors and increases the speed of gastrointestinal motility resulting in diarrhea. Elevated estrogen levels results in feminization and increased risk of some cancers. Elevated growth hormone causes gigantism and acromegaly. Hypoaldosteronism leads to elevated potassium levels.

4. B

Thyroid hormone is an amino acid derivative but works similarly to steroid hormones in that it directly alters gene transcription in cells. It is responsible for increasing the basal metabolic rate and would therefore increase the rate at which genes are transcribed by affected cells in the body. Peptide hormones such as ADH and insulin exert effects on cells via a second messenger, namely cyclic AMP. Phosphodiesterase moderates the response of the second messenger pathway.

5. B

T_4 is the main product of the thyroid gland; it is converted to T_3 by removing an iodine atom. This is done by deiodinases found in target organs. Adequate iodine-intake ensures that the thyroid gland makes enough T_4 for the body. Thryoperoxidase is an enzyme in the thyroid gland which synthesizes T_3 and T_4. Thryoglobulin is a protein in the thyroid gland which carries tyrosine molecules to be iodinated and released as thyroid hormones.

6. A

Serum calcium levels negatively feedback on the C cells of the thyroid in order to tightly control calcium concentrations. A seven-transmembrane G-coupled protein senses serum calcium levels and stimulates calcitonin release when levels rise via an intracellular, calcium mediated pathway.

7. D

Insulin causes the recruitment of $GLUT_4$ transporters to the surface of cells. The symportation of sodium and glucose into cells helps to drive the sodium/potassium ATPase also located on the cell membrane. Thus, the net effect of glucose and insulin administration is to relocate potassium and glucose intracellularly, while displacing sodium extracellularly.

8. D

Following ovulation, estrogen levels continue to remain elevated in order to maintain the thickness of the endometrial cavity in anticipation of embryo implantation. Progesterone, secreted by the corpus luteum, stimulates gland production within the endometrial lining also in preparation for implantation. During this phase, FSH levels begin to drop and do not play a role in endometrial maturation.

9. C

Glucocorticoids are widely used in medicine to temper inflammatory responses by inhibiting leukocyte movement and blood flow to the sight of injury. In addition, glucocorticoids increase the metabolism of proteins, fats and carbohydrates in the body in order to prepare to fight off stress and/or infection. Thus, blood sugar levels increase in response to elevated glucocorticoid levels and exacerbate hyperglycemia in poorly controlled diabetics. Pancreatic beta cell destruction occurs early in type I diabetes via an autoimmune process. Increased muscle mass is a side effect of anabolic steroid administration.

10. D

Thyroid hormone is a permissive hormone, in that it allows normal cellular function to occur and regulates systemic parameters such as basal metabolic rate and energy utilization of cells. Growth hormone a hormone required for growth of individual tissues as well as the body during development and childhood and thus directs utilization of body fuels including glucose. Estrogen is a hormone necessary for development and maintenance of secondary female sex characteristics as well as female fertility. It does not have a direct effect on glucose utilization in the body.

11. C

Iodine is halogen commonly found in seawater, which gets concentrated in the thyroid and incorporated into thyroid hormone. Thus, radioactive iodine (which emits beta particles that destroy tissue) can be employed to reduce the number of cells producing thyroid hormone, effectively treating some forms of hyperthyroidism.

12. D

Norepinephrine is made in parts of the brain, as well as in the presynaptic terminals of sympathetic nerves and in the adrenal medulla in response to stress requiring a physiologic adaptation. It is mainly in the adrenal medulla where phenylethanolamine N-methyltransferase converts norepinephrine into epinephrine. This also occurs at a lesser extent in the synaptic terminals that rely on norepinephrine as a neurotransmitter. It is not synthesized in the brain.

13. B

Estrogen and progesterone made from the placenta after the first trimester negatively feeds back on the anterior pituitary and prevents FSH and LH from being secreted, thus preventing ovulation and menstruation. The placenta does not secrete testosterone. Beta-HCG from the fetus is responsible for maintaining the corpus luteum in the first trimester of pregnancy. The uterine lining does not secrete estrogen at any point.

14. A

Parkinson's disease is characterized by a lack of dopaminergic neurons in the substantia nigra, leading to difficulty with movement and balance. Symptoms can be mimicked by use of anti-dopaminergic drugs such as typical anti psychotic medications. Dopamine negatively regulates secretion of prolactin from the anterior pituitary so dopamine antagonism would result in unstimulated lactogenesis. Dopamine can also increase blood pressure and is commonly used in emergency resuscitation.

15. B

Hyperaldosteronism is the presence of elevated aldosterone levels that are resistant to a negative feedback mechanism, usually from a source outside of the adrenal cortex. Aldosterone is a potassium-wasting entity in that it stimulates sodium retention and potassium excretion in the kidney. Increased sodium retention causes reflexive water retention and a relative increase in blood pressure. Elevated aldosterone does suppress the renin-angiotensin system and so one would expect low levels of angiotensin II in response to hyperaldosteronism.

16. B

TRH is made by hypothalamus and acts on the anterior pituitary to secrete TSH. TSH acts on receptors in the thyroid gland to secrete T_4 and to a lesser extent, T_3, which exists as bound and free form in the blood. Primary hyperthyroidism (A) is an isolated increase in thyroid hormone (T_4 and/or T_3) which feeds back to the hypothalamus and diminishes TRH secretion. Secondary hyperthyroidism (B) is an elevation in TSH levels causing an increase in thyroid hormone. TRH is once again suppressed by the negative feedback mechanism. Tertiary hyperthyroidism (C) is characterized by an elevated secretion of TRH from the hypothalamus. Primary hypothyroidism (D) would be evidenced by depressed thyroid hormone levels.

17. C

Estrogen exposure in a pre pubertal female would result in premature breast development. Since androgens and progesterone are not yet being synthesized by the body, one is unlikely to have a menstrual period (stimulated by a combination of estrogen and progesterone), axillary hair (stimulated by androgens), or coordinated uterine contractions (stimulated by progesterone).

18. D

Long-term daily administration of progesterone suppresses the hypothalamic-pituitary-ovarian axis, and in most cases, prevents estrogen secretion and thus ovulation. Ovulation may still occur in some cases. Thus, progesterone's effect on cervical mucus and the endometrial lining provide its main contraceptive benefit. Much like progesterone secretion following ovulation in a normal cycle, progesterone thickens cervical mucus to prevent the migration of sperm and causes a thickened endometrium to prepare for implantation. Without estrogen, however, the endometrial lining is not hospitable to a developing embryo and would not allow implantation.

19. D

While PTH acts on many sites in the body to increase serum calcium levels, it primarily uses calcium stored in bone. Calcium is not stored in the mucosal cells of the intestines as it is absorbed from food. PTH secretion is triggered by low serum calcium levels and is inhibited via a negative feedback loop.

HIGH-YIELD SIMILAR QUESTIONS

Menstrual Cycle

1. FSH is inhibited early in the follicular phase in order to prevent the development of multiple follicles.
2. Early in the follicular phase estrogen has a negative feedback on the anterior pituitary and prevents the release of FSH and LH. Late in the follicular phase (around day 12) estrogen has a positive feedback effect on the anterior pituitary and stimulates FSH and LH. Estrogen stimulates the LH surge which results in ovulation.
3. Ovulation can be prevented by manipulating the hormones involved in the menstrual cycle.

Birth control pills keep estrogen and progesterone levels high so that FSH and LH are inhibited. Because of this inhibition a follicle does not develop and the LH surge does not occur therefore preventing ovulation.

CHAPTER 12: NERVOUS SYSTEM

1. B

The other choices are all functions of myelin.

2. A

There is much more sodium outside of the cell than in it, which explains why there's an influx of sodium when the voltage gated sodium channels are opened. Therefore, E would be positive. (B), (C), and (D) are thus wrong.

3. C

The postsynaptic potential initiated at the cell body does proceed in all directions, including down towards the dendrites. While it may be true that action potential propagation is typically unidirectional because of the refractory periods of action potentials, this is not true of postsynaptic potentials that initiate the action potential at the axon hillock. (A) is a true statement when defining a "requisite" amount to be sufficient for action potential (not postsynaptic potential) propagation. (B) is wrong because myelin only speeds up the signal with a minimal loss of signal at the axon.

4. C

Pupil constriction does not occur during a sympathetic, flight-or-fight response, while all the other answer choices do.

5. B

Redirection of blood from digestive tract to muscles is activated in a sympathetic response. The other answer choices are all parasympathetic responses.

6. D

Once you see that (D) is correct, you would have been able to eliminate (B) regardless of your knowledge of interneurons.

7. A

At the beginning of the ascent, voltage-gated sodium channels begin to open while potassium channels stay closed and open later after some delay. A little time before the peak, potassium channels begin to open as sodium channels begin to inactivate. During the descent, more potassium channels open to repolarize while more sodium channels are inactivated.

8. B

(A), (C), and (D) are all reasonable conclusions.

9. A

The neurotransmitter is packaged inside the vesicles of the presynaptic neuron before it is released after the action potential reaches the voltage-gated calcium channels. Then, the neurotransmitter is released from the vesicle and presynaptic neuron into the synaptic cleft, where it binds to the receptors of the postsynaptic neuron. The receptors determine the excitatory or inhibitory nature of the postsynaptic response.

10. C

The iris gives eyes their color.

11. C

The fovea is the most likely area of injury due to the fovea having the role of relaying acute vision input as well as because it is the area of the retina which contains mostly cones.

12. B

Because sodium channels open faster in cardiac muscle, the potential rises steeply. The potassium channels opening slower also accounts for the less dramatic repolarization/downward-sloping.

13. A

Schwann cells are glial cells that provide myelination to the neurons. They essentially wrap themselves around the axons. Astrocytes are phagocytic cells within the central nervous system. Lymphocytes are peripheral immunocytes. Leukocytes are the broader category of immunocytes that not only include lymphocytes, but also granulocytes.

14. C

The ectoderm gives rise to the central nervous system. Remember that the retina is also a component of the central nervous system, so defects in the ectoderm may led to defects in the retina.

15. B

TPA will inhibit the Na/K pump. This will not affect the influx of Na or the efflux of K in the neuron. However, it will inhibit and retard (possibly cease) the return to resting potential. Hence, once the neuron fires, exciting the muscle fiber and inducing contraction, there will be an inability to relax afterward.

HIGH-YIELD SIMILAR QUESTIONS

Action Potential

1. At the highest point of the curve.
2. An action potential is all or nothing and therefore the speed of an action potential cannot be increased. Information coded in action potentials can be altered by the frequency of action potentials, but not by altering the speed of one action potential.
3. When a membrane is hyperpolarized it is further from threshold and would require a larger stimulus to create an action potential. Therefore hyperpolarizing a membrane would be a way to inhibit an action potential. Action potentials are also inhibited during the absolute refractory period, which occurs during an action potential.

CHAPTER 13: GENETICS

1. C

The probability that the man is a carrier of the disease gene is 50 percent. Based on the information given, Tay-Sachs disease can be either X-linked or autosomal recessive. Tay-Sachs is actually autosomal recessive and, therefore, his dead brother was homozygous recessive. That means the dead brother received a copy of a recessive allele from each parent. It can be concluded that both parents are heterozygous because, first, they must both have one recessive allele given the homozygous recessive requirement of the disease, and second, they cannot be homozygous because they would not survive past age six to reproduce. During a mating of two heterozygous individuals, the probability of having a heterozygous child is 50 percent.

2. B

Crossing-over occurs during prophase I of the meiotic division, when homologous chromosomes attach at chiasma and can exchange genetic material. During anaphase I, chiasma disappear and homologus chromosomes are pulled to opposite poles of the cell. During telophase I, two haploid daughter cells are formed. During anaphase II, single chromatids are pulled towards the opposite poles of the cell.

3. A

The probability of crossing-over will increase the farther the genes are located on the chromosome. The other answer choices contradict this statement. The number of genes on a chromosome does not affect the rate of crossing-over.

4. C

The only way a type I (O) mother can have children with blood types II (A) and III (B) is if the father has a type IV (AB) blood type. That way, the father can pass an allele for antigen A or an allele for antigen B which would determine the blood type of a child. A father of blood type II (A) does not have an allele for antigen B and thus cannot have a child with blood type III. A father of blood type III (B) does not have an allele for antigen A and thus cannot have a child with blood type II.

5. C

The gene encoding the ABO blood system has three primary alleles (A, B, and O) which can combine in different combinations responsible for the four blood types.

6. D

A donor with type III (B) blood has antigen B and anti-A antibodies, while the receiver with blood type II (A) has antigen A and anti-B antibodies. The agglutination reaction occurs between the antigens of the donor and the antibodies of a receiver. In this case, antigens B will clump with anti-B antibodies.

7. A

Each birth is an independent event, so the probability of a boy is 50 percent no matter how many boys were born earlier.

8. C

The question is asking to identify a test cross represented by a mating of the subject being tested with a homozygous recessive individual. Then if the black dog is heterozygous, there would be a 50 percent chance of progeny with the recessive color of the coat (homozygous recessive). In mating with a homozygous dominant individual, 100 percent of the progeny would be black, not helping the verification. In mating with another heterozygote, there is only 25 percent probability of seeing a different color progeny if the dog is not purebred.

9. B

The question asks you to determine the probability of a phenotypically (homozygous dominant or heterozygous) healthy child if both parents are heterozygotes. According to Punnett square analysis the probability is 75 percent. Fifty percent is the probability of having only heterozygous children. Twenty-five percent is the probability of having homozygous dominant children.

10. A

Penetrance gives the fraction of individuals who, while having a disease allele, will develop the disease. Only (A) is consistent with this explanation.

11. D

(D) is correct because pleiotropy is the condition when one gene has multiple phenotypic effects, as in this case. Full penetrance would mean that 100 percent of the population carrying the defective allele develops the disease. Codominance means that heterozygotes display the in-between phenotype when compared to homozygous dominant and homozygous recessive individuals. Imprinting explains the differences in phenotypes depending whether the mutation is of maternal or paternal origin.

12. A

Trisomy 21 is a result of nondisjunction, a condition where homologous chromosomes do not separate during meiotic division, and one of the gametes receives an extra copy of a chromosome resulting in three instead of two chromosomes. Other causes of mutations generally refer to nucleotide addition-insertion, elimination-deletion, reverse nucleotide sequence-inversion, making other answer choices wrong.

13. D

If a homozygous recessive man marries a heterozygous woman there is a 50 percent chance that each child is affected. To find out the probability that all four children are affected, use the multiplication rule for statistical probability: $(1/2)^4 = 1/16$.

14. C

If sons are affected by the X-linked recessive disorder, they must have received the disease allele from the mother, because the father must have provided a Y-chromosome in order for the offspring to be a son. Thus the mother has to have at least one mutant allele, making (B) and (D) wrong. It is not possible exclude the possibility that 50 percent of boys would be affected. This is due to the fact that there are not enough children to rule out the possibility of a heterozygous mother. The best answer is (C).

15. B

The pedigree shows an autosomal recessive mode of inheritance because phenotypically normal parents (carriers) have about a 25 percent probability of an affected child. Generally, one generation is skipped. In an autosomal dominant mode of inheritance one would expect to see much more affected children. In the case of an X-linked recessive disorder, only males are generally affected, and on the pedigree shown none of the males are affected. Mitochondrial inheritance transmits the disease through the mother's alleles, and all the offspring of an affected mother would be affected, which is in a disagreement with the pedigree shown.

16. C

The daughter in generation two is affected and has to be heterozygous because her mother (generation I) was homozygous recessive. The father in generation II is normal and has to be homozygous recessive. As a result, the test cross in generation II of a heterozygous and a homozygous recessive individual results in a 50 percent chance of having an affected child (heterozygote).

17. C

In mitochondrial inheritance all offspring of affected females have a disorder due to the fact that there are no mitochondria passed to the children from their fathers, because the female egg contains the cytoplasm of the zygote, while the sperm provides only genetic material. Thus, condition I is correct. Part of the explanation depends on the cytoplasmic location of a mitochondrion; condition III is correct. There is no information provided to conclude that this is an X-linked condition; condition II is wrong.

18. D

A mother in generation I has to be a carrier to have two sons affected, because the disorder is X-linked recessive, affecting mostly males when both parents are phenotypically normal (mother is a carrier). The disorder cannot be dominantly X-linked because the mothers would be affected as well. This is not an autosomal recessive condition because one would not expect to see the predominance of either sex in the children affected, and the probability of children with the condition would be smaller (25 percent in the second generation). The father in generation II cannot be a carrier as the disorder is X-linked, and the father can either be affected or have a healthy genotype.

19. D

An extra chromosome 18 is an example of trisomy. It is a specific case of aneuploidy, a condition where the chromosomal number is not a multiple of 23. Triploidy refers to three full sets of chromosomes or 69 chromosomes. Polyploidy refers to numerous sets of chromosomes $n \times 23$. Monosomy is a lack of one of the chromosomes in a pair.

20. C

The frequency of the disorder genotype is 1/10000. According to the Hardy-Weinberg principle, the frequency of the disease allele is the square root of 1/10000 or 0.01. Thus, the frequency of a healthy allele is 1 – 0.01 = 0.99.

HIGH-YIELD SIMILAR QUESTIONS

Genetics

1. Yes, as long as she had at least one child
2. 100%, 0%
3. 25%, 6.25% (presuming BO and AO genotypes)

CHAPTER 14: MOLECULAR GENETICS

1. B

A DNA primer is a short strand of DNA with a complementary sequence to a specific DNA sequence. Adenine matches with thymine, and guanine matches with cytosine. In the DNA double helix the strands are antiparallel, meaning they run in *opposite directions*. Standard notation requires writing from 5′ to 3′. Choice (B) is the only answer choice that obeys these rules. (A) is complementary to the sequence but not antiparallel. (C) is the same sequence as the target and is therefore not complementary.

2. D

RNA sequences can bind to specific complementary DNA sequences. However, in the case of RNA, thymine is replaced with uracil. Thefore, adenine matches with uracil, and guanine matches with cytosine. Just as with DNA primers, the RNA strand and its complementary DNA sequence will run antiparallel to each other. Given these rules, (D) is the only choice that fits. (A) describes the complementary DNA sequence. (B) and (C) are complementary but not antiparallel to the DNA sequence.

3. A

Point mutations exchange a single nucleotide for another. In the case of a point mutation in an intron, these mutations can usually have one of three possible effects: a nonsense mutation, a silent mutation, or a mutation that affects a splice site. Splicing, otherwise known as post-transcriptional processing, normally results in specific modifications to RNA products, usually involving the removal of introns and joining of exons. This process occurs in the cell's nucleus.

4. D

A point mutation results in the replacement of a single base nucleotide with another nucleotide. A frame-shift insertion involves the addition of one or more nucleotides, shifting the reading frame. A frame-shift deletion removes one or more nucleotides, shifting the reading frame. Each of these can introduce a premature stop codon.

5. C

Because host cell DNA polymerase is found only in the nucleus and mitochondrion, varicella virus, along with other DNA viruses that replicate in the cytoplasm, encodes for its own DNA polymerase.

6. D

While eukaryotic and prokaryotic DNA polymerases both have 3′ → 5′ polymerase activity, only Prokaryotic DNA polymerases have 5′ → 3′ exonuclease activity, a process used to remove primers. In eukaryotes, this is taken care of by specific RNase enzymes. Some eukaryotic DNA polymerases do have 3′ → 5′ exonuclease activity, which is used in proofreading and mismatch repair.

7. C

All eukaryotic DNA synthesis requires a primer. DNA synthesis involves the connection of the

5′ phosphate group to the 3′ hydroxyl group. DNA synthesis always occurs in the 3′ → 5′ direction.

8. A

The eukaryotic start codon codes for methionine. While some proteins undergo post-translation modification to remove the methionine, all proteins will have methionine as the first amino acid translated. The N-terminus is the beginning of a peptide chain and consists of a free amine group ($-NH_2$). The C-terminus is the end of a peptide chain and consists of a carboxyl group (–COOH)

9. C

Helicase is responsible for unwinding the DNA double helix, one of the first steps in initiating DNA synthesis. Topoisomerase acts to prevent tension from building up in the helix as it is unwound.

10. B

An insertion involves the addition of one or more basepairs to a sequence. A nonsense mutation A is a mutation that introduces a premature stop codon into a sequence. A frame-shift C changes the reading frame by adding or removing a multiple of one or two basepairs, shifting the reading frame. A silent mutation D involves the substitution of a basepair so that the sequence still codes for the same amino acid.

11. D

Ultraviolet ray exposure via sunlight can result in DNA damage (formation of pyramidine dimmers). Depending on the extent of the damage, a DNA repair pathway can be induced. Sunlight exposure can cause somatic cell DNA damage but does not result in germ cell damage.

12. D

Thymine and cytosine are pyramidines. Adenine and guanine are purines. The only purine-purine or pyramidine-pyramidine substitution listed is cytosine to thymine.

13. A

Macrolide antibiotics interfere with ribosomal translocation, which is necessary for peptide elongation. (B), (C), and (D) occur prior to ribosomal translocation.

HIGH-YIELD SIMILAR QUESTIONS

DNA Transcription

1. 3′–UAGGGUACGUACCUA–5′
2. The following segments will be produced:
   5′–CUUAUGGUCAUCAUAAACG–3′
   5′–GCUACUGAUCAAUCG–3′
   5′–GCAAUCG–3′

DNA Replication

1. 5′–ACGAGCTATGCTACTATATG–3′ (the same as the original strand)
2. 25% posses an unlabeled strand from the original DNA sample.

CHAPTER 15: EVOLUTION

1. B

Darwin believed that random genetic mutation, in combination with natural selection, is the basis of evolution. He believed, then, that chance was a component of evolution. Lamark, conversely, believed that traits are actively acquired. He believed animals "acquired" traits by using them more than others, and not by chance.

2. A

Punctuated equilibrium is an evolutionary theory that states that most populations experience very little change throughout their histories, and when change does occur, it occurs in relatively short and rapid burst. Darwin's theory of evolution and natural selection states that genes that improve the reproductive success of the organism will increase in frequency over time. Lamark's theory of acquired characteristics states that the frequency of genes that organisms use often in their lifetime will increase over time. Differential reproduction states that gene frequencies in a population change over time as a result of certain individuals in a population producing offspring than other individuals in that population, therefore passing on their genes more often.

3. C

Radiometric dating works on the principle that a given radioisotope decays at a consistent rate, unaffected by environmental factors. Elements can have many different isotopes; that is, an identical number of protons but different number of neutrons. Radioisotopes are isotopes that spontaneously decay, or, in other words, transform into a different isotope. The half-life of a radioisotope is the rate at which this decay occurs. Carbon-14 dating is radiometric dating specific to living organisms. It works on the principle that while animals and plants are alive, they breathe in carbon-14 through CO_2 in the atmosphere. Because their bodies stop incorporating carbon-14 once they pass away, measuring the stage of decay of carbon-14 in organic remains can tell us how much time has passed since an organism died. The one caveat with carbon-14 dating is that carbon has a short half-life of only 5,730 years; therefore, it is useful to measure time for around only 60,000 years. In this example, the bird fossil has been dated to 200,000 b.c. through reliable stratigraphic analysis. Carbon-14 data is invalid in such cases.

4. A

Founder's effect refers to an evolutionary phenomenon in which a small number of individuals with rare genetic traits become isolated from their population, and their descendants form a population with a high concentration of those traits. The swallows on Tree Island and on Juvialand are the same species. Any sexual selection (B) should exert the same effects, rather than produce two starkly different populations. Likewise, any natural selection (C) for red feathers over black feathers is unlikely; if that were the case, one would expect the swallows on Juvialand to have higher concentrations of red feathers. Codominance (D) is used incorrectly in this context; it refers to a sharing of dominance between two gene phenotypes. Codominance between a red feather color gene and a black feather color gene, for instance, refers to equal and simultaneous expression of the genes, producing a mixture of both colors.

5. A

The Bottleneck effect simply refers to the general isolation of a number of individuals from a population, which results in a change of gene frequencies in that population. This isolation could be caused by any number of factors: death, movement, disease, environmental change, and so on. The Founder effect is a specific instance of this; it refers to a bottleneck event caused by displacement of a small group of the population. Genetic drift (D) is a chance change in allele frequencies from generation to generation, and not a genetic frequency change due to a specific event. Genetic drift does not cause a major change in the characteristics of an organism. Note the contrast with genetic *shift*, which can drastically alter the phenotypic characteristics of the organism, resulting, for instance, in increased virulence.

6. D

Analogous structures are similar structures found in two species that evolved in parallel due to similar environmental or evolutionary pressures. (Homologous structures, on the other hand, are similar structures found in two species that result from a common ancestral line and genetic background.) If the red bird is a descendant of the blue bird, then its wings are homologous to the blue bird's wings. In (A), (B), and (C), the two birds do not share a common ancestor and thus the characteristic would be considered analogous.

7. D

Polyphyletic groups are groups that do not include a common ancestor. The group composed of Z and B does not include a common ancestor. Monophyletic groups (B) include a common ancestor and all of its descendants. Paraphyletic groups (A) include a common ancestor but not all of the descendants of that ancestor. Parsimonious (C) means that when constructing a cladogram to represent evolutionary relationships between species, the simplest possible cladogram is also the most likely.

8. C

Natural selection would simultaneously select for very small gophers adept at hiding in small crevices, as well as very large gophers able to intimidate the squirrels. This would cause the gopher population to evolve into two opposite extremes for the size trait; this is called disruptive selection. Stabilizing selection (A) is the opposite; it refers to evolutionary forces that favor middle-of-the-road incarnations of a trait, preventing a population from moving toward either extreme of a trait. Directional selection (B) refers to evolutionary forces that move the population toward one gene extreme. Finally, Hardy-Weinberg equilibrium (D) refers to an environment in which gene frequencies and gene ratios are stable and remain constant.

9. B

The ratio of allele A and allele B should equal 100 percent, which means their frequencies should add up to 1.

10. B

Small populations (A) are less likely to remain in Hardy-Weinberg equilibrium because they are more susceptible to random variations in allele frequencies or genetic drift. Migration (C) means that the gene pool is not in a stable state. The different populations could, for instance, be under slightly different selective pressures, and migration between populations would prevent an equilibrium. If increased mating were associated with specific traits (D), that would confer a reproductive advantage on those traits, thus changing the gene frequency. Only (B) is correct: When all genes in a population offer the same reproductive advantage, then no gene will be favored by natural selection and frequencies will remain constant.

11. C

A monophyletic group is by definition a single species and all of its descendants. Thus, species A and species B must be descendants of a common ancestor. While it's likely both species' beaks are homlogous structures (A), we cannot determine this conclusively. It is possible that somewhere in the ancestral line between species A and B, beaks disappeared and re-appeared analogously. For this same reason, we cannot conclusively determine that (B) is true.

12. A

Simply based on condition iii, you can deduce that only (A) is possible. Monophyletic groups contain a single species and all its descendents. Only in species A is this true of condition iii. Furthermore, condition i is true for all answer choices except for (C). Paraphyletic refers to a group sharing common ancestors, but the group does not have to include all descendants. Polyphyletic refers to a group of individuals that do not share a common ancestor.

13. C

(A) is true: Even though the two species share a common ancestor, on the evolutionary path from species A to species M, the trait was lost and then regained. Thus, it was not genetically passed on as a common ancestory normally suggests. (B) is also true: I and A are direct descendants of one another and they both have the wing trait. (D) is also true: D and G share the no-wing trait as well as a common ancestor.

14. C

The founder effect results from the isolation of a genetically abnormal subset of a larger population, causing a population to evolve with starkly different genetic frequencies from the original population. The founder effect causes one species to evolve in different directions.

15. A

Adaptive radiation refers to a diversifying lineage in response to an increase in environmental and ecological diversity. The density of population (D) is irrelevant.

16. B

Assortative mating is a phenomenon in which individuals show a preference for mates who are similar to themselves in some respect: size, color, and so on. This phenomenon has the evolutionary effect of decreasing the range of variation or trait variance.

17. C

The bottleneck effect refers to an evolutionary event that causes a large proportion of a population to be killed off or isolated from the rest. Graph C best illustrates a drop in population.

18. C

The group selection theory states that certain individuals are altruistic and will act to the detriment of their own reproductive success for the benefit of the group's overall reproductive success. This theory has been invalidated and replaced by the theory of kin selection., which claims that when individuals act altruistically, it is in fact indirectly favorable to individual reproductive success. Individuals only sacrifice direct reproductive success when it significantly increases indirect reproductive success via their kin who share many of the same genes. Inclusive fitness (A) refers to the sum of an individual's direct and indirect fitness.

19. C

Hardy-Weinberg equilibrium is a state in which genotypic frequencies of the population are not changing. If p represents frequency of allele 1 and q represents frequency of allele 2, then the frequency of the AA genotype should be p^2, while the frequency of the aa genotype should be q^2. Finally, the frequency of the Aa genotype should be $q \times p$, and the frequency of the aA genotype should be $p \times q$. The frequencies of these three genotype frequencies of one gene should add up to one. Therefore, at Hardy-Weinberg equilibrium, the following formula is true:

$$p^2 + 2pq + q^2 = 1$$

In this question supposing p represents allele A, and q represents allele B, then it follows that $p = 80\% = 0.80$ and $q = 20\% = 0.20$.

The frequency of recessive homozygotes, then, is $q^2 = 0.20^2 = 0.04 = 4\%$.

The frequency of dominant heterozygotes, then, is $2pq = 2 \times 0.20 \times 0.80 = 32\%$.

HIGH-YIELD SIMILAR QUESTIONS

Hardy-Weinberg

1. frequency of the recessive allele = 0.021; frequency of the dominant allele = 0.979; number of heterozygotes in the population = 8305 people
2. frequency of XX = 0.04; frequency of Xx = 0.32; frequency of xx = 0.64
3. 84% of individuals are phenotypically normal (assuming that the phenotype coded for by the dominant allele is "normal")

PRACTICE SECTIONS

PRACTICE SECTION 1

ANSWER KEY

1. A	19. D	36. A
2. D	20. D	37. B
3. A	21. A	38. A
4. C	22. D	39. D
5. C	23. A	40. D
6. B	24. D	41. C
7. C	25. B	42. C
8. C	26. B	43. B
9. A	27. D	44. B
10. B	28. C	45. D
11. A	29. A	46. B
12. B	30. D	47. D
13. B	31. D	48. B
14. D	32. A	49. C
15. D	33. B	50. A
16. B	34. B	51. A
17. A	35. A	52. A
18. B		

PASSAGE I

1. A

The null hypothesis is a hypothesis designed such that if it is refuted, then the actual hypothesis must be true. (B), (C), and (D) all present null hypotheses that if rejected, do not invalidate the actual hypothesis that hermit crab shell choice is influenced by color. If (B) is shown to be false, hermit crabs could prefer shells with the starkest color difference from their environment, and thus would still display color preference. If (C) is shown to be false, hermit crabs could prefer shells with the least color difference from their environment, and thus would still display color preference. If (D) is shown to be false, hermit crabs could prefer lighter-colored shells in certain instances, in which case color preference would still be an influence.

2. D

If the black paint was not actually black in practice, but a dark gray, this would not nullify the hypothesis that hermit crabs show shell preference based on color cues. There is still a color difference between the white shells and the dark-gray shells.

3. A

According to the data, the hermit crabs do choose the black shells over the white shells at a statistically significant rate, suggesting a preference for color. While in this particular experimental setup the hermit crabs always prefer the black shells, the experiment does not prove that this is always the case. For instance, the crabs could be choosing the black shells to stand out on the substrate such that their kin can find them easily. Perhaps on black substrate they would prefer white shells. It is also possible that they are choosing black shells because their natural environment is black. However, neither of these statements were proved conclusively in the experiment. It only demonstrates that a basic preference based on color.

4. C

(A), (B), and (D) present scenarios in which the visual cue—color—would affect hermit crab reproductive success. (C), however, presents a scenario in which color does not confer any advantage or disadvantage. Because hermit crabs show a preference for certain colors in the experiment, this suggests that certain colors confer reproductive advantages.

5. C

The experiment shows that crabs prefer dark-colored shells on white substrate, suggesting some kind of reproductive advantage for dark-colored shells in this environment. One would therefore expect evolutionary forces to select for crabs with dark shells in an environment of pure-white rocks, moving crabs in the direction of dark shells. Based on the experiment, one would also expect evolutionary forces to select for crabs with white shells in an environment of pure-black rocks. As evolutionary forces push the hermit crabs to fill different environmental niches, you will see selection in two opposite directions, also known as disruptive selection.

6. B

These findings do not strongly support the hypothesis that shell color affects hermit crab shell choice because the findings do not offer any indication as to why the crab population died out. Nor are the crabs in this population presented with a choice between different colored environments or shells. These findings do not conflict with the hypothesis either. Again, no evidence of preference or indifference to shell color is presented. Finally, the fact that the hermit crabs are not native to Jordan may suggest that the environment was likely suboptimal in many ways. However, it does not invalidate the fact that hermit crabs use color to help choose new shells.

7. C

Because these two species of hermit crabs are monophyletic, that means they share a common ancestor. As the species of hermit crabs used in the experiment show a strong preference for shells based on color, we can conclude that they are not colorblind. The trait must have arisen spontaneously in the second hermit crab species, or it must have been lost spontaneously in the first. In either case, because the trait is not shared between the two species, it can be neither analogous nor homologous. An analogous trait refers to a shared trait that arose separately through parallel evolutionary forces. A homologus trait refers to a shared trait that arose from shared genetic lines. (C), then, could be possible. The founder effect refers to new selective pressures affecting a population introduced to a new environment, which cause it to deviate from the rest of the species.

PASSAGE II

8. C

The disease allele is most likely recessive. While neither parent expresses the condition, one of the children is affected. In a dominant condition, one parent (at least) would need to be affected. There is no information in the text or pedigree to suggest codominance or a sex-linked trait. In the case of X-linked recessive inheritance, males are generally affected and that is not seen in this case.

9. A

If male 7, who is affected, marries a carrier, 50 percent of offspring would be affected and 50 percent would be carriers. A healthy noncarrier child cannot be born. It can be seen that male 7 is affected looking at the gel analysis. Male 7 has the same marker as an affected female 3 and no other marker to be heterozygous. It also makes sense as a smaller fragment with disease allele (due to deletion) migrates faster through the gel.

10. B

Expressivity, a term that refers to the degree of disease severity observed in affected individuals, varies according to the passage. It is mentioned that while some patients have mild respiratory difficulties, others have serious problems.

11. A

A mutation leading to cystic fibrosis can be classified as a deletion, as it results in a loss of three nucleotides. Inversion (C) would not change the number of nucleotides and would only affect their sequence. Insertion (D) would increase the number of nucleotides. Nondisjunction (B) refers to a failure of chromosomes to separate during meiosis; it does not deal with nucleotides.

12. B

Male 7 is homozygous recessive according to the gel electrophoresis results.

13. B

The fourth member alone is neither affected nor carrying a disease allele. On the gel, he has a larger fragment which migrated more slowly than the disease allele-containing fragment. It is the only fragment present, pointing to a homozygous condition.

14. D

A DNA fragment containing the disease allele would be shorter due to the deletion leading to cystic fibrosis; thus, it would move faster through the gel.

15. D

A mutation responsible for cystic fibrosis results in a deletion of three nucleotides. A nonsense mutation (B) introduces a stop code prematurely into the DNA sequence. A missense mutation (A) replaces one nucleotide with another, changing the peptide sequence of the encoded protein. A silent mutation (C) changes one of the nucleotides without affecting the type of amino acid in a sequence.

16. B

The frequency of the disease genotype is 1/100. The frequency of the disease allele, according to the Hardy-Weinberg principle, is the square root of 1/100 or 0.1.

17. A

Family member 5 is a carrier, as she has two types of DNA fragments: one for the wild type and one for the mutant allele. If member 5 marries another carrier, ¼ of their offspring on average will be affected.

QUESTIONS 18–21

18. B

(A) is a misuse of a detail; both rheumatic fever and type I diabetes occur initially in young populations, but co-occurence does not imply a similar etiology. (C) is a distortion; the specific hypersensitivity mechanism that causes rheumatic fever is cross-reactivity, where the immune system mistakes a body tissue for a foreign substance because they look similar. In an allergic reaction, the body has a response against a foreign substance that is too severe. In (D), although rheumatic fever causes a structural problem in the heart, the type of lesion mentioned in the passage occurs after infection, not at birth.

19. D

The question is intended to distract you with enzyme names that might seem intimidating. Nevertheless, the concept is simple: A kinase, when activated, phosphorylates its substrate. If the substrate is a metabolic enzyme, then this phosphorylation will take place at an allosteric site. Because this action activates PFK-1, the indicated process is an example of allosteric activation. (A) and (C) are wrong because the process causes an activation or agonistic effect, not an inactivation or antagonistic effect. Synergism (B) would require more than one enzyme with the same substrate to be present. This question presents two enzymes with different substrates.

20. D

The suffix kinase indicates that the function of the enzyme is to phosphorylate not isomerizes, thus eliminating (C). (A) is wrong because the indicated reaction does not occur. (B) is wrong because the indicated conversion would require two enzymes: an isomerase to convert glucose to fructose and a kinase to add the second phosphate group.

21. A

This question tests your ability to paraphrase the question and see the concept through the details. A good paraphrase is: Under what conditions does the breakdown of glucose stop with glycolysis and not proceed to form intermediates of the Krebs cycle? Since oxygen is the final electron acceptor of the electron transport chain, one could predict that low levels of oxygen would prevent aerobic metabolism. This is true and the accumulated pyruvate is converted to lactate under such conditions. (B) indicates a high concentration of oxidized substrates, implying an abundance of oxygen. (C) is wrong because while this would signal for an increase in the rate of glycolysis, it gives no information as to the oxygen levels of the cell and thus the ability of the cell to proceed into aerobic respiration. (D) is wrong because low levels of fructose-1,6-bisphosphate initiate the signal for gluconeogenesis, a separate metabolic pathway.

PASSAGE III

22. D

The passage describes that protons (H^+) are pumped across inner mitochondrial membrane into the intermembrane space making the intermembrane space more positive when compared to the matrix. pH drops in the intermembrane space as the proton concentration increases when compared to the matrix of mitochondria. (A) and (B) are only half right, and (C) is opposite the correct answer.

23. A

You're asked to choose one of the results that cannot be observed upon administration of antimycin A. According to the table, antimycin A blocks step 4 of the electron transport chain. The first figure shows that blocking step 4 will prevent the passage of electrons from cytochrome b to cytochrome c in the electron transport chain. As electrons don't travel further than cytochrome b, oxygen cannot remain the final acceptor of electrons (step 6 of ETC) and the transport is stopped at step 4 (choice A). (B) is wrong, as antimycin A indeed decreases the proton gradient, because when electrons travel only part of the transport chain less protons are pumped to the mitochondrial intermembrane space. This can be inferred from the passage that describes the buildup of proton gradient as electrons are passed from carrier to carrier. (C) is wrong: ATP synthesis is indeed stopped as the electrons never reach the final acceptor oxygen and the gradient would be lower than needed for ATP synthesis. This is inferred from the passage that mentions the specific gradient required. (D) is wrong as cytochrome b is indeed fully reduced and it can no longer pass its electrons to cytochrome c.

24. D

You're asked to use information in the passage and figures to determine which of the inhibitors will stop ATP synthesis without affecting the proton gradient. The table shows that oligomycin blocks the action of ATP synthase, which is responsible for ATP production. At the same time, as oligomycin does not affect any of the carriers in the chain, the electron gradient would be established and could not be dissipated as ATP synthase does not work (D). Choices (B) and (C) are wrong because both inhibitors interfere with electron transport along the chain, making the proton gradient less, even though ATP synthesis will come to a halt. (A) is wrong as 2, 4-dinitrophenol makes the inner mitochondrial membrane more permeable to protons that can escape from the intermembrane space back into the matrix without building up the gradient.

25. B

The question asks you to identify inhibitors that will interfere with the transport of electrons along the chain so that the final electron acceptor oxygen cannot receive electrons. Inhibitors listed in items II and III alone will interfere with the electron transport chain, while oligomycin does not disrupt the chain of carriers and blocks ATP synthase directly.

26. B

The question asks you to suggest what happens when the permeability of the inner mitochondrial membrane is increased. As the passage addresses the importance of building up a proton gradient across impermeable inner membrane, it can be inferred that if protons are allowed to pass, they will escape the intermembrane space—thus, decreasing the gradient. For (C), a lower proton gradient would decrease ATP synthesis, not increase ATP production.

27. D

The passage explains that, as protons pass through the ATP synthase into the mitochondrial matrix, ATP is made. As ADP and phosphates are needed for ATP production, it makes sense that they would be present in mitochondrial matrix. (A) is wrong because, as per the passage, ATP synthase is a transmembrane enzyme complex and embedded into the membrane, and thus not in the mitochondrial matrix.

28. C

Rotenone will not produce a fully reduced cytochrome a, as rotenone disrupts step 2 of ETC and electrons don't go beyond FMN, leaving cytochrome a oxidized. (A), (B), and (D) interfere with step 6 preventing cytochrome a from passing its electrons to oxygen. Thus cytochrome a would be left fully oxidized.

PASSAGE IV

29. A

The presence of pre-existing lung disease could have a negative effect on the inspiratory reserve volume of the individuals in the study. A patient with asthma, an obstructive pulmonary disease, an asbestosis, or a restrictive lung disease would likely have different inspiratory reserve volumes. Tidal volume should not impact this experiment because the amount of drug delivered is the same in each case; we look for radioactivity, not a concentration-dependent phenomenon. Sex will make no difference; male lungs would generally be larger, but the measurements are made per unit of lung tissue. Bronchodilators with zero order kinetics are metabolized independently of their concentration. Because these medications are delivered directly to the lungs and do not undergo metabolism before contacting their target tissue, the kinetics of metabolism will have no bearing on the results.

30. D

IgE is formed as a result of exposure to an allergen. The first time the allergen is present, the body will form IgE, but there will be no signs of allergy.

IgE circulates and 'docks' or 'connects' to mast cells via the Fc region of the antibody. When the antibody comes in contact again with its antigen, a conformation change takes place in the antibody and the mast cell degranulates, resulting in histamine release and contributing to asthma attack.

31. D

The key to this question is knowing that acetylcholine is the primary neurotransmitter of the parasympathetic response. During the parasympathetic response the body is relaxed; the heart rate decreases and blood flow to the gut is increased. Remember parasympathetic is to 'rest and digest.' The sympathetic response, in contrast, comes into play when being chased by a tiger. The body will need great airflow to support running away. An asthma attack, then, is the opposite of a sympathetic response; it causes relative bronchoconstriction. The use of an anticholinergic medication will promote the sympathetic system to open the airways.

32. A

This question just requires summing the values for each column. The largest total will be the most effective, on average, at delivering medication to the lungs.

QUESTIONS 33–35

33. B

Chylomicrons transport fats from the intestines to the circulation. With that, one can predict that with low levels of chlyomicrons, the lipids will not enter circulation (eliminating (C) and (D)) but will pass out with the stool. While diarrhea (A) is always possible in a metabolic disorder, it is not specific to abetalipoproteinemia.

34. B

Replication errors are the least severe if chemical class of the base isn't changed. That is a mutation from a purine to a purine is less severe than a mutation from a purine to a pyrimidine. Using this, we can predict that (B) is true since (A) and (C) involve the change from a purine, A, to a pyrimidine, C or T. (D) is wrong for two reasons: first is, again, a purine change, and second, uracil is found only in RNA. Its inclusion in a strand of DNA would indicate a serious replication error.

35. A

The central dogma of molecular biology is that the genetic information contained in DNA is first transcribed to RNA and then translated to a linear sequence of amino acids which comprise the primary structure of a protein. The central dogma does not make claims to the details of transcription, only that is transferred information between DNA and RNA (B), nor does it tell of the flow of information or the organelle subserving this function (C) and (D).

PASSAGE V

36. A

There are multiple ways with which parietal cells are stimulated to release H^+. (A) G cells, located in antrum of the stomach, releases gastrin. Gastrin thereby will stimulate the cholecystokinin-B (CCKb) receptor. (B) Histamine can stimulate the release of H^+ by activating the H_2 receptors located on the parietal cells. (C) Postganglionic neurons release acetylcholine, which will activate the muscarinic (M3) receptors of the parietal cells, causing an increase in production of H^+. (D) Somatostatin inhibits H^+ secretion.

37. B

There are a few ways that Zollinger-Ellison syndrome can cause malabsorption of dietary lipids. One way is inactivation of pancreatic enzymes. Pancreatic enzymes are inactivated at acidic pH. With the overproduction of H^+ caused by an oversecretion of gastrin, pancreatic enzymes are inactivated, causing impairment of dietary lipid absorption. Zollinger-Ellison syndrome does not affect the liver's ability to create bile salts (A). Celiac disease is an autoimmune disease of the small intestine in reaction to gluten(C). One of the major causes of peptic ulcer disease (PUD) is *H. pylori*, a flagellated bacteria associated with duodenal and gastric ulcers (D).

38. A

Acetylcholine (Ach), Histamine, and Gastrin ((B), (C), and (D)) all bind to different receptors on parietal cells, all three leading to an increase in H^+ secretion. Ach is released from the vagus nerves, Histamine is released from mastlike cells in the gastric mucosa, and gastrin is released from G cells in the stomach's antrum. (A) GIP (gastric inhibitory peptide) causes pancreatic beta cells to secrete insulin. GIP also inhibits gastric H^+ secretion.

39. D

Gastrin is secreted by G cells located in the antrum of the stomach. It is secreted when food is ingested. Gastrin can also be stimulated to secretion by local vagal reflexes. Following an action potential, neurocrines (peptides synthesized in GI tract neurons) are released onto the G cells. These neurocrines are called gastrin-releasing peptides (GRP) or bombesin. Gastrin has two main functions: first, to stimulate H^+ secretion by gastric parietal cells, and second, to stimulate gastric mucosa growth. Cholecystokinin (CCK) promotes fat digestion and absorption (A). CCK also slows down/inhibits gastric emptying (B) and increases gastric emptying time. Secretin increases the secretion of pancreatic and biliary HCO_3^- (choice C).

40. D

In some cases of Zollinger-Ellison syndrome, diarrhea may be the only presenting symptom. This results from an oversecretion of gastrin and gastric acid production. The high acid content damages intestinal villi, leading to malabsorption and frequent diarrhea. Motilin, produced by intestinal M cells, increases GI motility (C). Some studies suggest that motilin release is stimulated by an alkaline pH in the duodenum.

41. C

The physiologic control of gastrin, the gastric G cells, are under negative feedback control. Once the gastric contents have been properly acidified, gastrin secretion is inhibited. But in Zollinger-Ellison syndrome the tumor does not respond to gastric pH and gastrin is produced regardless.

PASSAGE VI

42. C

The free energy of the reaction is the same whether it is catalyzed or uncatalyzed. It is the difference between the starting energy (here 45 kJ/mol) and the final reaction energy (here 10 kJ/mol), yielding 35 kJ/mol. (A) is the uncatalyzed activation energy—final energy. (B) is the catalyzed activation energy—final energy. (D) is wrong because the final energy is much lower than the initial value.

43. B

The activation energy for the uncatalyzed reaction is 80 kJ/mol, and the catalyzed is 55 kJ/mol. $80 - 55 = 25$, and $25/85 \sim 32\%$. (A) is wrong because the enzyme by definition lowers the activation energy some amount. (C) is wrong because the activation energy required is still 66% of what it was originally; it only went down 33%. (D) is wrong because there is still clearly some activation energy required for the reaction to occur.

44. B

Estrogen is associated with conversion from fat to muscle, and therefore some of it is necessary in the body. In people with high fat content, however, the estrogen cannot 'keep up,' and its efficacy is reduced. (A) is wrong because velocity can never be higher than V_{max} in any individual. (C) is wrong because the aromatase is just as active (i.e., requires same activation energy) as in a healthy person, but is working over many more cells. (D) is wrong because the only thing that can make the enzyme structure change is an artificial chemical (i.e., drug), which is not the case here.

45. D

Noncompetitive inhibition is an irreversible form of inhibition where the inhibitor covalently binds to the enzyme and deactivates it permanently. No type of feedback mechanism would be effective here. (A) is wrong because there is no allosteric (remote) control in aromatase. (B) is wrong because there is no allosteric site and also because the enzyme is being inhibited, not activated. (C) is wrong because there is no feedback from the product (estrogen) in this type of inhibition.

46. B

Aromatase inhibition will decrease estrogen production, and therefore increase androgen availability. (A) is wrong because as the enzyme converts androgen to estrogen, activating aromatase will lead to even lower androgen counts. (C) is wrong because men do naturally have some aromatase in their bodies, and for the same reason as (A), androgen counts would decrease with artificial injection. (D) is wrong because aromatase (and the estrogen it produces) does affect men (by increasing libido, for instance) as well as women.

PASSAGE VII

47. D

It is impossible to ascertain what genotype the second sister (individual I-3) has; we can ascertain that she has passed the MIDD form of diabetes to her children through her mitochondrial DNA, which cannot be represented through the typical autosomal alleles. This eliminates (B) and (C) (even though heterozygosity would be correct for the first sister). Even if we could determine both genotypes, (A) would be wrong because MODY is autosomal dominant, and if homozygous dominant. all the children would present with the disease.

48. B

The individual could present with type II diabetes or MIDD. The age of onset means that the individual could not present with type I (juvenile) diabetes. Type II is the most likely option given his age, but MIDD is also possible; we do not have any information on his mother, and as a male he would not pass on the disease to his children. One could also argue that MODY is possible; if he had MODY, his wife would be homozygous recessive since she did not present with the disease, but each of his children has a 50 percent chance of developing the disease. The likelihood of all three offspring not developing the disease is low (1/8), but not zero. However, item III with MODY is unambiguously wrong.

49. C

This requires the determination that the MODY form of diabetes is present on the bloodline containing individual IV-2, and that it has autosomal dominant inheritance (stated in the passage introduction). This means that the mother, who has the disease, is heterozygous (homozygous dominant is extremely rare for such diseases, but this can be confirmed to not be the case by looking at the previous generations). With this deduction, a Punnett square could be made as follows.

	Mother	
Father	M	m
m	Mm	mm
m	Mm	mm

From this, the answer is clearly 50 percent. (A) would require both parents to be homozygous recessive, and this is not the case since the mother had young-onset diabetes. (B) is typical of autosomal *recessive* conditions, and the passage stem said that MODY is autosomal dominant. (D) requires both parents to be heterozygous, and in this case the father would also have diabetes.

50. A

These two individuals have no risk of developing a genetically-inherited form of diabetes (the only types that come before age 40). Their father has MIDD, but since this disease is mitochondrial, it will not be passed through him. The mother can be assumed to have type II diabetes, due to the late age of occurrence. (B) would have assumed that both offspring would have had a 25 percent chance of getting the disease, as is typical with autosomal recessive. (C) would have assumed both offspring had a 50 percent chance of developing the disease, as would have been the case with autosomal dominant. (D) is simply the chance of one individual getting it if it had been autosomal dominant.

51. A

Penetrance is the likelihood that a certain genotype will be expressed in the phenotype. There are three nondiabetic offspring in generation 2. If each of these offspring fall within the 15 percent chance of nonpenetrance, the overall probability of this happening is $(.15)^3 = 0.03$. (B) is $(.15)^2$, which would be for only two of the offspring. (C) is the chance that *any one* of the nondiabetic children is a carrier. (D) is the rate of penetrance for those who have diabetes.

52. A

ADM, from the question stem, is not insulin-dependent. MIDD is, but because the individual's father has MIDD, it will not be passed on to him through mitochondrial DNA. Therefore, the individual has no chance of developing insulin-dependent diabetes (and a 50 percent chance of developing ADM). (B) is the likelihood if one of the conditions was autosomal recessive. (C) would be correct if looking at the risk of developing any kind of diabetes. (D) is the chance if the mother, not the father, had MIDD.

PRACTICE SECTION 2

ANSWER KEY

1.	B	19.	D	37.	C
2.	C	20.	B	38.	A
3.	B	21.	B	39.	A
4.	B	22.	C	40.	B
5.	B	23.	C	41.	C
6.	C	24.	D	42.	B
7.	C	25.	D	43.	C
8.	B	26.	A	44.	A
9.	C	27.	D	45.	D
10.	C	28.	B	46.	A
11.	A	29.	A	47.	D
12.	D	30.	D	48.	A
13.	C	31.	A	49.	B
14.	C	32.	D	50.	C
15.	C	33.	C	51.	D
16.	D	34.	A	52.	C
17.	B	35.	A		
18.	A	36.	C		

PASSAGE I

1. B

The goal of this experiment, mentioned in the context of the two major classes of antiretroviral drugs that target reverse transcriptase, is to compare the two different mechanisms by which they act.

2. C

This question is asking which nucleotide pairs with adenine. The trick is to recognize that the parent strand in this case is RNA. Therefore, an adenine nucleotide (DNA) will pair with a uracil (RNA).

3. B

Drug C decreases the activity of the reverse transcriptase. This result, along with the information provided in the passage about drug mechanisms, means (B) is a possible mechanism (nonnucleoside reverse transcriptase inhibitor). (D) describes the mechanism of a nucleotide/nucleoside reverse transcriptase inhibitor, which based on the information in the passage, does not affect reverse transcriptase activity. (A) and (C) would not have any effect on reverse transcriptase activity.

4. B

The assay described in the passage is used to evaluate drugs that target reverse transcriptase. It is likely that drugs with other targets will not have an effect on the same variables as those examined in the assay used. Drug D is FDA approved and therefore should have an effect on the virus (A, C, and D).

5. B

Competitive inhibitors bind to the same active site that the substrate binds to, preventing the binding of the substrate. Noncompetitive inhibitors bind to the enzyme at a different site than the enzyme's active site. Given the description provided in the passage, non-nucleotide reverse transcriptase inhibitors act as noncompetitive inhibitors of reverse transcriptase.

6. C

As described in the passage, the mechanism of nucleoside/nucleotide reverse transcriptase inhibitors involves the early termination of transcription after their incorporation into the daughter DNA strand, implying that they cannot be removed. They do not affect translation (A). They are competitive inhibitors of reverse transcriptase (B). They act at the active site of reverse transcriptase (D).

7. C

Once a retrovirus integrates its DNA into the host DNA, it is called a provirus until its viral mRNA is transcribed. By definition, it will be found in the nucleus.

PASSAGE II

8. B

The most critical (and susceptible) stage of fetal development is considered to be the embryonic stage (weeks 3–8), when all organ morphogenesis is occurring. If the drug was ingested during fertizilation (C), the likely outcome would be termination of pregnancy before implantation. The later weeks (A) and (D) are considered less critical because all the organ systems have been formed.

9. C

Down syndrome is the excess of genetic code on the 21st chromosome. A typical human's karyotype is either 46 XY (typical male) or 46 XX (typical female). There are many ways for this to occur, via either a complete extra chromosome [trisomy 21 (47, XX, +21)] or a portion of (i.e., due to translocations). About 95 percent of Down syndrome is due to trisomy 21; in the majority of cases, nondisjunction occurs with the maternal gamete. Cystic fibrosis (A) is caused by a mutation in the CFTR (cystic fibrosis transmembrane conductance regulator) gene. Sickle cell disease (B) is an inherited blood disorder whereby red blood cells contain an abnormal type of hemoglobin. Polycythemia vera (D), a myeloproliferative disorder, is considered to be due to a mutation of the JAK2 protein, thereby allowing for unregulated control of blood cell production.

10. C

The first sign of gastrulation is the formation of the primitive streak, which arises from (C) epiblast cells, not (A) hypoblast cells. During normal embryonic development, the primitive streak will diminish in size and eventually become an insignificant structure that ultimately disappears by the end of the fourth week. But sometimes the remnants will persist and give rise to a sacrococcygeal teratoma. This is the most common tumor in newborns and most often occurs in females. Most of the tumors are benign, diagnosed on routine antenatal ultrasonography, and surgically removed. The prochordal plate (B) is composed of hypoblast cells that fused with epiblast cells to form a circular, midline thickening, and will be the future site of the mouth. The yolk sac is formed from a portion of the exocoelomic cavity (D), which is formed in part from hypoblast cells and the inner surface of the cytotrophoblast.

11. A

Medulloblastoma is a highly malignant primary brain tumor that originates in the cerebellum or posterior fossa. It manifests with increased intracranial pressure due to blockage of the fourth ventrcile. Craniopharyngioma (B) is a slow-growing tumor that develop from Rathke's pouch. It is the most common supratentorial tumor in childhood. The tumor may enlarge and compress the optic chiasm, resulting in blindness. Glioblastoma multiforme (C) is the most common primary brain tumor in adults. It is a rapidly growing, highly destructive tumor with death occurring within months. The tumor is associate with necrotic tissue because the tumor grows faster than new blood vessels can be developed to provide nourishment for the tumor cells. Optic nerve glioma (D) is the most common primary neoplasm of the optic nerve. Often diagnosed during childhood, about 10 percent of cases occur in association with neurofibromatosis type I. It is a tumor of the visual system and has been known to involve the optic nerve, optic chiasm, and/or optic tract.

12. D

Gastroschisis is a result of a defect lateral to the median plane of the anterior abdominal wall. This defect allows the intestines and sometimes other organs to develop outside the fetal abdomen without involving the umbilical cord. No parietal peritoneum covers the organs. Omphalocele (B) is an anterior abdominal defect that does involve the umbilical cord. During the eighth week of development, the fetal midgut undergoes a physiologic umbilical herniation, in which the organs extend out into the extraembryonic celom, occupying the proximal segment of the umbilical cord. It is believed that an omphalocele occurs when the bowel fails to return into the abdomen. Meckel diverticulum (C) is a small outpouching of the small intestine that is present at birth. It is the vestigial remnant of the omphalomesenteric duct (vitelline duct) and is considered to be the most common gastrointestinal tract malformation. Myeloschisis (A) is considered to be the most severe form of spina bifida. The spinal cord in this area remains open due to lack of complete neural tube fusion.

13. C

Triploidy is an abnormal chromosomal condition usually resulting from fertilization of an oocyte by two sperms (dispermy). Most triplod fetuses are aborted spontaneously or are stillborns, and some die shortly after birth. (A) and (B) are aneuploidy, (C) triploidy, and (D) tetraploidy.

14. C

An ectopic pregnancy occurs when the blastocyst implants within an abnormal location. Oftentimes, the woman has a history of endometriosis or pelvic inflammatory disease. The most common site is the ampulla portion of the fallopian tube (80–90%), isthmic (5–10%); cornual (1–2%), abdominal (1–2%), and cervix (less than 1%).

15. C

Pelvic inflammatory disease/disorder (PID) is a general term applied to inflammation of the female reproductive system (uterus, fallopian tube, and/or ovaries) that has progressed to scarring and adhesions to nearby tissues and organs. PID is often associated with STDs (sexually transmitted diseases). With each episode of infection, the chance of infertility increases. (C) Chlamydia trachomatis and Neisseria gonorrhoeae are considered the leading causes of PID. Patients testing positive for one are often tested for the other, as the two are often both present. Syphillis (A) is an STD caused by the spirochete, treponema pallidum. Untreated syphilis can lead to systemic dissemination and damage—especially of the heart, brain, eyes, and bones—and has even been fatal in some. Human papilloma virus (HPV) (B) is considered to be the most common sexually transmitted disease in the United States. There are over 100 subtypes and some are known to cause cancer, primarily cervical, anal, vulvar, and penile cancers. Herpes (D) simplex virus (HSV) type 1 (HSV-1) and type 2 (HSV-2) are known to cause herpes simplex. Although in the past, genital herpes was considered to have been caused by HSV-2, the rate of genital HSV-1 infections has increased dramatically. Typical manifestations are painfully inflamed papules and vesicles on the outer genital surface, as well as the inner thigh, buttocks, or anus.

16. D

Fetal erythroblastosis (aka hemolytic disease of the newborn) occurs when small amounts of fetal blood pass through the placental membrane and enters the maternal blood. If the mother is Rh negative, and the fetus is Rh positive, the mother may have anti-Rh IgG antibodies which will enter fetal circulation and attack fetal red blood cells. If severe, the infant may be stillborn or die shortly after birth. Rubella (aka German measles) (A) is caused by the rubella virus. The disease is usually mild in children and adults, but if a mother is infected within the first 20 weeks of pregnancy, the child may be born with congenital rubella syndrome (CRS), and that can lead to developmental deafness, blindness, congenital heart defects, and even infant death. Sickle cell anemia occurs when there is a point mutation on the beta-globin chain of haemoglobin (B), when glutamic acid is substituted by valine. This causes red blood cells to lose their elasticity and become sickle-shaped during low oxygen conditions. Cystic fibrosis is caused by mutation of the CFTR gene (cystic fibrosis transmembrane conductance regulator gene) (C). This gene produces a chloride ion channel that is issential in sweat glands, digestive juices, and mucus production.

17. B

A partial hydatidiform mole usually results from an oocyte fertilized by two sperms. Most partial moles are triploid (contain three chromosome sets). The embryo usually dies, and the chorionic villi form into cystic swellings which resemble bunches of grapes. The moles will produce an abnormally high amount of human chorionic gonadotropin. Dizygotic twins (A) are the result of fertilization of two oocytes. The two zygotes may be of the same or different sexes.

QUESTIONS 18–21

18. A

Translation refers to the production of protein from mRNA. Though the conversion of DNA to RNA is discussed, the idea here is that one initial piece of information gives rise to other secondary pieces.

You can predict, then, that only eukaryotes have alternate splicing. Prokaryotic DNA is monocistronic. Although in transcription prokaryotes do have multiple reading frames (as do eukaryotes), this is not true in translation; their genes are organized in an operon and thus groups of proteins are produced en masse on one mRNA transcript in tandem fashion.

19. D

Gram-negative bacteria do not take up the gram stain because they have an outer cell wall which impedes the movement of any polar or large substance into the periplasmic space. This could also be a barrier to drugs. Capsids (A) are found in viruses, not bacteria. Bacteria are prokaryotes and thus have no membrane-bound organelles (B). All bacteria have an inner cell wall (C).

20. B

Only the endoplasmic reticulum is directly connected to the nucleus. The nucleolus (A) resides in the nucleus. Neither (C) nor (D) is continuous with the nucleus.

21. B

This is a straight recall question. Plasma cells (C) do not secrete hormones; they function in the immune system. Beta cells of the islets of Langerhans in the pancreas secrete insulin. Delta cells secrete somatostatin, which is also secreted by the D cells of the gastric antrum.

PASSAGE III

22. C

The destructive phase (A) is another name for the menstrual phase. It is named as such because during this period, the uterine lining is destroyed and discarded. The secretory phase (B) is another name for the luteal phase. It is named as such because during this period, many hormones are secreted. The gestational phase (C) does not exist. Gestation refers to the period in which a woman carries an embryo in her womb. As menstruation refers to the cycle of events which lead up to gestation, it does not logically follow that one of its phases would occur during gestation. You may be thinking of the name *pregestational phase*, which is another name for the luteal phase. The proliferative phase (D) is another name for the follicular phase. It is called as such because during this period, follicules and the endometrium proliferate.

23. C

The passage tells us that the female menstrual cycle is a set of events which leads to ovulation. Ovulation is the release of ova into the uterus for fertilization. The chart shows us that Mary's menstrual cycle is 28 days long. This means that in a 365-day year, Mary would undergo 365/28 = 13 full menstrual cycles.

24. D

If fertilization fails to occur, the ovum is distentegrated through menses (A). It does not become the corpus luteum. The product of ovum and sperm fertilization is a zygote. The follicle before ovulation occurs is a follicle. It goes through different stages such as tertiary follicle and then Graafian follicle. What remains of the follicle following ovulation becomes the corpus luteum.

25. D

One would expect the conditions in (D) to increase the proportion of time a woman is susceptible to pregnancy, and in so doing, indirectly increase fertility. As for (A), about one-third of estrogen comes from fat. One needs very high levels of estradiol (an estrogen) to stimulate the LH surge necessary of ovulation. This is also why anorexic women often experience secondary ammenorhea. Progesterone (B) is actually used as a form of birth control. Low levels of estrogen (C) would exacerbate infertility, as explained in (A).

26. A

The combination pill is a mixture of progesterone and estradiol, in levels that mimic these hormones' levels during pregnancy. This tricks your body into believing it is pregnant, preventing the proliferative uterine phase and causing a lighter period.

27. D

The zygote is what is formed after the egg's fertilization by the sperm. If fertilization occurs, menses is prevented from occurring. Blood (A) is contained in menstrual discharge as a result of broken blood vessels in the endometrium. As the endometrium exits the body, it sloughs off some of the cells lining the vagina (B). The stratum functionalis (C) is the outer layer of the endometrium, and is the layer that is discharged.

28. B

FSH is inhibited by high estradiol levels. Estradiol levels increase until the midpoint of the follicular phase, and FSH increases until that time as well. FSH dips at the midpoint as a result of high levels of estradiol secreted by large follicles, inhibiting GnRH. GnRH from the hypothalamus controls FSH secretion by the pituitary.

29. A

In the beginning of the follicular phase, estradiol levels are low, and FSH and LH secretion is high due to the absence of negative feedback by estradiol on FSH and LH production. At about the middle of the follicular phase, estradiol levels are moderately high and begin to exert negative feedback on FSH and LH production. By the end of the follicular phase, very high estradiol levels are present, and at very high concentrations, estradiol stimulates FSH and LH production, resulting in an LH surge.

30. D

If you refer to the figure in the passage, you will see that (D) is true. The relationship between estradiol and progesterone levels controls gonadotropin release. Before the FSH and LH surge, there is high estradiol but low progesterone. After ovulation, there is high progesterone but low estradiol.

31. A

To prevent pregnancy, the couple needs to limit coitus in a way that prevents viable sperm from coming in contact with a viable ovum. We know from the passage that ova can remain viable for up to three days after ovulation (ovum disentegration typically begins 24 hours after ovulation but can begin as late as 72 hours later). We also know that male sperm can stay viable in the female reproductive tract for up to four days. A woman with the given menstrual cycle should limit coitus to three days after the basal temperature rise, and the following 21 days (four days before ovulation), choice (A).

PASSAGE IV

32. D

The experiment shows that the size of gene X in family 2 and the control group is the same. It is possible that there was a point mutation in gene X that affected its functional capability yet not the length of the gene. In mammals mtDNA encodes for 37 genes, so it is possible that the mtDNA mutation in family 2 affects one of the other genes. We know from the passage that family 2 has the clinical presentation of mitochondrial inheritance disorder, so item III is wrong. Items I and II are correct.

33. C

Since we know from the passage that gene X plays a role in aerobic respiration, we can predict the location of the gene X product. All proteins that play a role in aerobic respiration reside in the inner mitochondrial membrane and mitochondrial matrix. Because we know that the protein is a transmembrane protein, we can assume it is found in the inner membrane and not as a free protein in the matrix (D).

34. A

This question tests your ability to synthesize information from the passage with your knowledge about aerobic respiration. When oxygen is unavailable to accept electrons, pyruvate acts as the electron acceptor, forming lactic acid. It is unlikely that dysfunctions of aerobic respiration would cause an increase in phospholipids, alanine, or carbon dioxide.

35. A

As described in the passage and the subsequent experiment, mitochondrial inheritance disorders can take on multiple phenotypes (the visible appearance of a disease) and can be due to different mutations (different genotypes).

36. C

If a mitochondrial disorder were to be caused by a mutation in nuclear DNA, the mitochondria must rely somewhat on certain gene products from nuclear DNA. Mitochondria are only semi-autonomous and do not encode all their necessary genes in the mitochondrial DNA (D). Mitochondria are the only nonnuclear organelle to possess their own DNA (B).

37. C

Based on the passage and family tree illustration, we know that mitochondrial inheritance disorders have maternal inheritance of a mitochondrial genome that is separate from the nuclear genome. Maternal inheritance occurs because sperm cell mitochondria do not contribute to ova during fertilization. Items I, II, and III are correct.

38. A

Mitochondria have their own ribosomes separate from those made in the nucleus. Mitochondrial DNA is circular, but nuclear DNA is often found as linear chromosomes. mtDNA has maternal inheritance, whereas there are maternal and paternal inputs in nuclear DNA inheritance.

QUESTIONS 39–41

39. A

Lipase (B) breaks down fats, which are a different chemical class from polyscchartides. Pepsin (D) is a hormone, not an enzyme. Trypsinogen (C) is a zymogen, not a hormone. The rationale for eliminating these answer choices is guided by the prediction, garnered from the question stem, that the answer must be an enzyme which is specific for starches.

40. B

For remembering RNA mutations, hint 1: Like DNA, changes within a base chemical class produce less severe mutation than changes between chemical classes. Hint 2: With RNA questions, eliminate any answer choice that includes T, as RNA only has U. Hint 3: Remember the wobble position! The third position in any codon is always most subject to variation due to the structure of the tRNA-mRNA interface. Thus, the genetic code has evolved to tolerate this variation without adverse consequences. Using this knowledge, one sees that (B) is correct because the mutation is both in the wobble position and changes a purine for a purine. (D) is wrong because, although the mutation is in the wobble position, AAT is not a valid RNA codon (AAU would be).

41. C

This question tests your ability to critically evaluate what some consider an inflammatory statement. (A) and (B) have no basis in genetics. (D) assumes that a longer time for procreation will result in increased progeny. (C) is true because male gametes have more genetic variation than female gametes and thus have a higher chance of containing a mutation encoding a sexually advantageous trait.

PASSAGE V

42. B

The voltage-gated sodium channels that are affected by carbamazepine are very likely to be implicated as a mediator for a kindling-like mechanism which is voltage-dependant in action. The sodium channel activity does not necessarily support excitotoxicity, which is based on the toxicity of certain neurotransmitters in the synapse.

43. C

Excitotoxicity, not the kindling model, deals primarily with the toxicity of neurotransmitters that are found at the synapse, so (A) is wrong. Moreover, even though lots of sub-threshold potentials are shot and culminate at the synapse (leading to excitability of downstream neurons), (A) is wrong because the excitotoxicity model does deal with processes at the synapse. The kindling model, albeit in most instances with electrical stimulation, may use chemical stimulation as well to cause sensitization, so (B) is wrong.

44. A

In light of the excitotoxicity view, extracellular administration of an enzyme which degrades glutamate (A) is a suitable method for normal treatment of a chronically epileptic patient. (B), (C), and (D) would exacerbate the seizures.

45. D

(A), (B), and (C) are not true of glutamate.

46. A

By cutting off blood flow, metabolic nutrients for the maintenance and production of various enzymes and carriers are impaired. Nothing in the passage leads you to believe reasonably that trauma to the brain would cause an increase in Brownian motion of neurotransmitters (B). Nor does the passage suggest any impact on action potential propagation (C) by trauma to the brain.

47. D

(A) is not plausible because the kindling model does not gradually increase the stimulus; moreover, the "epileptic threshold" is lowered, whereas the threshold stimulus is raised in accommodation. (B) and (C) are concerned as well with a raising of the threshold, and in the case of absolute refractory period, to an infinitely high one.

48. A

The cerebellum is responsible for balance.

PASSAGE VI

49. B

The sodium/potassium pump releases three sodium ions for every two potassium ions, creating a ratio of 1.5. This same ratio must be matched by the water concentration in the cell; hence, it is 60 percent water within the cell and 40 percent out of it. (This could also be determined from the figure by counting the 18 K^+ ions in the cell and 12 Na^+ ions outside the cell.) A 50/50 water concentration (A) would lead to too much water outside the cell (hypotonicity). A 75/25 concentration puts too much water inside the cell (hypertonicity).

50. C

ATP is the energy source for the sodium-potassium pump, which is necessary to control the sodium level in the cell. NaCl (table salt) is wrong because the sodium has no chemical effect until it is a separate positive ion. Glucose is actually a worsening factor because its presence would force some water into the cell. Urea plays no role within the cell; its function is to excrete sodium from the body.

51. D

Vasopressin is released when the body is dehydrated and causes the body to conserve water. It also controls the menstrual cycle and is highest at the time of ovulation. Vasopressin interferes with the sodium potassium pump, causing a "misinforming" such that the body thinks it is dehydrated when there's actually an excess of water. There is no evidence that women consume any more water than men (A); in fact, it is likely that they consume less because they sweat less. Brain mass (B) is determined by size, not gender (children do have a higher likelihood of hyponatremia for this reason, however). Although estrogen (C) does contribute to water storage, testosterone (another sex hormone also found in women) can actually block the effect of vasopressin.

52. C

The myelin sheath is a phospholipid layer that protects the neurons; this is the same function as the phospholipid bilayer of the cell membrane within the cell. The neuron has its own nucleus (called the same), choice (A). Animal cells do not have cell walls (B). The cytoplasm (D) is the fluid portion of the cell.

PRACTICE SECTION 3

ANSWER KEY

1. A	19. D	36. C
2. D	20. E	37. C
3. C	21. D	38. B
4. A	22. A	39. C
5. D	23. B	40. D
6. B	24. D	41. B
7. B	25. D	42. C
8. A	26. B	43. A
9. D	27. C	44. A
10. A	28. C	45. A
11. A	29. A	46. C
12. C	30. A	47. D
13. C	31. D	48. B
14. A	32. A	49. D
15. A	33. D	50. D
16. A	34. B	51. B
17. A	35. A	52. C
18. D		

PASSAGE I

1. A

(A) allows both hypotheses 1 and 2 to be valid and their data accepted. Tyrosinase levels are not correlated with melanin levels; they are correlated with melanin levels and thus skin color. A logical synthesis of the two hypotheses would be that somehow after translation of the gene for tyrosinase, the actual enzyme's activity is changed to become more active to produce darker colorations. Gene alterations (B) would mean gene products would correlate with melanin synthesis—that gene product could only be tyrosinase. (C) bears no relation to the relevance of the hypotheses.

2. D

The table shows that the cooler temperature correlates with more active melanin production and hence, tyrosinase activity level. A lower temperature (A) means more activity. The table shows varying activity levels with different group temperatures (B). A small percentage of coloration is detected at 5° (C).

3. C

The limb is the coolest region of the body, since it is the farthest from the body's core. Thus, it will have the highest activity rate at lower temperatures based on the passage results.

4. A

The active site (A) is most sensitive and involved in the activity of any enzyme. The other areas are either not as involved or not real areas of an enzyme.

5. D

At tertiary or quaternary levels, the active site emerges and is most delicate and susceptible to temperature changes.

6. B

Allosteric inhibitor (B) would alter enzymatic activity after translation of the gene and the activity level of tyrosinase. (A) and (C) apply to tyrosinase levels and would refute hypothesis 1 because it is pre-translational. (D) is simply about pH, which is an unknown variable based upon the passage.

7. B

There is some coloration at 10°C indicating some level of activity (B). There is no complete denaturing at any level (A) and (D). Choice (C) is a distracter because an allosteric site would enhance enzymatic activity if it were denatured, but in this case, activity is only moderate at 25°C so it's less plausible than (B).

8. A

pH is often a physical factor regulating enzymatic activity. Pressure is not generally an issue in living systems' enzymatic metabolism.

PASSAGE II

9. D

The passage states that the glomerular filtration rate is equal to the clearance of inulin, which is neither secreted nor reabsorbed. Glucose is normally always reabsorbed from the proximal convoluted tubules.

10. A

Less of the solute has been excreted than has entered the Bowman's capsule.

11. A

GFR is best approximated by a solute that is neither secreted nor reabsorbed in the glomerulus.

12. C

Inulin is a polysaccharide, as the passage states. Inulin would not be able to filter into the Bowman's capsule if it were bigger than an erythrocyte (red blood cell) or albumin (A) and (B), both of which cannot be filtered.

13. C

Approximately 90 percent of PAH which enters the kidneys, whether via the glomerular apparatus or nephron vasculature, is excreted. (A) and (B) are wrong because PAH would not be able to be filtered if it were bigger than an erythrocyte and albumin.

14. A

Clearance is a measurement of the excretion flow rate and GFR is a flow rate measurement of all the volume of fluid, including the solute, which filters through all the glomeruli in the body.

15. A

PAH clearance is equal to RPF, and if you look at the graph, a plasma creatinine concentration of 4 mg/dL corresponds to about 30 mL/min. Thus, using the filtration fraction equation, you get 30 mL/min/550 mL/min.

16. A

PAH is equal to RPF, and if one remembers that plasma is a component of blood, renal blood flow should be greater than renal plasma flow.

PASSAGE III

17. A

Interferons are messenger proteins that cause upregulation of anti-infective genes in other cells. This means that the antiviral properties of interferons can be utilized only on pathogens located within the cell, such as viruses and a few bacteria. They have no effect on typical extracellular pathogens such as fungi and protozoa.

18. D

Interferon works to protect cells that have yet to be virally infected or which have yet to undergo viral uncoating inside the cell. Addition of interferon at this point in time would not be protective to the cells on the plate, and would thus cause the cytotoxic effect to clear the plate of viable cells.

19. D

Viral RNA is needed to produce proteins vital to viral proliferation, which includes the capsid protein. The viral envelope is obtained as the virus buds off of the infected cell and is not synthesized by genetic material contained in the virus. The cytotoxic burst is not a characteristic of every virus's replication cycle. Some viruses carry their own nucleic acid polymerase and thus do not need to penetrate the nucleus. The genetic material of the virus can be DNA or RNA; thus, the virus's inability to infect is not specific to the inhibition of viral RNA.

20. D

Stimulation of humoral, or B cell immunity, requires presentation of antigens to B cells, which then form antibodies specific to those antigens. Inflammation, phagocytosis, and histamine are mechanisms used by the non-specific and/or cell-mediated immune system. B lymphocytes may or may not be activated, depending on if they carry the immunoglobulin specific to the antigen being presented. Therefore, the most specific indication of B cell activation is the presence of immunoglobulins.

21. D

Cytotoxic T cells eliminate infected cells in three main ways: first, direct cytotoxicity via granzymes (B), second, indirect cytotoxicity via the FAS/FAS-L pathway (C), and third, interferon production, stimulating phagocytosis of the infected cell (D). Immunoglobulin production is a hallmark of the humoral immune system (A).

22. A

Recall that the thymus is the maturation site for T cells, the predominant lymphocyte in the bloodstream. Without this maturation process, T lymphocytes are quickly removed from circulation.

23. B

Oxygen is required for the synthesis of digestive enzymes used by macrophages. Poor perfusion leading to chronically hypoxic tissue tends to result in macrophages with a diminished ability to phagocytize foreign material and present antigens to stimulate the B cell response.

QUESTIONS 24–29

24. D

Insertional mutagenesis (A) describes site-directed mutagenesis. Nucleotide template-directed polymerization (B) describes the polymerase chain reaction (PCR). Plasmid-driven transcription (C) describes the creation of a knock-in mutant. This is a straight recall question.

25. D

This question requires that you recall the assumptions of the Hardy-Weinberg model. Rather than predicting an answer outright, it is easier to scan the answer choices and eliminate those that are not tenets of the model. (A) is a distortion because mating between species would introduce new genes into the pool and thus change the frequency of alleles in a population. However, you could be fooled by the phrase "set rate," which implies stability. (B) and (C) directly contradict the HW model.

26. B

This question requires you to reason through the renin-angiotensin-aldosterone (RAS) system. Renin is secreted by the juxtaglomerular apparatus (JGA) in response to low vascular volume (and hence low blood pressure). This causes the release of angiotensin, which in turn causes the release of aldosterone from the zona glomerulosa of the adrenal cortex. (A) causes the release of angiotensin. (C) is released in response to high serum calcium levels. (D) is released in response to TSH.

27. C

Stop: What do you have to know to answer this question? Think: How is the likelihood of inheritance of a trait determined? Predict: The second child's genotype is independent of the first. The genotype of the first child is unrelated to the odds of the second child having a given genotype. Using a Punnett square, with *C* as the normal gene and c as the gene for cystic fibrosis, the chances of the child inheriting the *cc* genotype, and thus having the disease, are 25 percent.

28. C

The formula for determining the number of genetically unique gametes for a given genotype with two possible alleles at each gene is 2^n, where n = 3. Therefore, there are a total of eight possible gametes.

29. A

Here you must know the role of the loop of Henle in the nephron. The question stem states that it maintains the osmotic gradient. It therefore allows the urine to become more concentrated, or hypertonic to the blood. (B) is wrong because a steeper osmotic gradient would allow more sodium to be excreted, not less. (C) is wrong because urine should be hypertonic to body fluids, to allow the body to clear waste without becoming dehydrated. (D) is wrong because the loop of Henle does not reabsorb blood proteins. In fact, blood proteins should not pass through the glomerulus at all; they are too large and their negative charge prohibits glomerular filtration.

QUESTIONS 30–36

30. A

(A) is correct because steroids are lipid-based and will pass into the cell readily. (B) is incorrect because peptides are generally negatively charged and thus would not move across the phospholipid membrane. (C) is incorrect because second messengers are molecules that work within the cell in response to activation from substance that bind to the cell membrane, rather than themselves originating from outside the cell. (D) is incorrect because glucose is a hydrophilic substance and a glucose analog would be unlikely to pass readily across the plasma membrane without a glucose transporter molecule.

31. D

Choice (A) is incorrect because there is no reason that the lungs would be uniquely suited to support the growth of mycobacteria. (B) is incorrect because although the lungs are the site for oxygen exchange, the digestive tract also has sufficient oxygen to support aerobic bacterial growth, such as the bacteria that causes stomach ulcers. (C) is incorrect because the bile salts are involved in fat emulsification, and would not likely prohibit bacterial growth. (D) is correct because it explains why the digestive tract is inhospitable to bacterial growth: most bacteria will not survive in the low pH of the stomach.

32. A

The question requires you to know that vasopressin (ADH) and oxytocin are the hormones released by the posterior pituitary gland. Because vasopressin increases fluid retention, a tumor causing increased vasopressin release could lead to hypertension. Plasma calcium levels are increased and decreased by parathyroid hormone and calcitonin, respectively, which are not related to the posterior pituitary, and thus choices (B) and (C) are incorrect. Choice (D), precocious puberty, can be triggered by a tumor forming on the anterior pituitary gland, which releases FSH and LH, but not the posterior gland.

33. D

To answer this question, you need to know that osteoclasts are responsible for reabsorbing bone into the blood. Choice (D), the macrophage, is a cell type that is also responsible for engulfing substances (such as infectious materials). Of choices (A), (B), and (C), red blood cells supply oxygen to the tissues, fibroblasts compose connective tissue and skin, and plasma cells produce antibodies as part of the immune response, but none of these cell types have roles in physiology analogous to that of an osteoclast.

34. B

(A) is incorrect because bronchiole constriction would decrease gas exchange, thus contributing to decreased running performance. Choice (B) is correct because increased surfactant would facilitate gas exchange by reducing surface tension on the alveoli, not reduce it. Choice (C) is incorrect because swollen epithelial linings would make it more difficult for gas exchange to occur. (D) is incorrect because these cilia normally beat continuously to remove excess fluids and foreign debris from the respiratory tract.

35. A

The question relies on your knowledge of the differences between prokaryotes and eukaryotes. Even if you do not remember which of the structures are found in prokaryotes such as bacteria, you can predict the answer based on your knowledge that prokaryotes lack membrane-bound organelles. Ribosomes lack membranes, so choice (A) is correct. (B), the mitochondrion, has the inner and outer membranes crucial to the electron transport chain. (C), the Golgi apparatus, has a single membrane. (D), the nuclear membrane, would not be present in a prokaryote, because it lacks a nucleus.

36. C

The question asks how coding for a functional protein could be retained in the presence of a genetic mutation. (A) is incorrect because mutations in DNA actually give rise to a wide array of illnesses. (B) is incorrect because codons are always the same size and would not expand to fill a gap; furthermore, there would be no physical gap to fill because the codons would still be linked normally in the DNA strand. (C) is correct because codons consist of three base pairs. If three base pairs were deleted, the reading frame would be conserved and a polypeptide would be created lacking one amino acid but otherwise normal; function might be retained. (D) is incorrect because back mutations resulting in restored function are extremely rare

PASSAGE IV

37. C

The bone marrow of centrally located bones such as the skull, sternum, vertebrae, and pelvis is primarily where hematopoiesis is located. The liver and spleen are sites of red cell production in the fetus, and occasionally in children and adults if the bone marrow is unable to keep up with demand for new red blood cells.

38. B

The kidney is the site of hydroxylation of vitamin D precursors into the most biologically active form, 1,25-dihydroxycholecalciferol. Folic acid and riboflavin (Vitamin B_2) are supplied by diet. Vitamin K is obtained from dietary sources as well as from the normal flora present in the large intestine.

39. C

EPO stimulates red blood cell formation in the bone marrow and is also thought to promote longevity of the red blood cell once it leaves the bone marrow. Thus lack of EPO would not result in abnormally sized or shaped cells unless an iron deficiency was also present. Schistocytes are the remnants of destroyed red blood cells in the circulation.

40. D

ELISA utilizes labeled antibodies which can be formulated to almost any moiety, including the manufactured sugars attached to exogenous EPO. Northern and Western blots are tests of RNA and protein expression, respectively. A peripheral smear would be used to examine the relative shapes and sized of blood cells. Spectrophotometry would not be sensitive in a blood sample.

41. B

Heme synthesis is dependent on iron stores in the body. Oxygen carrying capacity of red blood cells is dependent on the concentration of heme. Thus at chronically low states of oxygen, the body eventually loses the ability to compensate due to exhaustion of iron stores. At low oxygen states, one would expect elevated amounts of HIF, which the data confirms. Clumping of red blood cells would cause an increase in the expected red blood cell percentage.

42. C

HIF is thought to be an enhancer of EPO transcription in the cells of the kidney. Therefore a nonsense mutation would result in the loss of negative feedback regulation. HIF would not be hydroxylated and inactivated at high levels of oxygen. With this, one would expect that EPO production would remain constant at all levels of oxygen concentrations.

43. A

Red blood cells are anuclear—therefore, they do not reproduce by binary fission nor make proteins once they are matured and released into the bloodstream. The lack of a nucleus makes the cell particularly bendable, and thus able to navigate narrow capillaries. The structural proteins of the red blood cell allow it to fold down upon itself without losing its functional capacity to carry oxygen. The red blood cell membrane contains both cholesterol for structural stability and proteins to allow interactions with endothelial cells in capillaries.

44. A

HIF is active in its nonhydroxylated state to act as a transcription factor for EPO. The effect of EPO on erythropoiesis is mediated by the EPO receptor in the bone marrow. Heme precursors (amino acids and pyroxidine) become heme by a process dependent on iron stores. Increased red blood cell production leads to tissue oxygenation by improved oxygen carrying capacity of the blood per volume.

45. A

Epinephrine preferentially shunts blood away from the digestive and filtration systems of the body toward systems that facilitate escape from danger. The blood vessels supplying the kidneys vasoconstrict, thus exposing them to lower levels of oxygenated blood. In addition to increased EPO production, renin secretion also increases, as the vasoconstriction of the renal arterioles causes a sensation of volume depletion to the cells of the kidney. Epinephrine is normally regulated with a negative feedback mechanism. Prolonged exposure to exogenous epinephrine would shut down the body's normal production of it.

46. C

Methemoglobin reductase is responsible for converting Fe^{3+} back to Fe^{2+} in order to bind to oxygen. Fe^{3+} incorporated into heme is seen in 1–2 percent of molecules in a healthy individual. This percentage can increase with certain blood cell or metabolic diseases, leading to a chronic hypoxic state. The pneumonic OIL RIG (oxidation is loss, reduction is gain) can be used to remember how charges change.

PASSAGE V

47. D

Vitamin D is an important part of bone development. It can be synthesized from a precursor that is found in the skin. This precursor gets hydroxylated in the liver and again in the kidneys to become active. Vitamin D then acts at the kidney and intestine to increase reabsorption and absorption of calcium respectively. The development of the periosteum (A) will not be affected by a decrease in sunlight. Vitamin C (B) is important to the hydroxylation and cross-linking of collagen fibrils, not for bone development. Slight changes in barometric pressure (C) will not impact bone development.

48. B

Osteoclasts are responsible for breaking down bone so it can be remodeled or so calcium can be released into the serum. Osteoclast function is opposed by osteoblasts which lay down bone matrix that is subsequently calcified (remember osteoBlast Builds). Overactivity of osteoclasts will cause bone loss, known clinically as osteoporosis. Overactivity of T and B cells (C) and (D) can cause a variety of problems including autoimmunity, leukemia, and hypergammaglobulinemia, but will not directly contribute to bone loss.

49. D

Secondary healing is responsible for most of bone healing. It involves the presence of a large hematoma that forms at the site of a bone break. This hematoma becomes a callus, which is subsequently vascularized. Collagen is laid down by mesechymal cells that migrate to the callus from the periosteum and surrounding soft tissue. Over time, the collagen that is laid down is replaced by calcified bone. Primary healing (C) is the direct deposition of bone at the site of a fracture without the step of collagen deposition that is subsequently replaced by bone. Membranous ossification (B) is a process of bone development that is responsible for the development of flat bones like the pelvis and bones of the cranium. In these instances, no collagen skeleton is present before bone is produced. Endochondral ossification (A) involves the deposition of collagen. (A) and (B) are processes of embryologic bone development, not bone healing.

50. D

Calcium is crucial to the functioning of nervous and muscle contraction. The key to this question is to know that the parathyroid glands and cells producing calcitonin are ensheathed with the thyroid. If the thyroid is removed, parathyroid must be retained to maintain calcium homeostasis. Calcitonin (B) does not contribute nearly as much to calcium homeostasis, so no effort is made to preserve those cells. In this case, lack of PTH (A) leaves the serum calcium relatively unchecked, and the patient will have calcium in excess producing her symptoms.

51. B

Vitamin D is one of four fat-soluble vitamins; A, K, and E are also stored in the fat. The other common vitamins are water-soluble and are lost in the urine if they aren't used at the time of ingestion.

52. C

The thymus is an organ in the neck which is very active during development and childhood. T cells in the thymus undergo a process of clonal deletion; if, for example a T cell "recognizes" or seeks to attack antigens naturally present on body tissues, that T cell will be eliminated by the thymus so it does not proliferate and go into the body to attack "self" tissues. Clonal deletion may lead to autoimmune attacks, in which T cells attack body tissue that they believe is foreign material; the problem is that the T cells think the foreign material must be neutralized and removed from the body.

INDEX

E

F

G

M

N

O

P

R

S

T

MCAT®

PHYSICS

2009–2010 EDITION

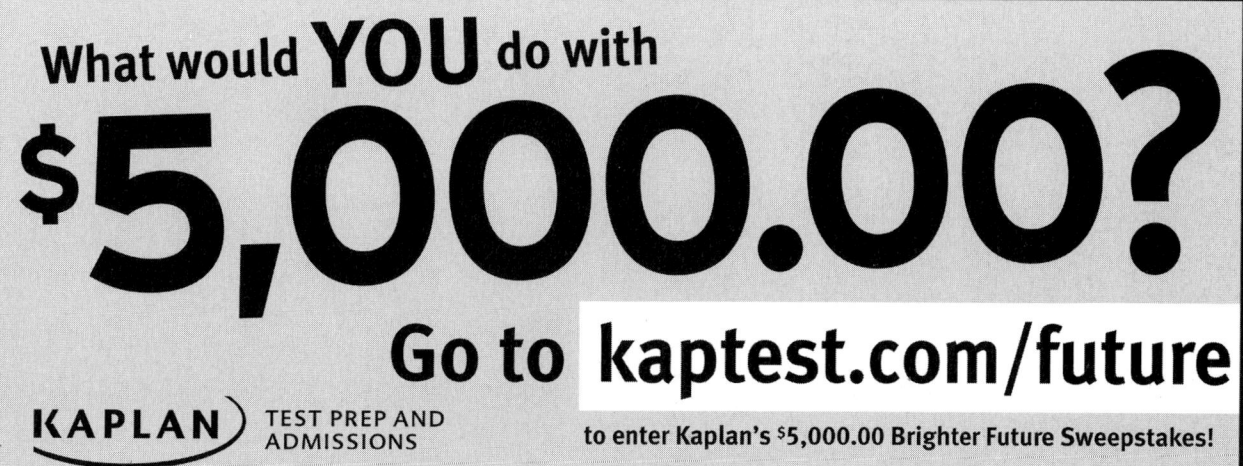

Related Titles

Kaplan MCAT Biology 2009–2010
Kaplan MCAT General Chemistry 2009–2010
Kaplan MCAT Organic Chemistry 2009–2010
Kaplan MCAT Verbal Reasoning and Writing 2009–2010

MCAT®

PHYSICS

2009–2010 EDITION

The Staff of Kaplan

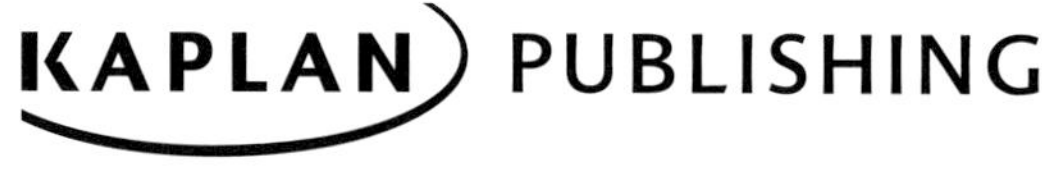

New York

Published by Kaplan Publishing, a division of Kaplan, Inc.
1 Liberty Plaza, 24th Floor
New York, NY 10006

Printed in the United States of America

10 9 8 7 6 5 4 3 2 1

ISBN: 978-1-4277-9875-6

Kaplan Publishing books are available at special quantity discounts to use for sales promotions, employee premiums, or educational purposes. Please email our Special Sales Department to order or for more information at kaplanpublishing@kaplan.com, or write to Kaplan Publishing, 1 Liberty Plaza, 24th Floor, New York, NY 10006.

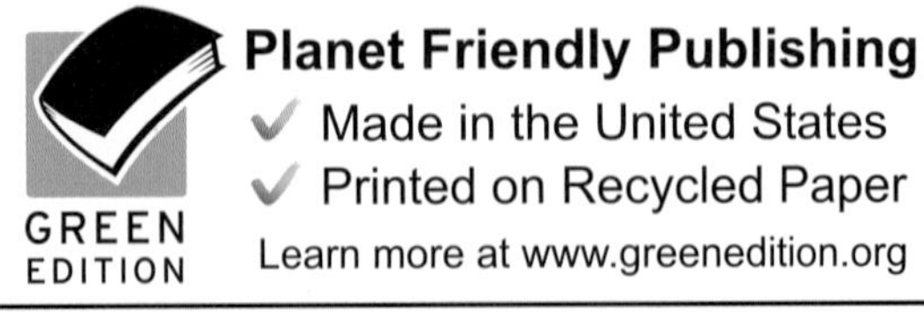
Planet Friendly Publishing
Made in the United States
Printed on Recycled Paper
GREEN EDITION
Learn more at www.greenedition.org

- Manufacturing books in the United States ensures compliance with strict environmental laws and eliminates the need for international freight shipping, a major contributor to global air pollution. Printing on recycled paper helps minimize our consumption of trees, water and fossil fuels.
- Trees Saved: 63 • Air Emissions Eliminated: 5,593 pounds
- Water Saved: 24,682 gallons • Solid Waste Eliminated: 2,429 pounds

Contents

How to Use this Book

Kaplan MCAT Physics, along with the other four books in our MCAT subject review series, brings the Kaplan classroom experience right into your home!

Kaplan has been preparing premeds for the MCAT for more than 40 years in our comprehensive courses. In the past 15 years alone, we've helped over 400,000 students prepare for this important exam and improve their chances of medical school admission.

TEACHER TIPS

Think of Kaplan's five MCAT subject books as having a private Kaplan teacher right by your side! We've created a team of the **top MCAT teachers in the country**, who have read through these comprehensive guides. On every page, they offer the same tips, advice, and Test Day insight as in their Kaplan classroom.

Pay close attention to **Teacher Tip** sidebars like this:

> **TEACHER TIP**
> While it's good to be aware of the various systems of measurement, the only system you are required to know for the MCAT is the SI system.

When you see these, you know what you're getting the same insight and knowledge that students in Kaplan MCAT classrooms across the country receive.

HIGH-YIELD MCAT REVIEW

At the end of several chapters, you'll find a special **High-Yield Questions** spread. These questions tackle the most frequently tested topics found on the MCAT. For each type of problem, you will be provided with a stepwise technique for solving the question and key directional points on how to solve for the MCAT specifically.

Included on each spread are two icons: the first, a sideways hand pointing toward equations, notes equations that you should memorize for the MCAT. The second, an open hand, indicates where in a problem you can stop without doing further calculation.

At the end of each topic you will find a "Takeaways" box, which gives a concise summary of the problem-solving approach; and a "Things to watch out for" box, which points out any caveats to the approach discussed above that usually lead to wrong answer choices. Finally, there is a "Similar Questions" box at the end so you can test your ability to apply the stepwise technique to analogous questions. You can find the answers in the Answers and Explanations section of this book.

We're confident that this guide, and our award-wining Kaplan teachers, can help you achieve your goals of MCAT success and admission into medical school!

Good luck!

EXPERT KAPLAN MCAT TEAM

Marilyn Engle

MCAT Master Teacher; Teacher Trainer; Kaplan National Teacher of the Year, 2006; Westwood Teacher of the Year, 2007; Westwood Trainer of the Year, 2007; Encino Trainer of the Tear, 2005

John Michael Linick

MCAT Teacher; Boulder Teacher of the Year, 2007; Summer Intensive Program Faculty Member

Dr. Glen Pearlstein

MCAT Master Teacher; Teacher Trainer; Westwood Teacher of the Year, 2006

Matthew B. Wilkinson

MCAT Teacher; Teacher Trainer; Lone Star Trainer of the Year, 2007

Introduction to the MCAT

THE MCAT

The Medical College Admission Test, affectionately known as the MCAT, is different from any other test you've encountered in your academic career. It's not like the knowledge-based exams from high school and college, whose emphasis was on memorizing and regurgitating information. Medical schools can assess your academic prowess by looking at your transcript. The MCAT isn't even like other standardized tests you may have taken, where the focus was on proving your general skills.

TEST TIP

The MCAT places more weight on your thought process. However you must have a strong hold of the required core knowledge. The MCAT may not be a perfect gauge of your abilities, but it is a relatively objective way to compare you with students from different backgrounds and undergraduate institutions.

Medical schools use MCAT scores to assess whether you possess the foundation upon which to build a successful medical career. Though you certainly need to know the content to do well, the stress is on thought process, because the MCAT is above all else a thinking test. That's why it emphasizes reasoning, critical and analytical thinking, reading comprehension, data analysis, writing, and problem-solving skills.

The MCAT's power comes from its use as an indicator of your abilities. Good scores can open doors. Your power comes from preparation and mindset, because the key to MCAT success is knowing what you're up against. That's where this section of this book comes in. We'll explain the philosophy behind the test, review the sections one by one, show you sample questions, share some of Kaplan's proven methods, and clue you in to what the test makers are really after. You'll get a handle on the process, find a confident new perspective, and achieve your highest possible scores.

ABOUT THE MCAT

Information about the MCAT CBT is included below. For the latest information about the MCAT, visit www.kaptest.com/mcat.

MCAT CBT

Format	United States—All administrations on computer International—Most on computer with limited paper and pencil in a few isolated areas
Essay Grading	One human and one computer grader
Breaks	Optional break between each section
Length of MCAT Day	Approximately 5.5 hours
Test Dates	Multiple dates in January, April, May, June, July, August, and September Total of 24 administrations each year.
Delivery of Results	Within 30 days. If scores are delayed notification will be posted online at www.aamc.org/mcat Electronic and paper
Security	Government-issued ID Electronic thumbprint Electronic signature verification
Testing Centers	Small computer testing sites

PLANNING FOR THE TEST

As you look toward your preparation for the MCAT consider the following advice:

Complete your core course requirements as soon as possible. Take a strategic eye to your schedule and get core requirements out of the way now.

Take the MCAT once. The MCAT is a notoriously grueling standardized exam that requires extensive preparation. It is longer than the graduate admissions exams for business school (GMAT, 3½ hours), law school (LSAT, 3¼ hours) and graduate school (GRE, 2½ hours). You do not want to take it twice. Plan and prepare accordingly.

> **KAPLAN EXCLUSIVE**
>
> Go online and sign up for a local Kaplan Pre-Med Edge event to get the latest information on the test.

THE ROLE OF THE MCAT IN ADMISSIONS

More and more people are applying to medical school and more and more people are taking the MCAT. It's important for you to recognize that while a high MCAT score is a critical component in getting admitted to top med schools, it's not the only factor. Medical school admissions officers weigh grades, interviews, MCAT scores, level of involvement in extracurricular activities, as well as personal essays.

In a Kaplan survey of 130 premed advisors, 84 percent called the interview a "very important" part of the admissions process, followed closely by college grades (83%) and MCAT scores (76%). Kaplan's college admissions consulting practice works with students on all these issues so they can position themselves as strongly as possible. In addition, the AAMC has made it clear that scores will continue to be valid for three years, and that the scoring of the computer-based MCAT will not differ from that of the paper and pencil version.

REGISTRATION

The only way to register for the MCAT is online. The registration site is: www.aamc.org/mcat.

You will be able to access the site approximately six months before your test date. Payment must be made by MasterCard or Visa.

Go to www.aamc.org/mcat/registration.htm and download *MCAT Essentials* for information about registration, fees, test administration, and preparation. For other questions, contact:

MCAT Care Team
Association of American Medical Colleges
Section for Applicant Assessment Services
2450 N. St., NW
Washington, DC 20037
www.aamc.org/mcat
Email: mcat@aamc.org

You will want to take the MCAT in the year prior to your planned start date. For example, if you want to start medical school in Fall 2010, you will need to take the MCAT and apply in 2009. Don't drag your feet gathering information. You'll need time not only to prepare and practice for the test, but also to get all your registration work done.

ANATOMY OF THE MCAT

TEST TIP

The MCAT should be viewed just like any other part of your application: as an opportunity to show the medical schools who you are and what you can do. Take control of your MCAT experience.

Before mastering strategies, you need to know exactly what you're dealing with on the MCAT. Let's start with the basics: The MCAT is, among other things, an endurance test.

If you can't approach it with confidence and stamina, you'll quickly lose your composure. That's why it's so important that you take control of the test.

The MCAT consists of four timed sections: Physical Sciences, Verbal Reasoning, Writing Sample, and Biological Sciences. Later in this section we'll take an in-depth look at each MCAT section, including sample question types and specific test-smart hints, but here's a general overview, reflecting the order of the test sections and number of questions in each.

Physical Sciences

Time	70 minutes
Format	• 52 multiple-choice questions: approximately 7–9 passages with 4–8 questions each • approximately 10 stand-alone questions (not passage-based)
What it tests	basic general chemistry concepts, basic physics concepts, analytical reasoning, data interpretation

Verbal Reasoning

Time	60 minutes
Format	• 40 multiple-choice questions: approximately 7 passages with 5–7 questions each
What it tests	critical reading

Writing Sample

Time	60 minutes
Format	• 2 essay questions (30 minutes per essay)
What it tests	critical thinking, intellectual organization, written communication skills

Biological Sciences

Time	70 minutes
Format	• 52 multiple-choice questions: approximately 7–9 passages with 4–8 questions each • approximately 10 stand-alone questions (not passage-based)
What it tests	basic biology concepts, basic organic chemistry concepts, analytical reasoning, data interpretation

TEST TIP

There's no penalty for a wrong answer on the MCAT, so NEVER LEAVE ANY QUESTION BLANK, even if you only have time for a wild guess.

The sections of the test always appear in the same order:

Physical Sciences

[optional 10-minute break]

Verbal Reasoning

[optional 10-minute break]

Writing Sample

[optional 10-minute break]

Biological Sciences

SCORING

Each MCAT section receives its own score. Physical Sciences, Verbal Reasoning, and Biological Sciences are each scored on a scale ranging from 1–15, with 15 as the highest. The Writing Sample essays are scored alphabetically on a scale ranging from J to T, with T as the highest. The two essays are each evaluated by two official readers, so four critiques combine to make the alphabetical score.

TEST TIP

The percentile figure tells you how many other test takers scored at or below your level. In other words, a percentile figure of 80 means that 80 percent did as well or worse than you did, and that only 20 percent did better.

The number of multiple-choice questions that you answer correctly per section is your "raw score." Your raw score will then be converted to yield the "scaled score"—the one that will fall somewhere in that 1–15 range. These scaled scores are what are reported to medical schools as your MCAT scores. All multiple-choice questions are worth the same amount—one raw point—and *there's no penalty for guessing*. That means that *you should always select an answer for every question, whether you get to that question or not!* This is an important piece of advice, so pay it heed. Never let time run out on any section without selecting an answer for every question.

Your score report will tell you—and your potential medical schools—not only your scaled scores, but also the national mean score for each section, standard deviation, national scoring profile for each section, and your percentile ranking.

WHAT'S A GOOD SCORE?

There's no such thing as a cut-and-dry "good score." Much depends on the strength of the rest of your application (if your transcript is first rate, the pressure to strut your stuff on the MCAT isn't as intense) and on where you want to go to school (different schools have different score expectations). Here are a few interesting statistics:

For each MCAT administration, the average scaled scores are approximately 8s for Physical Sciences, Verbal Reasoning, and Biological Sciences, and N for the Writing Sample. You need scores of at least 10–11s to be considered competitive by most medical schools, and if you're aiming for the top you've got to do even better, and score 12s and above.

You don't have to be perfect to do well. For instance, on the AAMC's Practice Test 5R, you could get as many as 10 questions wrong in Verbal Reasoning, 17 in Physical Sciences, and 16 in Biological Sciences and still score in the 80th percentile. To score in the 90th percentile, you could get as many as seven wrong in Verbal Reasoning, 12 in Physical Sciences, and 12 in Biological Sciences. Even students who receive perfect scaled scores usually get a handful of questions wrong.

It's important to maximize your performance on every question. Just a few questions one way or the other can make a big difference in your scaled score. Here's a look at recent score profiles so you can get an idea of the shape of a typical score distribution.

Physical Sciences		
Scaled Score	Percent Achieving Score	Percentile Rank Range
15	0.1	99.9–99.9
14	1.2	98.7–99.8
13	2.5	96.2–98.6
12	5.1	91.1–96.1
11	7.2	83.9–91.0
10	12.1	71.8–83.8
9	12.9	58.9–71.1
8	16.5	42.4–58.5
7	16.7	25.7–42.3
6	13.0	12.7–25.6
5	7.9	04.8–12.6
4	3.3	01.5–04.7
3	1.3	00.2–01.4
2	0.1	00.1–00.1
1	0.0	00.0–00.0
Scaled Score Mean = 8.1 Standard Deviation = 2.32		

Verbal Reasoning		
Scaled Score	Percent Achieving Score	Percentile Rank Range
15	0.1	99.9–99.9
14	0.2	99.7–99.8
13	1.8	97.9–99.6
12	3.6	94.3–97.8
11	10.5	83.8–94.2
10	15.6	68.2–83.7
9	17.2	51.0–68.1
8	15.4	35.6–50.9
7	10.3	25.3–35.5
6	10.9	14.4–25.2
5	6.9	07.5–14.3
4	3.9	03.6–07.4
3	2.0	01.6–03.5
2	0.5	00.1–01.5
1	0.0	00.0–00.0
Scaled Score Mean = 8.0 Standard Deviation = 2.43		

TEST TIP

The raw score of each administration is converted to a scaled score. The conversion varies with administrations. Hence, the same raw score will not always give you the same scaled score.

Writing Sample		
Scaled Score	Percent Achieving Score	Percentile Rank Range
T	0.5	99.9–99.9
S	2.8	94.7–99.8
R	7.2	96.0–99.3
Q	14.2	91.0–95.9
P	9.7	81.2–90.9
O	17.9	64.0–81.1
N	14.7	47.1–63.9
M	18.8	30.4–47.0
L	9.5	21.2–30.3
K	3.6	13.5–21.1
J	1.2	06.8–13.4
		02.9–06.7
		00.9–02.8
		00.2–00.8
		00.0–00.1
75th Percentile = Q 50th Percentile = O 25th Percentile = M		

Biological Sciences		
Scaled Score	Percent Achieving Score	Percentile Rank Range
15	0.1	99.9–99.9
14	1.2	98.7–99.8
13	2.5	96.2–98.6
12	5.1	91.1–96.1
11	7.2	83.9–91.0
10	12.1	71.8–83.8
9	12.9	58.9–71.1
8	16.5	42.4–58.5
7	16.7	25.7–42.3
6	13.0	12.7–25.6
5	7.9	04.8–12.6
4	3.3	01.5–04.7
3	1.3	00.2–01.4
2	0.1	00.1–00.1
1	0.0	00.0–00.0
Scaled Score Mean = 8.2 Standard Deviation = 2.39		

WHAT THE MCAT REALLY TESTS

It's important to grasp not only the nuts and bolts of the MCAT, so you'll know *what* to do on Test Day, but also the underlying principles of the test so you'll know *why* you're doing what you're doing on Test Day. We'll cover the straightforward MCAT facts later. Now it's time to examine the heart and soul of the MCAT, to see what it's really about.

THE MYTH

Most people preparing for the MCAT fall prey to the myth that the MCAT is a straightforward science test. They think something like this:

> *"It covers the four years of science I had to take in school: biology, chemistry, physics, and organic chemistry. It even has equations. OK, so it has Verbal Reasoning and Writing, but those sections are just to see if we're literate, right? The important stuff is the science. After all, we're going to be doctors."*

Well, here's the little secret no one seems to want you to know: The MCAT is not just a science test; it's also a thinking test. This means that the test is designed to let you demonstrate your thought process, not only your thought content.

The implications are vast. Once you shift your test-taking paradigm to match the MCAT modus operandi, you'll find a new level of confidence and control over the test. You'll begin to work with the nature of the MCAT rather than against it. You'll be more efficient and insightful as you prepare for the test, and you'll be more relaxed on Test Day. In fact, you'll be able to see the MCAT for what it is rather than for what it's dressed up to be. We want your Test Day to feel like a visit with a familiar friend instead of an awkward blind date.

THE ZEN OF MCAT

Medical schools do not need to rely on the MCAT to see what you already know. Admission committees can measure your subject-area proficiency using your undergraduate coursework and grades. Schools are most interested in the potential of your mind.

In recent years, many medical schools have shifted pedagogic focus away from an information-heavy curriculum to a concept-based curriculum. There is currently more emphasis placed on problem solving, holistic thinking, and cross-disciplinary study. Be careful not to dismiss this important point, figuring you'll wait to worry about academic trends until you're actually in medical school. This trend affects you right now, because it's reflected in the MCAT. Every good tool matches its task. In this case the tool is the test, used to measure you and other candidates, and the task is to quantify how likely it is that you'll succeed in medical school.

Your intellectual potential—how skillfully you annex new territory into your mental boundaries, how quickly you build "thought highways" between ideas, how confidently and creatively you solve problems—is far more important to admission committees than your ability to recite Young's modulus for every material known to man. The schools assume they can expand your knowledge base. They choose applicants carefully because expansive knowledge is not enough to succeed in medical school or in the profession. There's something more. It's this "something more" that the MCAT is trying to measure.

Every section on the MCAT tests essentially the same higher-order thinking skills: analytical reasoning, abstract thinking, and problem solving.

Most test takers get trapped into thinking they are being tested strictly about biology, chemistry, and so on. Thus, they approach each section with a new outlook on what's expected. This constant mental gear-shifting can be exhausting, not to mention counterproductive. Instead of perceiving the test as parsed into radically different sections, you need to maintain your focus on the underlying nature of the test: It's designed to test your thinking skills, not your information-recall skills. Each test section thus presents a variation on the same theme.

WHAT ABOUT THE SCIENCE?

With this perspective, you may be left asking these questions: "What about the science? What about the content? Don't I need to know the basics?" The answer is a resounding "Yes!" You must be fluent in the different languages of the test. You cannot do well on the MCAT if you don't know the basics of physics, general chemistry, biology, and organic chemistry. We recommend that you take one year each of biology, general chemistry, organic chemistry, and physics before taking the MCAT, and that you review the content in this book thoroughly. Knowing these basics is just the beginning of doing well on the MCAT. That's a shock to most test takers. They presume that once they recall or relearn their undergraduate science, they are ready to do battle against the MCAT. Wrong! They merely have directions to the battlefield. They lack what they need to beat the test: a copy of the test maker's battle plan!

> **TEST TIP**
>
> Don't think of the sections of the MCAT as unrelated timed pieces. Each is a variation on the same theme, because the underlying purpose of each section and of the test as a whole is to evaluate your thinking skills. Memorizing formulas won't boost your score. Understanding fundamental scientific principles will.

You won't be drilled on facts and formulas on the MCAT. You'll need to demonstrate ability to reason based on ideas and concepts. The science questions are painted with a broad brush, testing your general understanding.

TAKE CONTROL: THE MCAT MINDSET

In addition to being a thinking test, as we've stressed, the MCAT is a standardized test. As such, it has its own consistent patterns and idiosyncrasies that can actually work in your favor. This is the key to why test preparation works. You have the opportunity to familiarize yourself with those consistent peculiarities, to adopt the proper test-taking mindset.

> **TEST TIP**
>
> Those perfectionist tendencies that make you a good student and a good medical school candidate may work against you in MCAT Land. If you get stuck on a question or passage, move on. Perfectionism is for medical school—not the MCAT. You don't need to understand every word of a passage before you go on to the questions—what's tripping you up may not even be relevant to what you'll be asked.

The following are some overriding principles of the MCAT mindset that will be covered in depth in the chapters to come:

- Read actively and critically.
- Translate prose into your own words.

- Save the toughest questions for last.
- Know the test and its components inside and out.
- Do MCAT-style problems in each topic area after you've reviewed it.
- Allow your confidence to build on itself.
- Take full-length practice tests a week or two before the test to break down the mystique of the real experience.
- Learn from your mistakes—get the most out of your practice tests.
- Look at the MCAT as a challenge, the first step in your medical career, rather than as an arbitrary obstacle.

That's what the MCAT mindset boils down to: Taking control. Being proactive. Being on top of the testing experience so that you can get as many points as you can as quickly and as easily as possible. Keep this in mind as you read and work through the material in this book and, of course, as you face the challenge on Test Day.

Now that you have a better idea of what the MCAT is all about, let's take a tour of the individual test sections. Although the underlying skills being tested are similar, each MCAT section requires that you call into play a different domain of knowledge. So, though we encourage you to think of the MCAT as a holistic and unified test, we also recognize that the test is segmented by discipline and that there are characteristics unique to each section. In the overviews, we'll review sample questions and answers and discuss section-specific strategies. For each of the sections—Verbal Reasoning, Physical/Biological Sciences, and the Writing Sample—we'll present you with the following:

- **The Big Picture**
  You'll get a clear view of the section and familiarize yourself with what it's really evaluating.
- **A Closer Look**
  You'll explore the types of questions that will appear and master the strategies you'll need to deal with them successfully.
- **Highlights**
  The key approaches to each section are outlined, for reinforcement and quick review.

TEST EXPERTISE

The first year of medical school is a frenzied experience for most students. In order to meet the requirements of a rigorous work schedule, students either learn to prioritize and budget their time or else fall hopelessly behind. It's no surprise, then, that the MCAT, the test specifically designed to predict success in the first year of medical school, is a high-speed, time-intensive test. It demands excellent time-management skills as well as that sine qua non of the successful physician—grace under pressure.

It's one thing to answer a Verbal Reasoning question correctly; it's quite another to answer several correctly in a limited time frame. The same goes for Physical and Biological Sciences—it's a whole new ballgame once you move from doing an individual passage at your leisure to handling a full section under actual timed conditions. You also need to budget your time for the Writing Sample, but this section isn't as time sensitive. When it comes to the multiple-choice sections, time pressure is a factor that affects virtually every test taker.

TEST TIP

For complete MCAT success, you've got to get as many correct answers as possible in the time you're allotted. Knowing the strategies is not enough. You have to perfect your time-management skills so that you get a chance to use those strategies on as many questions as possible.

So when you're comfortable with the content of the test, your next challenge will be to take it to the next level—test expertise—which will enable you to manage the all-important time element of the test.

THE FIVE BASIC PRINCIPLES OF TEST EXPERTISE

On some tests, if a question seems particularly difficult you'll spend significantly more time on it, as you'll probably be given more points for correctly answering a hard question. Not so on the MCAT. Remember, every MCAT question, no matter how hard, is worth a single point. There's no partial credit or "A" for effort, and because there are so many questions to do in so little time, you'd be a fool to spend 10 minutes getting a point for a hard question and then not have time to get a couple of quick points from three easy questions later in the section.

TEST TIP

In order to meet the stringent time requirements of the MCAT, you have to cultivate the following elements of test expertise:

- Feel free to skip questions.
- Learn to recognize and seek out questions you can do.
- Use a process of answer elimination.
- Remain calm.
- Keep track of time.

Given this combination—limited time, all questions equal in weight—you've got to develop a way of handling the test sections to make sure you get as many points as you can as quickly and easily as you can. Here are the principles that will help you do that:

1. FEEL FREE TO SKIP AROUND

One of the most valuable strategies to help you finish the sections in time is to learn to recognize and deal first with the questions that are easier and more familiar to you. That means you must temporarily skip those that promise to be difficult and time-consuming, if you feel comfortable doing so. You can always come back to these at the end, and if you run out of time, you're much better off not getting to questions you may have had difficulty with, rather than not getting to potentially feasible material. Of course, because there's no guessing penalty, always put an answer to every question on the test, whether you get to it or not. (It's not practical to skip passages, so do those in order.)

This strategy is difficult for most test takers; we're conditioned to do things in order, but give it a try when you practice. Remember, if you do the test in the exact order given, you're letting the test makers control you. You control how you take this test. On the other hand, if skipping around goes against your moral fiber and makes you a nervous wreck—don't do it. Just be mindful of the clock, and don't get bogged down with the tough questions.

2. LEARN TO RECOGNIZE AND SEEK OUT QUESTIONS YOU CAN DO

Another thing to remember about managing the test sections is that MCAT questions and passages, unlike items on the SAT and other standardized tests, are not presented in order of difficulty. There's no rule that says you have to work through the sections in any particular order; in fact, the test makers scatter the easy and difficult questions throughout the section, in effect rewarding those who actually get to the end. Don't lose sight of what you're being tested for along with your reading and thinking skills: efficiency and cleverness.

Don't waste time on questions you can't do. We know that skipping a possibly tough question is easier said than done; we all have the natural instinct to plow through test sections in their given order, but it just doesn't pay off on the MCAT. The computer won't be impressed if you get the toughest question right. If you dig in your heels on a tough question, refusing to move on until you've cracked it, well, you're letting your ego get in the way of your test score. A test section (not to mention life itself) is too short to waste on lost causes.

TEST TIP

Every question is worth exactly one point, but questions vary dramatically in difficulty level. Given a shortage of time, work on easy questions and then move on to the hard ones.

TEST TIP

Don't let your ego sabotage your score. It isn't easy for some of us to give up on a tough, time-consuming question, but sometimes it's better to say "uncle." Remember, there's no point of honor at stake here, but there are MCAT points at stake.

3. USE A PROCESS OF ANSWER ELIMINATION

Using a process of elimination is another way to answer questions both quickly and effectively. There are two ways to get all the answers right on the MCAT. You either know all the right answers, or you know all the wrong answers. Because there are three times as many wrong answers, you should be able to eliminate some if not all of them. By doing so you either get to the correct response or increase your chances of guessing the correct response. You start out with a 25 percent chance of picking the right answer, and with each eliminated answer your odds go up. Eliminate one, and you'll have a $33\frac{1}{3}$ percent chance of picking the right one, eliminate two, and you'll have a 50 percent chance, and, of course, eliminate three, and you'll have a 100 percent chance. Increase your efficiency by actually crossing out the wrong choices on the screen using the strike-through feature. Remember to look for wrong-answer traps when you're eliminating. Some answers are designed to seduce you by distorting the correct answer.

4. REMAIN CALM

It's imperative that you remain calm and composed while working through a section. You can't allow yourself to become so rattled by one hard reading passage that it throws off your performance on the rest of the section. Expect to find at least one killer passage in every section, but remember, you won't be the only one to have trouble with it. The test is curved to take the tough material into account. Having trouble with a difficult question isn't going to ruin your score—but getting upset about it and letting it throw you off track will. When you understand that part of the test maker's goal is to reward those who keep their composure, you'll recognize the importance of not panicking when you run into challenging material.

5. KEEP TRACK OF TIME

Of course, the last thing you want to happen is to have time called on a particular section before you've gotten to half the questions. Therefore, it's essential that you pace yourself, keeping in mind the general guidelines for how long to spend on any individual question or passage. Have a sense of how long you have to do each question, so you know when you're exceeding the limit and should start to move faster.

So, when working on a section, always remember to keep track of time. Don't spend a wildly disproportionate amount of time on any one question or group of questions. Also, give yourself 30 seconds or so at the end of each section to fill in answers for any questions you haven't gotten to.

SECTION-SPECIFIC PACING

Let's now look at the section-specific timing requirements and some tips for meeting them. Keep in mind that the times per question or passage are only averages; there are bound to be some that take less time and some that take more. Try to stay balanced. Remember, too, that every question is of equal worth, so don't get hung up on any one. Think about it: If a question is so hard that it takes you a long time to answer it, chances are you may get it wrong anyway. In that case, you'd have nothing to show for your extra time but a lower score.

VERBAL REASONING

Allow yourself approximately eight to ten minutes per passage and respective questions. It may sound like a lot of time, but it goes quickly. Keep in mind that some passages are longer than others. On average, give yourself about three or four minutes to read and then four to six minutes for the questions.

> **TEST TIP**
>
> For Verbal Reasoning, here are some of the important time techniques to remember:
>
> - Spend eight to ten minutes per passage
> - Allow about three to four minutes to read and four to six minutes for the questions

PHYSICAL AND BIOLOGICAL SCIENCES

Averaging over each section, you'll have about one minute and 20 seconds per question. Some questions, of course, will take more time, some less. A science passage plus accompanying questions should take about eight to nine minutes, depending on how many questions there are. Standalone questions can take anywhere from a few seconds to a minute or more. Again, the rule is to do your best work first. Also, don't feel that you have to understand everything in a passage before you go on to the questions. You may not need that deep an understanding to answer questions, because a lot of information may be extraneous. You should overcome your perfectionism and use your time wisely.

> **TEST TIP**
>
> Some suggestions for maximizing your time on the science sections:
>
> - Spend about eight to nine minutes per passage
> - Maximize points by doing the questions you can do first
> - Don't waste valuable time trying to understand extraneous material

WRITING SAMPLE

You have exactly 30 minutes for each essay. As mentioned in discussion of the seven-step approach to this section, you should allow approximately five minutes to prewrite the essay, 23 minutes to write the essay, and two minutes to proofread. It's important that you budget your time, so you don't get cut off.

COMPUTER-BASED TESTING STRATEGIES

ARRIVE AT THE TESTING CENTER EARLY

Get to the testing center early to jump-start your brain. However, if they allow you to begin your test early, decline.

USE THE MOUSE TO YOUR ADVANTAGE

If you are right-handed, practice using the mouse with your left hand for Test Day. This way, you'll increase speed by keeping the pencil in your right hand to write on your scratch paper. If you are left-handed, use your right hand for the mouse.

KNOW THE TUTORIAL BEFORE TEST DAY

You will save time on Test Day by knowing exactly how the test will work. Click through any tutorial pages and save time.

PRACTICE WITH SCRATCH PAPER

Going forward, always practice using scratch paper when solving questions because this is how you will do it on Test Day. Never write directly on a written test.

GET NEW SCRATCH PAPER

Between sections, get a new piece of scratch paper even if you only used part of the old one. This will maximize the available space for each section and minimize the likelihood of you running out of paper to write on.

REMEMBER YOU CAN ALWAYS GO BACK

Just because you finish a passage or move on, remember you can come back to questions about which you are uncertain. You have the "marking" option to your advantage. However, as a general rule minimize the amount of questions you mark or skip.

MARK INCOMPLETE WORK

If you need to go back to a question, clearly mark the work you've done on the scratch paper with the question number. This way, you will be able to find your work easily when you come back to tackle the question.

LOOK AWAY AT TIMES

Taking the test on computer leads to faster eye-muscle fatigue. Use the Kaplan strategy of looking at a distant object at regular intervals. This will keep you fresher at the end of the test.

PRACTICE ON THE COMPUTER

This is the most critical aspect of adapting to computer-based testing. Like anything else, in order to perform well on computer-based tests you must practice. Spend time reading passages and answering questions on the computer. You often will have to scroll when reading passages.

Part I
Subject Review

CHAPTER 1

UNITS AND KINEMATICS

In this first chapter we will review some of the basic mathematics necessary for the study of MCAT physics, such as scientific notation, basic trigonometric functions, and vectors. In addition, the topic of units is presented with emphasis on the three systems of units that you need to be familiar with, *i.e.,* MKS, CGS, and FPS. Finally, the topic of kinematics, which is the study of motion, is discussed. Here, a review is given of the basic quantities of displacement, speed, velocity, and acceleration. These basic quantities are then applied to the study of motion with constant acceleration. The case of one-dimensional motion is discussed, including an example of free-fall. The case of projectile motion, which is motion in two dimensions, is also covered in a detailed example.

UNITS

A. FUNDAMENTAL MEASUREMENTS AND DIMENSIONS

Physics is the most basic of all the sciences. Everything in the world around us is subject to the laws of physics. In order to describe nature, physicists use the language of mathematics, in the form of equations, to make their quantitative descriptions.

These descriptions, however, mean nothing if they are not expressed in some kind of units. While explaining how you were pulled over on the highway doing seventy might mean something amongst friends, a scientist would ask whether your speed was 70 miles per hour or 70 kilometers per hour or some other speed. Scientists have developed systems of units that give meaning to all the numbers in the formulas. The British, or **FPS,** system is commonly used in America but virtually nowhere else in the world (not even in Britain). Basic units for length, weight, and time are the foot (ft), the pound (lb), and the second (s), respectively. The most common system of units is the metric system, the basic units of which include length, mass (instead of weight like in FPS), and time. The metric system comes in two main variations. One metric system uses meter (m), kilogram (kg), and second (s) as its base, and is referred to as **MKS** and

> **MCAT SYNOPSIS**
> Don't mix units! An answer with the correct number of *incorrect* units may be one of the choices.

MCAT SYNOPSIS

On the MCAT, conversion factors will be given when needed.

TEACHER TIP

While it's good to be aware of the various systems of measurement, the only system you are required to know for the MCAT is the SI system.

also **SI** (SI being the initials of the French abbreviation for the International System of Units). The other metric system uses centimeter (cm), gram (g), second (s) and is referred to as **CGS.** The SI system is becoming the standard.

The following chart lists some important units in the three systems

Some Important Units

Quantity	CGS	SI	FPS
Length	centimeter (cm)	meter (m)	foot (ft)
Mass	gram (g)	kilogram (kg)	slug (sl)
Force	dyne (dyn)	Newton (N)	pound (lb)
Time	second (s)	second (s)	second (s)
Work & Energy	erg	Joule (J)	foot-pound (ft•lb)
Power	erg/second	Watt (W)	foot-pound/sec

MCAT SYNOPSIS

Most Common Prefixes:

$m = 10^{-3}$, $k = 10^{3}$, $\mu = 10^{-6}$, $M = 10^{6}$, $n = 10^{-9}$

In atomic-sized systems, because of the extremely small scale of the interactions, some different scales are used that make the numbers a little easier to handle. Useful length units on the atomic scale include the angstrom (Å where 1 Å = 10^{-10} m) and the nanometer (nm), where 1 nm = 10^{-9} m. Also important at this level is the unit of energy called the electron–volt (eV), which is the energy acquired by an electron accelerating through a potential difference of one volt. Compared with the SI unit of energy, the joule, the electron–volt is very small (1 eV = 1.6×10^{-19} J).

Metric system prefixes are often added to units to make numbers easier to handle. The chart below lists prefixes sometimes encountered.

Multiples

factor	prefix	prefix abbreviation
10^{9}	giga	G (or B)
10^{6}	mega	M
10^{3}	kilo	k

Submultiples

factor	prefix	prefix abbreviation
10^{-2}	centi	c
10^{-3}	milli	m
10^{-6}	micro	μ
10^{-9}	nano	n
10^{-12}	pico	p

B. SCIENTIFIC NOTATION

Scientific notation is a convention for expressing numbers that simplifies computation and standardizes results. To express a number in scientific notation, convert it into a number between one and ten, then multiply it by 10 to the appropriate power.

Example: $123 = 1.23 \times 10^2$

1.23 is the **mantissa** and 2 is the **exponent** (power of ten)

Example: $0.042 = 4.2 \times 10^{-2}$

One can easily obtain products and quotients of numbers expressed in scientific notation. When multiplying, one simply multiplies the mantissas and adds the exponents to find the new mantissa and exponent of the answer. Some additional conversion may be necessary so that the new mantissa is again between one and ten as in the third example on this page.

Example: $(1.1 \times 10^6)(5.0 \times 10^{17}) = ?$

Solution: Multiply the mantissas 1.1 and 5.0, and add the exponents 6 and 17.

The answer is 5.5×10^{23}.

The quotient of two numbers expressed in scientific notation is obtained by dividing the mantissa in the numerator by the mantissa in the denominator, and subtracting the power of 10 in the denominator from the power of 10 in the numerator.

Example: $\dfrac{6.2 \times 10^5}{2.0 \times 10^{-7}}$

Solution: Divide 6.2 by 2.0 and subtract –7 from 5 (note that $5 - (-7) = 5 + 7 = 12$).

The answer is 3.1×10^{12}.

When a number expressed in scientific notation is raised to a power, the mantissa is raised to that power, and the exponent is multiplied by that number.

MCAT SYNOPSIS

Avoid excess calculating by seeing if the correct power of 10 is enough.

TEACHER TIP

Always look at your answer choices before diving into a problem. This will give you an idea of what you are actually solving for, as well as the scale of the answers. If your answer choices are all different by a power of 10 or more, you can make your work easier by rounding, without worrying that your rounded answer may be too close to another answer choice.

TEACHER TIP

Because the MCAT is a timed test without the use of a calculator, it is essential that you know how to do math quickly by hand. Rounding can often help, though it is possible to manipulate numbers without doing so. In the example here, if you change 6.2×10^5 to 62×10^4, you know that 62 divided by 2 is 31 and that 4 minus (–7) is 11. You can then change 31×10^{11} to 3.1×10^{12}. Make these changes only if it truly makes sense in your head; otherwise, you'll lose time.

Example: $(6.0 \times 10^4)^2$

Solution: Square the 6.0 and multiply the exponent by 2.

$(6.0)^2 \times 10^{4 \times 2} = 36.0 \times 10^8 = 3.6 \times 10^9$

(Note that when we move the decimal point one place to the left we must increase the power of 10 by one, from 8 to 9.)

When adding or subtracting numbers expressed in scientific notation they must have the **same** power of 10; when they do not, the appropriate conversion must be made first.

Example: $3.7 \times 10^4 + 1.5 \times 10^3 = ?$

Solution: First convert 1.5×10^3 to 0.15×10^4 so both numbers have the same exponent. Then $3.7 \times 10^4 + 0.15 \times 10^4 = 3.85 \times 10^4$ rounded to 3.9×10^4.

C. TRIGONOMETRIC RELATIONS

TEACHER TIP

Remember high school? SOH(so), CAH(ca), TOA(toe-a)

SOH = sin is opposite over hypotenuse
CAH = cos is adjacent over hypotenuse
TOA = tan is opposite over adjacent

For the right triangle, the trigonometric functions for angle θ are:

$$\sin\theta = \frac{y}{h} = \frac{\text{opposite side}}{\text{hypotenuse}}$$

$$\cos\theta = \frac{x}{h} = \frac{\text{adjacent side}}{\text{hypotenuse}}$$

$$\tan\theta = \frac{y}{x} = \frac{\text{opposite side}}{\text{adjacent side}}$$

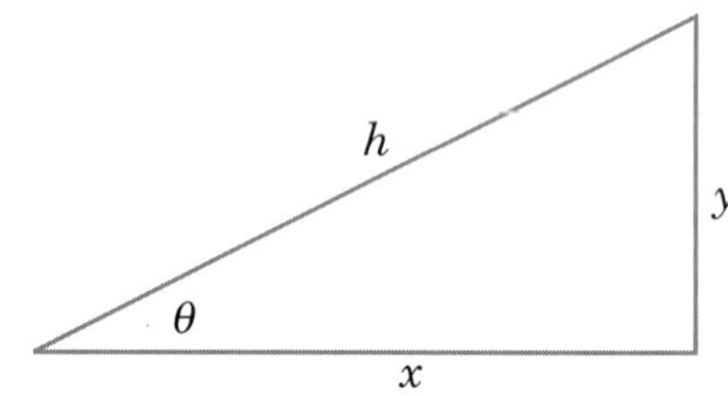

Some important values of the trigonometric functions:

TEACHER TIP

Because calculators are not permitted, you'll need to remember the functions in this table. Those that appear most frequently on the MCAT are the ones that work out to have nice clean numbers: sin of 0, 30, 90, 180, and cos of 0, 60, 90, 180.

π	sin π	cos π
0°	0°	1
30°	$\frac{1}{2}$	$\frac{\sqrt{3}}{2}$
45°	$\frac{\sqrt{2}}{2}$	$\frac{\sqrt{2}}{2}$
60°	$\frac{\sqrt{3}}{2}$	$\frac{1}{2}$
90°	1°	0
180°	0°	−1

D. VECTORS AND SCALARS

Scalars are those numerical quantities that have **magnitude** but no direction, such as distance, speed and mass. **Vector** quantities have **both magnitude and direction.** Some vector quantities are displacement, velocity, and force.

TEACHER TIP

It's important to know a scalar from a vector. Anything that can exist without a direction is a scalar. If you climb a mountain and reach 14,000 feet, the direction from which you approached doesn't matter, nor does the direction in which you are going. Regardless, you're at 14,000 feet. Elevation, then, is a scalar quantity.

1. Vector Representation

We can represent a vector by an arrow. The direction of the arrow corresponds to the direction of the vector. The length of the arrow **may or may not** be proportional to the magnitude of the vector. Common notations for a vector quantity are either an arrow or **boldface.** For example, vector A can be written as $\vec{A}$ or **A.** The magnitude of vector A can be represented as $|\vec{A}|$, **|A|,** or simply, A (no arrow or boldface).

MCAT SYNOPSIS

Scalars: speed, energy, magnitude of any vector.
Vectors: acceleration, force, momentum.

2. Vector Addition

The **sum** of two or more vectors is called the **resultant** of the vectors. The terms vector sum and resultant are interchangeable.

One method of finding the resultant A + B of the two vectors A and B is to place the tail of B at the tip of A (without changing the length or direction of either arrow). In this method of vector addition the lengths of the arrows **must** be proportional to the magnitudes of the vector. The vector sum A + B is the vector joining the tail of A to the tip of B and pointing towards the tip of B. For three or more vectors, proceed similarly (see Figure 1.1 below).

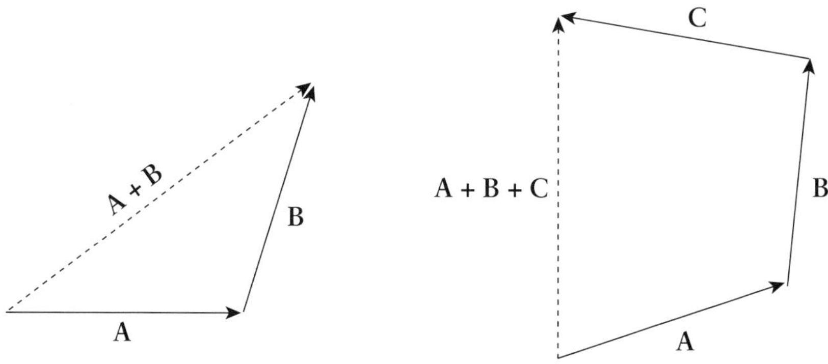

Figure 1.1

Another method more commonly used for finding the resultant of several vectors involves breaking each vector into perpendicular (*X* and *Y*) components. These components are often, but not always, horizontal and vertical.

MCAT SYNOPSIS

X and Y Components of V:
$V_x = V \cos \theta$, $V_y = V \sin \theta$

Given any vector **V**, we can find the **X** component and the **Y** component by drawing a right triangle with V as the hypotenuse (see Figure 1.2 below). If θ is the angle between V and the x direction, then $\cos \theta = X/V$ and $\sin \theta = Y/V$. In other words:

$$X = V \cos \theta$$

$$Y = V \sin \theta$$

Example: V = 10 m/s

θ = 30°

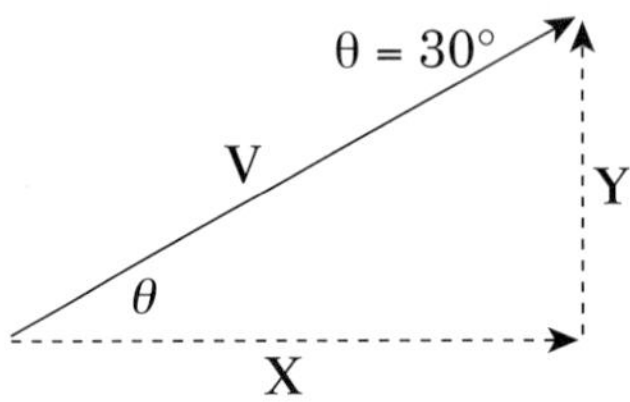

Figure 1.2

$$X = 10 \cos 30° = \frac{10\sqrt{3}}{2} = 5\sqrt{3} \text{ m/s}$$

$$Y = 10 \sin 30° = \frac{10}{2} = 5 \text{ m/s}$$

TEACHER TIP

Because calculators are not permitted, you'll be able to solve any of the problems with either the Pythagorean theorem or the values of sin and cos shown on the previous page. It is also to your advantage to know the most common Pythagorean triples such as 3:4:5 and 5:12:13.

Conversely, if we know X and Y, we can find V by using the Pythagorean theorem: $X^2 + Y^2 = V^2$; or $V = \sqrt{x^2 + y^2}$.

Example: X = 3 m/s

Y = 4 m/s

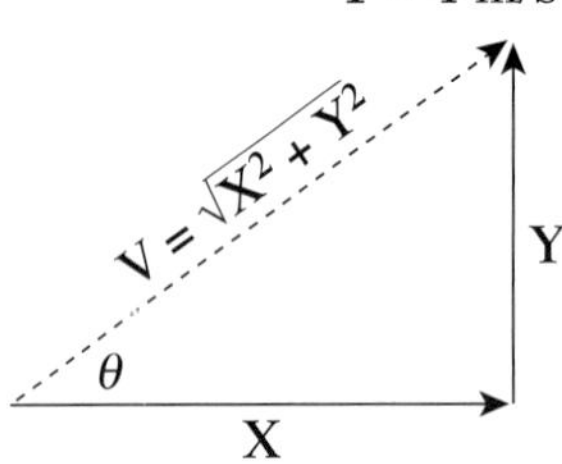

Figure 1.3

$$V = \sqrt{3^2 + 4^2} = \sqrt{25} = 5 \text{ m/s}$$

(Also note that we can find θ from $\tan \theta = Y/X$. In this example $\tan \theta = 4/3$, so $\theta = 53°$.)

The X component of the resultant vector is the sum of the X components of the vectors being added. Similarly, the Y component of the resultant vector is the sum of the Y components of the vectors being added.

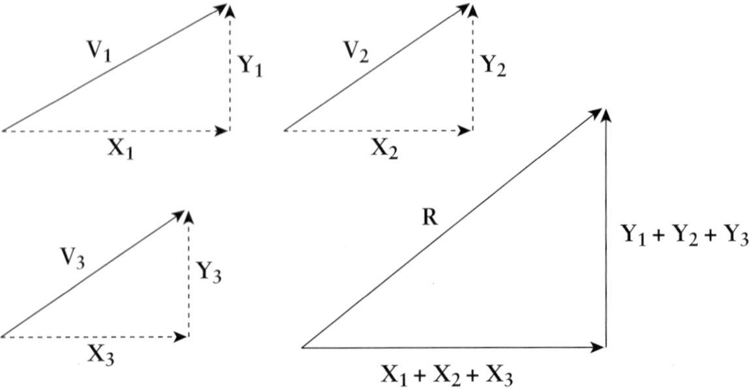

Figure 1.4

To find the resultant **(R)** using the components method:

1. Resolve the vectors to be summed into their X and Y components.
2. Add together the X components to get the X component of the resultant (R_x). In the same way, add the Y components to get the Y component of the resultant (R_y).
3. Find the magnitude of the resultant by using the Pythagorean theorem. If R_x and R_y are the components of the resultant then:

$$R = \sqrt{R_x^2 + R_y^2}$$

4. Find the direction (θ) of the resultant by using the relation $\tan\theta = \frac{R_y}{R_x}$. From the value of tan θ you can find θ, the angle R makes with the x direction.

TEACHER TIP

Remember, when adding vectors, *add tip to tail!*

MCAT SYNOPSIS

Magnitude of a vector V:

$V = \sqrt{Vx^2 + Vy^2}$

Example: Find the horizontal and vertical components of V.

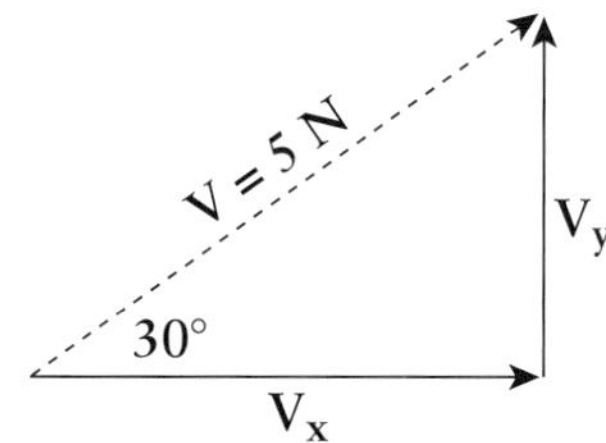

Figure 1.5

Solution: Let x be the horizontal direction and y be the vertical direction. Then:

$$V_x = V\cos\theta = 5\cos 30° = \frac{5\sqrt{3}}{2} = 2.5\sqrt{3}\text{ N} \approx 4.3\text{ N}$$

$$V_y = V\sin\theta = 5\sin 30° = \frac{5}{2} = 2.5\text{ N}$$

Example: Find the resultant of A, B, C, and D.

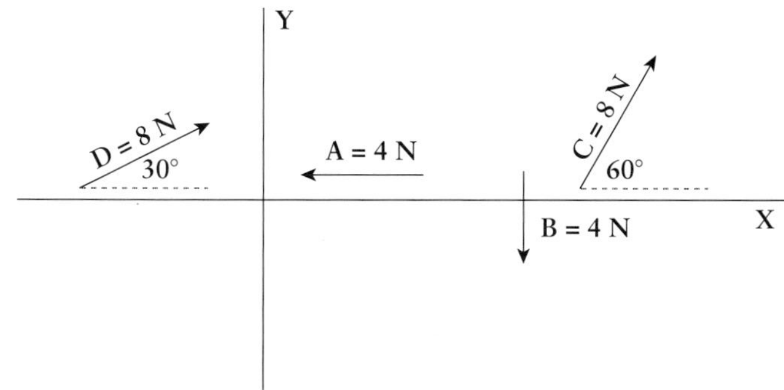

Figure 1.6

Solution: Resolve the vectors into their horizontal (x) and vertical (y) components. Note that we have x components going both left and right, and y components going both up and down. **In each case choose one direction as the positive direction. The other direction is then automatically the negative direction.** In this example we chose going to the right as the positive x direction (so to the left is negative), and up as the positive y direction (so down is negative). **A component in the positive direction is then positive and a component in the negative direction is then negative.**

a. $A_x = -4$ N

$B_x = 0$

$C_x = 8 \cos 60° = \frac{8}{2} = 4$ N

$D_x = 8 \cos 30° = \frac{8\sqrt{3}}{2} = 4\sqrt{3}$ N

b. $A_y = 0$

$B_y = -4$ N

$C_y = 8 \sin 60° = \frac{8\sqrt{3}}{2} = 4\sqrt{3}$ N

$D_y = 8 \sin 30° = \frac{8}{2} = 4$ N

Add together the components of A, B, C, and D to get the components of the resultant R:

a. $R_x = (-4) + 0 + 4 + 4\sqrt{3} = 4\sqrt{3}$ N

b. $R_y = 0 + (-4) + 4\sqrt{3} + 4 = 4\sqrt{3}$ N

Find the magnitude of the resultant:

$$R = \sqrt{R_x{}^2 + R_y{}^2}$$

$$R = \sqrt{(4\sqrt{3})^2 + (4\sqrt{3})^2} = \sqrt{96} = 4\sqrt{6} \text{ N}$$

Find the angle the resultant makes with the horizontal:

$$\tan\theta = \frac{4\sqrt{3}}{4\sqrt{3}} = 1;\ \theta = 45°$$

TEACHER TIP

Because X and Y are equal we know that it is a 45-degree angle without doing any work. Get in the habit of solving things quickly on the MCAT.

Thus, we have found that R is a vector of magnitude of $4\sqrt{6}$ N, making an angle of 45° with the horizontal. (In general, $\tan\theta = |R_y| / |R_x|$ where θ is the smallest angle with the x-axis.)

3. Vector Subtraction

Subtracting two vectors is exactly the same as adding the negative of the vector being subtracted. When expressed in a mathematical formula, the idea looks like this:

$$A - B = A + (-B)$$

By –B we mean a vector with the same magnitude as B, but pointing in the opposite direction.

TEACHER TIP

When we subtract vectors, we're simply flipping the direction of the vector being subtracted, and then following the same rules as normal: add tip to tail.

Example: What is the resultant of A – B as pictured below?

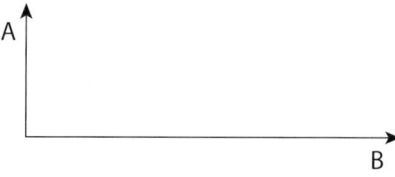

Figure 1.7

Solution: The first thing to do is make the vector –B. This is done by erasing the arrow head at the tip of B, and redrawing it where the tail used to be (see Figure 1.8a). Now, add this to A. To do this move the tip of A to the tail of –B, and join the tail of A to the tip of –B (see Figure 1.8b).

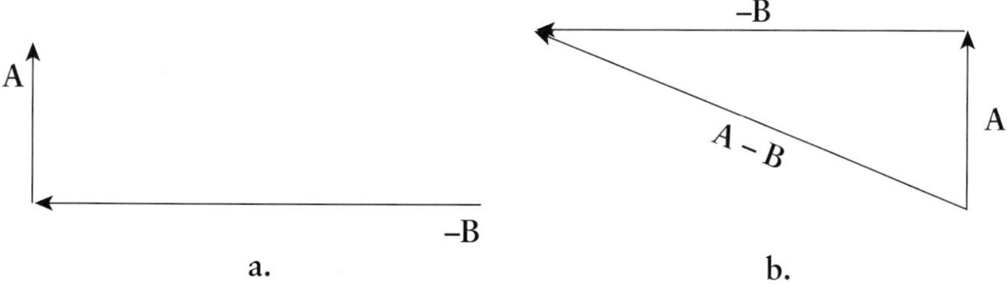

Figure 1.8

To find –B using the method whereby the vectors are broken up into their horizontal and vertical components, each vector component is multiplied by –1 before adding.

Example: If A has components $A_x = 3$ and $A_y = 4$ and B has components $B_x = 2$ and $B_y = 1$, then what is A – B?

Solution: First, remember A – B = A + (–B). Since B has components B_x and B_y, –B has components $-B_x$ and $-B_y$.

$$R_x = A_x - B_x = 3 - 2 = 1$$

$$R_y = A_y - B_y = 4 - 1 = 3$$

To get the magnitude of the final resultant vector R:

$$R = \sqrt{(3^2 + 1^2)}$$

$$= \sqrt{(9 + 1)} = \sqrt{10}$$

To get the direction:

$$\tan\theta = \frac{R_y}{R_x} = 3$$

$$\theta = 72^\circ$$

4. Multiplying a Vector by a Scalar

Now consider the case where a vector is multiplied by a scalar, B = nA. To find the magnitude of B simply multiply the magnitude of A by the absolute value of n, B = |n| A. If n is a positive number, then B and A are in the same direction. However, if n is a negative number, then B and A are in opposite directions. For example, if vector A is multiplied by +3, the resultant vector B will be three times as long as A and point in the same direction. However, if A is multiplied by –3, then B would again be three times as long as A, but it would point in the opposite direction.

TEACHER TIP

With kinematics questions, quickly sketch a picture of what is happening in the problem. This will keep everything relative, and help prevent common mistakes.

KINEMATICS

Kinematics is that branch of mechanics dealing with the description of motion. In physics, the **position** of an object or particle is defined on a three-dimensional coordinate axis. Most problems you will have to deal with concerning motion will involve only one or two dimensions.

A. DISPLACEMENT

The **displacement** (Δx) of an object is a vector quantity that describes the change in position. It goes (in a straight line) from the initial position to the final position without regard to the actual path taken. Because this is a vector quantity, displacement has both direction and magnitude.

Example: A man walks 2 km east, then 2 km north, then 2 km west, and then 2 km south. His actual total distance traveled is 8 km, because distance is a scalar. But his displacement is a vector quantity that is the change in position. In this case his displacement is zero, because the man ends up in the same place he started (see Figure 1.9).

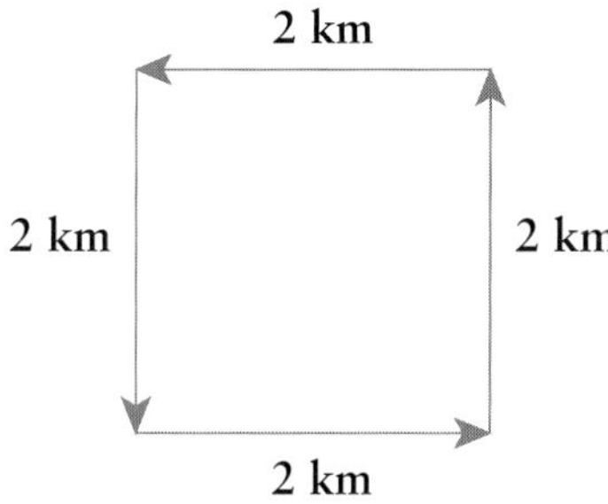

Figure 1.9

B. VELOCITY

1. Average Velocity

The **average velocity** of a particle is the ratio of the displacement vector over the change in time. It is a vector quantity.

$$\bar{\mathbf{v}} = \Delta\mathbf{x}/\Delta t$$

$\bar{\mathbf{v}}$ has the same direction as $\Delta\mathbf{x}$.

2. Instantaneous Velocity

The **instantaneous velocity** or **velocity** refers to a single instant of time. It is the average velocity as Δt approaches 0. This can be represented as:

$$v = \lim_{\Delta t \to 0} \Delta x/\Delta t$$

Graphically, this corresponds to the slope of the graph of the object's position with respect to time at the particular time t.

TEACHER TIP

The speedometer on a car does *not* indicate velocity. That is because the velocity changes every time the car changes direction. A car driving 30 mph in a circle has a constant speed of 30 mph, but a constantly changing velocity that is always tangential to the circle. This tangential velocity, as shown, is the instantaneous velocity.

Real-World Analogy

If a car goes 10 miles to the north and then drives 10 miles to the south, it will end it up where it started.

The $\Delta \mathbf{x} = 0$
The distance = 20 miles

In addition, if the car drives the 20 miles in 1 hour, then the speed is 20 m/hr, but the velocity is 0 m/hr.

3. Speed

The **average speed** is given by:

$$\bar{s} = d/\Delta t$$

where d is the actual distance traveled. It is a scalar. Because actual distance traveled is not always the same as the magnitude of the displacement vector, average speed is not always the same as the magnitude of the average velocity.

The **instantaneous speed** or **speed** is the magnitude of the instantaneous velocity vector. It is also a scalar.

C. ACCELERATION

1. Average Acceleration

Acceleration is the rate of change of an object's velocity. It is a vector quantity. **Average acceleration $\bar{\mathbf{a}}$** is the change in instantaneous velocity over the time period Δt:

$$\bar{\mathbf{a}} = \Delta\mathbf{v}/\Delta t$$

2. Instantaneous Acceleration

The **instantaneous acceleration**—the acceleration at one point of a particle's path—is defined the same way as instantaneous velocity, i.e., it is the average acceleration as Δt approaches 0.

$$\mathbf{a} = \lim_{\Delta t \to 0} \Delta\mathbf{v}/\Delta t$$

Graphically, this corresponds to the slope of the graph of the object's velocity with respect to time at the particular time t. The direction of the acceleration vector is not always along the direction of the velocity vector. The direction of **a** is the same as the direction of $\Delta\mathbf{v}$.

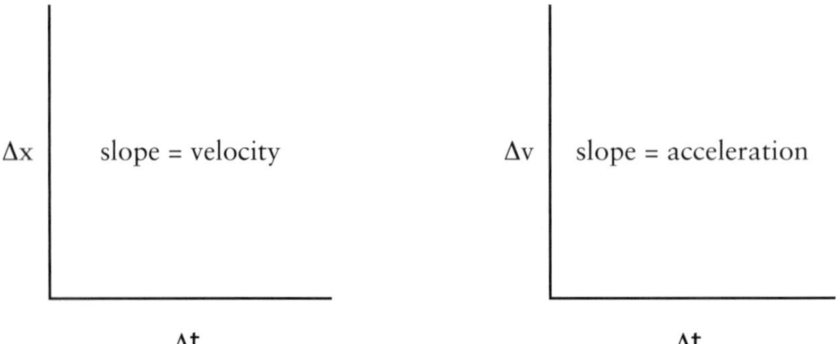

Figure 1.10

MOTION WITH CONSTANT ACCELERATION

The acceleration of a body is proportional to the force (see chapter 2) applied to that body. When a body is under the influence of a constant force, the acceleration is also constant. In the following sections it is assumed that the acceleration is constant.

TEACHER TIP

Newton's second law is one of the most important physics concepts on the MCAT, and is represented by F = ma. If you see force, think acceleration. If you see acceleration, think force.

A. LINEAR MOTION

In linear motion the acceleration and velocity vectors are along the line of motion. Note that the linear motion need not be in the horizontal direction. One-dimensional motion of this kind can be fully described by the following equations:

$$v = v_0 + at$$

$$x - x_0 = v_0t + \frac{at^2}{2}$$

$$v^2 = v_0^2 + 2a(x - x_0)$$

$$\bar{v} = \frac{(v_0 + v)}{2}$$

$$\Delta x = \bar{v}t = \left(\frac{v_0 + v}{2}\right)t$$

Notes:

1. v_0, x_0 are v and x at t = 0.
2. When the motion is vertical, we use y instead of x.
3. As illustrated below, in using these equations, we must remember that velocity and acceleration are vector quantities

By way of an example let's examine free-falling bodies. *Free-fall* means that the only force acting on a body is its own weight (gravity) and it neglects, for example, any force of air resistance. All objects in free-fall have the same acceleration called **the acceleration due to gravity (*g*),** which in SI units is 9.8 m/s^2. The following example demonstrates the use of the above equations in the analysis of free falling bodies.

Example: A ball is thrown vertically up into the air with an initial velocity of 10 m/s.

a. Find the position and velocity of the ball after 2 seconds.

b. Find the distance and time at which the ball reaches its maximum height.

Solution: a. Remember that velocity and acceleration are vector quantities. Taking the initial position of the ball $y_0 = 0$,

TEACHER TIP

When dealing with these types of problems, you can make "down" either positive or negative, thus making the force of gravity positive or negative. As long as you keep all forces upward and the opposite sign of all forces downward, you'll find the correct answer. For the sake of simplicity, we recommend always making *"up" positive* and *"down" negative.*

TEACHER TIP

Whenever an object reaches its maximum height, its velocity will be zero for the brief instant that it stops going "up" and starts falling "down." As soon as the ball leaves the person's hand, though, the only force acting on it will be gravity; thus, the ball's *acceleration* will be $-9.8 m/s^2$ the *entire* time it is in flight.

and taking "up" as positive, the initial velocity is v_0 = +10 m/s and the acceleration is $g = -9.8 m/s^2$. Notice g is negative because its direction is down, and we are taking "up" to be the positive direction. Velocity after two seconds can be found using the equation:

$$v = v_0 + at$$
$$= (+10) + (-9.8)(2)$$
$$= -9.6 \text{ m/s}$$

(Minus sign for v means that the ball is coming down).

After two seconds, the position of the ball is found using the equation:

$$y = v_0 t + \frac{at^2}{2} \quad (y_0 = 0)$$
$$= 10(2) + \frac{(-9.8)(2)^2}{2}$$
$$= 20 - 19.6$$
$$= +0.4 \text{ m}$$

b. When the ball is at its maximum height, the velocity, v, which has been decreasing on the way up, is zero. Using the following equation and plugging in values, we can find the maximum height the ball reaches above the ground:

$$v^2 = v_0^2 + 2ay$$
$$0 = (10)^2 + 2(-9.8)y$$
$$y = 5.1 \text{ m}$$

The time at which the ball reaches its maximum height can be found from the equation:

$$v = v_0 + at$$
$$0 = 10 + (-9.8)t$$
$$t = 1.0 \text{ s}$$

TEACHER TIP

The amount of time an object takes to get to its maximum height is the same time it takes for the object to fall back down. This fact makes solving problems easier; because you can solve for maximum height by setting your final velocity to zero, you can multiply your answer by two, giving you total time in flight. Because the only force acting on the object after it is launched is gravity, the velocity it has in the X direction will remain constant throughout its time in flight. By multiplying the time and the X velocity together, you can find the horizontal distance traveled.

B. PROJECTILE MOTION

Note again that we have been considering only linear motion in the above example. In the case of **projectile motion,** however, the object has velocity and position components in both the vertical and horizontal directions. The two components of the velocity vector v_x and v_y are

PAVLOV'S DOG

When you see projectile motion, think V_x is constant and $a_x = 0$.

independent, so the change in the vertical velocity v_y due to gravity does not affect and is not affected by the constant horizontal velocity v_x. The following example demonstrates how projectile motion is analyzed.

Example: A projectile is fired from ground level with an initial velocity of 50 m/s and an initial angle of elevation of 37°. Assuming $g = 10\ m/s^2$, find:

a. the projectile's total time in flight.

b. the maximum height attained.

c. the total horizontal distance traveled.

d. the final horizontal and vertical velocities just before it hits the ground.

(sin 37° = 0.6; cos 37° = 0.8)

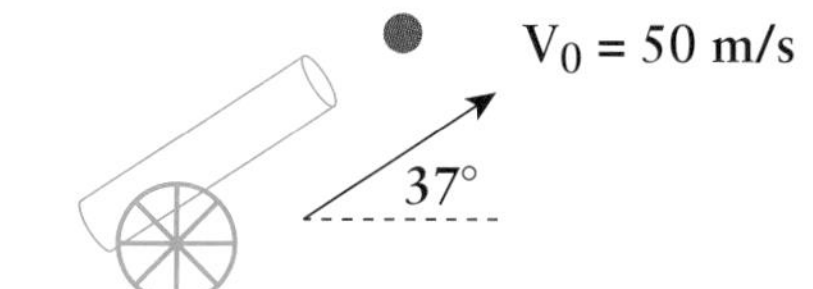

Figure 1.11

Solution: a. Let y equal the vertical height; let up be the positive direction.

$$a = -10\ m/s^2$$

$$y = v_{0_y}t + \frac{1}{2}at^2 \qquad (y_0 = 0)$$

$$v_{0_y} = v_0 \sin 37°$$

$$v_{0_y} = 50(0.6) = 30\ m/s$$

$$y = 30t - 5t^2$$

y = 0 both when the projectile is first fired and also when it hits the ground later. Its time in flight will be the difference between the values of t at the two points when y = 0.

$$30t - 5t^2 = 0$$

$$5t(6 - t) = 0$$

$$t = 0 \text{ (first fired)},\ t = 6 \text{ (hits the ground)}$$

Time in flight = 6 – 0 = 6 s

b. To find the maximum height attained:

$$v_y^2 = v_{0_y}^2 + 2ay$$

$$0 = 30^2 + 2(-10)(y) \ (v_y = 0 \text{ at highest point})$$

$$y = \frac{900}{20}$$

$$y = 45 \text{ m}$$

c. To find the horizontal distance traveled:

$$x = v_x t \quad (a_x = 0)$$

$$v_x = 50 \cos 37° = 40 \text{ m/s}$$

$$x = 40(6) = 240 \text{ m}$$

d. The horizontal velocity remains constant, so $v_x = 40$ m/s. To find the vertical velocity at impact:

$$v_y = v_{0_y} + at$$

$$v_y = 30 - 10(6)$$

$$v_y = 30 - 60$$

$$v_y = -30 \text{ m/s}$$

Because we chose up as positive, the minus sign means the vertical component of the velocity is directed down.

PRACTICE QUESTIONS

1. A computer monitor that weighs 10 kg is dropped from rest from a height of 50 meters. What is its speed as it hits the ground?

   A. –32 m/s
   B. –3.2 m/s
   C. 3.2 m/s
   D. 32 m/s

2. A rifle is held by a man whose arms are 1.5 m above the ground. He fires a bullet at 100 m/s at an angle of 30° with the horizontal. After 2.0 seconds, how far has the object traveled in the horizontal direction?

   A. 87 m
   B. 140 m
   C. 174 m
   D. 175.5 m

3. A hang gilder runs off a cliff, with a speed of 3 m/s. What is its overall velocity after 5 seconds?

   A. 3 m/s
   B. –5 m/s
   C. 5 m/s
   D. 10 m/s

4. A bored tennis player decides to set his ball machine on the edge of his school's roof and point it such that its barrel is completely perpendicular to the roof. A ball leaves the machine that is even with the rooftop fencing, with an upward speed of 30 m/s. On its way back down, it misses the building. How long does it take the ball to reach its maximum height?

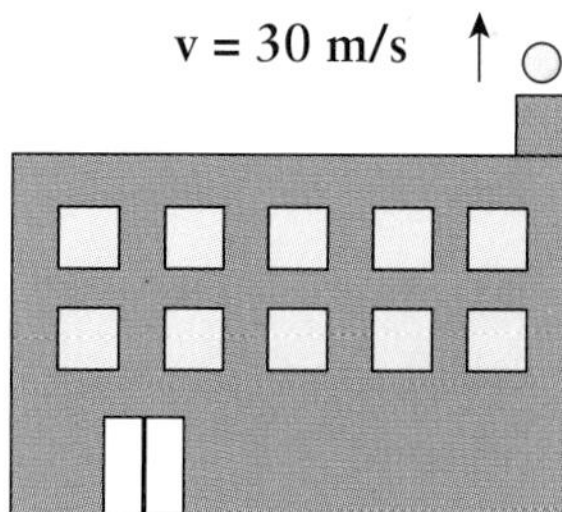

   A. 3 s
   B. 6 s
   C. 9 s
   D. 15 s

5. A student driver is asked to drive straight on a residential road. To determine how steadily she can control the car while following directions, her instructor tracks her speed and determines that her velocity at any time can be determined by the equation below. What is her average acceleration between 1 and 4 seconds?

   $$v = (0.5\ \text{m/s}^3)t^2 + 10\ \text{m/s}$$

   A. 0 m/s^2
   B. 0.5 m/s^2
   C. 2.5 m/s^2
   D. 7.5 m/s^2

6. A player mistakenly hits a ball much too high while playing a game. After he hits it, the ball moves with a speed of 50 m/s at an angle of 30° with the horizon. An observer notices that the ball reaches an apex directly above his head. How far above the ground is the ball at this point?

A. 2.5 m
B. 25 m
C. 26 m
D. 31 m

7. What two terms represent a vector quantity and the scalar quantity of the vector's magnitude?

A. Displacement and distance
B. Weight and force
C. Speed and time
D. Acceleration and velocity

8. A bike rider is training on a closed course. At point A, she passes her friend who has stopped on the side of the road and who notices that she is going 1 m/s at that point (see below). After passing her friend, she decides to accelerate at a pace of 0.5 m/s². She also notes that her friend's bike is 50 m from the start of the course. How far from the start is she when she has reached a speed of 3 m/s?

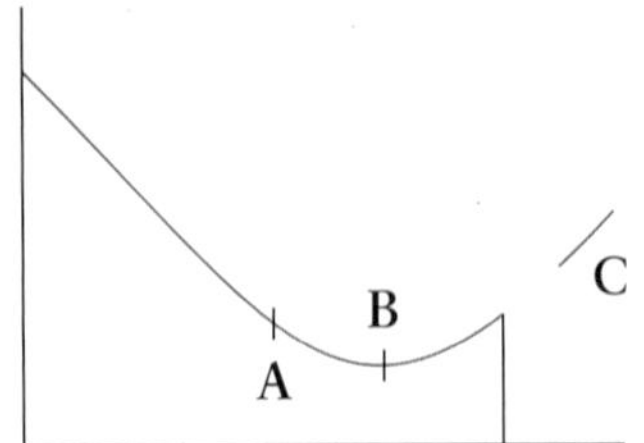

A. 3 m
B. 8 m
C. 54 m
D. 58 m

9. A, a rock, (m = 2 kg) is shot up vertically at the same time that B, a ball, (m = 0.5 kg) is projected horizontally. If both start from the same height,

A. A and B will reach the ground at the same time.
B. A will reach the ground first.
C. B will reach the ground first.
D. More information is required.

10. Two concurrent forces have a maximum resultant of 45 N and a minimum resultant of 5 N. What is the magnitude of each of these forces?

A. 0 N, 45 N
B. 0 N, 50 N
C. 5 N, 9 N
D. 20 N, 25 N

11. A ball is thrown horizontally with an initial velocity of 35 m/s from the top of a tower 125 m high. What is the horizontal velocity of the ball just before it reaches the ground?

A. 10 m/s
B. 20 m/s
C. 35 m/s
D. 60 m/s

12. Which of the following is a vector quantity?

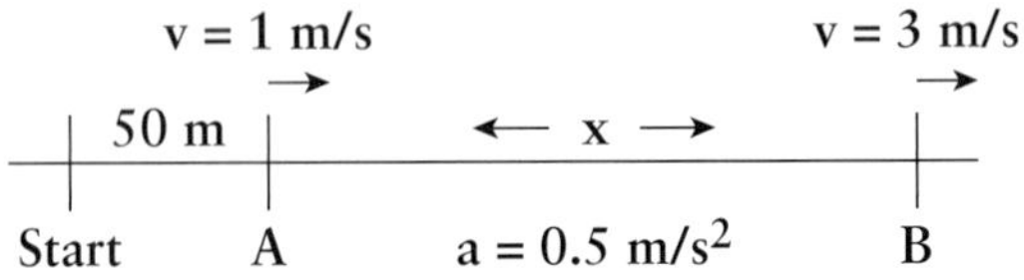

A. Charge of an electron moving toward a proton
B. Mass of a brick thrown to the right
C. Potential energy of a roller coaster at the top of a hill
D. Gravitational field strength of Saturn

13. A girl throws a ball horizontally from the top of a building with an initial velocity of 12 m/s. At that exact moment, her brother drops a rock from rest from the top of a building 20 m away and 15 m higher than that of his sister. The two balls will have the same

A. initial vertical velocity.
B. initial horizontal velocity.
C. path as they fall.
D. final velocity as they reach the ground.

14. A boy throws a basketball from the top of a set of bleachers, down to his friend who waits on the ground below. The bleachers are 19 m above the ground, the boy's arm is 1 m above the ground, and the ball is thrown horizontally at 25 m/s. If his friend catches the ball, how far is he from the base of the bleachers when he catches the ball?

A. 1 m
B. 2 m
C. 25 m
D. 50 m

15. A projectile is fired from a gun near the surface of a planet where the acceleration due to gravity is equal to that on Earth. The initial velocity of the projectile has a vertical component of 100 m/s and a horizontal component of 50 m/s. How long will it take the projectile to reach the highest point in its path?

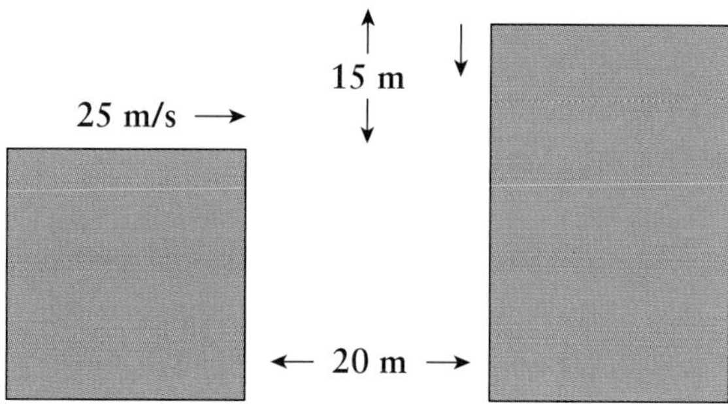

A. 0 s
B. 5 s
C. 7.5 s
D. 10 s

16. A golf ball leaves a club with a starting velocity of 40 m/s and leaves the tee at an initial angle of 30° to the horizontal. What is the total horizontal distance traveled by the golf ball during the first 2.5 seconds of flight?

A. 50 m
B. 70 m
C. 87.5 m
D. 100 m

17. A punter is told by his coach to kick a football over a goalpost, which is 28 m away from him. As he kicks the ball, it has an initial speed of 20 m/s and leaves his foot at an angle of 45°. The low post on the goal is 2.5 meters high. When the football has reached the level of the low post, how far above or below is the ball?

A. 3.25 m under
B. 3.25 m over
C. 5.75 m under
D. 5.75 m over

18. A penny that weighs 3.0 g is dropped off the top of the tallest building in the city, which reaches 380 m. What is the speed of the penny after it has passed the window of the CEO of the biggest company in town? The bottom of his window is 350 m from the sidewalk.

A. 6 m/s
B. 24 m/s
C. 60 m/s
D. 277 m/s

19. Refer to the following table illustrating velocity versus time for a small child observed by a scientist. How far had the child wobbled after the first seven minutes?

Time (seconds)	Velocity (m/s)
1	3
2	3
3	3
4	6
5	5
6	4
7	3
8	0.5
9	2
10	4

A. 21.5 m
B. 25.5 m
C. 30 m
D. 42 m

CHAPTER 2

NEWTONIAN MECHANICS

This chapter covers the most important area of MCAT physics, namely Newton's laws of motion. Basic to the study of Newton's laws are the fundamental concepts of force and mass, which are discussed along with the distinction between mass and weight and a detailed example of obtaining the resultant of two or more forces. The classic example of a block sliding down a frictionless incline is presented as an exercise for applying Newton's second law in a situation where there are forces in two directions. Translational and rotational equilibrium are discussed as examples of cases where the net force or net torque respectively vanishes. The real-world problem of motion in the presence of friction is briefly discussed qualitatively, followed by a detailed numerical example. Lastly, the topic of circular motion is discussed along with the associated concepts of tangential and centripetal acceleration, and centripetal force.

NEWTON'S THREE LAWS

A. FORCE

Force is a vector quantity. Forces are observed as the push or pull on an object. Forces can either be exerted between bodies in contact (such as the force a person exerts to push a box across the floor), or between bodies not in contact (such as the force of gravity holding the earth in its orbit around the sun). The unit for force in SI is the newton (N), and is equivalent to kilogram•meter/second_2.

TEACHER TIP

If there is no acceleration then there is no net force on the object. This means that any object with a constant velocity has no net force acting on it.

B. MASS AND WEIGHT

The mass of an object should not be mistaken for the weight of an object. **Mass (m)** is a scalar quantity that measures a body's inertia, while **weight (W)** is a force vector that measures a body's gravitational attraction to the earth. The two are related by the equation:

$$\mathbf{W} = m\mathbf{g}$$

where **g** is the acceleration due to gravity. The unit for weight is the same as for any other force, the newton (N).

MCAT FAVORITE

g decreases with height above the earth and increases the closer you get to the earth's center of mass. Near the earth's surface, use $g = 10\ \text{m/s}^2$.

MCAT FAVORITE

First law: No change in motion unless a net force acts.

When one of the forces acting on a body is its own weight, the entire force due to gravity can be thought of as applied at a single point, called the center of gravity. For a homogeneous body the center of gravity is at its geometric center.

C. NEWTON'S LAWS OF MOTION STATED

Mechanics is the study of bodies in motion and at rest. Newtonian mechanics is a way of describing the effect forces have on macroscopic bodies. In order to carry out such a description, it is first necessary to have an understanding of Newton's three laws of motion and how to apply them to various situations. Newton's three laws are:

TEACHER TIP

The best way to visualize Newton's first law is to picture an asteroid flying through space. It will continue at its current velocity for an eternity unless it is acted upon by the gravitational force of another celestial object.

TEACHER TIP

The net force is the sum of all forces acting on an object. Even though the force of gravity is always acting on us, the net force on our bodies will be zero unless there is no ground below us pushing back up against gravity.

1. A body either at rest or in motion with constant velocity will remain that way unless a net force acts upon it.
2. A net force applied to a body of mass m will result in that body undergoing an acceleration in the same direction as the net force. The magnitude of the body's acceleration is directly proportional to the magnitude of the net force and inversely proportional to the body's mass. This can be expressed in general terms as:

   $$F_{net} = \sum F = ma$$

   or in components as:

   $$\sum F_x = ma_x$$
   $$\sum F_y = ma_y$$

   Note that the acceleration in the x-direction depends only on the forces (or components of forces) in the x-direction (and the same is true for the y-direction).

3. If body A exerts a force F on body B, then B exerts a force –F back on A (equal in magnitude and opposite in direction). In Newton's words, "to every action there is always an opposed but equal reaction."

   $$F_B = -F_A$$

PAVLOV'S DOG

When you see $F_{net} = 0$, think $a = 0$ and vice versa.

D. FREE-BODY DIAGRAM

Another concept useful in force problems is the **free-body diagram,** which helps to clarify what forces are acting and what their directions are. The following examples demonstrate the use of this technique.

Example: Three people are pulling on ropes tied to a tire with forces of 100 N, 150 N, and 200 N, as shown in Figure 2.1. Find the magnitude and direction of the resultant force.

TEACHER TIP

When solving these types of problems, *always* break each force that is not *only* in the X- or Y-direction into its X- and Y-component parts, using trigonometry.

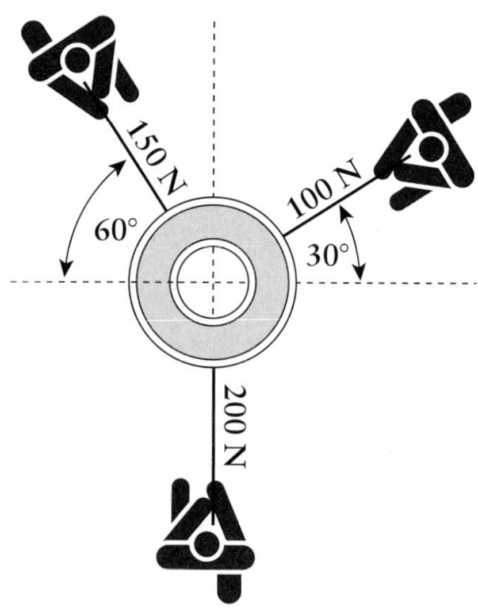

Figure 2.1

MCAT SYNOPSIS

Forces must be added as vectors.

Solution: First we draw a free-body diagram that shows the forces acting on the tire. Its purpose is to identify and better visualize the acting forces.

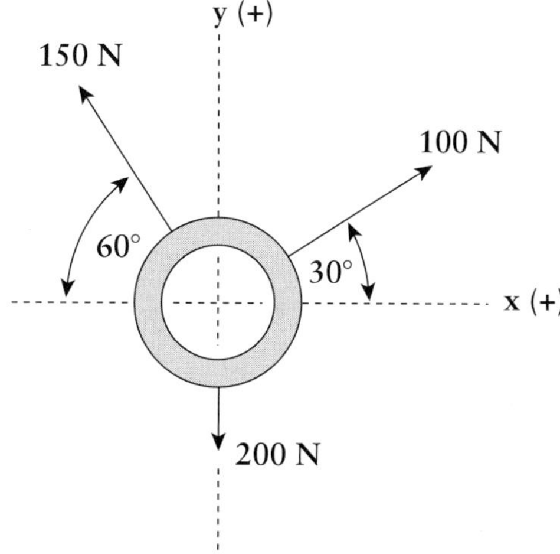

Figure 2.2

The resultant force is simply the sum of the forces. To find the resultant force vector, first we need the sum of the force components:

$$R_x = \sum F_x = 100 \cos 30° - 150 \cos 60°$$
$$= 86.6 - 75$$
$$= 11.6 \text{ N (positive x-direction, to the right)}$$
$$R_y = \sum F_y = 100 \sin 30° + 150 \sin 60° - 200$$
$$= 50 + 129.9 - 200$$
$$= -20.1 \text{ N (negative y-direction, down)}$$

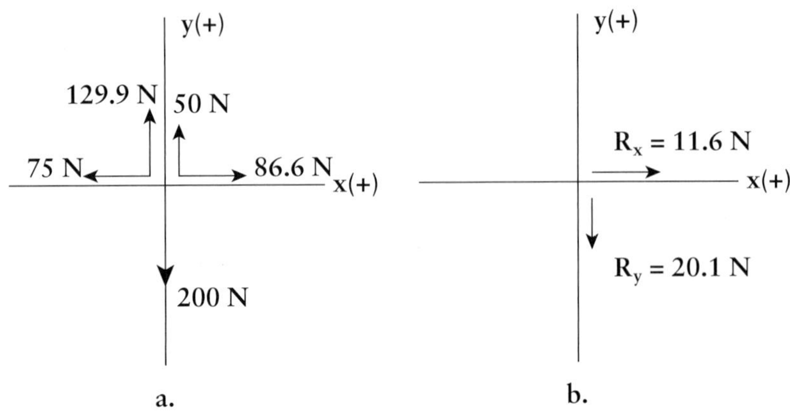

TEACHER TIP

Looking at the forces, we know there is more force in the negative y-direction than there is in the positive x-direction. Before doing the math, see if one of the answer choices has an angle that puts the vector closer to the negative y than to the positive x. This would translate as an angle between 45° and 90° below the x-axis.

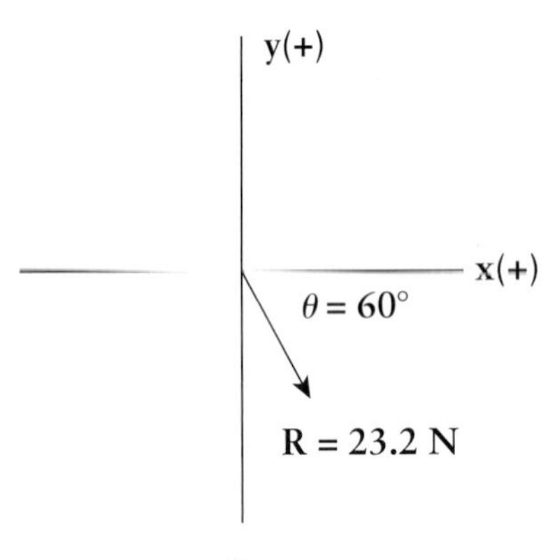

Figure 2.3

$$R = \sqrt{(11.6)^2 + (-20.1)^2}$$
$$= 23.2 \text{ N}$$
$$\tan \theta = \frac{-20.1}{11.6}$$
$$\theta = -60° \text{ (R is in the 4th quadrant)}$$

Example: Starting from rest, a 5 kg block takes 4 s to slide down a frictionless incline. Find the normal force, the acceleration of the block, and the vertical height h the block starts from, if the plane is at an angle of 30°.

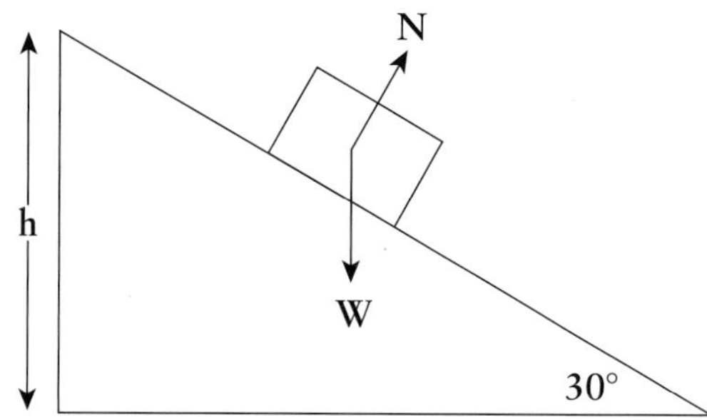

Figure 2.4

MCAT SYNOPSIS

A block on a frictionless incline feels two forces: gravity downwards and the normal force perpendicular to the incline.

Solution: It is usually best to choose the x- and y-axes such that one of the axes is parallel to the surface, even when the surface is not horizontal. This is what we will do here. The force that the surface exerts on the block is broken up into two components, one perpendicular to the surface called the **normal force (N)**, and the other parallel to the surface, called the **friction force** (f). In this problem the incline is frictionless (i.e., no **f**), so we have only the normal force **N.** The block's weight **W** is, of course, vertically down. We need to find the components of W parallel and perpendicular to the inclined surface (i.e., the components of W in the x- and y-directions, W_x and W_y).

TEACHER TIP

If you ever lose track of your angles, use this trick: Drawing out vectors, create a right triangle out of the vectors $W_{gravity}$, W_x, and W_y. Because you are breaking gravity into its component parts, it will be the largest value, making it the hypotenuse. W_y, which goes perpendicular to the incline, will be equal to the normal force. Final force W_x goes parallel to the sliding of the block down the incline. The angle theta will equal the angle between the force of gravity and the normal force. By plugging W_x into F = ma, solve for the acceleration of the block in the x-direction.

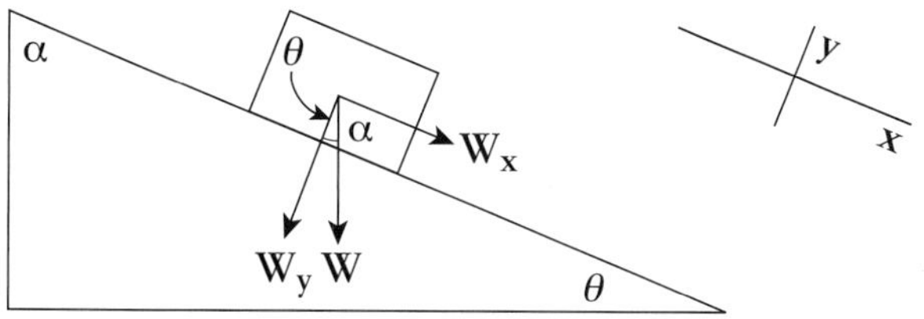

Figure 2.5

MCAT SYNOPSIS

The angle of the incline equals the angle between the force of gravity and the line perpendicular to the incline.

Note that in Figure 2.5 the angle W makes with the x-axis is α, and we would normally use this angle in expressing the components of W; $W_x = W \cos \alpha$ and $W_y = W \sin \alpha$. However, it is more useful to express the components of W in terms of the angle θ which the inclined surface makes with the horizontal. In terms of θ the components of W are:

$$W_x = W \sin \theta = mg \sin \theta \quad (W = mg)$$

$$W_y = W \cos \theta = mg \cos \theta$$

So let the x-axis be parallel to the inclined surface, and let the y-axis be perpendicular to it. The motion is along

MCAT SYNOPSIS

Resolve the weight, mg, into its components parallel to and perpendicular to the incline.

TEACHER TIP

Because the block is neither breaking through the incline nor floating off it, the normal force and the W_y must be equal and opposite, meaning the net force in the y-direction is zero.

MCAT SYNOPSIS

When there are forces in two directions, apply Newton's second law to each direction separately.

the inclined surface, in other words, along the x-axis. Therefore, any acceleration is only in the x-direction, and a_y is automatically zero.

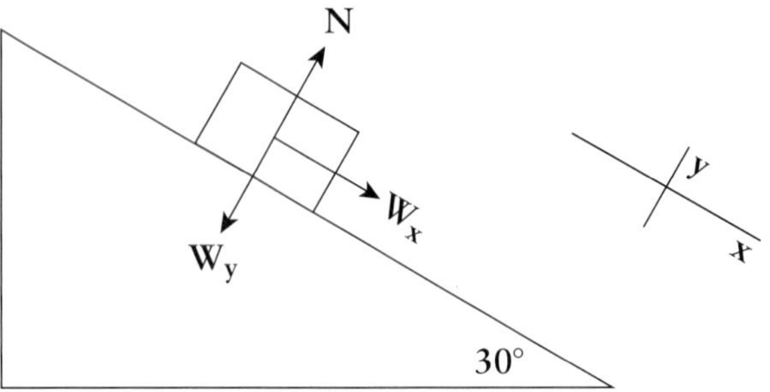

Figure 2.6

Only the forces in the x-direction affect the motion of the block. Because there is no acceleration in the y-direction, the sum of those forces equals zero.

$$\Sigma F_x = W_x = (5)(9.8) \sin 30° = 24.5 \text{ N} = ma_x$$

$$\Sigma F_y = ma_y = N - W_y = 0$$

From the second equation we can solve for N:

$$N = (5)(9.8) \cos 30° = 42.4 \text{ N}$$

From the first equation we can solve for a_x: (Note that $a_x = a$ since $a_y - 0$.)

$$a = \frac{F}{m} = \frac{245}{5} = 4.9 \text{ m/s}^2$$

The length d of the incline from where the block started can now be found using:

$$d = \frac{at^2}{2} \qquad (V_0 = 0)$$

$$= \frac{(4.9)(4)^2}{2}$$

$$= 39.2 \text{ m}$$

From trigonometry, the vertical height h is readily available:

$$\sin 30° = \frac{h}{d}$$

$$h = 39.2 \sin 30°$$

$$= 19.6 \text{ m}$$

E. GRAVITY

Gravity is an attractive force that is felt by all forms of matter. The magnitude of the **gravitational force (F)** is given as:

$$F = \frac{Gm_1m_2}{r^2}$$

where G is the gravitational constant (6.67×10^{-11} N•m²/kg²), m_1 and m_2 are the masses of the two objects, and r is the distance between their centers.

> **TEACHER TIP**
>
> Newton's third law states that the force of gravity on m_1 from m_2 is equal and opposite to the force of gravity on m_2 from m_1. This means that the force of gravity on you from the earth is equal and opposite to the force of gravity from you on the earth. This may sound strange but with Newton's second law we can make sense of it. Because the forces are equal but the masses are very different, we know that the accelerations must also be very different, from F = ma. Because our mass compared to the earth is very small, we experience a large acceleration from it; because the earth is very massive and it feels the same force, it experiences only a *tiny* acceleration from us.

Example: Find the gravitational attraction between an electron and a proton at a distance of 10^{-11} m. (Proton mass = 10^{-27} kg; electron mass = 10^{-30} kg)

Solution: Using Newton's law of gravitation:

$$F = \frac{Gm_1m_2}{r^2}$$

$$= \frac{(6.67 \times 10^{-11})(10^{-27})(10^{-30})}{(10^{-11})^2}$$

$$= 6.67 \times 10^{-46} \text{ N}$$

EQUILIBRIUM

If several forces act on an object simultaneously, their vector sum may cancel, leaving the motion of the body unchanged. This balancing phenomenon is called **equilibrium.**

A. TRANSLATIONAL EQUILIBRIUM

An unbalanced force acting on an object accelerates the object in the direction of the force. For an object to be in **translational equilibrium,** the sum of the forces pushing the object through space in one direction must be counterbalanced by the sum of the forces acting in the opposite

> **TEACHER TIP**
>
> Just because the net forces equal zero *does not mean* the velocity equals zero. This an extremely important concept.

MCAT SYNOPSIS

Translational equilibrium implies two equations: $\sum F_x = 0$ and $\sum F_y = 0$.

direction. This is called the first condition of equilibrium and can be written as:

$$\sum F = 0 \text{ (vector sum)}$$

or, if the vectors are resolved into their x and y components:

$$\sum F_x = 0 \qquad \sum F_y = 0$$

Example: A block of mass 20 kg is supported as shown in the diagram. Find the tensions T_1 and T_2.

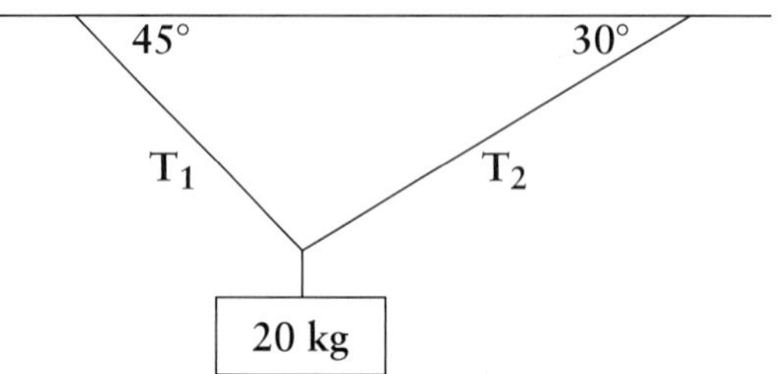

Figure 2.7

Solution: A free-body diagram at the point of intersection of the three cords will help solve this problem. Cords, strings, and the like can only exert pulling forces, and these are in the direction of each cord. Note also that the tension in the vertical cord is equal to the weight of the 20 kg mass, as shown in the other free-body diagram on the right.

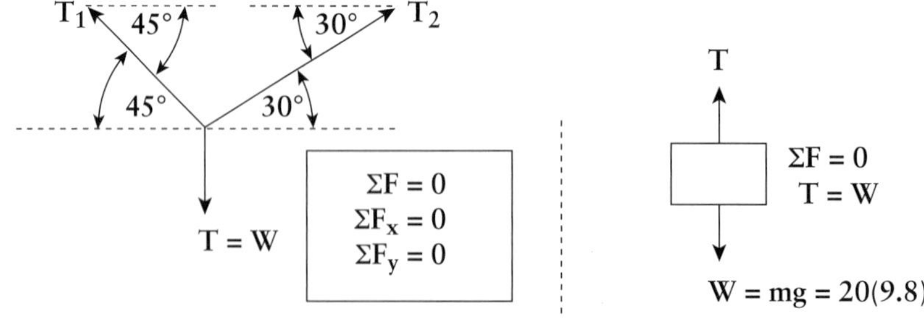

Figure 2.8

The force components are:

$$\sum F_x = 0 = T_2 \cos 30° - T_1 \cos 45°$$

$$\sum F_y = 0 = T_1 \sin 45° + T_2 \sin 30° - 20(9.8)$$

Solve the second equation for T_1:

$$T_1 = \frac{20(9.8) - T_2 \sin 30°}{\sin 45°}$$

$$= \frac{20(9.8) - T_2/2}{\sqrt{2}/2}$$

$$= \frac{196(2) - (T_2/2)2}{\sqrt{2}}$$

$$= \frac{392 - T_2}{\sqrt{2}}$$

Substitute this into the first equation:

$$\frac{T_2\sqrt{3}}{2} - \frac{\sqrt{2}}{2}\left(\frac{196 - T_2}{\sqrt{2}}\right) = 0$$

$$T_2(\sqrt{3} + 1) = 196$$

$$T_2 = \frac{196}{\sqrt{3} + 1}$$

$$= 71.7 \text{ N}$$

And now T_1 follows from this:

$$T_1 = \frac{196 - 71.7}{\sqrt{2}}$$

$$= 87.9 \text{ N}$$

B. ROTATIONAL EQUILIBRIUM

Unlike translational motion, rotational motion depends not only on the magnitude and direction of the force, but also on the distance from the force to the axis of rotation. The greater the distance, the greater the change in rotational motion that will be produced by a given force. (As an example, try closing a door first by pushing on it a few inches from the hinge, then by pushing far from the hinge. You'll find it's much easier to close the door when you push farther from the hinge because the distance between the axis and the force is greater.)

TEACHER TIP

Sin 90° equals 1. This means that torque is greatest when the force applied is 90° (perpendicular) to the length of the lever arm. Knowing the sin 0 equals 0 tells us that there is no torque when the force applied is parallel to the lever arm.

MCAT SYNOPSIS

Maximum torque when $\theta = 90°$ (τ_{max} = rF), minimum torque when $\theta = 0°$ (τ_{min} = 0).

The quantity that causes rotation is called the **moment of the force** or the **torque** τ, and is given by:

$$\tau = rF \sin \theta$$

where F is the magnitude of the force, r is the distance between the axis and the force (also called the lever arm), and θ is the angle between F and r.

Torque can act in two directions about a pivot point, clockwise and counterclockwise. Counterclockwise is the positive direction and clockwise the negative direction. For **rotational equilibrium** to occur, the sum of the torques in both these directions must be equal. Because torques causing a rotation in the clockwise direction are negative and torques causing counterclockwise rotations are positive, we can also say that the sum of all the torques must be zero:

MCAT SYNOPSIS

Clockwise torques are negative, while counterclockwise torques are positive.

$$\sum \tau = 0$$

This is called the second condition of equilibrium.

REAL-WORLD ANALOGY

A balanced seesaw has $\sum \tau = 0$, and $\sum F = 0$. Choose fulcrum as the pivot point for calculating torques.

Example: A seesaw with a mass of 5 kg has one block of mass 10 kg two meters to the left of the fulcrum and another block 0.5 m to the right of the fulcrum. If the seesaw is in equilibrium,

a. find the mass of the second block.
b. find the force exerted by the fulcrum.

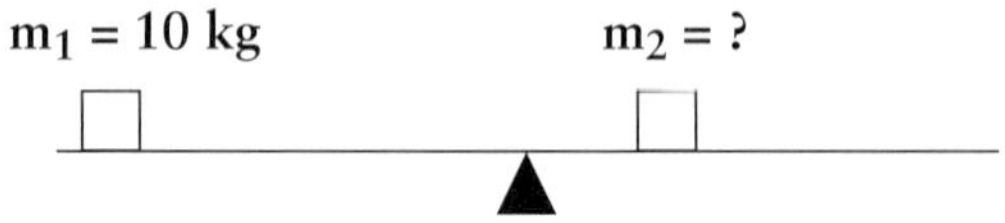

$m_1 = 10$ kg $\qquad m_2 = ?$

Figure 2.9

Solution: a. To find τ take the point of the fulcrum as the pivot point. This way, both the normal force and the weight of the seesaw will be eliminated from the equation (r = 0). Let's call the 10 kg mass object 1 and the block whose mass we are trying to find object 2.

TEACHER TIP

Before jumping into the math, approximate what the mass should be so you can eliminate some answers choices straight away. Because the mass is much closer to the fulcrum, we know that the m_2 must be more massive.

$$\sum \tau = 0 = m_1 g d_1 - m_2 g d_2$$

$$m_2 = \frac{m_1 d_1}{d_2} = \frac{10(2)}{0.5} = 40 \text{ kg}$$

b. To find the normal force, N, exerted by the fulcrum, $\sum F_y = 0$. There is the upward force exerted by the fulcrum and the downward weights of the seesaw and the two masses. Don't forget that W = mg. Taking up as positive:

$$N - 5(9.8) - 10(9.8) - 40(9.8) = 0$$

$$N = 49 + 98 + 392 = 539 \text{ N}$$

MOTION

A. TRANSLATIONAL MOTION

Translational motion is defined as motion in which there is no rotation. An example of translational motion is a block sliding on an inclined plane. With Newton's three laws and enough initial conditions, any translational motion problem can be solved.

B. FRICTION

Whenever two objects are in contact, their surfaces rub together creating a friction force. **Static friction f_s** is the force that must be overcome to set an object in motion. Its equation is:

$$0 \le f_s \le \mu_s N$$

where μ_s is the **coefficient of static friction** and N is the normal force. Note that static friction can have any value up to some maximum $\mu_s N$. For example, to send a book that is at rest sliding across a table, a force greater than the maximum static friction force is required. Once the book starts to slide, though, the friction force is not quite as strong. This new friction force is called **kinetic friction f_k**, and its equation is:

$$f_k = \mu_k N$$

where μ_k is the **coefficient of kinetic friction** and N is the normal force. Remember that friction always acts to oppose motion.

Example: Two blocks are in static equilibrium as shown in Figure 2.10.

a. If block A has a mass of 15 kg and the coefficient of static friction μ_s equals 0.20, then find the maximum mass of block B.

b. If an extra 5 kg are added to B find the acceleration of A and the tension T in the rope. (μ_k equals 0.14)

TEACHER TIP

The maximum coefficient of static friction will always be larger than the coefficient of kinetic friction. It's always harder to get an object to start sliding than it is to *keep* an object sliding.

MCAT SYNOPSIS

An object at rest on a real surface requires a force greater than $\mu_s N$ to start moving.

TEACHER TIP

The force of static friction changes according to the strength of the force being applied to the object. It will increase as increasing force is applied (if the force of friction were greater than the force being applied, it would push back against the person, something that is quite impossible), until the object starts moving and there is no longer static friction. Then, kinetic friction has taken over.

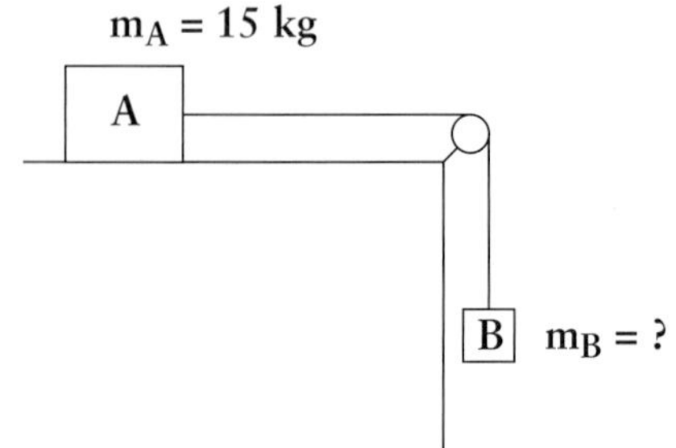

Figure 2.10

Solution: a.

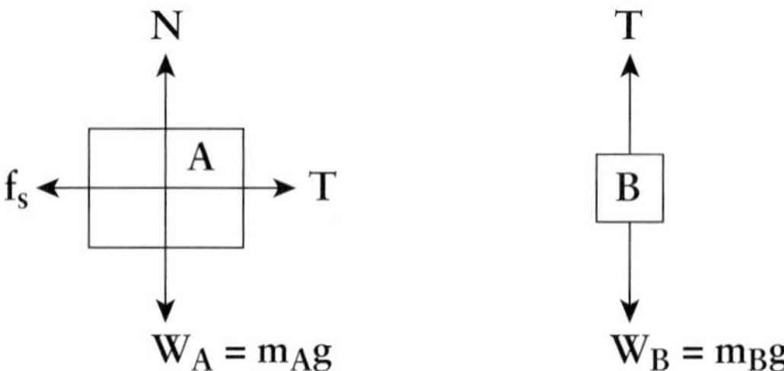

Figure 2.11

For block B:

$$\Sigma F_y = 0 = T - W_B$$
$$T = W_B = m_B g$$

For block A:

Asking for the maximum mass of block B means that the coefficient of static friction holding block A is at its maximum, $f_s = \mu_s N$.

$$\Sigma F_y = 0 = N - W_A$$
$$N = W_A = m_A g$$
$$\Sigma F_x = 0 = T - \mu_s N$$
$$T = \mu_s m_A g$$
$$T = (0.2)(15)(9.8)$$
$$T = 29.4 \text{ N}$$

Since block B is in static equilibrium, the tension in the rope must equal the weight of the block, so we have:

$$m_B g = 29.4$$
$$m_B = 3 \text{ kg}$$

b.

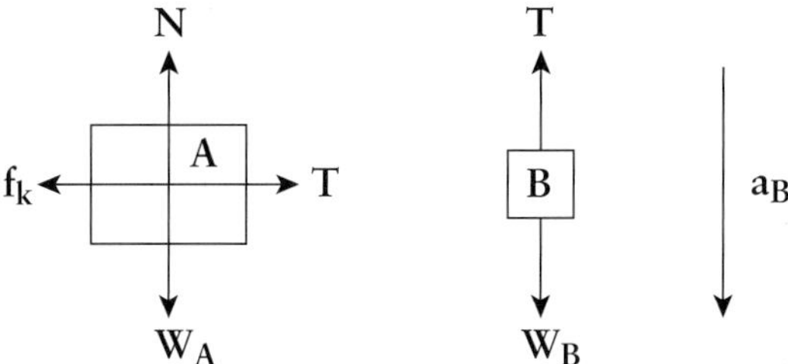

Figure 2.12

We found the maximum mass of B for the system to be in static equilibrium. Adding an extra 5 kg to B means that the system is now in motion.

For block B:

$$\Sigma F_y = m_B g - T = m_B a_B$$

For block A:

$$\begin{aligned} \Sigma F_x &= T - \mu_k N \\ &= T - \mu_k m_A g \\ &= m_A a_A \end{aligned}$$

Since the blocks are connected by the string, the magnitude of the acceleration for both of them is the same:

$$a_A = a_B = a$$

and

$$\begin{aligned} m_B g - T &= m_B a \\ T - \mu_k m_A g &= m_A a \end{aligned}$$

Adding the two equations gives:

$$m_B g - T + T - \mu_k m_A g = (m_A + m_B)a$$

Solving for a:

$$\begin{aligned} a &= \frac{(m_B - \mu_k m_A)g}{(m_A + m_B)} \\ &= \frac{(8 - (0.14)(15))9.8}{(15 + 8)} \\ &= 2.5 \text{ m/s}^2 \end{aligned}$$

Substituting this value into the equation $m_A a = T - \mu_k m_A g$ and solving for the tension gives:

$$\begin{aligned} T &= m_A(\mu_k g + a) \\ &= 15(0.14(9.8) + 2.5) \\ &= 58.1 \text{ N} \end{aligned}$$

MCAT SYNOPSIS

Centripetal acceleration only causes a change in direction of velocity.

CIRCULAR MOTION

The velocity vector is always tangent to the circular path. In general, the acceleration vector can be broken into radial and tangential components as shown in Figure 2.13.

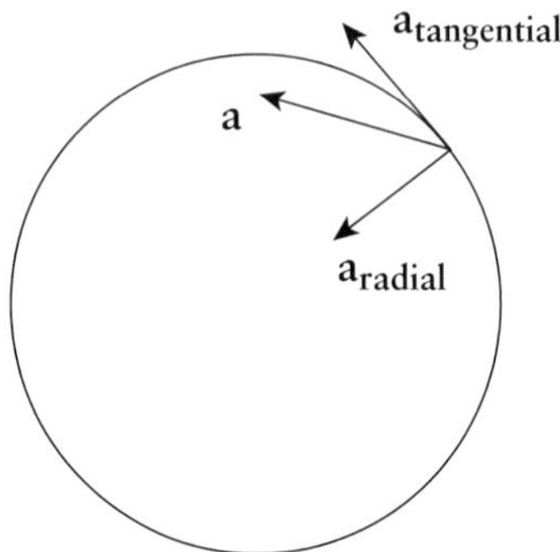

Figure 2.13

PAVLOV'S DOG

When you see uniform circular motion, think centripetal acceleration and thus centripetal force.

In uniform circular motion, the speed of the object remains constant. When uniform circular motion is assumed, there is no tangential acceleration. The radial component of the acceleration is always directed towards the center of the circle and is called **centripetal acceleration.** Its magnitude is given by:

$$a = \frac{v^2}{r}$$

TEACHER TIP

The centripetal force is not a force in itself; it must be applied by something. Gravity in the motion of a satellite applies centripetal force, as does tension in an object being spun on a string. It is the force that keeps the object from flying off tangentially.

The centripetal acceleration towards the center of the circle must be the result of some force also directed towards the center. Whatever the particular force happens to be, it is called the **centripetal force.** Using the relationship $a = v^2/r$ for the centripetal acceleration, the magnitude of the centripetal force on a particle in circular motion is given by:

$$F = ma = \frac{mv^2}{r}$$

In nonuniform circular motion, the speed of the object changes. In this case there is a tangential component of acceleration, and therefore the resultant acceleration is not directed toward the center of the circle. Instead its direction is given by the resultant of the radial component of the acceleration and the tangential component of the acceleration.

Consider a mass tied to a string, moving with circular motion. To keep the mass moving in a circular path, the string must constantly pull the object toward the center. In this case, the force exerted by the string is the centripetal force. If at some point the string breaks, the inward force no longer acts, and the mass flies off along a path tangential to the circle.

There is always some force that causes circular motion. As another example, consider a planet in orbit around the sun. In this case, the centripetal force is the force of gravity.

PRACTICE QUESTIONS

1. As a rocket accelerates, it burns fuel and emits gas at a constant rate. Which of the following diagrams best illustrates the force of propulsion of the rocket as related to time?

A.
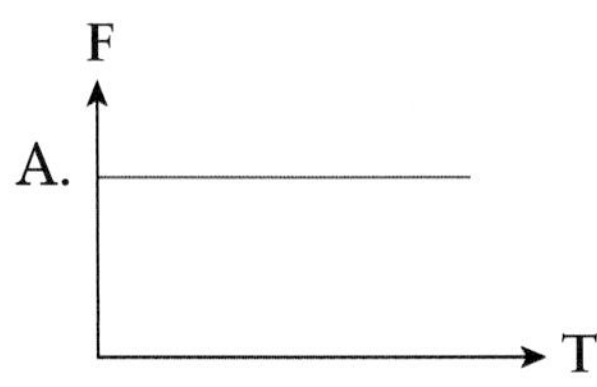

B.
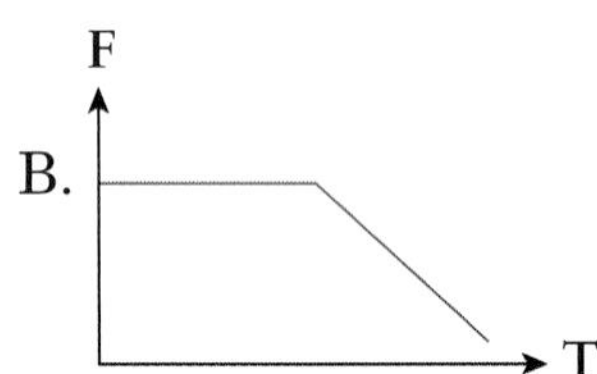

C.
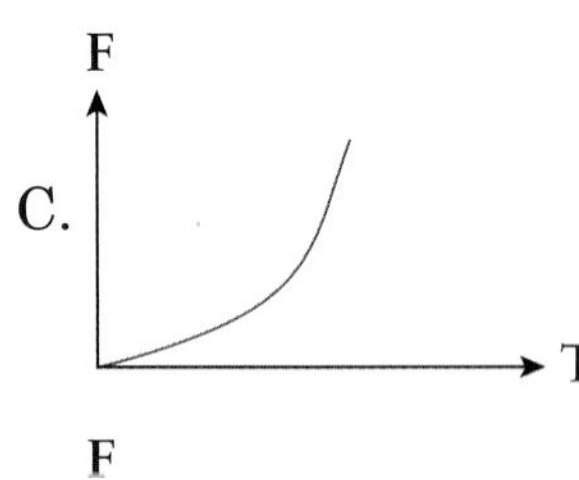

D.
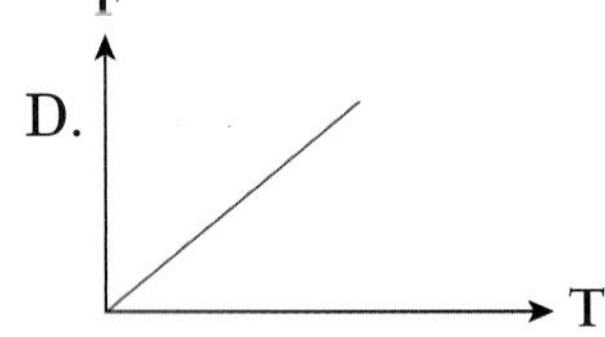

2. A train is accelerating east at 4 m/s^2. A 5 kg lamp is attached to a rope hanging off the ceiling. What is the tension in the rope?

A. 50 N up
B. 45 N
C. 55 N
D. 10 N

3. Force is applied to move a 5 kg box connected to a pulley system along a homogenous surface, shown below:

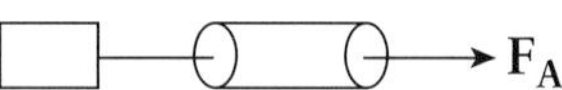

If the coefficient of static friction is 0.8 and the coefficient of kinetic friction is 0.5, what is the force that is required to start the movement of the box?

A. 0 N
B. 4 N
C. 25N
D. 40 N

4. Using the same conditions as in the previous question, what is the force required to keep the box moving at constant velocity?

A. 12.5 N
B. 20 N
C. 25 N
D. 40 N

5. A triangular ramp is accelerating to the left. A rectangular box is placed on top of it and there is no friction between the surfaces (see below). What is the acceleration of the box down the ramp?

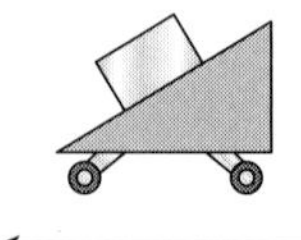

A. Less than the value of g
B. Greater than the value of g
C. Directed up the ramp
D. More information is needed

6. An elevator is accelerating down at 4 m/s^2. How much does a 10 kg fish weigh if measured inside the elevator?

A. 140 N
B. 100 N
C. 60 N
D. 50 N

7. A knight points a sword 120° from the vertical direction. His hands are placed 10 cm from the base of the 1 m, 10 kg sword. What is the magnitude of the upward force required to maintain the sword in this position?

A. 100 N
B. 500 N
C. 667 N
D. 240 N

8. What is the average force required to stop a 70 kg parachutist, falling at 50 m/s, over a period of 10 s? Neglect force of air resistance.

A. 70 N
B. 700 N
C. 1050 N
D. 1400 N

9. A 1 kg arrow is held by a man so that the string of the bow is stretched 50 cm from its equilibrium point. When he lets go, the arrow begins to accelerate at 10 m/s^2. In its stretched position, the string makes an angle of 30° from the line parallel to the arrow. Assume the string of the bow is like a spring, with a constant of 19.5 N/m. What is the force applied by the man in order to hold the arrow?

A. 5 N
B. 8.7 N
C. 10 N
D. 17.5 N

10. If 100 N of force is required to rip apart a towel, what is the minimum amount of force applied to the left side of the towel when it's pulled apart in opposite directions?

A. 50 N
B. 100 N
C. 180 N
D. 200 N

QUESTIONS 11–12 USE THE FOLLOWING INFORMATION:

A 1 kg ball with a radius of 20 cm rolls down a 5 m high inclined plane, below. Its speed at the bottom is 8 m/s.

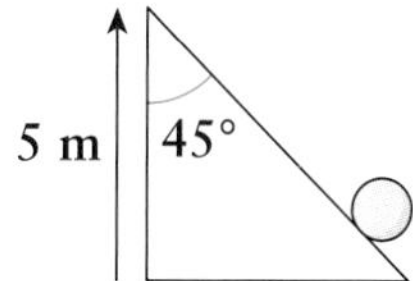

11. How many revolutions per second is the ball making when at the bottom of the plane?

A. 6 rev/sec
B. 12 rev/sec
C. 20 rev/sec
D. 23 rev/sec

12. What is the force of friction acting on the ball?

A. Static, up the incline
B. Static, down the incline
C. Kinetic, up the incline
D. Kinetic, down the incline

13. If the coefficient of friction between the ramp and the ball in the previous questions were increased during subsequent experiments, then the ball would

A. start to slip, and the speed will increase.
B. continue to roll, and its speed will stay the same.
C. start to slip, and its speed will decrease.
D. continue to roll, and its speed will decrease.

14. A 1,000 kg satellite traveling at speed v maintains an orbit of radius R around the earth. What should be its speed if it is to develop a new orbit of radius 4R?

A. ¼ v
B. ½ v
C. 2 v
D. 4 v

15. A 100 kg elevator accelerates up at rate $\bar{a}$. What is the average force acting on the elevator if it covers a distance x over a period of 10 s?

A. $2x + 1{,}000$
B. $100(\bar{a} + 1)$
C. $2\bar{a} + 1{,}000$
D. $2\bar{a}\,x$

16. A train is moving east at a constant velocity. A man inside the train also decides to run east. Which of the following statements are true about the movement of the train?

I. A nonzero net force east causes the train to move forward.
II. The runner supplies a nonzero force east on the train.
III. The train starts to decelerate as the runner starts to accelerate.

A. I only
B. III only
C. I and III only
D. II and III only

17. If the period of the earth orbit around the sun suddenly increased, then

A. velocity would double and the radius would triple.
B. velocity would be halved and the radius would quadruple.
C. velocity would stay the same and the radius would increase.
D. velocity would decrease and the radius would stay the same.

CHAPTER 3

WORK, ENERGY, AND MOMENTUM

In this chapter we will review the fundamental concepts of energy and momentum and the associated concepts of work and impulse. Essentially, you can think of work as responsible for changing the energy of an object and impulse as responsible for changing the momentum of an object. Regarding energy and momentum, the great laws of conservation of energy and conservation of momentum are discussed along with concrete examples of problems that make use of these laws for their solution. The topic of collisions is discussed in detail as the most common example on the MCAT of the application of conservation of momentum. The concept of work is applied to the problem of pulley systems resulting in the definition of the efficiency of a simple machine. The chapter closes with a review of the equivalent concepts of center of mass and center of gravity.

WORK

A. WORK DEFINED

As was shown in chapter 2, solving mechanics problems using Newtonian methods involves analyzing the forces acting on a system. In this chapter, energy and momentum considerations, rather than forces, will be used to solve problems. Before we undertake a discussion of energy, though, it is important that we first talk about work. For a constant **force** F acting on an object which moves through a distance d, the **work** W is:

$$W = Fd \cos \theta$$

where θ is the angle between F and d. Units for work (and energy) are the joule (**J**) in SI (1 joule = 1 newton•meter) and the foot•pound in FPS. Only the component of the force parallel to the path, F cos θ, is relevant. For a force perpendicular to the motion, W = 0 ($\theta = 90°$, thus cos 90° = 0). Note that for a force opposite to the motion ($\theta > 90°$), the work will be negative (cos $\theta < 0$).

TEACHER TIP

To conceptualize this formula, think of pushing a large box. Pushing straight into the box means you are pushing parallel to the ground, and thus parallel to its *displacement*, producing the ideal result. Remembering your trig, the cos of 0° is 1, meaning that all the force is going into the work. If you were to change the angle and push downward at 60°, then only half your force would go into the work. In other words, if you want to move the box a certain distance, it would take double the force to move it at 60° than at zero, though the same amount of *work* would be done.

Example: A block weighing 100 N is pushed up a frictionless incline over a distance of 20 m to a height of 10 m. Find:

a. the minimum force required to push the block.
b. the work done by the force.
c. the force required and the work done by the force if the block were simply lifted vertically 10 m.

Solution:

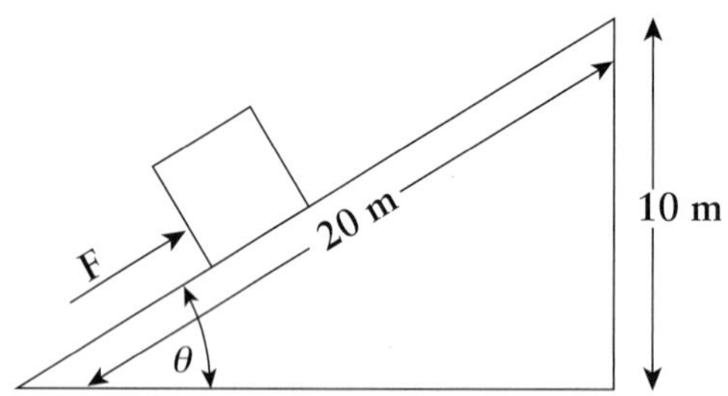

Figure 3.1

a. A free-body diagram of the forces acting on the block:

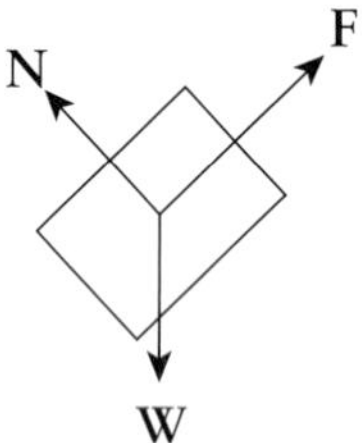

Figure 3.2

The minimum force needed is a force parallel to the plane that will push the block with no acceleration. Since $a = 0$, $\sum F = 0$:

$$\sum F = 0 = F - mg \sin \theta$$

$$F = mg \sin \theta$$

$mg = 100$ N; $\sin \theta = 10/20$. Therefore:

$$F = 100 \frac{10}{20}$$

$$= 50 \text{ N}$$

b. The work done by F is:

$$W = Fd \cos \theta$$

In this case θ is the angle between the force vector and the displacement vector. Since they are parallel, $\theta = 0$, therefore $\cos\theta = 1$. Substituting the numbers into the equation:

$$W = 50(20)(1)$$
$$= 1{,}000 \text{ J}$$

c. To raise the block vertically, the force should also be vertical and equal to the object's weight.

$$F = mg$$
$$= 100 \text{ N}$$

The work done by the lifting force is:

$$W = Fd\cos\theta$$
$$= 100(10)(1)$$
$$= 1{,}000 \text{ J}$$

The same amount of work is required in both cases, but twice the force is needed to raise the block vertically compared with pushing it up the incline.

MCAT SYNOPSIS

The force needed to lift an object equals the weight of the object.

B. POWER

Often, the amount of work required to perform an operation is less important than the amount of time required to do the work. The rate at which work is done is called **power** (P), and is given as:

$$P = \frac{W}{t}$$

Units of power are the watt (W) in SI (1 watt = 1 joule/sec) and foot•pound/sec in FPS.

TEACHER TIP

Power is used in many different situations (as we will see in the discussion of circuits), though it always refers to the amount of "something" PER UNIT TIME.

PAVLOV'S DOG

When you see "rate of work" or "rate of change of energy," think power!

Example: Find the power required to raise the block (of the previous example) in four seconds in each case.

Solution: When lifted up the incline, power is:

$$P = \frac{W}{t}$$
$$= \frac{1{,}000}{4}$$
$$= 250 \text{ W}$$

When lifted straight up, the power equals:

$$P = \frac{1{,}000}{4} = 250 \text{ W}$$

ENERGY

A. KINETIC ENERGY

TEACHER TIP

Kinetic energy is incredibly important on the MCAT. Any time that an object has a velocity, think about kinetic energy and thus, conservation of energy.

A body in motion possesses energy. This energy of motion is called **kinetic energy,** and is defined for a body of mass m and velocity v as:

$$KE = \frac{mv^2}{2}$$

Units for kinetic energy are joules (J) in SI.

Example: A 15 kg block, initially at rest, slides down a frictionless incline and comes to the bottom with a velocity of 7 m/s. What is the kinetic energy at the top and at the bottom?

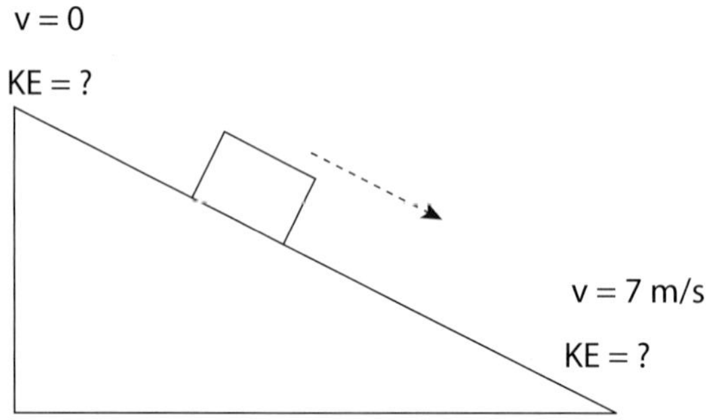

Figure 3.3

Solution: At the top v = 0, so kinetic energy is:

$$KE = \frac{mv^2}{2} = \frac{15(0)}{2} = 0$$

At the bottom:

$$KE = \frac{15(7)^2}{2} = 367.5 \text{ J}$$

B. POTENTIAL ENERGY

Another form of energy a body can possess is **potential energy.** Unlike kinetic energy, which depends upon a body's motion, potential energy depends upon a body's **position.** One example of potential energy is the gravitational potential energy an object has when it is raised to a height h. Objects on the earth possess greater potential energy the higher they are from the surface. Gravitational potential energy (U) is given as:

$$U = mgh$$

where m is the mass of the body, g is the acceleration due to gravity, and h is the height of the body. Just as for work and kinetic energy, potential energy's units are joules (J).

TEACHER TIP

The height used in the potential energy equation is relative to whatever the question states. However, it will often be the distance to the ground because all objects are actually falling toward the center of the earth. It does not need to be relative to the ground. Just listen to the question stem and use the height that is discussed.

MCAT SYNOPSIS

The equation mgh for potential energy means the ground (h = 0) is the zero of potential energy.

MCAT SYNOPSIS

Potential energy in a stretched or compressed spring is $1/2kx^2$. (See chapter 9.)

Example: An 80 kg diver leaps from a 10 m cliff into the sea. Find the diver's potential energy at the top of the cliff and just as he hits the water (set height equal to zero at sea level).

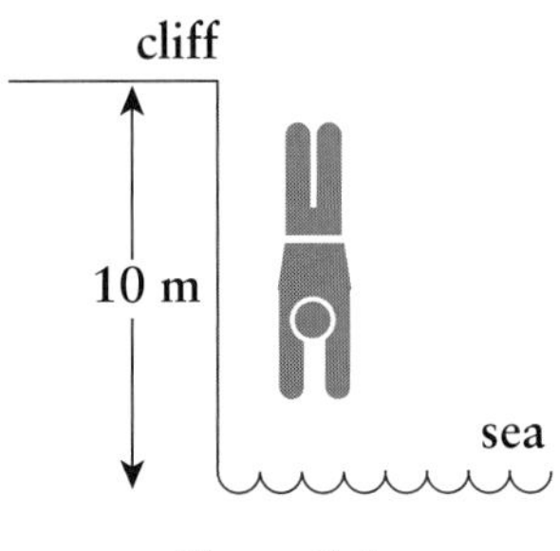

Figure 3.4

Solution: At the top of the cliff:

$$\begin{aligned} U &= mgh \\ &= 80(9.8)(10) \\ &= 7{,}840 \text{ J} \end{aligned}$$

At the water's surface:

$$\begin{aligned} U &= 80(9.8)(0) \\ &= 0 \end{aligned}$$

C. TOTAL MECHANICAL ENERGY

Kinetic and potential energy are both forms of mechanical energy. The total mechanical energy (E) is the sum of the kinetic and the potential energies:

$$E = KE + U$$

TEACHER TIP

To visualize this relationship, imagine a skateboarder in a half-pipe. When she is at the top of the pipe, all of her energy is potential. As she careens down the wall, her energy is being converted to kinetic energy. When she reaches the bottom, all of her potential energy is gone and has been converted into kinetic energy. At this point, her velocity is greatest.

MCAT SYNOPSIS

Δk always means $k_{final} - k_{initial}$.

where KE is the kinetic energy of a system and U is the potential energy. Mechanical energy is conserved when the sum of the potential and kinetic energies remains constant. Mechanical energy is not always conserved, though. For example, when friction is present, mechanical energy is drained away in the form of heat.

CONSERVATION OF ENERGY

A. WORK-ENERGY THEOREM

The work-energy theorem relates the work performed by **all** the forces acting on a body in a certain time interval to the change in kinetic energy during that time. In equation form, the theorem is:

$$W = \Delta KE$$

Example: A baseball of mass 0.25 kg is thrown straight up in the air with an initial velocity of 30 m/s. Assuming no air resistance, find the work done by the force of gravity when the ball is at its maximum height.

Solution: Neglecting air resistance, the only force acting on the ball is gravity. Because the ball's speed is 0 at its maximum height, using the work-energy theorem:

$$\begin{aligned} W &= \Delta KE \\ &= 0 - \frac{mv^2}{2} \\ &= \frac{-(0.25)(30)^2}{2} \\ &= -112.5 \text{ J} \end{aligned}$$

B. CONSERVATIVE AND NONCONSERVATIVE FORCES

Conservative forces have associated potential energies (e.g., gravity). There are two equivalent tests that are used to determine whether a force is conservative or not:

MCAT SYNOPSIS

Conservative forces: gravity, spring forces, electrostatic force.
Nonconservative forces: friction.

1. If the work done to move a particle in any round-trip path is zero, the force is conservative.
2. If the work needed to move a particle between two points is the same regardless of the path taken, then the force is conservative.

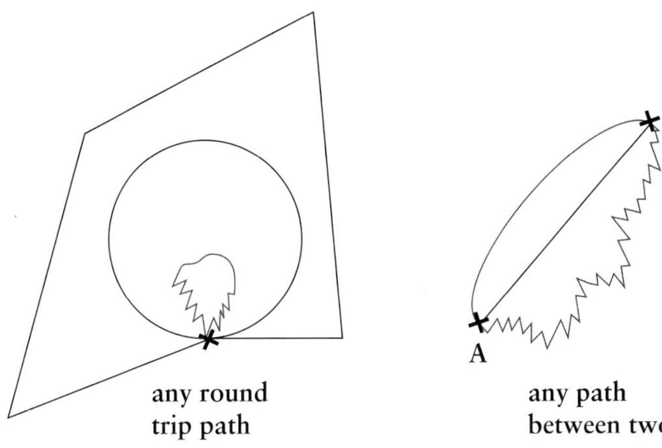

Figure 3.5

For our purposes we will simply use the following rule of thumb: A force that has an associated potential energy (e.g., gravity) is conservative. An object's weight is just another name for the gravitational force on the object, so an object's weight is a conservative force.

C. CONSERVATION OF ENERGY

When the work done by the nonconservative forces is 0 (or when there are no nonconservative forces, for example, an object falling without air resistance), the total mechanical energy remains constant, and we have **conservation of energy**:

$$E = KE + U = \text{constant}$$

or equivalently:

$$\Delta E = \Delta KE + \Delta U = 0$$

TEACHER TIP

To continue with the skateboarder example on the previous page, if the track was frictionless (meaning there were no nonconservative forces), we would have a good example of conservation of energy. When the skateboarder gets back to the top of the half-pipe, she would have the exact same potential energy with which she started. Her total energy remains constant throughout the trip; it is simply converted from potential into kinetic and back into potential again.

However, when nonconservative forces such as friction or air resistance are present, mechanical energy is **not** conserved. The equation for a nonconservative system is:

$$W' = \Delta E = \Delta KE + \Delta U$$

MCAT SYNOPSIS

In the presence of friction: $E_{initial} > E_{final}$, and the lost energy goes into heat.

where **W′ is the work done by the nonconservative forces only.** Note that if the work done by the nonconservative forces is zero (which is automatically true if there aren't any such forces), $W' = 0 = \Delta E = \Delta KE + \Delta U$ and we have conservation of energy.

Example: A baseball of mass 0.25 kg is thrown in the air with an initial speed of 30 m/s, but because of air resistance the ball returns to the ground with a speed of 27 m/s. Find the work done by air resistance.

Solution: Air resistance is a nonconservative force. To do this problem, the energy equation for a nonconservative system is needed. The work done by air resistance is W′.

$$W' = \Delta E = \Delta KE + \Delta U$$

Since $\Delta U = 0$ (final height = initial height):

$$\begin{aligned} W' &= \Delta KE \\ &= \frac{mv_f^2}{2} - \frac{mv_i^2}{2} \\ &= \frac{1}{2}(0.25)[(27)^2 - (30)^2] \\ &= -21.4 \text{ J} \end{aligned}$$

PULLEYS

Pulley systems allow heavy weights to be lifted using a much smaller force. Consider first the heavy block in Figure 3.6, suspended from two ropes. The force that the block exerts downwards is equaled by the sum of the tensions in the two ropes. For a symmetrical system, the tensions in the two ropes are the same and are equal to half the weight of the block.

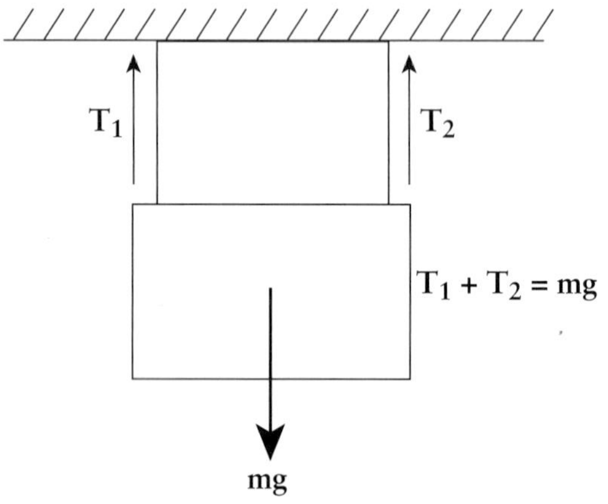

Figure 3.6

Now consider the pulley setup in Figure 3.7, with the block being held stationary. The tension in both vertical ropes will be equal; if they were different, then the pulleys would turn until the tensions on both sides were equal. Because the tensions are equal, each rope supports half the total weight of the block. This means that the force required to raise the block is now only half the total weight of the block. Though only half the force is now required to lift the block, the length of rope that must be pulled through is twice the distance that the block moves upwards. This can be visualized more clearly in considering a case when a block is raised 5 meters. For this to happen, both sides of the supporting rope have to shorten 5 meters, and the only way to accomplish this is by pulling through 10 meters of rope.

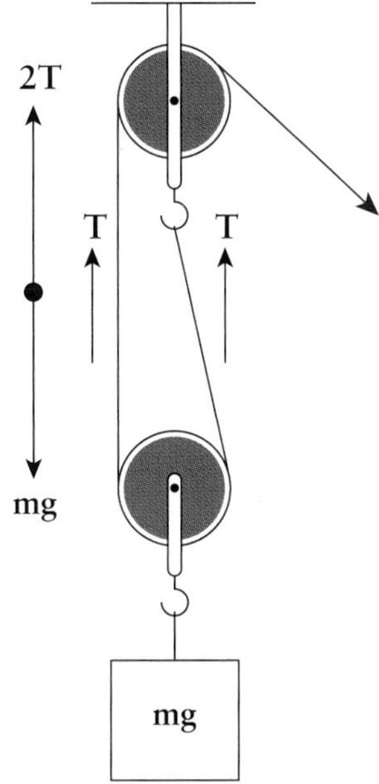

Figure 3.7

MCAT SYNOPSIS

Pulleys don't give you something for nothing. The force is reduced at the expense of exerting the force over a greater distance, i.e., the work done is the same with or without the pulley.

TEACHER TIP

On the MCAT, you'll almost certainly be given a massless frictionless pulley system.

In a frictionless pulley system in which the pulleys themselves have no mass, the work expended pulling the rope and the potential energy gained by the mass would be equal. However, no pulley system has these properties, because the pulleys do have mass and are not frictionless. This implies that no real pulley system is 100 percent efficient. At this point it is worth defining some terms. The weight of the object being lifted is the **load,** and the distance it rises is the **load distance.** The force exerted on the rope when lifting the load is known as the **effort,** and the distance through which the effort is exerted is the **effort distance.** It has been mentioned previously that work is force multiplied by the distance that the force moves an object through. Work input is, therefore, the product of the effort and the effort distance, and work output is the product of the load and the distance the load moves through. A measure of the **efficiency** of the system is given by the ratio of the work output to the work input, and is given by

$$\text{Efficiency} = \frac{W_{out}}{W_{in}} = \frac{\text{Load} \times \text{Load distance}}{\text{Effort} \times \text{Effort distance}}$$

Efficiencies are often spoken of as percentages (multiply decimal by 100 to get percent), but in doing calculations efficiencies have to be decimals or fractions (divide percentage by 100 to get a decimal). The efficiency gives a measure of the amount of work a person puts into a machine that comes out as useful work.

Consider the pulley system in Figure 3.8. By increasing the number of pulleys, it is possible to reduce the effort still further. In this case, the load has been divided among six strands of the rope, so the effort required is now only one sixth the load. However, it is important to note that, generally speaking, as the number of pulleys increases, the efficiency decreases. This decrease in efficiency is caused by the added weight of each pulley as well as the increase in frictional forces.

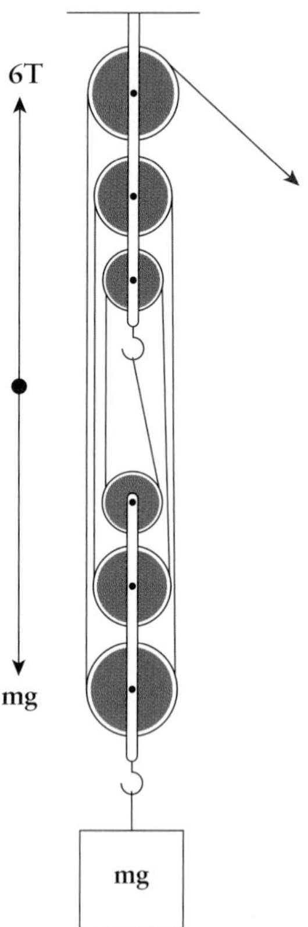

Figure 3.8

Example: The pulley system of Figure 3.8 has an efficiency of 80 percent and a person is required to lift 200 kg. Find:

a. the distance through which the effort must move to raise the load a distance of 4 m.
b. the effort required to lift the load.

c. the work done by the person lifting the load through a height of 4 m.

Solution:

a. For the load to move through a vertical distance of 4 m, all six of the supporting ropes must shorten 4 m also. This may only be accomplished by pulling 6 × 4 = 24 m of rope through. So the effort must move through a distance of 24 m.

b. To calculate the effort required, the equation for efficiency must be used. The load is the weight of the object being lifted and is equal to the mass times the acceleration due to gravity g. Since g is approximately 10 m/s² and all the other parameters except the effort are known, it is possible to substitute into this equation to calculate the effort:

$$\text{Efficiency} = \frac{\text{Load} \times \text{Load distance}}{\text{Effort} \times \text{Effort distance}}$$

$$0.80 = \frac{(200)(10)(4)}{(\text{Effort})(24)}$$

$$\text{Effort} = \frac{(2{,}000)(4)}{(0.80)(24)}$$

$$= 417 \text{ N}$$

c. The work done is given by:

$$\text{Work done} = \text{Effort} \times \text{Effort distance}$$

$$= 417 \times 24$$

$$= 10{,}000 \text{ J}$$

CONSERVATION OF MOMENTUM

A. MOMENTUM

In nonrelativistic physics, **momentum p** means the product of mass and velocity. Momentum, like velocity, is a vector quantity. In equation form it is given as:

$$p = mv$$

For two or more objects, the total momentum is the vector sum of the individual momentums.

TEACHER TIP

On the MCAT, momentum is almost always tested with a collision.

MCAT FAVORITE

Total momentum is vector sum of individual momenta. Keep track of velocity directions!

B. IMPULSE

Applying a force to an object over time will cause that object's momentum to change. The product of the force applied F and the time it was applied for t is a vector quantity, and is given the name **impulse J.** For constant forces, impulse and momentum are related by the equation:

$$J = Ft = mv - mv_0 = \Delta p$$

TEACHER TIP

If the problem is two-dimensional, then you'll have to use trigonometry as discussed in chapter 1.

In one-dimensional problems the forces and velocities are either in the positive or the negative direction, and the equation becomes a single scalar equation:

$$J = Ft = mv - mv_0$$

(In this equation, J, F, v, and v_0 are positive or negative depending on whether the corresponding vectors are in the positive or the negative direction.)

Example: A 7 kg bowling ball initially at rest is acted on by a 110 N force for 3.5 s. Find the final speed of the ball.

Solution: From the equation for impulse:

$$Ft = mv - mv_0$$
$$v = v_0 + \frac{Ft}{m}$$
$$= 0 + \frac{110(3.5)}{7}$$
$$= 55 \text{ m/s}$$

C. CONSERVATION OF MOMENTUM

MCAT SYNOPSIS

Conservation of momentum means $p_{initial} = p_{final}$ (p's are total initial and final momentum).

Those forces that one part of a system exerts on another are called **internal forces.** Those forces that are exerted on any part of a system from outside the system are called **external forces.** The principle of **conservation of momentum** states that when the net impulse of the external forces acting on a system is zero, the total momentum of the system remains constant. This condition is automatically satisfied when there are no external forces, or when their vector sum is zero.

D. COLLISIONS

One of the most common applications of conservation of momentum occurs when two objects collide in an idealized collision: one that occurs instantaneously at a specific location. Because there are no external forces, conservation of momentum applies. Conservation of momentum means that the total momentum before the collision equals the total momentum after the collision. For a collision between two objects a, and b, this is given by:

$$p_{ai} + p_{bi} = p_{af} + p_{bf}$$

where p_{ai}, p_{bi} are the momenta before the collision, and p_{af}, p_{bf} are the momenta after the collision. Because momentum has been defined previously as p = mv, the conservation of momentum equation may be written as:

$$m_a v_{ai} + m_b v_{bi} = m_a v_{af} + m_b v_{bf}$$

where v_{ai}, v_{bi} are the velocities before the collision, and v_{af}, v_{bf} are the velocities after the collision.

In one-dimensional problems, velocities are either in the positive direction or in the negative direction, and the conservation of momentum equation becomes a simple scalar equation:

$$m_a v_{ai} + m_b v_{bi} = m_a v_{af} + m_b v_{bf}$$

v_{ai}, v_{bi}, v_{af}, and v_{bf} are the magnitudes of the respective velocity vectors. They have positive signs if the velocities are in the positive direction, and negative signs if the velocities are in the negative direction. The positive direction is chosen arbitrarily.

MCAT SYNOPSIS

In collision problems, choose one direction as positive; the other is then the negative direction.

Example: Figure 3.9 shows two bodies moving toward each other on a frictionless air track. Body A has a mass of 2 kg and a speed of 4 m/s, body B has a mass of 3 kg and has a speed of 1 m/s. After the bodies collide, body A moves away with a velocity of 2 m/s to the left. What is the final velocity of body B?

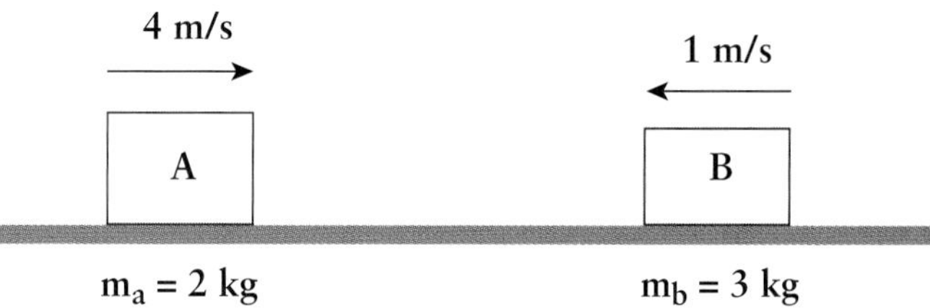

Figure 3.9

MCAT SYNOPSIS

The sign of velocity, positive or negative, determines its direction.

Solution: This problem may be solved by equating the total momentum before the collision with the total momentum after

TEACHER TIP

There are three types of collisions, two of which will be discussed here. In all collisions on the MCAT, momentum is conserved. In both completely inelastic collisions (objects stick together) and elastic collisions (objects don't stick together), kinetic energy is *not* conserved though momentum is. In completely elastic collisions (objects don't stick together), we have a perfect collision in which both momentum and kinetic energy are conserved.

the collision. Let the final velocity of body B be v_{bf}. Taking the right as positive (and therefore the left as negative):

$$m_a v_{ai} + m_b v_{bi} = m_a v_{af} + m_b v_{bf}$$

$$2(4) + 3(-1) = 2(-2) + 3(v_{bf})$$

$$v_{bf} = \frac{8 - 3 + 4}{3}$$

$$v_{bf} = 3 \text{ m/s}$$

The fact that the solution is positive means that body B is moving to the right after the collision.

MCAT FAVORITE

In inelastic collisions: (total kinetic energy before collision) > (total kinetic energy after collision). Lost energy is converted to heat.

In many typical one-dimensional problems the velocities before the collision are known, and **both** velocities after the collision are unknown. The two most common types of such problems are **completely inelastic collisions** and **completely elastic collisions.**

1. Completely Inelastic Collisions

A completely inelastic collision is one in which the colliding bodies stick together after the collision. This means that the final velocities of the two bodies are equal, and hence:

$$v_{af} = v_{bf} = v_f$$

MCAT SYNOPSIS

In inelastic collisions, only conservation of momentum applies.

Thus, there is only one unknown final velocity. This can be combined with the principle of the conservation of momentum to give:

$$m_a v_{ai} + m_b v_{bi} = (m_a + m_b) v_f$$

Example: Two rail freight cars are being hitched together. The first car has a mass of 15,750 kg and is moving at a speed of 4 m/s toward the second car which is stationary and which has a mass of 19,250 kg. Calculate the final velocity of the two cars.

Solution: Using the modified equation above for the conservation of momentum:

$$m_a v_{ai} + m_b v_{bi} = (m_a + m_b) v_f$$

$$v_f = \frac{m_a v_{ai} + m_b v_{bi}}{m_a + m_b}$$

Taking the direction of the initial velocity of the car as the positive direction:

$$v_f = \frac{15,750(4) + 19,250(0)}{(15,750 + 19,250)}$$

$$v_f = 1.8 \text{ m/s}$$

The fact that v_f is positive means that after the collision, the two cars together are moving in the direction that the first car was moving initially.

2. Completely Elastic Collisions

A completely elastic collision is one in which kinetic energy is conserved. The final velocities are not necessarily equal. If neither is given, then from the conservation of momentum equation there is one equation and two unknowns. However, in a completely elastic collision, the kinetic energy is conserved. That is to say, the sum of the kinetic energies just after the collision equals the sum of the kinetic energies just before the collision. This provides the needed second equation.

MCAT SYNOPSIS

Use conservation of energy and conservation of momentum in elastic collisions.

Conservation of momentum:

$$m_a v_{ai} + m_b v_{bi} = m_a v_{af} + m_b v_{bf}$$

TEACHER TIP

The equations for momentum and kinetic energy are both immensely important. *Remember them.*

Conservation of kinetic energy:

$$\frac{1}{2}m_a v_{ai}^2 + \frac{1}{2}m_b v_{bi}^2 = \frac{1}{2}m_a v_{af}^2 + \frac{1}{2}m_b v_{bf}^2$$

Example: Using the results obtained from the example accompanying Figure 3.9, establish whether the collision was completely elastic.

Solution: For the collision to be completely elastic, both the kinetic energy and the momentum must be conserved. The second condition has already been satisfied. Now the kinetic energy before the collision and the kinetic energy after the collision must be calculated, and only if these values are equal can it be said that the collision was completely elastic.

The kinetic energy before the collision is:

$$\frac{1}{2}m_a v_{ai}^2 + \frac{1}{2}m_b v_{bi}^2$$

$$= \frac{1}{2}(2)(4)^2 + \frac{1}{2}(3)(-1)^2$$

$$= 17.5 \text{ J}$$

MCAT FAVORITE

In elastic collisions: (total kinetic energy before collision) = (total kinetic energy after collision).

The kinetic energy after the collision is:

$$\frac{1}{2}m_a v_{af}^2 + \frac{1}{2}m_b v_{bf}^2$$

$$= \frac{1}{2}(2)(-2)^2 + \frac{1}{2}(3)(3)^2$$

$$= 17.5 \text{ J}$$

Because the kinetic energy is not changed by the collision, it can be said that the collision was completely elastic.

CENTER OF MASS

TEACHER TIP

Homogenous objects have their center of mass at the center of the object.

Every object has a special point known as the **center of mass.** Consider a tennis racket being thrown into the air. Each part of the racket moves in its own way, so it's not possible to represent the motion of the racket as a single particle. However, there will be one point along the axis of the racket that moves in a simple parabolic path, very similar to the flight of a tennis ball. It is this point that is known as the center of mass. This is shown more clearly in Figure 3.10.

MCAT SYNOPSIS

Real objects can rotate about their center of mass, as the center of mass moves along a simple parabolic trajectory.

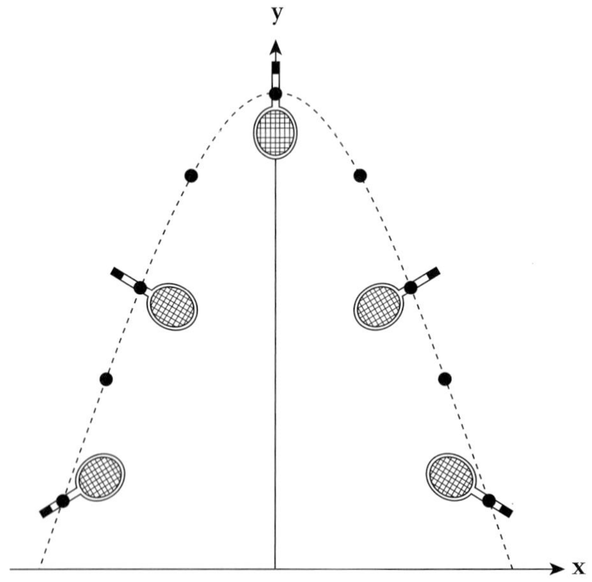

Figure 3.10

For a system of two masses m_1, m_2 lying along the x-axis at points x_1 and x_2 respectively, the center of mass is:

$$X = \frac{m_1x_1 + m_2x_2}{m_1 + m_2}$$

For a system with several masses strung out along the x-axis, the center of mass is given by

$$X = \frac{m_1x_1 + m_2x_2 + m_3x_3 + \cdots}{m_1 + m_2 + m_3 + \cdots}$$

For a system in which the particles are distributed in all three dimensions, the center of mass is defined by the three coordinates:

$$X = \frac{m_1x_1 + m_2x_2 + m_3x_3 + \cdots}{m_1 + m_2 + m_3 + \cdots}$$

$$Y = \frac{m_1y_1 + m_2y_2 + m_3y_3 + \cdots}{m_1 + m_2 + m_3 + \cdots}$$

$$Z = \frac{m_1z_1 + m_2z_2 + m_3z_3 + \cdots}{m_1 + m_2 + m_3 + \cdots}$$

The **center of gravity** is the point at which the entire force due to gravity can be thought of as acting. It is found from similar formulas:

$$X = \frac{w_1x_1 + w_2x_2 + w_3x_3 + \cdots}{w_1 + w_2 + w_3 + \cdots}$$

$$Y = \frac{w_1y_1 + w_2y_2 + w_3y_3 + \cdots}{w_1 + w_2 + w_3 + \cdots}$$

$$Z = \frac{w_1z_1 + w_2z_2 + w_3z_3 + \cdots}{w_1 + w_2 + w_3 + \cdots}$$

Since W = mg, the center of gravity and the center of mass will be the same point as long as g is constant.

Example: Find the center of mass with respect to the x- and y-axes of two uniform metal cubes that are attached to each other as shown in the figure below. One cube has a mass of 2 kg and is 0.4 m on its side, the other has a mass of 0.5 kg and is 0.2 m on its side.

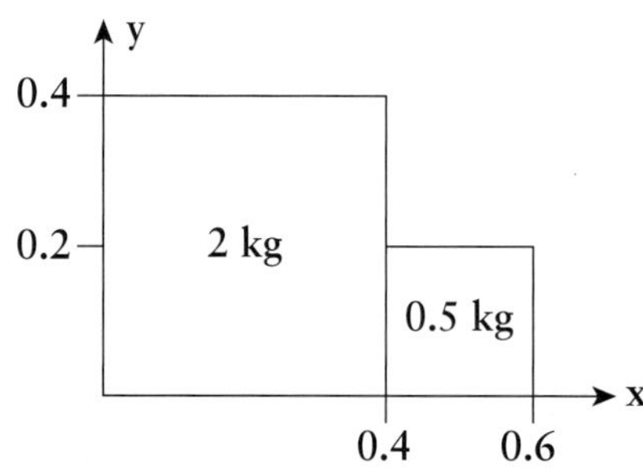

Figure 3.11

MCAT SYNOPSIS

The force of gravity on an object acts through the center of gravity.

Solution: The fact that the cubes are uniform implies that the center of mass for each cube is located at the center of that cube. Therefore, the problem becomes finding the center of mass of two point masses; one is a 2 kg mass located at 0.2 m along the *x*-axis and 0.2 m along the *y*-axis, and the other is a 0.5 kg mass located at 0.5 m along the *x*-axis and 0.1 m along the *y*-axis.

Let's consider the *x*-coordinate first. The *x* component of the center of mass can be determined by the following formula:

$$X = \frac{m_1x_1 + m_2x_2 + m_3x_3 + \cdots}{m_1 + m_2 + m_3 + \cdots}$$

Taking m_1 as 2 kg, x_1 as 0.2 m, m_2 as 0.5 kg, and x_2 as 0.5 m:

$$X = \frac{m_1x_1 + m_2x_2}{m_1 + m_2}$$

$$= \frac{2(0.2) + 0.5(0.5)}{2 + 0.5}$$

$$= \frac{0.65}{2.5}$$

$$= 0.26 \text{ m}$$

The *y* component of the center of mass can be determined by the following formula:

$$Y = \frac{m_1y_1 + m_2y_2 + m_3y_3 + \ldots}{m_1 + m_2 + m_3 + \ldots}$$

Taking m_1 as 2 kg, y_1 as 0.2 m, m_2 as 0.5 kg, and y_2 as 0.1 m:

$$Y = \frac{m_1y_1 + m_2y_2}{m_1 + m_2}$$

$$= \frac{2(0.2) + 0.5(0.1)}{2 + 0.5}$$

$$= \frac{0.45}{2.5}$$

$$= 0.18 \text{ m}$$

PRACTICE QUESTIONS

1. Tom, whose mass is 80 kg, sits at the rear of a 2 meter long, 50 kg boat. Becky, whose mass is 50 kg, sits at the front. Suddenly, Tom jumps at Becky. Where will the boat move?

   A. It will not move, because that would violate the law of conservation of momentum.
   B. It will move toward the stern to conserve momentum by moving in the direction opposite to Tom's movement.
   C. It will move toward the bow but will conserve momentum by stopping as soon as Tom stops moving.
   D. It will move toward the bow, and it will continue moving by inertia without violating Newton's first law or the law of conservation of momentum.

2. Tom, whose mass is 80 kg, jumps off a bench that is 1 meter off the ground. Immediately after landing on the ground with both feet, he jumps 1 meter up into the air. What is the average force on his left foot if the time of contact with the ground is 0.2 seconds?

   A. 800 N
   B. 1,520 N
   C. 2,200 N
   D. 4,400 N

3. A 4 kg object and a 2 kg object are attached by a pulley and held at rest (figure below). What is the acceleration of the rope after it is released?

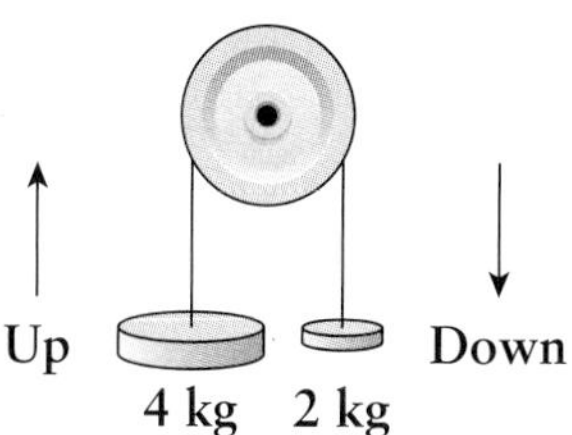

   A. 10 m/s^2
   B. 6.7 m/s^2
   C. 3.3 m/s^2
   D. Zero; the heavier weight will descend at a constant rate.

4. A 100 kg elevator starts from rest and accelerates downward at 4 m/s^2. What is the average power generated by the motor over a span of 5 seconds?

   A. 30 kW
   B. 15 kW
   C. 9 kW
   D. 6 kW

5. How much work is done by a parachute to bring a 60 kg skydiver from his terminal velocity of 60 m/s down to 10 m/s, over a period of 10 s?

   A. 90,000 J
   B. 105,000 J
   C. 210,000 J
   D. 270,000 J

6. A 70 kg pilot is cruising at 200 m/s. He then performs a hook maneuver by flying a lower semicircle at 100 m/s and an upper semicircle at 200 m/s. The radius of the circle is 500 m and the pilot ends up at his original position (figure below). What is the total amount of work done on the pilot?

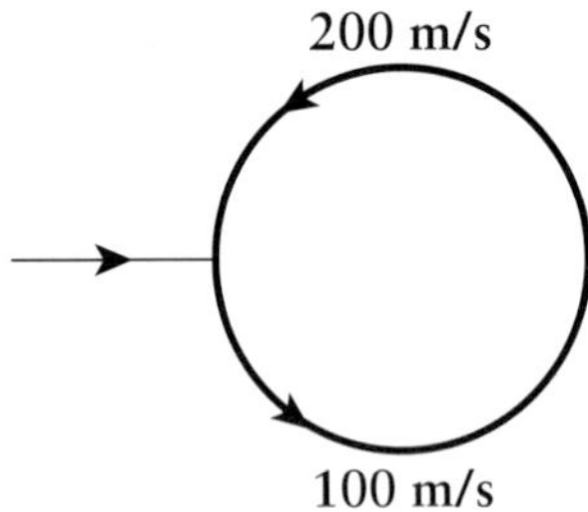

A. 0 kJ
B. 700 kJ
C. 1,050 kJ
D. 1,750 kJ

7. A 1,000 ton asteroid is directly approaching a planet. The asteroid reaches its terminal velocity of 1 km/s when it is 18,000 km above the surface of the planet. At 12,000 km above the surface, it is vaporized. The radius of this planet is 6,000 km. What portion of the asteroid's initial gravitational potential energy is converted into heat?

A. 100%
B. 75%
C. 33%
D. 25%

8. Which of the following are elastic collisions?

I. A planet breaks into several fragments
II. Two balls collide and then move away from each other with the same speed but reverse directionality
III. A volleyball hits the net, slows down, then jumps back with one half of the initial speed

A. I only
B. II only
C. II and III only
D. I, II, and III

9. An oxygen molecule vibrates so that the distance between its intramolecular bonds changes from 1 Angstrom to 3 Angstrom; this change occurs 1,000 times every second. If the average speed of the movement is 100 m/s and the weight of the molecule is 32 amu or 10^{-26} kg, how much energy is produced by these vibrations?

A. 0 J
B. 1×10^{-21} J
C. 5×10^{-21} J
D. 1×10^{-22} J

10. A 1 kg cart travels down an inclined plane at 5 m/s and strikes two billiard balls, which start moving in opposite directions perpendicular to the initial direction of the cart. Ball A has a mass of 2 kg and moves away at 2 m/s, while ball B has a mass of 1 kg and moves away at 4 m/s. Which of the following statements is true?

A. The cart will stop to a halt in order to conserve momentum.
B. The cart will slow down.
C. The cart will continue moving as before, while balls A and B will convert the gravitational potential energy of the cart into their own kinetic energy.
D. These conditions are impossible because they violate either the law of conservation of momentum or the law of conservation of energy.

11. Tom, whose mass is 80 kg, and Mary, whose mass is 50 kg, jump off a 20 meter tall building and land on a fire net. The net compresses and they bounce back up at the same time. Which of the following statements is NOT true?

A. Mary will bounce higher than Tom.
B. The magnitude of the change in momentum for Tom is 3,200 kg × m/s.
C. Tom will experience greater force upon impact than Mary.
D. The energy in this event is converted from potential to kinetic to elastic to kinetic.

12. A man holds a 1 kg arrow as depicted below. Initially, the angle between the string and the arrow is a bit over 50°, as shown. At the moment when the arrow leaves the bow, the angle is 90°. When the man lets go off the arrow, it starts accelerating at 24 m/s^2. Assuming that the string of the bow is like a spring with a constant of 100 N/m, what is the momentum of the arrow as it leaves the bow?

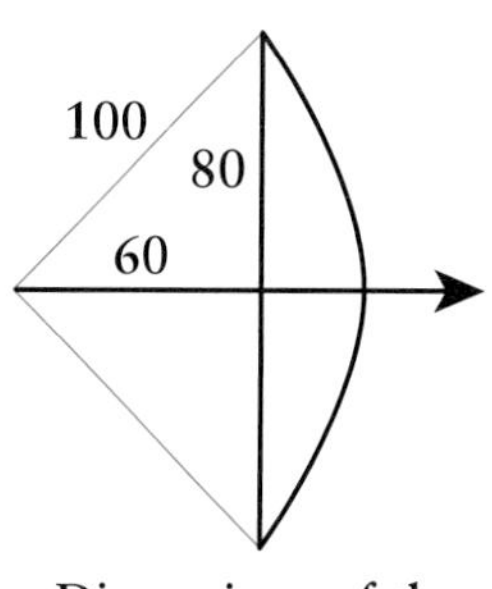

Dimensions of the bow in cm

A. 2 kg × m/s
B. 2.8 kg × m/s
C. 25 kg × m/s
D. 50 kg × m/s

13. A 1,000 kg torpedo travels through the water at a constant speed of 100 m/s. The movement of the torpedo is generated by a combustible engine, which burns 100 kJ of fuel every second and works at 20% efficiency. The resistance of water is proportional to the speed of the moving torpedo. If fuel consumption per second is doubled, then the new momentum and kinetic energy of the torpedo will be

A. unchanged.
B. doubled.
C. doubled and quadrupled, respectively.
D. increased by a factor $\sqrt{2}$ and doubled, respectively.

14. What is the acceleration of a 20 kg box if a force of 100 N is applied, as depicted in the ramp and pulley system shown below?

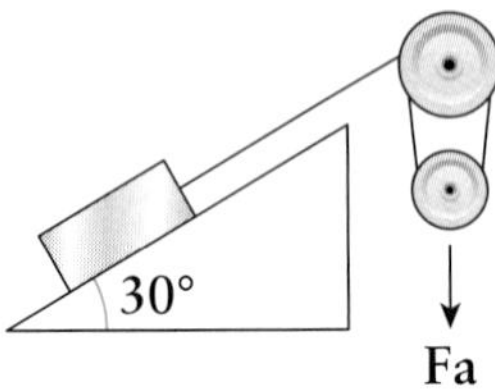

A. 3 m/s^2 down the ramp
B. 5 m/s^2 down the ramp
C. 3 m/s^2 up the ramp
D. 5 m/s^2 up the ramp

15. Two identical molecules, A and B, move with the same horizontal velocities but opposite vertical velocities. Which of the following statements is always NOT true after the two molecules collide?

A. The sum of the kinetic energies of the molecules after collision is less than the sum of the kinetic energies of the molecules before the collision is.
B. Molecule A will have greater momentum after the collision than molecule B will.
C. The sum of the kinetic energies of the molecules after the collision is greater than the sum of the kinetic energies of the molecules before the collision is.
D. Molecule A will have greater vertical velocity than molecule B will.

POWER AND ENERGY

The electricity for a certain industrial-strength space heater costs \$1.50 for 40 minutes. The electric company charges 2 cents per kWh. How long would a light with a 100 W lightbulb have to run continuously to use the same amount of energy as the heater uses in 40 minutes?

1) Determine the energy used by the heater.

$$\frac{\$1.50}{(\$0.02/\text{kWh})} = 75\ \text{kWh}$$

A kWh is a unit of energy, because 1 kW = 1 kJ/s, so 1 kWh = 1 (kJh/s).

---

2) Determine the power of the heater.

$$40\ \text{minutes} = \frac{2}{3}\ \text{hour}$$

$$75\ \text{kWh} = 75\ (\text{kJh/s})$$

$$p = \frac{75(\text{kjh/s})}{\left(\frac{2}{3}\ \text{h}\right)} = 112.5\ \text{kJ/s} = 112.5\ \text{kW}$$

Power is always energy (or work) divided by time, so divide the energy from step 1 by the time. Pay attention to the units here—the time must be in hours!

---

3) Determine the time for which the lightbulb could run on the same amount of power.

$$\frac{112.5\ \text{kW}}{100\ \text{W}} = 1{,}125$$

$$\left(\frac{2}{3}\ \text{h}\right) \times 1{,}125 = 750\ \text{h}$$

Divide the power of the heater by the power of the lightbulb. This tells you that the heater uses 1,125 times as much energy every second as the lightbulb does. Then, multiply the time that the heater operated to use 75 kWh of energy by this factor to determine the time for the lightbulb to use that much energy.

SIMILAR QUESTIONS

1) How much heat is given off by a 60 W lightbulb in 1 hour if only 99% of the energy is released thermally?
2) How much heat is dissipated in 10 minutes by a 2 kΩ resistor with a current of 25 mA?
3) A certain laser beam delivers 10,000 J of energy to a sample in 5 minutes, and 10% of the laser energy is lost in transit to the sample. What is the power of this laser?

KEY CONCEPTS

Power

Energy

Dimensional analysis

TAKEAWAYS

This problem essentially tests your understanding of the units for energy and power. Many students think that kWh is a unit of power, not energy, because of the presence of W in the units. These questions become easy points on Test Day when you use dimensional analysis to get the correct answer!

THINGS TO WATCH OUT FOR

The relationship between power and energy can be tested in many different scenarios, including electrical circuits, mechanical devices, electrical appliances, or efficiency questions.

KEY CONCEPTS

Conservation of energy

Centripetal acceleration

Gravitational potential energy: $U = mgh$ (J)

Kinetic energy: $KE = \left(\frac{1}{2}\right)mv^2$ (J)

$E_i = mgh$ (J)

TAKEAWAYS

The key to this problem is knowing that the normal force is zero at the top of the loop in the case where the block is just about to fall.

Notice that the loop problem follows the same process as any other conservation of energy problem, but with the added aspect of centripetal acceleration. Draw a free-body diagram and solve for the velocity. After this, your goal is the same as always: 1) write expressions for the energy at two points; and 2) set them equal and solve for the unknown quantity.

CIRCULAR LOOPS

A 1 kg block slides down a ramp and then around a circular loop of radius 10 m, as shown in the diagram below. Assuming that all surfaces are frictionless, what is the minimum height of the ramp so that the block makes it all the way around the loop without falling?

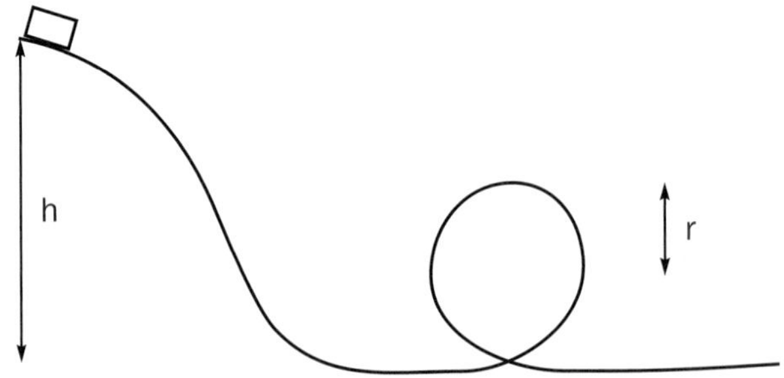

1) Write an expression for the initial energy of the system.

☞ $E_i = mgh$

At the top of the ramp, the block has only potential energy given by the formula $PE = mgh$.

Remember: *Leaving the expressions in terms of variables will save time and reduce the chance of calculation error.*

---

2) Write an expression for the energy of the system at the top of the loop.

$E_{loop} = mg(2R) + 1/2mv^2$

At the top of the loop, the block has both potential energy and kinetic energy. The height of the block at the top of the loop is $2R$. Add these to get the total energy.

---

3) Draw a free-body diagram of the block at the top of the loop.

There are two forces acting on the block at the top of the loop: the weight of the block (equal to mg) and the normal force (labeled F_n). Note that the normal force is acting down because the track is above the mass.

Remember: *The normal force is always perpendicular to the surface and points from the surface to the object.*

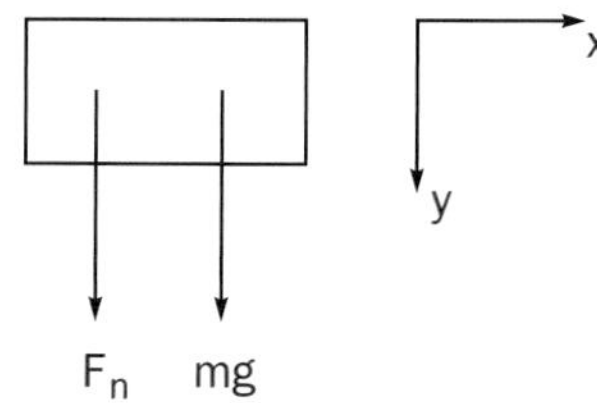

4) Add the forces in the *y* direction.

$\Sigma F_y = ma_y = mg + F_n$

There are no forces acting in the *x*-direction, so add the forces in the *y*-direction only.

5) Set the normal force equal to zero.

$F_n = 0 \rightarrow ma_y = mg$

If the block falls off of the ramp at the top of the loop, the normal force will become zero because the ramp is no longer touching the block. By setting the normal force equal to zero, we are solving for the case where the block just starts to fall off.

6) Identify the acceleration as centripetal.

$$a_y = \frac{v^2}{R} \rightarrow \frac{mv^2}{R} = mg$$

$$v = (gR)^{\frac{1}{2}}$$

Because the block is traveling in a circle, it has an acceleration directed towards the center of the circle, which is called centripetal acceleration. The magnitude of this acceleration is given by the formula $a_c = v^2/R$. Plug this into the equation from step 5 and solve for *v*.

7) Set the energy expressions equal and solve.

$$E_i = E_{loop}$$

$$mgh = mg(2R) + \frac{1}{2}mv^2$$

$$mgh = mg(2R) + \frac{1}{2}m((gR)^{\frac{1}{2}})^2$$

$$mgh = mg(2R) + \frac{1}{2}m(gR)$$

$$mgh = 2.5mgR$$

$$h = 2.5R = 25m$$

Due to the conservation of energy, we can set the energy at any two points equal. Do this and set the velocity at the top of the loop equal to the value from step 6. Then solve for *h*. Because we have set the velocity equal to that at which the block starts to fall off the ramp, we have solved for the minimum height of the ramp.

THINGS TO WATCH OUT FOR

Other variations to this problem include solving for the normal force at various points on the loop, adding friction to the ramp, or having multiple changes in elevation. They are all solved using the same process.

SIMILAR QUESTIONS

1) What is the normal force at the bottom of the loop if the height of the ramp is four times that of the radius of the loop?
2) How fast does the block need to be going at the bottom of the ramp so that the acceleration of the block at the top of the loop is 4 g?
3) What is the speed of the block as it exits the loop if the normal force at the top of the loop was 80 N?

KEY CONCEPTS

Momentum: $p = mv$

Conservation of momentum: $\Sigma p_i = \Sigma p_f$

Collisions

Vector addition

$m_1v_1 + m_2v_2 = (m_1 + m_2)v_f$

TAKEAWAYS

Conservation of momentum will get you through any collision problem on the MCAT. Remember to break motion down into *x*- and *y*-components if an angle is involved.

CONSERVATION OF MOMENTUM

A rugby player with a mass of 80 kg is running due north with a speed of 4 m/s. He is hit by a 90 kg rival at 5 m/s at an angle 30° from the south. The two players move together with an unknown velocity before falling to the ground. Find their combined speed and direction.

1) Determine the type of collision.

The question stem states that the two players move together after impact. This indicates an inelastic collision. Energy is lost in an inelastic collision due to heat, sound, deformation, and so on, so that we cannot use the equation for conservation of kinetic energy. We can, however, use the equation for conservation of momentum.

---

2) Draw vectors representing the collision.

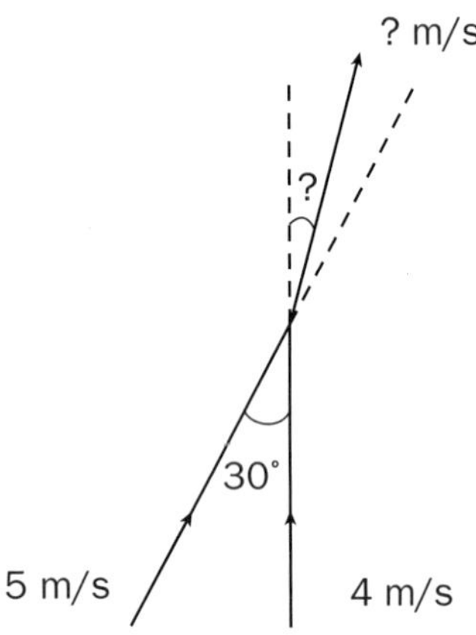

Because we are dealing with angles, we'll need to break the velocity vector down into *x*- and *y*-components. First we need to sketch what those components will be.

Remember: *Think critically. If the second player hits the first at a 30° angle, the final angle should be between 0 and 30° from the north. Even if the second player had a significantly greater momentum, the final angle could not be greater than the initial one!*

---

3) Break the vectors into x- and y-components.

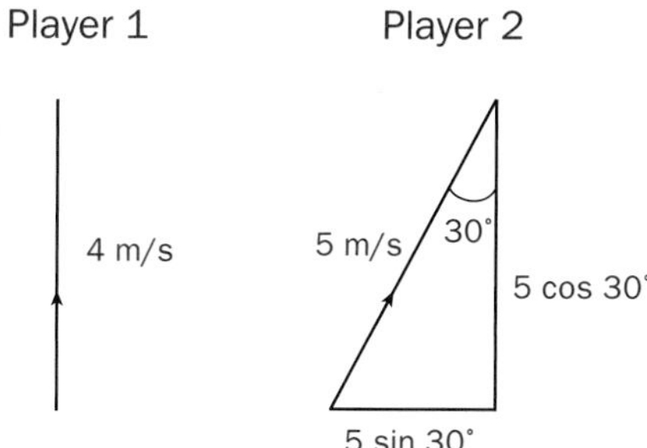

Player one is moving due north, so all 4 m/s of his speed are oriented upward. Player two, however, is moving at an angle. We must consider how much of his momentum moves right and how much moves up. Break his velocity into x- and y-components.

Remember: *The mnemonic SOH CAH TOA will help you remember which trigonometric function to use for each component.*

---

4) Apply the equation for conservation of momentum.

$p_{before} = p_{after}$

☞ $m_1v_1 + m_2v_2 = (m_1 + m_2)v_f$ y: $80(4) + 90(5 \cos 30°) = (80 + 90)(v_f \cos \theta) \rightarrow (320 + 389.7)/170 \approx 4.17 = v_f \cos \theta$

x: $80(0) + 90(5 \sin 30°) = (80 + 90)(v_f \sin \theta) \rightarrow 225/170 \approx 1.32 = v_f \sin \theta$

In both elastic and inelastic collisions, momentum is conserved. This means that we can set the momentum of the system before the collision equal to the momentum of the system after the collision. In this case, we are dealing with a totally inelastic collision. This means that the two masses stick together after impact and move off as a unit. Thus, the momentum of the system before the collision is $m_1v_1 + m_2v_2$, and afterwards it is $(m_1 + m_2)v_f$. Because this problem deals with two dimensions, we must break the velocity vectors down into x- and y-components and then apply the equation for conservation of momentum to each. We end up having two equations with two variables, v_f and θ, where θ is the angle from north.

---

5) Use the relationship between sinusoidal functions to solve for θ.

$1.32/4.17 = (v_f \sin \theta) \div (v_f \cos \theta)$

$[(\sin \theta) \div (\cos \theta) = \tan \theta]$

$1.32/4.17 = \tan \theta$

$\tan^{-1}(0.316) = 17.6°$

THINGS TO WATCH OUT FOR

If you are given a situation in which two objects collide with two angles, it may prove far easier to reorient the axes of the situation so that you only have to deal with one set of vector components.

SIMILAR QUESTIONS

1) A 1,980 kg car moving at 13 m/s is brought to a stop in 2 seconds when it collides with a wall. If a new model of this car has a longer crumple zone, the passengers experience a 3,217.5 N force upon impact. By what percentage has the period of impact been increased? Has the impulse on the car and its passengers changed?
2) A curler slides a stone across an ice rink towards the center of a target with an initial speed of 3 m/s. It strikes a second stone that then hits a third stone. All stones have a mass of 44 kg and are hit head on. If the second and third stones move with individual final velocities of 1 m/s, find the velocity of the first stone after it collides with the second.
3) A 4.2 g bullet is fired into a stationary, 5 kg block of wood. If the bullet lodges in the block, knocking it back with a speed of 0.81 m/s, find the speed of the bullet prior to impact.

In order to find θ, we need to get rid of v_f temporarily. Divide the x-equation by the y-equation. v_f cancels out, and the components allows us to find θ with the arc tangent.

Remember: *Use the mnemonic SOH CAH TOA if you forget how sine and cosine are related to tangent. If you divide sine by cosine, you end up with (O/H)/(A/H) = O/A, the definition of tangent. This is yet another example of simple dimensional analysis.*

---

6) Use θ to find the final speed.

y: $80(4) + 90(5 \cos 30°) = (80 + 90)(v_f \cos 17.6°) \rightarrow v_f = 4.17 \div (\cos 17.6°) \approx 4.37$ m/s

x: $80(0) + 90(5 \sin 30°) = (80 + 90)(v_f \sin 17.6°) \rightarrow v_f = 1.32 \div (\sin 17.6°) \approx 4.37$ m/s

Plug 17.6° back into either the x- or y-equation. In both cases, we find v_f = 4.37 m/s. If we find different values with these equations, we should take a very careful look for our mistake.

---

7) Alternate solution.

$$p_x = p_{1x} + p_{2x} = mv_{1x} + mv_{2x} = 0 + (90)5 \sin 30° = 225$$

$$p_y = p_{1y} + p_{2y} = mv_{1y} + mv_{2y} = (80)4 + (90)5 \cos 30° = 709.7$$

$$p = (p_x + p_y)^{\frac{1}{2}} = (225^2 + 709.7^2)^{\frac{1}{2}} = 744.5$$

$$p = (m_1 + m_2)v_f \rightarrow v_f = p/(m_1 + m_2) = 744.5 \div (90 + 80) = 4.37 \text{ m/s}$$

$$\alpha = \tan^{-1}(p_y \div p_x) = \tan^{-1}(709.7/225) = 72.4° \rightarrow \theta = 90° - 72.4° = 17.6°,$$

where α is the angle from east an θ is the angle from north.

An alternate solution is to calculate the x- and y-components of the momentum directly by adding the x- and y-components of the momentum of the system before the collision. Then, use the Pythagorean theorem to calculate the magnitude of the vector. Because momentum is conserved, set this equal to the momentum of the system after the collision and solve for v_f. To find the angle, use trigonometry, and note that to find the angle relative to the horizontal, you must find the complementary angle.

ELASTIC COLLISIONS

A circus performer weighing 700 N steps off a platform 9 m high. She lands on a seesaw to launch her 630 N partner straight into the air. Compare the landing and launching velocities. Find the height her partner achieves. Ignore the height of the seesaw and any dissipative forces.

1) Find the potential energy of the first performer.

☞ $U = mgh$

$U = (700 \text{ N})(9 \text{ m}) = 6300 \text{ N·m}$

Gravitational potential energy is given by the equation $U = mgh$. Because weight is the product of mass and gravitational acceleration, we need only multiply the performer's weight by her height.

Remember: *A Joule is defined as a Newton-meter.*

---

2) Find the landing velocity of the first performer.

☞ $E = U + KE$

☞ $KE = \left(\frac{1}{2}\right)mv^2$

$E = 6{,}300 \text{ N·m}$

$6{,}300 \text{ N·m} = \left(\frac{1}{2}\right)(70 \text{ kg})v^2 \rightarrow v \approx 13.4 \text{ m/s}$

Because gravity is a conservative force, the total energy is the sum of the potential and kinetic energies. When the performer is atop the platform, all her energy is potential. Thus, $E = 6{,}300$ N·m. Just before the performer hits the seesaw, all of her energy is kinetic. The equation $KE = \left(\frac{1}{2}\right)mv^2$ is used to find her landing velocity.

Remember: *On the MCAT, you will use 10 m/s² for the acceleration due to gravity, as used in the solution to this question.*

---

3) Find the launching velocity of the second performer.

$6{,}300 \text{ N·m} = \left(\frac{1}{2}\right)(63 \text{ kg})v^2 \rightarrow v \approx 14.1 \text{ m/s}$

All of the first performer's kinetic energy is transferred to the second performer. Thus, she also has 6,300 J. She has a smaller mass, so it makes sense that her velocity is increased.

KEY CONCEPTS

Gravitational potential energy: $U = mgh$ (Nm: kgm²/s²)

Kinetic energy: $KE = \left(\frac{1}{2}\right)mv^2$ (kgm²/s²)

Collisions

Conservation of mechanical energy: $E_i = E_f$

TAKEAWAYS

Gravity is a conservative force, and at any point, the total energy is found by adding the gravitational and potential energies. In an elastic collision, kinetic energy (as well as momentum) is conserved.

THINGS TO WATCH OUT FOR

Dissipative forces such as air resistance, heat, and sound reduce the total mechanical energy of the system such that $E_f < E_i$.

4) Find the maximal height of the second performer.

$6{,}300\ \text{N}\cdot\text{m} = (630\ \text{N})h \rightarrow h = 10\ \text{m}$

After being launched into the air, the second performer's kinetic energy is transferred back to potential energy. Compare the total energy of the system with her weight to find the maximal height she reaches.

---

5) Here is an alternate solution.

$U_i = U_f$

$U = mgh = Wh$

$(700\ \text{N})(9\ \text{m}) = (630\ \text{N})h \rightarrow h = 10\ \text{m}$

At any point, $E = U + KE$. When the first performer hits the seesaw, all of her energy is kinetic. It is transferred to her partner, and as the second performer goes higher in the air, her energy increasingly becomes potential. Thus, we can simply equate the potential energy of the first performer with the second.

SIMILAR QUESTIONS

1) The first step in the fusion reaction that occurs on the sun is $^1H + {}^1H \rightarrow {}^2H +$ antielectron + neutrino. This step is rarely ever successful. If an unsuccessful collision of hydrogen nuclei is considered to be elastic, and they each have a mass of 1.008 amu, how do their kinetic energies compare before and after the collision?
2) A frictionless, vertical wire has two metal beads upon it. The beads are held 30 cm apart by horizontal magnets. If the top magnet is removed, the first bead falls under the force of gravity and strikes the second. The first bead bounces back up to a height of 10 cm, and the second is knocked free of the magnet and falls downward. If the two beads each have a mass of 49.7 g, what is the kinetic energy of the second immediately after impact?
3) Two adult bighorn rams butt heads in an elastic collision. The alpha male (136 kg) moves slower than his challenger (113 kg). If the challenger collides at 8 m/s and is repelled at 6 m/s, find the kinetic energy of the system and the percent increase in speed that the alpha male experiences.

COLLISIONS AND ENERGY

A 10 kg block starts from rest at a height of 20 meters and slides down a frictionless, semicircular track. The block collides with a stationary object of 50 kg at the bottom of the track. If the objects stick together upon collision, what is the maximum height that the block-object system could reach?

1) Draw a rough sketch of the collision.

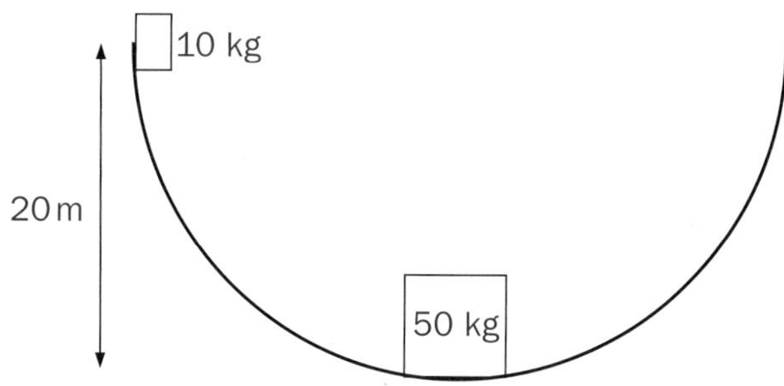

Once you draw the semicircle, draw two objects: one along the top of the semicircle and one at the bottom of the semicircle. Both objects start at rest. The 10 kg block will travel down and reach a velocity *v* before impact with the object. The objects will stick together and travel up the semicircle to a maximum height *h*. The question asks you to find *h*.

---

2) Write an expression for the initial energy of the falling block.

$E_i = PE_i + KE_i$

☞ $PE = mgh$

☞ $KE = \frac{1}{2}mv^2$

$E_i = mgh_i + \frac{1}{2}mv_i^2$

$E_i = mgh_i$

Write an expression for the energy of the falling block. The total energy of the block is its kinetic energy plus its potential energy. The block is initially at rest, so it has no kinetic energy.

---

3) Write an expression for the final energy of the falling block.

$E_f = PE_f + KE_f$

$E_f = 0 + \frac{1}{2}mv_f^2$

KEY CONCEPTS

Kinetic energy

Potential energy

Momentum

Collision

$PE = mgh$ (Nm: kg · m²/s²)

$KE = \left(\frac{1}{2}\right)mv^2$ (Nm: kg · m²/s²)

$p = mv$ (kg · m/s)

Conservation of energy

Conservation of momentum

TAKEAWAYS

This problem combines a conservation of energy problem with a conservation of momentum problem. Remember that the conservation of energy is useful for finding velocities or distances, whereas momentum is used exclusively to find the conditions after a collision.

This is an inelastic collision. Momentum is conserved while energy is not. Therefore, the maximum height reached should be significantly less than the initial height of the block.

THINGS TO WATCH OUT FOR

Momentum is conserved in all types of collisions in all cases! Energy is conserved only in elastic collisions.

SIMILAR QUESTIONS

1) In the above question, determine the height reached by each object if the collision were inelastic and the falling mass rebounded back with a speed of 1 m/s.
2) A man of mass 140 kg standing on a frictionless surface throws a 10 kg rock horizontally away from himself. What is the momentum of the system immediately after the throw?
3) Two baseballs undergo a head-on collision. Ball 1 is twice as heavy as ball 2. Ball 1 was traveling at an initial speed of v_1, while ball 2 had an initial speed of v_2. The type of collision was elastic. If ball 1 travels at a speed of $\frac{7}{5}v_1$ after impact, what is the speed of ball 2?

Write an expression for the energy of the falling block just before it collides with the other block. At this point it has no potential energy; it has only kinetic energy.

---

4) Set the expressions equal and solve for velocity.

$$E_f = E_i$$

$$mgh_i = \frac{1}{2}mv_f^2$$

$$v_f = (2gh_i)^{\frac{1}{2}} = 19.8 \text{ m/s}$$

Due to the conservation of energy, we can set the energy at any two points equal and solve. Use the energy found in steps 1 and 2 to solve for the velocity of the block just before impact.

---

5) Write an expression for the momentum of the system before the collision.

$$p_{\text{before}} = m_1v_1$$

Before the collision, only mass 1 is moving. The momentum of the system is entirely due to mass 1.

---

6) Write an expression for the momentum of the system after the collision.

$$p_{\text{after}} = (m_1 + m_2)v_2$$

After the collision, both masses are stuck together and move with the same velocity.

---

7) Set the expressions equal and solve for velocity.

$$p_{\text{after}} = p_{\text{before}}$$

$$m_1v_1 = (m_1 + m_2)v_2$$

$$v_2 = \frac{m_1v_1}{(m_1+m_2)} = \frac{10(19.8)}{(10+50)} = 3.3 \text{ m/s}$$

Due to the conservation of momentum, we can set the momentum of the system before the collision equal to that after the collision. Solve for the velocity.

Remember: *Momentum is conserved in all types of collisions: elastic, inelastic, or perfectly inelastic. Energy is only conserved in elastic collisions (perfect bouncing). Because this is not an elastic collision, you cannot use energy to calculate the velocity after impact.*

---

8) Write an expression for the energy of the system just after the collision.

$$E_a = PE_a + KE_a$$

$$E_a = 0 + \frac{1}{2}(m_1 + m_2)v_a^2$$

The energy of the system after the collision is due to the kinetic energy of the two blocks moving together.

---

9) Write an expression for the energy of the system at the top.

$E_t = PE_t + KE_t$

$E_t = (m_1 + m_2)gh + 0$

When the blocks get to the top, they stop moving briefly (before falling back down), so their kinetic energy is zero.

---

10) Set the expressions equal and solve for height.

$E_a = E_t$

$\frac{1}{2}(m_1 + m_2)v_a^2 = (m_1 + m_2)gh$

$\frac{1}{2}v_a^2 = gh$

$h = \frac{1}{2}v_a^2/g = 0.56 \text{ m}$

CHAPTER 4

THERMODYNAMICS

Thermodynamics is the study of heat and its effects. Primary to this study are the concepts of temperature, heat, pressure, volume, work, internal energy, and entropy. As applications of these concepts, we will review thermal expansion, heat transfer processes, the notion of specific heat, heat of transformation (latent heat), and p-v diagrams, including the relationship between work, pressure, and volume. The first law of thermodynamics, or conservation of energy in the presence of heat transfer, is reviewed as is the second law of thermodynamics along with the associated concept of entropy.

TEMPERATURE

A. TEMPERATURE

All bodies possess a property called **temperature.** In common usage, temperature is the relative measure of how hot or cold something is. In the study of thermodynamics, however, temperature must be measured quantitatively on a defined scale. There are three scales used to make these measurements of temperature on a thermometer: the **Fahrenheit** (°F), the **Celsius** (°C), and the **Kelvin** (K) scales. Absolute zero and the boiling and freezing points of water for the three scales are listed in the table below.

MCAT SYNOPSIS

Temperature is a measure of the random kinetic energy of the molecules of a substance.

Temperature Scales

Situation	K	°C	°F
absolute zero	0	–273	–460
freezing point of water	273	0	32
boiling point of water	373	100	212

TEACHER TIP

Kelvin is a scale based around "absolute zero," which is the temperature at which all random atomic motion stops. This occurs at 0° Kelvin.

The Kelvin scale is most commonly used for scientific measurements and is a base unit in SI. The Celsius scale is convenient for everyday usage because of its phase change points for water. The Kelvin degree

TEACHER TIP

Don't worry about Fahrenheit on the exam; conversions will be provided.

MCAT SYNOPSIS

A change of 1K = a change of 1°C. 0°C = 273 K.

and Celsius degree are the same size. The following formulas are used to convert from one scale to another:

$$T_C = T_K - 273$$
$$T_F = \frac{9}{5}T_C + 32$$

where T_C stands for degrees Celsius, T_K stands for degrees Kelvin, and T_F stands for degrees Fahrenheit.

Example: If the weatherperson says that the temperature will reach a high of 303 K today, what will be the temperature in °C and in °F?

Solution: To convert from Kelvin to Celsius use:

$$T_C = T_K - 273$$
$$= 303 - 273$$
$$= 30°C$$

Now to convert from Celsius to Fahrenheit use:

$$T_F = \frac{9}{5}T_C + 32$$
$$= \frac{9}{5}(30) + 32$$
$$= 86°F$$

B. THERMAL EXPANSION

TEACHER TIP

It is because of this property that bridges and sidewalks have gaps between their segments; they allow for thermal expansion without damaging the integrity.

Rising temperatures cause most solids to increase in length. The amount of expansion, known as **thermal expansion,** is proportional to the length of the solid and the increase in temperature:

$$\Delta L = \alpha L \Delta T$$

PAVLOV'S DOG

When you see the symbol Δ in front of a quantity, think final minus initial value. The symbol delta means change.

where ΔL is the change in length, L is the original length, and ΔT is the change in temperature. The **coefficient of linear expansion** α is a constant that characterizes how a specific material's length changes as the temperature changes. This usually has units of K^{-1}, though it may sometimes be quoted as $°C^{-1}$. Note that since a change of 1 K is the same as a change of 1°C, α quoted in units of K^{-1} is absolutely equal to α quoted in units of $°C^{-1}$.

Example: A metal rod of length 2 m and a coefficient of expansion of 11×10^{-6} K^{-1} is heated from 30°C to 1,080°C. By what amount does the rod expand?

Solution: By using the information given in the problem, we can substitute directly into the thermal expansion formula:

$$\Delta L = \alpha L \Delta T$$
$$= (11 \times 10^{-6})(2)(1{,}080 - 30)$$
$$= 0.023 \text{ m}$$

Liquids also expand when heated, but in their case the only meaningful parameter of expansion is **volume expansion.** The formula that governs this expansion for both solids and liquids is:

$$\Delta V = \beta V \, \Delta T$$

where $\beta = 3\alpha$.

MCAT SYNOPSIS

Percentage change in length or volume is $\Delta L/L$ or $\Delta V/V$, $(\Delta L/L)100$ or $(\Delta V/V)100$ respectively.

Example: Assume that a thermometer with 1 ml of mercury is taken from a freezer with a temperature of –25°C and placed near an oven at 225°C. If the coefficient of volume expansion of mercury is 1.8×10^{-4} K^{-1}, by how much will the liquid expand?

Solution: Using the information given:

$$\Delta V = \beta V \, \Delta T$$
$$= (1.8 \times 10^{-4})(1)(225 - (-25))$$
$$= 0.045 \text{ ml}$$

HEAT

As was stated in the earlier section, all macroscopic objects have a property called temperature. What exactly does a body's temperature say about that body? The answer is that a body's temperature is related to the internal energy of that body. At constant volume, an increase in temperature indicates an increase in internal energy, and a decrease in temperature indicates a decrease in internal energy.

When two objects that are at different temperatures are brought into contact, the object with a higher temperature will give off **heat** energy to the cooler body until both objects have the same temperature. Heat can be defined as the energy transferred between two objects as a result of a difference in temperature. Note that heat can never be transferred from a cooler body to a warmer body without doing work on the system.

MCAT SYNOPSIS

Heat transferred to a body means the random kinetic energy of the molecules of the body increases.

A. HEAT TRANSFER

Heat energy can be transferred by conduction, convection, or radiation (or any combination of these processes). **Conduction** is the direct transfer of energy from molecule to molecule through molecular collisions.

MCAT SYNOPSIS

Heat Transfer Processes

Conduction: heat transfer through collisions.

Convection: heat transfer through mass motion of heated material.

Radiation: heat transfer via electromagnetic waves.

Metals are the best heat conductors, because mobile electrons play a role in heat transfer from one molecule to the next. Gases tend to be the poorest heat conductors. An example of heat transfer through conduction is the heat that is rapidly conducted to your finger when you touch a hot stove.

Convection is the transfer of heat by the physical motion of the heated material. Because convection involves a flow of material, it can take place only in fluids (liquids and gases). During convection, heated portions of fluid rise from the source of heat, while colder portions sink. Thus, convection involves the transfer of heat through a flow of material.

Radiation is the transfer of energy by electromagnetic waves, which can travel through a vacuum. An example of this form of heat transfer is the warming effect the sun has on the earth.

REAL-WORLD ANALOGY

Why is it that thermos bottles have a shiny surface on the inside? The shiny surface acts to reflect electromagnetic radiation back into the liquid in the thermos, thus retarding one of the primary mechanisms of heat loss from the liquid to the environment.

B. UNITS

Units of heat are either the **calorie** (cal) for SI, or the **British thermal unit** (Btu) for English units. Note that the calorie defined here (lowercase c) and the term **calorie** used in nutrition (uppercase C) are not the same. One food Calorie is equal to one thousand calories.

TEACHER TIP

One calorie (little c) is the amount of heat it takes to raise 1 g (1mL) of water one degree Celsius. One Calorie (big C) is the amount of heat it takes to raise 1 kg of water one degree Celsius.

Because heat is equivalent to energy, the **joule** is also suitable.

The conversion factors among the heat units are as follows:

$$1 \text{ Cal} = 10^3 \text{ cal} = 3.97 \text{ Btu} = 4{,}184 \text{ J}$$

C. SPECIFIC HEAT

The heat Q gained or lost by an object and the change in temperature of that object ΔT are related by the equation:

$$Q = mc\,\Delta T = mc(T_f - T_i)$$

where m is the mass of the object and c is a proportionality constant called the **specific heat.** The specific heat can be defined as the amount of heat required to raise 1 kg of a substance 1 K or 1°C, and depends solely on the material of the object. This formula applies provided that the phase of the object—solid, liquid, or gas—does not change.

D. HEAT OF TRANSFORMATION

The formula previously discussed, $Q = mc\,\Delta T$, applies only when there is no change of phase. During a phase change the temperature remains constant and the heat gained or lost is related to the amount of material which changes phase. The amount of heat needed to change the phase of 1 kg of a substance is the **heat of transformation** L. The total amount of heat gained or lost by a substance during a phase change is given by:

$$Q = mL$$

where Q is the heat gained or lost, m is the mass of the substance, and L is the heat of transformation of the substance.

The phase change from liquid to solid, or solid to liquid, occurs at the melting point temperature. The corresponding heat of transformation is often referred to as the **heat of fusion.** On the other hand, the phase change from liquid to gas, or gas to liquid, occurs at the boiling point temperature. Here the heat of transformation is often referred to as the **heat of vaporization.**

Example: Silver has a melting point of roughly 1,000°C and a heat of fusion of 1×10^5 J/kg. The specific heat of silver is roughly 250 J/kg•°C. Approximately how much heat is required to completely melt a 1 kg silver chain, whose initial temperature is 20°C?

Solution: Before melting the chain, we must first get the temperature of the chain to the melting point. To figure out how much heat is required, we use the formula:

$$\begin{aligned} Q &= mc(T_f - T_i) \\ &= 1(250)(1{,}000 - 20) \\ &= 245{,}000 \text{ J} \\ &= 245 \text{ kJ} \end{aligned}$$

This tells us we have to add 245 kJ of heat to the chain just to get the chain's temperature to the melting point. The chain is still in the solid phase. To melt it (change its

MCAT FAVORITE

In the equation $Q = mc\Delta T$, $Q > 0$ means heat gained, $Q < 0$ means heat lost. Only apply this equation in a temperature region where no phase transition occurs.

MCAT SYNOPSIS

Temperature is constant during a phase transition, i.e., when melting ice at 0°C, all of the ice must melt before the temperature increases.

TEACHER TIP

It is because of the heat of transformation that sweating is so efficient. When the sweat evaporates, the heat of transformation is lost from the surface of the body. This is why heat seems so much worse when it is very humid outside. The sweat is less likely to evaporate due to the dampness of the environment, so less heat will be lost from the surface of the skin through sweating.

TEACHER TIP

Know the following phase changes: sublimation (solid to gas), deposition (gas to solid), fusion (solid to liquid), freezing (liquid to solid), condensation (gas to liquid), and vaporization (liquid to gas).

phase to liquid), we must continue to add heat in accordance with the formula:

$$Q = mL$$
$$= 1(1 \times 10^5)$$
$$= 100{,}000 \text{ J}$$
$$= 100 \text{ kJ}$$

The total heat needed to melt the solid silver chain is 245 kJ + 100 kJ = 345 kJ.

FIRST LAW OF THERMODYNAMICS

TEACHER TIP

The first law of thermodynamics is that energy is neither created nor destroyed. This means that the energy of a closed system (such as the universe) will always remain constant.

A. PRESSURE

Consider a gas contained in a box. The gas particles move in a random direction and some of them hit the wall of the box. As the gas particles hit the wall of the box, they impart a force to the wall. If many particles hit the wall, the net force on the wall increases. The force per unit area is the **pressure** of the gas:

MCAT SYNOPSIS

Pressure of a gas on its container is due to the forces of the individual molecules of the gas on the walls of the container.

$$P = \frac{F}{A}$$

The SI unit of pressure is the pascal (Pa). The pascal is equivalent to a Newton/meter^2. Because this unit is a relatively low pressure, you will often see the pressure quoted in kilopascals (kPa) where 1 kPa = 10^3 Pa. The pressure at sea level can also be used as a unit. This is called an atmosphere (atm), and one atm is equal to 1.013×10^5 Pa.

TEACHER TIP

Another unit of pressure you may see on the exam is mmHg, in which 760 mmHg is equal to 1 atm.

B. WORK

When dealing with the various problems of thermodynamics, the concept of a system is used. To describe a physical process there are two things to take into account: the system whose behavior is being observed and everything else (the environment).

MCAT SYNOPSIS

Work done by a gas on its surroundings (positive work) increases the volume of a gas. Work done on a gas (negative work) decreases the volume of the gas.

A good example of a system is a gas contained in a cylinder with a piston that is able to move up when the gas expands and down when the gas is compressed. When the piston moves up, a force is exerted by the gas inside the cylinder to physically expand the system. Because the volume of the system has increased because of a pressure applied by it, work is said to have been done *by* the system. When the piston is compressed, causing the system's volume to decrease, work is done *on* the system by the environment. This implies that work, in thermodynamics problems, depends on pressure and volume.

During any thermodynamic process, a system goes from some initial state with an initial pressure and volume to some other state with a different pressure or volume. These thermodynamic processes are often represented in graphical form with volume on the x-axis and pressure on the y-axis [see Figure 4.1(a)–4.1(d)]. There are an infinite number of paths between an initial and final state. Different paths require different amounts of work. You can calculate the work done on or by a system by finding the area under the pressure-volume curve. Note that if volume doesn't change, then there can be no work done because there is no area to calculate. On the other hand, if pressure remains constant, the area under the curve is a rectangle of length P and width ($V_f - V_i$) or ΔV. Thus, for processes in which the pressure remains constant,

$$W = P\,\Delta V$$

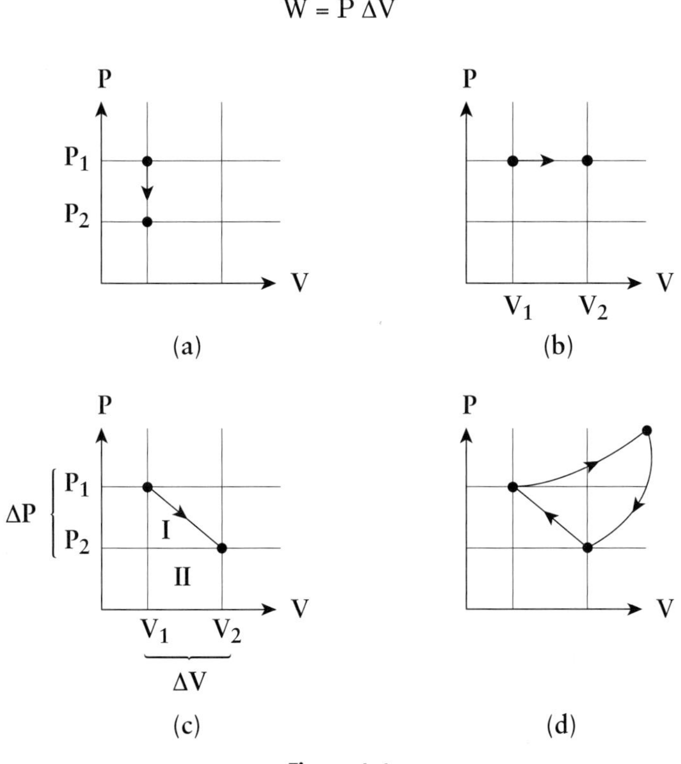

Figure 4.1

TEACHER TIP

From the work equation we see that it takes much more work to change volume at high pressures. Think of a pressurized cylinder. To put more gas into an already pressurized cylinder would take an incredible amount of work. Conversely, when a pressurized cylinder is broken, it quickly does a *great deal* of work on its environment.

Figure 4.1(a) shows that the system undergoes a decrease in pressure from P_1 to P_2. The work done in this process is zero, because volume is constant. In Figure 4.1(b) the system expands from V_1 to V_2 at constant pressure. When the pressure remains constant, the process is called **isobaric.** Here the work done is found using the formula shown above.

The work in this case is positive. Figure 4.1(c) shows a case in which neither pressure nor volume is held constant. The total area under the graph (regions I and II) gives the work done. Region I is a triangle whose base is ΔV and whose height is ΔP and so the area is:

$$A_I = \frac{1}{2}\Delta V \Delta P$$

Region II is a rectangle with base ΔV and height P_2 so its area is:

$$A_{II} = P_2 \Delta V$$

Work now is the sum of region I and II:

$$W = A_I + A_{II}$$

Figure 4.1(d) shows a closed cycle in which, after certain interchanges of work and heat, the system returns to its initial state. Here, the work done is the area enclosed by the curve.

MCAT SYNOPSIS

The internal energy of a system is the sum of all the potential and kinetic energies of the molecules of the system.

C. FIRST LAW OF THERMODYNAMICS

Internal energy (U) is the measure of all the energy, potential and kinetic, possessed by molecules in a system. The internal energy of a system can be increased by doing work on it or by adding heat to it. This change in internal energy ΔU is calculated from the **First Law of Thermodynamics**:

$$\Delta U = Q - W$$

TEACHER TIP

Remember that when work is done on a system, the work is noted as negative. Looking at the equation here, we can see that when work is done on the system, we increase the internal energy of the system.

where Q is the heat energy transferred to the body and W is the work done by the system. Note, we have chosen to use the more common letter U to represent internal energy; however, you may see it also represented by E. Also, note the following **sign convention**: Work done by the system is positive, but work done on the system is negative; heat flow into the system is positive, but heat flow out of the system is negative. The table below gives some special cases of the First Law:

MCAT SYNOPSIS

Internal energy increases ($\Delta U > 0$) when heat is absorbed ($Q > 0$) or when work is done on the system ($W < 0$). Internal energy decreases ($\Delta U < 0$) when heat is lost ($Q < 0$) or when work is done by the system ($W > 0$).

Some Special Cases of the First Law of Thermodynamics

Process	First Law Becomes
Adiabatic ($Q = 0$)	$\Delta U = -W$
Constant Volume ($W = 0$)	$\Delta U = Q$
Closed Cycle ($\Delta U = 0$)	$Q = W$

Example: A gas in a cylinder is kept at a constant pressure of 3.5×10^5 Pa while 300 kJ of heat are added to it, causing the gas to expand from $0.9\ m^3$ to $1.5\ m^3$. Find:

a. the work done by the gas.
b. the change in internal energy of the gas.

Solution: a. The pressure is held constant through the entire process so the work can be found using the equation:

$$\begin{aligned} W &= P\Delta V \\ &= (3.5 \times 10^5)(1.5 - 0.9) \\ &= 2.1 \times 10^5 \text{ J} \end{aligned}$$

b. The change in internal energy can be found from the First Law of Thermodynamics:

$$\begin{aligned} \Delta U &= Q - W \\ &= 3 \times 10^5 - 2.1 \times 10^5 \\ &= 0.9 \times 10^5 \\ &= 9 \times 10^4 \text{ J} \end{aligned}$$

ENTROPY AND THE SECOND LAW OF THERMODYNAMICS

Entropy can be defined as the measure of disorder of a system. One way to picture entropy is to imagine a pool divided in two by an impermeable barrier; one side is filled with water, and the other with ink. This system is highly ordered because the ink molecules and water molecules are physically separated. The position of a particular ink molecule is limited to one half of the pool; therefore, there is some degree of certainty as to where a given ink molecule can be found. If someone were to remove the barrier, however, the water and ink would mix until there was no discernible difference between them. The position of a particular ink molecule is less certain now because it has access to the entire pool, as opposed to half of it. Therefore, the order of the system has decreased and its entropy has increased.

The Second Law of Thermodynamics states that in any thermodynamic process that moves from one equilibrium state to another, the entropy of the system and environment together will either increase or remain unchanged. The entropy of the system and environment together will not change during a totally reversible process, but the entropy will increase

TEACHER TIP

The universe is a closed expanding system, so we know that the entropy of the universe is always increasing. The more space that appears with the expansion of the universe, the more space there is for all of the molecules to move around in, hence the more chaos (entropy).

MCAT SYNOPSIS

The entropy of an isolated system increases for all real (irreversible) processes. The entropy of a system (not isolated) can decrease as long as the entropy of its surroundings increases by at least as much (refrigerators are examples of such a system).

in an irreversible process. Reexamination of the pool previously described shows that it is perfectly acceptable for the ink and water to diffuse and mix together, but it is a violation of the Second Law for the mixture to spontaneously separate into two distinct sections of water and ink.

Isothermal processes are processes in which the temperature remains constant throughout. For reversible isothermal processes, the change in entropy of the system or of the environment can be found from:

$$\Delta S = \frac{Q}{T}$$

where T is the constant temperature of the system or environment in Kelvins.

Example: If, in a reversible process, 6.66×10^4 J of heat is used to change a 200 g block of ice to water at a temperature of 273 K, what is the change in the entropy of the system? (The heat of fusion of ice = 333 kJ/kg.)

Solution: We know that during a change of phase the temperature is constant, in this case 273 K. From the information given,

$$\Delta S = \frac{Q}{T}$$

$$= \frac{6.66 \times 10^4}{273}$$

$$= 244 \text{ J/K}$$

Note that we did not need to know the mass.

PRACTICE QUESTIONS

1. Which of the following changes would definitely cause an increase in a particle's kinetic energy?

   A. Isobaric temperature increase
   B. Isobaric volume increase
   C. Isothermal pressure increase
   D. Isothermal volume increase

2. At a temperature of 0 K, the molecules in a substance

   A. are in solid form.
   B. have no internal energy.
   C. are incapable of reacting with other molecules.
   D. are not moving.

3. Changes in temperature lead to changes in size for which of the following?

   I. Gases
   II. Liquids
   III. Solids

   A. I only
   B. I and II only
   C. II and III only
   D. I, II, and III

4. The internal energy of an object increases in an adiabatic process. Which of the following is definitely true regarding this process?

   A. The kinetic energy of the system is changing.
   B. The potential energy of the system is changing.
   C. Work is done on the system.
   D. Heat flows into the system.

5. Different arrangements of molecules are shown below. Which arrangement is likely to have the most entropy?

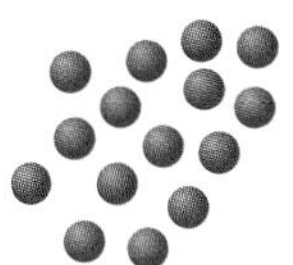

A.

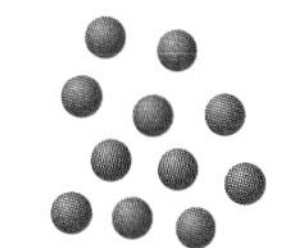

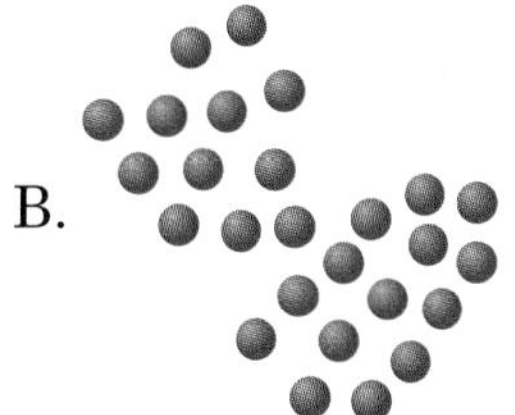

B.

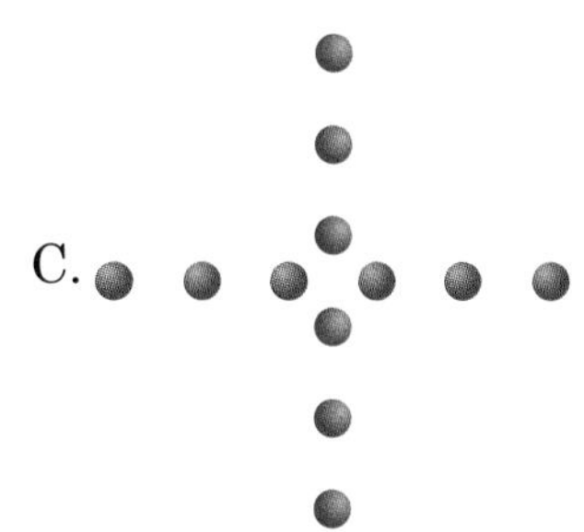

C.

D.

6. A certain object emits heat into space along the lines depicted in the figure below. This heat transfer is an example of

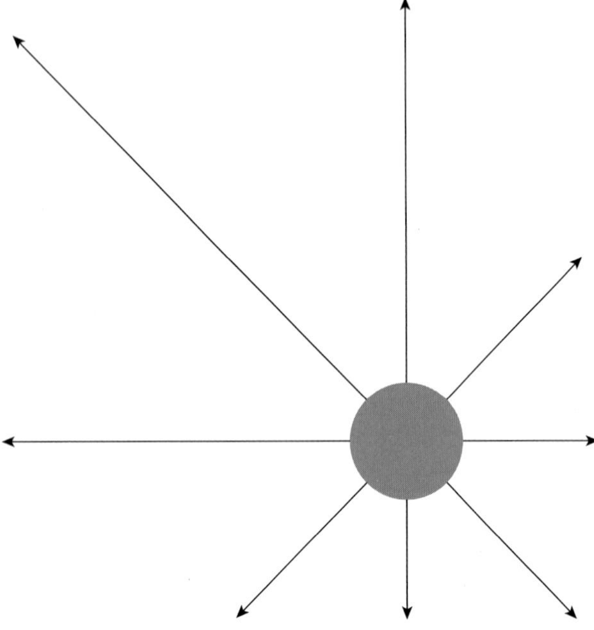

A. conduction.
B. convection.
C. radiation.
D. work.

7. A certain substance has a specific heat of 1 J/(mol*K) and a melting point of 350 K. If one mole of the substance is currently at a temperature of 349 K, how much energy must be added in order to melt it?

A. Greater than 1 J
B. Exactly 1 J
C. Less than 1 J, but greater than 0 J
D. Less than 0 J

8. Which of the following is always true when an object is frozen as a part of an isothermal reaction?

A. The pressure of the system is increased.
B. The change in enthalpy of the system is negative.
C. The temperature of the system is decreased.
D. The volume of the system is decreased.

9. A total of 400 J of heat is added to a pot on a stove. The resulting expansion of air inside the pot causes the pot's lid to be propelled upward. If the lid does 100 J of work during this process, what is the total change in energy of the pot?

A. –300 J
B. 300 J
C. –100 J
D. 100 J

10. When an object is cooled in a refrigerator, its entropy and internal energy can both decrease while the entropy and energy of the refrigerator remain constant. Which of the following explains this phenomenon?

A. The entropy and energy of the object are transferred to the environment around the refrigerator.
B. The entropy of the object is transferred to the environment around the refrigerator, while the energy is dissipated because of the low temperature.
C. The energy of the object is transferred to the environment around the refrigerator, while the entropy is dissipated because of the low temperature.
D. The entropy and energy of the system can decrease because they have undergone an irreversible process.

11. The following graphs depict the change in pressure and volume of a gas. Which graph most likely represents a process in which work is done by the gas as the process moves from point A to point B?

A.
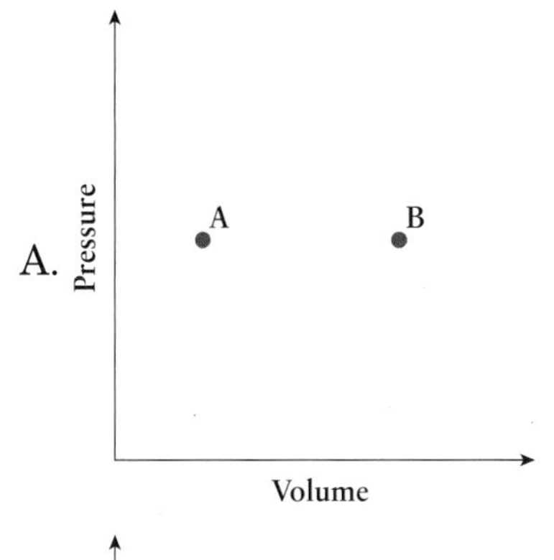

B.
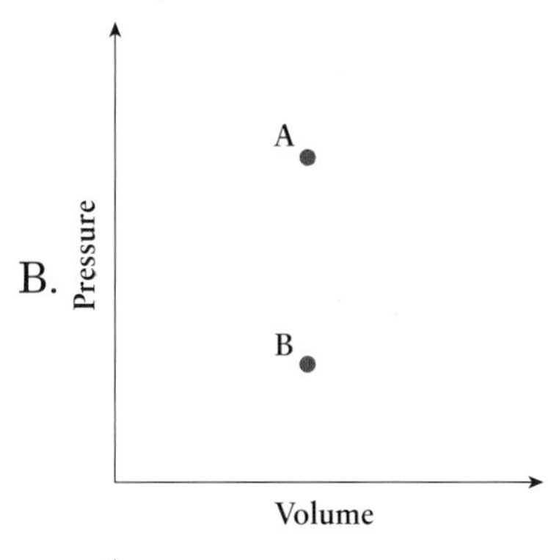

C.
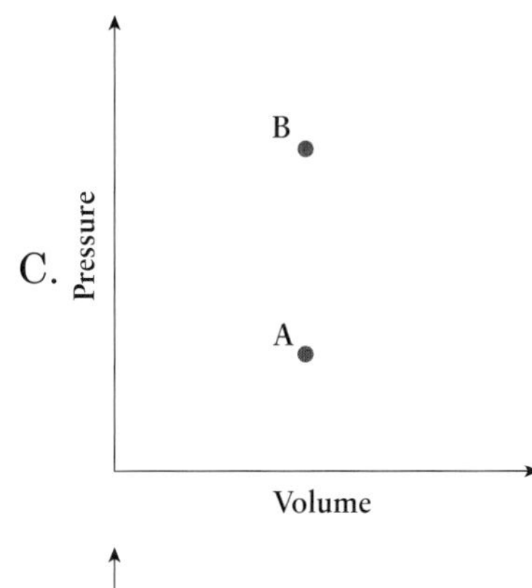

D.
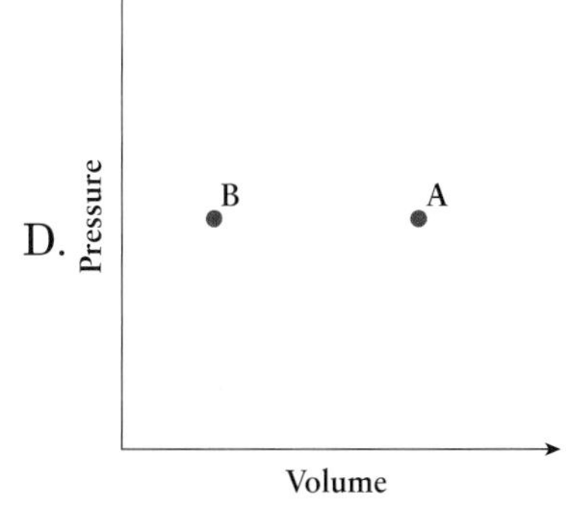

12. The figure below depicts a thick metal container with two compartments. Compartment A is full of a hot gas, while compartment B is full of a cold gas. What is the primary mode of heat transfer in this system?

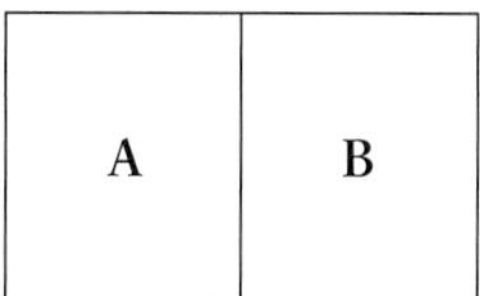

A. Radiation
B. Convection
C. Conduction
D. Enthalpy

13. Substances A and B have the same freezing and boiling points. If solid samples of both substances are heated in the exact same way, substance A boils before substance B. Which of the following would NOT explain this phenomenon?

A. Substance B has a higher specific heat.
B. Substance B has a higher heat of vaporization.
C. Substance B has a higher heat of fusion.
D. Substance B has a higher internal energy.

14. In experiment A, a student mixes ink with water and notices that the two liquids mix evenly. In experiment B, the student mixes oil with water; in this case, the liquids separate into two different layers. The entropy change is

A. positive in experiment A and negative in experiment B.
B. positive in experiment A and zero in experiment B.
C. negative in experiment A and positive in experiment B.
D. zero in experiment A and negative in experiment B.

15. In the diagram below, object A applies a force F on object B. The cross-sectional area of object A is equal to a, the cross-sectional area of object B is equal to b, and the cross-sectional area of object C is equal to c. How much pressure is applied to object C?

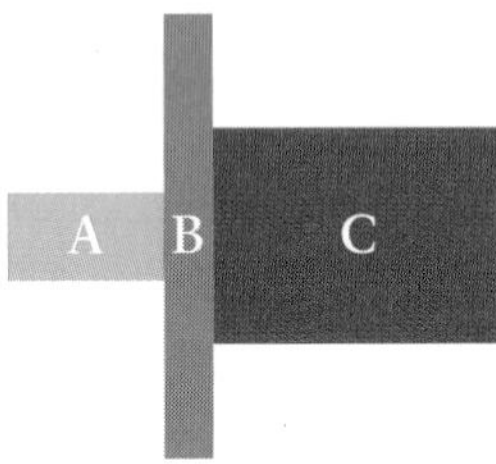

A. F/a
B. F/b
C. F/c
D. F/(a + b)

16. The figure below depicts two rigid containers that are capable of storing equal volumes of gas. One mole of a certain gas at 300 K is placed in each container. Which of the following is true about the pressure of the two systems at equilibrium?

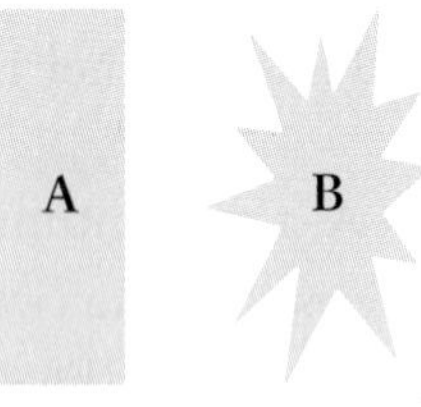

A. Container A experiences more pressure because of its smaller surface area.
B. Container B experiences more pressure because the gas particles are more likely to collide with the container's walls.
C. Both containers experience the same amount of pressure because their contents are identical.
D. Both containers experience the same amount of pressure because they are rigid.

17. The length of a metal rod is 300 cm at 300 K. When heated to a temperature of 500 K, the length of the rod increases to 302 cm. What is its length at 700 K?

A. 303 cm
B. 304 cm
C. 306 cm
D. 310 cm

18. A process with a positive entropy change is always which of the following?

I. Spontaneous
II. Irreversible
III. Exothermic

A. II only
B. I and III only
C. II and III only
D. I, II, and III

19. Which of the following changes will always result when work is done on a closed system?

A. Heat will be released by the system.
B. The temperature of the system will increase.
C. The pressure of the system will increase.
D. The volume of the system will decrease.

20. Which of the following processes is LEAST likely to be accompanied by a change in temperature?

A. The kinetic energy of a gas is increased through a chemical reaction.
B. Energy is transferred to a solid via electromagnetic waves.
C. A boiling liquid is heated on a hot plate.
D. A warm gas is mixed with a cold gas.

21. A certain substance has a specific heat of 1 J/(g * K), a heat of fusion of 120 J/g, and a melting point of 300 K. How much heat is required to bring 10 grams of the substance from 250 K to 350 K?

A. 420 J
B. 1,000 J
C. 2,200 J
D. 4,200 J

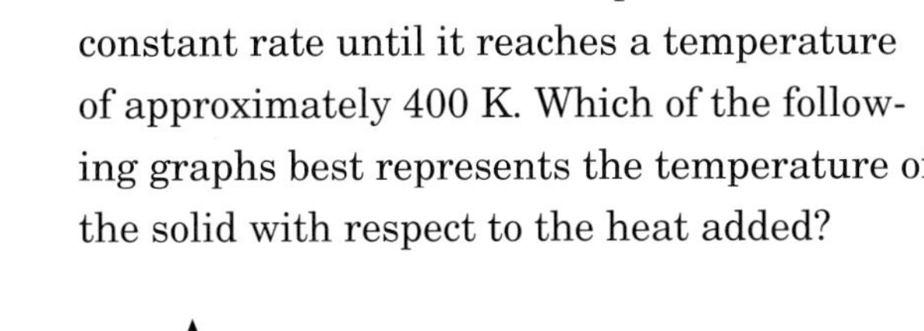
22. Heat is transmitted to a sample of ice at a constant rate until it reaches a temperature of approximately 400 K. Which of the following graphs best represents the temperature of the solid with respect to the heat added?

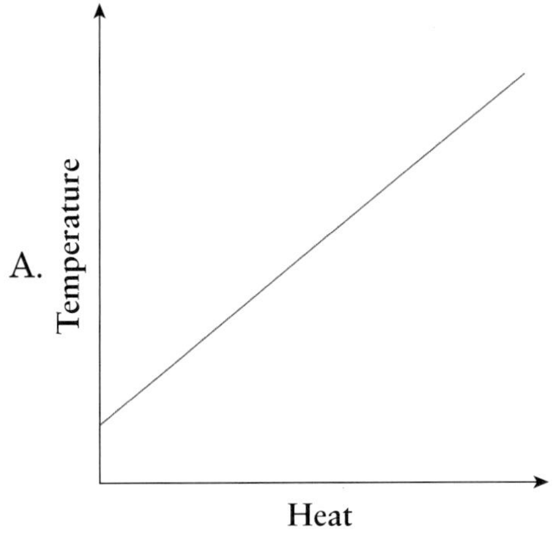

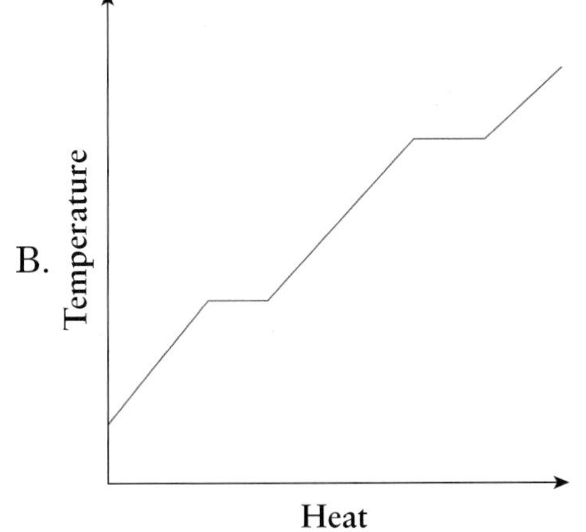

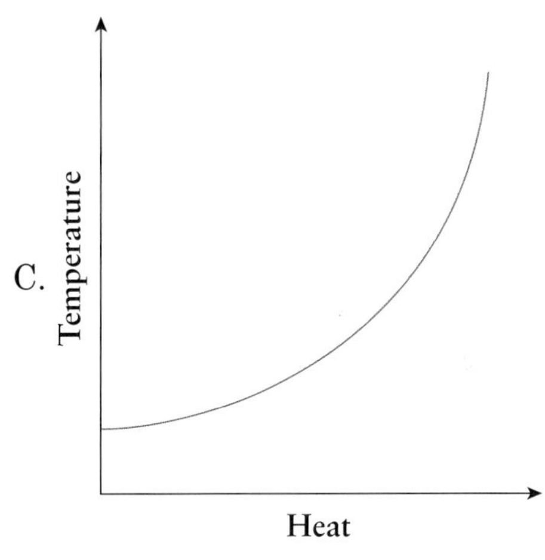

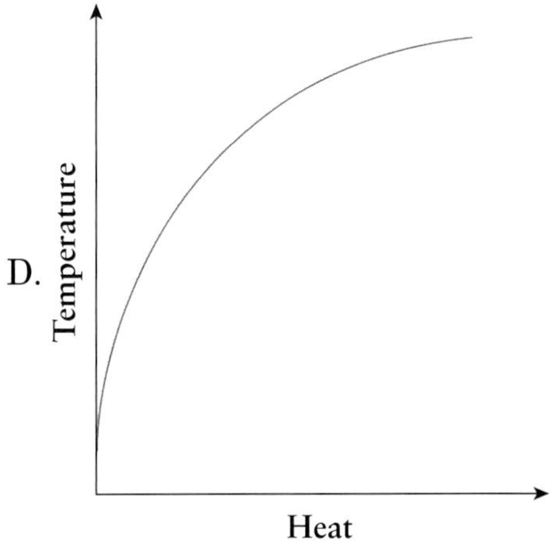

23. In the system shown below, the cross-sectional diameter of piston A is twice the cross-sectional diameter of piston B. If the force applied by piston A is doubled and piston B is replaced by a piston with the same diameter as piston A, then the force applied to the new piston B

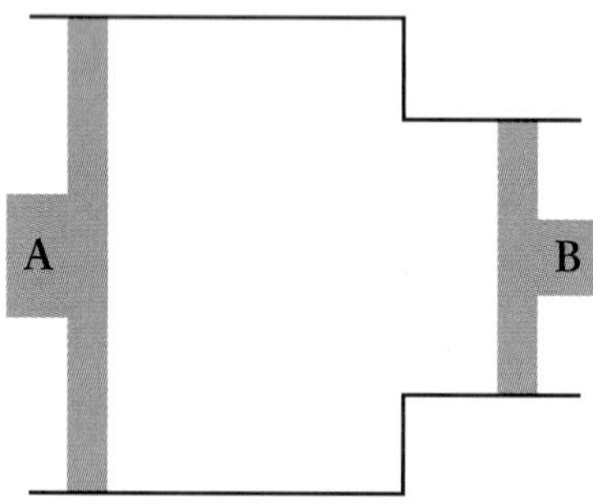

A. decreases by a factor of 2.
B. remains constant.
C. increases by a factor of 2.
D. increases by a factor of 4.

24. Which of the following thermodynamic constants is always the same for every material, regardless of temperature and phase?

A. Thermal expansion coefficient
B. Specific heat capacity
C. Internal energy
D. Heat of vaporization

CHAPTER 5

FLUIDS AND SOLIDS

In this chapter we review the physics of both fluids and solids. The basic concepts of density and pressure are covered as well as the applied concept of the pressure as a function of depth in a fluid. Hydrostatics, or the study of fluids at rest, is presented from the point of view of the two dominant concepts of hydrostatics: Pascal's principle and Archimedes' principle. Hydrodynamics, or the study of fluids in motion, takes us into a discussion of the continuity equation and Bernoulli's equation, as well as a brief discussion of the viscosity and behavior of real fluids. Finally, the elastic properties of solids are discussed along with the associated concepts of stress, strain, Young's Modulus, Shear Modulus, and the Bulk Modulus.

A. FLUIDS AND SOLIDS

Both liquids and gases are classified as fluids; solids are not. Fluids are characterized by their ability to flow and to conform to the boundaries of any container they are put in. Solids, however, are characterized by their rigidity. While both fluids and solids can exert forces perpendicular to their surfaces, only solids can withstand shear (tangential) forces.

MCAT Synopsis

Different materials have different densities. Density is independent of the size of an object.

B. DENSITY AND PRESSURE

Density ρ is a scalar quantity that is defined as mass m per unit volume V. In equation form:

$$\rho = \frac{m}{V}$$

The units of density are kg/m^3 (SI). From the definition of density, the weight of an object can be expressed as the product of its density, volume, and the acceleration due to gravity:

$$W = mg$$
$$m = \rho V$$
$$W = \rho V g$$

The density of water is $10^3\ kg/m^3$ (= 1 gm/cm^3). The ratio of the density of a substance to the density of water is called **specific gravity.** Because it is a ratio, specific gravity has no units.

Teacher Tip

All we need to know about specific gravity is that if our specific gravity is greater than 1, then it is more dense than water. If it is less than 1, then it is less dense than water.

Example: Find the specific gravity of benzene, given that the density of benzene is 879 kg/m³.

Solution: The ratio of the density of benzene to the density of water is the specific gravity.

$$\text{specific gravity} = \frac{\rho_{\text{benzene}}}{\rho_{\text{water}}} = \frac{879}{1{,}000} = 0.879$$

MCAT SYNOPSIS

The same force exerted over a smaller area generates a greater pressure, i.e., spiked heels (greater pressure) versus flat ones (less pressure).

Pressure P is also a scalar quantity. It is defined as the magnitude of the normal force F per unit area A. As an equation it reads:

$$P = \frac{F}{A}$$

The SI unit of pressure is the newton per square meter, also called the pascal (1 Pa = 1 N/m²). Another commonly used unit of pressure is the atmosphere, which is the average atmospheric pressure at sea level. It is related to the SI unit of pressure by:

$$1 \text{ atm} = 1.013 \times 10^5 \text{ Pa}$$

TEACHER TIP

If you forget the units of a value, you can derive it from the equation. We know that Pressure equals Force over Area. Because we know the units of Force (N) and Area (m²), we can solve for the units of Pascals by plugging our units into the equation (N/m²).

Example: The window of a skyscraper measures 2.0 m by 3.5 m. If a storm passes by and lowers the pressure outside the window to 0.997 atm while the pressure inside the building remains at 1 atm, what net force is pushing the window out?

Solution: The forces acting inside and outside the building are needed. However, before the forces may be calculated, the values of the pressure both inside and outside the building must be converted from atmospheres to pascals.

$$1 \text{ atm} = 1.013 \times 10^5 \text{ Pa}$$
$$0.997 \text{ atm} = (0.997)(1.013 \times 10^5) = 1.010 \times 10^5 \text{ Pa}$$

Using the equation for pressure, the force inside pushing out is:

$$F_i = P_i A$$
$$F_i = (1.013 \times 10^5)(7.0) = 7.091 \times 10^5 \text{ N}$$

and the force outside pushing in is:

$$F_o = P_oA$$
$$F_o = (1.010 \times 10^5)(7.0)$$
$$= 7.070 \times 10^5 \text{ N}$$

The net force is the difference of these two:

$$F_{net} = 7.091 \times 10^5 - 7.070 \times 10^5$$
$$= 2{,}100 \text{ N}$$

To find the **absolute pressure P** in a fluid due to gravity somewhere below the surface use the equation:

$$P = P_0 + \rho gh$$

where P_0 is the pressure at the surface, ρ is the density of the fluid, g is the acceleration due to gravity, and h is the depth. In many applications the pressure at the surface is atmospheric pressure, $P_0 = P_{atm} = 1.013 \times 10^5$ Pa. More common in everyday usage than the absolute pressure is what is called the **gauge pressure.** Automobile tire pressure is, for example, reported as gauge pressure. Gauge pressure P_g, is simply the difference between the absolute and atmospheric pressure. The equation for gauge pressure is:

$$P_g = P - P_{atm}$$

Note that if $P_0 = P_{atm}$, then $P_g = \rho gh$ at a depth h.

TEACHER TIP

Many students forget to use the density of the *fluid*—not the object—with this equation. The same mistake is also made when dealing with buoyancy. Make sure to use the density of the fluid itself.

MCAT SYNOPSIS

Pressure increases linearly with depth below the surface of a liquid, and depends on the density of the liquid but not on the density of the object in the liquid.

Example: A diver in the ocean is 20 m below the surface.

a. What is the absolute pressure he experiences? (Density of sea water = 1,025 kg/m^3.)

b. What is the gauge pressure?

Solution: a. Using the equation for absolute pressure in a liquid:

$$P = P_{atm} + \rho gh$$
$$= 1.013 \times 10^5 + (1{,}025)(9.8)(20)$$
$$= 3.02 \times 10^5 \text{ Pa}$$

b. Using the equation for gauge pressure:

$$P_g = P - P_{atm}$$
$$= (3.02 - 1.013) \times 10^5$$
$$= 2.01 \times 10^5 \text{ Pa}$$

HYDROSTATICS

A. PASCAL'S PRINCIPLE

Pascal's principle deals with the transmission of pressures in enclosed fluids. The principle states:

> A change in the pressure applied to an enclosed fluid is transmitted undiminished to every portion of the fluid and to the walls of the containing vessel.

For example, a fluid in a tube exerts pressure on an object at any depth below the surface of the fluid. When the pressure on the fluid is increased, pressure will be increased throughout the fluid and on any submerged object in the fluid.

Pascal's principle is the basis of the hydraulic lever (see Figure 5.1). Consider the case when an external force of magnitude F_1 is applied to the left-hand piston of area A_1. To keep the system in equilibrium, a force of magnitude F_2 must be applied to the right-hand piston of area A_2.

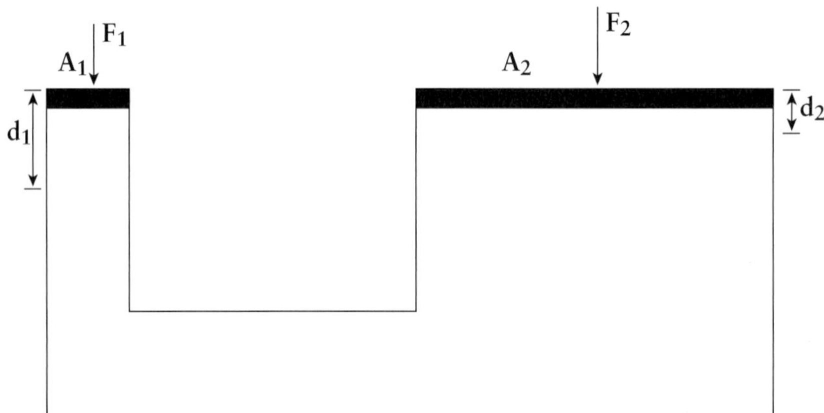

Figure 5.1

TEACHER TIP

With Pascal's principle, remember the following: The larger the area, the larger the force, though this force will be generated over a smaller distance.

Pascal's principle states that a change in pressure is transmitted to every portion of the fluid. Because the system remains in equilibrium as the pressure changes, the change in pressure in both pistons must be equal and is given by:

$$\Delta P = \frac{F_1}{A_1} = \frac{F_2}{A_2}$$

$$F_2 = \frac{F_1 A_2}{A_2}$$

This equation shows that F_2 can be made larger if $A_2 > A_1$.

When piston 1 is moved down a distance d_1, piston 2 moves up a distance d_2. If the fluid is incompressible, then the volume in the system must remain constant. This implies that:

$$V = A_1d_1 = A_2d_2$$

$$d_2 = d_1\frac{A_1}{A_2}$$

By combining the above two equations the expression below is obtained:

$$F_1d_1 = F_2d_2 = W$$

where work W is the product of force and distance. This shows that no additional work is being done by the greater force; the greater force is moving through a smaller distance.

Example: A hydraulic press has a piston of radius 5 cm, which pushes down on an enclosed fluid. A 45 kg weight rests on this piston. The other piston has a radius of 20 cm. Taking g = 10 m/s^2, what force is needed on the larger piston to keep the press in equilibrium?

Solution: Using Pascal's principle:

$$\frac{F_2}{A_2} = \frac{F_1}{A_1}$$

$$F_2 = \frac{F_1A_2}{A_1}$$

Since F_1 = mg, and A = πr^2, it is possible to solve for F_2:

$$F_2 = \frac{45(10)\pi(0.2)^2}{\pi(0.05)^2}$$

$$= 7{,}200 \text{ N}$$

B. ARCHIMEDES' PRINCIPLE

Archimedes' principle deals with the buoyancy of objects when placed in a fluid. It explains why ships float and why objects seem lighter when underwater. The principle states:

> A body wholly or partially immersed in a fluid will be buoyed up by a force equal to the weight of the fluid that it displaces.

In other words, when any object is placed in a fluid, it displaces some of that fluid, and the weight of the displaced fluid equals the magnitude

TEACHER TIP

One way to conceptualize the buoyant force is to imagine that it is the force of the liquid trying to return to the place from where it was displaced, thus pushing the object up and out of the water. This is an important concept because the buoyant force is due to the liquid itself, not the object. Two objects with different masses but the same volumes will experience the exact same buoyant force (assuming that both objects have the same volume submerged).

of the upward buoyant force that the fluid exerts on the object. If the volume of fluid displaced by the object has a weight greater than the object's weight, then the object will float. If the weight of fluid displaced is less than the object's weight, then the object will sink deeper until the weight of the displaced fluid exceeds its own weight. If the weight of the displaced fluid is less than the object's weight even when fully submerged, then the object will sink. In terms of density, if the average density of the object is less than that of the surrounding fluid, then the object will float. However, if the average density of the object is greater than that of the surrounding fluid, then the object will sink.

Example: A wooden block floats in the ocean with half its volume submerged. Find the density of the wood ρ_b. (The density of seawater is 1,024 kg/m^3.)

Solution: The weight of the block of total volume V_b is:

$$W_b = m_b g = \rho_b V_b g$$

The weight of the displaced seawater is the buoyant force and is given by:

$$W_w = F_{buoy} = m_w g = \rho_w V_w g$$

where ρ_w is the density of seawater (1,024 kg/m^3) and V_w is the volume of displaced water, which is also the volume of that part of the block which is submerged. Because the block is floating, the buoyant force equals the block's weight:

$$W_b = F_{buoy}$$
$$\rho_b V_b g = \rho_w V_w g$$

We are given that half the block is submerged, so $V_w = V_b/2$.

$$\rho_b V_b g = \frac{1}{2}\rho_w V_b g$$
$$\rho_b = \frac{1}{2}\rho_w$$
$$\rho_b = \frac{1}{2}(1{,}024)$$
$$= 512 \text{ kg/m}^3$$

C. SURFACE TENSION

There are two types of forces that the molecules of a liquid experience. The first type is **adhesion,** which is the attractive force that a molecule of the liquid feels toward the molecules of some other substance. For example, the adhesive force causes water droplets to stick to the windshield of a car even though gravity is pulling them downward.

The second type of force experienced by the molecules in a liquid is **cohesion.** Cohesion is the attractive force that a molecule of the liquid feels toward the other molecules of the liquid. Below the surface of the liquid, the cohesive forces cancel out because any one molecule is surrounded on all sides by the other molecules of the liquid. However, on the surface, the molecules feel an unbalanced force pulling them back toward the liquid. This causes the surface to behave like a skin and results in what is known as the **surface tension.** An example of the force of the surface tension is the fact that an insect can float on water even though its density is greater than that of water.

MCAT SYNOPSIS

The surface of a liquid has a tension, just like a stretched rubber sheet.

TEACHER TIP

Cohesion occurs between molecules with similar properties. "Like dissolves like." In a container of both water and oil, the water molecules will be attracted only to other water molecules, and the oil will be attracted only to other oil molecules.

HYDRODYNAMICS

A. STREAMLINES

When talking about the steady, nonturbulent flow of fluids, it is helpful to use streamlines. Streamlines are the paths followed by tiny fluid elements (sometimes called fluid particles) as they move. The velocity of a fluid particle will always be tangent to the streamline at that point. It is important to note that streamlines may never cross.

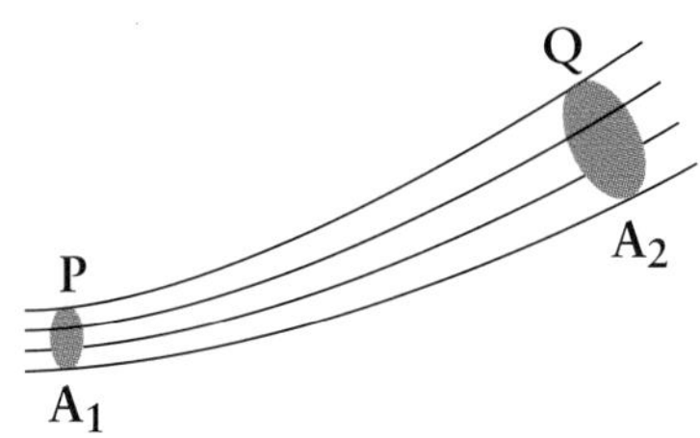

Figure 5.2

Figure 5.2 shows a tube of flow defined by streamlines that form its boundary. Mass flows from cross sectional area A_1 to A_2. The mass of fluid flowing per second through cross sectional area A is given by $Av\rho$, where v is the velocity and ρ is the density. Because matter is conserved, the mass flow rate of fluid must remain constant from one cross-section to another. It is also assumed that the fluid is incompressible, which implies that the densities are equal. Therefore, canceling the density, we find that the volume flow rate is given by:

$$v_1A_1 = v_2A_2 = \text{constant}$$

which is known as the **continuity equation.** This equation states that in narrow passages the flow is faster than in wide passages.

B. BERNOULLI'S EQUATION

The continuity equation, stated previously, results from the conservation of the mass of the fluid. This equation is a statement of the fluid's incompressibility as it flows from one point to another. Energy is also conserved as the fluid flows, and Bernoulli formulated this fact into the following equation that bears his name:

$$P_1 + \frac{\rho v_1^2}{2} + \rho g y_1 = P_2 + \frac{\rho v_2^2}{2} + \rho g y_2 = \text{a constant}$$

where P is the absolute pressure of the fluid, ρ is the density of the fluid, v is the velocity of the fluid, g is the acceleration due to gravity, and y is the height of the fluid relative to some reference height. Like the continuity equation, the Bernoulli equation also refers to two distinct points along the fluid flow labeled by subscripts 1 and 2, respectively. An important relation is derived for the case in which the height of the fluid doesn't change from point 1 to point 2 ($y_1 = y_2$). The pressure of the fluid then decreases as the velocity of the fluid increases and vice versa.

MCAT Synopsis

Fluid velocity vs. cross-section: decreased cross-section means increased velocity, and increased cross-section means decreased velocity.

MCAT Synopsis

For constant height ($y_1 = y_2$), Bernoulli's equation says: increased velocity means decreased pressure, and decreased velocity means increased pressure.

Teacher Tip

The effects of velocity on pressure can be a bit counterintuitive: increasing the velocity of the fluid results in a decrease in pressure, which the fluid exerts on the walls of the container. In other words, the water is being pushed through the container so quickly that it isn't given enough time to interact with the walls of the container. Imagine an approaching tornado. As it approaches the velocity of the air, molecules outside increase greatly. This causes an outdoor *decrease* in pressure, meaning that if the windows are closed they will explode *outward*. That is why one should crack the windows if a tornado is approaching.

Example: An office building with a bathroom 40 m above ground has its water enter the building through a pipe at ground level with an inner diameter of 4 cm. If the flow velocity when entering is 3 m/s and at the top is 8 m/s, find the cross-sectional area of the pipe at the top and the pressure needed at the bottom so that pressure in the bathroom is 3×10^5 Pa.

Solution: The cross-sectional area of the pipe in the bathroom is calculated using the continuity equation, where point 1 is the ground level and point 2 is the bathroom:

$$A_2 = A_1 \frac{V_1}{V_2}$$

$$= \pi(0.02)^2 \frac{3}{8}$$

$$= \pi(1.5 \times 10^{-4})$$

$$= 4.71 \times 10^{-4}\ \text{m}^2$$

The pressure can be found from Bernoulli's equation:

$$P_1 + \frac{1}{2}\rho v_1^2 + \rho g y_1 = P_2 + \frac{1}{2}\rho v_2^2 + \rho g y_2$$

$$P_1 = P_2 + \frac{1}{2}\rho(v_2^{\,2} - v_1^{\,2}) + \rho g(y_2 - y_1)$$
$$= 3 \times 10^5 + \frac{1}{2}(1 \times 10^3)((8)^2 - (3)^2) + (1 \times 10^3)(9.8)(40)$$
$$= 7.2 \times 10^5 \text{ Pa}$$

C. VISCOSITY

Viscosity η is a measure of the internal friction of a fluid. Because of viscosity, a force must be exerted to cause one layer of fluid to slide past another. Both liquids and gases have viscosity, though the viscosity of gases is much lower than that of liquids because a gas has a much lower density. Consider a person moving a hand through air. Little effort is required to move the air out of the way. Hence the viscosity of air is very low. However, for the same person to move the same hand through a tub of water is much more difficult. This is because water has a much higher viscosity than air, and so a greater force is required to move the water out of the way.

TEACHER TIP

Viscosity is a nonconservative force.

The SI unit of viscosity is the newton•second/meter^2 (N•s/m^2). The CGS unit is the dyne•second/centimeter^2 (dyn•s/cm^2), also called the poise. 1 N•s/m^2 = 10 poise.

D. LAMINAR AND TURBULENT FLOW

The simplest type of flow in a tube is **laminar flow**: thin layers of liquid sliding over one another. However, when the velocity of a fluid flowing in a tube exceeds a certain critical velocity v_c (dependent on the properties of the fluid and the diameter of the tube), the nature of the flow becomes very complex. In this case laminar flow occurs only in a very thin layer adjacent to the walls, called the boundary layer. The flow velocity is zero at the tube walls and increases uniformly throughout the layer. Beyond the boundary layer, the motion is highly irregular. Here, random local circular currents called vortices develop within the fluid, and this results in a large increase in resistance to flow. This type of flow is known as **turbulent flow.**

For a fluid flowing through a tube of diameter D, a critical velocity v_c exists below which the flow is laminar and above which it is turbulent. This critical velocity can be calculated from the properties of the fluid flow and is given by:

$$v_c = \frac{N_R \eta}{\rho D}$$

where N_R is a dimensionless constant called the Reynolds number, η is the viscosity of the fluid, ρ is the density of the fluid, and D is the diameter of the tube.

ELASTIC PROPERTIES OF SOLIDS

A. YOUNG'S MODULUS

MCAT Synopsis

Stress is just pressure.

Teacher Tip

Both Young's modulus and the shear modulus represent the same relationship STRESS/STRAIN. Both express stress in the same way as Pressure (F/A), though it is the way that they represent strain that distinguishes them.

The elasticity of a solid is characterized by a number of different quantities called **moduli.** When subjected to a stretching or tensile force F, a material will stretch a length ΔL. Defining a modulus in terms of F and ΔL is difficult because two bodies made of the same substance might require differing forces to yield the same ΔL. This ambiguity is eliminated by defining the tensile stress as the force per unit area, where the force is perpendicular to the area. Similarly, the change in length ΔL may vary for identical materials of different starting lengths L. This ambiguity is also eliminated by defining a quantity called the **strain,** which is the elongation per unit length $\Delta L/L$. It is assumed that upon termination of the stress, the material returns to its original length. **Young's modulus** Y is then defined as the quotient of stress over strain and is given by:

$$Y = \frac{(F/A)}{(\Delta L/L)}$$

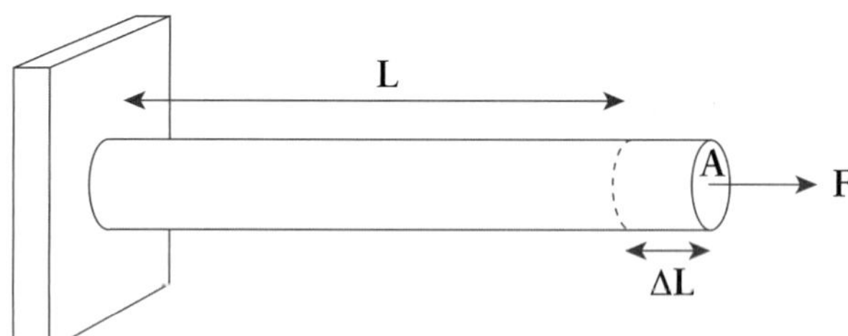

Figure 5.3

Yield strength is the point beyond which a material will not return to its original dimensions once the force is removed. If more stress is applied, eventually the ultimate strength is reached. Beyond that point, rupture occurs.

B. SHEAR MODULUS

Another type of deforming stress is **shearing,** which is measured in units of force per unit area. However, in this case the force vector lies parallel to the area as shown in Figure 5.4. The corresponding deformation or strain is x, the movement in the direction of the force, divided by h. The **shear modulus** is defined as the ratio of the stress to the strain and is given by:

$$S = \frac{(F/A)}{(x/h)}$$

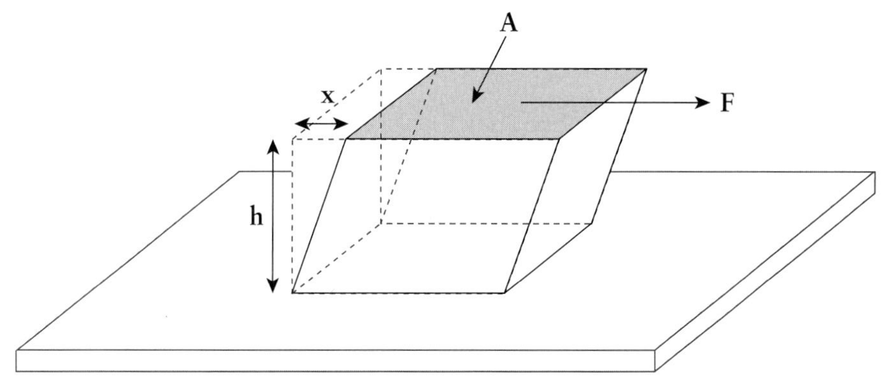

Figure 5.4

TEACHER TIP

In all three moduli, a *large* number represents a more rigid material, while a *small* number represents a more malleable material.

C. BULK MODULUS

The **bulk modulus** relates the change in pressure acting on the surfaces of a solid or fluid to the change in volume that is produced. The stress is the change in pressure ΔP and the strain is $\Delta V/V$, where V is the original volume and ΔV is the decrease in volume. This leads to the following equation for the bulk modulus:

$$B = \frac{\Delta P}{\Delta V/V}$$

PRACTICE QUESTIONS

1. A student is testing the strength of a non-absorbent polymer in fresh and salt water. Which of the following is most consistent with the likely observations of the student?

   A. The polymer will demonstrate a larger bulk modulus in fresh water.
   B. The polymer will demonstrate a larger bulk modulus in salt water.
   C. The polymer will have a similar bulk modulus in fresh and salt water.
   D. The polymer will have no bulk modulus in salt or fresh water.

2. Two women push a wheeled cart up a 30° incline. The second woman pushes with half the force of the first. Over how much area must the second woman apply force to equal pressure exerted by the first woman?

   A. Twice as much area
   B. Half as much area
   C. Same amount of area
   D. The pressure is independent of area.

3. Human lung tissue is very elastic; it prefers to recoil and collapse against itself. However, cells produce surfactant molecules in the lung to prevent this from happening. What parameter is reduced by the presence of surfactant in the lung?

   A. Capacitance
   B. Force
   C. Surface tension
   D. Negative thoracic pressure

4. Laminar flow transitions to turbulent flow at a value known, as the critical velocity of the fluid. Which of the following accurately describes the relationship between resistance and flow of the same fluid?

   A. Resistance in laminar flow is increased, compared to turbulent flow.
   B. Resistance in laminar flow is decreased, compared to turbulent flow.
   C. Resistance in laminar flow is initially higher than turbulent flow but then decreases as the velocity increase.
   D. Resistance in laminar flow is initially higher than turbulent flow and remains higher.

5. Per unit volume, gold is 50 percent as dense as iron. Gravitational pull on Mars is 75 percent that of Earth. By how much will the weight of gold on Earth differ from the weight of iron on Mars?

   A. 25%
   B. 37.5%
   C. 50%
   D. 0%

6. An oddly shaped water-filled sculpture is designed to allow water levels to change depending on a force applied at the top of the tank as shown below. If a force, F_1, of 4 N is applied to a square flexible cover where A_1= 16, and the area A_2 = 64, what force must be applied to A_2 to keep the water levels from changing?

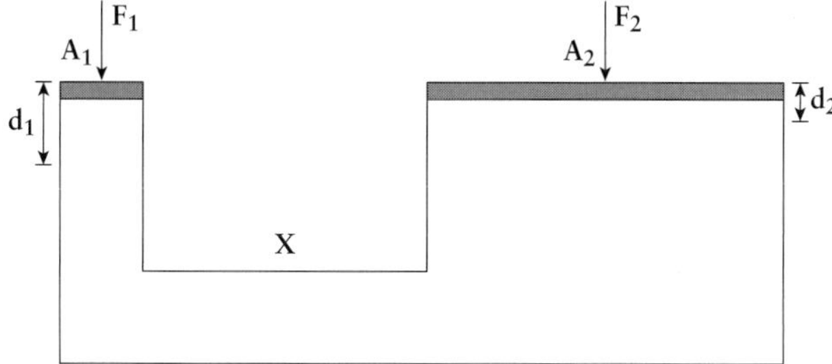

A. 4N
B. 16N
C. 32 N
D. No force

7. A heater is placed at point x in the figure above. Which liquid will boil first?

A. Salt water
B. Fresh water
C. Both salt and fresh water at the same time
D. More information is needed

8. Balls A and B of equal mass are placed in a swimming pool, as in the figure below. Which will produce a greater buoyant force?

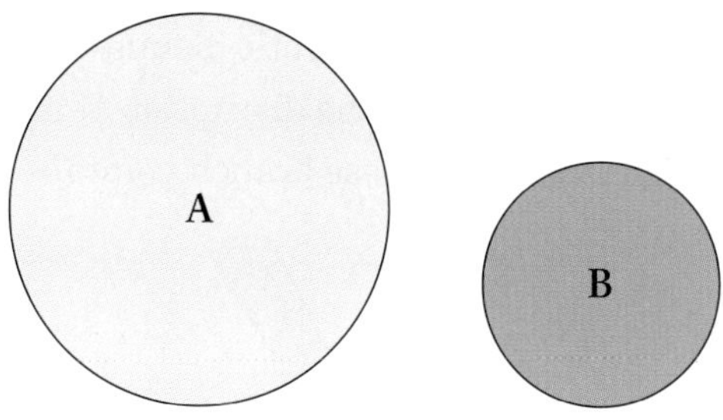

A. Ball A
B. Ball B
C. Force will be equal
D. Impossible to know without knowing the volume of each ball

9. One thousand grams of water is dropped from the top floor of a plank 10 meters high. Assume acceleration due to gravity is 10 m/s^2. What will be the approximate speed of the water when it first hits the pavement?

A. 10 km/h
B. 23 km/h
C. 7 km/h
D. 0.7 km/h

10. Atherosclerotic plaques are collections of oxidized cholesterol and other lipids which form in the lining of arteries. Branch points in arteries, as the one shown below, are often the location of severe atherosclerotic plaques. What concept may explain the disruption of arterial lining integrity at these branch points?

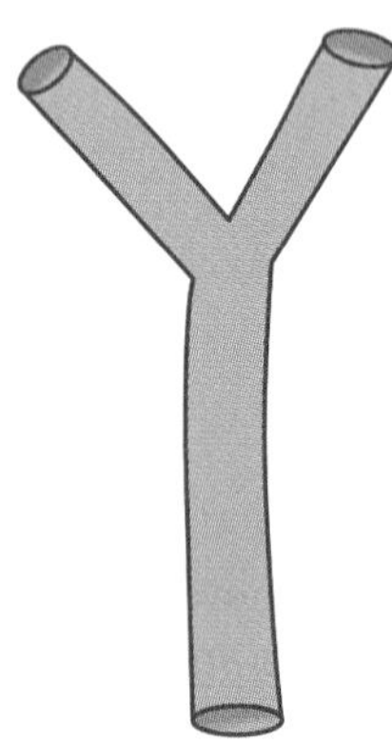

A. Cohesion
B. Laminar flow
C. Surface tension
D. Agglutination

11. Bernoulli's principle is the reason for the upward force that permits a lift force to cause airflight. What statement best summarizes the principle's relationship to flight?

A. The speed of airflow is equal on the top and bottom of a wing, resulting in non-turbulent flight.
B. The speed of airflow is greater over the curved top of the wing, resulting in less pressure on the top of the wing, and the production of a net upward force on the wing, resulting in flight.
C. The speed of airflow on the flat bottom of the wing is greater than over the curved top of the wing, resulting in less pressure below the wing and the production of a net upward force on the wing, resulting in flight.
D. The weight of the wing is directly proportional to the weight of air it displaces.

12. The viscosity of water at increasing temperatures is shown below. Which of the following explains why viscosity changes as temperature changes?

Temperature [°C]	Viscosity [Pa·s]
10	1.308×10^{-3}
20	1.003×10^{-3}
30	7.978×10^{-4}
40	6.531×10^{-4}
50	5.471×10^{-4}
60	4.668×10^{-4}
70	4.044×10^{-4}
80	3.550×10^{-4}
90	3.150×10^{-4}
100	2.822×10^{-4}

I. Increased movement of water molecules
II. Equilibrium shifts to more molecules being present as gas
III. Viscosity is a colligative property

A. I only
B. II only
C. III only
D. I and II only

13. Bulk modulus is defined as the pressure increase needed to cause a given relative decrease in volume (B = dP/(dV/V)). How will bulk modulus relate to Young's modulus in a solid?

A. Bulk modulus is the inverse of Young's modulus.
B. Bulk modulus relates to solids, and Young's modulus relates to liquids.
C. They are identical.
D. Bulk modulus is an extension of Young's modulus to three dimensions.

14. A low pressure weather system can decrease the atmospheric pressure from 1 atm to 0.990 atm. By what percent will this decrease the force bearing on a rectangular window, 6 m by 3 m? The glass is 3 cm thick.

A. 1%
B. 10%
C. 1/3%
D. 3%

15. Laminar-turbulent transition is governed by which constant?

A. Bernoulli's
B. Reynolds
C. Magnetic constant
D. Pascal's

16. Two fluids, one of density x and one of density 2x, are tested independently to assess absolute pressure at varying depths (see table). At what depths will the pressure below the surface of these two fluids be equal?

Depth	Density of Fluid A	Density of Fluid B	Po	Absolute Pressure, Fluid A	Absolute Pressure, Fluid B
2	x	2x	2		
4	x	2x	2		
6	x	2x	2		
8	x	2x	2		

A. Wherever the depth of fluid A is 4 times that of fluid B
B. Whenever the depth of fluid A equals depth of fluid B
C. Whenever the depth of fluid A is 2 times that of fluid B
D. They will never be equal

17. The vapor pressure of a solid

A. increases as the volume of the solid increases.
B. decreases as the temperature of the solid increases.
C. increases as the temperature of the solid increases.
D. decreases as the volume of the solid increases.

18. A water tower operator is interested in increasing the pressure of a column of water that is applied to a piston. She hopes that increasing the pressure will increase the force being applied to the piston. The only way to increase the pressure is to alter the speed of the water as it flows through the pipe previous to the piston. How should the velocity of the water change to increase the pressure and force?

A. Increase the speed
B. Decrease the speed
C. Speed of the water will not change the pressure at the piston
D. Water will release intermittently against the pipe

19. The water tower operator from the previous question decreases the velocity of the water so that the pressure at the piston increases to four times the pressure that was experienced at the previous water velocity. This pressure is to be transmitted between two pipes, one of diameter = 1 m and one of diameter 0.5m. How will the pressure in pipes A and B differ?

A. Pressure will be equal in pipes A and B
B. Pressure in pipe A will be greater than pipe B
C. Pressure in pipe A will be less than pipe B
D. Pressure will be different initially, and the same by the end of the pipe

20. Solid balls of iron and lead are released into a pool of water. How will the pressure beneath the surface on each ball differ when the depth is 15 m?

A. The pressure on iron will be greater.
B. The pressure on lead will be greater.
C. The pressure will be equal in both cases.
D. More information is needed

SPECIFIC GRAVITY

A cube, composed of substance X and having a side length of 5 cm, hangs from a string while fully submerged in saltwater ($\rho = 1.1$ g/cm^3). The tension in the string is 11 N. What is the specific gravity of substance X?

1) Find the volume of the cube.

$V = (\text{side})^3 = (5\text{ cm})^3 = 125\text{ cm}^3$

The volume of a cube is the side length cubed.

---

2) Find the buoyant force on the cube.

☞ generic: $F_B = \rho_{fluid} g V_{submerged}$

$(\rho_{fluid} = \rho_{saltwater} = 1.1\text{ g/cm}^3 = 1.1 \times 10^{-3}\text{ kg/cm}^3)$

$F_B = (1.1 \times 10^{-3}\text{ kg/cm}^3)(9.8\text{ m/s}^2)(125\text{ cm}^3) = 1.35\text{ N}$

The buoyant force depends on the density of the fluid, acceleration due to gravity, and volume of the object submerged. Convert the density of saltwater to kg/cm^3 so that the buoyant force will be in newtons.

---

3) Draw a free-body diagram of the cube.

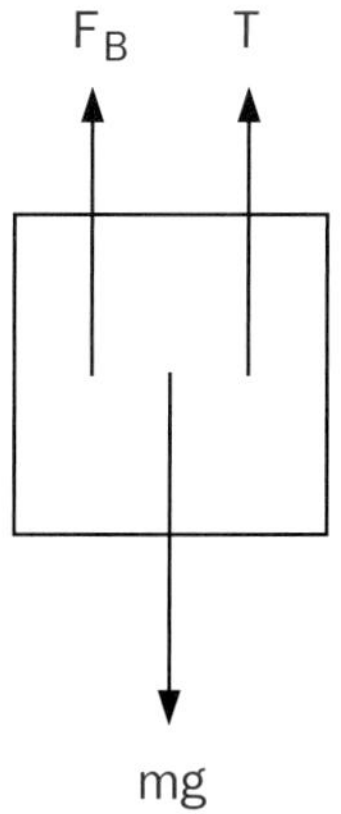

There are three forces acting on the block: the weight of the block (which equals mg), the tension in the string (labeled T), and the buoyant force (labeled F_B).

Remember: *The buoyant force always acts upward.*

Key Concepts

Buoyant force

Archimedes' principle

Newton's laws

Specific gravity

Density

Takeaways

Unit conversion is common in problems dealing with buoyancy, specific gravity, or density. Use dimensional analysis to assist you. Specific gravity is an often-forgotten quantity, but one that is easily calculated.

☞ $\rho_{water} = 1\text{ g/cm}^3 = 1{,}000\text{ kg/m}^3$

Things to Watch Out For

The buoyant force depends on the density of the fluid, *not* the density of the object. This is a common misconception.

SIMILAR QUESTIONS

1) What is the specific gravity of a substance that weighs 40 N and has a volume of 4 cm^3?
2) Three liters of a certain fluid weighs twice as much as 2 liters of water. What is the specific gravity of the fluid?
3) The specific gravity of a block is 5.6. When fully submerged, what is the buoyant force, in water, on this 2 kg block?

4) Add the forces in the *y* direction and solve for the mass.

$$\Sigma F_y = ma_y = T + F_B - mg$$

$$a_y = 0 \rightarrow T + F_B - mg = 0$$

$$m = \frac{(T + F_B)}{g} = \frac{(11 + 1.35)}{9.8} = 1.26 \text{ kg}$$

Every time you draw a free-body diagram, the next step is to add the forces in a direction and set them equal to mass times acceleration in that direction. Because the cube is not moving, the acceleration is zero. Solve for mass.

---

5) Find the density of the cube.

$$1.26 \text{ kg} = 1{,}260 \text{ g}$$

$$\rho = m/V = \frac{(1{,}260 \text{ g})}{(125 \text{ cm}^3)} = 10.08 \text{ g/cm}^3$$

The density of the cube is needed to find the specific gravity. Find the density in g/cm^3 because we know that the density of water is 1 g/cm^3. Density is mass divided by volume.

---

6) Find the specific gravity of the cube.

$$\text{specific gravity} = \frac{\rho_{material}}{\rho_{water}} = \frac{(10.08 \text{ g/cm}^3)}{(1 \text{ g/cm}^3)} = 10.08$$

The specific gravity of a substance is the density of that substance divided by the density of water. When working in g/cm^3, this is a simple calculation because the density of water is 1.

HYDRAULIC LIFT

An automobile hydraulic lift consists of two circular pistons, one with a radius of 25 cm and the other with a radius of 75 cm. They are connected via a tube filled with an incompressible fluid. A constant force is applied to the smaller piston in order to raise a car with a mass of 2,000 kg to a height of 0.5 m. What is the minimum force applied to the smaller piston? How far is the smaller piston compressed?

1) Find the work performed.

☞ $W = mgh = (2{,}000)(9.8)(0.5) = 9{,}800$ J

The amount of work performed is simply the change in potential energy of the automobile, which equals the potential energy of the automobile at 0.5 meters. It is common to think that there is a more complex relationship due to the hydraulic lift being used, but the idea is that the hydraulic lift has 100 percent efficiency, and thus all of the work put into it is used to raise the car.

---

2) Find the force on the larger piston.

☞ $W = Fd$

$9{,}800\ J = F(0.5)$

$F = 19{,}600$ N

The work performed is equal to the force times the distance. You can solve for the force from this formula. However, it is simpler to realize that the minimum force is the weight of the car, which equals *mg*. Realizing this will save you a step of calculation!

---

3) Find the area of the pistons.

$A_1 = \pi r_1^2 = \pi(0.25)^2 = 0.196\ \text{m}^2$

$A_2 = \pi r_2^2 = \pi(0.75)^2 = 1.77\ \text{m}^2$

A hydraulic lift is useful because the force is multiplied by the ratio of the areas of the pistons. Any time you see a hydraulic lift problem, count on needing to calculate the areas. You will see in step 4 that explicit calculation of the area is generally not needed.

KEY CONCEPTS

Pascal's principle

Work: $W = Fd$ (Nm)

Gravitational potential energy: $U = mgh$ (Nm)

$p = \dfrac{F}{A}$ (N/m²)

TAKEAWAYS

Every time you see hydraulics problems, get ready to set up ratios involving the areas of the cylinders in order to calculate forces, distances, or volumes. All of the same rules of work and energy apply to hydraulics, and 100% efficiency is assumed. Remember: the less force used, the greater the distance.

THINGS TO WATCH OUT FOR

There are multiple ways to solve hydraulics problems. To avoid confusion, pick a plan at the beginning and stick with it.

SIMILAR QUESTIONS

1) A hydraulic lift has a cylinder with a radius of 5 cm. What should be the radius of the other cylinder so that the force applied to the first cylinder is multiplied by a factor of 10?
2) The small piston in a hydraulic lift with a piston radius ratio of 10:1 is compressed by 50 cm. How far does the large piston move?
3) What is the volume of fluid moved when the large piston of a hydraulic press is moved 0.2 m (the radii of the pistons are 20 cm and 80 cm)?

4) Set the pressure in the pistons equal to each other and solve.

$$P_1 = \frac{F_1}{A_1} = P_2 = \frac{F_2}{A_2}$$

$$F_1 = \left(\frac{A_1}{A_2}\right)F_2 = \frac{[\pi(0.25)^2]}{[\pi(0.75)^2]} \times 19{,}600 = \left(\frac{0.25}{0.75}\right)^2 \times 19{,}600$$

$$F_1 = \left(\frac{1}{3}\right)^2 \times 19{,}600 = \left(\frac{1}{9}\right) \times 19{,}600 = 2{,}178 \text{ N}$$

Pascal's principle states that the pressure on both pistons must be equal. Set them equal and solve, using $P = \frac{F}{A}$, the general formula for pressure. Note that the calculation can be simplified somewhat by leaving the expressions for area in terms of π. This type of thinking will save you time on Test Day.

---

5) Calculate the compression of the small piston.

$$V_1 = V_2$$

$$d_1A_1 = d_2A_2$$

$$d_1 = \left(\frac{A_2}{A_1}\right)d_2 = (9) \times 0.5 = 4.5 \text{ m}$$

Fluid is pushed through the tube, and none is allowed to escape; nor is it compressed. This means that the volume of fluid moved by each piston must be the same. Set them equal to each other and solve.

This highlights a drawback of hydraulic lifts—even though the force is greatly reduced, the distance is increased. This is because the amount of work performed, given by $W = Fd$, is the same for both pistons:

$$W_1 = F_1d_1 = (2178)(4.5) = 9{,}800 \text{ J}$$

(Thus, another way to calculate distance is to set the work done by one pistion equal to the work by the other piston.)

GAUGE PRESSURE

A certain saltwater solution has a density 10 percent greater than that of water. At what depth in this solution does the gauge pressure equal 2.5 times atmospheric pressure? (ρ_{water} = 1 g/cm^3, P_{atm} = 101 kPa)

1) Find the density of the saltwater solution.

$\rho_{saltwater} = \rho_{water} \times 1.1 = 1.1 \text{ g/cm}^3$

$1.1 \text{ g/cm}^3 \times (1 \text{ kg}/1{,}000 \text{ g}) \times (100 \text{ cm/m})^3 = 1{,}100 \text{ kg/m}^3$

The density of the solution is 10 percent greater than that of water. This is a factor of 1.1. Convert this density to kg/m^3 because these are SI units.

2) Write the expression for pressure.

$P_{total} = P_{atm} + \rho_{fluid}gz$

$P_{gauge} = P_{total} - P_{atm} = \rho_{fluid}gz$

The gauge pressure of a solution is the total pressure minus atmospheric pressure. This is simply $\rho_{fluid}gz$, where z is the depth in the solution.

3) Solve for the depth.

$2.5\,(101{,}000) = 1{,}100\,(9.8)(z)$

$z = 2.5\,\dfrac{(101{,}000)}{[1{,}100(9.8)]} = 23.4 \text{ meters}$

Set the gauge pressure equal to 2.5 times atmospheric pressure. Solve for z.

KEY CONCEPTS

Gauge pressure

Density

Atmospheric pressure

$P_{total} = P_{atm} + \rho_{fluid}gz$

TAKEAWAYS

The gauge pressure of a solution is the pressure due only to the weight of the solution pushing down from above. It does not include the effect of the atmosphere pushing down.

SIMILAR QUESTIONS

1) The gauge pressure of a solution at a depth of 1 m equals twice the atmospheric pressure. What is the density of this solution?
2) What is the pressure at a depth of 50 m below the surface of a pool of freshwater?
3) By what factor does the gauge pressure increase in going from a depth of 30 m to a depth of 40 m in pure water?

KEY CONCEPTS

Archimedes' principle: F_B = weight of the displaced water

Buoyancy

Newton's laws

$F_B = \rho_{fluid} g V_{submerged}$

TAKEAWAYS

When confronting this problem, it may seem that not enough information has been given to you to solve it because you are not given the mass, density, or total size of the raft. You must use two commonly forgotten facts about buoyancy: 1) if something is floating, the buoyant force must equal the weight of that object; and 2) the buoyant force depends on the volume of the part of the object that is submerged.

When in doubt on how to start a buoyancy problem, write the buoyant force formula and see where it leads you. Remember that the buoyant force is a force just like any other: draw it in free-body diagrams and apply Newton's laws.

HYDROSTATICS

A raft of area 2 m^2 floats on water with the bottom 2 cm of the raft submerged. Assuming a thick raft, to what depth is the raft submerged when a brick of mass 3 kg is placed on top of the raft?

1) Determine the volume of the submerged part of the raft.

$V_{submerged}$ = area × height = (2 m^2) × (0.02 m) = 0.04 m^3

The part of the raft that is submerged has the shape of a rectangular prism with a height of 2 cm (0.02 m) and a base area of 2 m^2. In any buoyancy problem, the volume of the portion of the object that is submerged is a useful quantity, so this is a good starting point even if you do not know where to begin.

---

2) Determine the buoyant force on the raft.

$F_B = \rho_{fluid} g V_{submerged}$

$F_B = (1{,}000\ \text{kg/m}^3)(9.8\ \text{m/s}^2)(0.04\ \text{m}^3) = 392\ \text{N}$

The buoyant force is given by the formula $F_B = \rho_{fluid} g V_{submerged}$. Because the raft is floating (not sinking), the net force on the raft must be zero. This means that the buoyant force equals the weight of the raft. This is the connection that most people will not make on Test Day.

MCAT Pitfall: *The buoyant force depends on the density of the fluid,* not *the density of the object. Also, it depends on the submerged volume of the object,* not *the total volume (unless the whole object is submerged).*

---

3) Find the new buoyant force with the added mass.

$F_B = \text{weight}_{raft} + \text{weight}_{brick} = 392 + m_{brick} g = 392 + (3)(9.8) = 421.4\ \text{N}$

This buoyant force is the force required to support the weight of the raft and the brick.

---

4) Find the volume of the submerged part of the raft.

$F_B = \rho_{fluid} g V_{submerged}$

$$V_{submerged} = \frac{F_B}{(\rho_{fluid} g)} = \frac{(421.4\ \text{N})}{(1{,}000\ \text{kg/m}^3 \times 9.8\ \text{m/s}^2)} = 0.043\ \text{m}^3$$

Use the buoyant force found in step 3 in the buoyancy formula. The only unknown is the new submerged volume.

---

5) Find the submerged depth of the raft.

$$V = Az$$

$$z = V/A = \frac{(0.043 \text{ m}^3)}{(2 \text{ m}^2)} = 2.15 \text{ cm}$$

Once again, we are considering the volume of a rectangular prism with a base area of 2 m^2.

THINGS TO WATCH OUT FOR

A very common pitfall for buoyancy problems is to try to use the density of the object to determine the buoyant force.

SIMILAR QUESTIONS

1) A block of mass 5 kg and density 3 g/cm^3 is hung from a string while submerged in water. What is the tension in the string?
2) A cube of side length 3 cm floats in water ($\rho = 1$ g/cm^3) with 1 cm floating above the water. What is the density of this cube?
3) A piece of cork ($\rho = 0.2$ g/cm^3) with mass 5 grams is held underwater. When the cork is released, what is its initial acceleration?

KEY CONCEPTS

Pressure

Density

Bernoulli's equation: $P + (1/2)\rho v^2 + \rho gh$ = constant (N/m^2)

Continuity equation: Av = constant

TAKEAWAYS

Bernoulli's equation looks complicated, but it is really just a statement of the conservation of energy. The process is the same for every problem: 1) write Bernoulli's equation at the two points of interest; 2) eliminate any variables if possible (often via the continuity equation); and 3) solve for the unknown quantity.

THINGS TO WATCH OUT FOR

A common use of Bernoulli's equation is with no change in height, so that $P + 1/2\rho v^2$ = constant. In this situation, a decrease in pressure causes an increase in velocity. This is known as the Bernoulli Effect and is responsible for balls curving in flight, windows exploding during hurricanes, and (partially) for airplane wings experiencing lift.

HYDRODYNAMICS

A water storage tank is located 300 m away from a water outlet, as shown in the diagram below. The empty space in the water tank is held at a pressure of 3 atm. The storage tank has a diameter of 5 m, and the outlet has a diameter of 1 cm. What is the speed of the water exiting the outlet?
(1 atm = 101 kPa, ρ_{water} = 1,000 kg/m^3)

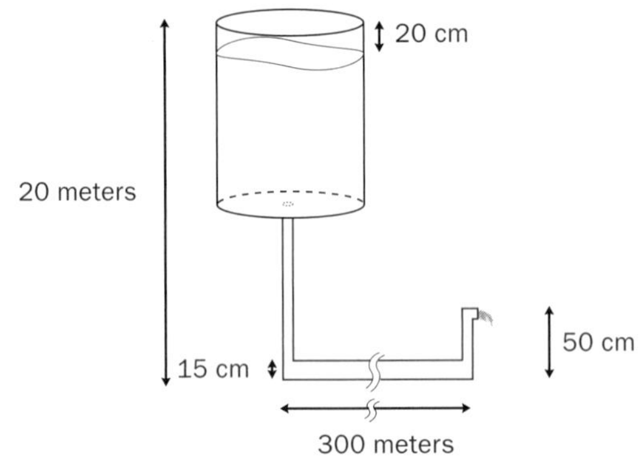

1) Write an expression using Bernoulli's equation.

generic: $P + \left(\frac{1}{2}\right)\rho v^2 + \rho gh = \text{constant}$

$$P_1 + \left(\frac{1}{2}\right)\rho v_1^2 + \rho gh_1 = P_2 + \left(\frac{1}{2}\right)\rho v_2^2 + \rho gh_2$$

Bernoulli's equation is a statement of the conservation of energy for fluids. It has three terms: one analogous to kinetic energy, one analogous to potential energy, and one for pressure (a form of stored energy).

Write the expression for Bernoulli's principle at the two points of interest, just as you would write the total energy of a mechanical system at two points. For this problem, the two points are the top of the water level in the storage tank and the outlet.

---

2) Use the continuity equation.

generic: Av = constant

$A_1 >> 0$, so $v_1 \approx 0$.

$$P_1 + \rho gh_1 = P_2 + \left(\frac{1}{2}\right)\rho v_2^2 + \rho gh_2$$

In almost all of Bernoulli's equation applications, you will need to eliminate some of the terms in order to solve. A common one here is velocity. The continuity equation relates fluid-flow velocity to area. It states that the product of the area and velocity is a constant. Because the storage tank has a very large area, we can approximate the velocity as zero. Think about this: the level of the water tank is moving down very slowly. This simplifies the equation.

---

3) Plug in the given information and solve.

$P_1 = 3\ (1\ \text{atm}) = 3\ (101\ \text{kPa}) = 303{,}000\ \text{Pa}$

$P_2 = 1\ \text{atm} = 101{,}000\ \text{Pa}$

$h_1 = 20 - 0.2 = 19.8\ \text{m}$

$h_2 = 50\ \text{cm} = 0.5\ \text{m}$

$\rho = 1{,}000\ \text{kg/m}^3$

$$P_1 + \rho g h_1 = P_2 + \left(\frac{1}{2}\right)\rho v_2^2 + \rho g h_2$$

$$v_2^2 = 2(P_1 + \rho g h_1 - P_2 - \rho g h_2)/\rho$$

$$v_2^2 = \frac{2 \times [(303{,}000) + (1{,}000)(9.8)(19.8) - (101{,}000) - (1{,}000)(9.8)(0.5)]}{1{,}000}$$

$v_2^2 = 782.3$

$v_2 = 28.0\ \text{m/s}$

The pressure inside the tank is 3 atm. Convert this to pascals, the SI unit for pressure. The pressure at the outlet is 1 atm because the outlet is exposed to outside air, and there is always 1 atm of pressure outside. Plug in the pressures, heights, and density and solve for *v*.

Remember: *Any pipe that is exposed to the outside will have a pressure of 1 atm. When using Bernoulli's equation, though, remember to convert this to pascals! Don't get bogged down with arithmetic: estimate whenever possible.*

SIMILAR QUESTIONS

1) The pressure at one point in a horizontal pipe is triple the pressure at another point. How do the fluid velocities compare at these two points?
2) Pipe *A* has twice the radius of pipe *B*. Both pipes are placed horizontally and are subjected to a fluid pressure of 1.6 atm. What is the ratio of fluid velocities in these two pipes?
3) A water storage tank is open to air on the top and has a height of 1 meter. If the tank is completely full, and a hole is made at the center of the wall of the tank, how fast will the water exit the tank?

CHAPTER 6

ELECTROSTATICS

Electrostatics is the study of stationary or static charges and the forces between them. In this chapter we will review Coulomb's law, which gives the electrostatic force between two charges and then discuss the concept of the electric field, which gives the electrostatic force per unit charge. The topic of electric potential energy is discussed along with the related topic of the electric potential, which is electric potential energy per unit charge. One can think of the electric potential being related to the electric potential energy in the same way as the electric field is related to the electric force. Associated with the electric field and electric potential are the concepts of field lines and equipotential lines which are reviewed separately. Finally, a detailed discussion of the electric dipole is presented with a worked example of a real-life dipole, the H_2O molecule.

CHARGES

Charge may be either positive or negative. A positive charge and a negative charge attract one another; positive repels positive; and negative repels negative. To summarize: **unlike charges attract, like charges repel.** The force that exists between stationary charges is known as the **electrostatic** force.

TEACHER TIP

While many of the particles we discuss in electrostatics are very, very tiny, they are still particles meaning they have mass. You can still use equations such as the kinetic energy equation when solving these problems.

Net charge can appear on a macroscopic object due to friction. If a glass rod is rubbed on a piece of silk, electrons, which are negatively charged, flow from the glass rod to the silk cloth. This results in the glass rod being positively charged and the silk cloth being negatively charged. The rod and cloth then attract each other; this is known as static cling.

The SI unit of charge is the **Coulomb** and the **fundamental unit of charge** is:

$$e = 1.60 \times 10^{-19}\ C$$

Both protons and electrons have this amount of charge, though protons are positively charged ($q = +e$), and electrons are negatively charged ($q = -e$).

MCAT SYNOPSIS

Coulomb's law gives the magnitude of the force of q_1 on q_2 = the force of q_2 on q_1. This is analogous to Newton's law of gravity which gives force of m_1 on m_2 = force of m_2 on m_1.

TEACHER TIP

Notice how this equation is basically the same as the gravitational force equation, only using different terms. While Coulomb's equation deals with electrostatic force between two charges, the other deals with the gravitational force between two bodies of mass.

MCAT FAVORITE

When the distance between two charges is doubled, the force is reduced to 1/4 of the original force, i.e., $F \propto 1/r^2$.

COULOMB'S LAW

Coulomb's law gives the magnitude of the electrostatic force F between two charges, q_1 and q_2, whose centers are separated by a distance r:

$$F = k\frac{q_1 q_2}{r^2}$$

where k is called **Coulomb's constant** or the **electrostatic constant,** and is a number that depends on the units used in the equation. In SI units $k = 1/4\pi\varepsilon_0 = 8.99 \times 10^9\ \text{N} \bullet \text{m}^2/\text{C}^2$, where $\varepsilon_0 = 8.85 \times 10^{-12}\text{C}^2/\text{N} \bullet \text{m}^2$ and is called the **permittivity of free space**.

Coulomb's law in SI units is therefore:

$$F = k\frac{q_1 q_2}{r^2} = \frac{1}{4\pi\varepsilon_0}\frac{q_1 q_2}{r^2} = 8.99 \times 10^9 \frac{q_1 q_2}{r^2}$$

where the force F is in newtons, the charges q_1 and q_2 are in coulombs, and the distance r is in meters. The direction of the force may be obtained by remembering that unlike charges attract and like charges repel. The force always points along the line connecting the centers of the two charges.

Example: A positive charge is attracted to a negative charge a certain distance away. The charges are then moved so that they are separated by twice the distance. How has the force of attraction changed between them?

Solution: Coulomb's law states that the force between two charges varies as the inverse of the square of the distance between them. Therefore, if the distance is doubled, the square of the distance is quadrupled and the force is reduced to 1/4 of what it was originally. Note that it was not necessary to know the distance or the units being used, but only the fact that the distance was doubled and that the relation was an inverse square law.

Example: Negatively charged electrons are electrostatically attracted to positively charged protons (together they form hydrogen atoms). Because electrons and protons have mass, they will be gravitationally attracted to each other as well. Compare the two forces using Coulomb's law and Newton's law of gravitation. (Use $m_p = 1.67 \times 10^{-27}$ kg, $m_e = 9.11 \times 10^{-31}$ kg, and a Bohr radius separation between the electron and proton so that r = 5.29×10^{-11}m.)

Solution: Both Coulomb's law and Newton's law state that the attractive forces between the electron and proton vary as the inverse of the square of the distance between them. As calculated in chapter 2, the gravitational attractive force is:

$$F_N = \frac{Gm_pm_e}{r^2}$$

$$= \frac{(6.67 \times 10^{-11})(1.67 \times 10^{-27})(9.11 \times 10^{-31})}{(5.29 \times 10^{-11})^2} F$$

$$= 3.63 \times 10^{-47}\ \text{N} \approx 10^{-47}\ \text{N}$$

On the other hand, the magnitude of the electrostatic attractive force is:

$$F_c = \frac{1}{4\pi\varepsilon_0}\frac{q_pq_e}{r^2}$$

$$= \frac{(8.99 \times 10^9)(1.60 \times 10^{-19})(1.60 \times 10^{-19})}{(5.29 \times 10^{-11})^2}$$

$$= 8.22 \times 10^{-8}\ \text{N} \approx 10^{-7}\ \text{N}$$

Note that the electrostatic attraction between the electron and proton is stronger than the gravitational attraction by a factor of approximately 10^{40}.

ELECTRIC FIELD

Every electric charge sets up a surrounding **electric field.** The electric field can be detected by the force it exerts on other electric charges. It is defined as the force on a stationary positive test charge q_0 divided by the charge. It is therefore a vector quantity given by:

$$E = \frac{F}{q_0}$$

The electric field E points in the direction of the force F on the positive test charge q_0. In SI units, E is measured in newtons/coulomb, which equals volts/meter. The volt will be defined in the next section where the electric potential is discussed.

MCAT SYNOPSIS

The Electric field is a vector with units given by $E = \frac{F}{q_0}$ = newtons/coulomb.

MCAT SYNOPSIS

A positive charge in an electric field feels a force in the direction of the field. A negative charge in an electric field feels a force in the direction opposite the field.

Given an electric field E in some region of space, any charge q placed in the field experiences a force F given by:

$$F = qE$$

In this vector equation we keep the sign of the charge, so that the force F is in the direction of qE: that is, in the same direction as E itself if q is positive, but in the opposite direction to E if q is negative.

The force on a positive test charge q_0 placed a distance r from a charge q is given by Coulomb's law:

$$F = k\frac{qq_0}{r^2}$$

Using this equation and the fact that the electric field $E = F/q_0$, we get an equation for the electric field at any distance r from a charge q:

$$E = k\frac{q}{r^2}$$

MCAT SYNOPSIS

The electric field of a positive charge points radially outward from the charge. The electric field of a negative charge points radially inward towards the charge.

MCAT SYNOPSIS

The electric field strength is stronger where the field lines are closer together and weaker where the field lines are farther apart. Electric field lines NEVER cross.

The **direction** of the electric field vector is such that it points away from q if q is a positive charge, but it points towards q if q is a negative charge. In order to visualize the direction and magnitude of the electric field vector over a wide number of points, it is helpful to think of **field lines.** Field lines, or **lines of force,** as they are sometimes called, are imaginary lines that represent how a positive test charge would be accelerated in the electric field. For example, the field lines for a negatively charged particle such as an electron would point radially toward the charge, because the positive test charge would be attracted toward a negative charge. Similarly, the field lines point radially away from a positive charge, such as a proton, because the positive test charge would be repelled away from another positive charge.

The direction of the electric field, at a given point, is always tangent to the field line at that point and in the same direction. Field lines also indicate the relative strength of the electric field. Where the field lines are closer together the electric field is stronger; where the field lines are farther apart the electric field is weaker.

MCAT SYNOPSIS

Electric fields of separate charges add as vectors.

For a collection of charges, the total electric field at a point in space is the **vector sum** of the electric field due to each charge:

$$E_{total} = E_{q_1} + E_{q_2} + E_{q_3} + \cdots \text{ (vector sum)}$$

The vector sum must be carried out using the rules of vector addition, as shown in the following example.

Example: A positive charge of $+1 \times 10^{-5}$ C is located one meter away from another positive charge of $+2 \times 10^{-5}$ C. At what point along the line between the two charges is the electric field equal to zero?

Solution: In order for the sum of two vectors to be zero, they must be equal in magnitude and opposite in direction. Because both of the charges are positive, the electric field vector of each charge points away from the charge. Along the line between the two charges the two electric field vectors point in opposite directions. If the charges were equal in magnitude, the point at which the two fields have the same magnitude (and therefore where the resultant field is zero) would be exactly halfway between them. However, the charges are not equal, since one charge is half the charge of the other. Let x be the distance from the $+1 \times 10^{-5}$ C charge. The distance from the other charge is the total distance of one meter minus x, or $(1 - x)$.

Setting the magnitudes of the two fields equal to each other to find the distance x that will make them equal, we have:

$$k\frac{(1 \times 10^{-5})}{x^2} = k\frac{(2 \times 10^{-5})}{(1 - x^2)}$$

$$\frac{1}{x^2} = \frac{2}{(1-x)^2}$$

$$2x^2 = (1-x)^2$$

$$\sqrt{2}\,x = 1 - x$$

$$x(1 + \sqrt{2}) = 1$$

$$x = \frac{1}{\sqrt{2} + 1}$$

$$x = 0.41 \text{ m}$$

As might be expected, this point is closer to the smaller charge because the field of the larger charge is stronger.

TEACHER TIP

The electric potential or voltage equation is very similar to the electric field equation, though instead of r^2 it is simply r. The difference between these two is that while electric field is a vector, the electric potential is a scalar.

MCAT SYNOPSIS

The electric potential, V, has units of Volts and is electric potential energy per unit charge, so:

volt = joule/coulomb.

MCAT SYNOPSIS

The electric potentials of separate charges add as scalars (numbers).

ELECTRIC POTENTIAL

Just as work is required to lift an object against the earth's gravitational field, work must be done to move an electric charge in an electric field. The **electric potential** at a point is defined as the amount of work needed to move a positive test charge q_0 from infinity to that point divided by the test charge q_0:

$$V = \frac{W}{q_0}$$

In SI units electric potential is measured in **volts** (V) where 1 volt = 1 joule/coulomb.

The electric potential at a distance r from a point charge q is:

$$V = k\frac{q}{r}$$

V is a scalar quantity whose sign is determined by the sign of the charge q. For a positive charge V is positive, but for a negative charge V is negative. For a collection of charges, the total electric potential at a point in space is the **scalar sum** of the electric potential due to each charge:

$$V_{total} = V_{q_1} + V_{q_2} + V_{q_3} + \cdots \text{ (scalar sum)}$$

Potential difference (voltage) is the difference in potential between two points. If V_a and V_b are the electric potentials at points a and b, then the potential difference between a and b is $V_b - V_a$. From the definition of electric potential, it follows that the potential difference between a and b can be expressed as:

$$V_b - V_a = \frac{W_{ab}}{q_0}$$

where W_{ab} is the work needed to move a test charge q_0 through an electric field from a to b. The work depends only on the potentials at the two points a and b, and is independent of the path. This means that like the gravitational force in chapter 3, the electrostatic force is a conservative force.

Typical voltages encountered in medical research range from the millivolt (e.g., the 70 to 90 millivolt potential across a cell membrane), to 10 volts (the approximate pulse voltage of a pacemaker), to the tens of billions of volts (gigavolts or GV) used to accelerate protons for nuclear medicine purposes (as in the preparation of radioisotopes).

EQUIPOTENTIAL LINES

An **equipotential line** is one for which the potential at every point is the same. The potential difference between any two points on an equipotential line is zero. From the above equation it follows that no work is done when moving a test charge q_0 from one point to another on an equipotential line. Work will be done in going from one line to another, but the **work depends only on the potential difference of the two lines and not on the path.**

> **TEACHER TIP**
>
> Because the work does not depend on the path, we know that we're dealing with conservative forces here.

Example: In Figure 6.1 an electron goes from point a to point b in the vicinity of a very large positive charge. The electron could be made to follow any of the paths shown. Which path requires the least work to get the electron charge from a to b?

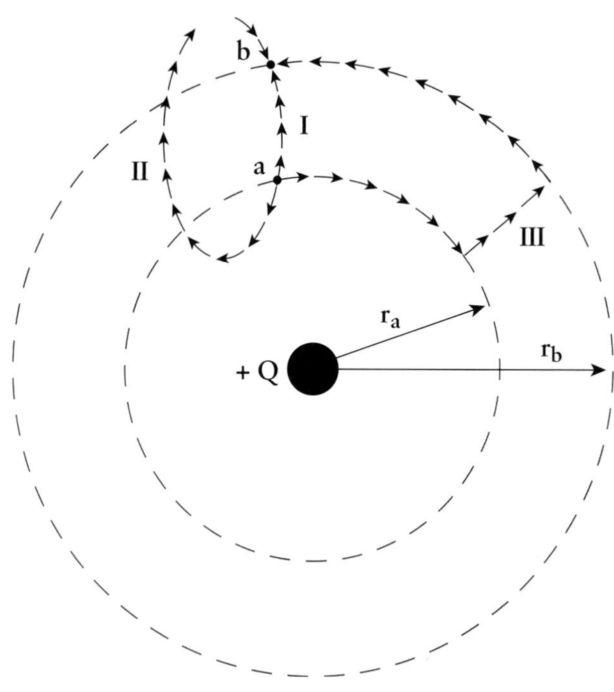

Figure 6.1

> **TEACHER TIP**
>
> Once again, the electric potential energy relates to our other equations. It is similar to electrostatic force in that it deals with the potential energy between two charges, though the radius is not squared so we're dealing with a scalar quantity.

Solution: As stated, the **work depends only on the potential difference and not on the path,** so any of the paths shown would require the same amount of work in moving the electron from a to b, namely:

$$W_{ab} = q_e(V_b - V_a)$$

$$= q_e\left(k\frac{Q}{r_b} - k\frac{Q}{r_a}\right)$$

> **MCAT SYNOPSIS**
>
> The amount of work necessary to move a charge in an electric field depends only on the potential difference. Recall that in the case of gravity, the work required to move a mass depends only on the difference in height.

So paths I, II, and III all require the same amount of work to move the electron. (Note that W_{ab} is positive in this example because $r_a < r_b$ and $q_e = -e$).

ELECTRIC POTENTIAL ENERGY

MCAT SYNOPSIS

Electric potential energy, U, equals charge times electric potential: U = qV. Change in electric potential energy equals charge times change in electric potential: $\Delta U = q\Delta V$.

We have already defined the electric potential V at a point in space as the amount of work W required to move a positive test charge q_0 from infinity to that point divided by q_0. We now define the electric potential energy U of an arbitrary charge q at that point in space to be the amount of work needed to move it from infinity to the point. Using the definition of the electric potential we get:

$$U = W = qV$$

where V is the electric potential due to the other charges. Note that the sign of U depends on the signs of q and V. Since U = qV, it may be said that V = U/q; electric potential can also be thought of as electric potential energy per unit charge. When V is due to just one other charge Q, V is given by kQ/r, and U may be rewritten as:

$$U = k\frac{qQ}{r}$$

$$= \left(\frac{1}{4\pi\varepsilon_0}\right)\frac{qQ}{r}$$

TEACHER TIP

We have dealt with a lot of equations in this chapter, though in reality it's only four equations that have different relationships. The distinguishing factors are the number of charges (one or two) and the radius (is it squared or not). All the other equations we have discussed can be derived from these four.

$F = (kq_1q_2)/r^2$	$U = (kq_1q_2)/r$
$E = (kq_1)/r^2$	$V = (kq_1)/r$

The main task you have as an MCAT student is to know how these equations relate and when to use them. Say you were trying to solve for the velocity of a charged particle. Because none of these equations has velocity in them, we need one that does, such as kinetic energy. Using the equation for potential energy (U), we can solve for kinetic energy once we know that all the potential energy has been converted into kinetic.

If the charges are both positive or both negative (in other words, like charges), U will be positive, but if one charge is positive and the other negative (that is, unlike charges), U will be negative.

Example: If a charge of +2e and a charge of −3e are separated by a distance of 3 nm, what is the potential energy of the system? (e is the fundamental unit of charge equal to 1.6×10^{-19} C.)

Solution:

$$U = k\frac{qQ}{r}$$

From the question stem we know that q = +2e, Q = −3e, and r = 3nm = 3×10^{-9}m. So, putting these numbers into the equation, and approximating k as 9.0×10^9:

$$U = (9 \times 10^9)\frac{(2)(1.6 \times 10^{-19})(-3)(1.6 \times 10^{-19})}{3 \times 10^{-19}}$$

$$= -4.6 \times 10^{-19}\,\text{J}$$

THE ELECTRIC DIPOLE

Two equal and opposite charges a small distance d away from each other form what is called an **electric dipole.** Suppose there is a dipole with charges +q and –q, as shown in Figure 6.2.

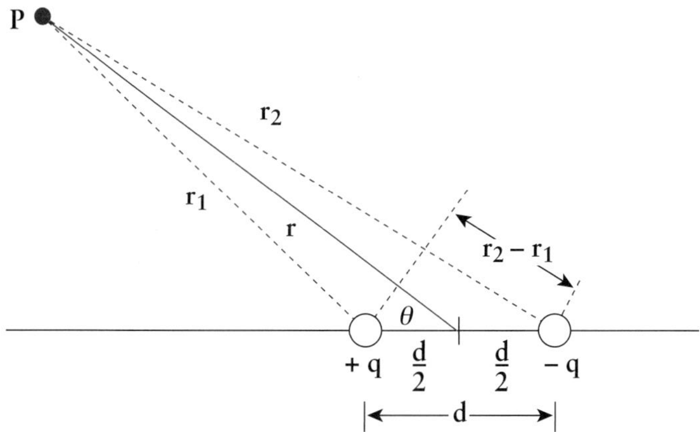

Figure 6.2

TEACHER TIP

This concept will be essential to understanding reactions in organic chemistry. Make sure you have the concept down solid.

MCAT SYNOPSIS

An electric dipole consists of two charges of equal magnitude and opposite sign separated by a small distance.

The potential at any point P is given by the sum of the two potentials:

$$V = k\frac{q}{r_1} - k\frac{q}{r_2}$$

$$= kq\left(\frac{r_2 - r_1}{r_1 r_2}\right)$$

For points relatively far from the dipole (compared to d), $r_1 r_2 \cong r^2$ and $r_2 - r_1 \cong d\cos\theta$. With these approximations the potential becomes:

$$V = k\frac{qd}{r^2}\cos\theta$$

The product of qd is defined as the **dipole moment p** with SI units of C • m. This is a vector quantity. Its magnitude is equal to the product qd, and its direction lies along the line connecting the charges (dipole axis) and points from the negative charge toward the positive charge. (Beware! Chemists often reverse this convention, having p point from the positive toward the negative charge.) In terms of dipole moment, one can rewrite the dipole potential as:

$$V = k\frac{p}{r^2}\cos\theta$$

Note that the potential is zero for $\theta = 90°$ and that this is the plane that lies halfway between +q and –q (called the perpendicular bisector of the dipole).

The electric field produced by the dipole at any point is the vector sum of each of the individual fields due to each of the two charges. Along the perpendicular bisector of the dipole the magnitude of the electric field can be approximated as:

$$E = \frac{1}{4\pi\varepsilon_0}\frac{p}{r^3}.$$

The field will point in the opposite direction to p.

Example: The H_2O molecule has a dipole moment of 1.85 D, where D = Debye unit = 3.34×10^{-30} C • m. Calculate the electric potential due to an H_2O molecule at a point 89 nm away along the axis of the dipole. (Use $k = 9 \times 10^9$ N • m^2/C^2.)

Solution: Since the question asks for the potential along the axis of the dipole, the angle θ is given by 0°. Substituting the values into the equation for the dipole potential and multiplying 1.85 D by 3.34×10^{-30} to convert it to C•m:

$$\begin{aligned} V &= k\frac{p}{r^2}\cos\theta \\ &= 9 \times 10^9 \frac{(1.85)(3.34 \times 10^{-30})(\cos\ 0°)}{(89 \times 10^{-9})^2} \\ &= 7 \times 10^{-6}\ V \end{aligned}$$

Now consider the case when an electric dipole is placed in a uniform external electric field. If there is no field present, the dipole moment will assume any random orientation. With a uniform external electric field present, however, each of the equal but opposite charges that make up the dipole will feel a force exerted on it by the external electric field. The net force will be zero, because the force on each charge is equal in magnitude but opposite in direction. The dipole therefore feels no translational force. However, there will be a nonzero torque about the center:

$$\begin{aligned} \tau &= F\frac{d}{2}\sin\theta + F\frac{d}{2}\sin\theta \\ &= Fd\sin\theta \\ &= qEd\sin\theta \\ &= (qd)E\sin\theta \\ &= pE\sin\theta \end{aligned}$$

where p is the magnitude of the dipole moment (p = qd), E is the magnitude of the uniform external electric field, and θ is the angle the dipole moment makes with the electric field. This torque will cause the dipole to reorient itself by rotating, so that its dipole moment, p, aligns with the electric field E. This is shown in Figure 6.3.

TEACHER TIP

This is a good example of what the MCAT would test conceptually. Is there translational motion, is there rotational motion, and in what direction would the dipole rotate?

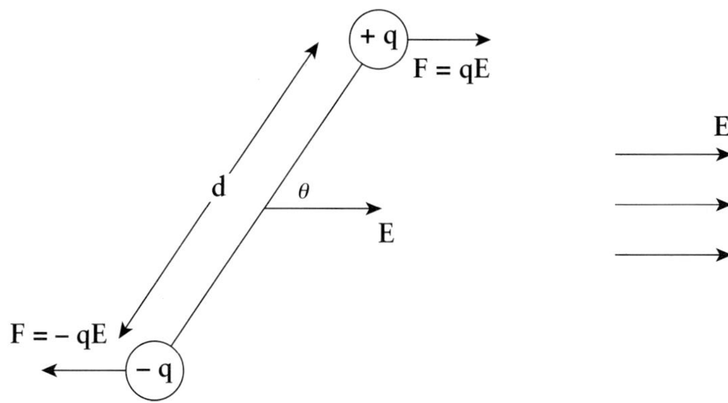

Figure 6.3

PRACTICE QUESTIONS

1. Two protons in a vacuum exhibit a repulsive force F_1. An independent pair of electrons is separated by a distance d and features a repulsive force of $4F_2$. What is the distance between the two protons?

A. 2d C. d/2

B. 4d D. d/4

2. An unknown particle is found to carry an electric potential energy of approximately 10–19 J. Which of the following is definitely NOT true?

A. The particle is a proton.
B. The particle is an electron.
C. The particle is a positron.
D. The particle is a quark.

3. Which of the following is always true about the electric dipole in the figure? *p* represents a positron (a positively charged electron), *e* represents an electron, and *a* represents a point halfway between the two.

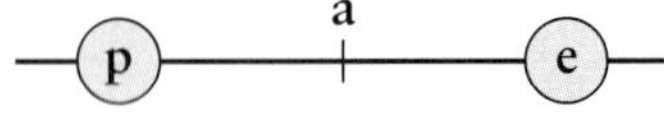

A. A particle at point *a* experiences an electric field of zero.
B. If no external field is present, then a charged particle at point *a* will move in an unpredictable direction.
C. A particle directly above point *a* is subject to an electric potential that is weaker than the potential at point a.
D. A particle directly above point *a* is subject to an electric potential that is stronger than the potential at point a.

4. Continuing with the same figure and conditions from the previous question, an external field causes the electron to move downward. How does this affect the rest of the system?

A. The positron moves upward, while point a remains stationary.
B. Point *a* moves downward, while the positron remains stationary.
C. Point *a* and the positron both move downward.
D. Point *a* and the positron both remain stationary.

5. The electric potential applied to a certain electron is increased by a factor of 4. The velocity of the electron will increase by

A. a factor of 16.
B. a factor of 8.
C. a factor of 4.
D. a factor of 2.

6. Which of the following accurately depicts the field lines around a proton that is moving toward the right of this page?

A.

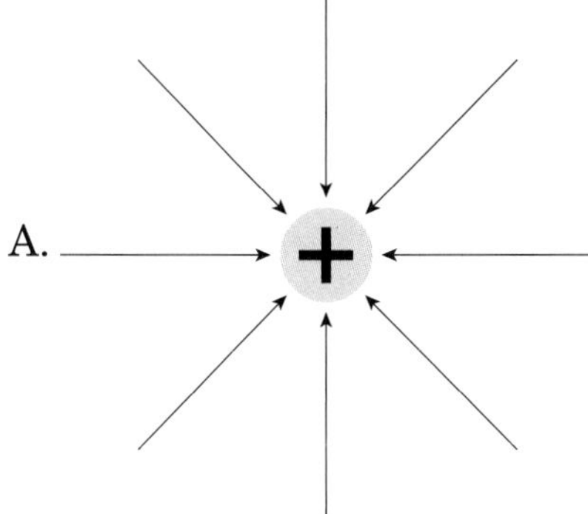

B.

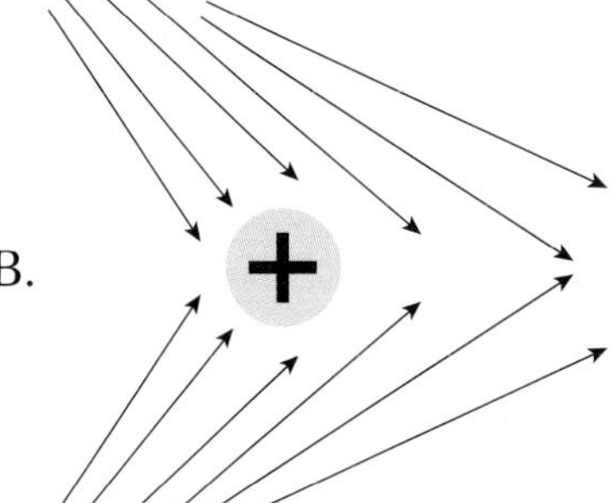

C.

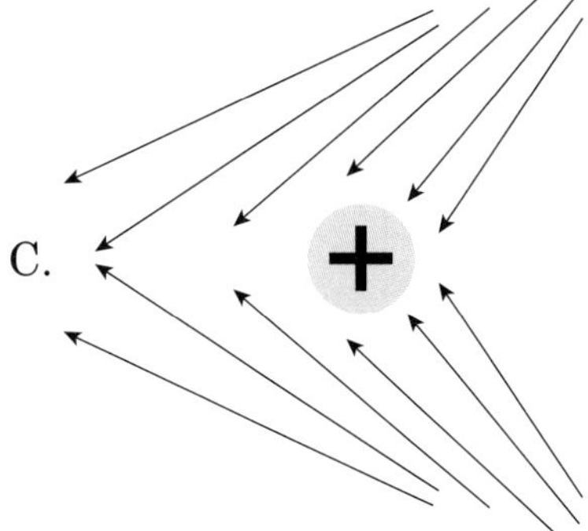

D.

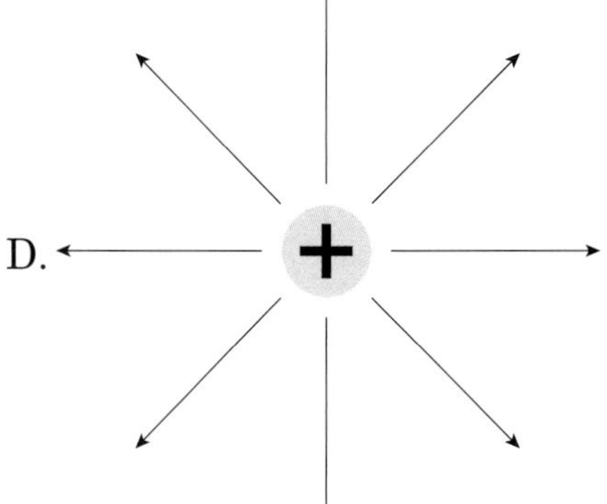

7. A positively charged particle is moving horizontally toward the right. What is the direction of the electrostatic force?

A. Left
B. Right
C. Up
D. Down

8. A certain 9V battery is used as a power source to move a 2C charge. How much work is done by the battery?

A. J
B. 9 J
C. 18 J
D. 36 J

9. For the figure below, which of the following is NOT a true statement regarding the differences in electric potentials?

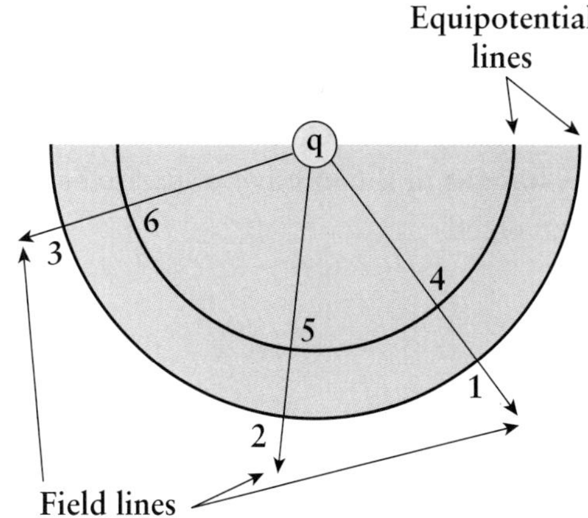

A. $V_1 - V_6 < 0$
B. $V_2 - V_3 = 0$
C. $V_5 - V_2 < 0$
D. $V_4 - V_6 = 0$

10. Continue with the same figure from the previous question. Starting at point 6, electron A travels to point 1, electron B travels to point 3, and electron C travels to point 4. Which of the following is true?

A. The work done on electron A is greater than the work done on electron B.
B. The work done on electron B is greater than the work done on electron C.
C. The work done on electron B is greater than the work done on electron A.
D. The work done on electron C is greater than the work done on electron A.

11. Which of the following does NOT affect the value of the net electrostatic force within a system?

A. Changes in the charge of the particles involved
B. Changes in the distance between the particles
C. Changes in the value of Coulomb's constant for the system in question
D. Changes in the number of particles involved

12. Consider the figure below. The four particles along the circumference of the circle (q_1, q_2, q_3, and q_4) carry a charge of 1 C, 2 C, 3 C, and 4 C, respectively. The distance d is equal to 2 m. If Coulomb's constant is equal to k, what is the potential at point p?

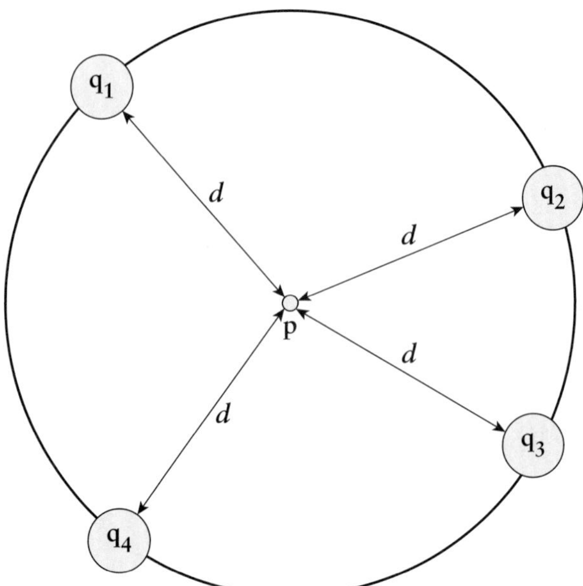

A. 5 k
B. 2.5 k
C. 1.25 k
D. 0.625 k

13. A proton and an alpha particle (a helium nucleus) repel each other with a force of F while they are 20 nm apart. If each particle combines with three electrons, what is the new force between them?

A. 9 F
B. 3 F
C. F
D. $F/9$

14. The diagram below represents the field lines for two charges of equal magnitude. What are the signs on each charge?

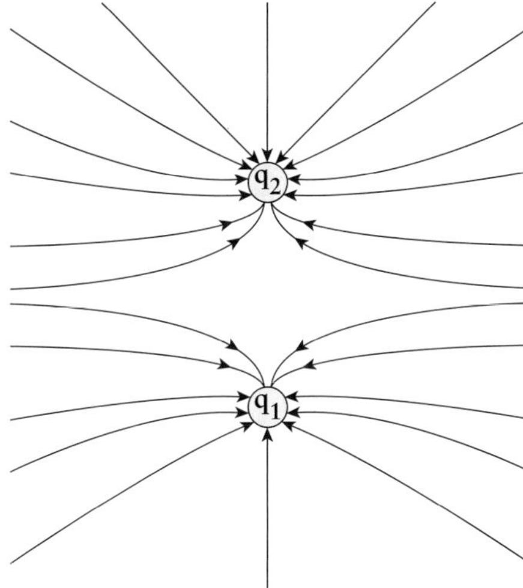

A. q_1 is positive, q_2 is negative
B. q_1 is negative, q_2 is positive
C. q_1 and q_2 are both positive
D. q_1 and q_2 are both negative

15. In the figure below, P is a positively charged particle that is equidistant from four known charges. What position vector represents the net force acting on particle *p*?

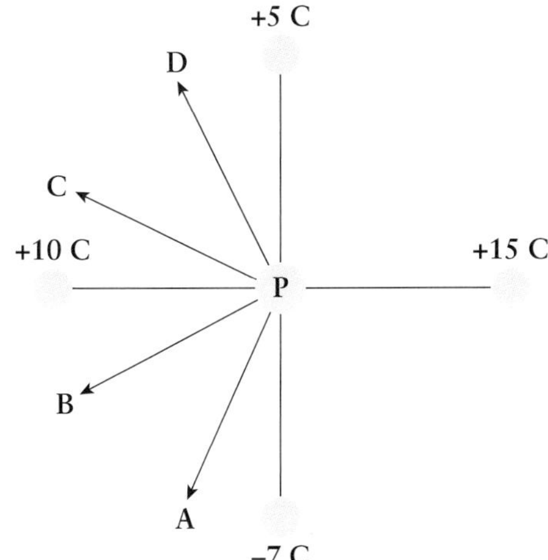

A. A
B. B
C. C
D. D

16. Continuing with the same figure and conditions from the previous question, what is the magnitude of the net charge?

A. 2 C
B. 5 C
C. 12 C
D. 13 C

17. A certain 10 kg object carries a charge of –5 C. When the object is placed in an electric field, it is accelerated directly upward at a rate of 5 m/s^2. If the acceleration due to gravity is –10 m/s^2, what is the magnitude and direction of the electric field?

A. 30 V, upward
B. 30 V, downward
C. 10 V, upward
D. 10 V, downward

18. When an electron collides with a positron (a particle with identical mass and a positive charge), the two particles are converted completely into energy; this is called an annihilation reaction. Which of the following is true immediately before the annihilation reaction?

I. There is no electric field at the point halfway between the positron and the electron.
II. The system is an electric dipole.
III. The particles move toward each other at a constant acceleration.

A. I only
B. II only
C. I and II only
D. II and III only

KEY CONCEPTS

Electric field: $E = kq/r^2$ (N/C)

Dipoles

$E = V/d$ (V/m) (parallel plate capacitor)

Capacitors

Vector addition

TAKEAWAYS

To find the net electric field (or magnetic field), find the effect of each source separately and then add them together. Remember that fields are vectors, so you have to add them like vectors: break the vectors into *x*- and *y*-components and add the components separately. Then use trigonometry and the Pythagorean theorem to find the net field.

THINGS TO WATCH OUT FOR

Most multiple-charge problems will have a geometry that allows you to cancel out certain components of the fields. Always look for an opportunity to do so, because this will save you time on Test Day.

NET ELECTRIC FIELD WITH MULTIPLE SOURCES

The diagram below shows an apparatus assembled by a physicist, using a 120 V battery and a capacitor with 10-cm plate separation. First, switch S was closed for a long time, fully charging the plates of the capacitor. Then, switch S was opened and a dipole with charges of 1 pC and –1 pC and a separation of 2 mm was placed between the plates of the capacitor, oriented with its positive end on the right-hand side. The dipole is held in a fixed position. What is the magnitude and direction of the electric field at a point 1 mm below the center of the dipole? ($k = 9 \times 10^9$ Nm^2/C^2)

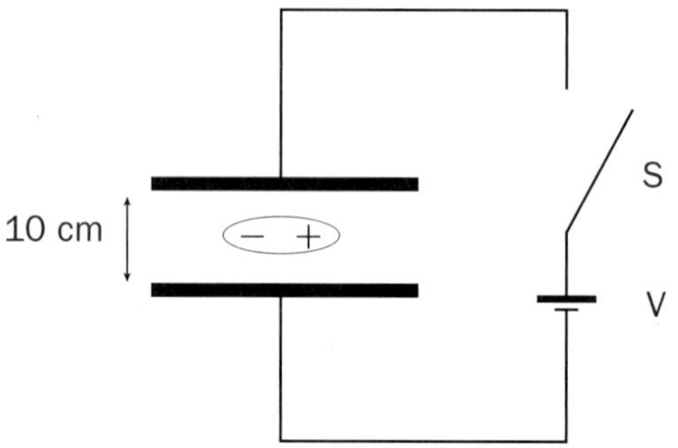

1) Find the electric field due to the plates.

☞ $E = V/d = 120/(0.1) = 1{,}200$ V/m

The electric field due to a potential difference inside a parallel plate capacitor is given by $E = V/d$. The voltage on the plates is the same as the voltage on the battery because the capacitor is fully charged. The top plate of the capacitor is positively charged because it was attached to the positive terminal of the battery (which is always the side with the longer line). Thus, the electric field points vertically from the top plate to the bottom plate.

---

2) Draw the electric field due to the dipole.

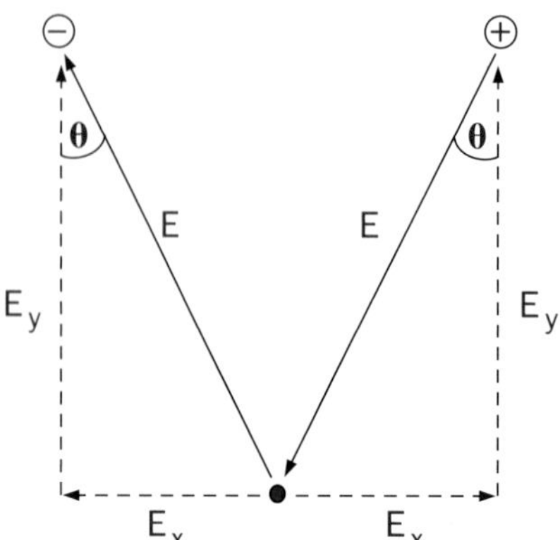

The two charges of the dipole are best treated simultaneously because their effect partially cancels out. The electric field points away from the positive charge and towards the negative charge. Find the *x*- and *y*-components of the field for both charges. Note that the *y*-components cancel each other out and that the *x*-components are equal and in the same direction. Thus, the electric field due to the dipole is twice the *x*-component of the electric field due to either dipole. The *x*-component of the electric field is E sin(θ).

---

3) Calculate the electric field due to the dipole.

$\theta = \tan^{-1}(1/1) = 45°$

$r = (1^2 + 1^2)^{1/2} = 1.41 \text{ mm}$

$E_x = E\cos(\theta)$

☞ $E = kq/r^2$

$E = (kq/r^2)\sin(\theta) = \left(\dfrac{(9\times10^9)(1\times10^{-12})}{(1.41\times10^{-3})^2}\right)\sin(45°)$

$= 3{,}201 \text{ V/m}$

$E_{dipole} = 2E_x = 6{,}402 \text{ V/m}$

Find the angle θ from trigonometry. Find *r*, the distance from the charges to the point, using the Pythagorean theorem. Then calculate E_x using the formula for electric field due to a point charge. The net electric field is twice E_x, and is directed to the left.

---

4) Find the net electric field.

$E_{net}^2 = E_x^2 + E_y^2$

$E_{net}^2 = (6{,}402)^2 + (1{,}200)^2 = 4.243 \times 10^7$

$E_{net} = 6{,}514 \text{ V/m}$

$\theta = \tan^{-1}(E_y/E_x) = 10.6°$

The net electric field is the vector sum of the electric field due to the plates and the dipole. Because one is in the *x*-direction and the other is in the *y*-direction, they form two sides of a right triangle. The length of the hypotenuse of the triangle is the magnitude of the net electric field and is given by the Pythagorean theorem. Find the angle ϕ from the horizontal using trigonometry.

SIMILAR QUESTIONS

1) What is the electric field halfway in between two protons separated by a distance of 1 mm?
2) A proton and an electron are separated by 1 μm. Is there a point directly between them at which the electric field is zero?
3) Three protons are positioned at the corners of an equilateral triangle with sides 2 mm in length. What is the electric field at the center of one of the edges of the triangle? ($e = 1.6 \times 10^{-19}$ C)

KEY CONCEPTS

Work: $W = q\Delta V$

Electrostatics

Electric potential energy, U

TAKEAWAYS

To find the work required to assemble a distribution of charges, find the work required to place each charge individually and then add. The work to place the first charge is always zero.

THINGS TO WATCH OUT FOR

It is common to make sign errors on these types of problems. Keep this in mind to check your work: like charges increase in potential energy as they are brought closer; unlike charges decrease in potential energy as they are brought together.

CHARGE DISTRIBUTION AND WORK

Three charges are lined up along the x axis. Charge 1 has a charge of +1 μC. Charge 2 has a charge of −2 μC. Charge 3 has a charge of +4 μC. The charges are all 1 mm away from each other. How much work was required to assemble this distribution of charge, assuming that the charges were initially very far apart? ($k = 9 \times 10^9$ Nm^2/C^2)

1) Find the work required to place charge 1.

$W = \Delta U = q\Delta V$

$W = 0$

The work done to move a charge equals the charge times the change in electric potential. The work done to place charge 1 is zero because there is no change in electric potential.

Remember: *As a matter of convention, the work to place the first charge is always zero.*

---

2) Find the work required to place charge 2.

$W = \Delta U = q\Delta V = q_2(V_f - V_i)$

$V_i = 0$

$V_f = \left(\frac{kq_1}{r_{12}}\right)$

generic: $V = \frac{kq}{r}$

$$W = q_2\left[\left(\frac{kq_1}{r_{12}}\right) - 0\right]$$

$$W = (-2 \times 10^{-6})\left[\frac{(9 \times 10^9)(1 \times 10^{-6})}{1 \times 10^{-3}}\right] = -18\text{ J}$$

The same formula is used in this step as in step 1. Here, charge 2 has an initial electric potential of zero because it is very far away from charge 1. The final electric potential is given by the formula $V = \frac{kq}{r}$, where q is the charge of the stationary charge and r_{12} is the distance between charges 1 and 2.

---

3) Find the work required to place charge 3.

$$W = \Delta U = q\Delta V = q_3(V_f - V_i)$$

$$V_i = 0$$

$$V_f = \left(\frac{kq_1}{r_{13}}\right) + \left(\frac{kq_2}{r_{23}}\right)$$

$$W = q_3\left[\left(\frac{kq_1}{r_{13}}\right) + \left(\frac{kq_2}{r_{23}}\right) - 0\right]$$

$$W = 4\times10^{-6}\left\{\left[\frac{(9\times10^9)(1\times10^{-6})}{2\times10^{-3}}\right]\right.$$

$$\left.+\left[\frac{(9\times10^9)(-2\times10^{-6})}{(1\times10^{-3})}\right]\right\} = 18 - 72 = -54\text{ J}$$

Much like step two, the work to place charge 3 equals the magnitude of charge 3 times the change in electric potential. Once again, the initial electric potential is 0. The final potential is the potential due to charge 1 plus the potential due to charge 2. Be careful, because the distances must be from charge 1 to charge 3 (call this r_{13}) and from charge 2 to charge 3 (call this r_{23}), respectively.

---

4) Add the work from steps 1, 2, and 3.

$$W_{net} = 0 - 18\text{ J} - 54\text{ J} = -72\text{ J}$$

Add the work from steps 1, 2, and 3 to find the net work. The net work is negative, meaning that the potential energy of the system has been lowered.

SIMILAR QUESTIONS

1) A 1μC charge sits 1 cm from a –2μC charge. How much work is done in tripling the distance between these charges?
2) How much work is done in assembling a square-shaped charge distribution with a side length of 1 μm if all of the charges have a charge of 5 nC?
3) Charges 1, 2, and 3 are lined up, in that order, at 1 mm intervals along the *y* axis. Three charges are lined up along the *y* axis. Charge 1 has a charge of +4 μC. Charge 2 has a charge of –2 μC. Charge 3 has a charge of –3 μC. What is the change in potential energy of the system if charge 1 is removed?

KEY CONCEPTS

Voltage

Mechanical energy

$U = qV$ (J: CV)

$E = U + KE$

$KE = \frac{1}{2}mv^2$

TAKEAWAYS

This problem appears complex due to the unusual situation, but it is solved the same way as any other energy problem: 1) write expressions for the total energy of the system at two points; 2) set the expressions equal; and 3) solve.

THINGS TO WATCH OUT FOR

Many students do not realize that problems involving charged particles and voltages can be solved most easily using the conservation of energy.

VOLTAGE AND ENERGY

A dipole sits at the center of a large wire circle of radius 50 cm that is sitting horizontally in a plane. A small, –2 C charge with a mass of 4 kg is constrained to slide with no friction along the loop. The potential of the dipole is given as $V = V_o \cos(\theta)$, where V_o is 5 and θ measures the angle from the vertical. The point charge's initial position on the loop is directly above the dipole ($\theta = 0$) of the loop and is given an initial speed of 3 m/s. How fast is the point charge moving at the point corresponding to $\theta = 90°$?

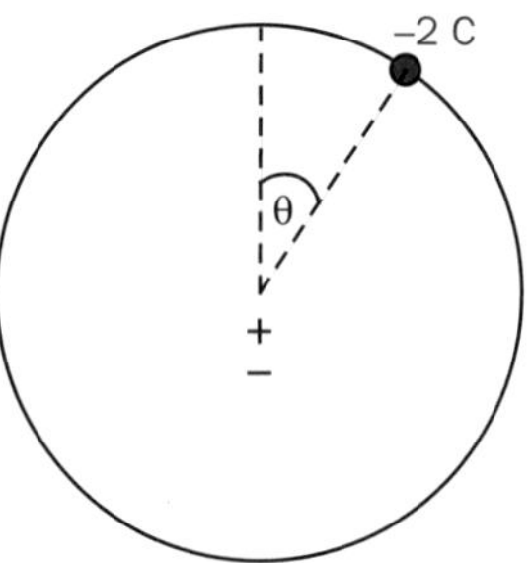

1) Write an expression for the initial energy of the system.

$E_i = U_i + KE_i$

☞ $U_i = qV_i = qV_o \cos(\theta_i)$

☞ $KE_i = \frac{1}{2}mv_i^2$

$E = qV_o \cos(\theta_i) + \frac{1}{2}mv_i^2$

The energy of the system is the sum of the potential energy and the kinetic energy. The potential energy is given by $U = qV$, where the formula for V is given in the question.

---

2) Write an expression for the final energy of the system.

$E_f = U_f + KE_f$

☞ $U_f = qV_f = qV_o \cos(\theta_f)$

$E = qV_o \cos(\theta_f) + \frac{1}{2}mv_f^2$

Much like step 1, the energy of the system is the sum of the potential energy and the kinetic energy.

---

3) Set the energy expressions equal to each other and solve.

$E_i = E_f$

$qV_0 \cos(\theta_i) + \frac{1}{2}mv_i^2 = qV_0 \cos(\theta_f) + \frac{1}{2}mv_f^2$

$\theta_i = 0 \rightarrow \cos(\theta_i) = 1$

$\theta_f = 90° \rightarrow \cos(\theta_f) = 0$

$qV_0 + \frac{1}{2}mv_i^2 = \frac{1}{2}mv_f^2$

$(-2)(5) + \frac{1}{2}(4)(3)^2 = \frac{1}{2}(4)v_f^2$

$8 = 2v_f^2$

$v_f = 2$ m/s

Due to the conservation of energy, we can set the initial and final energies as equal. This allows us to solve for v_f. Plug in the angles, mass, charge, and initial velocity to find v_f.

SIMILAR QUESTIONS

1) How fast does a 1 kg ball move after falling from a height of 10 meters if the ball is thrown down with a speed 2 m/sec?
2) An alpha particle, starting from rest, travels through a potential difference of 200 V. What is the final speed of the particle? ($e = 1.6 \times 10^{-19}$ C)
3) Two protons (mass = 1.66×10^{-27} kg) initially are at rest at a distance of 10 nm from each other. They are released and accelerate away from each other. How fast are they both going after they are very far apart? ($k = 9 \times 10^9$ Nm^2/C^2)

KEY CONCEPTS

Voltage

Electrical potential energy

Conservation of energy

ELECTROSTATICS AND VELOCITY

A particle with a mass of 1 g and a charge of +1 μC is released from rest at a distance of 20 cm from another particle with a charge of +20 μC, which is held fixed. How fast is the moving particle traveling when it is 150 cm away from the fixed particle? ($k = 9 \times 10^9$ Nm²/C²)

1) Determine the electrical potential energy at the points of interest.

point 1: $U_1 = \frac{kq_1q_2}{r_1} = \frac{(9\times10^9)(20\times10^{-6})(1\times10^{-6})}{(0.2)} = 0.9\text{ J}$

point 2: $U_2 = \frac{kq_1q_2}{r_2} = \frac{(9\times10^9)(20\times10^{-6})(1\times10^{-6})}{(1.5)} = 0.12\text{ J}$

☞ Generic: $U = \frac{kq_1q_2}{r}$

Potential energy can only be defined as a relative value, but in these types of problems, it is easiest to use the definition that the potential energy is zero at infinite distance. This way, you can use the formula $U = \frac{kq_1q_2}{r}$, which saves time as compared to using $\Delta U = q\Delta V$ by bypassing the step of first calculating V.

---

2) Determine the change in potential energy and kinetic energy.

$\Delta U = U_2 - U_1 = -0.78\text{ J} = -\Delta KE$

$\Delta KE = 0.78\text{ J}$

There is a negative change in potential energy. From the conservation of energy, this means that there must be a positive change in kinetic energy because the total energy must remain constant. In these types of problems, $\Delta U = -\Delta KE$.

---

3) Determine the velocity of the particle from the kinetic energy.

$\Delta KE = \frac{1}{2}mv_2^2 - \frac{1}{2}mv_1^2$; ($v_1 = 0$, so $\Delta KE = \frac{1}{2}mv_2^2$)

$0.78\text{ J} = \frac{1}{2}(1 \times 10^{-3})v^2$

$v^2 = \frac{0.78(2)}{(1\times10^{-3})} = 1{,}560$

$v = 39.50\text{ m/s}$

Because the initial velocity is 0, the change in kinetic energy equals the kinetic energy that the particle has at point 2. Set them equal and solve.

TAKEAWAYS

Problems involving charged particles that move around near other charged particles (or in electric fields) are solved most easily using the conservation of energy. Do these problems just as you would for gravity. Find the change in potential energy, set that equal to the negative of the change in kinetic energy, and solve for the quantity of interest.

THINGS TO WATCH OUT FOR

These problems can be presented in several different ways. If you are given the potential at two points, simply multiply by the magnitude of the charge in motion to determine the electrical potential energy at those points. A common mistake is to multiply by the source charge. Remember, the q in the equation $U = qV$ refers to the charge that is moving. Work is often tested with these problems, so remember that work is equal to the change in kinetic energy. For problems involving point charges and speed, you will always use the work energy theorem.

SIMILAR QUESTIONS

1) A proton initially at rest is accelerated through a potential difference of 100 V. What is the proton's final speed? ($e = 1.6 \times 10^{-19}$ C, $m_p = 1.67 \times 10^{-27}$)
2) How much work is done in moving an electron from a distance of 1 nm to a distance of 10 nm away from a hydrogen nucleus?
3) What voltage is required to accelerate protons to a speed of 10^4 m/s?

KEY CONCEPTS

Coulomb's law

Vector addition

$F = \frac{kq_1q_2}{r^2}$

ELECTRIC FORCE

Find the net force exerted on point charge a by the other two point charges depicted in the diagram below. (k = 8.99 × 10⁹ Nm²/C²)

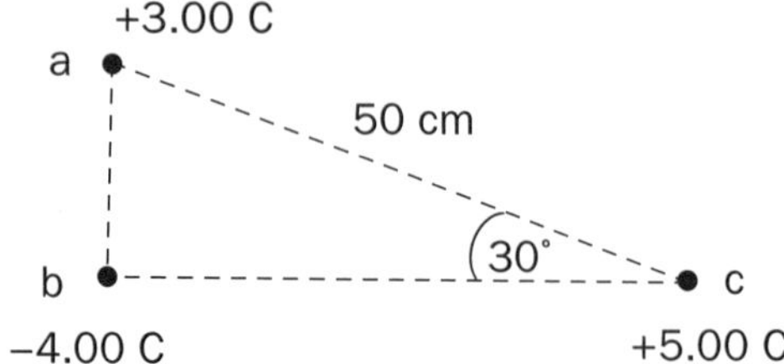

1) Find the distance from charge a to charge b.

sin 30° = r_{ab}/50 cm

r_{ab} = 50 cm × sin 30°

r_{ab} = 25 cm

To find the distance between points *a* and *b*, use sine. Sine of angle 30 is the hypotenuse over opposite.

TAKEAWAYS

To find the net force on an object:

(1) Choose positive directions for your *x*- and *y*-axes.

(2) Break each of the individual forces on the object into *x*- and *y*-components.

(3) Add the *x*-components of the individual forces to obtain the *x*-component of the net force on the object; add the *y*-components of the individual forces to obtain the *y*-component of the net force.

(4) To find the magnitude of the net force, apply the Pythagorean theorem to the *x*- and *y*-components of the net force.

(5) To find the direction of the net force (measured as an angle from the *x*-axis), take the inverse tangent of the y-component of the net force divided by the *x*-component of the net force.

2) Find the force exerted by charge *b* on charge *a*.

☞ $F = \frac{kq_1q_2}{r^2}$

$F_{ab} = \frac{kq_aq_b}{r_{ab}^2}$

$F_{ab} = \frac{(8.99 \times 10^9 \text{ Nm}^2/\text{c}^2)(3.00 \text{ c})(-4.00 \text{ c})}{(.250 \text{ m})^2}$

$F_{ab} = -1.73 \times 10^{12}$ N

Start with Coulomb's law. Plug in the charges located at points *a* and *b*. r_{ab} is the distance between points *a* and *b*.

Remember: *The negative sign for the force means that there is an attraction (unlike charges). Because point charge* a *is positive whereas* b *is negative, the direction is straight down toward charge* b.

---

3) Find the force exerted by charge *c* on charge *a*.

$F = \frac{kq_1q_2}{r^2}$

$F_{ac} = \frac{kq_aq_b}{r_{ac}^2}$

$F_{ac} = \frac{(8.99 \times 10^9 \text{ Nm}^2/\text{c}^2)(3.00 \text{ c})(5.00 \text{ c})}{(0.500 \text{ m})^2}$

$F_{ac} = 5.39 \times 10^{11}$ N

Start with Coulomb's law. Plug in the charges located at points *a* and *c*. r_{ac} is the distance between points *a* and *c*.

Remember: *The positive sign for the force means that there is repulsion (like charges). This means that the direction of the force is away from point charge* c.

---

4) Draw the force diagram and separate into vectors.

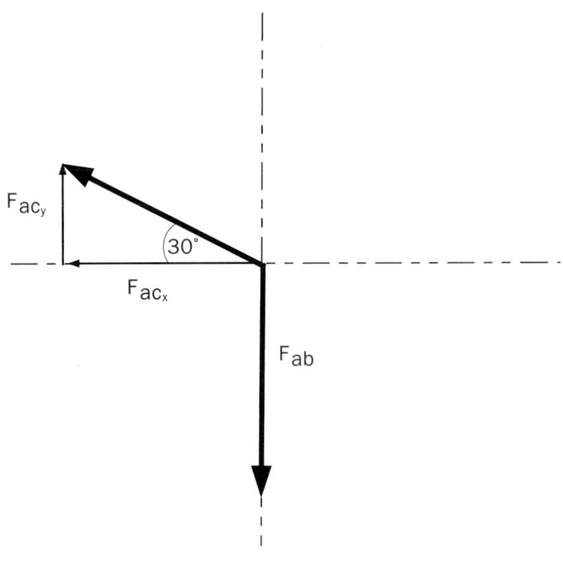

$F_{ab,\,x} = 0$ N

$F_{ab,\,y} = -1.73 \times 10^{12}$ N

$F_{ac,\,x} = F_{ac} \times (-1)\cos(30°)$

$= (5.39 \times 10^{11}\text{ N}) \times (-.866) = -4.67 \times 10^{11}$ N

$F_{ac,\,y} = F_{ac} \times \sin(30°) = (5.39 \times 10^{11}\text{ N}) \times (0.5)$

$= 2.70 \times 10^{11}$ N

F_{ab} points towards point *b*, which is straight down. Thus, F_{ab} has no *x*-component—only a *y*-component.

F_{ac} points away from point *c*, which is 30° above the horizontal to the left. F_{ac} has both a horizontal and vertical component. Find the *x*- and *y*-components by using the cosine and sine of 30°, respectively.

Remember: *F_{ab} is pointing down, so the* x*-vector component should be 0 while the* y*-vector component should be negative.* F_{ac} *is pointing up and to the left, so the* x*-vector component should be negative while the* y*-vector component should be positive.*

THINGS TO WATCH OUT FOR

This problem shows the nature of the coulomb. One coulomb is a huge charge. Usually you will deal with microcoulombs. Even when you solve for inverse tangent, be sure the angle measurement is pointing in the right direction. Draw force diagrams to confirm.

SIMILAR QUESTIONS

1) Two point charges, the first with a charge of $+1.97 \times 10^{-6}$ C and the second with a charge of -5.01×10^{-6} C, are separated by 25.5 cm. Find the magnitude of the electrostatic force experienced by the positive charge.
2) Point charge *a* has a charge of 3.693×10^{-7} C whereas point charge *b* has a charge of 1.75×10^{-6} C. They exert an electrostatic force of magnitude 36.1×10^{-3} N on each other. Find the separation between the point charge *a* and point charge *b*.
3) Point charge *a* has a charge of 3.693×10^{-7} C and exerts a force of 36.1×10^{-3} N on point charge *b*. If the two charges are separated by a distance of 0.025 m, find the charge of point charge *b*.

5) Add the vector components.

X-components:

$$F_x = F_{ab,x} + F_{ac,x} = 0 + -4.67 \times 10^{11}\text{ N}$$
$$= -4.67 \times 10^{11}\text{ N}$$

Y-components:

$$F_y = F_{ab,y} + F_{ac,y} = -1.73 \times 10^{12}\text{ N} + 2.70 \times 10^{11}\text{ N}$$
$$= -1.46 \times 10^{12}\text{ N}$$

$$F_a^2 = F_x^2 + F_y^2$$
$$F_a^2 = (-4.67 \times 10^{11}\text{ N})^2 + (-1.46 \times 10^{12}\text{ N})^2$$
$$F_a = 1.53 \times 10^{12}\text{ N}$$

Add the *x*- and *y*-components separately. To find the magnitude, take the square root of the sum of the squares of each component (the Pythagorean theorem).

---

6) Solve for the magnitude and direction.

Magnitude $F_a^2 = (-4.67 \times 10^{11}\text{ N})^2 + (-1.46 \times 10^{12}\text{ N})^2$

$F_a = 1.53 \times 10^{12}$ N

$$\text{Direction} = \tan^{-1}\left(\frac{F_y}{F_x}\right)$$

$$= \tan^{-1}\left(\frac{-1.46\times10^{12}\text{ N}}{-4.67\times10^{11}\text{ N}}\right)$$

$$= 72.3°$$

To solve for the magnitude, take the square root of the sum of the squares of each component. To solve for direction, take the tan inverse of the *y*-component over the *x*-component. The net force exerted on point charge *a* is 1.53×10^{12} N exerted at 72.3° south of west.

ELECTRON BETWEEN CHARGED PLATES

A charged particle of mass 1 μg and charge 10 mC with velocity 2,000 m/s enters the center of the gap in a parallel-plate capacitor as shown below. The capacitor holds a charge of 2 C and has a capacitance of 5 mF. How far away from the center of the gap is the electron when it exits the capacitor?
(plate sep = 2 mm, L = 10 cm)

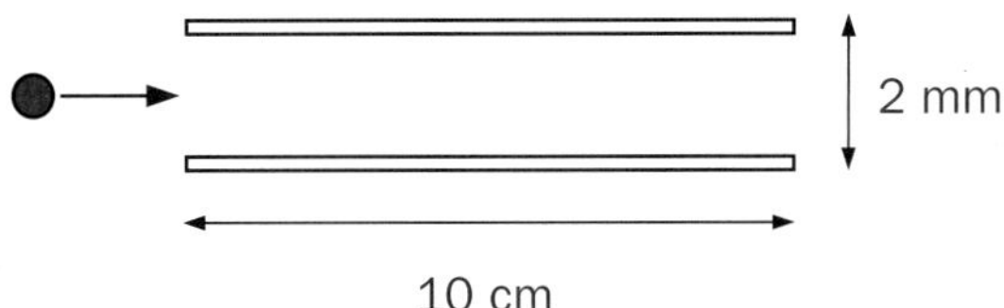

1) Find the voltage across the capacitor.

$$C = \frac{Q}{V} \rightarrow V = \frac{Q}{C} = \frac{(2)}{(5 \times 10^{-3})} = 400 \text{ volts}$$

The capacitance of a capacitor is related to the charge and voltage across the capacitor by $C = \frac{Q}{C}$. Solve for V.

2) Find the electric field in between the plates.

$$V = Ed \rightarrow E = \frac{V}{d} = \frac{400}{(2 \times 10^{-3})} = 200{,}000 \text{ V/m}$$

The magnitude of the electric field inside a parallel plate capacitor is given by the formula $E = \frac{V}{d}$.

3) Find the acceleration of the particle.

$$a = \frac{F}{m}$$

$$F = qE \rightarrow a = \frac{qE}{m} = \frac{(10 \times 10^{-9})(200{,}000)}{(1 \times 10^{-9})} = 2{,}000{,}000 \text{ m/s}^2$$

Remember to convert the mass to SI units (kg).

4) Find the time that the particle is between the plates.

$$\Delta x = V_{ox}t + \frac{1}{2}a_x t^2$$

$$a_x = 0 \rightarrow \Delta x = v_{ox}t$$

$$t = \frac{\Delta x}{v_{ox}} = \frac{(0.1)}{2{,}000} = 5 \times 10^{-5} \text{ s}$$

Use the standard kinematics formula to find the amount of time it takes the particle to travel the distance across the capacitor. Note that there is no force in the x-direction, so there is no acceleration in the x-direction. Solve for time.

KEY CONCEPTS

$C = \frac{Q}{V}$ (C/V)

$F = ma$ (N: kg · m/s²)

$F = qE$ (N)

$\Delta y = v_{oy}t + \frac{1}{2}a_y t^2$

Capacitance

Kinematics

Electrostatics

Voltage

Electric field

Electric force

$E = V/d$ (V/m) (parallel plate capacitor)

TAKEAWAYS

This is a combination between a capacitor problem, an electrostatics problem, and a kinematics problem. Use the properties of capacitors to find the voltage, which leads you to the force and acceleration of the particle. After you have the acceleration, this problem is no different than a standard free-fall or projectile problem.

THINGS TO WATCH OUT FOR

There are several equations you must have memorized to solve this problem.

5) Find the deflection of the particle.

$$\Delta y = v_{oy}t + \frac{1}{2}a_y t^2$$

$$v_{oy} = 0 \rightarrow \Delta y = \frac{1}{2}a_y t^2 = \frac{1}{2}(2{,}000{,}000)(5 \times 10^{-5})^2$$

$$= 2.5 \times 10^{-6} \text{ m} = 2.5 \text{ mm}$$

Use the standard kinematics formula to find the movement in the *y*-direction based on the acceleration, time, and initial velocity. Note that initially there is no velocity in the *y*-direction.

SIMILAR QUESTIONS

1) An electron starts from rest at one plate of a parallel-plate capacitor and accelerates to the other plate. The plate separation is 2 mm, and it takes 1 ms for the electron to travel from one side to the other. What is the capacitance of this capacitor if there are 2 C of charge stored on the plates? ($m_e = 9.11 \times 10^{-31}$ kg, $e = 1.6 \times 10^{-19}$ C)
2) An electron is brought to rest by a potential difference of 1 kV. What was the initial velocity of the electron?
3) A proton experiences a force of 10 mN as it travels between the plates of a parallel plate capacitor, parallel to the plates. If the capacitor holds 1 mC of charge and has a potential of 10 V, what is the separation between the plates?

ELECTROSTATIC IMPULSE

A +2e charge is sitting on the negative plate of a parallel-plate capacitor. A mechanical error accidentally reverses the charge on the plates such that the test charge is accelerated towards the other plate. In the 7 s that it takes for the technician to correct this mistake, the test charge traverses the entire 20 mm distance between the plates. If the test charge loses 3.2×10^{-16} J of potential energy, what was the impulse created by the electric force? ($1\ e = 1.6 \times 10^{-19}$ C)

1) Find the potential difference for the drop in electric potential.

☞ $\Delta V = \dfrac{\Delta U}{q_o}$

$$\Delta V = \frac{(3.2 \times 10^{-16}\ \text{J})}{(2)(1.6 \times 10^{-19}\ \text{C})} = 1{,}000 \text{ volts}$$

The +2e charge is equal to two fundamental units of charge. Thus, the test charge q_o is 3.2×10^{-19} coulombs.

---

2) Find the electric field between the plates.

☞ $\Delta V = Ed$

$1{,}000\ \text{V} = E(0.02\ \text{m}) \rightarrow E = 5 \times 10^4\ \text{V/m}$

Once again, we need only plug in the data to the appropriate equation.

---

3) Find the electric force.

☞ $F = Eq_o$

$F = (5 \times 10^4\ \text{V/m})(3.2 \times 10^{-19}\ \text{C}) = 1.6 \times 10^{-14}\ \text{N}$

Substitute for the relevant quantities and constants.

Remember: *Use dimensional analysis to check your work. In this case, we see that $F/q_o = E$. From the previous step, we found the electric field to have the unit V/m. However, looking at the equation here, we see that the electric field will also have the unit N/C. This means that V/m = N/C. Recognizing this allows us to find alternative ways of defining the units V and C, for instance.*

---

4) Find the impulse.

☞ $I = F_{av}\Delta t$

$I = (1.6 \times 10^{-14}\ \text{N})(7\ \text{s}) = 1.12 \times 10^{-13}\ \text{N·s}$

KEY CONCEPTS

Electric potential energy: $\Delta U = \Delta V q_o$ (V · C)

Potential difference (voltage): $V = Ed$ (V: Nm/C) (parallel plate capacitor)

Impulse: $I = F_{av}\Delta t$ (kg · m/s)

Electric field

$F = q_o E$

TAKEAWAYS

Memorizing a few equations can make even complex-sounding problems simple. Even if you are given several of these equations on Test Day, the familiarity from memorizing them and the comfort from using them will decrease the amount of time that questions like this will take.

THINGS TO WATCH OUT FOR

Typically, the math isn't too difficult if you round the numbers. Be careful with the scientific notation.

Plug and chug.

Remember: *The impulse on an object is equal to the change in the object's momentum. It is similar to work, as in the equation* $W = P\Delta t$.

SIMILAR QUESTIONS

1) Three positive charges, +1e, +2e, and +3e, are sitting in a row with 5 mm between them. What is the potential energy of the system? ($k = 9 \times 10^9$ Nm^2/C^2)
2) A −6e charge experiences an electric force upwards when it is fired through a parallel-plate capacitor. If the potential difference experienced by the test charge is 1,000 V and the plates are 2 cm apart, what is the force?
3) If a +1e test charge loses 1 J of electric potential energy in moving from equipotential line *a* to *b*, which is closer to the positive point charge that creates the field, V_a or V_b?

PHOTOELECTRIC EFFECT

A beam of monochromatic light of wavelength 550 nm and power of 5 W is incident on a metal wire with work function 1.1 eV. Assuming 60 percent efficiency, what is the maximum possible current produced in the wire? (1 eV = 1.6×10^{-19} J, e = 1.6×10^{-19} C, h = 6.6×10^{-34} Js)

KEY CONCEPTS

Photoelectric effect

Efficiency

Properties of light

$P = E/t$ (W: J/s)

1) Find the energy of the incident photons.

550 nm = 5.5×10^{-7} m

$$E = hf = \frac{hc}{\lambda} = \frac{(6.6\times10^{-34})(3\times10^{8})}{(5.5\times10^{-7})}$$

$$E = \left[\frac{(6.6)(3)}{(5.5)}\right] \times \left[\frac{(10^{-34})(10^{8})}{(10^{-7})}\right] = 3.6\times10^{-19}\ \text{J}$$

The energy of a photon depends only on the frequency of that photon and Planck's constant, h. They are related by the formula $E = hf$. The speed, c, wavelength, λ, and frequency, f, of light are related by the formula $c = f\lambda$. Substitute to find the energy in terms of wavelength.

TAKEAWAYS

If the work function were greater than the energy of the photons, there would be no current produced, regardless of the power of the light source. This is a major source of confusion for most test takers.

The energy (and thus frequency or wavelength) determines whether the photoelectric effect will occur.

The power (or intensity) is related to the number of photons arriving per second, and thus determines how many electrons will be generated.

Problems involving the photoelectric effect often involve tricky, unfamiliar units. Use dimensional analysis to your advantage.

---

2) Convert units.

$$1\ \text{eV} = 1.6 \times 10^{-19}\ \text{J} \rightarrow 1.1\ \text{eV} \times \left(\frac{1.6\times10^{-19}\ \text{J}}{1\ \text{eV}}\right) = 1.76 \times 10^{-19}\ \text{J}$$

Convert the work function of the metal to joules using the conversion factor given in the question. If it is more comfortable, you could work this problem in terms of eV as well.

---

3) Compare photon energy to work function.

$3.6 \times 10^{-19}\ \text{J} > 1.76 \times 10^{-19}\ \text{J}$

The work function is the amount of energy required to completely free one electron from an atom. The energy of the photons is greater than the work function. This means that each photon has enough energy to liberate an electron from an atom. Any energy above the level of the work function is given to the electron in the form of kinetic energy.

---

4) Calculate the number of photons arriving per second.

☞ $P = E/t = 5\ \text{W} = 5\ \text{J/s}$

$$5\ \text{J/s} \times \left(\frac{1\ \text{photon}}{3.6\times10^{-19}\ \text{J}}\right) = 1.39 \times 10^{19}\ \text{photons/s}$$

The power given in the question tells us that 5 J/s arrive at the wire. Calculate the number of photons in 5 J using dimensional analysis. There are 1.39×10^{19}

THINGS TO WATCH OUT FOR

Light energy can be converted into electrical energy, which can then also be converted to mechanical energy via a generator with a certain efficiency. In that case, you would multiply the electrical energy by the efficiency of the generator to find the useful mechanical work output of the entire system.

photons hitting the wire each second. Because each photon produces a free electron, there are 1.39×10^{19} free electrons produced each second.

---

5) Calculate the charge produced each second (the maximum current).

$$I = \frac{\Delta q}{\Delta t}$$

1.39×10^{19} electrons/s $\times$ (1.6×10^{-19} C/electron) = 2.22 C/s = 2.22 A

Current equals charge per time, not electrons per time. Use dimensional analysis to find the amount of charge contained in 1.39×10^{19} electrons. This amount of charge per second is the current.

---

6) Calculate the real current.

$I = 2.22 \text{ A} \times (0.6) = 1.33 \text{ A}$

The efficiency is only 60 percent, so multiply the current from step 5 by 0.6 to find the real current.

SIMILAR QUESTIONS

1) What is the minimum frequency that a photon can have to induce a current in a metal with work function 2 eV?
2) What is the kinetic energy of an electron ejected from an atom of work function 0.5 eV when it is struck by a photon of wavelength 100 nm?
3) What power and frequency of incident radiation must be used to strike a metal (of work function 1×10^{-18} J) to produce 10,000 electrons per second?

CHAPTER 7

MAGNETISM

In this chapter we will review the subject of magnetism. Unlike with electrostatics, where electric charges create electric fields that exert forces on other electric charges, magnetism has no fundamental magnetic charges. Instead, magnetic fields are created by moving charges, currents in wires, and permanent magnets. These magnetic fields, in turn, exert magnetic forces on the very things that create them, *i.e.,* moving charges, currents in wires, and permanent magnets.

MCAT Synopsis

Magnetic fields are created by moving charges and permanent magnets, and in turn exert forces on moving charges and permanent magnets.

The first half of the chapter is concerned with the determination of the magnetic force due to a given magnetic field. Because force is a vector, both the magnitude and direction of the magnetic force are considered. The second half of the chapter then examines sources of magnetic fields, including a brief review of magnetic materials, and also a discussion of the two most common current configurations, the straight wire and the loop of wire.

THE MAGNETIC FIELD

Teacher Tip

Have you heard the term electromagnetism before? These two phrases are combined into a single concept: a changing magnetic field produces an electric field and a changing electric field produces a magnetic field. It is this interconnectedness that causes both to be part of a single, fundamental force.

In discussing the magnetic force on moving charges and on current-carrying wires, we will assume the presence of a fixed and uniform magnetic field **B.** Of course, this field must be produced by some external source such as a magnet or arrangement of current-carrying wires, but for our purposes we are concerned only with the strength and direction of this field.

Like all physical quantities, magnetic fields have units. The SI unit of the magnetic field is the tesla (T) where $1\ \text{T} = 1\frac{\text{N}\bullet\text{s}}{\text{m}\bullet\text{C}}$. Small magnetic fields are sometimes measured in gauss where 1 tesla = 10^4 gauss.

MCAT Favorite

When a charge moves parallel to ($\theta = 0°$) or antiparallel to ($\theta = 180°$) a magnetic field, the magnetic force is zero.

A. FORCE ON A MOVING CHARGE

When a charge moves in a magnetic field, a magnetic force is exerted on it. This force, like all forces, is a vector. The **magnitude** of F is given by:

$$F = qvB \sin \theta$$

In this formula, θ is the smallest angle between the vectors qv and B (more on qv below), q is the charge of the moving particle, v is the particle's speed, and B = |**B**| is the magnitude of the magnetic field vector.

TEACHER TIP

Similar to electrostatic problems, magnetic problems always assume a positive test charge. Both magnetic and electric fields describe the direction in which a positive charge would travel. If you are ever given a negative charge, solve it in the standard way but change your answer to the "opposite" as your last step (i.e., right to left or up to down).

Right-Hand Rule for the Direction of the Magnetic Force on a Moving Charge

Turning our attention to the **direction** of the magnetic force, we should first note that qv is a vector that depends on the velocity vector v and the sign of the charge q. If q is nonzero and positive (positive charge), then qv points in the same direction as v. If q is nonzero and negative (negative charge), then qv points in the opposite direction as v. (If q or v is zero, then the magnetic force will be zero.) The direction of the magnetic force will be **perpendicular** to the plane defined by qv and B, but this could be either of two directions. To find the correct direction, let the thumb of the **right hand** (left-handed people must be careful to use the correct hand) point in the direction of the vector qv (that is, parallel to v if q is positive and antiparallel to v if q is negative). Let the remaining fingers of the **right hand** point in the direction of B. Your **palm** now points in the direction of F, the magnetic force on q.

TEACHER TIP

Another version of the right-hand rule (depicted on the next page) is to let your thumb be the direction of velocity, your index finger the magnetic field, and the palm the direction of force. Whatever method works for you, use it.

(Note: The right-hand rule as stated above may differ from what you have previously learned. A different version would have the right index finger in the direction of qv and right middle finger in the direction of B and, holding the thumb perpendicular to these two fingers, the right thumb points in the direction of F. It is important only to get the direction correct no matter which rule you use. **If you have committed to memory another version of the rule, and it works, then use it.)**

MCAT SYNOPSIS

The symbol 'x' means the magnetic field direction is into the page, and the symbol '•' means the magnetic field direction is out of the page.

Because of the three-dimensional nature of problems involving magnetic fields, scientists have chosen the following conventions to denote magnetic fields going into the page, or coming out of the page. The symbol 'x' represents a field going into the page. The x represents the tail end of an arrow travelling into the page. The symbol '•' represents a field coming out of the page. The • represents the tip of an arrow coming out of the page.

Example: Suppose a proton, whose charge is $+1.6 \times 10^{-19}$ C, is moving with a speed of 15 m/s in a direction parallel to a uniform magnetic field of 3.0 T. What is the magnitude and direction of the magnetic force on the proton?

Solution: Because the proton is positively charged, the vector qv is in the same direction as v, which is the same direction as B as stated in the problem. Because qv and B are pointing in the same direction, the angle between the vectors is zero. Because sin 0° = 0 and F = qvB sin θ, the magnetic force on the proton is zero, too. Note that if the charge had been negative (an electron, for example), the angle between qv and B would have been 180° and because sin 180° = 0, the magnetic force on a negative charge moving parallel to a uniform magnetic field would be zero as well. In general, the magnetic force on a moving charge will be zero if the charge is moving parallel or antiparallel to the magnetic field.

TEACHER TIP

Sin of 0° and 180° = zero
This means that any charge moving parallel or antiparallel to the direction of the magnetic field will experience no force from the magnetic field.

MCAT SYNOPSIS

The magnetic force on a moving charged particle is always perpendicular to both the velocity of the charge and the magnetic field direction. Thus, a magnetic force does no work. (See chapter 3.)

Example: Suppose a proton whose charge equals $+1.6 \times 10^{-19}$ C is moving with a speed of 15 m/s toward the top of the page and through a uniform magnetic field of 3.0 T directed into the page [see Figure 7.1(a)]. What is the magnitude and direction of the magnetic force on the proton?

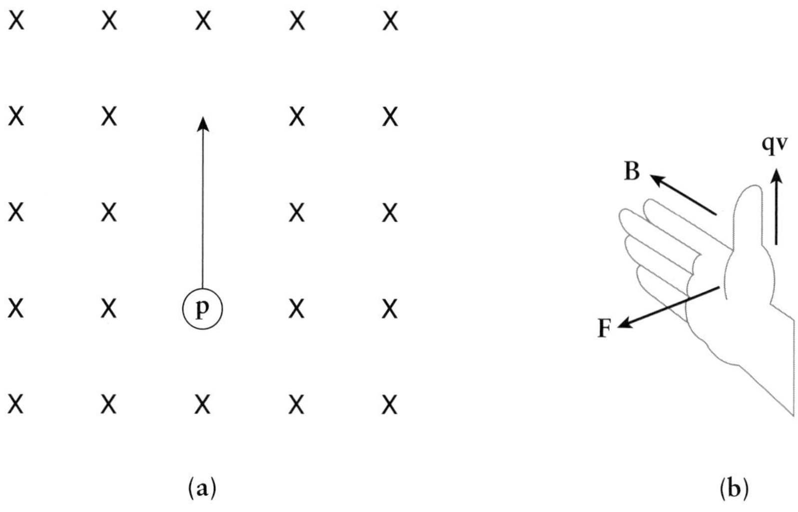

Figure 7.1

Solution: Because the proton is positively charged, the vector qv is in the same direction as v, which is perpendicular to B as stated in the problem. (B is perpendicular to the plane of the page.) Because qv and B are perpendicular, the angle between the vectors is $\theta = 90°$, and because sin 90° = 1, the magnetic force on the proton is:

$$F = qvB \sin \theta$$
$$= qvB$$
$$= (1.6 \times 10^{-19})(15)(3.0)$$
$$= 7.2 \times 10^{-18} \text{ N}$$

MCAT SYNOPSIS

A charged particle moving perpendicular to a constant, uniform magnetic field, undergoes uniform circular motion. The centripetal force in this case is the magnetic force on the charge.

By holding the thumb of the **right hand** so that it is directed toward the top of the page, then holding the remaining fingers of the **right hand** so that they point towards (into) the page, one's **right hand** palm points to the left [see Figure 7.1(b)]. Hence, the proton is deflected to the left on its upward journey. As the velocity of the proton changes, so does the magnetic force that it experiences. Note that if the charge had been negative (an electron, for example), the angle between qv and B still would have been 90°, but the right-hand rule would have required that **qv** point toward the bottom of the page, meaning that one's right-hand palm would point to the right. Hence, an electron is deflected to the right on its upward journey. One can readily see that the direction of the magnetic force on a negative charge moving through a magnetic field is opposite to the direction of the magnetic force acting on a positive charge moving in the same direction.

When a charged particle moves **perpendicular** to a **constant, uniform magnetic field,** the resulting motion is circular motion with constant speed in the plane perpendicular to the magnetic field. A centripetal force is always associated with circular motion. In this case, the centripetal force is the magnetic force (F = qvB). Because the centripetal force equals mv^2/r, we get:

$$F = qvB = \frac{mv^2}{r}$$

From this equation one can solve for the orbit radius, the magnetic field, and so on:

$$r = \frac{mv}{qB} \qquad B = \frac{mv}{qr}$$

Example: Suppose the proton of the previous example is allowed to circle (counterclockwise) in the same perpendicular magnetic field of 3.0 T with the same speed of 15 m/s [as in Figure 7.2(a)]. What is the orbit radius r? (The mass of a proton is 1.67×10^{-27} kg.)

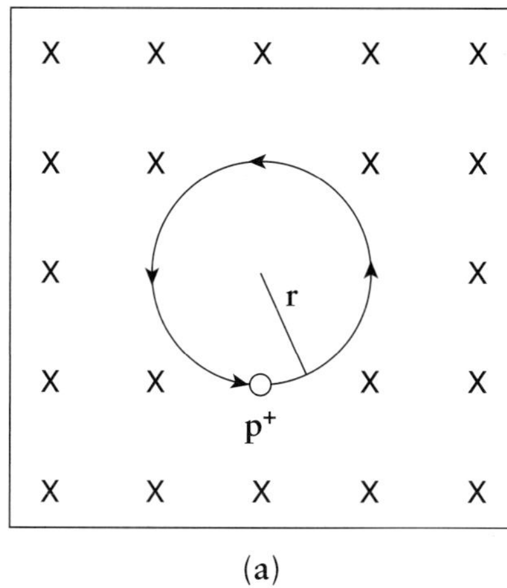

(a)

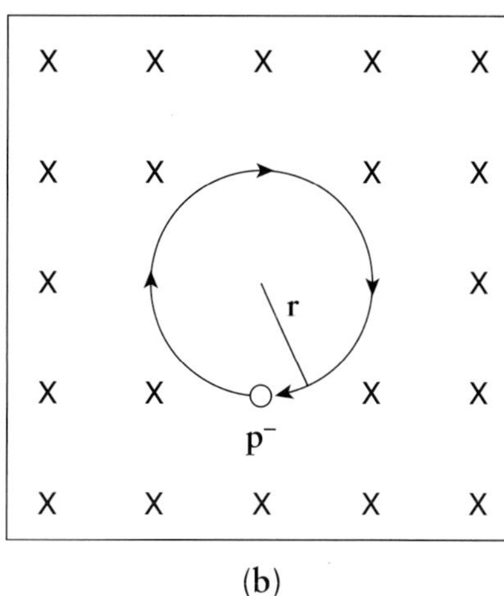

(b)

Figure 7.2

MCAT SYNOPSIS

To determine sense of rotation (clockwise or counterclockwise) of a charged particle undergoing uniform circular motion, apply the right-hand rule for magnetic force on the particle.

Solution: By equating the centripetal force to the magnetic force and solving for the orbit radius as shown above:

$$r = \frac{mv}{qB}$$

$$= \frac{(1.67 \times 10^{-27})(15)}{(1.6 \times 10^{-19})(3)}$$

$$= 5.2 \times 10^{-8}\,\text{m}$$

Note that the direction of the magnetic force on a negative charge moving through a uniform magnetic field is opposite to the direction of the magnetic force acting on a positive charge moving in the same direction. Therefore, if the charge had been negative (an antiproton, for example, which has the mass of the proton but is negatively charged), it would have circled in the **clockwise** direction with the same orbit radius. [See Figure 7.2 (b).]

B. CURRENT

Electric current will be discussed more completely in chapter 8. However, it is important to realize that when two points at different electric potentials are connected with a conductor (such as a metal wire), charge flows between the two points. The flow of charge is called an **electric current.** The magnitude of the current i is the amount of charge Δq passing through the conductor per unit time Δt, or in the form of an equation:

$$i = \frac{\Delta q}{\Delta t}$$

TEACHER TIP

Think of current in wire as you would current in a river. It is a measurement of how much moves through per unit time. In a river, it's the number of water molecules; in a wire it's the amount of charge.

MCAT SYNOPSIS

Current is in the direction that positive charges would flow.

MCAT SYNOPSIS

A current in a magnetic field behaves similarly to a positive charge moving in a magnetic field because current is a collection of moving positive charges.

The SI unit of current is the ampere (1 A = 1 coulomb/second).

Charge is transmitted by a flow of electrons in a conductor. Because electrons are negatively charged, they go from lower potentials to higher potentials. But, **by convention,** the direction of **current** is the direction in which **positive charge** would flow, or from high to low potential. **Thus the direction of current is opposite to the direction of electron flow.**

C. FORCE ON A CURRENT-CARRYING WIRE

Because moving charge is subject to magnetic forces and electric current is a flow of charge, it is no surprise that magnetic forces can act on a current-carrying wire. For a straight wire of length L carrying a current i in a direction that makes an angle θ with a uniform magnetic field B, the magnitude of the magnetic force on the current-carrying wire is:

$$F = iLB \sin \theta$$

TEACHER TIP

A current-carrying wire will itself generate a magnetic field.

The direction of the force is given by a simple right hand rule, the **right-hand rule for the magnetic force on currents.** The force will be **perpendicular** to the plane defined by B and the direction of the current flow, but this could be either of two directions. To find the correct direction, let the thumb of the right hand (left-handed people must be careful to use the correct hand) point in the direction of the current i. Now let the remaining fingers of the right hand point in the direction of B. The palm of the right hand now points in the direction of F, the magnetic force on the current-carrying wire. (Note: This rule is virtually the same as the rule given above for moving charges. Again, you should feel free to use any right-hand rule that you have committed to memory and that gives the correct direction.)

Example: Suppose a wire of length 2.0 m is conducting a current of 5.0 A toward the top of the page and through a 30 gauss uniform magnetic field directed into the page [see Figure 7.3(a)]. What is the magnitude and direction of the magnetic force on the wire?

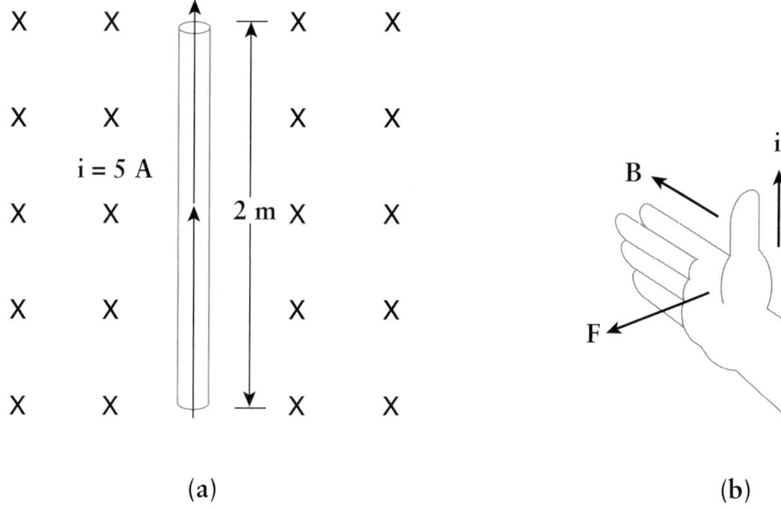

Figure 7.3

MCAT SYNOPSIS

For direction of magnetic force on a current, use same right-hand rule as for charges, but replace velocity direction with current direction.

Solution: Since 1 T = 10^4 gauss, 1 gauss = 10^{-4} T, 30 gauss = 30×10^{-4} T = 3×10^{-3} T. The wire is conducting current toward the top of the page, and the magnetic field points into the page; therefore, the current is perpendicular to B. The angle between them is $\theta = 90°$, and since sin 90° = 1, the magnetic force on the wire is:

$$F = iLB \sin\theta = iLB$$
$$= 5.0(2.0)(3.0 \times 10^{-3})$$
$$= 3.0 \times 10^{-2}\ N = 0.03\ N$$

By holding the thumb of the right hand so that it is directed toward the top of the page, then holding the remaining fingers towards (into) the page, the palm of the right hand points to the left. Hence the force on the wire is to the left.

MCAT SYNOPSIS

Wires are electrically neutral, so there's no magnetic force if the wire simply moves through a magnetic field with no current in the wire.

SOURCES OF MAGNETIC FIELD

The previous section dealt with the magnetic force on a moving charge and a current-carrying wire, but it did not discuss how the field was generated. Any moving charge creates a magnetic field. Magnetic fields may be set up by the "flow" of charge in permanent magnets, or electric currents, or simply by individual moving charges (e.g., an electron moving through space). This section deals only with permanent magnets and current-carrying wires, but it is important to realize that each of these sources of magnetic

FLASHBACK

Magnetic field lines are analogous to electric field lines, i.e., the magnetic field is tangent to the magnetic field line at any point.

Teacher Tip

Like electric field lines, magnetic field lines never cross.

field has, in one sense or another, a flow of charge or a current—it is the movement of charge that gives rise to the magnetic field.

As with electric fields, magnetic **field lines** can be used to visualize the magnetic field. At any point along a field line the magnetic field itself is in the tangential direction.

Teacher Tip

The magnetic field of the earth is created by the movement of molten metals under the earth's surface.

A. MAGNETIC MATERIALS

Materials are classified as diamagnetic, paramagnetic, and ferromagnetic. In a **diamagnetic material** the individual atoms have no net magnetic field. Diamagnetic materials will be repelled from the pole of a strong bar magnet, so they are sometimes called weakly antimagnetic. In **paramagnetic** and **ferromagnetic** materials the individual atoms do have a net magnetic field, but normally these individual atomic fields are randomly oriented so the material itself exhibits no net magnetic field. In a paramagnetic material under certain conditions, some degree of alignment of the individual atomic magnetic fields can occur. Paramagnetic materials will be attracted toward the pole of a strong bar magnet, so they are sometimes called weakly magnetic. In a ferromagnetic material a special effect takes place when the temperature drops below a critical value that allows a high degree of alignment of the magnetic fields of the individual atoms to occur. Above this critical temperature, called the Curie temperature, the material is paramagnetic. Ferromagnetic materials are sometimes called strongly magnetic and include iron, nickel, and cobalt. When the Curie temperature is above room temperature, ferromagnetic materials are permanently magnetized at room temperature (for example, the familiar bar magnet).

MCAT Synopsis

Magnetic field lines come out of north poles and go into south poles. Opposite magnetic poles attract and like poles repel.

When a paper with iron filings is placed on top of a permanent bar magnet, the iron filings tend to form lines connecting the top of the magnet to the bottom of the magnet. The iron filings are showing the **magnetic field lines.** All bar magnets have a **north** and **south** pole. The north pole is the place where the magnetic field lines emerge; the south pole is where they enter. Given two bar magnets, opposite poles attract each other, like poles repel.

B. CURRENT-CARRYING WIRES

Teacher Tip

The radius we use is the distance from the wire, not the radius of the wire itself.

A current-carrying wire will produce a magnetic field in its vicinity. The magnetic field of a current carrying wire is the vector sum of the magnetic fields due to the individual moving charges that comprise the current. The final result depends on the shape of the wire. Special cases include a **long straight wire** and the **center of a circular loop of wire.**

At a perpendicular distance r from an infinitely long and straight current-carrying wire the magnitude of the magnetic field produced by the current i in the wire is given by:

$$B = \frac{\mu_0 i}{2\pi r}$$

where μ_0 is the **permeability of free space** = $4\pi \times 10^{-7}$ tesla • meter/ampere = 1.26×10^{-6} T • m/A. The above equation shows that for a long straight wire, the field strength drops off with distance.

The magnetic field lines are concentric perpendicular circles about the wire. You can use a **right-hand rule to find the direction of the magnetic field produced by a long straight wire.** This rule differs from the previous ones. In this rule your **right thumb** points in the direction of the current. Your remaining **right fingers** mimic the circular magnetic field lines and curl around the wire. Your fingers now show you the direction of the magnetic field lines and the direction of B itself at any point. Note that this rule differs from the previous two in that it gives the direction of the field lines produced by the current instead of starting with a given direction of B to find the direction of a force. Also note that, as shown in a later example, this rule may be applied to current loops as well as straight wires.

MCAT SYNOPSIS

Magnetic field lines encircle currents. Use the right-hand rule (different from the rule for magnetic force on a moving charge) to find the field direction.

Example: A straight wire carries a current of 5 A toward the top of the page [see Figure 7.4(a)]. What is the magnitude and direction of the magnetic field at point P, which is 10 cm to the left of the wire? What is the magnitude and direction of the magnetic field at point Q, which is 2 cm to the right of the wire?

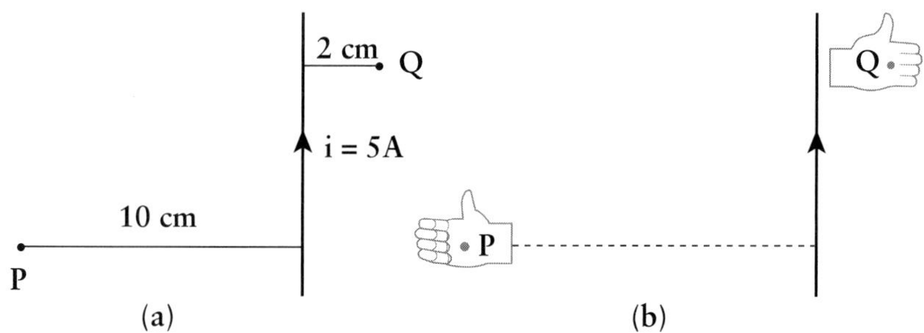

Figure 7.4

MCAT SYNOPSIS

For a wire in the plane of the page, the field lines will go into the page on one side of the wire and come out of the page on the other side of the wire.

Solution: To find the magnitude at point P:

$$B = \frac{\mu_0 i}{2\pi r}$$

$$= \frac{(4\pi \times 10^{-7})(5)}{2\pi(0.1)}$$

$$= 10^{-5}\ T = 0.1\ \text{gauss}$$

To find the magnitude at point Q:

$$B = \frac{(4\pi \times 10^{-7})(5)}{2\pi(0.02)}$$

$$= 5 \times 10^{-5}\ T = 0.5\ \text{gauss}$$

Now to get the direction of the field for each of these points, we use the right-hand rule. Hold your **right thumb** towards the top of the page. Now curl your fingers around the wire. At Q your fingers should point into the page. Keep curling around and you notice that at point P your fingers come out of the page. [See Figure 7.4 (b).] So your answer should be: B (at P) = 0.1 gauss, pointing out of the page, and B (at Q) = 0.5 Gauss, pointing into the page. Note that as we move farther from the wire the magnitude of magnetic field decreases.

MCAT SYNOPSIS

For a circular loop of wire, the equation $\frac{\mu_0 i}{2r}$ only gives the magnetic field at one point in space, the point at the center of the loop.

The magnitude of the magnetic field at the center of a circular loop of current-carrying wire of radius r is:

$$B = \frac{\mu_0 i}{2r}$$

TEACHER TIP

Know when to use each of these equations; you will likely see magnetism problems on the exam.

Notice that these two laws for magnetic fields look similar. For the long straight wire, r refers to the perpendicular distance from the wire and gives B for any point away from the wire. However, r in the second case is the radius of the loop and the expression gives the magnetic field at the loop's center point only. The following example illustrates how to find directions.

Example: Suppose a wire is formed into a loop that carries current clockwise (that is, electrons flow counterclockwise) as in Figure 7.5(a). Find the direction of the magnetic field produced by this loop:

a. within the loop.

b. outside of the loop.

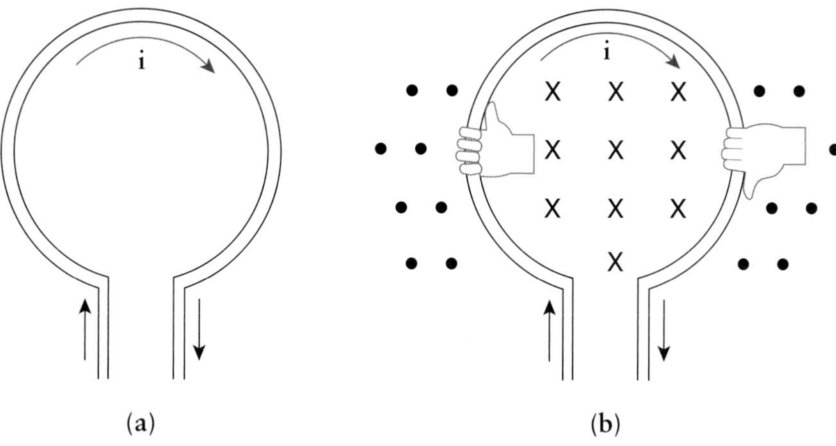

Figure 7.5

MCAT SYNOPSIS

The magnetic field circles around a current, so it will be into the page on one side of a current loop (inside or outside) and out of the page on the other side.

Solution: Look at Figure 7.5(b). By holding your right thumb anywhere around the loop in the direction of current flow (clockwise) and encircling the wire with the remaining fingers of the right hand, your right fingers should point:

a. into the page. Thus the magnetic field within the loop points into the page.

b. out of the page. Thus the magnetic field outside the loop points out of the page.

PRACTICE QUESTIONS

1. A uniform magnetic field points into the page. The direction of a magnetic force felt by the electron moving to the right is

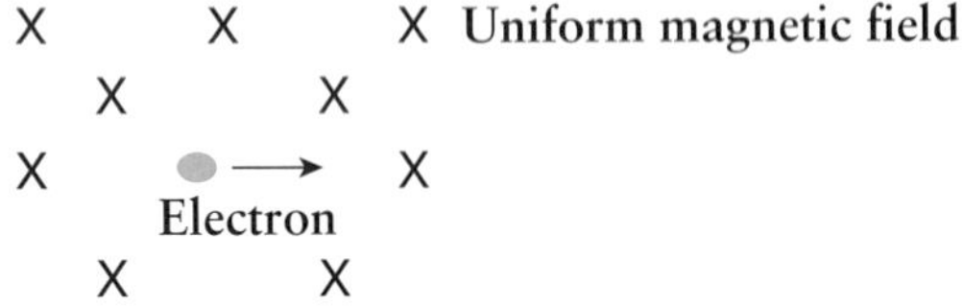

A. down.
B. to the left.
C. up.
D. to the right.

2. A positive charge of 5 C is positioned on a table. One can conclude that the magnetic force due to the magnetic field generated by the charge is

A. constant.
B. zero.
C. changing with time.
D. decreasing.

3. A straight wire is carrying a current of 3 A. Motionless charges A 3 C and B 10 C are located away from the wire as shown below. We can logically infer that

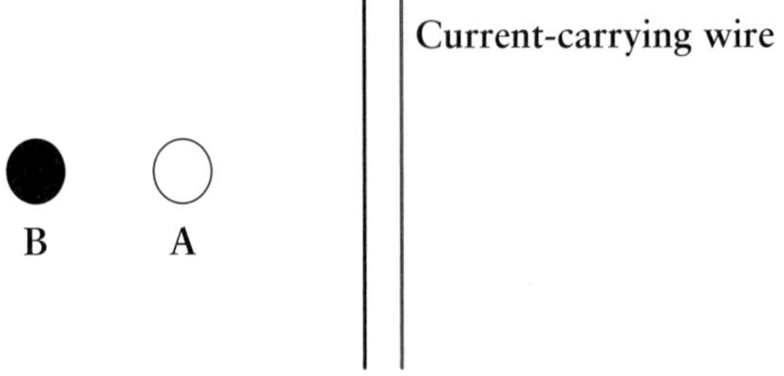

A. charge B is experiencing a stronger magnetic field than charge A is.
B. charge A is experiencing a stronger magnetic field than charge B is.
C. both charges experience the same strength of magnetic field.
D. neither charge experiences a magnetic field as they are motionless.

4. A negative charge is located above a current-carrying wire. The direction of the 5 A current in the wire is to the left, as shown below. Determine the direction of the magnetic field experienced by the negative charge.

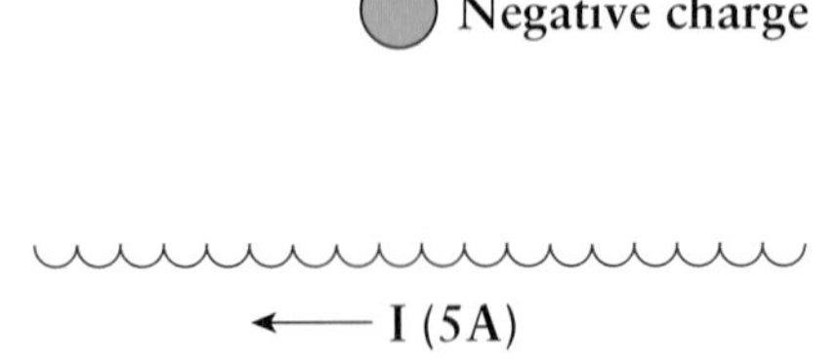

A. Into the plane of the page
B. Out of the plane of the page
C. To the left
D. To the right

5. Two positive charges are traveling in opposite directions parallel to the uniform magnetic field. It can be inferred that the magnetic force on both charges

A. is equal in magnitude and opposite in direction.
B. has the same direction but different magnitudes.
C. is zero.
D. is different in both magnitude and direction.

6. An electron is ejected straight up into a uniform magnetic field of 3 T pointing out of the page. What can be most reasonably assumed about the electron's path?

A. The electron's trajectory will deflect to the left.
B. The electron will continue traveling straight.
C. The electron's trajectory will deflect to the right.
D. The electron will reverse the direction of its movement.

7. Current flows to the right in a wire 2 meters in length. The wire is located in an external magnetic field of 5 T directed into the page. Knowing that the wire is connected to an energy source of 6 V and has 2 resistors of 6 Ω and 3 Ω in parallel, calculate the magnetic force experienced by the wire portion.

A. 7 N
B. 15 N
C. 120 N
D. 30 N

8. A negatively charged particle of 2 C and 0.005 g is spinning in a uniform magnetic field along the circle with a radius of 8 cm. Knowing that the strength of magnetic field is 5 T, calculate the speed of the particle.

A. 13×10^{-3} m/s
B. 160 m/s
C. 16×10^{4} m/s
D. 13×10^{-6} m/s

9. A magnetic force of 5 N is acting on an electron moving perpendicular to the uniform magnetic field. Knowing that the electron covers the distance of 25 cm, calculate the work done by the magnetic force.

A. 0 J
B. 125 J
C. 12.5 J
D. 1.25 J

10. In the figure below, the loop of wire is carrying a current of 10 A in the direction shown. With the uniform magnetic field coming out of the page, it can be inferred that

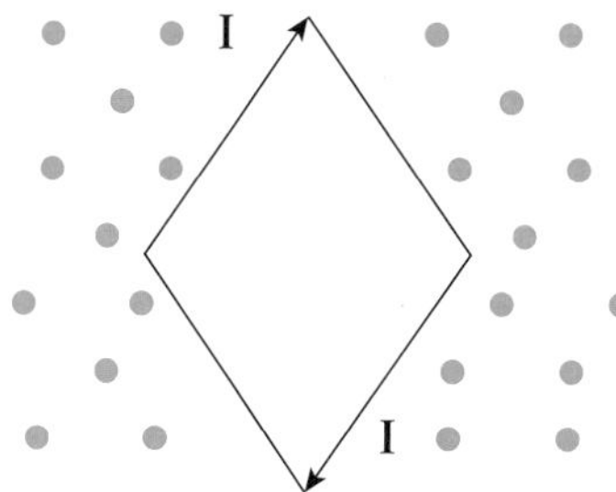

A. there is no net magnetic force.
B. the net magnetic force is to the right.
C. the net magnetic force is to the left.
D. the net magnetic force cannot be determined.

11. While very weakly magnetic, most substances—including water, gases, and organic compounds—will repel from a pole of a strong magnet. This is an example of which of the following?

A. Paramagnetism
B. Diamagnetism
C. Ferromagnetism
D. Torque

12. A power cable, stretched 8 m above the ground, is carrying 50 A of current. Determine the magnetic field produced by the current at the ground level under the wire if μ*, the permeability of free space, is 1.26×10^{-6} Tm/A.

A. 1.26×10^{-6} T
B. 4.5×10^{-6} T
C. 33×10^{6} T
D. 0.5×10^{6} T

13. A researcher is interested in creating a particle accelerator that can spin particles in the uniform magnetic field at the highest possible speed. This can be achieved by all of the following EXCEPT

A. increasing magnetic field strength.
B. increasing mass of the particles.
C. increasing orbital radius.
D. increasing charge of the particle.

14. A triangular loop of a current-carrying wire is suspended in the uniform magnetic field. What can be determined about the magnetic force acting on the portion BC of the wire loop?

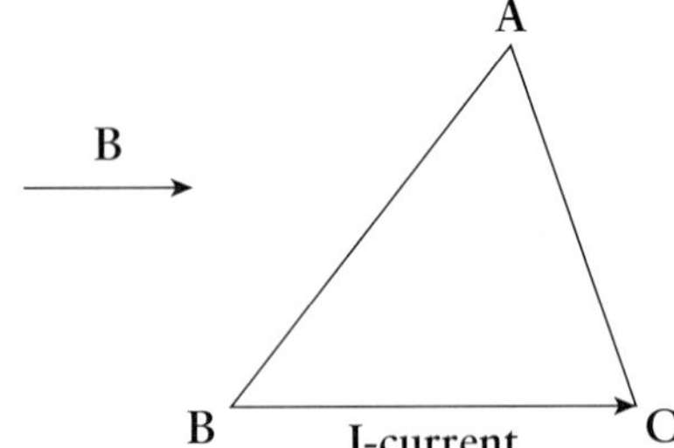

A. Magnetic force on the portion BC of the wire is out of the page.
B. Magnetic force on the portion BC of the wire is pointing up.
C. Magnetic force on the portion BC of the wire is into the page.
D. There is no magnetic force on the portion BC.

15. Proton and electron are traveling in the uniform magnetic field with identical velocities. If the movement of both particles is perpendicular to the magnetic field lines, which of the following are NOT true?

I. The acceleration of the proton is greater than that of electron.
II. The proton will experience a greater kinetic energy change than the electron does.
III. The magnetic force on both particles is zero.

A. III only
B. I and III only
C. II and III only
D. I, II, and III

16. A velocity filter is used to detect charged particles moving with specific speed, by using electric and magnetic fields of constant magnitude. The filter is most likely to be ineffective in selecting which of the following particles?

A. Electron
B. Neutron
C. Proton
D. Alpha particle

17. Two long straight wires are running parallel to each other and carrying identical amounts of current in opposite directions. The magnetic fields produced by each wire result in a repulsive force between the wires, which can be calculated by the formula $F = \mu_0 I^2/2\pi r$, where μ_0 = the permeability of free space, r = the distance between wires, and I = the current through each wire. A researcher interested in keeping the repulsive force the same, would first double the amount of current through each wire and then

A. decrease the permeability of free space.
B. halve the distance between wires.
C. double the distance between wires.
D. increase by four the distance between wires.

18. A velocity filter detects particles of particular speed at the point when electric force F = Eq and magnetic force F = qvB produced by the filter are equal. It can be reasonably assumed that, in order to select a particle with a higher speed, one should increase

A. the electric field.
B. the charge of the particle.
C. the magnetic field.
D. both electric and magnetic fields.

19. What is most likely true about a square loop of wire with clockwise direction of current in the uniform magnetic field pointing upward?

A. The wire square would remain still.
B. There are no magnetic forces acting on the wire square.
C. The square would rotate top over bottom.
D. The square would rotate bottom over top.

KEY CONCEPTS

Magnetic field

Right-hand rule

Vector addition

$B = \frac{\mu_0 I}{2\pi r}$ (T)(long straight wire)

$B = \frac{\mu_0 I}{2r}$ (T)(center of loop of wire)

TAKEAWAYS

This problem is another example of considering the sources of a field separately and then adding their effects. This is the same process you use to find the net electric field due to multiple charges.

THINGS TO WATCH OUT FOR

Many students confuse the right-hand rule, but the rule is essential to getting the correct answer on any magnetic field problem.

MAGNETIC FIELD

A current of 2 A flows down a long wire with a loop of radius 50 cm in it. The current flows around the loop counterclockwise, as shown in the diagram below. What is the magnitude and direction of the of the magnetic field at the center of the loop?
($\mu_o = 4\pi \times 10^{-7}$ T·m/A)

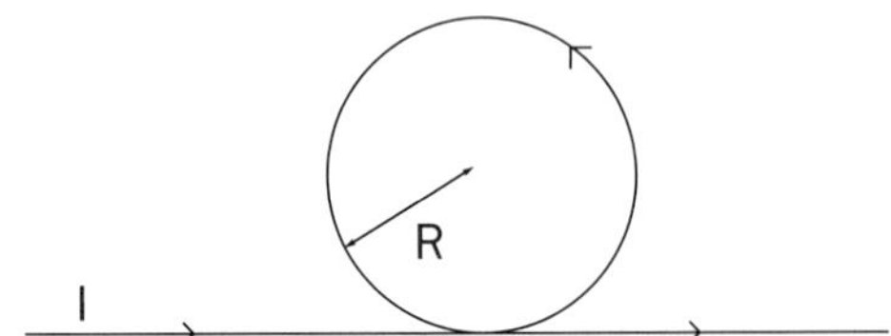

1) Find the magnetic field due to the straight section.

☞ $B_{straight} = \frac{\mu_0 I}{2\pi r} = \frac{(4\pi \times 10^{-7})(2)}{[2\pi(0.5)]} = 8 \times 10^{-7}$ T

The magnetic field due to the straight section is given by the formula $B = \mu_o I/2\pi r$.

---

2) Find the magnetic field due to the circular section.

☞ $B_{circular} = \frac{\mu_0 I}{2r} = \frac{(4\pi \times 10^{-7})(2)}{[2(0.5)]} = 2.5 \times 10^{-6}$ T

The magnetic field due to the circular section is given by the formula $B = \mu_o I/2r$.

---

3) Determine the direction of each of the magnetic fields.

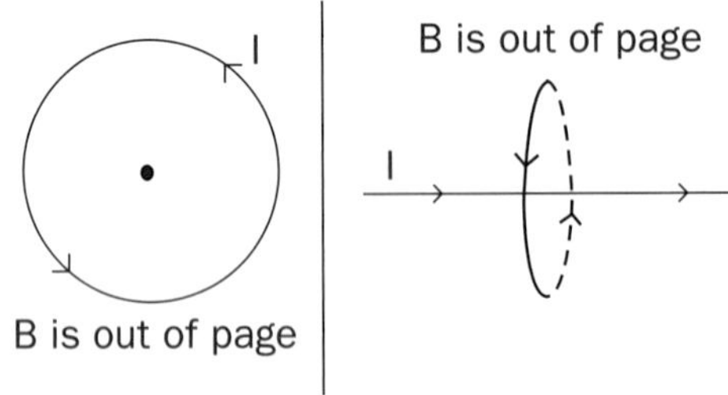

Determine the direction of the magnetic field produced by each source separately. To determine the direction of a magnetic field we use a right-hand rule—essentially the same right-hand rule for a long straight wire as for a circular loop: (i) Grasp a section of the wire, with your thumb pointing in the direction of the current through that section. (ii) Your fingers will now curl in the direction of the magnetic field. To find the direction of the magnetic field at a particular location, position your fingertips at that location (while still gripping the wire with your thumb pointing in the direction from step (i)); your fingertips will now point in the direction of the magnetic field at that location.

MCAT Pitfall: There are two different right-hand rules, one for finding the direction of a magnetic field and one for finding the direction of a magnetic force. Don't confuse them!

To determine the direction of the field generated by the loop: (i) Let's say you grasp the bottom of the loop. Then you should point your thumb to the right. (ii) Your fingers will now curl in the direction of the magnetic field around the bottom of the loop. We want to know the direction of the field inside the loop; therefore, position your fingertips inside the loop. Your fingertips will now be pointing out of the page; therefore, the direction of the magnetic field inside the loop is out of the page.

To determine the direction of the field generated by the straight wire: (i) Grasp the wire, pointing your thumb to the right. (ii) Your fingers will now curl in the direction of the magnetic field. We want to know the direction of the field above the wire; therefore, position your fingertips above the loop. Your fingertips will now be pointing out of the page; therefore, the direction of the magnetic field above the wire is out of the page.

---

4) Find the net magnetic field.

$$B_{net} = B_{straight} + B_{circular} = 8 \times 10^{-7} + 2.5 \times 10^{-6}$$
$$= 3.3 \times 10^{-6}\ \text{T}$$

Because the magnetic fields are pointed in the same direction, simply add their magnitudes to find the net field. If they were pointed in opposite directions, you would need to subtract one from the other.

SIMILAR QUESTIONS

1) For a long wire with a loop in it as in the previous problem, at what point(s) is there no net magnetic field?
2) Two parallel, straight wires, each carrying a current of 10 mA in the same direction, are located 10 cm apart. What is the net magnetic field halfway between the two wires?
3) Two circular loops of wire are concentric. They both carry a current of 50 mA, but in opposite directions. If the radii of the loops are 10 cm and 30 cm, and the inner loop carries a clockwise current, what is the magnitude and direction of the magnetic field at the center of the loops?

KEY CONCEPTS

Magnetic field

Magnetic force

Alpha particles

TAKEAWAYS

From the force relationship above, it can be deduced that the units of magnetic field are $\frac{N \cdot s}{C \cdot m}$ or $\frac{N}{A \cdot m}$. This unit is named the tesla. It is a large unit, and the smaller unit, gauss, is used for small fields like the Earth's magnetic field. A tesla is 10,000 gauss.

THINGS TO WATCH OUT FOR

The force is perpendicular to both the velocity (v) of the charge (q) and the magnetic field (B). The magnetic force on a stationary charge or a charge moving parallel to the magnetic field is zero. The direction of the force is given by the right-hand rule.

MAGNETIC FORCE

The speed of an alpha particle is 4.5×10^4 m/s and the magnitude of the magnetic force is 7.5×10^{-15} N. What is the magnitude of the magnetic field, if the particle is traveling perpendicular to the field?
($e = 1.6 \times 10^{-19}$ C)

1) Determine the charge of the object that the force is acting upon.

$2 \times 1.6 \times 10^{-19}$ C = 3.2×10^{-19} C

The magnetic field is acting upon an alpha particle. An alpha particle has two protons and two neutrons. Because the charge of one proton is 1.6×10^{-19} C, multiply that by 2.

Remember: *The sign of the charge will depend on the particle. If you have an electron, the charge is negative. If you are dealing with a proton, the charge is positive.*

---

2) Set up the force equation.

☞ $F = qvB \sin \theta$

In this formula, F is the magnitude of the magnetic force on the moving charge; q is the magnitude of the charge; v is the magnitude of the velocity of the moving charge; B is the magnitude of the magnetic field; and θ is the angle between the magnetic field and the velocity of the charge. The question states that the particle is moving perpendicular to the field, so θ is 90°.

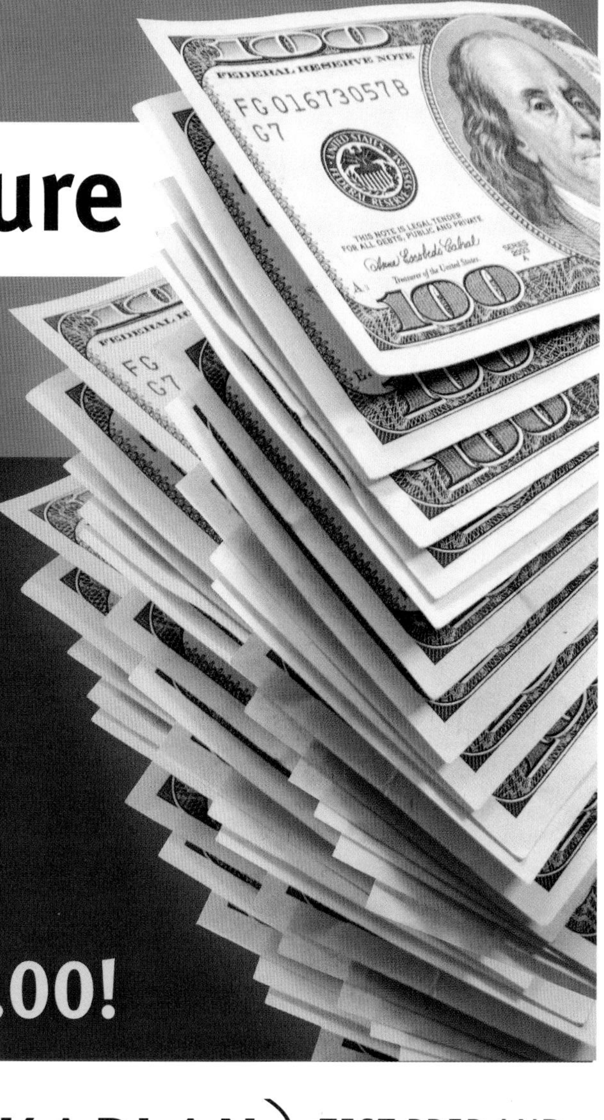

3) Solve for the magnitude of the magnetic field.

$$B = \frac{F}{qV}$$

$$= \frac{7.5 \times 10^{-15}\ \text{N}}{(3.2 \times 10^{-19}\text{C} \times 4.5 \times 10^{4}\text{m/s})}$$

$$= 0.521\ \text{T}$$

Solve for B in the equation from step 2 and plug in values.

SIMILAR QUESTIONS

1) A beam of electrons moves at right angles to a 0.60-T field. The electrons have a velocity of 2.5×10^{7} m/s. What force acts on the electrons? What force acts if the beam of electrons moves at an angle of 45° to the field?
2) What is the force felt from a magnetic field where the speed of an electron is 5×10^{3} m/s, the magnitude of the magnetic field is 1.5 T, and the particle travels at a 30° angle to the field?
3) A proton moves at right angles to a 0.003-T field directed out of the page. The proton moves from right to left with a speed of 5×10^{6} m/s. What is the magnitude and direction of the force that the proton experiences?

CHAPTER 8

DC AND AC CIRCUITS

Electric circuits pervade our everyday world, existing in myriad forms in the various necessities of modern day living, most notably, televisions, VCRs, and stereos. In this chapter we will review the essentials of DC circuits, touching only briefly and qualitatively on the subject of AC circuits. Included are the usual topics of DC circuit theory: emf, resistance, power dissipated by resistors, Kirchhoff's laws, parallel and series resistor circuits, capacitors, parallel and series capacitor circuits, and a brief discussion of dielectrics. Although the topic of DC circuits can be a place to encounter a substantial amount of algebra when solving complicated circuits, the emphasis on the MCAT and in this chapter is on the essential concepts involved and on applying those concepts in simple situations. Let's begin with a short review of conductors and insulators, the essential materials of the wires of any circuit.

Some materials allow electric charge to move freely within the material. These materials are called electrical **conductors.** Metal atoms can easily lose one or more of their outer electrons, which are then free to move around in the metal. This makes most metals good electrical conductors. In most conductors, the positive ions remain fixed and the liberated electrons are free to move.

BRIDGE

In that the divisions of science are all related, this is a perfect bridge to General Chemistry. Remember that the metals on the periodic table are on the left side. These are the atoms that are the least electronegative, thus it is easiest for them to lose electrons. Due to this weak hold on their electrons, metals have a proverbial "sea of electrons" that can move back and forth between metal atoms, conducting electrical charges.

In other materials electric charge is bound to the constituent atoms and is not free to move. These materials severely retard the flow of electricity and are called **insulators.** Most nonmetals are good insulators.

The wires to most appliances have a conducting core of copper wire perhaps, with an insulating sheath of some plastic. The copper wire conducts the electricity to the appliance from the wall socket. The insulating sheath protects you from touching the wire and getting an electric shock.

DIRECT CURRENT

A. CURRENT AND CIRCUIT VOLTAGE

The flow of charge is called an **electric current.** The magnitude of the current i is the amount of charge Δq passing a given point per unit time Δt, and is given by:

$$i = \frac{\Delta q}{\Delta t}$$

MCAT SYNOPSIS

Current flows from higher potential (positive terminal), to lower potential (negative terminal), analogous to masses, which naturally fall (flow) from higher potential energy to lower potential energy.

The SI unit of current is the **ampere** (1 A = 1 coulomb/second). The two basic types of current flow are **direct current** (DC), where the charge flows in one direction only, and **alternating current** (AC), where the flow changes direction periodically. AC current will be discussed later.

When two points at different electric potentials are connected by a conductor (such as a metal wire), charge flows between the two points. In a conductor, only negatively charged electrons are free to move. These act as the charge carriers, and move from low to high potentials. By convention, however, the direction of the **current** is taken as the direction in which **positive charge** would flow, from high to low potential. **Thus the direction of current is opposite to the direction of electron flow.**

TEACHER TIP

Voltaic cells are also called galvanic cells. Standard batteries used in flashlights or remote controls are voltaic cells.

A voltage (potential difference) can be produced by an electric generator, a voltaic cell, or by a group of cells wired into a battery. **Electromotive force** (emf or ε) is the name given to the voltage across the terminals of a cell when no current is flowing. Electromotive force should not be confused with a force or an electric field; it is a potential difference and is measured in volts.

TEACHER TIP

Most batteries dealt with on the MCAT are considered "perfect batteries," and you do not have to accommodate for their internal resistances.

Because cells typically have a small internal resistance R_{int} of their own, the voltage they actually furnish to a circuit is reduced by iR_{int}, where i is the current supplied by the cell. The voltage V across the terminals of the cell when current is flowing out, is given in terms of the cell's emf and internal resistance by:

$$V = \varepsilon - iR_{int}$$

Note: If the cell is supplying no current (i = 0), or if the cell has no internal resistance ($R_{int} = 0$), then $V = \varepsilon$. For cases in which the current supplied is greater than zero and the internal resistance is not negligible, then $V < \varepsilon$. When a cell is supplying current (discharging), the current flows out of the positive terminal and into the negative terminal. When a cell is being recharged, current from another source is sent into the positive terminal.

B. RESISTANCE

1. Resistance and Ohm's Law

Resistance R can be thought of as the opposition within a conductor to the flow of an electric current. This opposition takes the form of an energy loss or drop in potential. **Ohm's law** states that the voltage drop across a resistor is proportional to the current it carries, with R being the proportionality constant:

$$V = iR$$

This equation applies to a single resistor within a circuit, to any part of a circuit, or to an entire circuit (provided one knows how to add resistances in series and parallel). Note that the current is unchanged as it passes through the resistor. This is because no charge is lost inside the resistor. Therefore, the current that is supplied to several resistors wired in series must all flow through each resistor. The SI derived unit of electrical resistance is the **Ohm (Ω).**

TEACHER TIP

Though any appliance functions as a resistor. the most common resistors you'll see on the exam are lightbulbs.

2. Resistance of a Conductor

The resistance of an object depends on its size, the type of material from which it is made, and its temperature. Specifically the resistance depends on:

a. Length (L)

Resistance is directly proportional to length. A longer conductor means greater resistance, because there is a longer path that current-carrying electrons must travel. For example, two wires, identical in every respect except that one is twice as long as the other, will have different resistances. The longer one will have twice the resistance of the shorter one.

MCAT SYNOPSIS

- The resistance of a wire increases with increased length.
- The resistance of a wire decreases with increased cross-sectional area.

b. Cross-sectional area (A)

The resistance of a conductor is inversely proportional to its cross-sectional area. An increase in cross-sectional area causes a decrease in resistance. This is because there is an increase in the number of conduction paths electrons can follow. For example, two wires, identical in every respect except that one has twice the cross-sectional area of the other, will have different resistances. The thinner wire will have twice the resistance of the thicker wire.

TEACHER TIP

Using the 'river is a current' analogy, the wider the river, the more current can flow through. The same holds true for a wire; the bigger the cross-sectional area, the more current can flow through.

c. Resistivity of the conductor (ρ)

Some materials are intrinsically better conductors of electricity than others. For example, copper conducts electricity much better than does glass. The number that characterizes the intrinsic resistance to current flow in a material is called the **resistivity** (ρ), where the SI unit of resistivity is the Ohm•meter. The resistivity

MCAT SYNOPSIS

Resistivity, ρ, is a measure of the intrinsic resistance of a type of material, independent of length and cross-sectional area.

is therefore defined as the proportionality constant relating a conductor's resistance to the ratio of its length over its cross-sectional area:

$$R = \rho \frac{L}{A}$$

d. Temperature

Most conductors have greater resistance at higher temperatures. This is due to increased thermal oscillations of atoms in the conductor which produce a greater resistance to electron flow. The resistivity can then be thought of as a function of temperature. A few materials, such as glass, pure silicon, and most semiconductors are exceptions to this general rule.

MCAT SYNOPSIS

P = iV means P = (charge/second) × (energy/charge). So P = energy/second, as power always does.

TEACHER TIP

$P = i^2R$ solves for power *lost* during transmission. Think of a power company that sends electricity down its power lines. Because power equals voltage times current, the company can manipulate these two values while keeping power constant. One option is to increase current, which results in a decrease in voltage. The other option is to increase voltage, thus decreasing the current. *High voltage* means the company used high voltage lines to keep the current smaller (based on $P = i^2R$, which indicates how much power is *lost* in the line). Because the current is squared in this relationship, having a large current exponentially increases the amount of power lost in the line.

TEACHER TIP

Once again, think of a river: There are a certain amount of water molecules in a river, and at any junction that number has to go in one of the two directions. Nothing magically appears or disappears. The same holds true for the amount of current at any junction.

3. Power Dissipated By a Resistor

Electric potential is electric potential energy per unit positive charge. Because current is a flow of charge, it should come as no surprise that through a current-carrying resistor there is a **flow of energy.** In a resistor, this electric energy is converted into heat. The **rate** at which the energy loss occurs is equal to the power dissipated by the resistor and is given by:

$$P = iV$$

where i is the current flowing through the resistor and V is the potential drop across the resistor. Using Ohm's law this expression can be rewritten as:

$$P = i^2R = V^2/R$$

C. CIRCUIT LAWS

An electric circuit is a conducting path that usually has one or more voltage sources (such as a cell) connected to one or more **passive circuit elements** (such as resistors). This subsection deals primarily with voltages, resistances, and currents in DC circuits.

1. Kirchhoff's Laws

a. At any point or junction in a circuit the sum of currents directed into that point equals the sum of currents directed away from that point. This is a consequence of the **conservation of electric charge.**

Example: Three wires (a, b, and c) meet at a junction point P, as in Figure 8.1. A current of 5 A flows into P along wire a, and a current of 3 A flows away from P along wire b. What is the magnitude and direction of the current along wire c?

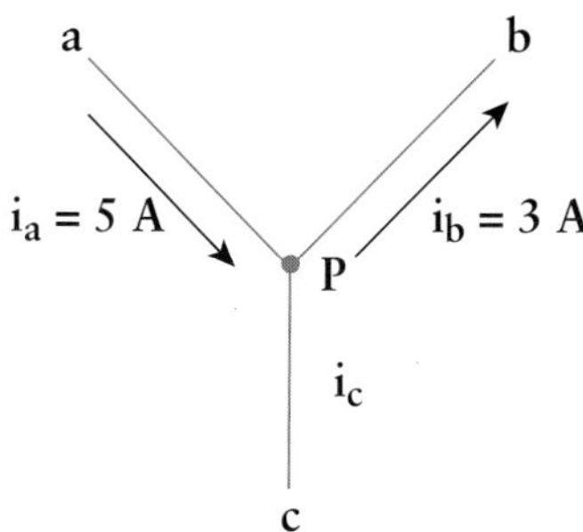

Figure 8.1

Solution: The sum of currents entering P must equal the sum of the currents leaving P. Assume for now that i_c flows out of P. If we find that it is negative, then we know that it flows into P.

$$i_a = i_b + i_c$$
$$i_c = 5 - 3$$
$$i_c = 2 \text{ A}$$

Thus a current of 2 A flows out of P along wire c. Note that the total current into and out of P is then zero.

MCAT SYNOPSIS

Energy is conserved in one complete loop of a circuit. Energy lost in the resistors is gained back in the battery.

b. **The sum of voltage sources is equal to the sum of voltage (potential) drops around a closed circuit loop.** This is a consequence of the conservation of energy: All the electrical energy supplied by a source gets fully used up by the rest of the circuit. No excess energy appears or disappears. (But remember that voltage is energy per unit charge not just energy.)

TEACHER TIP

If all the voltage weren't "used up" in each loop of the circuit, then it would build after each trip around the circuit—something that is quite impossible.

2. Resistors in Series

It has already been mentioned that the same current flows through all the resistors in series and from the laws here we can deduce that voltage drops add in series. Therefore, using Ohm's law we find that resistances add in series (see Figure 8.2). That is:

$$R_s = R_1 + R_2 + R_3 + \cdots + R_n$$

TEACHER TIP

When resistors are in series, the current *must* pass through every one; that is why we find the total resistance by adding together every resistor.

MCAT SYNOPSIS

Each additional resistor in a series of resistors increases the total resistance and thus decreases the total current.

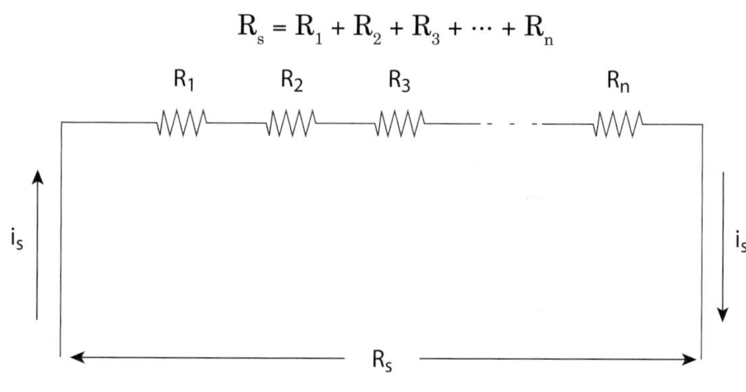

Figure 8.2

Example: A circuit is wired with one cell supplying 5 V (neglect the internal resistance of the cell) in series together with three resistors of 3 Ω, 5 Ω, and 7 Ω also wired in series as shown in Figure 8.3. What is the resulting voltage across, and current through, each resistor of this circuit, as well as the entire circuit?

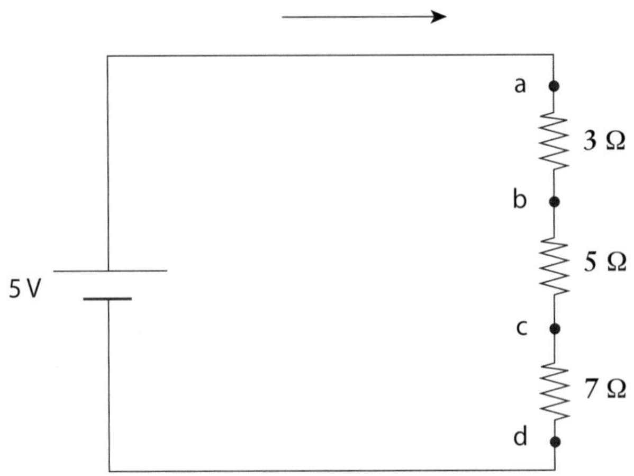

Figure 8.3

Solution: The total resistance of the resistors is:

$$R_s = R_1 + R_2 + R_3$$
$$= 3 + 5 + 7$$
$$= 15\ \Omega$$

Now use Ohm's law to get the current through the entire circuit (because everything is in series this is also the current through each element):

$$i_s = \frac{V_s}{R_s} = \frac{5}{15} = \frac{1}{3}\text{A}$$

Now use Ohm's law for each of the resistors in turn. From a to b the voltage drop across R_1 is:

$$iR_1 = (1/3)(3)$$
$$= 1.0\text{ V}$$

From b to c the voltage drop across R_2 is:

$$iR_2 = (1/3)(5)$$
$$= 1.67\text{ V}$$

From c to d the voltage drop across R_3 is:

$$iR_3 = (1/3)(7)$$
$$= 2.33\text{ V}$$

TEACHER TIP

When there is only one path for the current to take, the current will be the same at every point in the line, including through every single resistor. Once we know the current, we can use V = iR to solve for the voltage drop across each resistor (assuming we know the resistances of the resistors).

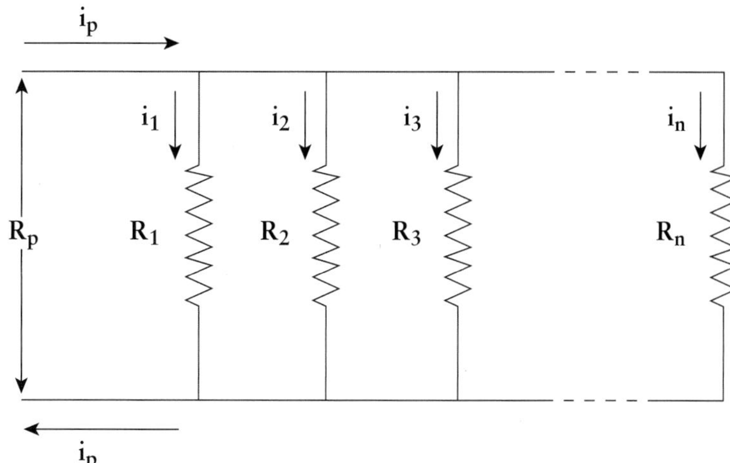

Figure 8.4

3. Resistors in Parallel

When resistors are wired in parallel, they are all wired with a common high potential terminal and a common low potential terminal (see Figure 8.4). The effect of **adding resistors in parallel** is the same as that of increasing the cross-sectional area of a conductor. It increases the paths by which current can flow and thereby **decreases resistance** (there is also the analogy to viscous blood flow through capillaries—flow resistance is reduced when several capillaries are arranged in parallel). The rule for combining resistances in parallel is a bit more complicated than the previous rules. It states that the reciprocal of the equivalent resistance equals the sum of the reciprocals of their individual resistances. In equation form this may be written as:

$$\frac{1}{R_p} = \frac{1}{R_1} + \frac{1}{R_2} + \frac{1}{R_3} + \cdots + \frac{1}{R_n}$$

MCAT SYNOPSIS

Each additional resistor added in parallel acts to decrease the total resistance and thus increase the current.

When resistors are in parallel, the voltage drop across each is the same and is equal to the voltage drop across the entire combination:

$$V_p = V_1 = V_2 = V_3 = \cdots V_n$$

TEACHER TIP

Remember Kirchhoff's second law: If every resistor is in parallel, then the voltage drop across each pathway must be the voltage of the entire circuit.

Example: Consider two equal resistors wired in parallel. What is the equivalent resistance of the two?

Solution: The equation for summing resistors in parallel is:

$$\frac{1}{R_p} = \frac{1}{R_1} + \frac{1}{R_2}$$

MCAT SYNOPSIS

Parallel resistors experience the same voltage drop.

Find the common denominator of the right-hand side and take the inverse to find:

$$R_p = \frac{R_1 R_2}{(R_1 + R_2)}$$

Since $R_1 = R_2$ in this special case, let $R = R_1 = R_2$:

$$R_p = \frac{R^2}{2R} = \frac{R}{2}$$

In the above example, it is seen that the total resistance is **halved** by wiring two identical resistors in parallel. More generally, when n identical resistors are wired in parallel, the total resistance is given by R/n. Note that the voltage across each of the parallel resistors is equal and, that for equal resistances, the current flowing through each of the resistors is also equal.

TEACHER TIP

When approaching circuit problems, you first need to find the total values: total voltage (almost always given as the voltage of the battery), total resistance, and total current. To find the total current, first determine the total resistance of the circuit.

Example: Consider two resistors wired in parallel with $R_1 = 5\ \Omega$ and $R_2 = 10\ \Omega$. If the voltage across them is 10 V, what is the current through each of the two resistors?

Solution: First the current flowing through the whole circuit must be found. To do this, the combined resistance must be determined:

$$\frac{1}{R_p} = \frac{1}{R_1} + \frac{1}{R_2}$$

$$= \frac{1}{10} + \frac{1}{5}$$

$$= \frac{3}{10}$$

$$R_p = \frac{10}{3}\ \Omega$$

Using Ohm's law to calculate the current flowing through the circuit gives:

$$i_p = \frac{V_p}{R_p}$$

$$= \frac{10}{(10/3)}$$

$$= 3\ \text{A}$$

Three amps flow through the combination R_1 and R_2. Since the resistors are in parallel $V_p = V_1 = V_2 = 10$ V. Apply Ohm's law to each resistor individually:

$$i_1 = \frac{V_p}{R_1} = \frac{10}{5} = 2\text{ A}$$

$$i_2 = \frac{V_p}{R_2} = \frac{10}{10} = 1\text{ A}$$

As a check, note that $i_p = 3\text{ A} = i_1 + i_2 = 2 + 1 = 3$ A. More current flows through the smaller resistance. In particular note that R_1 with half the resistance of R_2 has twice the current. Once i_p was found to be 3 A, the problem could have been solved by noting that because R_1 is half of R_2, $i_1 = 2i_2$, and $i_1 + i_2 = 3$ A.

D. CAPACITORS AND DIELECTRICS

1. Capacitors and Capacitance

When two electrically neutral plates of metal are connected to a voltage source, positive charge builds up on the plate connected to the positive terminal, and an equal amount of negative charge builds up on the plate connected to the negative terminal. The two plate system stores charge and is called a **capacitor.** It is important to remember that charge collects on a capacitor any time there is a potential difference between the plates. The **capacitance** C of a capacitor is defined as the ratio of charge stored (meaning the absolute value of the charge on one plate) to the total potential difference across the capacitor. So, if a voltage difference V is applied across the plates of the capacitor and a charge Q collects on it (with +Q on the positive plate and –Q on the negative plate), then the capacitance is given by:

$$C = \frac{Q}{V}$$

The SI unit of capacitance is the **farad** (where 1 F = 1 coulomb/volt). Because one coulomb is such a large amount of charge, one farad is a very large capacitance. Capacitances are therefore quoted in submultiples of the farad such as microfarads ($1\ \mu F = 10^{-6}$ F), or nanofarads (1) nF = 10^{-9} F), or picofarads (1 pF = 10^{-12} F). Note also that the farad should not be confused with the faraday, the unit of charge equal to the charge on a mole of elementary charges (= 9.65×10^4 coulombs).

TEACHER TIP

In practice, capacitors are used to release a lot of energy from a small energy source. They store energy from a power source over time, and then release that energy all at once. The perfect example of a capacitor is in a disposable camera. By pushing the button on the camera the small internal battery starts to release energy. This energy is stored by the capacitor until the capacitor is fully charged. Once it is charged, the energy will be released by the lightbulb in an instantaneous bright flash when the picture is taken.

MCAT SYNOPSIS

The total charge on a capacitor is zero, +Q on one plate, and –Q on the other.

TEACHER TIP

On the MCAT, you need only remember the faraday as 105 coulombs.

TEACHER TIP

If you look back to the equations discussed at the end of the last chapter, we can see that this equation can be derived from the four fundamental electrostatics equations. The only difference between V and E is that E has radius (or distance, it means the same thing) squared in the denominator; we can derive E from V, by simply dividing V by distance, making the distance in the denominator squared.

TEACHER TIP

A dielectric material can never decrease the capacitance, thus K can never be less than one.

MCAT SYNOPSIS

Dielectrics are insulators that increase the capacitance when inserted between the plates of a charged capacitor.

The capacitance of a capacitor is dependent on the geometry of the two conducting surfaces. For the simple case of the parallel plate capacitor, the capacitance is given by:

$$C = \varepsilon_0 \frac{A}{d}$$

where ε_0 is the **permittivity of free space** ($\varepsilon_0 = 8.85 \times 10^{-12}$ F/m), A is the area of overlap of the two plates, and d is the separation of the two plates. The separation of charges sets up an electric field between the plates of the capacitor. The electric field between the plates of a parallel plate capacitor is a uniform field whose magnitude at any point is given by:

$$E = \frac{V}{d}$$

The direction of the electric field at any point between the plates is toward the negative plate and away from the positive plate.

2. Dielectric Materials

When an insulating material (such as glass, plastic, or certain metal oxides) is placed between the plates of a charged-up capacitor, the voltage across the capacitor decreases. Such insulating materials are called **dielectrics.** By lowering the voltage across the charged-up capacitor the dielectric has "made room for" even more charge, hence, the capacitance of the capacitor is increased. Dielectric materials are characterized by a dimensionless number called the **dielectric constant K,** which tells by what factor the capacitance of a capacitor is increased:

$$C' = KC$$

where C' is the new capacitance with the dielectric, and C is the original capacitance.

Example: The voltage across the terminals of an isolated 3 μF capacitor is 4 V. If a piece of ceramic having dielectric constant K = 2 is placed between the plates, find:

a. the new charge on the capacitor.
b. the new capacitance of the capacitor.
c. the new voltage across the capacitor.

Solution: a. The introduction of a dielectric by itself has no effect on the charge stored on the isolated capacitor. There is no new charge, so the charge is the same as before. The charge stored is therefore given by:

$$\begin{aligned} Q' &= Q \\ &= CV \\ &= (3 \times 10^{-6})(4) \\ &= 12 \times 10^{-6} \text{ C} \\ &= 12\ \mu\text{C} \end{aligned}$$

b. By introducing a dielectric with a value of 2, the capacitance of the capacitor is doubled ($C' = KC$). Hence the new capacitance is 6 μF.

c. Using the relationship $V' = Q'/C'$, the new voltage across the capacitor may be determined. Putting numbers into the equation gives:

$$\begin{aligned} V &= \frac{12 \times 10^{-6}}{6 \times 10^{-6}} \\ &= 2 \text{ V} \end{aligned}$$

Example: The voltage across the terminals of a 3 μF capacitor is 4 V. Now suppose a piece of ceramic having dielectric constant $K = 2$ is placed between the plates **and the voltage is held constant** (e.g., by a battery). What is the new charge on the capacitor?

Solution: By introducing the dielectric ceramic the capacitance of the capacitor has been altered. But because the voltage was held constant, the charge on the capacitor plates must have been altered. From the definition of dielectric constant and the above example it is clear that the new capacitance is:

$$\begin{aligned} C' &= KC \\ &= 6\ \mu\text{F} \end{aligned}$$

But the new voltage is still 4 V, so the new charge must be:

$$\begin{aligned} Q' &= C'V' \\ &= (6 \times 10^{-6})(4) \\ &= 24 \times 10^{-6} \text{ C} \\ &= 24\ \mu\text{C} \end{aligned}$$

Because the original charge was $Q = CV = (3 \times 10^{-6})(4) = 12\ \mu$C, by keeping the voltage constant the battery had to supply an additional +12 μC of charge to the positive plate and 12 μC to the negative plate.

TEACHER TIP

Resistors and capacitors add oppositely. Adding resistors in parallel *decreases* overall resistance, while adding capacitors in parallel *increases* overall capacitance.

MCAT SYNOPSIS

Each capacitor added in parallel acts to increase the total capacitance of the combination.

TEACHER TIP

The sum of the voltage drops across any combination of resistors or capacitors will always equal the voltage of the entire system (the voltage of the battery).

MCAT SYNOPSIS

As with resistors, the voltage across each parallel capacitor is the same.

MCAT SYNOPSIS

Each capacitor added in series acts to decrease the total capacitance of the combination.

3. Capacitors in Parallel

When wired in parallel, capacitors can be added directly. The capacitors wired in parallel can be thought of as combining to form a single capacitor with increased capacitance. Since the wire from one capacitor to the next is a conductor and an equipotential surface, the potential of all plates on one side are the same (see Figure 8.5).

$$C_p = C_1 + C_2 + C_3 + \cdots + C_n$$

The voltage across each parallel capacitor is the same, and is equal to the voltage across the entire combination:

$$V_p = V_1 = V_2 = V_3 = \cdots = V_n$$

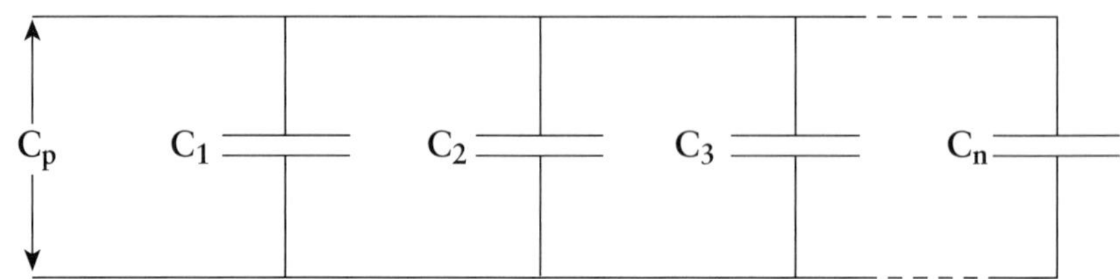

Figure 8.5

4. Capacitors in Series

Each additional capacitor added in series decreases the total capacitance of the circuit, so just as for resistors in parallel, the reciprocal of the total capacitance in series is equal to the sum of the reciprocals of the individual capacitances (see Figure 8.6).

$$\frac{1}{C_s} = \frac{1}{C_1} + \frac{1}{C_2} + \frac{1}{C_3} + \cdots + \frac{1}{C_n}$$

For capacitors in series, the total voltage is the sum of the individual voltages:

$$V_s = V_1 + V_2 + V_3 + \cdots + V_n$$

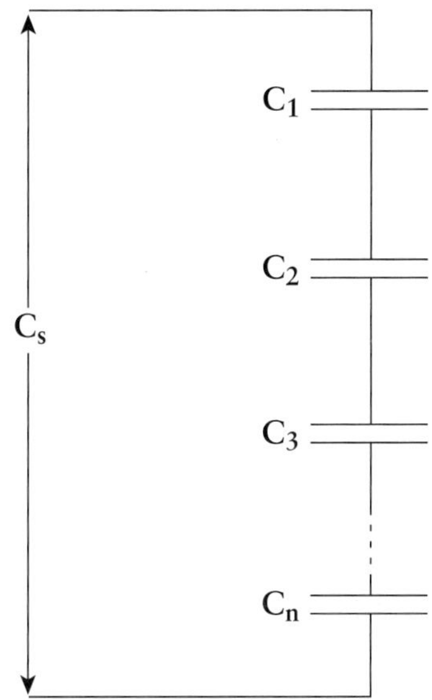

Figure 8.6

MCAT SYNOPSIS

As with resistors, the total voltage drop across a series of capacitors is the sum of the voltage drops across each separately.

E. A SUMMARY OF CIRCUIT ELEMENT ADDITION

SERIES

$$R_s = R_1 + R_2 + R_3 + \cdots + R_n$$

$$\frac{1}{C_s} = \frac{1}{C_1} + \frac{1}{C_2} + \frac{1}{C_3} + \cdots + \frac{1}{C_n}$$

PARALLEL

$$\frac{1}{R_p} = \frac{1}{R_1} + \frac{1}{R_2} + \frac{1}{R_3} + \cdots + \frac{1}{R_n}$$

$$C_p = C_1 + C_2 + C_3 + \cdots + C_n$$

ALTERNATING CURRENT

A. ALTERNATING CURRENT

Alternating current (AC) changes its direction of flow periodically. The most common form of AC current oscillates in a sinusoidal way as shown in Figure 8.7. Note that for half of the cycle the current flows in one direction, and for the other half of the cycle the current flows in the opposite direction. Such a current can be described by the equation

$$\begin{aligned} i &= I_{max} \sin(2\pi f t) \\ &= I_{max} \sin \omega t \end{aligned}$$

TEACHER TIP

On the MCAT, AC currents are largely tested qualitatively.

where i is the instantaneous current at the time t, I_{max} is the maximum current, f is the frequency, and $\omega = 2\pi f$ is the angular frequency.

The most common sinusoidal current is the ordinary AC house current that oscillates with a frequency f of 60 Hz. In some countries, such as England, the frequency is 50 Hz.

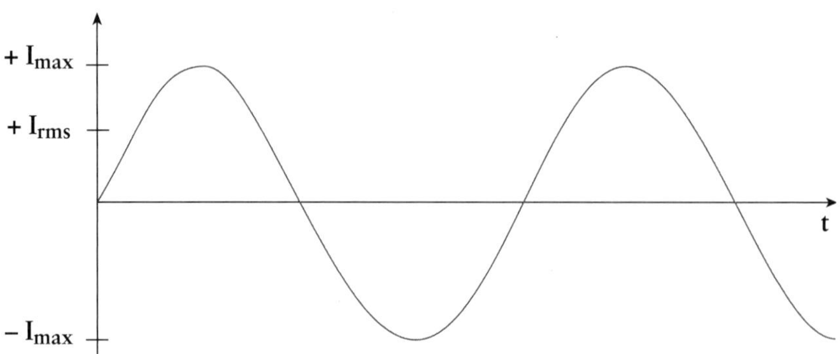

Figure 8.7

TEACHER TIP

The only AC equations to remember are those for I_{rms} and V_{rms}. Just realize that these two equations state the exact same thing for both current and voltage, so in reality there is only one AC equation we need to know.

B. RMS CURRENT

In alternating current circuits the magnitude of the current varies from a maximum positive value to a minimum negative value. A problem arises when one tries to calculate the average current for sinusoidal AC currents: for one cycle, the sum of the positive current flowing in one direction is exactly canceled by the sum of the negative current that flows in the other direction. Yet there is AC current; it delivers power. Consider the power dissipated in a resistor R that carries an AC current i. It is given by the equation $P = i^2R$. Therefore, in order to find the average power dissipated we must find the average of i^2 over one period. This is equal to $I_{rms}^{\ 2}$, where I_{rms} is the root-mean-square (rms) current given by:

MCAT SYNOPSIS

The average value of an AC current is zero because half the time it's positive and the other half of the time it's negative by the same amount.

$$I_{rms} = \frac{I_{max}}{\sqrt{2}}$$

MCAT SYNOPSIS

Average power in an AC circuit is not zero because $P = i^2R$ and i^2 is always positive.

Example: What is the rms current of an AC signal that will produce a maximum current of 1.00 A?

Solution:

$$I_{rms} = \frac{I_{max}}{\sqrt{2}}$$
$$= \frac{1.00}{\sqrt{2}}$$
$$= \frac{1.00}{1.41}$$
$$= 0.71 \text{ A}$$

C. RMS VOLTAGE

Voltage in AC circuits, like current, is sinusoidal and changes sign back and forth over time. It can be described by an equation similar to the equation for sinusoidal current. So just as for current, one can calculate an **rms voltage**:

$$V_{rms} = \frac{V_{max}}{\sqrt{2}}$$

Example: The AC current used in a home is frequently called "120 V AC." Assuming that this refers to the rms voltage, what is the maximum voltage?

Solution: Using the above equation gives:

$$V_{max} = \sqrt{2}V_{rms}$$
$$= \sqrt{2}\,(120)$$
$$= 170 \text{ V}$$

PRACTICE QUESTIONS

1. Which of the following will increase the resistance of a copper wire?

    I. Increased length
    II. Increased cross-sectional area
    III. Increased temperature

    A. I only
    B. I and III only
    C. II and III only
    D. I, II, and III

2. Which of the following materials has the highest resistivity?

    A. Tin
    B. Aluminum
    C. Copper
    D. Glass

3. A certain battery delivers 4 A of current at a potential of 6 V. How much energy can this battery deliver in 10 seconds?

    A. 24 J
    B. 240 J
    C. 1.5 J
    D. 15 J

4. In the figure below, six charges meet at point P. What is the magnitude and direction of the current between points P and X?

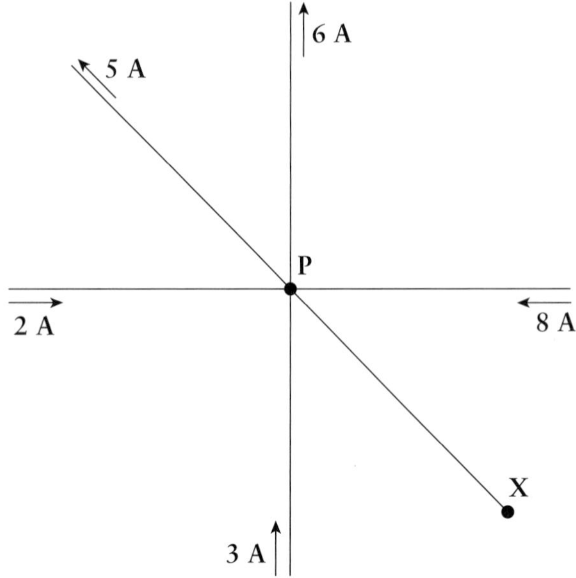

    A. 2 A, toward X
    B. 2 A, toward P
    C. 10 A, toward X
    D. 10 A, toward P

5. In the figure below, R_1 and R_2 are equal to 2 Ω. Assuming zero resistance in the wire, how much power is used up by object X?

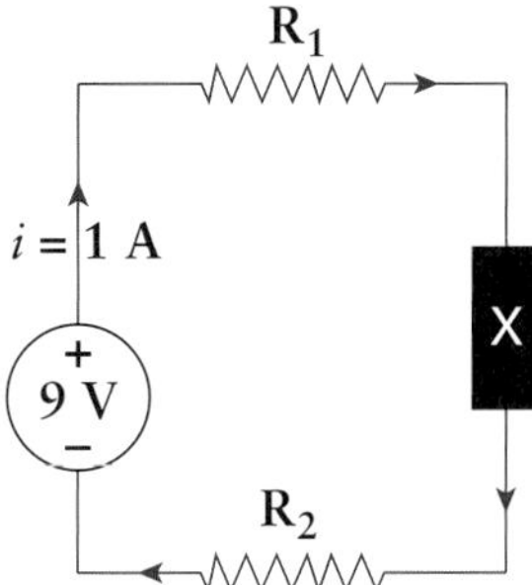

A. 2 W
B. 4 W
C. 5 W
D. 7 W

6. Continuing with the figure from the previous question, if the resistance of object X is 3 Ω, which of the following is most likely true?

A. The current increases after the charge passes through object X.
B. The total potential of the circuit decreases after the charge passes through object X.
C. The wire has a high resistivity.
D. The wire has a high cross-sectional area.

7. Which of the following would have an effect most similar to that of increasing the cross-sectional area of the wire around a resistor?

A. Adding more resistors in parallel
B. Adding more resistors in series
C. Increasing the current delivered to the resistor
D. Increasing the potential delivered to the resistor

8. Two electrically neutral metal plates are connected to a voltage source as illustrated below. If these plates are found to have a capacitance of 80 μF, how much charge are they capable of storing?

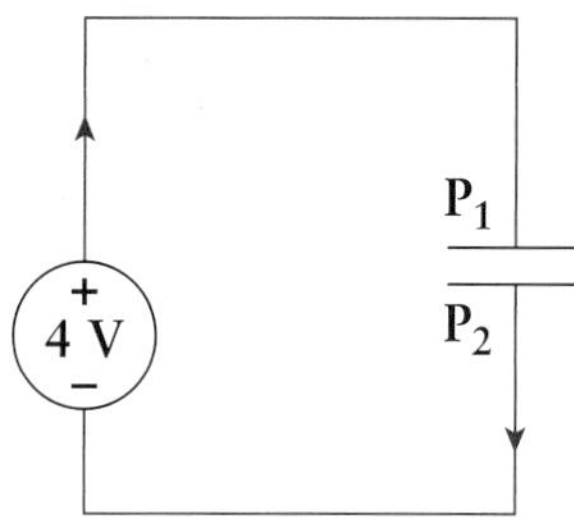

A. 2.0×10^{-5} C
B. 3.2×10^{-4} C
C. 20 C
D. 320 C

9. Which of the following will most likely increase the electric field between the plates of a parallel plate capacitor?

A. Adding a resistor that is connected to the capacitor in series
B. Adding a resistor that is connected to the capacitor in parallel
C. Increasing the distance between the plates
D. Adding an extra battery to the system

10. A certain material has a dielectric constant of 2.0. What will be the effect of placing this material between the plates of a parallel plate capacitor?

A. Capacitance is increased by a factor of 2
B. Capacitance is decreased by a factor of 2
C. Capacitance is increased by a factor of 4
D. Capacitance is decreased by a factor of 4

11. A capacitor is continuously charged and discharge Which of the following graphs describes the current flowing through the capacitor with respect to time?

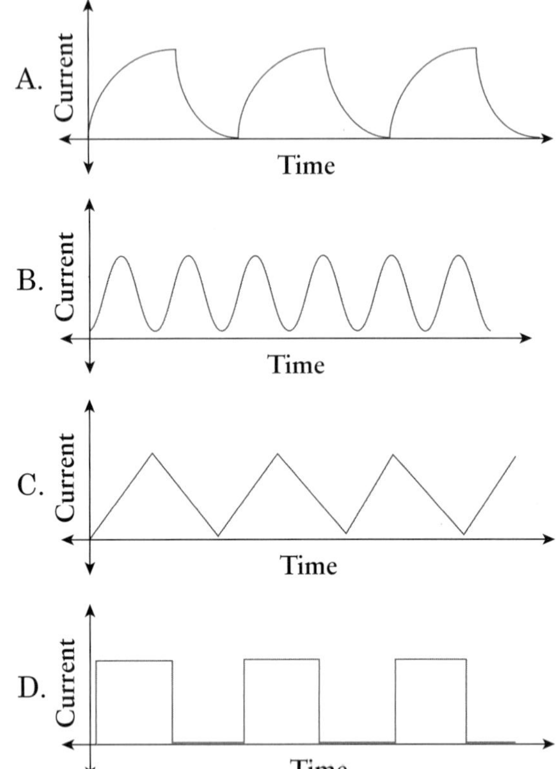

12. The following pairs of plates are made of the same materials. Which pair is likely to store the greatest total charge when fed from the same battery?

A.

B.

C.

D.

13. A certain AC signal is described by the equation $I = (14\ A) \sin (4\pi t)$. What is the approximate root-mean-square (rms) current of the signal?

A. 5 A
B. 7 A
C. 10 A
D. 14 A

14. A newly discovered element readily loses one electron. Which of the following is most likely true about the element's electrical properties?

A. The element is an insulator
B. The element is a conductor
C. The element forms dielectric materials
D. The element has a high resistivity

15. Each of the resistors below carries an individual resistance of 4 Ω. Assuming negligible resistance in the wire, what is the overall resistance of the circuit?

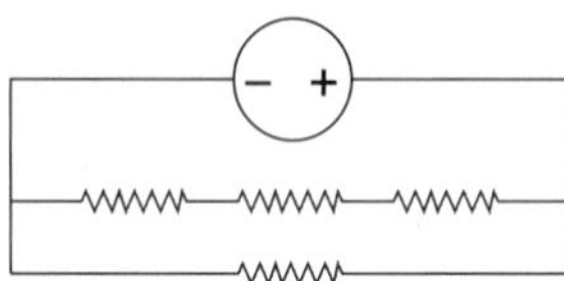

A. 16 Ω
B. 8 Ω
C. 4 Ω
D. 3 Ω

16. A student has an AC circuit with a total resistance of 2 Ω and a current described by the following graph. What is the approximate average value of the current in the circuit?

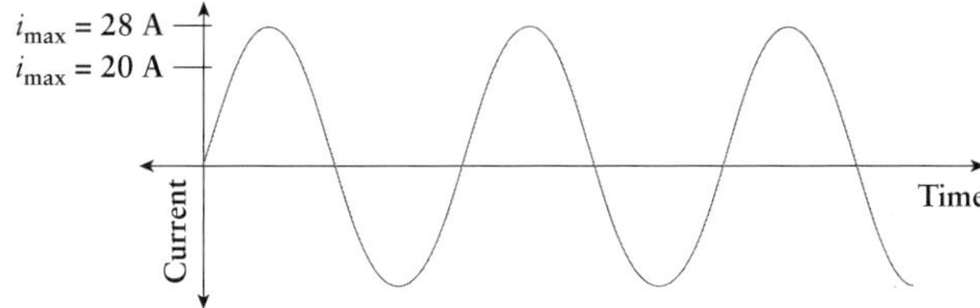

A. 0 A
B. 14 A
C. 20 A
D. 28 A

17. Continuing with the conditions from the previous question, what is the approximate average value of the power dissipated by the circuit?

A. 0 W
B. 400 W
C. 800 W
D. 1,600 W

18. Which of the following solids is likely to have the highest dielectric constant?

A. Copper
B. Aluminum
C. Silicon
D. Iodine

19. In the circuit below, each capacitor has a capacitance of 3 F. What is the maximum amount of charge that the system is capable of storing?

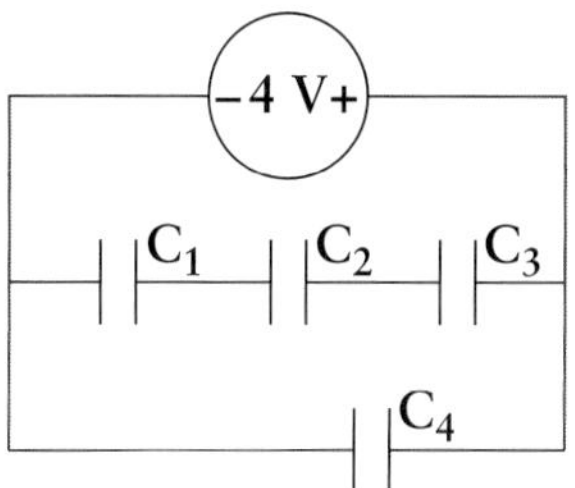

A. 1 C
B. 2.25 C
C. 4 C
D. 16 C

20. Which of the following always remains constant in an AC circuit?

I. Charge per second of time
II. Charge per volt of potential
III. Charge per joule of energy

A. I only
B. II only
C. I and II
D. II and III

CHAPTER 9

PERIODIC MOTION, WAVES, AND SOUND

OSCILLATIONS

Oscillating systems are those that continuously show repetitive movement of some kind. There are many different examples of oscillatory motion in the natural world, from the waves in the ocean to the waves of light that illuminate our world to the waves of sound that literally bring music to our ears. In this chapter, we will first lay the foundation for understanding wave phenomena by reviewing the subject of simple harmonic motion. General properties of waves are then introduced including the concepts of amplitude, wavelength, frequency, wave speed, and resonance. The superposition of two waves is discussed along with the related concepts of constructive versus destructive interference and the production of standing waves, both in strings and open and closed pipes. The subject of sound is reviewed as a subject that is rich in wave-related phenomena, such as beats and the Doppler effect. A brief summary is also given of sound production by musical instruments.

A. SIMPLE HARMONIC MOTION

A very important type of oscillation, or periodic motion, is **simple harmonic motion** (SHM). In SHM, a particle or mass oscillates about an equilibrium point subject to a linear restoring force. A linear restoring force has two characteristics: (i) it is always directed back toward the equilibrium position, and (ii) its magnitude is directly proportional to the displacement from the equilibrium position. By Newton's second law, the particle's acceleration is also proportional to the displacement from equilibrium:

$$F = -kx$$
$$a = -\omega^2 x$$

where the angular frequency ω is given by:

$$\omega = \sqrt{k/m}$$

A mass attached to a spring, and a simple pendulum (provided the angle of swing is not too large) are two examples of simple harmonic oscillators.

MCAT SYNOPSIS

The minus sign in $F = -kx$, means that the restoring force is in the opposite direction to the displacement.

TEACHER TIP

The angular frequency equation tells us the stiffer the spring (the larger the value of k) or the smaller mass attached, the faster the spring will oscillate.

MCAT SYNOPSIS

A larger spring constant, k, means a stronger or stiffer spring.

A stretched or compressed spring exerts a linear restoring force, where the constant k is called the **spring constant** (or force constant), and the equation $F = -kx$ is called **Hooke's law**. k is a measure of the stiffness of the spring. Figure 9.1(a) shows a spring-mass system with the mass at the equilibrium position. Figure 9.1(b) shows the same system with the mass displaced a distance x from the equilibrium position.

For other systems that execute SHM, k may be related to other properties of the system. In the case of a simple pendulum, $k = mg/L$ where m is the mass, and L is the length of the pendulum. Figure 9.1(c) shows a simple pendulum displaced at an angle θ with the vertical.

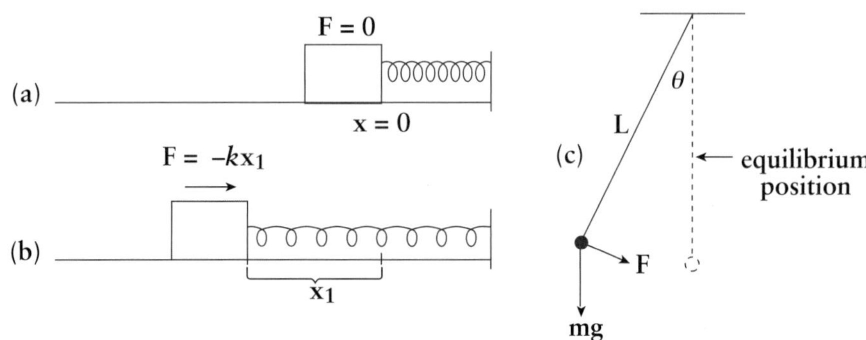

Figure 9.1

MCAT SYNOPSIS

The amplitude is the maximum displacement.

Let X be the particle's amplitude (maximum displacement x from the equilibrium position). Then assuming the particle has a maximum displacement at t = 0, the equation that describes the particle's displacement x is:

$$x = X \cos(\omega t)$$

where t is the time and ω is the angular frequency. ($\omega = 2\pi f = 2\pi/T$, where f is the frequency and T is the period.)

TEACHER TIP

The frequency describes the number of oscillations per second. The period describes how many seconds it takes for one oscillation to occur. These two are inverse to each other.

One final consideration in simple harmonic motion is energy. If the forces are conservative and the system is frictionless, by the conservation of energy:

$$E = K + U = \text{constant}$$

where K is the kinetic energy and U is the potential energy. Kinetic energy for both the mass attached to the spring and the pendulum mass is given by:

$$K = \frac{1}{2}mv^2$$

For the pendulum, the potential energy is the gravitational potential energy (mgh) as it swings up. For the spring, the potential energy is given by:

$$U(\text{spring}) = \frac{1}{2}kx^2$$

When the mass is at the equilibrium position, the potential energy is zero and the kinetic energy is a maximum given by $E = K_{max}$. However, when the oscillation reaches its maximum displacement the mass has zero speed. At this point the kinetic energy is zero and the potential energy is a maximum given by $E = U_{max}$.

The chart below gives important information on both the mass-spring system and the simple pendulum and shows the similarities between them. Note that when talking about a simple pendulum we commonly refer to the angle θ, which it makes with the vertical.

NOTE: Period (T) is the time to complete 1 cycle, frequency (f) is the number of cycles completed in 1 second, and angular frequency $\omega = 2\pi f = 2\pi/T$. In SHM the frequency and period are independent of the amplitude.

	mass-spring	simple pendulum
force constant k	spring constant k	mg/L
period T	$2\pi\sqrt{m/k}$	$2\pi\sqrt{L/g}$
ang. freq. ω	$\sqrt{k/m}$	$\sqrt{g/L}$
frequency f	1/T or ω/2π	1/T or ω/2π
kinetic energy K	$\frac{1}{2}mv^2$	$\frac{1}{2}mv^2$
K_{max} occurs at	x = 0	θ = 0 (vertical position)
potential energy U	$\frac{1}{2}kx^2$	mgh
U_{max} occurs at	x = ±X	max value of θ
max acceleration at	x = ±X	max value of θ

Example: What is the length of a pendulum that has a period of one second?

Solution: Using our equation for the period of a simple pendulum we can find the length:

$$T = 2\pi\sqrt{L/g}$$
$$L = T^2g/4\pi^2$$
$$= g/4\pi^2$$
$$= 0.25 \text{ m}$$

MCAT SYNOPSIS

For a pendulum, potential energy is mgh where h is the height above the lowest point.

MCAT SYNOPSIS

Potential energy is zero and kinetic energy is maximum at the equilibrium point. Potential energy is maximum and kinetic energy is zero at the points of maximum displacement.

TEACHER TIP

Notice how there are only two factors that affect frequency in both situations. In springs it is mass and spring constant. In pendulums it is gravity and the length of the pendulum.

This means that on a swing set, every person will swing at exactly the same frequency, as long as the length of the swing is the same, regardless of how large his amplitude. Other than changing the length, the only other way to change frequency is by changing gravity, something that can be simulated by accelerating either up or down on an elevator. Remember that if you are going upward but slowing down, it means that you're accelerating in the downward direction.

MCAT SYNOPSIS

Maximum acceleration occurs where there is maximum force, and maximum force occurs at maximum displacement ($F = kx$). At equilibrium there is no force on the object, thus it has no acceleration.

TEACHER TIP

Angular frequency is measured in radians: one full rotation equals 2ð radians or 360°.

B. UNIFORM CIRCULAR MOTION AND SHM

Consider a particle moving around a circular path at constant angular frequency ω. If the path were projected onto a line adjacent to the circle (Figure 9.2), it is obvious that the particle is oscillating back and forth between +X and –X and obeying the laws of SHM. This fact helps give some insight as to where the idea of angular frequency comes from.

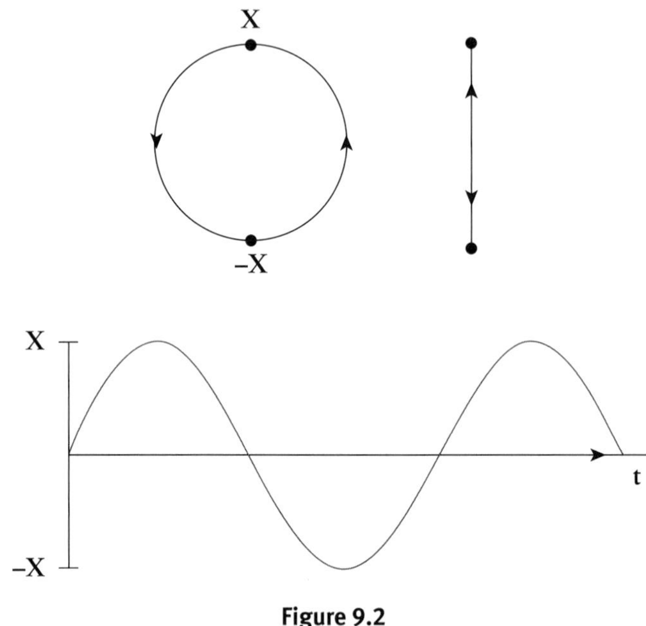

Figure 9.2

TEACHER TIP

Most waves we see are transverse waves (even "the wave" at sporting events is a transverse wave). The only longitudinal waves we're likely to see are sound waves.

GENERAL WAVE CHARACTERISTICS

A. TRANSVERSE AND LONGITUDINAL WAVES

MCAT SYNOPSIS

When a sinusoidal wave propagates through a medium, the particles in the medium oscillate back and forth, like masses on springs.

This chapter will be primarily concerned with sinusoidal waves. In such waves the individual particles oscillate back and forth with simple harmonic motion. In the case of **transverse waves** the particles oscillate perpendicular to the direction of the wave motion as shown in Figure 9.3(a). The oscillating string elements are moving at right angles to the direction of travel of the wave. In the case of **longitudinal waves** the particles oscillate along the direction of the wave motion, and this is illustrated in Figure 9.3(b). In this case, the longitudinal wave created by the person moving the piston back and forth consists of oscillating air molecules that move parallel to the direction of motion of the wave.

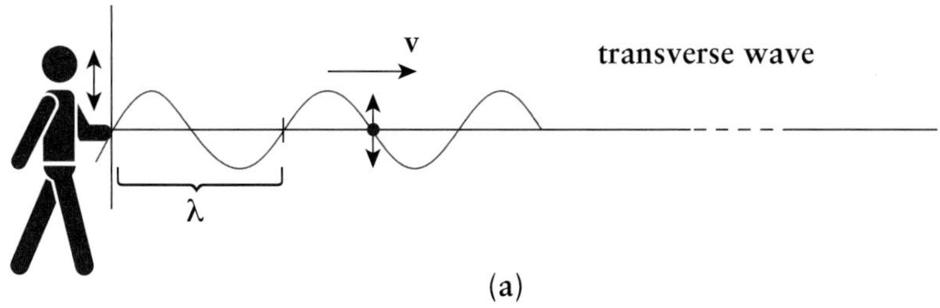

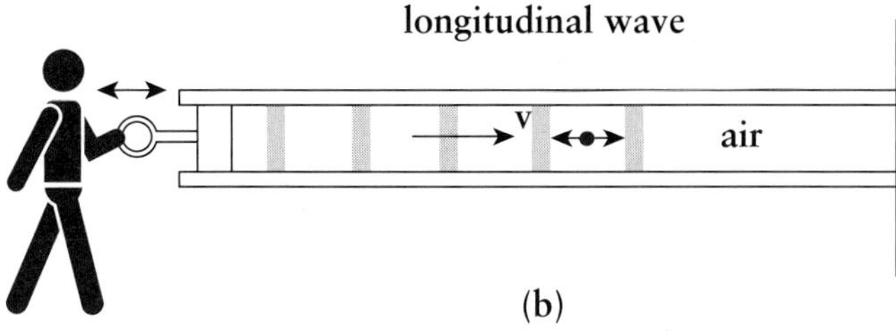

Figure 9.3

B. DESCRIBING WAVES

The displacement y of a particle may be plotted at each point x along the direction of the wave's motion. It is given mathematically by:

$$y = Y \sin (kx - \omega t)$$

where Y is the amplitude (maximum displacement), k is the wave number (not to be mistaken with the *k* of Hooke's law), ω is the angular frequency, and t is the time.

The distance from one maximum (crest) of the wave to the next is the wavelength λ. The frequency f is the number of wavelengths passing a fixed point per second (cycles per second (cps) or hertz (Hz)). The speed of the wave v is related to the frequency and wavelength by the very important equation:

$$v = f\lambda$$

The following relations define k and ω:

$$k = \frac{2\pi}{\lambda}$$

$$\omega = 2\pi f = \frac{2\pi}{T}$$

MCAT SYNOPSIS

The maximum displacement or amplitude is Y, because the maximum of the sin function is 1.

TEACHER TIP

As long as velocity remains constant, frequency and wavelength are inverse to each other. A large wavelength will have a small frequency and a small wavelength will have a large frequency.

MCAT FAVORITE

Frequency and period are reciprocals of one another:

$f = 1/T$, $T = 1/f$.

where the period T is the time for the wave to move one wavelength ($f = 1/T$). The following relationships for the velocity of the wave follow from the above definitions:

$$v = f\lambda = \frac{\omega}{k} = \frac{\lambda}{T}$$

TEACHER TIP

It is the differences in phase that result in interference. If the two waves have different but similar frequencies, they will periodically go in and out of phase, resulting in "beats."

Example: If a wave on a string were described by the equation $y = (0.01) \sin (2x - 10t)$, find the frequency, wavelength, and speed of the wave. (Assume units of meters and seconds.)

Solution: Everything that is needed to find the frequency, wavelength, and speed is given in the wave's equation, $y = Y \sin (kx - \omega t) = (0.01) \sin (2x - 10t)$. Remembering that frequency is given by $f = 1/T$ and that $T = 2\pi/\omega$:

$$\begin{aligned} f &= \omega/2\pi \\ &= 5/\pi \\ &= 1.59 \text{ Hz} \end{aligned}$$

The wavelength is given by:

$$\begin{aligned} \lambda &= 2\pi/k \\ &= 2\pi/2 \\ &= \pi \\ &= 3.14 \text{ m} \end{aligned}$$

and the speed:

$$\begin{aligned} v &= f\lambda \\ &= (5/\pi)\pi \\ &= 5 \text{ m/s} \end{aligned}$$

MCAT SYNOPSIS

A phase difference between two waves means that the crests (or troughs) don't occur at the same points in space.

C. PHASE

When comparing two waves, we often speak about a **phase difference.** This phase difference describes how "in step" two waves are with each other. Let's take two separate waves that have the same frequency, amplitude, and wavelength. If the waves are perfectly in phase, the maxima and minima of each wave coincide, i.e., they occur at the same point. In this case, the phase difference is zero. However, if the two waves are out of phase, then one wave is shifted with respect to the other by some definite fraction of a cycle. This phase difference is usually expressed as an angle. In Figure 9.4(a), waves y_1 and y_2 are nearly in phase; their phase difference is approximately 0°. In Figure 9.4(b), wave y_2 is shifted nearly one-half wavelength with respect to y_1. The phase difference in this case is almost 180°.

MCAT SYNOPSIS

When two waves are in phase and interfere, the resultant amplitude is the sum of the two separate amplitudes.

D. PRINCIPLE OF SUPERPOSITION

The principle of superposition states simply that when waves interact with each other the result is a sum of the waves. When the waves are in phase, the amplitudes add together **(constructive interference),** but when waves are 180° out of phase, the resultant amplitude is the difference between interacting amplitudes **(destructive interference).** Figures 9.4(a) and (b) show the interference between two waves when they are nearly in phase and when they are nearly 180° out of phase.

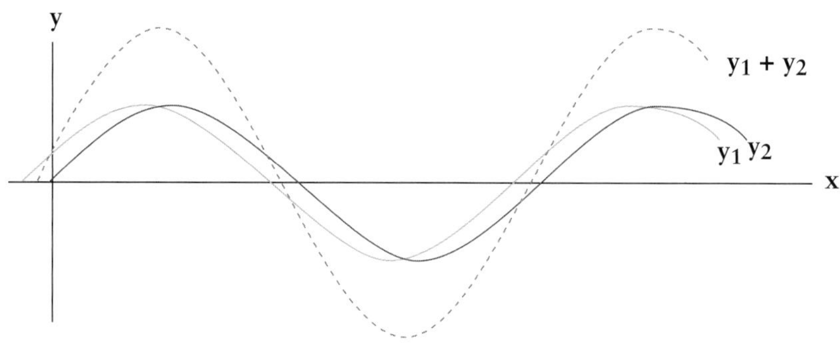

Figure 9.4(a)

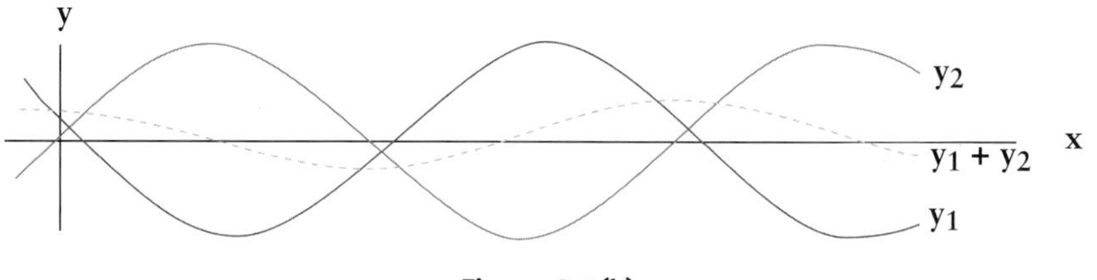

Figure 9.4(b)

TEACHER TIP

If the two waves were exactly 180° out of phase, then the resultant wave would have zero amplitude; thus, there would be no wave.

E. TRAVELING AND STANDING WAVES

If a string fixed at one end is moved from side to side, it is seen that a wave travels or propagates down the string. Such a wave is known as a **traveling wave.** When the wave reaches the fixed boundary it is reflected and inverted (see Figure 9.5). If the free end of the string is continuously moved from side to side, there will then be two waves: the original wave moving down the string and the reflected wave moving the other way. These waves will then interfere with each other.

MCAT SYNOPSIS

Standing waves occur because of the interference of two or more waves.

MCAT SYNOPSIS

Nodes are points where the displacement is always zero.

Antinodes are points where the displacement oscillates between a crest and a trough with the same frequency as the wave frequency.

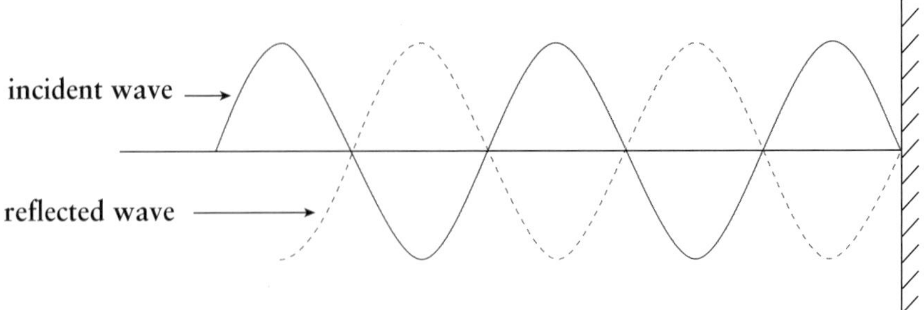

Figure 9.5

TEACHER TIP

Put this into practice. Get a rope, have one person hold one end still and another person shake the free end. By manipulating the frequency of the shaking, standing waves of varying wavelength can be seen.

Consider now the case when both ends of the string are fixed and traveling waves are excited in the string. Certain wave frequencies can result in a waveform remaining in a stationary position, while the amplitude fluctuates. These waves are known as **standing waves.** Points in the wave that remain at rest are known as **nodes,** and points that are midway between these nodes are known as **antinodes.** Antinodes are points that fluctuate with maximum amplitude.

It is also possible to set up standing waves in pipes in much the same way as in a string. Standing waves in strings and pipes are discussed in more detail later in this chapter.

MCAT SYNOPSIS

The resonance frequency of a pendulum is just the natural frequency $f = \frac{1}{2\pi}\sqrt{g/L}$.

The resonance frequency of a mass on a spring is $f = \frac{1}{2\pi}\sqrt{k/m}$.

F. RESONANCE

In any oscillatory system there will be one or more **natural frequencies** (normal modes) of vibration; that is to say that the system will oscillate at one of these natural frequencies if there are no external forces involved (in the case of the free-swinging pendulum there is only one natural frequency, whereas a stretched string will have an infinite number of natural frequencies).

TEACHER TIP

It may sound strange that a pendulum has a resonant frequency, but if you've ever pushed someone on a swing, you've experienced it for yourself. The best results for pushing someone on a swing are obtained when you push with the same tempo at which the swing is already moving. By pushing faster or slower you actually end up slowing the swing down. The natural tempo at which the swing is moving is the resonant frequency, and when you push at that frequency, maximum amplitude is obtained.

If a periodically varying force is applied to the system, the system will then be driven at a frequency equal to the frequency of the force. This is known as a **forced oscillation.** The amplitude of this motion will generally be small. However, if the frequency of the applied force is close to that of the natural frequency of the system, then the amplitude becomes much larger.

If the frequency of the periodically varying force is equal to a natural frequency of the system, then the system is said to be **resonating,** and the amplitude of the oscillation is a maximum. If the oscillating system were frictionless, then the periodically varying force would continually add energy to the system, and the amplitude would increase indefinitely. However, because no system is completely frictionless, there is always some damping that results in a finite amplitude of oscillation.

SOUND

Sound is transmitted by oscillation of particles along the direction of motion of the sound wave. It is therefore a longitudinal wave. More generally, sound is a mechanical disturbance propagated through a deformable medium, and so it can be transmitted through solids, liquids, and gases, but *not* through a vacuum. The relative speed of sound in a medium is determined by the spacing of adjacent particles. The smaller the spacing between the particles, the faster sound will travel in that medium. For this reason, sound travels faster in a solid than in a liquid, and faster in a liquid than in a gas.

MCAT SYNOPSIS

Sound propagates through liquids, solids, and gases, but NOT through a vacuum (empty space).

This section will be primarily concerned with waves that, when they strike the ear, produce the sensation we call sound. For humans, such waves are called **audible waves** and have frequencies ranging from 20 Hz to 20,000 Hz. Waves whose frequencies are below 20 Hz are called **infrasonic waves,** and those whose frequencies are above 20,000 Hz are called **ultrasonic waves.** For sound waves in air at 0°C, the speed of sound is 331 m/s.

A. CHARACTERISTICS OF SOUND

Intensity is defined as the average rate per unit area at which energy is transported across a perpendicular surface by the wave. In other words, the intensity is the power transported per unit area. In SI it has units of W/m^2. The amplitude of the sound wave is a measure of its energy. The total power P carried across a surface area (such as an eardrum) equals the product of the intensity I and the surface area A, when the intensity is uniformly distributed. Mathematically, one can write:

MCAT SYNOPSIS

Intensity is always power/area and is simply energy per unit time per unit area.

$$P = IA$$

The **sound level**, β, is measured in decibels and is defined as:

$$\beta = 10 \log \frac{I}{I_0}$$

where I_0 is a reference intensity of 10^{-12} W/m^2, corresponding to the faintest sound that can be heard by humans.

TEACHER TIP

We use logarithms with scales that have an extremely large range but on the exam you will see primarily logs with a base of 10. For instance, the log10 of 1,000 equals 3 because 10 to the power of three equals 1000; the log10 of 1 equals 0 because 10 (and every other number) to the power of 0 equals 1.

Example: A detector with a surface area of 1 square meter is placed 1 meter from an operating jackhammer. It measures the power of the jackhammer's sound to be 10^{-3} W. Find:

a. the intensity and the sound level of the jackhammer.
b. the ratio of the intensities of the jackhammer and a jet engine (assume β_{jet} = 130 dB).

Solution: a. Intensity is equal to power divided by area.

$$I = \frac{P}{A} = \frac{10^{-3}}{1} = 10^{-3} \text{ W/m}^2$$

The sound level is given by:

$$\beta = 10 \log \frac{I}{I_0} = 10 \log\left(\frac{10^{-3}}{10^{-12}}\right) = 10 \log 10^9 = 90 \text{ dB}$$

b. The ratio of 2 intensities of sound can be found from the difference of their sound levels:

$$\beta_{jet} - \beta_{jack} = 10 \log\left(\frac{I_{jet}}{I_{jack}}\right)$$

$$130 - 90 = 10 \log\left(\frac{I_{jet}}{I_{jack}}\right)$$

$$4 = \log\left(\frac{I_{jet}}{I_{jack}}\right)$$

$$10{,}000 = \left(\frac{I_{jet}}{I_{jack}}\right)$$

Thus the jet engine's sound is 10,000 times more intense than the jackhammer's.

Another characteristic of sound is **pitch.** This refers to the sensation of sound that enables one to classify the frequency of a note.

TEACHER TIP

To get rid of a log on one side of the equation, raise the entirety of each side of the equation as the exponent over 10. The log cancels out on one side of the equation and the other side is changed into 104.

B. PRODUCTION OF SOUND

For sound to be produced, there must be a longitudinal oscillation of air molecules. This oscillation can be produced by the vibration of a solid object that sets adjacent air molecules into motion, or by means of an acoustic vibration in an enclosed space.

MCAT SYNOPSIS

The frequency of sound produced by a guitar string, violin string, or piano string is the frequency of vibration of the string.

Sound produced by the vibration of a solid object includes sound that is created by string and percussion instruments such as the guitar, violin, and piano. In this case, a string or several strings are set into motion and vibrate at their normal mode frequencies. Because the strings are very thin, it makes them ineffective in transmitting their vibration to the surrounding air. For this reason a solid body is employed to provide a better coupling to the air. In the case of a guitar, the vibration is transmitted through the bridge to the body of the instrument, which vibrates at the same frequency as the string.

Sound created by acoustic vibration includes sound from instruments such as organ pipes, the flute, and the recorder. There are no moving parts, and sound is produced by a vibrating motion of air within the instrument. In the case of an organ pipe, the pitch is determined by the length of the pipe. However, instruments such as the recorder and the flute are able to generate more than one pitch by the opening and closing of holes.

In the case of the human voice, sound is created by passing air between the vocal cords. The pitch is controlled by varying the tension of the cords. This is very similar to the production of sound in wind instruments such as the oboe and the clarinet, but these use a reed instead of vocal cords. Pitch in this case is controlled both by the opening and closing of holes and by varying the tension across the reed.

C. BEATS

Beats are heard when two waves that have nearly equal frequencies are superimposed. By the principle of superposition, the two waves add together, and what results is a periodic variation in loudness called beats. The beat frequency is:

TEACHER TIP

These beats can be heard as periodic increases in loudness when an orchestra is tuning.

$$f_{beat} = f_1 - f_2$$

Example: Two tuning forks are sounded. One has a frequency of 250 Hz while the other has a frequency of 245 Hz. What is the frequency of the beats?

Solution: The frequency of the beats is the difference of the frequencies of the interacting waves:

$$f_{beat} = f_1 - f_2 = 250 - 245 = 5 \text{ Hz}$$

D. DOPPLER EFFECT

A qualitative description of the **Doppler effect** is that when a source emitting sound and the detector of that sound are moving relative to each other along the line joining them, the perceived frequency of the sound received f′ differs from the actual frequency emitted f. If the source and detector are moving toward each other, the observed frequency increases, and if the source and detector are moving away from each other, the observed frequency decreases. This can be seen from the following equation:

$$f' = f\frac{(v \pm V_D)}{(v \pm V_S)}$$

where v is the speed of sound in the medium, V_D is the speed of the detector relative to the medium, and V_S is the speed of the source relative to the medium. The upper sign on V_D (V_S) is used when the detector (source) moves toward the source (detector), while the lower sign is used when it moves away.

Example: The siren of a police car cruising at 144 km/hr is sounding while the car is in pursuit of a speeding motorist. Assume that the speed of sound is 330 m/s. The siren emits sound at a frequency of 1450 Hz. What is the frequency heard by a stationary observer when:

a. the police car is moving towards the observer?
b. the police car has passed the observer?

Solution: a. To do this problem the speed of the police car must first be converted to m/s.

$$\frac{144 \text{ km}}{\text{hr}} \cdot \frac{10^3 \text{m}}{\text{km}} \cdot \frac{\text{hr}}{3{,}600 \text{ s}} = 40 \text{ m/s}$$

Because the police car is moving toward the stationary observer, the denominator is $v - V_S$, and the numerator is simply v (since $V_D = 0$). This gives:

TEACHER TIP

The easiest way to approach this equation is to approach the detector and the source separately. Note that either one moving toward the other will increase the frequency, so you want to see if each object is working toward increasing or decreasing the frequency. Because the detector is in the numerator, if it is working to increase the frequency then we will add, making a larger number. Because the source is in the denominator, if it is working to increase the frequency then we will subtract, resulting in a larger number after dividing.

TEACHER TIP

The Doppler effect works with any waves, including light. This means that if a source of light is moving toward a detector, the observed frequency will increase "blue shift." If the source is moving away from a detector, the frequency will decrease "red shift." (The electromagnetic spectrum will be further discussed in chapter 10). It is for this reason that scientists believe the universe is expanding. Observing any distant galaxy, we can see that every single one is red shifted, meaning that every single galaxy is moving away from our own. In addition, the further away the galaxy, the more red shifted it is. This indicates not that we're at the center of an expanding universe, but rather that the space itself between every galaxy is itself expanding.

MCAT SYNOPSIS

When the source and observer are moving with the same speed and in the same direction, there is no frequency shift.

$$f' = f\frac{v}{v - V_s}$$

$$= \frac{1,450(330)}{330 - 40}$$

$$= 1,650 \text{ Hz}$$

b. In this part of the question the police car is now moving away from the observer, so the denominator is $v + V_S$. The numerator remains unchanged because the observer is still stationary.

$$f' = f\frac{v}{v + V_s}$$

$$= \frac{1,450(330)}{330 + 40}$$

$$= 1,293 \text{ Hz}$$

This example shows precisely why the pitch of a siren changes when an ambulance or police car passes you on the street. In this case, when the police car is moving toward the observer the perceived frequency is 1,650 Hz, whereas when the car has passed the observer the perceived frequency has decreased to 1,293 Hz.

MCAT SYNOPSIS

The first harmonic or fundamental is n = 1. The mth harmonic is n = m.

E. STANDING WAVES

1. Strings

Consider a string fixed rigidly at both ends. Because the string is fixed at both ends, each end must be a node (a point in a wave that remains at rest). This implies that if the string is to support a standing wave, the string's length L must be equal to some integer multiple of half a wavelength (e.g., $\lambda/2$, $2\lambda/2$, $3\lambda/2$, and so on). This string will be able to support standing waves with wavelengths:

$$\lambda = 2L, \frac{2L}{2}, \frac{2L}{3}, \ldots \frac{2L}{n} \qquad (n = 1, 2, 3, \ldots)$$

From the relationship that f = v/l, where v is the speed of the wave, the possible frequencies are:

$$f = \frac{v}{2L}, \frac{2v}{2L}, \frac{3v}{2L} \ldots = \frac{nv}{2L} \qquad (n = 1, 2, 3, \ldots)$$

MCAT SYNOPSIS

Higher harmonics have shorter wavelengths and higher frequencies, but the same wave speed.

MCAT SYNOPSIS

For the nth harmonic on a string, n half wavelengths exactly fit along the length of the string.

TEACHER TIP

For strings attached at both ends, the number of antinodes present will indicate which harmonic is present.

The lowest frequency that the string can support is given by v/2L and is known as the **fundamental frequency (first harmonic).** The frequency given by n = 2 is known as the first overtone (second harmonic) and so on. All the possible frequencies that the string can support are said to form a **harmonic series.** The waveforms of the first three harmonics are shown in Figure 9.6 below. (Note: N stands for node and A for antinode.)

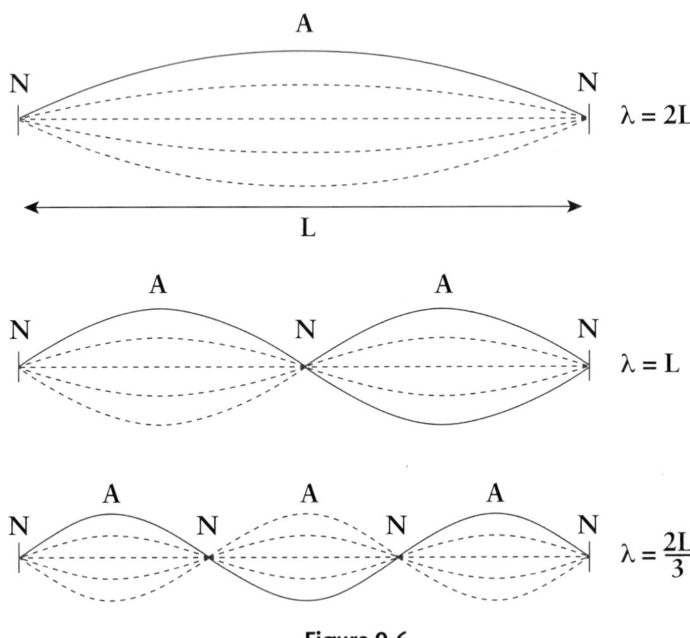

Figure 9.6

MCAT SYNOPSIS

Just as for strings, the higher harmonics in pipes (open and closed) have higher frequency, shorter wavelengths, and the same wave speed.

2. Pipes

Whereas strings are typically fixed at both ends, pipes may be open or closed at each end. In pipes the standing waves (if they occur) are sound waves originating in the air column. A closed end of a pipe corresponds to a fixed end of a string, and if standing waves occur a node will be at a closed end. On the other hand, at an open end of a pipe there will be an antinode. One end of the pipe will typically be open to allow air to enter. The pipe is then called open or closed depending on whether the other end is open or closed. The rules for the wavelengths and frequencies of the possible standing waves in a pipe of length L depend on whether the pipe is open (both ends are open) or closed (one end is open and the other end is closed).

Open pipes

An open pipe supports standing waves with antinodes at both ends. It is more difficult to illustrate the standing wave patterns in a pipe, because a sound wave is longitudinal. However, Figure 9.7 gives a symbolic representation, and it can be seen that this produces the same rule as for the string:

$$\lambda = \frac{2L}{n} \qquad (n = 1, 2, 3, \ldots)$$

$$f = \frac{nv}{2L} \qquad (n = 1, 2, 3, \ldots)$$

where v is the speed of the waves.

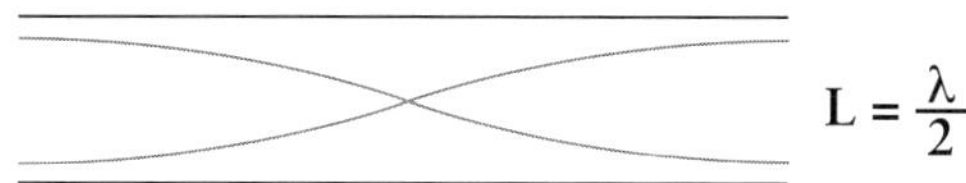
$L = \frac{\lambda}{2}$

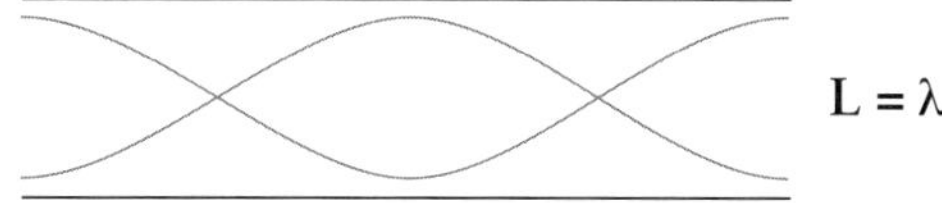
$L = \lambda$

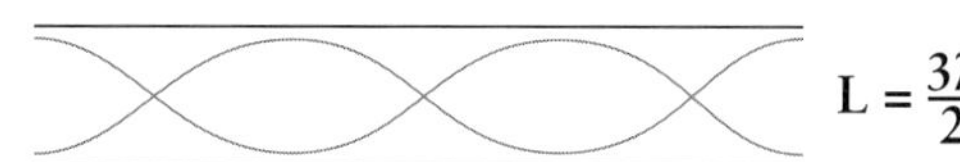
$L = \frac{3\lambda}{2}$

Figure 9.7

TEACHER TIP

For pipes with two open ends, the number of nodes present will indicate which harmonic is present.

Closed pipes

In the case of a pipe open at one end but closed at the other, there is a node at the closed end. As in the case of the open pipe, the open end has an antinode. A symbolic representation of the standing wave patterns for a closed pipe is shown in Figure 9.8.

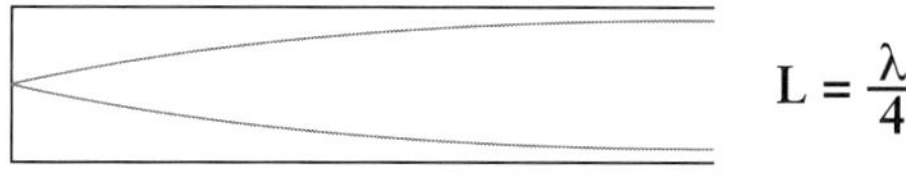
$L = \frac{\lambda}{4}$

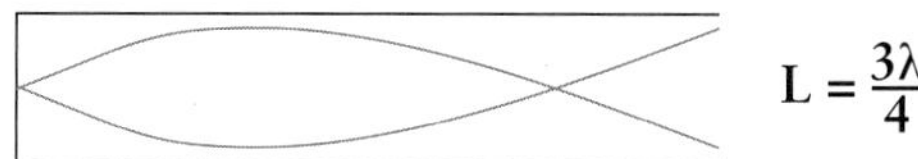
$L = \frac{3\lambda}{4}$

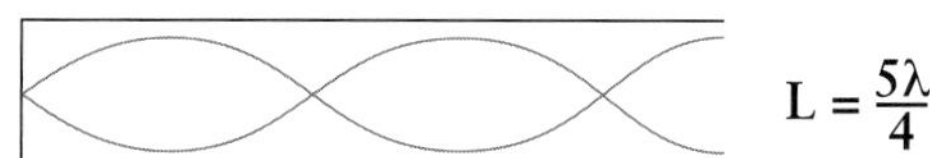
$L = \frac{5\lambda}{4}$

Figure 9.8

TEACHER TIP

Finding the harmonic for pipes with one open end works in the same manner as pipes with two open ends, with one important difference. Because the pipe only has one open end, the sound must go through the pipe, bounce off the wall, and go out again. Each sound wave, as a result, will travel double the length of the pipe. This is why the equations for these pipes have four in the denominator instead of two. By counting the number of nodes through which the sound wave passes (accounting for both passes), you'll know which harmonic is present.

It can be seen that in this case, because the wave goes from a node to an antinode, the length of the pipe needed to produce the fundamental frequency needs to be a quarter-wavelength long. The first overtone occurs when the pipe is 3/4λ; the next at 5/4λ; and so on. This can be represented by the general expression:

$$\lambda = \frac{4L}{n} \qquad (n = 1, 3, 5, \ldots \text{odd integers only})$$

$$f = \frac{nv}{4L} \qquad (n = 1, 3, 5, \ldots \text{odd integers only})$$

PRACTICE QUESTIONS

1. In simple harmonic motion, if the spring constant k is doubled and the mass is tripled, the angular frequency is

A. 2/3 of its original value.
B. $\sqrt{(2/3)}$ of its original value.
C. $\sqrt{(3/2)}$ of its original value.
D. 3/2 of its original value.

2. The figure below has mass m on a pendulum oscillating under simple harmonic motion. A student wants to double the period of the system. He can do this by which of the following?

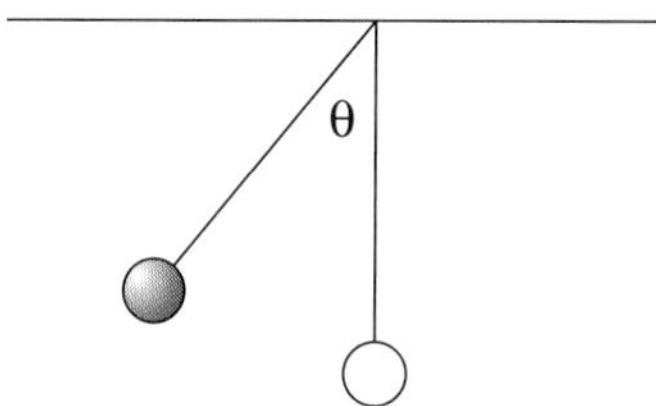

I. Increasing the mass
II. Dropping the mass from a higher height
III. Increasing the length of the string

A. I only
B. III only
C. II and III only
D. I and III only

3. A student plans to launch a 50 g ball vertically from a spring. After compressing the spring (k = 5 N/m) to a vertical length that is 2 meters shorter than its original length, he releases it and records the height of the ball's trajectory. He then decides that he wants the ball to fly up twice as high (figure below). He can do this by

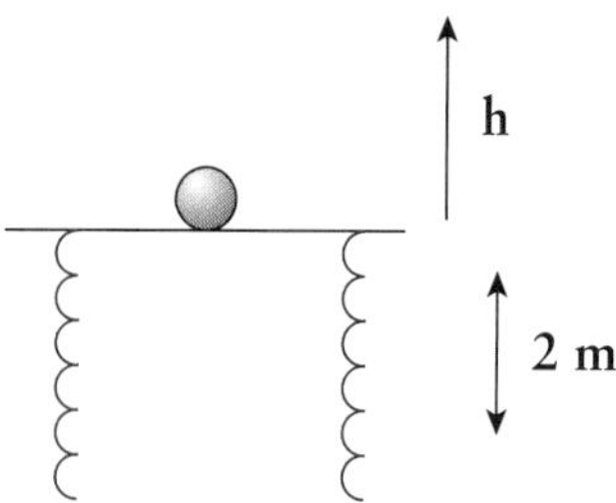

A. doubling the mass of the ball and halving the compression of the spring.
B. doubling the mass of the ball and halving the spring constant.
C. halving the spring constant and doubling the compression of the spring.
D. halving the mass of the ball and doubling the spring constant.

4. What is the frequency of a pendulum with a length of 2 meters?

A. 0.3 s^{-1}
B. 1 s^{-1}
C. 3 s^{-1}
D. 10 s^{-1}

5. As an officer approaches a student who is studying with his radio playing loudly beside him, he experiences the Doppler effect. Which of the following statements remains true as the officer moves closer to the student?

I. The apparent frequency of the music increases.
II. The exactly same effect will be produced if the officer were stationary and the student approached him.
III. The apparent velocity of the waves increases.

A. I only
B. II only
C. I and III only
D. I, II, and III

6. A police car's siren emits a wave with a frequency of 60 Hz. If the speed of sound is 300 m/s and the car is moving at 50 m/s, what is the approximate wavelength of the wave behind the car?

A. 4.3 m
B. 5 m
C. 6 m
D. 10 m

7. A student fixes one end of a string to a hook and vibrates the other end vertically. As the student vibrates the string, the

A. wave travels up and down and the string displacement points left and right.
B. wave travels left to right and the string displacement points up and down.
C. wave travels up and down and the string displacement points up and down.
D. wave travels left to right and the string displacement points left to right.

8. A guitar player is playing the third harmonic of a string, whose frequency he measures to be 600 Hz. If he adjusts the guitar string and plays the first harmonic with a frequency of 600 Hz, the string's length is now

A. 1/3 times the original length.
B. three times the original length.
C. 2/3 times the original length.
D. 3/2 times the original length.

9. A physicist generates the fundamental harmonic in a tube that is open on both ends. He now wants to generate the fourth harmonic. Which of the following should he expect in the new sound wave while he calibrates his equipment?

I. Increased frequency
II. Decreased velocity
III. More antinodes

A. I only
B. I and II only
C. I and III only
D. I, II, and III

10. A seesaw attached to a machine undergoes simple harmonic motion. The frequency is measured as 5 Hz and the amplitude is 2 cm (see figure). How long does it take the see-saw to travel from x = 0 to x = –2cm?

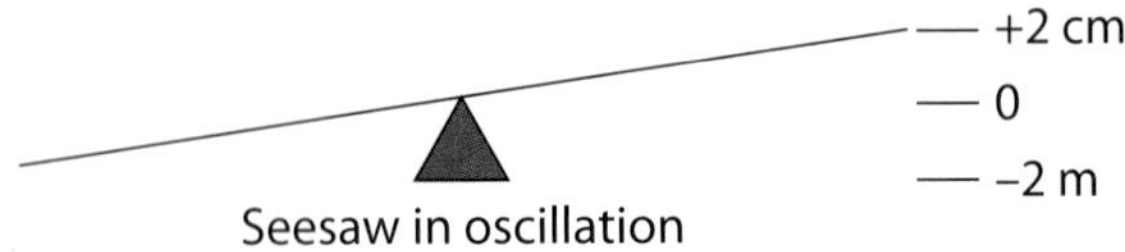

Seesaw in oscillation

A. 0.1 seconds
B. 0.5 seconds
C. 2 seconds
D. 4 seconds

11. A sound detector with a surface area of 5 m^2 measures the power of a stereo to be 10^{-4} W at a distance of 4 m. What is the intensity of the radio?

A. 2.5×10^{-5} W/m^2
B. 1.25×10^{-5} W/m^2
C. 4×10^{4} W/m^2
D. 1.6×10^{5} W/m^2

12. The frequency of tuning fork A is 450 Hz, while the frequency of tuning fork B is unknown. If the two forks are struck simultaneously, wavering sound is observed five times per second. The frequency of the unknown tuning fork is

A. 440 Hz, assuming it has a higher pitch than the 450 Hz tuning fork.
B. 445 Hz, assuming it has a lower pitch than the 450 Hz tuning fork.
C. 450 Hz, assuming it has a higher pitch than the 450 Hz tuning fork.
D. 455 Hz, assuming it has a lower pitch than the 450 Hz tuning fork.

13. Two speakers emit in-phase waves. A point *P* exists whose distance from the first speaker is $\lambda/2$ wavelengths longer than its distance from the second speaker. The two speakers will produce

A. constructive interference because the two sound waves are in phase.
B. destructive interference because the two sound waves are in phase.
C. destructive interference because the difference between their wavelengths is not a whole integer.
D. constructive interference because the difference between their wavelengths is not a whole integer.

14. A child is playing with a wire whose two ends are A and B. She flicks end A vertically, generating an upright transverse wave, which travels to the other end. Which of the following is true?

A. The wave is reflected right-side up if end B is free.
B. The wave is reflected right-side up if end B is fixed.
C. The wave is absorbed and no wave will be reflected back, regardless of whether end B is fixed or not.
D. The wave will be reflected upright, regardless of whether end B is fixed or not.

15. Given the two waves below, which of the following statements is true? Assume all units are the same between the waves.

$$X_1 = 2 \times \text{Cos}(5t - \pi)$$
$$X_2 = 5 \times \text{Cos}(3t + \pi/2)$$

A. The first wave has a greater period than the second wave and its y-intercept is below the second wave's y-intercept.
B. The first wave has a smaller frequency than the second wave has and its y-intercept is below the second wave's y-intercept.
C. The first wave has a smaller frequency than the second wave has and its y-intercept is above the second wave's y-intercept
D. The first wave has a smaller period than the second wave has and its y-intercept is above the second wave's y-intercept.

16. Two sine waves approach each other as shown below. They intersect at the midpoint of the rope, point M, and continue through the rope. If the rope were cut in half and the experiment were reproduced, then

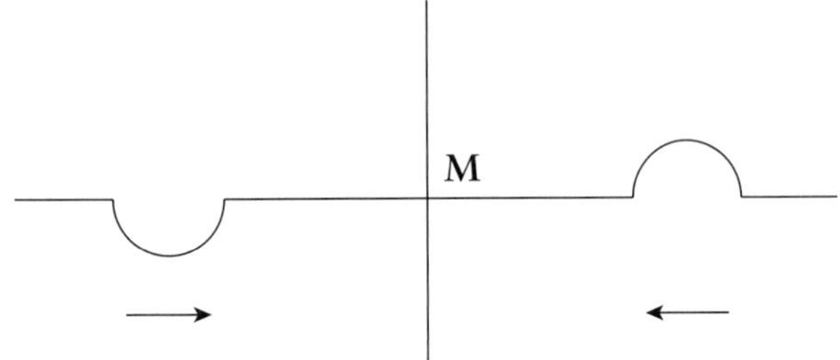

A. the inverted wave would come back from point M inverted, regardless of whether point M is fixed or not.
B. the inverted wave would come back from point M right-side up, as if it were attached to a fixed ring.
C. the inverted wave would come back from point M inverted, as if it were attached to a fixed ring.
D. Not enough information is given about the physical properties of the rope.

17. If the frequency of a pendulum is four times greater on an unknown planet than it is on Earth, then the gravitational constant on that planet is

A. 16 times greater.
B. 4 times greater.
C. 4 times lower.
D. 16 times lower.

18. A young physicist is using his computer for a simple harmonic motion experiment. The values from the computer tell him that the spring constant is 10 N/m, the amplitude of the wave is 3 cm, and the mass of the traveling object is 100 grams. Which of the following equations could describe the position of the wave with respect to time?

A. $x(t) = 3 \times \cos(7t + \pi)$
B. $x(t) = 0.03 \times \sin(10t)$
C. $x(t) = 0.03 \times \cos(10t - \pi)$
D. $x(t) = 0.03 \times \cos(3t)$

ENERGY AND SPRINGS

A block of mass 2 kg falls from a height of 3 meters onto a spring, and the spring reaches a maximum compression of 20 cm. What is the spring constant for this spring? When the block bounces off of the spring, how fast is it going?

1) Write an expression for the initial energy of the system.

$E_i = mg(h + x)$

The initial energy of the system is the gravitational potential energy of the block at a height of 3 meters. However, recognize that the block will fall 3 meters, plus an additional distance due to the spring compressing. Let $h = 3$ meters and $x =$ the compression of the spring. By doing so, we are saying that the gravitational potential energy of the system is 0 when the spring is fully compressed.

Remember: *You can set the potential energy to be zero at whatever point is most convenient, but you must be consistent through the entire problem.*

---

2) Write an expression for the final energy of the system.

☞ spring $U = \frac{1}{2}kx^2$

$\rightarrow E_f = \frac{1}{2}kx^2$

When a spring is stretched or compressed, potential energy is stored in the spring. This energy is given by the formula: $U = \frac{1}{2}kx^2$. As we saw in step 1, there is no gravitational potential energy at this point.

---

3) Set the final energy equal to the initial energy and solve for *k*.

$mg(h + x) = \frac{1}{2}kx^2$

$mgh + mgx = \frac{1}{2}kx^2$

$(2)(9.8)(3) + 2(9.8)(0.2) = \frac{1}{2}(k)(0.2)^2$

$58.8 + 3.92 = 0.02k$

$k = 3{,}136$ N/m

Due to the conservation of energy, we can set the total energy of the system at any two points equal to each other. Set the initial energy equal to the final energy and solve for *k*.

KEY CONCEPTS

Conservation of energy

Springs

Gravitational potential energy: $U = mgh$ (J)

Spring potential energy: $U = \frac{1}{2}kx^2$ (J)

Kinetic energy $KE = \frac{1}{2}mv^2$ (J)

TAKEAWAYS

This problem is solved in the same way as every conservation of energy problem: write expressions for the total energy of the system at two points, set them equal, and solve for the unknown quantity.

THINGS TO WATCH OUT FOR

Variations on this problem could include questions about work required to compress a spring, compression along an incline, or the introduction of nonconservative forces. Apply the process for solving conservation of energy problems and you will succeed!

SIMILAR QUESTIONS

1) A spring is compressed vertically 10 cm, and a 5 kg block is placed on top of it. The spring has a spring constant of 50 N/m. If the system is released from rest, what is the maximum height achieved by the block?
2) A spring has a spring constant of 100 N/cm. How much work is required to alter the spring from a compression of 10 cm to a compression of 50 cm?
3) A 5 kg mass and a 2 kg mass are placed on two identical springs (k = 1.3 kN/m). What is the ratio of the maximum compressions of these two springs?

4) Write an expression for energy of the system at the point that the block bounces up.

$$E_3 = \frac{1}{2}mv^2 + mgx$$

As the block bounces off of the spring, it has kinetic energy equal to $\frac{1}{2}mv^2$. It also has potential energy equal to mgx, because it is now at a height of x. The total energy is the sum of these two amounts.

---

5) Set the energies equal and solve for *v*.

$$mg(h + x) = \frac{1}{2}mv^2 + mgx$$

$$mgh + mgx = \frac{1}{2}mv^2 + mgx$$

$$gh + gx = \frac{1}{2}v^2 + gx$$

$$gh = \frac{1}{2}v^2$$

$$v = (2gh)^{-\frac{1}{2}} = 7.7 \text{ m/s}$$

Much like step 3, we can set the total energy of the system at any two points equal to each other. The numbers look easier to deal with for the energy expression from step 2, so choosing this one will save some time. (Note that the velocity is the same when it first hits the spring as when it rebounds up off of the spring. There is no difference in the energy expression for these two points.)

ACCELERATION OF A PENDULUM

A small ball, of mass 1 kg, is tied to a string. The string is fed through a small hole as shown in the diagram below. If the ball is held at a 60 degree angle, as shown, and is then released from rest as the string is pulled with a constant force of 10 N at the same angle, what is the initial acceleration (magnitude and direction) of the ball?

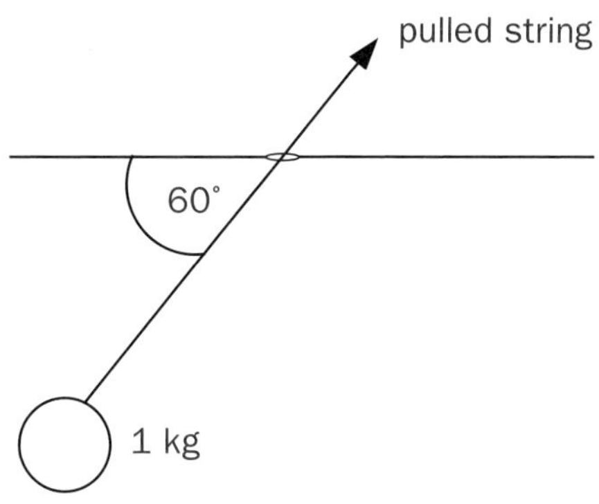

1) Draw a free-body diagram.

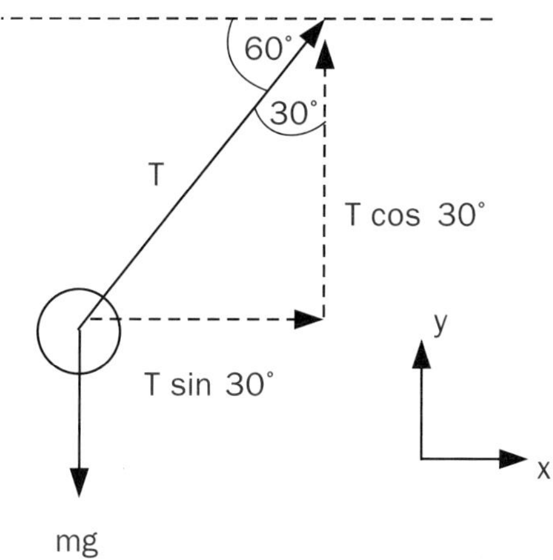

There are two forces acting on the ball: the tension in the string (labeled T) and the weight of the ball (which equals mg). If we use a standard *x*-*y*-axis, the tension in the string must be broken into its *x*- and *y*-components using trigonometry.

2) Add the forces in the *x* and *y* directions.

$\Sigma F_x = ma_x = \text{T} \sin 30° = (10)(0.5) = 5 \text{ N}$

$\Sigma F_y = ma_y = \text{T} \cos 30° - mg = (10)(0.866) - (1)(9.8)$
$= -1.14 \text{ N}$

KEY CONCEPTS

Newton's laws

Tension

Weight

$F = ma$ (N: kg · m/s²)

TAKEAWAYS

This problem seems complicated at first because it is an unusual setup, and the motion of the ball seems like it would take a very complicated path. Do not be scared off, because the same problem-solving process applies to this as to any other force/acceleration problem: 1) draw the free-body diagram; 2) add up the forces in each direction; and 3) solve.

THINGS TO WATCH OUT FOR

Keeping track of signs is important in these problems. If you had reversed the sign of F_y in calculating the angle, you would have gotten a positive angle instead, and those sorts of mistakes are always included among the answer choices.

SIMILAR QUESTIONS

1) A car drives around a circular track of radius 100 m at a speed of 120 m/s. What is the magnitude and direction of the acceleration of the car?
2) A 20 kg block is pushed from the east with a force of 100 N, from the west with a force of 20 N, and from the south with a force of 150 N. In what direction does the block travel?
3) A 10 kg sled is pulled at an angle of 35° east of north by a force of 100 N and with a force of 150 N directed due east. A friction force of 50 N acts as well. What is the acceleration (both magnitude and direction) of the sled?

Add the forces in the *x*- and *y*-directions separately. The net force in a direction always equals the mass times the acceleration in that direction. This is Newton's second law.

---

3) Find the magnitude and direction of the net force.

$F_x = 5$ N

θ

$F_y = 1.14$ N

F

$$F^2 = F_x^2 + F_y^2$$

$$F = (F_x^2 + F_y^2)^{\frac{1}{2}} = (5^2 + (-1.14)^2)^{\frac{1}{2}} = 5.13\,\text{N}$$

$$\theta = \tan^{-1}\left(\frac{F_y}{F_x}\right) = \tan^{-1}\left(\frac{-1.14}{5}\right) = -12.8^\circ$$

In step 2, we found the *x*- and *y*-components of the net force. These two vectors form the sides of a right triangle. To find the magnitude of the net force, use the Pythagorean theorem. To find the angle of the net force, use trigonometry.

---

4) Find the acceleration.

$$F_{net} = ma \rightarrow a = \frac{F_{net}}{m} = \frac{5.13}{1} = 5.13\,\text{m/s}^2$$

$$\theta = -12.8^\circ$$

Use Newton's second law to determine the acceleration from the net force. The direction of the acceleration is the same as the direction of the net force. This is always true.

DAMPENED HARMONIC MOTION

A vertical spring-mass system is submerged in oil. The spring has a stiffness coefficient of 3 N/m, and the mass is 1 kg. If the dampened angular frequency ω_d of oscillation is 0.866 Hz, find the damping coefficient b for the oil and how long it takes the spring to reach 50 percent of its original amplitude.

$$\omega_d = \sqrt{\omega^2 - \left(\frac{b}{2m}\right)^2}$$

$$A = A_0 e^{-\left(\frac{b}{2m}\right)t}$$

1) Find the angular frequency of the spring.

$$\omega = 2\pi f = \sqrt{\left(\frac{k}{m}\right)}$$

$$\omega = \sqrt{\left(\frac{3}{1}\right)} \approx 1.73 \text{ Hz}$$

If the spring-mass system were free of nonconservative forces, it would oscillate indefinitely with an angular frequency of ω. Looking at the equation for dampened frequency ω_d, we see that we're basically adjusting ω for friction by subtracting a quantity specific to the damping coefficient and mass.

Remember: *Use dimensional analysis whenever possible to check your work. In this case, we know that the frequency of oscillation needs to be in Hz or* s^{-1}*. The spring constant k is in N/m and the mass m is in kg. Even if we forget whether k goes on top or on bottom in this equation, thinking critically and using dimensional analysis allows us to find the right equation. If you are uncomfortable using the unit of Newton, think back to Newton's second law:* $F = ma$*. A newton is simply kg(m/s*^{2}*).*

---

2) Use the first equation to find the damping coefficient.

$$\omega_d = \sqrt{\omega^2 - \left(\frac{b}{2m}\right)^2}$$

$$0.866 = \sqrt{(1.73)^2 - \left[\frac{b}{2(1)}\right]^2} \rightarrow 0.75 \approx (3) - \left(\frac{b^2}{4}\right) \rightarrow (0.75-3)4 = -b^2 \rightarrow b = 3 \text{ kg/s}$$

KEY CONCEPTS

Dimensional analysis

Harmonic motion

Friction

Angular frequency
$\omega = 2\pi f (s^{-1})$

Springs

TAKEAWAYS

Use dimensional analysis to check your work.
Get comfortable with algebraic manipulations.

THINGS TO WATCH OUT FOR

Don't be thrown by situations that seem novel or overly complex. Nearly all of the information you need to solve this problem is given explicitly. Keep your units straight! In this example, both the spring constant and the damping constant have the same scalar value, but their units are different.

SIMILAR QUESTIONS

1) By what percentage does the frequency diminish in a horizontal spring-mass system where $k = 1 \times 10^3$ N/m and $m = 4$ kg if the motion is dampened by a frictional force that has a damping coefficient of 2 kg/s?
2) A military cannon has a hard recoil that is absorbed by a friction spring with a natural length of 1.5 m. The spring has a dampening constant of 1 kg/s and can be compressed to 0.2 m. Determine the spring constant for a friction spring that stops a 30,000 lb force in 0.01 s. Use the equation $F = -k(x - x_0) - bv$.
3) What is the period of oscillation of a curled filament with a mass of 100 g and a spring constant of 15 N/m? When heated to 113°C, the filament undergoes a spontaneous exothermic reaction to dissipate the heat. If the new dampening coefficient is 5 → 10^{-3} kg/s, how much energy is lost in 1.5 minutes? Use the equation $E = E_0 e^{-\left(\frac{b}{m}\right)t}$.

Here we are being tested with algebra. Square both sides of the equation to get rid of the square root on the right side. Solve for b. Dimensional analysis in the penultimate step shows us that we are multiplying angular frequency with mass. The individual units, respectively, are s^{-1} and kg, so our product, the damping coefficient, must have that unit. (Try using dimensional analysis to prove to yourself that b can also be recorded in N · s/m.)

---

3) Use the second equation to see how the amplitude of oscillation diminishes with time.

$$A = A_0 e^{-\left(\frac{b}{2m}\right)t}$$

$$0.5A_0 = A_0 e^{-\left(\frac{3}{2(1)}\right)t} \rightarrow$$

$$0.5 = e^{-\left(\frac{3}{2(1)}\right)t} \rightarrow$$

$$\ln 0.5 = -\left(\frac{3}{2(1)}\right)t \rightarrow$$

$$-2(-0.69) \div 3 = t \rightarrow$$

$$0.46 \text{ s} = t \rightarrow$$

This, too, is a test of our algebraic skills. We are asked to find the time needed to reach 50 percent of the original amplitude of oscillation. Thus, $A = 0.5A_0$. Plug into the equation and cancel the A_0 term. To find t, we need to get rid of the number e. Take the natural log of both sides (because $\ln(e^x) = x$) to drop t into a workable domain. Then solve for t. Dimensional analysis of the exponent on e reinforces our units are correct. The exponent overall should have no units, so to cancel out s/kg, we need b to have the unit kg/s.

Remember: *On the MCAT, you will not be expected to take natural logs. You should, however, be able to estimate logarithms to the base 10. Occasionally, you will be given the conversion factor between ln and log.*

DOPPLER EFFECT

KEY CONCEPTS

Doppler effect

Wavelength

Frequency

Two cars, car A and car B, are moving towards each other at 50 m/s when car B starts to beep its 475 Hz horn. Assuming that the speed of sound is 343 m/s, what is the wavelength of the horn as perceived by the driver of car A?

1) Identify this as a Doppler effect problem and determine the source and detector of the wave.

The source is the object that's emitting the wave: car B.

The detector or observer is the object that detects the wave: the person in car A.

Whenever you are given two objects with one emitting a wave and are asked to determine a perceived frequency or wavelength, the Doppler effect is involved.

---

2) Determine the effect of the velocity of the observer on the perceived frequency.

Every Doppler effect problem can be solved using the Doppler effect equation, which states that:

$$F_0 = F_s\left[\frac{1 \pm \frac{V_0}{V}}{1 \mp \frac{V_s}{V}}\right]$$

where F_0 is the frequency observed, F_s is the frequency emitted by the source, V is the speed of the wave, V_0 is the speed of the observer, and V_s is the speed of the source.

$$F_0 = F_s\left[\frac{1 + \frac{V_0}{V}}{1 \mp \frac{V_s}{V}}\right]$$

***Remember:** Isolate the Doppler effect into two parts: effect of velocity of source and effect of velocity of detector. When solving for what's asked, disregard the other variable.*

In this problem, the observer is moving toward the source (car A is moving toward car B) and we are not concerned with the motion of the source, car B. Therefore, the observed frequency (F_0) must be greater than the emitted frequency (F_s) and the numerator must be greater than 1, so we must use the positive sign in the numerator of the problem.

TAKEAWAYS

As the detector approaches the source, the observed frequency will be higher than the emitted frequency and when the detector moves away from the source, the observed frequency will be smaller than the emitted frequency. The same rule applies to the motion of the source. Therefore, when determining the right form of the Doppler equation, use the sign in the equation that will yield the appropriate observed frequency.

3) Determine the effect of the velocity of the source on the perceived frequency.

$$F_0 = F_s\left[\frac{1+\frac{V_0}{V}}{1-\frac{V_s}{V}}\right]$$

The source is also moving toward the detector (car B is moving toward car A). This should also make the perceived frequency greater than the emitted frequency. Thus, in order for F_0 to be greater than F_s, the denominator must be smaller than 1, hence we must use the negative sign in the denominator.

Alternate Method: If you look at the equation in step one, you will notice that in the denominator, the order of plus and minus signs is switched from the order in the numerator. This is written this way for a specific reason. When an object moves toward another object, the first sign is used. When an object moves away from an object, the second sign is used. In our case, because both the observer and source are moving toward each other, we used the first sign in both the numerator and the denominator.

---

4) Plug the values for the emitted frequency and the different velocities into the Doppler effect equation.

$$F_0 = 475\left[\frac{1+\frac{50}{343}}{1-\frac{50}{343}}\right] = 637\ s^{-1}$$

---

5) Convert frequency to wavelength.

☞ $V = f\lambda$

$\lambda = V/f$

$\lambda = \frac{(343\ m/s)}{(637\ s^{-1})}$

$\lambda = 0.54\ m$

THINGS TO WATCH OUT FOR

Always separate Doppler questions into two parts, the effect of the source and the effect of the observer. Be careful in problems where the object and the source are moving in the same direction. If the source is ahead of the detector, the source will be moving away from the detector while the detector is moving toward the source regardless of their speed. If the detector is ahead of the source, the detector will be moving away from the source while the source is moving toward the detector.

SIMILAR QUESTIONS

1) Suppose a policeman traveling at 5 m/s is firing his gun at a rate of 20 bullets per minute while chasing a bank robber who is peddling his Huffy at 50 m/s. At what rate do the bullets reach the bank robber (use 500 m/s for the speed of a bullet)?
2) A bungie jumper yells in triumph at 350 Hz as he falls off a bridge toward a river at a rate of 20 m/s. What are the frequencies heard by the observers on the bridge and a boat on the river (the speed of sound is 343 m/s)?

CHAPTER 10

LIGHT AND OPTICS

In this chapter we will review the basics of optics, which is the study of the reflection and transmission of light through material media and through constrictions such as apertures and slits. Our review will cover the two main areas of optics. The first is termed geometrical optics because we treat light as moving in a straight-line path and can apply simple geometry to determine its behavior. Geometrical optics pertains to the study of mirrors and lenses along with the concepts of reflection and refraction. The second topic is concerned with the wave nature of light and particularly how light behaves when it is passed through apertures and slits. In these instances the light doesn't simply travel in straight-line paths to the wave; concepts of superposition and interference are needed to understand the behavior. A brief review is also provided of the physical nature of light itself, i.e., the electromagnetic wave.

ELECTROMAGNETIC SPECTRUM

A. ELECTROMAGNETIC WAVES

A changing magnetic field can cause a change in the electric field, and a changing electric field can cause a change in the magnetic field. Because changing electric fields affect changing magnetic fields which affect changing electric fields (and so on and so on), we can begin to see how **electromagnetic waves** occur in nature. One field affects the other, totally independent of matter, and electromagnetic waves can travel through a vacuum.

Electromagnetic waves are transverse waves because the oscillating electric and magnetic field vectors are perpendicular to the direction of propagation. Furthermore, the electric field and the magnetic field are perpendicular to each other. This is illustrated in Figure 10.1.

TEACHER TIP

This perpendicular relationship is described by the right hand and was discussed in chapter 7.

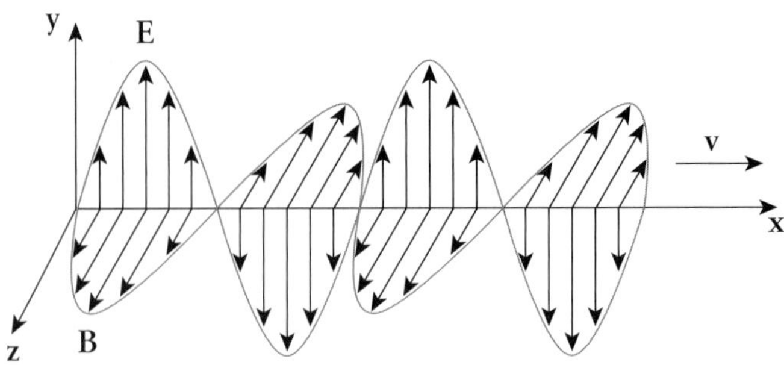

Figure 10.1

MCAT SYNOPSIS

The electric field, magnetic field, and direction of propagation are all mutually perpendicular in an electromagnetic wave.

The **electromagnetic spectrum** is a term used to describe the full range in frequency and wavelength of electromagnetic waves. The following prefixes are often used when quoting wavelength: 1 mm = 10^{-3} m, 1 μm = 10^{-6} m, 1 nm = 10^{-9} m, and 1 Å = 10^{-10}m. The full spectrum is broken into many regions which, in descending order of wavelength, are: radio (10^9 m to 1 mm), infrared (1 mm to 700 nm), visible light (700 nm to 400 nm), ultraviolet (400 nm to 50 nm), X ray (50 nm to 10^{-2} nm), and gamma ray (smaller than 10^{-2} nm). These regions have arbitrary boundaries, and some authors quote slightly different values. For example, one person will call 50 nm "short wavelength ultraviolet," while another may call it "long wavelength X ray."

Electromagnetic waves can vary in frequency or wavelength, but in a vacuum all electromagnetic waves travel at the same speed, called the **speed of light**. This constant is represented by the letter c and is equal to: 3.00×10^8 m/s. To a first approximation, electromagnetic waves also travel in air with this velocity. Now the familiar equation $v = f\lambda$ becomes:

$$c = f\lambda$$

for all electromagnetic waves in a vacuum and, to a first approximation, in air.

TEACHER TIP

The wavelengths of the visible spectrum appear frequently on the MCAT. Remember the boundaries.

B. COLOR AND THE VISIBLE SPECTRUM

We just mentioned that the electromagnetic spectrum is broken up into many regions. The visible part of the spectrum is the only part that is perceived as light by the human eye. Within this region different wavelengths induce sensations of different colors, with violet at one end of the visible spectrum (400 nm) and red at the other end of the visible spectrum (700 nm).

FLASHBACK

Like any wave, light has a frequency and wavelength related to speed by $v = \lambda f$. In vacuum, $v = c$. (See chapter 9.)

Light that contains all the colors in equal intensity is seen as white. The color of an object that does not emit its own light is dependent on the color of light that it reflects. So an object that appears red is one that absorbs all light except red. This implies that a red object receiving green light will appear black, because it absorbs the green light and has no light to reflect.

GEOMETRICAL OPTICS

When light travels through a single homogeneous medium it travels in a straight line. This is known as rectilinear propagation. The behavior of light at the boundary of a medium or interface between two media is described by the theory of geometrical optics.

MCAT SYNOPSIS

Reflection occurs even when light passes through a transparent medium, i.e., most of the light passes through but some is reflected.

A. REFLECTION

Reflection is the rebounding of incident light waves at the boundary of a medium.

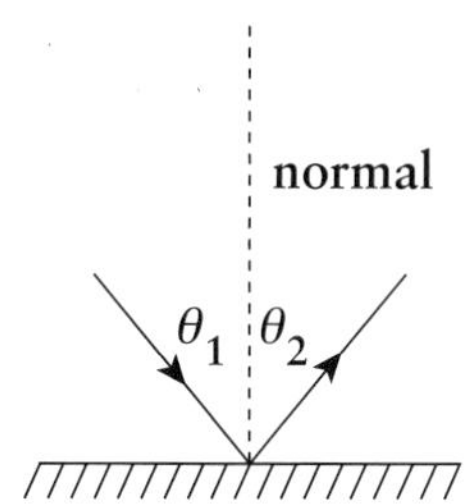

Figure 10.2

The law of reflection is:

$$\theta_1 = \theta_2$$

Important note: In optics, angles are always measured from a line drawn perpendicular to the boundary of a medium, often referred to as the **normal.**

1. Plane Mirrors

Parallel incident rays remain parallel after reflection from a plane mirror. In general, images created by a mirror can be either real or virtual. An image is said to be **real** if the light actually converges at the position of the image. An image is **virtual** if the light only *appears* to be coming from the position of the image but does not converge there.

Plane mirrors always create virtual images. In a plane mirror the image appears to be the same distance behind the mirror as the object's distance in front of it. Because the reflected light remains in front of the mirror but the image is behind the mirror, the image is virtual.

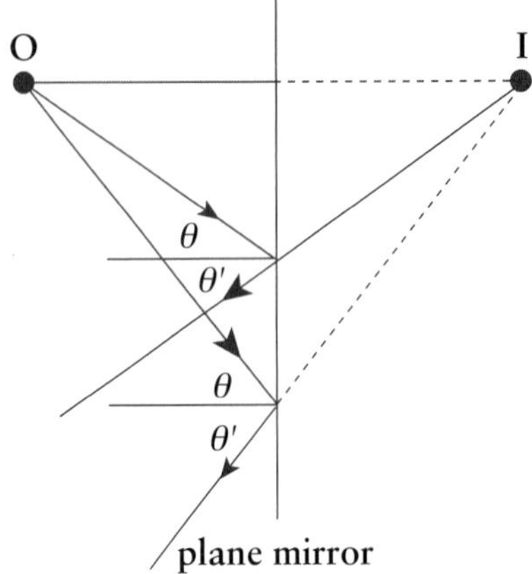

Figure 10.3

2. Spherical Mirrors

Spherical mirrors come in two varieties, **concave** and **convex.** The word *spherical* implies that the surface of the mirror has the shape of a sphere. In other words, if you had a sphere made out of a mirrorlike material, a spherical mirror would be a small portion cut out of that sphere. Therefore, spherical mirrors have a **center of curvature** C and a **radius of curvature** r associated with them.

EXCLUSIVE

You can recognize a conCAVE surface because it appears caved in when you're looking at it straight on.

TEACHER TIP

The side mirrors on a car are convex; the small circular mirrors used for applying makeup are concave.

If you were to look from the inside of a sphere to its surface, you would see a concave surface. However, if you were to look from outside the sphere you would see a convex surface. The **focal length** f is the distance between the focal point and the mirror. For all spherical mirrors $f = r/2$. For a convex surface the center of curvature and the focal point are behind the mirror. Concave mirrors are called **converging mirrors** and convex mirrors are called **diverging mirrors.**

MCAT SYNOPSIS

Concave (converging) mirrors have a positive focal length. Convex (diverging) mirrors have a negative focal length.

TEACHER TIP

The focal point of converging mirrors (and converging lenses) will always be positive. The focal point of diverging mirrors (and diverging lenses) will always be negative.

There are several important distances associated with mirrors. The focal length f is the distance between the focal point F and the mirror; the radius of curvature r is the distance between C and the mirror (remember that $r = 2f$); the distance of the object from the mirror is o; the distance of the image from the mirror is i. There is a simple relation satisfied by these distances:

$$\frac{1}{o} + \frac{1}{i} = \frac{1}{f} = \frac{2}{r}$$

While it is not important which units of distance are used in this equation, it is important that all values used have the same units, be they centimeters, meters, or whatever.

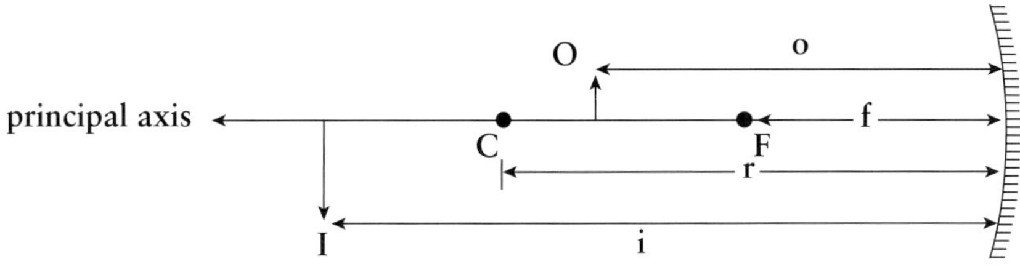

Figure 10.4

TEACHER TIP

Any time the object is at the focal point, the reflected rays will be parallel, and the image will be at infinity.

Often you will use this equation to calculate the image distance. If the image has a positive distance, it is a real image, which implies that the image is in front of the mirror. If the image has a negative distance, it is virtual and thus located behind the mirror. Note also that for a plane mirror $r = f = \infty$, and the equation becomes $1/o + 1/i = 0$ or $i = -o$ (virtual image).

MCAT SYNOPSIS

Real images have positive image distances, and virtual images have negative image distances.

The **magnification** (m) is a dimensionless value that is the ratio of the image's height to the object's height. Following the sign convention given below, the orientation of the image compared with the object can also be determined. A negative magnification signifies an inverted image, while a positive value means the image is upright.

$$m = -\frac{i}{o}$$

If $|m| < 1$ the image is reduced, if $|m| > 1$ the image is enlarged, and if $|m| = 1$ the image is the same size as the object.

MCAT SYNOPSIS

Upright images have positive magnification, and inverted images have negative magnification.

Figure 10.5 shows ray diagrams for a concave spherical mirror with the object at three different points. A ray diagram is useful for getting an approximation of where the image is. In general, there are three important rays to draw. For a concave mirror, a ray that strikes the mirror parallel to the horizontal is reflected back through the focal point. A ray that passes through the focal point before reaching the mirror is reflected back parallel to the horizontal. A ray that strikes the mirror right where the normal intersects it gets reflected back with the same angle (measured from the normal).

MCAT SYNOPSIS

Rays that come in parallel to principal axis reflect through the focal point. Rays that pass through the focal point, reflect back parallel to principal axis.

TEACHER TIP

To find the location of the image, draw the rays and find a point at which any two of them intersect. This point of intersection will show us where the image is.

A single diverging mirror forms only a virtual erect image, regardless of the position of the object. The image formed by a single converging mirror depends on the position of the object, demonstrated by Figure 10.5. When the object is farther away from the mirror than the focal point, the image is real and inverted. By moving the object to the focal point, the image disappears as the light rays reflect off the mirror parallel to each other and never converge. Moving the object closer to the mirror than the focal length makes an image that is virtual and erect.

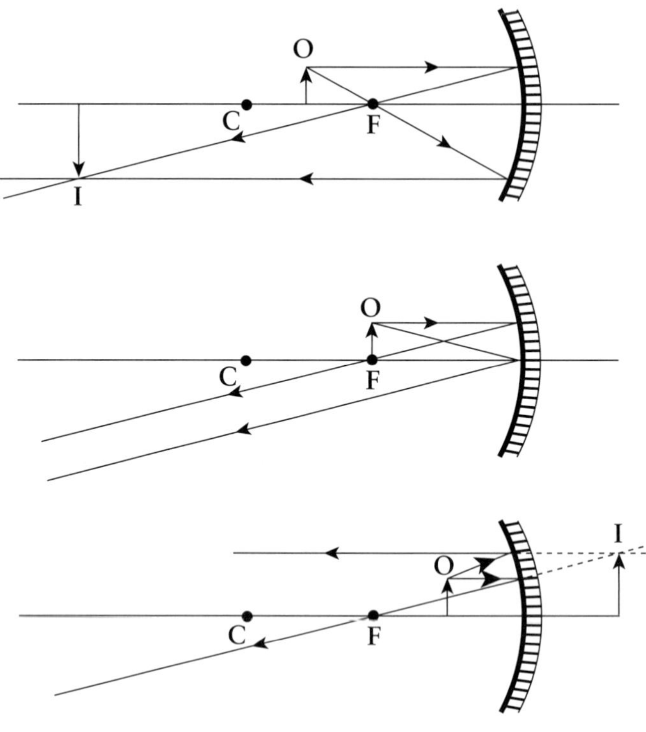

Figure 10.5

TEACHER TIP

Concave mirrors and convex lenses are both converging and thus have similar properties. Similarly, convex mirrors and concave lenses have similar properties and are both diverging.

3. Sign Convention

The following chart gives the proper signs for various instances when dealing with single mirrors. Note that R side is used to denote Real side, which for mirrors is in front of the mirror. Similarly, V side stands for Virtual side, which is behind the mirror.

Sign Chart for Single Mirrors

Symbol	Positive	Negative
o	object is in front of mirror (R side)	object is behind mirror (V side)
i	image is in front of mirror (R side)	image is behind mirror (V side)
r	concave mirrors	convex mirrors
f	concave mirrors	convex mirrors
m	image is upright (erect)	image is inverted

Note that in almost all problems the object will be in front of the mirror, and thus the object distance o will be positive.

TEACHER TIP

The only time the object is behind the mirror is when the object is the image from another mirror or lens. This will be discussed later in the chapter.

Example: An object is placed 7 cm in front of a concave mirror that has a 10 cm radius of curvature. Determine the image distance, the magnification, whether the image is real or virtual, and whether it is inverted or upright.

Solution: Using the mirror equation:

$$\frac{1}{i} + \frac{1}{o} = \frac{2}{r}$$

$$\frac{1}{i} = \frac{2}{r} - \frac{1}{o}$$

$$\frac{1}{i} = \frac{2}{10} - \frac{1}{7}$$

$$i = +17.5 \text{ cm}$$

The magnification m is:

$$m = -\frac{i}{o}$$

$$= -\frac{17.5}{7}$$

$$= -2.5$$

The image is in front of the mirror (i is positive) and therefore real. The image is inverted (m is negative) and 2.5 times larger ($|m| = 2.5$).

B. REFRACTION

1. Snell's Law

When light is not in a vacuum, its speed is less than c. (As previously noted, when light is in air, $v \cong c$.) For a given medium:

$$n = \frac{c}{v}$$

MCAT SYNOPSIS

Light travels more slowly in material media (like glass) than in a vacuum. The wavelength changes accordingly while the frequency remains constant.

where c is the speed of light in a vacuum, v is the speed of light in the medium, and n is a dimensionless quantity called the **index of refraction** of the medium. Because $v < c$, $n > 1$. For air, to a first approximation, $v = c$ and $n = 1$.

Refracted rays of light obey **Snell's law** as they pass from one medium to another:

$$n_1 \sin \theta_1 = n_2 \sin \theta_2$$

n_1 and θ_1 are for the medium the light is coming from, and n_2 and θ_2 are for the medium the light is going into. Note that θ is measured with respect to the perpendicular (normal) to the boundary.

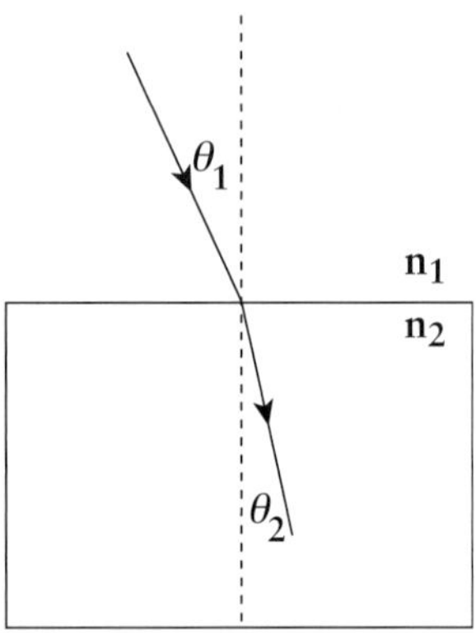

Figure 10.6

TEACHER TIP

When light enters a medium with a higher index of refraction, it bends toward the normal. When light enters a lower index of refraction, it bends away from the normal.

In general, when light enters a medium with a higher index of refraction ($n_2 > n_1$) it bends towards the normal so that $\theta_2 < \theta_1$. Conversely, if the light travels into a medium where the index of refraction is smaller ($n_2 < n_1$), the light will bend away from the normal so that $\theta_2 > \theta_1$.

Example: A penny sits at the bottom of a pool of water ($n = 1.33$) at a depth of 3.0 m. If an observer 1.8 m tall stands 30 cm away from the ledge, how close to the side can the penny be and still be visible?

TEACHER TIP

It may seem counterintuitive to make the light come from the water, but we want the light traveling toward the observer's eye.

Solution: First draw a picture of the situation as in Figure 10.7. Note that the light is coming from the water ($n_1 = 1.33$) and going into the air ($n_2 = 1$), so the light is bent away from the normal ($\theta_2 > \theta_1$).

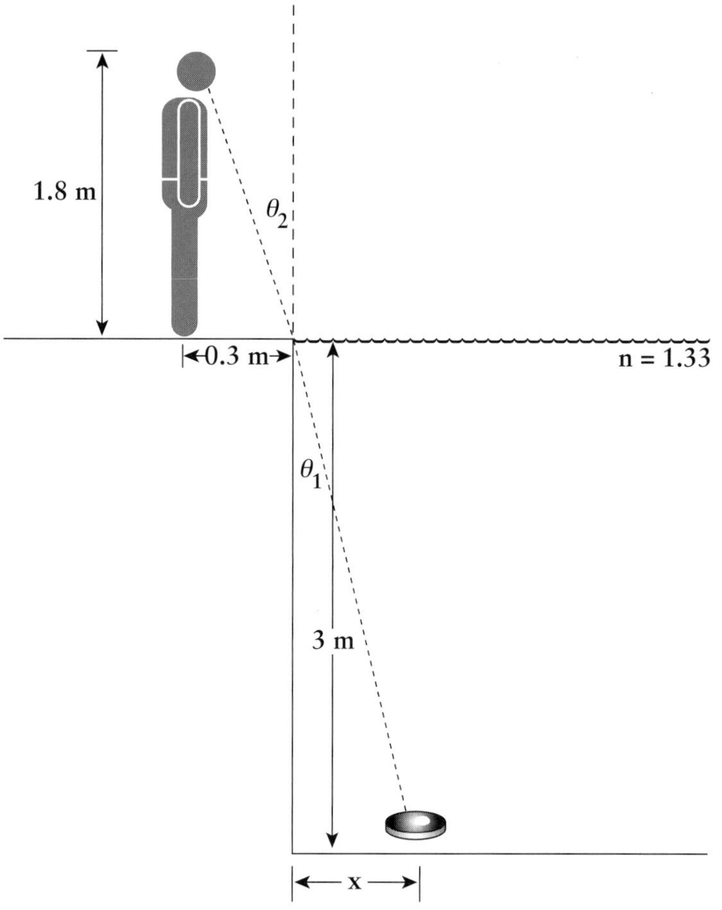

Figure 10.7

TEACHER TIP

It is this property of water that makes spear fishing so difficult. This fish is actually closer than it looks.

MCAT SYNOPSIS

Refraction (bending of light) can cause optical illusions.

We need to find the angles that the light rays make with the normal to the water's surface:

$$\tan \theta_2 = \frac{0.3}{1.8}$$
$$\theta_2 = 9.5^\circ$$

Using Snell's law we can solve for θ_1:

$$\sin \theta_1 = \frac{n_2}{n_1} \sin \theta_2$$
$$= \frac{0.165}{1.33}$$
$$\theta_1 = 7.1^\circ$$

We can find x using trigonometry:

$$x = 3 \tan \theta_1$$
$$= 0.37 \text{ m}$$
$$= 37 \text{ cm}$$

TEACHER TIP

Remember that the sin of 90° equals 1. This is why the second theta cancels out.

MCAT SYNOPSIS

Total internal reflection can only occur when going from a medium of greater index of refraction to one of lesser index of refraction.

2. Total Internal Reflection

When light travels from a medium with a higher index of refraction to a medium with a lower index of refraction, the refracted angle is larger than the angle of incidence ($\theta_2 > \theta_1$). As the angle of incidence is increased, a special angle is reached, called the **critical angle** (θ_c), where for this value of θ_1 the refracted angle θ_2 equals 90°. The critical angle can be found from Snell's law:

$$n_1 \sin \theta_1 = n_2 \sin \theta_2$$

$$n_1 \sin \theta_c = n_2 \sin 90° = n_2$$

$$\sin \theta_c = \frac{n_2}{n_1}$$

Total **internal reflection,** a condition in which all the light incident on a boundary is reflected back into the original material, results for any angle of incidence greater than θ_c.

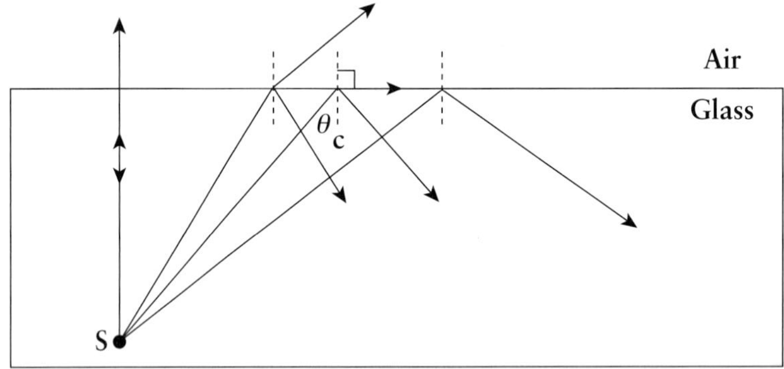

Figure 10.8

Example: From the previous example, suppose another penny is 10 times farther out than the first one. Will a light ray going from this penny to the top edge of the pool emerge from the water?

Solution: First find the critical angle:

$$\sin \theta_c = \frac{n_2}{n_1} = \frac{1}{1.33}$$

$$\theta_c = 48.8°$$

The angle made by the second penny's light ray is:

$$\tan \theta_1 = \frac{0.37 \times 10}{3} = 1.23$$

$$\theta_1 = 51°$$

$\theta_1 > \theta_c$, therefore the light ray will be totally internally reflected and will not emerge.

3. Thin Spherical Lenses

There is an important difference between lenses and mirrors aside from the obvious fact that lenses refract light while mirrors reflect it. When working with lenses, you are dealing with *two* surfaces that affect the light path. For example, a person wearing glasses sees light that travels from an object through the air into the glass lens (first surface). Then the light travels through the glass until it reaches the other side, where again it travels out of the glass into the air (second surface).

MCAT SYNOPSIS

Mirrors reflect light, whereas lenses refract light. The refraction occurs at both surfaces of the lens.

A thin lens is a lens whose thickness can be neglected. Because light can be coming from either side of a lens, a lens has two focal points (one on each side of the lens) and two focal lengths (see Figure 10.9). For thin spherical lenses the focal lengths are equal, and so we speak of the focal length.

MCAT SYNOPSIS

Converging lenses cause parallel rays to converge at the focal point and rays from the focal point to emerge parallel.

Figure 10.9(a) also illustrates that a **converging lens** is always thicker at the center, while Figure 10.9(b) illustrates that a **diverging lens** is always thinner at the center.

TEACHER TIP

Converging lenses are needed for those who are far-sighted; these tend to be reading glasses. They are similar to magnifying glasses in that they magnify the wearer's eyes. Diverging lenses are needed for those who are near-sighted (those who "can see near").

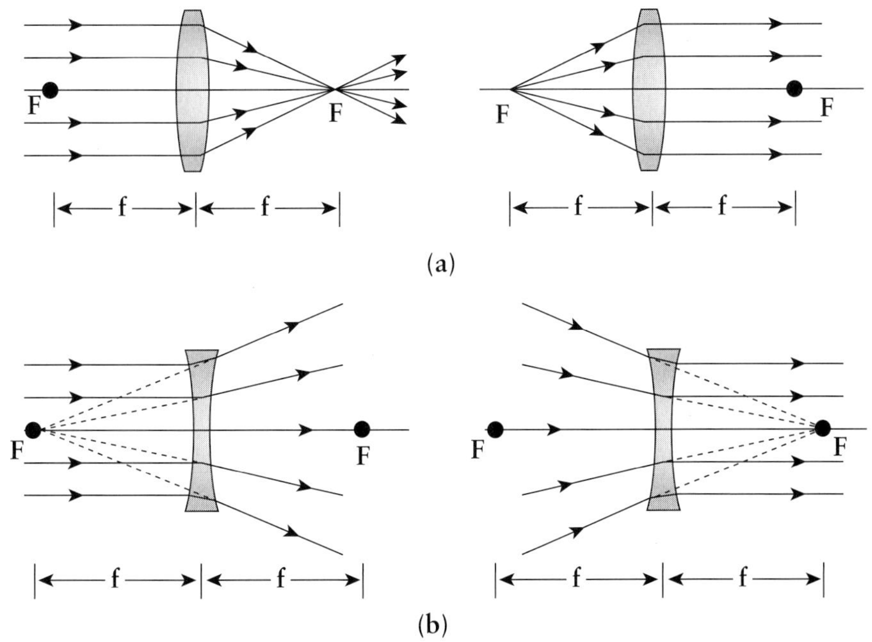

F F F F

f f f f

(a)

TEACHER TIP

If the rays you draw do not intersect, reflect the rays back to the side of the lens from which the light came, causing a virtual image.

F F F F

f f f f

(b)

Figure 10.9

MCAT SYNOPSIS

Positive images are always on the side that the light actually goes to; same side as object for mirrors, and opposite side to object for lenses.

The basic formulas for finding image distance and magnification for spherical mirrors (except r = 2f,) also apply to lenses. The object distance o, image distance i, focal length f, and magnification m, are related by:

$$\frac{1}{o}+\frac{1}{i}=\frac{1}{f}$$

$$m=-\frac{1}{o}$$

For lenses whose thicknesses cannot be neglected, the focal length is related to the curvature of the lens surfaces and the index of refraction of the lens by the **Lensmaker's equation**:

$$\frac{1}{f}=(n-1)\left(\frac{1}{r_1}-\frac{1}{r_2}\right)$$

where r_1 is the radius of curvature of the first lens surface and r_2 is the radius of curvature of the second lens surface.

Note that sign conventions change slightly for lenses. (Sign conventions are the trickiest part to optics.) For both lenses and mirrors, positive magnification means upright images and negative magnification means inverted images. Also, for both lenses and mirrors, a positive image distance means that the image is real and is located on the R side, whereas a negative image distance means that the image is virtual and located on the V side.

TEACHER TIP

Consider whether the image is on the side it's supposed to be on. Mirrors reflect light back and lenses let light pass through. If the image is on the wrong side, then it's a virtual image.

However, where to place the R side and V side confuses most people because it is different for mirrors and lenses. To place the R side, remember that the R side is where the light really goes after interacting with the mirror or lens. For mirrors, light is reflected and therefore stays in front of the mirror. The image may either appear in front of or behind the mirror, but the light rays always remain in front of the mirror. Since the R side is in front of the mirror, the V side is behind the mirror. For lenses, it is different: Light travels through the lens and comes out on the other side. The light really travels to the other side of the lens, and therefore, for lenses, the R side is on the opposite side of the lens from where the light came from. Thus the V side must be the side of the lens that the light came from. Although the object of a single lens is on the V side, this does not make the object virtual. Objects are real, with a positive object distance, unless they are in certain multiple lens systems.

Focal lengths have a simple sign convention. For both mirrors and lenses, converging lenses and mirrors have positive focal lengths and diverging mirrors and lenses have negative focal lengths. For radii of curvature you have to remember that a lens has two surfaces, each with its own radius of curvature (r_1 and r_2, where the surfaces are numbered in the order that they are encountered by the traveling light). For both mirrors and lenses, a radius of curvature is positive if the center of curvature is on the R side and negative if the center of curvature is on the V side.

Sign Chart for single lenses

Symbol	Positive	Negative
o	object on side of lens light is coming from	object on side of lens light is going to
i	image on side of lens light is going to (R side)	image on side of lens light is coming from (V side)
f	converging lens	diverging lens
m	image erect	image inverted
r	when on R side (convex surface as seen from side the light is coming from)	when on V side (concave surface as seen from side the light is coming from)

Optometrists often describe a lens in terms of its **power** (P). This is measured in **diopters** when f is in meters and is given by the equation:

$$p = \frac{1}{f}$$

P has the same sign as f and is therefore positive for a converging lens and negative for a diverging lens.

4. Multiple Lens Systems

Lenses in contact are a series of lenses with negligible distances between them. These systems behave as a single lens with equivalent focal length given by:

$$\frac{1}{f} = \frac{1}{f_1} + \frac{1}{f_2} + \cdots$$

$$(P = P_1 + P_2 + \cdots)$$

A good example is the eye.

For **lenses not in contact** the image of one lens is used to make the object of another lens. The image from the last lens is the image of the system. Microscopes and telescopes are good examples. The magnification for the system is $M = m_1 \times m_2 \times m_3 \times \cdots$

MCAT SYNOPSIS

For multiple lenses, the image from one lens becomes the object for the next.

TEACHER TIP

Because the MCAT is a timed exam, you'll be asked about a multiple lens system in more of a conceptual way than a detailed way.

Example: An object is 15 cm to the left of a thin diverging lens with a 45 cm focal length as shown below. Find:

a. where the image is formed, if it is upright or inverted, and if it is real or virtual.

b. the radii of curvature assuming the lens is symmetrical and made of glass (n = 1.50).

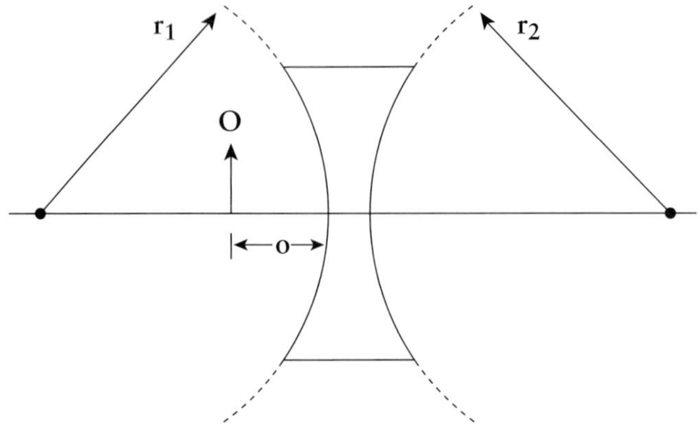

Figure 10.10

Solution: a. The image distance (i) is found using the equation:

$$\frac{1}{i} + \frac{1}{o} = \frac{1}{f}$$

$$\frac{1}{i} = \frac{1}{f} - \frac{1}{o}$$

Because the lens is diverging the focal length takes a negative sign, f = –45 cm. The object (like all objects in a single lens system) has a positive sign, o = 15 cm. Solving for i:

$$\frac{1}{i} = \frac{-1}{45} - \frac{1}{15}$$

$$= \frac{-1}{45} - \frac{3}{45}$$

$$= \frac{-4}{45}$$

$$i = -11.25 \text{ cm}$$

The negative sign indicates that the image is on the left side of the lens and therefore virtual (the light went through the lens and is on the right side). To find out whether the image is upright or inverted we need to calculate the magnification:

$$m = -\frac{i}{o}$$

$$= -\frac{-11.25}{15}$$

$$= \frac{11.25}{15}$$

$$= 0.75$$

Since the magnification is positive, the image is upright. Furthermore, since $|m| < 1$, the image is smaller than the object.

b. Because the lens is symmetrical, the radii are equal but opposite in sign. They can be found from the Lensmaker's equation:

$$\frac{1}{f} = (n-1)\left(\frac{1}{r_1} - \frac{1}{r_2}\right)$$

As the light progresses from left to right, the first surface of the lens is concave (r_1 negative) and the second surface of the lens is convex (r positive). So:

$$\frac{1}{f} = (n-1)\left(\frac{1}{-r} - \frac{1}{r}\right)$$

$$= (n-1)\left(-\frac{2}{r}\right)$$

We know that f = –45 cm (diverging lens). Therefore:

$$-\frac{1}{45} = (1.5-1)\left(-\frac{2}{r}\right)$$

$$= \frac{-1}{r}$$

$$r = 45 \text{ cm}$$

C. DISPERSION

As noted earlier, the speed of light for all wavelengths in a vacuum is the same. However, when light travels through a medium, different wavelengths travel at different velocities. This fact also implies that the index of refraction of a medium is a function of the wavelength, since the index of refraction is related to the velocity of the wave by $n = c/v$. When the speed of the wave varies with wavelength a material exhibits

TEACHER TIP

Remember the relative wavelengths and frequencies of the visible colors, and the order of the colors. Violet has the largest frequency and thus the smallest wavelength. Red has the smallest frequency and thus the largest wavelength.

dispersion. The most common example of dispersion is the splitting of white light into its component colors using a prism.

If a source of white light is incident on one of the faces of a prism, the light emerging from the prism is spread out into a fan shaped beam, as shown in Figure 10.11. The light has been dispersed into a spectrum. This occurs because violet light "sees" a greater index of refraction than red does and so is bent to a greater extent.

MCAT SYNOPSIS

A prism splits white light into its component colors (wavelengths) because each wavelength has a different index of refraction.

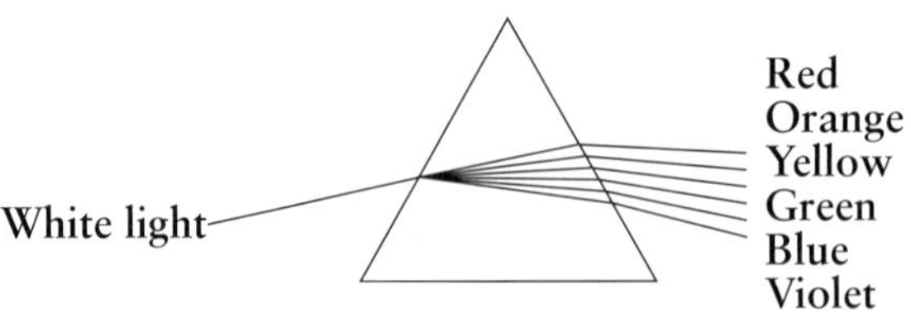

Figure 10.11

DIFFRACTION

When we first began discussing geometrical optics, we asserted that light travels in straight lines. But there are situations in which this is not strictly true. For example, when light passes through a narrow opening (an opening whose size is on the order of wavelengths), the light waves seem to spread out as is seen in Figure 10.12. As the slit narrows, the light is spread out more. This spreading out of light as it passes through a narrow opening is called **diffraction.**

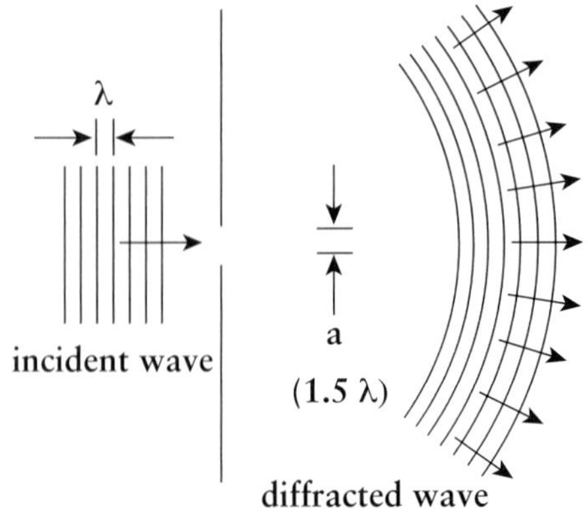

Figure 10.12

If a lens is placed between a narrow slit and a screen, a pattern is observed consisting of a bright central fringe with alternating dark and bright fringes on each side (see Figure 10.13). The central bright fringe is twice as wide as the bright fringes on the sides, and as the slit becomes narrower the central maximum becomes wider. The location of the dark fringes is given by the following formula:

$$a \sin \theta = n\lambda \quad (n = 1, 2, 3, \ldots)$$

where a is the width of the slit, λ is the wavelength of the incident wave, and θ is the angle made by the line drawn from the center of the lens to the dark fringe and the line perpendicular to the screen. Note that bright fringes are halfway between dark fringes.

TEACHER TIP

Because light is similar to other wave forms, it observes constructive and destructive interference. This interference is seen as light and dark fringes.

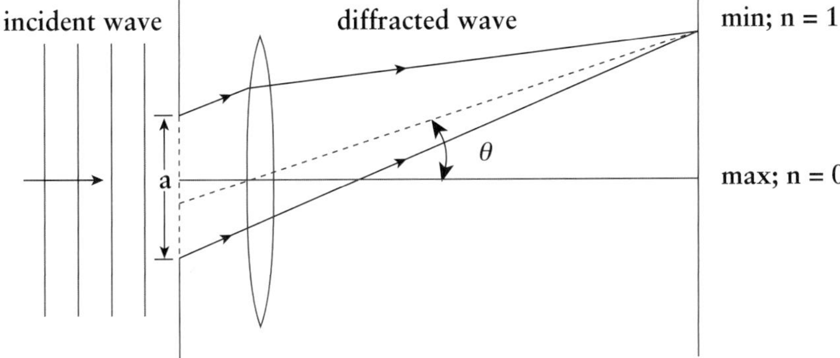

Figure 10.13

INTERFERENCE

By the superposition principle, when waves interact with each other, the amplitudes of the waves add together in a process called **interference** (see chapter 9). Young's experiment showed that two light waves can interfere with one another, and this contributed to the wave theory of light. Figure 10.14(a) shows the typical setup for Young's double slit experiment. When monochromatic light illuminates the slits, an interference pattern is observed on a screen placed behind the slits. Monochromatic light is light that consists of just one wavelength, and coherent light consists of light waves whose phase difference does not change with time. Regions of constructive interference between the two light waves appear as regions of maximum light intensity on the screen. Conversely, in regions where the light waves interfere destructively, the light is at a minimum intensity and the screen is dark. An interference pattern produced by a double slit setup is shown in Figure 10.14(b).

MCAT SYNOPSIS

Monochromatic light is light of a single frequency and thus a single wavelength.

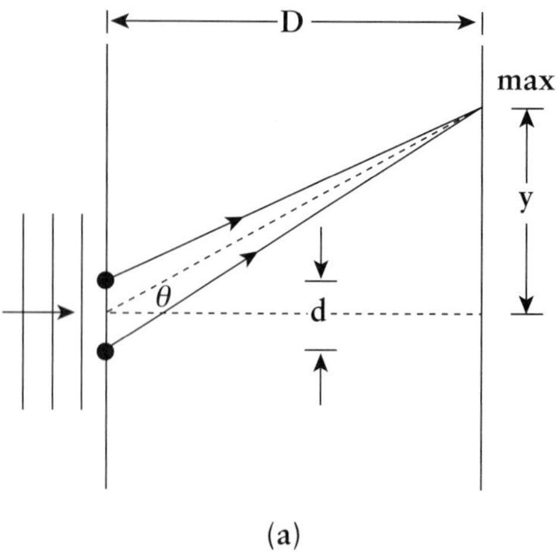

(a)

Zeroth fringe

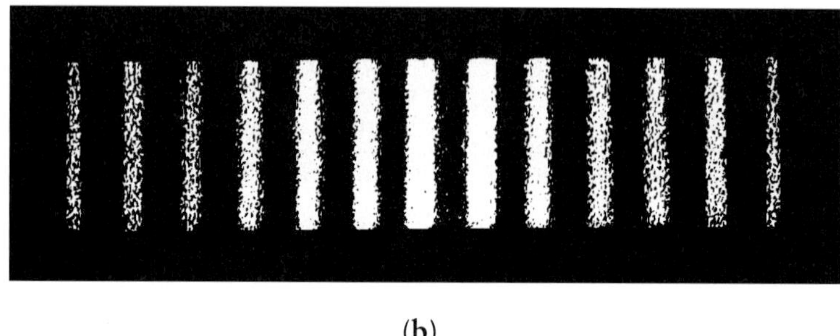

(b)

Figure 10.12

MCAT SYNOPSIS

When one refers to the second order maximum or fourth order minimum, one simply substitutes m = 2 or m = 4 into the appropriate equation.

The position of maxima and minima on the screen can be found from the following equations:

(maxima) $d \sin \theta = m\lambda$ $m = 0, 1, 2, \ldots$

(minima) $d \sin \theta = (m + \frac{1}{2})\lambda$ $m = 0, 1, 2, \ldots$

where d is the distance between the slits, θ is the angle between the dashed lines shown in Figure 10.14a, λ is the wavelength of the light, and m is an integer representing the order.

Example: What is the linear distance y, between the sixth and eighth maxima on the screen? The wavelength λ is 550 nm, the slits are separated by 0.14 mm, and the screen is 70 cm from the slits.

Solution: Using the small angle approximation $\sin \theta \approx \tan \theta \approx \theta$, the equation for the distance between maxima is derived as follows:

$$\sin\theta = \frac{m\lambda}{d}$$

$$\tan\theta = \frac{y}{D} \approx \frac{m\lambda}{d}$$

$$\Delta y \approx \frac{\Delta m\lambda D}{d}$$

where Δm is the difference between fringe numbers. Substituting the numbers gives:

$$y = \frac{2(550 \times 10^{-9})(0.70)}{0.14 \times 10^{-3}}$$

$$= 5.5 \text{ mm}$$

TEACHER TIP

Lightwaves exist as a wave in all three dimensions, meaning it osculates in all 360°. Polarizing light will limits the light into only two dimensions.

POLARIZATION

Plane-polarized light is light in which the electric fields of all the waves are oriented in the same direction, i.e., their electric field vectors are parallel. It is true that their magnetic fields vectors are also parallel, but convention dictates that the plane of the electric field identifies the plane of polarization.

MCAT SYNOPSIS

Plane-polarized light means electric field vector is always in the same direction.

Unpolarized light corresponds to a random orientation of the electric field vectors. Sunlight is a prime example. However, there are filters called polarizers, often used in cameras and sunglasses, which allow only light whose electric field is pointing in a particular direction to pass. If you hold one polarizer out the window, it will let through only that portion of the daylight that has a given E vector orientation. If you now hold up another polarizer and slowly turn it, you will see the light transmitted through the two polarizers vary from total darkness to the level of the original polarizer alone. When both the first and second polarizer are polarizing in the same direction, all the light that passed through the first also passes through the second. When the second polarizer is turned so that it polarizes in a direction perpendicular to the first, no light gets through at all.

MCAT SYNOPSIS

Unpolarized light means electric field vector points in randomly changing directions.

TEACHER TIP

Try this yourself with polarized sunglasses and an iPOD, iPhone, or even the digital display on a gas pump. Hold the sunglasses in front of the device and try rotating the glasses 360°. Whenever the two are oriented 90° or 270° relative to each other, no light will pass through.

PRACTICE QUESTIONS

1. A student shines monochromatic light on a pair of narrow slits in a diffraction experiment. If the intensity of that light is steadily increased, the spacing between maxima will

A. remain the same.
B. increase.
C. decrease.
D. increase or decrease depending on frequency.

2. Which of the following can only be true when we consider the wave-like nature of visible light?

A. The vibrations of electric and magnetic fields are both longitudinal.
B. The vibrations of electric and magnetic fields are both transverse.
C. The vibrations of an electric field are transverse while those of a magnetic field are longitudinal.
D. The vibrations of an electric field are longitudinal while those of a magnetic field are transverse.

3. An object that has a height of 4 m is placed 6 m to the left of an industrial-sized converging lens with a focal length of 4 m. A second converging lens with a focal length of 3 m is placed 18 m to the right of the first lens. The image produced by the two lenses together is located

A. 3 m to the left of the second lens.
B. 3 m to the right of the second lens.
C. 12 m to the left of the first lens.
D. 12 m to the right of the first lens.

4. Which of the following are able to produce a virtual image?

I. Convex lens
II. Concave lens
III. Plane mirror

A. I only
B. III only
C. II and III only
D. I, II, and III

5. Total internal reflection can occur between two transparent media if their relative index of refraction (first medium : second medium) is

A. less than 1.0.
B. equal to 1.0.
C. greater than 1.0.
D. This phenomenon is not possible.

6. A stuffed bear is placed 10 m from a giant unknown object. A student rests her head 22.5 m away from the opposite side of the object and looks toward the stuffed bear. A screen exists between the object and the student. She is able to observe the image of the teddy bear (figure below). The unknown object could be which of the following?

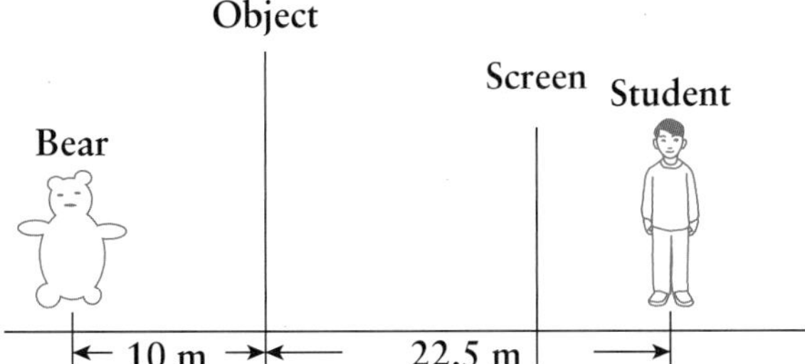

I. A convex mirror with a focal length of 5 m
II. A concave mirror with a focal length of 5 m
III. A convex lens with a focal length of 5 m
IV. A concave lens with a focal length of 5 m

A. III only
B. I and II only
C. III and IV
D. I, II, III, and IV

7. Imagine that blue light (wavelength of 460 nm) is allowed to shine through a double slit. What pattern will result?

A. A continuous spectrum
B. Alternate blue and black bands
C. Two bands of blue light
D. Bands of blue light and violet fringing

8. Monochromatic red light is allowed to pass between two different media. If the angle of incidence in medium 1 is 30° and the angle of incidence in medium 2 is 45°, what is the relationship between the speed of light in medium 2 compared to that in medium 1?

A. v2 = 1.4 v1
B. 1.4 v2 = v1
C. v2 = 1.7 v1
D. 1.7 v2 = v1

9. The figure below shows a light to one side of a solid wall with slits in it. Some distance from this wall is another wall, without slits, on which a pattern appears. What is the difference in path length of the light waves from the two slits at the center of the first bright fringe above the central maximum?

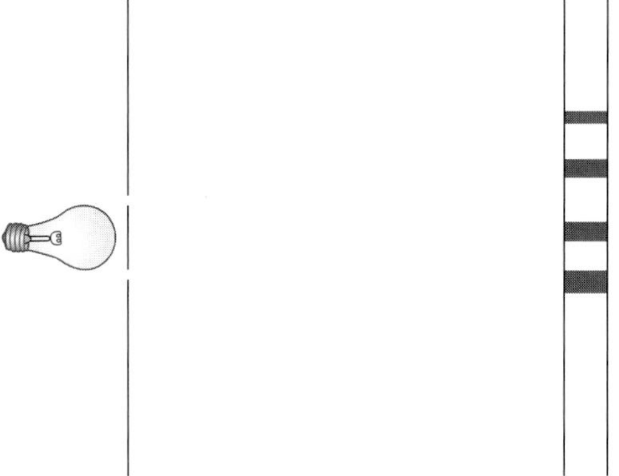

A. 0
B. ½ λ
C. λ
D. 3/2 λ

10. The near point of one of your eyes is 100 cm. You wish to see your friend's face clearly when she stands 50 cm in front of you. If you use a contact lens to adjust your eyesight, what must be the radius of curvature and power of the contact lens?

A. r = 33 cm, P = 3 diopters
B. r = 67 cm, P = 3 diopters
C. r = 100 cm, P = 2 diopters
D. r = 200 cm, P = 1 diopter

11. Imagine that a beam of monochromatic light originates in air and is allowed to shine upon the flat surface of a piece of glass at an angle of 60° with the horizontal. The reflected and refracted beams are perpendicular to each other. What is the index of refraction of the glass?

A. 0.58
B. 1
C. 1.7
D. This scenario is not possible.

12. A beam of monochromatic light with a frequency of 5.09 × 1,014 Hz passes through layers of glycerol (n = 1.47), medium A, and then medium B. The angle of incidence in glycerol is \°, in medium A it is \ –10°, and coming out of A into B, the angle of refraction is \° (see figure). What could media A and B be, respectively?

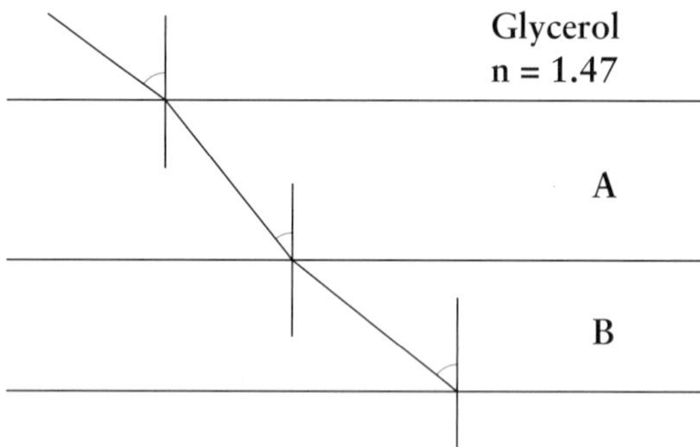

A. A could be flint glass (n = 1.66) and B could be corn oil (1.47).
B. A could be water (1.33) and B could be glycerol (1.47).
C. A could be corn oil (1.47) and B could be flint glass (1.66).
D. A could be flint glass (1.66) and B could be water (1.33).

13. What changes are observed when light originating in air is allowed to pass through a greenhouse?

A. Wavelength is longer, speed increases, and frequency remains the same
B. Wavelength is longer, speed increases, and frequency decreases
C. Wavelength is shorter, speed decreases, and frequency remains the same
D. Wavelength is shorter, speed decreases, and frequency increases

14. A cubic zirconium stud (n = 1.9) is placed on a table while an orange light with a wavelength of 620 nm is allowed to shine through it. What is the wavelength of this light while it is in the stud?

A. 310 nm
B. 322 nm
C. 620 nm
D. 1200 nm

15. A ray of light enters a prism in the shape of an isosceles right triangle perpendicular to its surface. The light enters through one of the legs and the index of refraction of the prism's constituents is 1.4. Where will the light go as it enters the prism? (sin 30° = 0.50 and sin 45° = 0.71)

A. It will not penetrate the prism.
B. It will penetrate the prism but cannot leave.
C. It will penetrate, continue through and hit the hypotenuse, and go through the second leg.
D. It will penetrate, continue through and hit the hypotenuse, and immediately leave through the hypotenuse.

16. A student sets up a double-slit opening and a screen and shines light of different colors through it. What light will create the greatest spacing between bands?

A. Red (3.5 × 1,014 Hz)
B. Orange (5.0 × 1,014 Hz)
C. Blue (6.4 × 1,014 Hz)
D. Violet (7.0 × 1,014 Hz)

KEY CONCEPTS

Refraction

Snell's law: $n_1 \sin \theta_1 = n_2 \sin \theta_2$

SNELL'S LAW

A gold doubloon rests on a rock 1 m below the surface of the ocean. A glass-bottom boat passes over the area and a passenger spots the coin at a 60° angle from the normal. If the glass layer is 3 cm thick, find the apparent depth of the coin. The indices of refraction are as follows: air: $n = 1$, glass: $n = 1.5$, salt water: $n = 1.34$.

1) Sketch the situation.

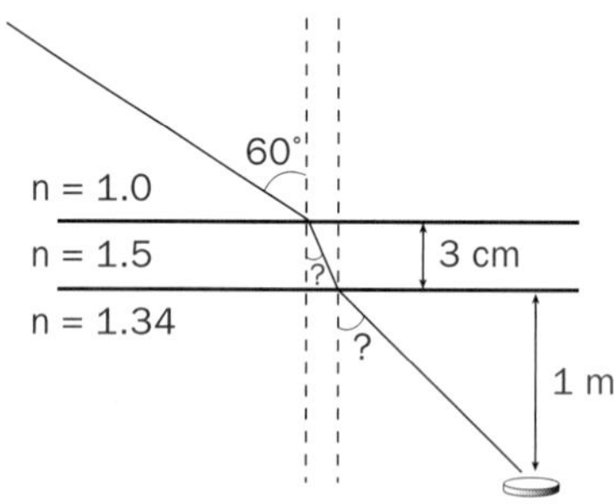

Light bends toward the normal when going from a medium with a lower refractive index to one with a higher refractive index.

Remember: *Our sketch need not be to scale; we use it to approximate what is going on and to keep track of the important data.*

TAKEAWAYS

Complex problems can be solved with a little bit of ingenuity. Snell's law is a simple concept and is likely to be one of the first steps in any problem dealing with the refraction of light. When light passes through multiple layers, the final angle can be determined merely by comparing the first and final media.

2) Apply Snell's law.

$n_1 \sin \theta_1 = n_2 \sin \theta_2$

$n_{air} \sin (\theta_a) = n_{glass} \sin (\theta_g)$

$(1) \sin 60° = 1.5 \sin (\theta_g)$

$\frac{[(1) \sin 60°]}{1.5} = \sin \theta_g \rightarrow \sin^{-1} 0.577 = \theta_g \approx 35°$

$\frac{[(1.5) \sin 35°]}{1.34} = \sin \theta_w \rightarrow \sin^{-1} 0.642 = \theta_w \approx 40°$

OR

$n_{air} \sin (\theta_a) = n_{water} \sin (\theta_w)$

$(1) \sin 60° = 1.34 \sin (\theta_w)$

$\frac{[(1) \sin 60°]}{1.34} = \sin \theta_w \rightarrow \sin^{-1} 0.646 = \theta_w \approx 40°$

Snell's law shows that light bends towards the normal (decreasing the angle) when it enters a medium with a higher refractive index. Here, we "plug-and-chug" through the formula to find the angles of light entry and exit for the two other substances.

THINGS TO WATCH OUT FOR

Light reflects off of media boundaries, too. Because of this, the refracted ray of light is less intense than the incident ray. Different wavelengths also have slightly different indices of refraction—this difference is what causes dispersion.

To do this more quickly, realize that when light passes through multiple layers, the final angle can be determined merely by comparing the first and final media. The glass in this example alters the distance that the light travels in the x-direction but has no bearing on the final angle because the light enters and exits the glass at the same angle.

---

3) Use trigonometry to determine how far the light goes.

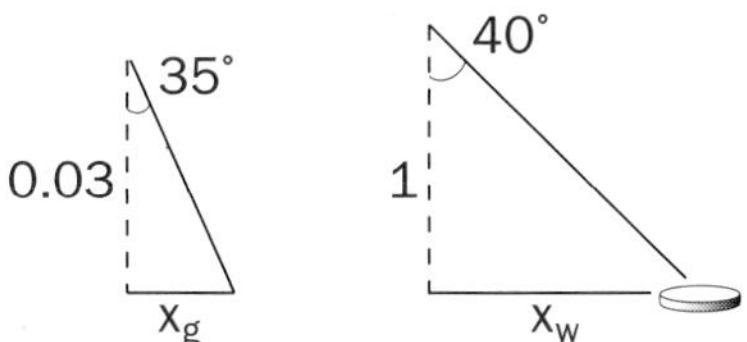

We know the thickness and depth of the glass and water, respectively, so we can use that information to determine how far the coin is from the ray of light the passenger sees. Light travels through a total of three media, but the distance of the observer from the glass doesn't actually matter. As long as he is looking 60° from the normal, he will see the coin. The trigonometry here is direct, using the relationship tan θ = opposite/adjacent or, in this case, $\frac{x}{y}$. The triangle in the glass, then, is $\tan 35° = \frac{x_g}{0.03}$, and $x_g \approx 0.02$. The triangle in the water is solved the same way, and $x_w = 0.85$. The ray of light escapes the water and glass 0.87 meters from the coin.

---

4) Find the object's image.

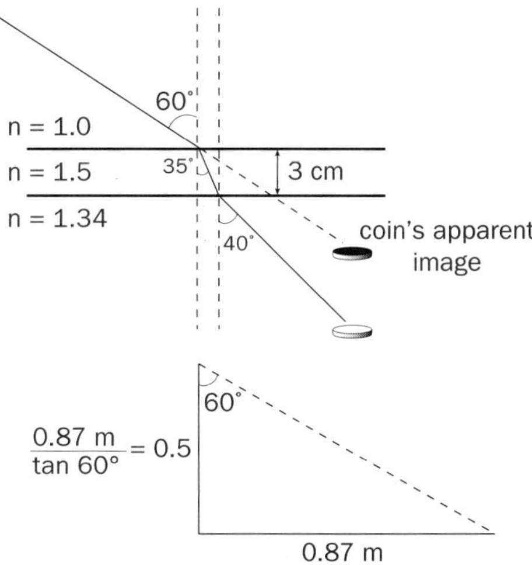

When the passenger sees the coin, his brain interprets light as a straight line. In other words, his brain doesn't consider the bending of light due to the refractive indices, and he perceives the coin to be closer than it actually is. We previously determined the x component of the light ray to be 0.87 m. The observer sees the coin at a 60° angle from the normal, so set up a new triangle with this angle. We are trying to find the depth of the coin—the y component of this triangle. Solving $\tan 60° = \frac{0.87}{y}$ gives us $y = 0.50$ m.

SIMILAR QUESTIONS

1) A fireman shines his flashlight through a smoky room at a 45° angle to a window. What angle does the beam of light make with the pane of glass on the outside? The indices of refraction are as follows: air: $n = 1$, glass: $n = 1.5$, smoke: $n = 1.1$.
2) A piece of gallium phosphide is frozen in ice. A beam of light is directed downward through the ice-gallium phosphide boundary at a 25° angle from the normal. The light emerges from the gallium phosphide 12.25 mm away from where it would have had the solid been pure ice. Find the thickness of the gallium phosphide layer. Gallium phosphide has the highest known optical density (3.5), and ice has the third lowest (1.31).
3) A jeweler is appraising the stone on a ring. He aims a beam of light 35° from the normal at a flat edge of the gem. What angle would he observe in the gem if the stone were diamond ($n = 2.4$)? What angle would he observe if the stone were zircon ($n = 1.9$)?

KEY CONCEPTS

Snell's law

Index of refraction

$n_1 \sin \theta_1 = n_2 \sin \theta_2$

REFRACTION

Light is refracted as it travels from a liquid into air unless the angle of incidence is greater than or equal to 51°, otherwise no light is refracted. What is the index of refraction of the liquid?

1) Write Snell's law.

$$n_1 \sin \theta_1 = n_2 \sin \theta_2$$
$$n_{liquid} \sin \theta_1 = n_{air} \sin \theta_2$$

Use Snell's law to write an equation relating the indices of refraction in the two media to the angles in those media. The angles, θ_1 and θ_2, are measured relative to the surface normals.

---

2) Set $\theta_2 = 90°$.

$$n_{liquid} \sin \theta_1 = n_{air} \sin \theta_2$$
$$n_{liquid} \sin \theta_{critical} = n_{air}$$
$$n_{liquid} = \frac{n_{air}}{\sin \theta_{critical}}$$

When no light is refracted, total internal reflection is occuring. The critical angle is the angle at which light experiences total internal reflection. That is when θ_2 (the exit angle) is 90°. In this case, $\theta_1 = \theta_{critical}$. Solve for n_{liquid}.

---

3) Plug in values.

$$n_{liquid} = \frac{n_{air}}{\sin \theta_{critical}}$$
$$n_{liquid} = \frac{1}{\sin 51°}$$
$$n_{liquid} = 1.29$$

The index of refraction of air is almost 1. Because the critical angle is less than 90°, the sine of the critical angle will be less than 1. Any number divided by a number less than 1 will lead to a larger result.

TAKEAWAYS

Snell's law gives the relationship between angles of incidence and refraction for a wave striking an interface between two media with different indices of refraction.

Observe that total internal reflection only occurs when the wave is passing from a medium with a higher index of refraction (lower speed) to a medium with a lower index of refraction (higher speed). This is true because the sine cannot be greater than 1.

THINGS TO WATCH OUT FOR

The angles in Snell's law are always measured relative to the surface normal.

SIMILAR QUESTIONS

1) A light ray is incident on crown glass ($n = 1.52$) at an angle of 30° to the normal. It is incident from air. What is the angle of refraction?
2) What is the critical angle for a diamond ($n = 2.42$) to air boundary?
3) A light ray passes from air into an unknown substance. The incident angle is 23° and the refracted angle is 14°. What is the index of refraction of the unknown substance?

TOTAL INTERNAL REFLECTION

KEY CONCEPTS

Refraction

Reflection

Total internal reflection

Snell's law

Light is directed from air (n = 1) into a glass tube (n = 1.3). A section is shown below. What is the maximum angle x that ensures that no light escapes the horizontal sides of the tube?

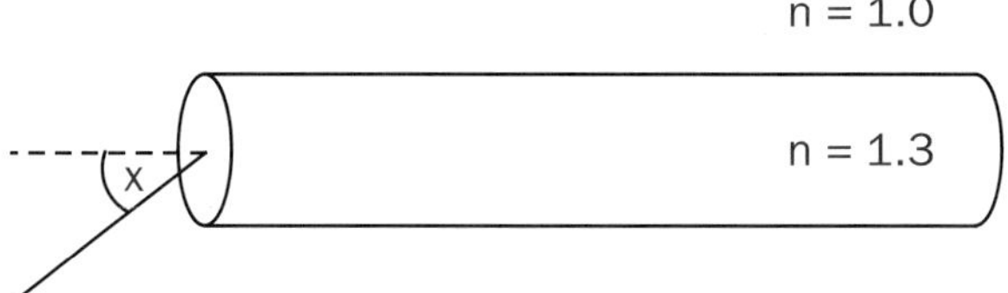

1) Draw a diagram of the ray traveling through the tube.

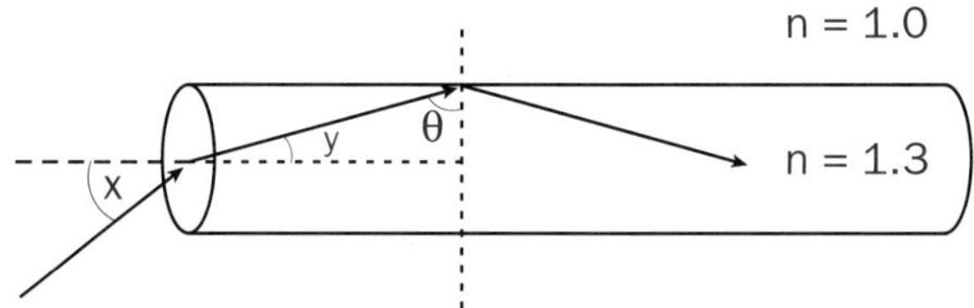

Draw a diagram of the ray entering the tube and reflecting off of the horizontal side. Draw the normal to each surface where the ray strikes, because the formulas for refraction are always in terms of the angles measured from the normal. Label the angles θ and *y*.

***Remember:** Light bends in toward the normal when entering a region of higher index of refraction.*

TAKEAWAYS

Drawing a diagram is key to solving this problem. The angles must be measured relative to the normal.

Note that the formula for a critical angle can be derived from Snell's law by setting $\theta_2 = 90°$.

---

2) Set θ equal to the critical angle.

$$\theta = \theta_c = \sin^{-1}\left(\frac{n_2}{n_1}\right) = \sin^{-1}\left(\frac{1}{1.3}\right) = 50.3°$$

If no light escapes from the horizontal side of the tube, then θ must be greater than or equal to the critical angle for the tube. This is referred to as Total Internal Reflection. The critical angle is given by $\theta_c = \sin^{-1}\left(\frac{n_2}{n_1}\right)$, where n_2 is the index of refraction outside of the tube and n_1 is the index of refraction inside the tube.

***Remember:** Total internal reflection can only occur when going from a high index to a low index of refraction.*

---

3) Find y from θ.

$\theta + y + 90 = 180$

$y = 90 - \theta = 39.7°$

θ and y are two angles of a right triangle. The sum of the angles of a triangle is 180°. Solve for angle y.

---

4) Use Snell's law to find *x*.

☞ generic: $n_1 \sin(\theta_1) = n_2 \sin(\theta_2)$
$(1)\sin(x) = (1.3)\sin(39.7°)$
$x = \sin^{-1}(1.3 \sin(39.7°)) = 56.1°$

Snell's law relates the indices of refraction for the two materials to the angles (measured relative to the normal) on both sides of the interface. This law is used to determine what happens when a light ray refracts. Plug in the value for y from step 3 and solve for x.

SIMILAR QUESTIONS

1) The critical angle for a certain interface is 35°. If the index of refraction of one material is 1.6, what is the index of refraction of the other material?
2) Light from air strikes a translucent plastic material. If the light strikes at an angle of 30° to the material and bends by 15°, what is the index of refraction of the plastic?
3) Light enters a glass slab ($n = 1.33$) from a vacuum. After traveling through the glass, it travels through a fluid ($n = 1.6$), through another section of glass, and then back into a vacuum. The two glass and fluid sections are parallel to each other. If the light enters the first glass slab at an angle of 35° to the normal, at what angle does it leave the final glass slab?

CONVERGING LENS

You have a 30 cm focal length converging lens with which to project an image onto a screen, such that the image is 5 times as large as the object. How far should the object be away from the screen?

1) Write the formula for magnification.

☞ $m = -\frac{i}{o} = -5$

For a single-lens system, the magnification is always the negative of the image distance over the object distance. The image is to be cast onto a screen, meaning that it cannot be a virtual image; it must be a real image. Virtual images cannot be projected, which explains why they are called virtual. Because a single lens can either create a virtual, erect image or a real, inverted image, the image must be real and inverted. This means that $m = -5$.

Remember: *A negative magnification indicates an inverted image.*

---

2) Write the lens formula.

☞ $\frac{1}{f} = \frac{1}{o} + \frac{1}{i}$

$\frac{1}{30} = \frac{1}{o} + \frac{1}{i}$

Understanding the sign conventions of this formula is the most important thing in this problem. Always make o, the distance from the object to the lens, a positive number; f is positive for converging lenses, negative for diverging lenses.

For a real (and thus inverted) image, i is always positive, and thus m is always negative (as long as you have taken o to be positive).

For a virtual (and thus erect) image, i is always negative and thus m is always positive.

If i is positive, the image is on the other side of the lens from the object. If i is negative, the image is on the same side as the object.

---

3) Solve the magnification formula and substitute it into the lens formula.

$-\frac{i}{o} = -5$

$i = 5o$

$\frac{1}{30} = \frac{1}{o} + \frac{1}{(5o)}$

KEY CONCEPTS

Lenses

$\frac{1}{f} = \frac{1}{o} + \frac{1}{i}$

$m = -\frac{i}{o}$

TAKEAWAYS

This question is posed in an unusual way—it does not ask for the object or image distance specifically. However, you should realize that on almost all quantitative lens (or mirror) problems, you will need to solve for the object or image distance, or both. When in doubt, write the magnification formula and lens formula and try to combine them.

Ray diagrams, although helpful conceptually, cannot be used to find exact values. A thorough understanding of the mathematical basis for these problems is essential.

THINGS TO WATCH OUT FOR

The biggest mistake on this problem is sign errors caused by a misunderstanding of the sign convention for these formulas. Know it well. Practice!

Many test takers do not understand the physical difference between a real and virtual image: a virtual image cannot be projected. To project an image, we would have to place a screen where the outgoing light rays converge. For a virtual image, though, the outgoing light rays never converge—they only *appear* to converge at the image location.

Also, many test takers do not realize that a single lens cannot produce a virtual, inverted image, nor can it produce a real, erect image. Use these facts to your advantage.

$$\frac{1}{30} = \frac{6}{(5o)}$$

$$\frac{5(o)}{6} = 30$$

$$o = \frac{180}{5} = 36 \text{ cm}$$

Remember: *We know that we are looking for a positive object distance. If you get a negative number here, you have made an error somewhere along the line.*

MCAT Pitfall: *We are not done. The questions asks for the distance between the object and the screen, not the object and the lens. We need to do more calculations to get the answer.*

---

4) Solve for the image distance.

$$m = -\frac{i}{o}$$

$$-5 = -\frac{1}{36}$$

$$i = 180 \text{ cm}$$

Use the expression for magnification from step 1 with the object distance we solved for in step 3.

Remember: *We know that we have to get a positive image distance. If you get a negative number here, you have made an error somewhere along the line.*

---

5) Add the image and object distance.

$$o + i = 36 + 180 = 216 \text{ cm}$$

The question asks for the distance between the object and the screen, or in other words, the distance between the object and image location. This is simply $o + i$.

Remember: *A real image always appears on the other side of the lens than the object. A virtual image appears on the same side as the object.*

SIMILAR QUESTIONS

1) What is the focal length of a lens that produces a real, inverted image 45 cm away from the lens for an object placed 20 cm from the lens?
2) A 2-cm-tall slide is placed 10 cm in front of a diverging lens with a focal length of 20 cm. What are the location and size of the resulting image?
3) What type and focal length of a lens should be used to produce an image that is the same size as the object, but flipped over, when the object is placed 20 cm away from the lens?

CHAPTER 11

ATOMIC PHENOMENA

Toward the end of the 19th century and throughout the 20th, research has shown that different sets of laws take effect at short distances, due to the wave nature of the discrete bits of matter. The theory that was developed to explain such phenomena is known as quantum mechanics. This chapter will primarily cover particular applications of quantum mechanical ideas to atomic physics but will not cover the formal theory of quantum mechanics. The first two topics covered here, blackbody radiation and the photoelectric effect, provided a first look at the quantum or discrete aspects of nature at the atomic level, particularly the discrete or particle nature of light. The quantum theory was later applied to the structure of the hydrogen atom, thus uncovering the discrete nature of the electron energies in hydrogen. This theory of the hydrogen atom, Bohr's theory, is reviewed along with a discussion (also due to Bohr) of the interaction of electromagnetic quanta (photons) with atoms. The application of quantum mechanics to nuclear physics is discussed in chapter 12.

MCAT Synopsis

Because all matter has temperature above absolute zero, all matter emits electromagnetic radiation.

THERMAL BLACKBODY RADIATION

At any temperature above absolute zero, matter will emit electromagnetic radiation. The amount of radiant energy emitted at a given wavelength depends on the temperature of the emitter. In addition, different materials may emit different amounts of radiant energy at a particular wavelength due to the differences in their atomic structure. Because of these complications, physicists at the turn of the century turned their attention to an **ideal radiator** known as a **blackbody** (because of the fact that any ideal radiator is also an ideal absorber and would appear totally black if it were at a lower temperature than its surroundings). In practice, a blackbody radiator can be approximated rather closely by radiation produced in a cavity within a hot object. Hence blackbody radiation is approximated by what is called **cavity radiation.**

Teacher Tip

Absolute zero is 0° Kelvin, at this temperature all random atomic movement stops.

Physicist Max Planck developed the theoretical derivation of the blackbody spectrum. His radiant spectrum for two blackbodies at different

TEACHER TIP

The only constant you'll need to know on this page is Planck's constant.

temperatures is shown in Figure 11.1. In the derivation Planck had to use a number called **Planck's constant** (h) whose value is given by:

$$h = 6.63 \times 10^{-34}\ J \cdot s = 4.14 \times 10^{-15}\ eV \cdot s$$

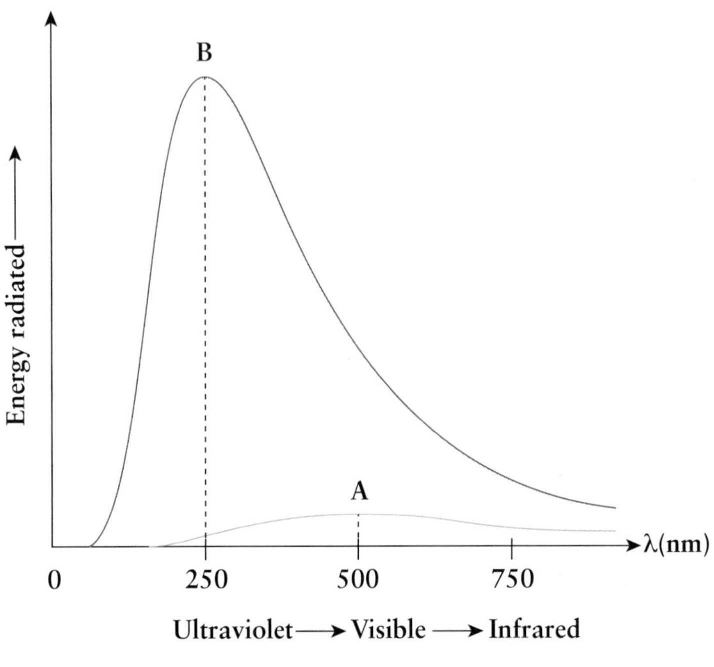

Figure 11.1

MCAT SYNOPSIS

The blackbody curve or spectrum shows the amount of energy radiated as a function of wavelength.

An analysis of Planck's formula for the blackbody spectrum shows that for a blackbody there is one wavelength at which the maximum amount of energy is emitted (λ_{peak}). This wavelength depends on the absolute temperature of the blackbody in a relation known as **Wien's displacement law,** which is expressed mathematically as:

$$\lambda_{peak} T = \text{constant}$$

The value of the constant is 2.90×10^{-3} m•K. Note that λ_{peak} is the wavelength at which more energy is emitted than any other wavelength. λ_{peak} **does not** refer to the maximum wavelength emitted.

Also, according to the **Stefan-Boltzmann law,** the total energy being emitted per unit area per second is proportional to the fourth power of the absolute temperature:

$$E_T = \sigma T^4$$

where σ is the Stefan-Boltzmann constant (5.67×10^{-8} J/s•m^2•K^4).

Example: In Figure 11.1 the radiant spectrum for two blackbodies is plotted. The first body is at temperature T_a, and the second body is at temperature T_b. How do the temperatures of the two blackbodies compare?

Solution: From the plots we find that $\lambda_{peak-a} = 2_{\lambda peak-b}$, and from Wien's law we know that $T_b = 2T_a$. [By the Stefan-Boltzmann law the emitted energy per unit area per second of blackbody b is $2^4 = 16$ times greater than that of blackbody a.]

PHOTOELECTRIC EFFECT

When light of a sufficiently high frequency (typically, blue or ultraviolet light) is incident on a metal in a vacuum, the metal emits electrons. This phenomenon, first discovered by Heinrich Hertz in 1887, is called the **photoelectric effect.** The minimum frequency of light that accomplishes this ejection of electrons is known as the **threshold frequency** f_T. The threshold frequency depends on the type of metal being exposed to the light. Einstein's explanation of these results was that the light beam consists of an integral number of light quanta, called photons, with the energy of each photon proportional to the frequency f of the light:

$$E = hf$$

The constant of proportionality h is Planck's constant.

It should also be noted that by knowing the frequency of the light you can easily find the wavelength λ via the relation:

$$\lambda = \frac{c}{f}$$

where c is the speed of light (3.00×10^8 m/s). These relations predict that shorter wavelength means higher frequency and therefore higher energy photons (toward the blue and ultraviolet end of the spectrum). Longer wavelength means lower frequency and therefore lower energy photons (toward the red and infrared end of the spectrum). Common units used for wavelength include nanometers (1 nm = 10^{-9} m) and Angstroms (1 Å = 10^{-10} m).

In the photoelectric effect, if the frequency of a photon incident on a metal is at the threshold frequency for the metal, the electron barely escapes

TEACHER TIP

The energy of a photon increases with increasing frequency. The reason we only discuss electrons being ejected from metals is due to the weak hold that metals have on their valence electrons. Metals are elements with very small electronegativities on the left side of the periodic table.

MCAT FAVORITE

The energy, E, of a quantum of light (photon) of frequency f is: E = hf.

MCAT SYNOPSIS

Wavelength and frequency of light in vacuum are related to speed of light by c = λf, just as wavelength, frequency, and velocity of any wave are related by v = λf.

MCAT SYNOPSIS

$E = hf = hc/\lambda$, which says that higher frequency or shorter wavelength light has higher energy, and lower frequency or longer wavelength light has lower energy.

TEACHER TIP

The photon's energy is converted into ejecting the electron (the amount required by the work function will be given in the question) and any excess energy is converted into the kinetic energy of the electron. This concept appears often on the MCAT.

MCAT SYNOPSIS

A photon can liberate an electron from a metal surface (photoelectric effect) only if the energy of the photon, $E = hf$, is greater than or equal to the work function, W, of the metal.

from the metal. However, if the frequency of an incident photon is above the threshold frequency of the metal, the photon will have more than enough energy to eject a single electron, and the excess energy will be converted to kinetic energy of the ejected electron. The maximum kinetic energy can be calculated from the formula:

$$K = hf - W$$

where W is the **work function** of the metal in question (the minimum energy required to eject an electron) which is related to the threshold frequency of that metal by:

$$W = hf_T$$

So for $f > f_T$ the photon will eject electrons with the excess energy appearing as kinetic energy (K). For $f < f_T$ the photon does not carry enough energy to eject an electron from the metal.

We can think of all of the electrons liberated from the metal by the photoelectric effect as producing a net charge flow per unit time, or a current. Provided that a light beam's frequency is above the threshold frequency of the metal, light beams of greater intensity produce greater current. This is because the higher the intensity of the beam, the greater the number of photons per unit time that fall on an electrode, producing a greater number of electrons per unit time liberated from the metal. When the light's frequency is above threshold frequency, the current is directly proportional to the intensity of the light beam.

Example: If the work function of a metal is 2.00 eV and blue light of frequency 6.00×10^{14} Hz is incident on the metal, will there be photo ejection of electrons? If so, how much kinetic energy will an electron carry away?

Solution: If the photons have a frequency of 6.00×10^{14} Hz, each photon has an energy given by:

$$\begin{aligned} E &= hf \\ &= (4.14 \times 10^{-15})(6.00 \times 10^{14}) \\ &= 2.48 \text{ eV} \end{aligned}$$

Clearly then, any given photon has more than enough energy to get an electron in the metal to overcome the 2.00 eV barrier. In fact, the excess kinetic energy carried away by the electron turns out to be:

$$\begin{aligned} K &= hf - W \\ &= 2.48 - 2.00 \\ &= 0.48 \text{ eV} \end{aligned}$$

THE BOHR MODEL OF THE HYDROGEN ATOM

A. ENERGY LEVELS

The hydrogen atom consists of an electron in orbit about a single, more massive, proton. As such, it is the simplest atom to describe and is a proving ground for any atomic theory. Before a more complete quantum mechanical description was developed, Niels Bohr proposed a model of the hydrogen atom consisting of the single electron in discrete circular orbits about the proton. It was necessary for Bohr to resort to new quantum ideas, because a classical model of hydrogen would require the electron to continuously radiate electromagnetic waves, thereby losing energy and spiraling into the proton. Bohr postulated that there were **specific stable, or allowed, orbits** of quantized (discrete) energy in which electrons did not radiate energy. This led him to deduce an **energy level formula.**

> **MCAT SYNOPSIS**
>
> The lowest energy (ground state) of an electron in hydrogen is negative. Higher energy bound states are also negative in energy but progressively smaller in magnitude.

The Bohr energy corresponding to the closest allowed orbit to the nucleus or the **ground state** (n = 1), is –13.6 eV. The energies corresponding to orbits farther away from the nucleus (n = 2,3,4,...) are less negative and therefore greater, until the electron is given so much energy that it is free from the electrostatic (coulomb) pull of the nucleus and can have any positive energy **(ionization).** An electron occupying one of these higher energy orbits or energy levels, but still bound to the proton, is said to be in an **excited state.** The quantum energy levels in the Bohr model of the hydrogen atom can be arranged from lowest to highest, each with an associated **principal quantum number** (n) that is a positive integer from n = 1 to n = ∞. The energy levels for hydrogen are given in electronvolts by the formula:

> **TEACHER TIP**
>
> The higher the principal quantum number, the more energetic the electron. Quantum numbers are an essential topic on the MCAT.

> **MCAT SYNOPSIS**
>
> Ionization means the electron ends up with an energy of at least 0 eV and is unbound (free).

$$E_n = \frac{-13.6}{n^2} \quad \text{(hydrogen)}$$

ELECTRON ENERGY LEVELS IN HYDROGEN

Principal quantum number n	Energy level E_n
1	$\frac{-13.6}{1}$ eV = −13.6 eV
2	$\frac{-13.6}{4}$ eV = −3.40 eV
3	$\frac{-13.6}{9}$ eV = −1.51 eV
4	$\frac{-13.6}{16}$ eV = −0.85 eV
•	• •
•	• •
•	• •
∞	$\frac{-13.6}{\infty}$ eV = 0 eV

Positive energy states have no principal quantum number, because the electron is not bound to the proton. It is in a free electron state and can have any positive energy.

B. EMISSION AND ABSORPTION OF LIGHT

It was found from experiments that hydrogen atoms radiate light only at particular frequencies. Bohr put forward a set of postulates that form the basis of his model. The postulates are:

1. Energy levels of the electron are stable and discrete. They correspond to specific orbits.
2. An electron emits or absorbs radiation **only** when making a transition from one energy level to another (from one allowed orbit to another).
3. To jump from a lower energy (inner orbit) to a higher energy (outer orbit), an electron must **absorb** a photon of precisely the right frequency such that the photon's energy (hf) equals the energy difference between the two orbits.

TEACHER TIP

Bohr's model will be sufficient for any of the calculations you will need.

MCAT SYNOPSIS

Conservation of energy applies to absorption and emission. For absorption, energy of photon absorbed equals increase in energy of electron. For emission, loss of electron energy equals energy of photon emitted.

4. When jumping from a higher energy (outer orbit) to a lower energy (inner orbit), an electron **emits** a photon of a frequency such that the photon's energy (hf) is exactly the energy difference between the two orbits.

Bohr's initial ideas were replaced with the advent of full quantum mechanical theories of atomic structure. In contemporary theories, the electron is not envisioned as following a circular or elliptical path like the planets do in orbiting the sun. However, the Bohr model is still useful for certain calculations.

MCAT FAVORITE

Absorption yields color. Emission yields fluorescence.

An electron in the lowest allowed energy level (n = 1 or ground state) cannot emit any more energy (though it could absorb radiation and jump up to a higher energy level). An electron occupying an **excited state** can either emit radiation when it jumps down to a lower energy level or absorb radiation when it jumps up to a higher energy level.

Bohr's third and fourth postulates can be used to find the frequency of radiation emitted or absorbed by an electron in going from energy level E_i to energy level E_f. The change in the electron's energy is $\Delta E = E_f - E_i$. Because bound state energy levels are negative, if ΔE is negative then the electron has jumped from a higher, less negative energy state (less tightly bound state) to a lower, more negative energy state (more tightly bound state). There is then an **emission** of a photon of frequency f where:

TEACHER TIP

An excited state is any orbit higher than the electron's ground state; thus, it has more energy than the ground state.

$$\Delta E < 0$$
$$hf = -\Delta E \text{ (emission)}$$

On the other hand, if ΔE is positive, then the electron has **absorbed** a photon and jumped from a lower, more negative energy state to a higher, less negative energy state. The absorbed photon has a frequency f where:

$$\Delta E > 0$$
$$hf = \Delta E \text{ (absorption)}$$

Example: What wavelength of light is emitted by a hydrogen electron going from the n = 5 to the n = 2 energy levels?

Solution: For hydrogen, the energy for a given principle quantum number n is given in electron-volts by

$$E = \frac{-13.6}{n^2}$$

Since the electron goes **from** n = 5 **to** n = 2, the initial energy level is:

$$E_i = E_5 = \frac{-13.6}{25} = -0.544 \text{ eV}$$

MCAT SYNOPSIS

Use E = hf to find frequency of photon given energy of photon.

The final energy level is:

$$E_f = E_2 = \frac{-13.6}{4} = -3.40 \text{ eV}$$

Therefore:

$$\begin{aligned}\Delta E &= E_f - E_i \\ &= -3.40 + 0.544 \\ &= -2.856 \text{ eV}\end{aligned}$$

TEACHER TIP

There is no such thing as a negative frequency, so don't worry about what sign ÄE signifies when calculating the frequency.

The negative value of ΔE confirms that the light is emitted. The frequency is found by:

$$\begin{aligned}f &= \frac{|\Delta E|}{h} \\ &= \frac{2.856}{4.14 \times 10^{-15}} \\ &= 6.90 \times 10^{14} \text{ Hz}\end{aligned}$$

Now we can easily find the wavelength (and convert to different units for comparison):

MCAT SYNOPSIS

Use c = λf to find wavelength of photon from frequency of photon or vice versa.

$$\begin{aligned}\lambda &= \frac{c}{f} \\ &= \frac{3.00 \times 10^{8}}{6.90 \times 10^{14}} \\ &= 4.35 \times 10^{-7} \text{ m} \\ &= 435 \text{ nm} \\ &= 4350 \text{ Å}\end{aligned}$$

Example: What wavelength of light is needed to free an electron from the ground state of hydrogen?

Solution: As previously mentioned, the electron in the ground state (n = 1) of hydrogen has an energy of –13.6 eV. Negative energies mean a bound state; positive energies mean a free state. It would take a photon of at least +13.6 eV to free the electron. Find the frequency:

$$f = \frac{E}{h} = \frac{13.6}{4.14 \times 10^{-15}} = 3.29 \times 10^{15} \text{ Hz}$$

Now the wavelength is given by:

$$\lambda = \frac{c}{f} = \frac{3.00 \times 10^{8}}{3.29 \times 10^{15}} = 9.12 \times 10^{-8} \text{ m} = 91.2 \text{ nm} = 912 \text{ Å}$$

FLUORESCENCE

Fluorescence refers to the process in which certain substances emit visible light when excited by other radiation, usually ultraviolet radiation. Photons corresponding to ultraviolet radiation have relatively high frequencies (short wavelengths). After being excited to a higher energy state by the ultraviolet radiation, the electron returns to its original state in two or more steps. By returning in two or more steps, each step involves less energy. In each step a lower frequency (longer wavelength) photon is emitted, whose wavelength may fall in the visible portion of the spectrum. This is the principle of the fluorescent light.

MCAT SYNOPSIS

An excited electron may make one large jump back to the ground state, or a number of smaller jumps, i.e. an electron in n = 4 may jump from 4 to 1 or from 4 to 2 to 1, and so on.

PRACTICE QUESTIONS

1. Planck's constant is equal to which of the following?

    I. Minimum energy of one photon
    II. Ratio of a particle's kinetic energy to its wavelength
    III. Ratio of a photon's energy to its frequency

    A. I only
    B. III only
    C. II and III only
    D. I, II, and III

2. The temperature of a household halogen light is slowly increased. The apparent color of the light

    A. approaches violet/ultraviolet.
    B. approaches red/infrared.
    C. remains constant.
    D. remains outside the visible spectrum.

3. Radiation is emitted from a small window in a large furnace. When the temperature of the furnace is doubled, the peak emitted energy

    A. remains constant.
    B. increases by a factor of 2.
    C. increases by a factor of 4.
    D. increases by a factor of 16.

4. The diagram below illustrates the energy from the radiation emitted by a black body at four different temperatures. What curve represents the body at the highest temperature?

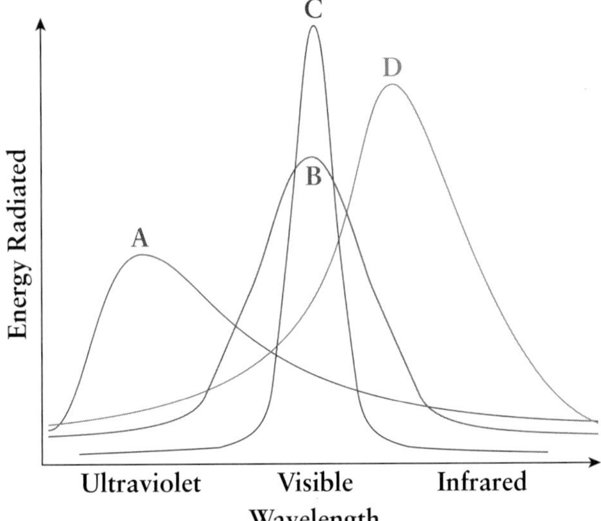

    A. A
    B. B
    C. C
    D. D

5. An electron in a metal object is struck by a photon whose energy is exactly equal to the metal's work function. The electron will

    A. be ejected from the atom and will move faster than its previous velocity.
    B. be ejected from the atom and move at its previous velocity.
    C. be ejected from the atom and move slower than its previous velocity.
    D. not be ejected from the atom, but will be accelerated to a greater velocity.

6. The figure below illustrates an electron with initial energy of –10 eV moving from point A to point B. What change accompanies the movement of the electron?

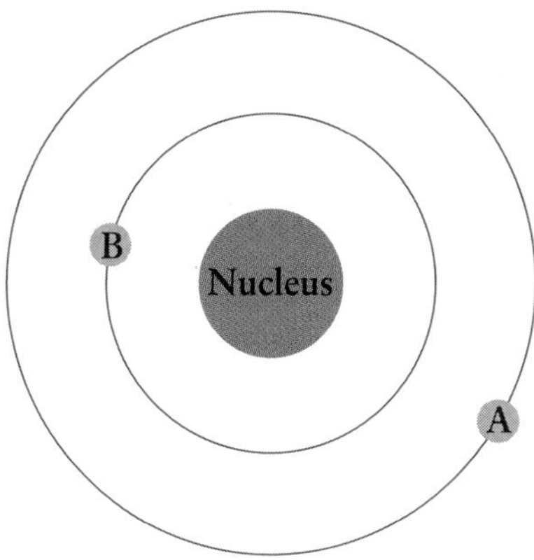

A. Absorption of a photon
B. Emission of a photon
C. Decrease in the atom's work function
D. Increase in the atom's total energy

7. Continuing with the figure from the previous question, what is the magnitude of the change in energy during the process?

A. 10 eV
B. 20 eV
C. 30 eV
D. 40 eV

8. Which of the following is NOT true about an electron that moves from its ground state to its excited state?

A. It carries more kinetic energy.
B. It is more likely to be affected by ionizing radiation.
C. It is more likely to be ejected in the photoelectric effect.
D. It feels a stronger electrostatic force with the nucleus.

9. After moving freely for some time, an electron falls into orbit in an atom that was previously missing an electron. Which of the following diagrams best represents the Bohr energy of the electron before and after it falls into orbit?

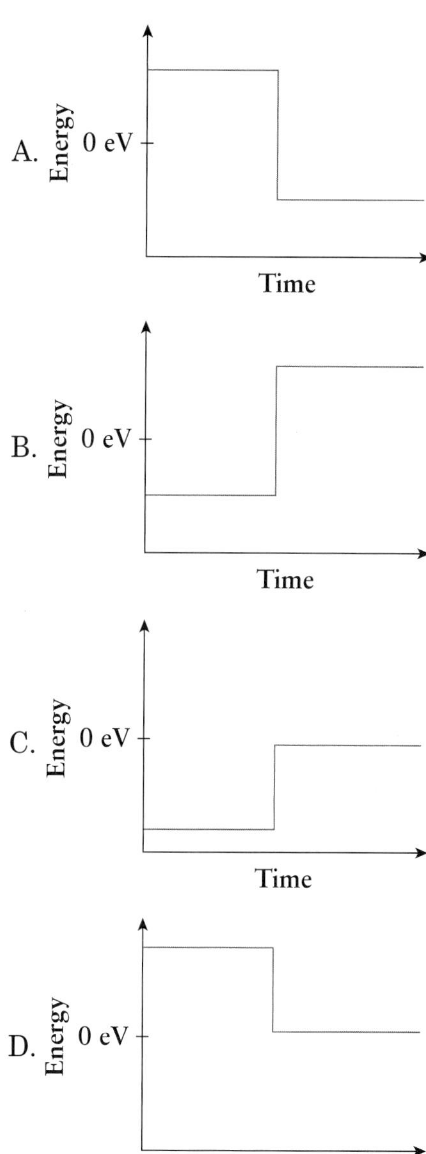

10. In a certain atom, the energy of electrons in the first energy level is equal to –20 eV. When one of these electrons is struck by a photon carrying 10 eV of energy, the electron

A. absorbs the photon and moves to the second energy level.
B. absorbs the photon and moves with a faster velocity within the same energy level.
C. absorbs the photon and is ejected from the atom.
D. does not absorb the photon.

11. A material is exposed to radiation in order to excite its electrons. When the electrons return to ground state, which of the following types of energy will be released?

A. Heat
B. Fluorescent light
C. X-rays
D. Colored-light spectrum

12. An excited electron residing in the third energy level of an atom carries an energy of –2 eV. What is the maximum frequency of light that it can emit? Let h equal Planck's constant in terms of eV·s.

A. $16/h$ Hz
B. $6/h$ Hz
C. $4/h$ Hz
D. $2/h$ Hz

13. Most of Niels Bohr's atomic model is still intact today. Which of the following theories is NOT an accepted premise in the accepted atomic model?

A. Every atom contains discrete energy levels.
B. Unless energy is added or removed, an electron will not change its energy level.
C. Electrons in a certain energy level will remain in a circular or elliptical orbit around the nucleus.
D. The energy of an electron can only change if the electron changes energy levels.

14. Ultraviolet light is more likely to cause a photoelectric effect than visible light. This is because photons of ultraviolet light

A. have a longer wavelength.
B. have a higher velocity.
C. are not visible.
D. have a higher energy.

15. A line appears on the emission spectrum for every possible photon that can be emitted by an atom. How many lines are on the emission spectrum for an atom with two possible excited states?

A. 1
B. 2
C. 3
D. 4

16. In the diagram below, what transition involves the release of a photon with the longest wavelength?

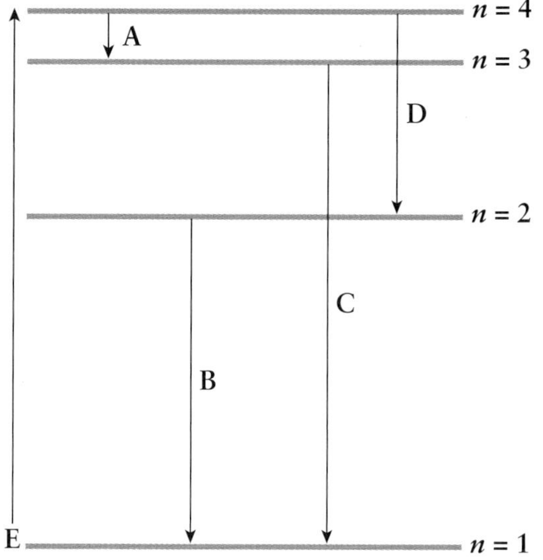

A. A
B. B
C. C
D. D

17. Infrared light is incident on a metal with a relatively high work function. An electron in the object will most likely

A. be ejected immediately.
B. be ejected after the light shines on the metal for a sufficient amount of time.
C. be ejected only if the intensity of the light is high.
D. not be ejected.

18. Which of the following properties of hydrogen does NOT explain why it is the simplest proving ground for most atomic theories?

A. It cannot gain an electron.
B. It typically contains no neutrons.
C. It typically contains only one energy level.
D. It contains a minimum number of protons and electrons.

19. The energy of a photon is increased. Which of the following could NOT have occurred?

A. The frequency of the photon was increased.
B. The color of the light was changed.
C. The photon was accelerated.
D. The wavelength of the light was decreased.

20. The figure below depicts the energy levels for a certain metal. If an electron in the second energy level is struck by a photon, it will be ejected from the atom if

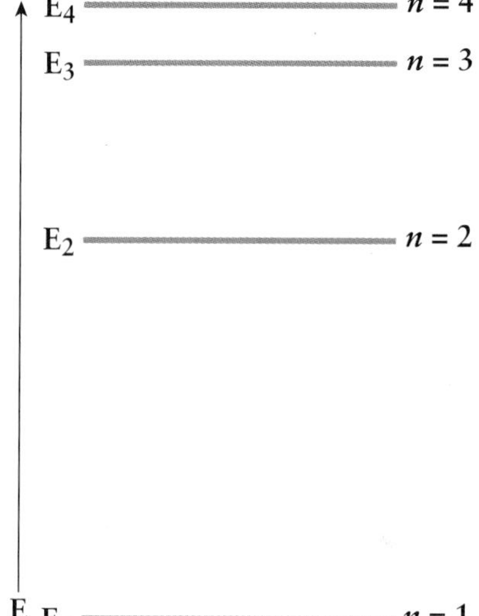

A. $E_{photon} > E4$.
B. $E_{photon} + E2 > 0$.
C. $E_{photon} < E2$.
D. $E_{photon} > E4 - E2$.

KEY CONCEPTS

Review notes chapter 11

Energy levels in hydrogen atoms

Wavelength/frequency

Energy units

ENERGY EMISSION FROM ELECTRONS

An electron in a hydrogen atom moves from the third energy level to the ground state. What is the wavelength of the emitted photon? (1 eV = 1.6×10^{-19} J, $h = 6.63 \times 10^{-34}$ J · s)

1) Determine the difference in energy between the energy levels.

For hydrogen, $E = \dfrac{-13.6 \text{ eV}}{n^2}$

$$E_1 = \frac{-13.6}{(1)^2} = -13.6 \text{ eV}$$

$$E_3 = \frac{-13.6}{(3)^2} = -1.51 \text{ eV}$$

$$\Delta E = E_3 - E_1 = 12.09 \text{ eV}$$

The energy values for hydrogen energy levels are given by $E = \dfrac{-13.6 \text{ eV}}{n^2}$, where E will be in electron-volts (eV). The ground state of the atom corresponds to $n = 1$. As the principle quantum number n increases, so does the energy of the electron. As the limit n goes to infinity, note that $E = 0$. Physically, this represents an atom that is completely ionized.

***Remember:** One eV is the amount of energy required to move an electron through a potential difference of 1 volt. Remember that it is related to Joules by the charge of an electron, 1.6×10^{-19}.*

TAKEAWAYS

Remember that the energy of the photon must be equal to the energy lost by the electron. This comes from the conservation of energy. Alternately, when a photon is absorbed by an atom, the gain in energy of the electron is the energy of the photon.

---

2) Find the wavelength of the photon from the energy lost by the electron.

$E = hf = \dfrac{hc}{\lambda}$.

Combination of the equations $E = hf$ and $\lambda f = c$

hc = 1,240 eV-nm,

Therefore,

$$\lambda = \frac{1{,}240 \text{ eV-nm}}{12.09 \text{ eV}}$$

$$\lambda = 103 \text{ nm}$$

On Test Day, you can quickly relate photon energy and wavelength by remembering that harmless radio waves with low energy have very large wavelengths, thus the inverse relationship.

For any photon, the energy is related to the frequency by $E = hf$. The energy of the photon must be equal to the energy lost by the electron in the transition. Use $c = f\lambda$ to convert to wavelength. Remember that for any photon, $E = \dfrac{1{,}240}{\lambda}$, when E is in eV and λ is in nm. Knowing this will drastically reduce your time spent on these problems.

THINGS TO WATCH OUT FOR

Remember that "completely ionized" means that an electron has an energy equal to zero (this corresponds to an infinite quantum number n).

SIMILAR QUESTIONS

1) What energy level is occupied by an electron, which was initially in the ground state, of a hydrogen atom when a photon of wavelength 55 nm is absorbed by the atom?
2) A photon of frequency 6×10^{14} Hz is ejected from an atom when an electron changes energy states. What was the change in energy of the electron, in joules?
3) What is the maximum wavelength that a photon must have to cause a ground-state electron in a hydrogen atom to be completely ejected from the atom?

CHAPTER 12

NUCLEAR PHENOMENA

The subject of this final chapter is the nucleus and nuclear phenomena, and it begins with a review of some of the standard terminology used in nuclear physics. The concept of binding energy and the equivalent concept of the mass defect are then introduced. Briefly, an amount of energy, called the binding energy, is required to break up a given nucleus into its constituent protons and neutrons. That energy is converted to mass via Einstein's $E = mc^2$, resulting in a larger mass for the constituent protons and neutrons than that of the original nucleus, the difference being called the mass defect. The remainder, and bulk, of the chapter is concerned with a brief discussion of nuclear reactions (fission and fusion) and an extended treatment of radioactive decay, which itself is presented in two distinct parts. The first deals with the four different types of radioactive decay and a discussion of the reaction equations that describe them. The second covers the general problem of determining the number of nuclei that have not decayed as a function of time, along with the associated concept of the half-life of a decay process.

NUCLEI

At the center of an atom lies its nucleus, consisting of one or more **nucleons** (protons or neutrons) held together with considerably more energy than the energy needed to hold electrons in orbit around the nucleus. The radius of the nucleus is about 100,000 times smaller than the radius of the atom. Some common nuclear properties are:

Teacher Tip

Protons and neutron have the same mass; the only difference is that protons have a positive charge while neutrons are neutral.

A. ATOMIC NUMBER (Z)

Z is always an integer, and is equal to the **number of protons** in the nucleus. Each element has a unique number of protons; therefore the atomic number Z identifies the element. Z is used as a presubscript to the chemical symbol in **isotopic notation.** The chemical symbols and the atomic numbers of all the elements are given in the periodic table.

MCAT Synopsis

Each element is defined by its atomic number Z (number of protons in the nucleus).

Atomic Numbers of the Chemical Elements

Atomic number Z	Chemical symbol	Element name
1	H	hydrogen
2	He	helium
3	Li	lithium
.	.	.
.	.	.
92	U	uranium
.	.	.
.	.	.
.	.	.

MCAT SYNOPSIS

Protons and neutrons are both referred to as nucleons.

B. MASS NUMBER (A)

A is an integer equal to the total **number of nucleons** (neutrons and protons) in a nucleus. Let N represent the number of neutrons in a nucleus. The equation relating A, N, and Z is simply:

$$A = N + Z$$

In isotopic notation, A is a presuperscript to the chemical symbol.

TEACHER TIP

Looking at the periodic table we can see that many elements have a mass number that is a noninteger. That's because the periodic table shows atomic weight, which is the average mass of all known isotopes.

Examples: ${}^{1}_{1}H$ —a single proton; the nucleus of ordinary hydrogen.

${}^{4}_{2}He$ —the nucleus of ordinary helium, consisting of 2 protons and 2 neutrons. It is also known as an alpha particle (α-particle).

${}^{235}_{92}U$ —a fissionable form of uranium, consisting of 92 protons and 143 neutrons.

C. ISOTOPE

The nucleus of a given element can have different numbers of neutrons and hence different mass numbers. For a nucleus of a given element with a given number of protons (atomic number Z), the various nuclei with different numbers of neutrons are called **isotopes** of that element. The term *isotope* is also used in a generic sense to refer to any nucleus. The term ***radionuclide*** is another generic term used to refer to any radioactive isotope, especially those used in **nuclear medicine.**

MCAT SYNOPSIS

All isotopes of a given element have the same value of Z, but different values of N and A.

Example: The three isotopes of hydrogen are:

^1_1H —a single proton; the nucleus of ordinary hydrogen.

^2_1H —a proton and a neutron together often called a **deuteron**; the nucleus of one type of heavy hydrogen called **deuterium.**

^3_1H —a proton and two neutrons together often called a **triton**; the nucleus of a heavier type of heavy hydrogen called **tritium.**

TEACHER TIP

The only difference between hydrogen, deuterium, and tritium is the number of neutrons. All still have one proton and one electron.

D. ATOMIC MASS AND ATOMIC MASS UNIT

Atomic mass is most commonly measured in **atomic mass units** (abbreviated amu or simply u). By definition, 1 amu is exactly one-twelfth the mass of the neutral carbon-12 atom (not just the nucleus—the atom includes the nucleus and all six electrons). In terms of more familiar mass units:

$$1 \text{ amu} = 1.66 \times 10^{-27} \text{ kg} = 1.66 \times 10^{-24} \text{ g}$$

E. ATOMIC WEIGHT

Because isotopes exist, atoms of a given element can have different masses. The atomic weight refers to a weighted average of the **masses** (not the weights) of an element. The average is weighted according to the natural abundances of the various isotopic species of an element. The atomic weight can be measured in amu.

Example: Of hydrogen, 99.985499% occurs in the common ^1H isotope with a mass of 1.00782504 u. About 0.0142972% occurs as deuterium with a mass (including the electron) of 2.01410 u, and about 0.0003027% occurs as tritium with a mass of 3.01605 u. The atomic weight of hydrogen $A_r(H)$ is the sum of the mass of each isotope multiplied by its natural abundance (x):

$$\begin{aligned} A_r(H) &= m_{1H}x_{1H} + m_{2H}x_{2H} + m_{3H}x_{3H} \\ &= (1.00782504)(0.99985499) \\ &\quad + (2.01410)(0.000142972) \\ &\quad + (3.01605)(0.000003027) \\ &= 1.00797 \text{ amu} \end{aligned}$$

MCAT SYNOPSIS

The mass of a nucleus is always less than the combined masses of its constituent protons and neutrons.

NUCLEAR BINDING ENERGY AND MASS DEFECT

Every nucleus (other than ${}^{1}_{1}H$) has a smaller mass than the combined mass of its constituent protons and neutrons. The difference is called the **mass defect.** Scientists had difficulty explaining why this mass defect occurred until Einstein discovered the equivalence of matter and energy, embodied by the equation $E = mc^2$. The mass defect is a result of matter that has been converted to energy. This energy, called **binding energy,** holds the nucleons together in the nucleus. (Note: The binding energy per nucleon peaks at iron, which implies that iron is the most stable atom. In general, intermediate-sized nuclei are more stable than large and small nuclei.)

TEACHER TIP

In the equation, m stands for mass and c stands for the speed of light.

The mass defect and binding energy of ${}^{4}He$ are calculated in the following example.

Example: Measurements of the atomic mass of a neutron and a proton yield these results:

$$\text{proton} = 1.00728 \text{ amu}$$
$$\text{neutron} = 1.00867 \text{ amu}$$

A measurement of the atomic mass of a ${}^{4}He$ nucleus yields:

$${}^{4}He = 4.00260 \text{ amu}$$

${}^{4}He$ consists of 2 protons and 2 neutrons which should theoretically give a ${}^{4}He$ mass of:

$$\begin{aligned} Z(m_p) + N(m_n) &= 2(1.00728) + 2(1.00867) \\ &= 4.03190 \text{ amu} \end{aligned}$$

What is the mass defect and binding energy of this nucleus?

Solution: The difference $4.03190 - 4.00260 = 0.02930$ amu is the mass defect for ${}^{4}He$, and is interpreted as the conversion of mass into the binding energy of the nucleus. The rest energy of 1 amu is 932 MeV, so using $E = mc^2$ we find that $c^2 = 932$ MeV/amu. Therefore the binding energy of ${}^{4}He$ is:

$$\begin{aligned} \text{B.E.} &= \Delta m\, c^2 \\ &= (0.02930)(932) \\ &= 27.3 \text{ MeV} \end{aligned}$$

TEACHER TIP

Another way to approach this problem without knowing the rest energy of 1 amu would be to convert mass from amu into kilograms. Then you could simply multiply the mass by c^2, which is $(3 \times 108 \text{ m/s})^2$. Doing this would produce an answer in joules instead of MeV.

NUCLEAR REACTIONS AND DECAY

Nuclear reactions such as fusion, fission, and radioactive decay involve either combining or splitting the nuclei of atoms. Because the binding energy per nucleon is greatest for intermediate-sized atoms, when small atoms combine or large atoms split a great amount of energy is released.

MCAT SYNOPSIS

Fusion: combine smaller nuclei into larger nucleus.

Fission: split larger nucleus into smaller nuclei.

Both fusion and fission release energy because initial mass > final mass.

A. FUSION

Fusion occurs when small nuclei combine into a larger nucleus. As an example, many stars, including the Sun, power themselves by fusing four hydrogen nuclei to make one helium nucleus. By this method, the sun produces 4×10^{26} J every second. Here on Earth, researchers are trying to find ways to use fusion as an alternative energy source.

B. FISSION

Fission is a process by which a large nucleus splits into smaller nuclei. Spontaneous fission rarely occurs. However, by the absorption of a low energy neutron, fission can be induced in certain nuclei. Of special interest are those fission reactions that release more neutrons, because these other neutrons will cause other atoms to undergo fission. This, in turn, releases more neutrons, creating a chain reaction. Such induced fission reactions power commercial nuclear electric-generating plants.

Example: A fission reaction occurs when uranium-235 (U-235) absorbs a low energy neutron, briefly forming an excited state of U-236, which then splits into xenon-140, strontium-94, and x more neutrons. In isotopic notation form the reactions are:

$$^{235}_{92}\text{U} + ^{1}_{0}\text{n} \longrightarrow ^{236}_{92}\text{U} \longrightarrow ^{140}_{54}\text{Xe} + ^{94}_{38}\text{Sr} + x^{1}_{0}\text{n}$$

How many neutrons are produced in the last reaction?

Solution: The question is asking "What is x?" By treating each arrow as an equal sign, the problem is simply asking to balance the last "equation." The mass numbers (A) on either side of each arrow must be equal. This is an application of **nucleon** or **baryon number conservation,** which says that the total number of neutrons plus protons remains the same, even if neutrons are converted to protons and vice versa, as they are in some decays. Since 235 + 1 = 236, the first arrow is indeed balanced. To find the number of neutrons solve for x in the last equation (arrow):

$$\begin{aligned} 236 &= 140 + 94 + x \\ x &= 236 - 140 - 94 \\ &= 2 \end{aligned}$$

TEACHER TIP

With these types of problems, count the number of protons and neutrons. Oftentimes wrong answer choices will simply have an error with the number of protons.

MCAT SYNOPSIS

Total mass number, A, remains unchanged in nuclear reactions.

So there are two neutrons produced in this reaction. These neutrons are free to go on and be absorbed by more ^{235}U and cause more fissioning, and the process continues in a chain reaction. Note that it really was not necessary to know that the intermediate state $^{236}_{92}\text{U}$ was formed.

Some radioactive nuclei may be induced to fission via more than one **decay channel** or **decay mode.** For example, a different fission reaction may occur when uranium-235 absorbs a slow neutron and then immediately splits into barium-139, krypton-94, and three more neutrons with no intermediate state:

$$^{235}_{92}\text{U} + ^{1}_{0}\text{n} \longrightarrow ^{139}_{56}\text{Ba} + ^{94}_{36}\text{Kr} + 3^{1}_{0}\text{n}$$

C. RADIOACTIVE DECAY

Radioactive decay is a naturally occurring spontaneous decay of certain nuclei accompanied by the emission of specific particles. It could be classified as a certain type of fission. Radioactive decay problems are of three general types:

- The integer arithmetic of particle and isotope species
- Radioactive half-life problems
- The use of exponential decay curves and decay constants

1. Isotope Decay Arithmetic and Nucleon Conservation

Let the letters X and Y represent nuclear isotopes, and let us further consider the three types of decay particles and how they affect the mass number and atomic number of the **parent isotope** $^{A}_{Z}\text{X}$ and the resulting **daughter isotope** $^{A'}_{Z'}\text{Y}$ in the decay:

$$^{A}_{Z}\text{X} \longrightarrow ^{A'}_{Z'}\text{Y} + \text{emitted decay particle}$$

a. **Alpha decay** is the emission of an α-particle, which is a ^{4}He nucleus that consists of two protons and two neutrons. The alpha particle is very massive (compared to a beta particle) and doubly charged. Alpha particles interact with matter very easily; hence they do not penetrate shielding (such as lead sheets) very far.

MCAT SYNOPSIS

An α-particle is a helium nucleus with 2 protons and 2 neutrons, i.e., ^{4}He. Alpha particles do not have any electrons so they carry a charge of +2.

The emission of an α-particle means that the daughter's atomic number Z will be 2 less than the parent's atomic number and the daughter's mass number will be 4 less than the parent's mass number. This can be expressed in two simple equations:

α decay

$$Z_{daughter} = Z_{parent} - 2$$
$$A_{daughter} = A_{parent} - 4$$

The generic alpha decay reaction is then:

$${}^{A}_{Z}X \longrightarrow {}^{A-4}_{Z-2}Y + \alpha$$

Example: Suppose a parent X alpha decays into a daughter Y such that:

$${}^{238}_{92}X \longrightarrow {}^{A'}_{Z'}Y + \alpha$$

What are the mass number (A′) and atomic number (Z′) of the daughter isotope Y?

Solution: Since $\alpha = {}^{4}_{2}He$, balancing the mass numbers and atomic numbers is all that needs to be done:

$$238 = A' + 4$$
$$A' = 234$$
$$92 = Z' + 2$$
$$Z' = 90$$

So A′ = 234 and Z′ = 90. Note that it was not necessary to know the chemical species of the isotopes to do this problem. However, it would have been possible to look at the periodic table and see that Z = 92 means X is uranium-238 (${}^{238}_{92}U$) and that Z = 90 means Y is thorium-234 (${}^{234}_{90}Th$).

b. **Beta decay** is the emission of a β-particle, which is an electron given the symbol e^- or β^-. Electrons do not reside in the nucleus, but are emitted by the nucleus when a neutron in the nucleus decays into a proton and a β^- (and an antineutrino). Because an electron is singly charged, and about 1,836 times lighter than a proton, the beta radiation from radioactive decay is more penetrating than alpha radiation. In some cases of induced decay, a positively charged antielectron known as a **positron** is emitted. The positron is given the symbol e^+ or β^+.

MCAT SYNOPSIS

A β^--particle is also called a β-particle and is just an electron.

β^- decay means that a neutron disappears and a proton takes its place. Hence, the parent's mass number is unchanged and the parent's atomic number is increased by 1. In other words, the daughter's A is the same as the parent's, and the daughter's Z is one more than the parent's.

In positron decay, a proton (instead of a neutron as in β^- decay) splits into a positron and a neutron. Therefore, a β^+ decay means that the

MCAT SYNOPSIS

A β^+-particle is positron, which is a particle with same mass as electron but opposite charge.

parent's mass number is unchanged and the parent's atomic number is decreased by 1. In other words, the daughter's A is the same as the parent's, and the daughter's Z is one less than the parent's. In equation form:

β^- decay

$$Z_{daughter} = Z_{parent} + 1$$
$$A_{daughter} = A_{parent}$$

β^+ decay

$$Z_{daughter} = Z_{parent} - 1$$
$$A_{daughter} = A_{parent}$$

TEACHER TIP

Both types of beta decay require conservation of charges. If a negative charge is created, a positive charge must be created as well (via neutron changed into a proton). Conversely, if a positive charge is created, a negative charge must be created as well (via proton changed into neutron).

Remember negative beta decay creates a negative beat particle and positive beta decay creates a positive beta particle.

The generic negative beta decay reaction is:

$$^{A}_{Z}X \longrightarrow {}^{A}_{Z+1}Y + \beta^-$$

The generic positive beta decay reaction is:

$$^{A}_{Z}X \longrightarrow {}^{A}_{Z-1}Y + \beta^+$$

Example: Suppose a cobalt-60 nucleus beta-decays:

$$^{60}Co \longrightarrow {}^{A'}_{Z'}Y + e^-$$

What is the element Y and what are A′ and Z′?

Solution: Again, balance mass numbers:

$$60 = A' + 0$$
$$A' = 60$$

Now balance the atomic numbers, taking into account that cobalt has 27 protons (you learn this by consulting the periodic table) and that there is one more proton on the right-hand side:

$$27 = Z' - 1$$
$$Z' = 28$$

Look at the periodic table to find that Z′ = 28 is nickel:

$$Y = {}^{60}_{28}Ni$$

TEACHER TIP

While gamma particles are dangerous, they are the easiest problems on the MCAT. No changes happen: parent and daughter are the same.

c. **Gamma decay** is the emission of γ–particles, which are high energy photons. They carry no charge and simply lower the energy of the emitting (parent) nucleus without changing the mass number or the atomic number. In other words, the daughter's A is the same as the parent's, and the daughter's Z is the same as the parent's.

γ decay

$$Z_{parent} = Z_{daughter}$$
$$A_{parent} = A_{daughter}$$

The generic gamma decay reaction is thus:

$$^{A}_{Z}X' \longrightarrow {}^{A}_{Z}X + \gamma$$

Example: Suppose a parent isotope $^{A}_{Z}X$ emits a β^+ and turns into an excited state of the isotope $^{A'}_{Z'}Y'$, which then γ decays to $^{A''}_{Z''}Y$, which in turn α decays to $^{A'''}_{Z'''}W$. If W is ^{60}Fe, what is $^{A}_{Z}X$?

Solution: Since the final daughter in this chain of decay is given, it will be necessary to work backward through the reactions. By looking at the periodic table one finds that W = Fe means $Z''' = 26$; hence the last reaction is the following α decay:

$$^{A''}_{Z''}Y \longrightarrow {}^{60}_{26}Fe + {}^{4}_{2}He$$

By balancing the atomic numbers you find:

$$Z'' = 26 + 2 = 28$$

A balancing of the mass numbers implies:

$$A'' = 60 + 4 = 64$$

The second-to-last reaction is a γ decay that simply releases energy from the nucleus but does not alter the atomic number or the mass number of the parent. That is: $Z' = Z'' = 28$ and $A' = A'' = 64$. So the second reaction is:

$$^{64}_{28}Y' \longrightarrow {}^{64}_{28}Y + \gamma$$

The first reaction was a β^+ decay that must have looked like:

$$^{A}_{Z}X \longrightarrow {}^{64}_{28}Y' + e^+$$

Again, balance the atomic numbers:

$$Z = 28 + 1 = 29$$

You carry out a balancing of mass numbers by taking into account that a proton has disappeared on the left and reappeared as a neutron on the right, leaving mass number unchanged:

$$A = 64 + 0 = 64$$

MCAT SYNOPSIS

γ-particles are high energy photons. γ-decay releases energy but doesn't change A or Z.

TEACHER TIP

Work backward on these types of questions.

By looking at the periodic table, you find that Z = 29 means that X is Cu. A = 64, so that means that the solution is:

$${}^{A}_{Z}X = {}^{64}_{29}Cu$$

Even though the problem did not ask for it, it is possible again to look at the periodic table to find that Z′ = Z″ = 28 means Y′ = Y = Ni. The total chain of decays can be written as:

$${}^{64}_{29}Cu \longrightarrow {}^{64}_{28}Ni' + \beta^{+}$$

$${}^{64}_{28}Ni' \longrightarrow {}^{64}_{28}Ni + \gamma$$

$${}^{64}_{28}Ni \longrightarrow {}^{60}_{26}Fe + \alpha$$

d. Electron capture

Certain unstable radionuclides are capable of capturing an inner (K or L shell) electron that combines with a proton to form a neutron. The atomic number is now one less than the original, but the mass number remains the same. Electron capture is a rare process that is perhaps best thought of as an inverse β^{-} decay.

MCAT SYNOPSIS

(fraction of original nuclei remaining after n half-lives) = $(1/2)^n$.

2. Radioactive Decay Half-Life ($T_{1/2}$)

In a collection of a great many identical radioactive isotopes, the **half-life** ($T_{1/2}$) of the sample is the time it takes for half of the sample to decay.

Example: If the half-life of a certain isotope is 4 years, what fraction of a sample of that isotope will remain after 12 years?

Solution: If 4 years is 1 half-life, then 12 years is 3 half-lives. During the first half-life—the first 4 years—half of the sample will have decayed. During the second half-life (years 4 to 8), half of the remaining half will decay, leaving one-fourth of the original. During the third and final period (years 8 to 12), half of the remaining fourth will decay, leaving one-eighth of the original sample. Thus the fraction remaining after 3 half-lives is $(1/2)^3$ or (1/8).

TEACHER TIP

Half-life questions are common on the MCAT. Make sure draw them out; it's easy to lose your place when doing them in your head.

3. Exponential Decay

Let n be the number of radioactive nuclei that have not yet decayed in a sample. It turns out that the **rate** at which the nuclei decay

($\Delta n/\Delta t$) is proportional to the number that remain (n). This suggests the equation:

$$\frac{\Delta n}{\Delta t} = -\lambda n$$

where λ is known as the **decay constant.** The solution of this equation tells us how the number of radioactive nuclei changes with time. The solution is known as an **exponential decay**:

$$n = n_0 e^{-\lambda t}$$

where n_0 is the number of undecayed nuclei at time t = 0. (The decay constant is related to the half-life by $\lambda = \frac{\ln 2}{T_{1/2}} = \frac{0.693}{T_{1/2}}$).

Example: If at time t = 0 there is a 2 mole sample of radioactive isotopes of decay constant 2 $(\text{hour})^{-1}$, how many nuclei remain after 45 minutes?

Solution: Since 45 minutes is 3/4 of an hour, the exponent is:

$$\lambda t = 2\left(\frac{3}{4}\right) = \frac{6}{4} = \frac{3}{2}$$

The exponential factor will be a number smaller than 1:

$$e^{-\lambda t} = e^{-3/2} = 0.22$$

So only 0.22 or 22 percent of the original 2-mole sample will remain. To find n_0 multiply the number of moles we have by the number of particles per mole (Avogadro's number):

$$n_0 = 2(6.02 \times 10^{23}) = 1.2 \times 10^{24}$$

From the equation that describes exponential decay, you can calculate the number that remain after 45 minutes:

$$\begin{aligned} n &= n_0 e^{-\lambda t} \\ &= (1.2 \times 10^{24})(0.22) \\ &= 2.6 \times 10^{23} \text{ particles} \end{aligned}$$

MCAT SYNOPSIS

(number of nuclei that have decayed in time t) = ($n_0 - n$), where $n = n_0 e^{-\lambda t}$.

PRACTICE QUESTIONS

1. The mass of a proton is about 1.007 amu and the mass of a neutron is about 1.009 amu. The mass of a helium nucleus is

   A. less than 4.032 amu.
   B. exactly 4.032 amu.
   C. greater than 4.032 amu.
   D. impossible to determine from the information given.

2. A nucleus with mass m dissociates into only protons (mass mp) and neutrons (mass mn). What is the overall change in energy?

   A. $[\, m - (mp + mn) \,] \times 932$ MeV/amu
   B. $[\, (mp + mn) - m \,] \times 932$ MeV/amu
   C. $[\, m - (mp + mn) \,] \times 932$ MeV
   D. $[\, (mp + mn) - m \,] \times 932$ MeV

3. Which of the following reactions will NOT be accompanied by the release of energy?

   A. 21H + 31H → 42He + 10 n
   B. 23592U + 10 n → 2 10 n + 14054Xe + 9438Sr
   C. 23892U → 23490Th + α
   D. 6428Y′ → 6428Y

4. A certain carbon nucleus dissociates completely into α particles. How many particles are formed?

   A. 1
   B. 2
   C. 3
   D. 4

5. 116C → 115B + 0.96 MeV + other particles
   The above reaction is an example of

   A. α decay.
   B. β decay.
   C. γ decay.
   D. x-ray decay.

6. Which of the following is always accompanied by a decrease in the mass number of the parent nuclide(s)?

   A. β decay
   B. γ decay
   C. Fusion
   D. Fission

7. In an annihilation reaction, an electron collides with a positron and both particles are destroyed. If the mass of an electron is me and both particles initially moved with a velocity of v, how much energy is released?

   A. $m_e c^2$
   B. $2m_e c^2$
   C. $m_e c^2 + \frac{1}{2} m_e v^2$
   D. $2m_e c^2 + m_e v^2$

8. The half-life of 14C is approximately 5,730 years, while the half-life of 12C is essentially infinite. If the ratio of 14C to 12C in a certain sample is 25 percent less than the normal ratio in nature, how old is the sample?

   A. Less than 5,730 years
   B. Approximately 5,730 years
   C. Significantly greater than 5,730 years, but significantly less than 11,460 years
   D. Approximately 11,460 years

9. Which of the following graphs best represents the activity of a radionuclide with respect to time?

A.

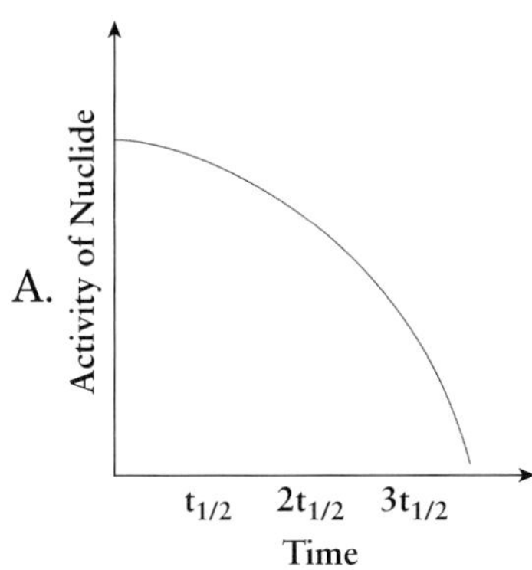

B.

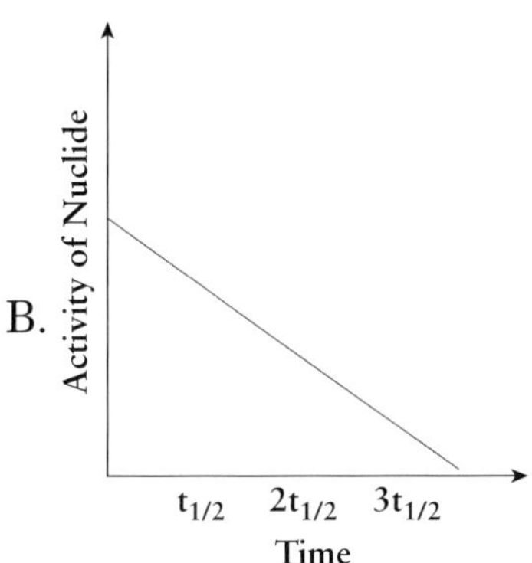

C.

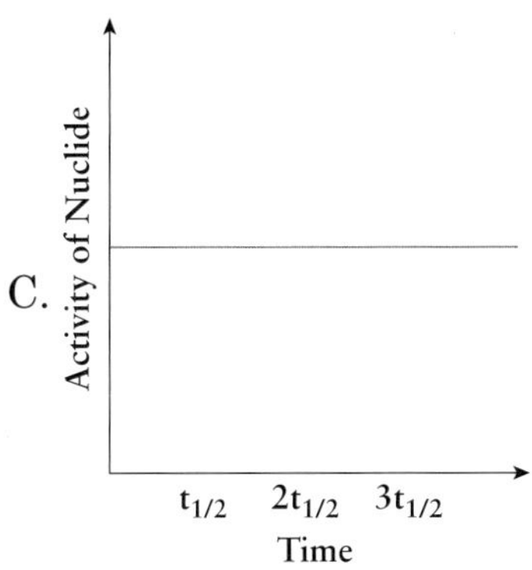

D.

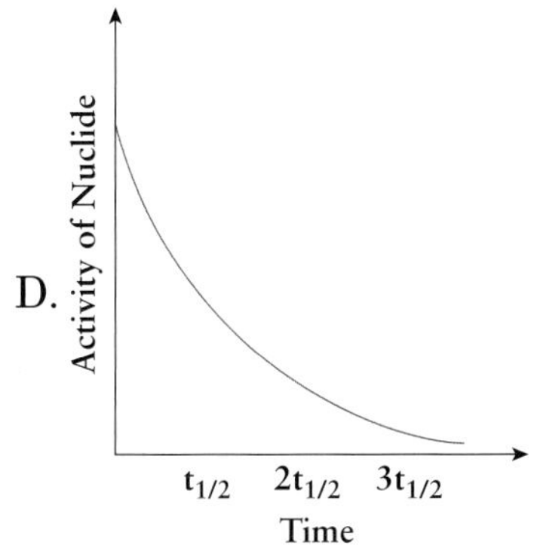

10. A nuclide undergoes 2 alpha decays, 2 positron decays, and 2 gamma decays. What is the difference between the atomic number of the parent nuclide and the atomic number of the daughter nuclide?

A. 0
B. 2
C. 4
D. 6

11. Outlined below is a certain element's change in concentration in a stable mixture. What is the half-life of the element?

Time (hours)	Concentration (mol/L)
0	8
3	3
6	1
9	0.4

A. 1 hour
B. 2 hours
C. 3 hours
D. 4 hours

12. An unknown stable nucleus fuses with three hydrogen nuclei to produce nuclide X. Which of the following is the LEAST likely path for the conversion of X into a daughter nuclide Y?

A. $X \rightarrow Y + \alpha$
B. $X \rightarrow Y + \beta^+$
C. $X \rightarrow Y + \beta^-$
D. $X + {}^1_0n \rightarrow Y$

13. What is the approximate decay rate of a 1 mol sample of ^{32}P ($t_{1/2}$ = 14 days)?

A. $-\frac{1}{2}$ mol/day

B. $-\frac{1}{7}$ mol/day

C. $-\frac{1}{14}$ mol/day

D. $-\frac{1}{20}$ mol/day

14. If a neutron spontaneously combines with a positron, the mass of the resulting particle is

A. higher than the mass of the neutron.

B. equal to the mass of the neutron.

C. lower than the mass of the neutron.

D. impossible to determine from the information given.

15. A helium nucleus fuses with a hydrogen nucleus and then captures an electron. What is the identity of the daughter nuclide?

A. ^{5}He

B. $^{5}He^{+}$

C. ^{5}Li

D. $^{5}Li^{+}$

16. A lead sheet is bombarded with α particles, β^{+} particles, β^{-} particles, and γ particles. Which type of particle is most likely to be deflected back after interacting with the lead?

A. α

B. β^{+}

C. β^{-}

D. γ

MASS DEFECT

Calculate the nuclear mass defect of cesium-137 if it has a mass of 136.87522 amu. (m_e = 5.5 × 10^{-4} amu, m_p = 1.00728 amu, m_n = 1.00867 amu)

1) Tally the number of protons, electrons, and neutrons for cesium.

55 protons + 55 electrons
# of neutrons = 137 − 55 = 82

To find the number of protons, look up cesium on the periodic table. It is element number 55. This means that it has 55 protons. We assume that it is a neutral atom, which means there are also 55 electrons. The 137 indicates that the number of protons plus neutrons is 137. Subtract 55 from 137 to find the number of neutrons.

---

2) Add up the components.

55 × 1.00728 amu
55 × 0.00055 amu
+ 82 × 1.00867 amu
138.14159 amu

Find the total mass of the components of the atom using the masses for each particle given in the question.

---

3) Calculate mass defect.

mass defect = sum of components − mass of atom = 138.14159 amu − 136.87522 amu = 1.26637 amu

The mass defect is the difference between the mass of the components and the actual mass of the atom.

Remember: *The mass defect will always be a positive value because the sum of the components is greater than the mass of the isotope.*

KEY CONCEPTS

Mass defect

TAKEAWAYS

The mass defect is the mass converted into energy when the atom is made from its components. A larger mass defect creates a larger binding energy. The greater the binding energy per nucleon, the more stable the nucleus.

SIMILAR QUESTIONS

1) Calculate the mass defect of strontium-84 at 83.9134 amu.
2) Calculate the mass defect of mercury-204 at 203.9735 amu.
3) Calculate the mass defect of tin-122 at 121.9034 amu.

Part II
Practice Sections

INSTRUCTIONS FOR TAKING THE PRACTICE SECTIONS

Before taking each Practice Section, find a quiet place where you can work uninterrupted. Take a maximum of 70 minutes per section (52 questions) to get accustomed to the length and scope.

Keep in mind that the actual MCAT will not feature a section made up of Physics questions alone, but rather a Physical Sciences section made up of both Physics and General Chemistry questions. Use the following three sections to hone your Physics skills.

Good luck!

PRACTICE SECTION 1

Time—70 minutes

QUESTIONS 1–52

Directions: Most of the questions in the following Physics Practice Section are organized into groups, with a descriptive passage preceding each group of questions. Study the passage, then select the single-best answer to the question in each group. Some of the questions are not based on a descriptive passage; you must also select the best answer to these questions. If you are unsure of the best answer, eliminate the choices that you know are incorrect, then select an answer from the choices that remain.

PASSAGE I (QUESTIONS 1–9)

Valence electrons are much more likely to be ejected from an atom than are inner electrons. In the rare cases where an inner electron is ejected, it leaves a hole in the energy level where it originally resided. This hole is quickly filled by an electron from one of the outer energy levels, which drops to a lower energy level and releases the excess energy in the form of an c-ray photon. Occasionally this photon strikes another electron and causes it to be ejected; this second electron is known as an *Auger electron* (figure below).

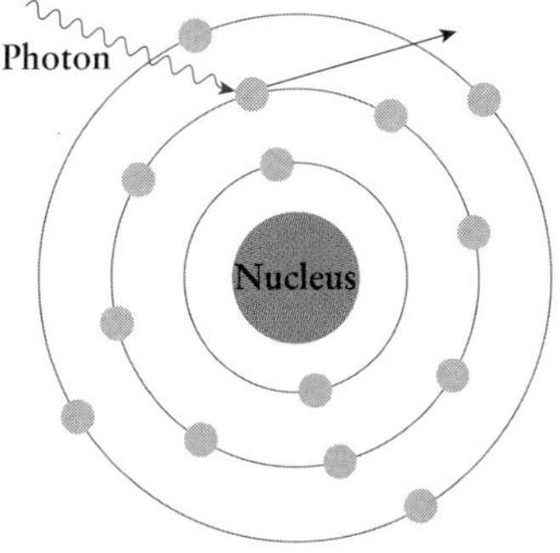

1. Ejection of inner electron

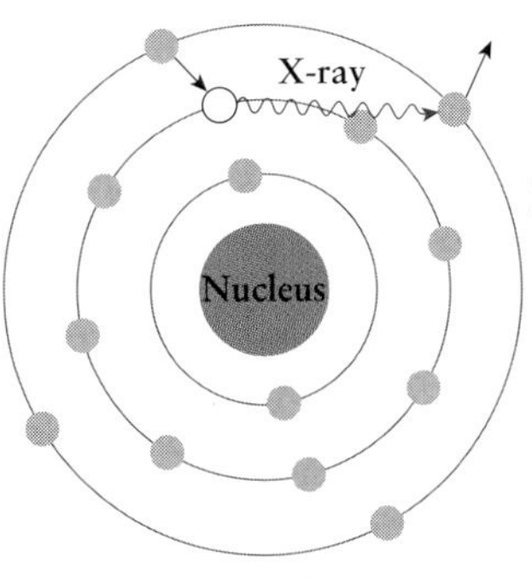

2. Formation of X-ray, ejection of Auger electron

Until the 1950's, Auger electrons were considered as little more than a source of noise in x-ray measurements. In recent years, however, scientists have used Auger electron spectroscopy (AES) to identify an element by measuring the energy of its Auger electrons. AES is effective for this purpose because each element features a unique spectrum of Auger emissions.

1. Inner electrons are more difficult to eject than outer electrons are because the Bohr energy of outer electrons is

   A. closer to the energy of the photon.
   B. closer to zero.
   C. a larger positive value.
   D. a larger negative value.

2. Whenever a hole is created by ejected lower-energy electrons, higher-energy electrons drop down to fill this hole because the

   A. emission of an x-ray causes a decrease in the electron's energy.
   B. atom must retain a net neutral charge.
   C. electron is naturally attracted by the gravitational force of the nucleus.
   D. electron is more stable at lower energy.

3. Which of the following transitions is most likely to produce an Auger electron?

A.

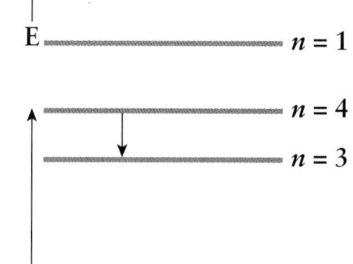

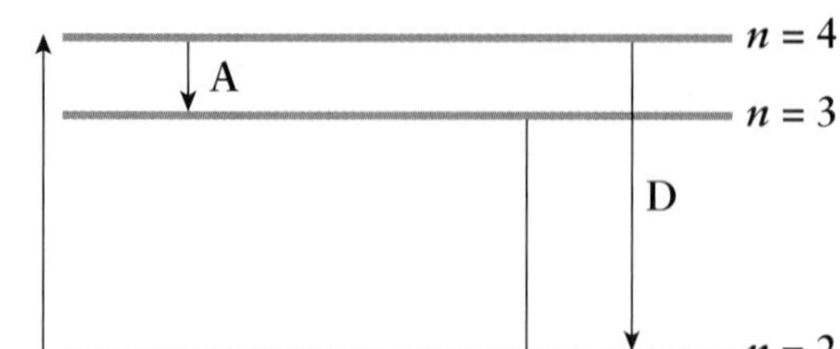

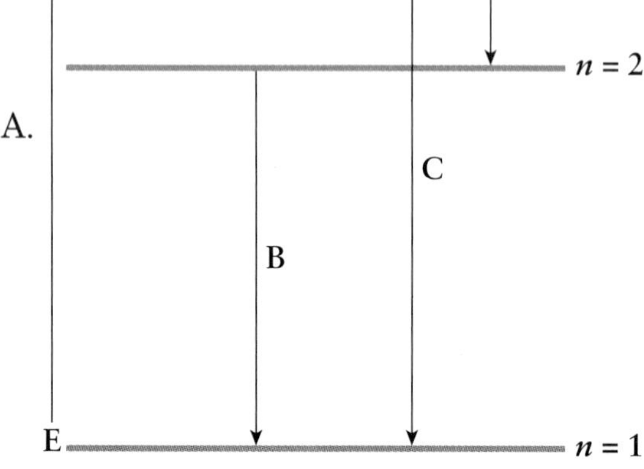

C.

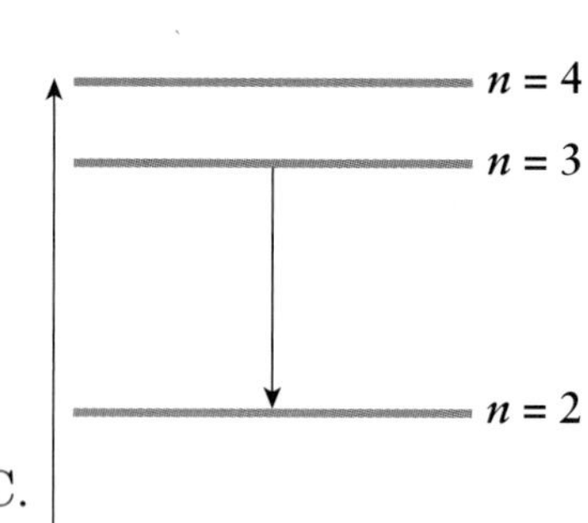

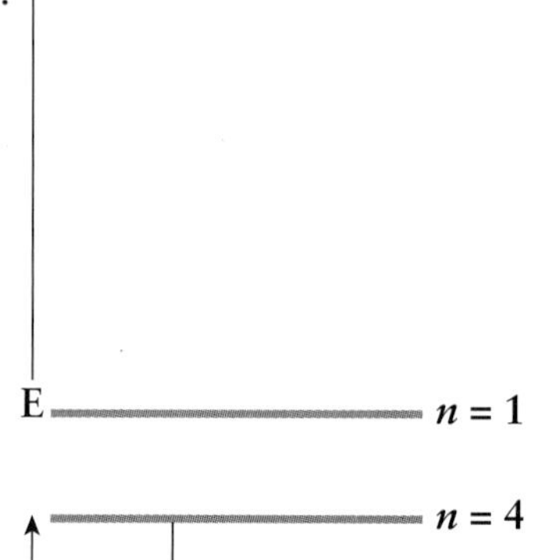

B.

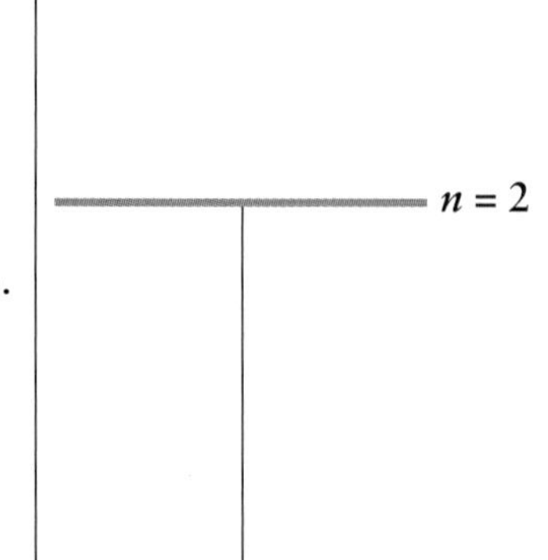

D.

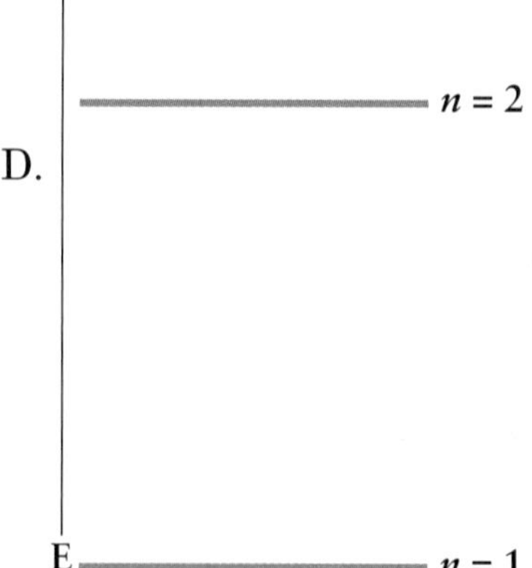

4. An electron carrying 10 eV of energy moves from point A to point B. What is the energy of the accompanying x-ray photon?

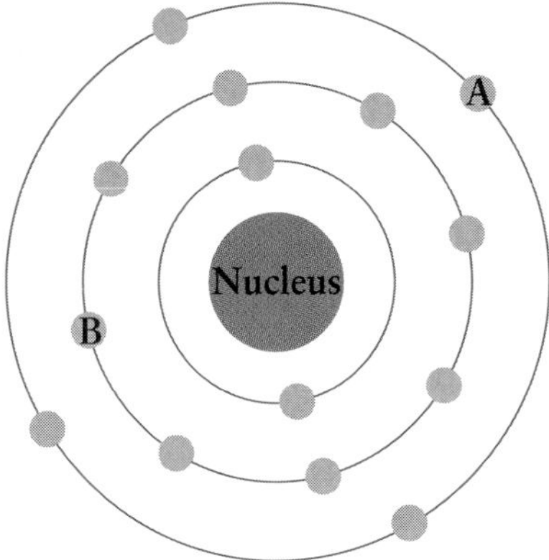

A. 15 Ev
B. 10 Ev
C. 7.5 Ev
D. 5 Ev

5. If scientists discovered a new technique to eliminate Auger electrons, how would this most likely impact the measurement of the energy of x-rays?

A. Decreased error in measurements
B. Decreased variability in measurements
C. Improved sensitivity of equipment
D. Improved resolution in readings

6. Samples A and B both contain the same number of energy levels. On average, the Auger electrons produced by sample A carry more energy than those produced by sample B. Which of the following is most likely true about sample A?

A. It contains more electrons per atom.
B. It contains fewer electrons per atom.
C. It carries a positive charge.
D. It carries a negative charge.

7. Which of the following elements cannot be detected accurately by AES?

A. Helium
B. Lithium
C. Beryllium
D. Sodium

8. Which of the following graphs (not to scale) most accurately describes the number of x-rays and Auger electrons produced when an inner electron is struck by photons of various energies?

A.

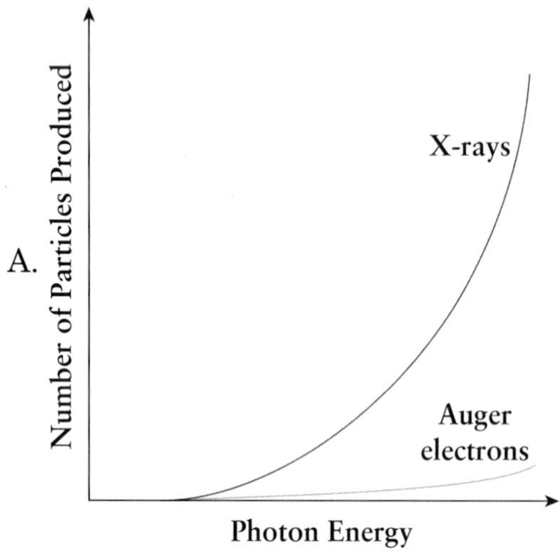

B.

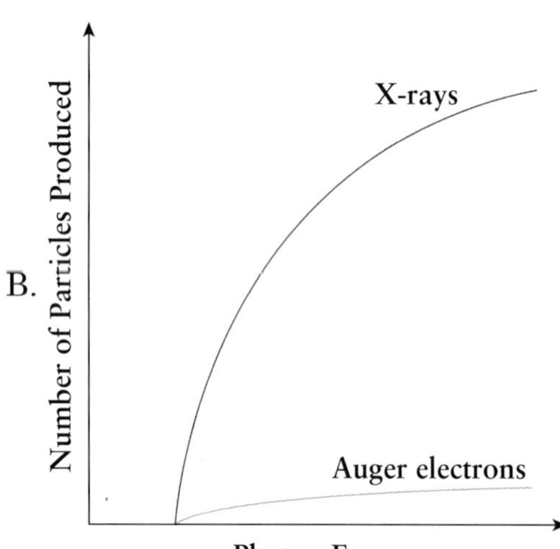

C.

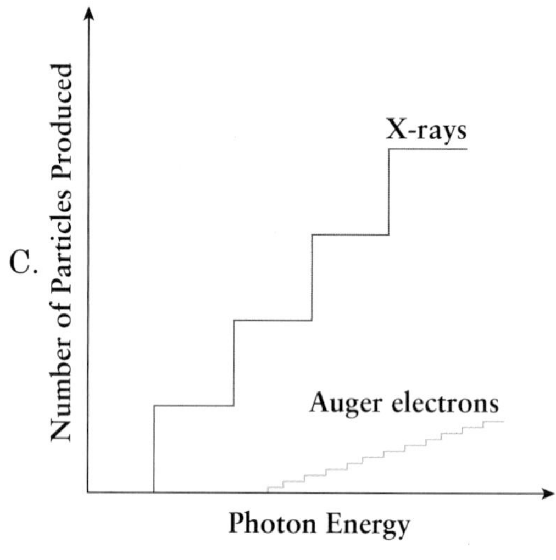

D.

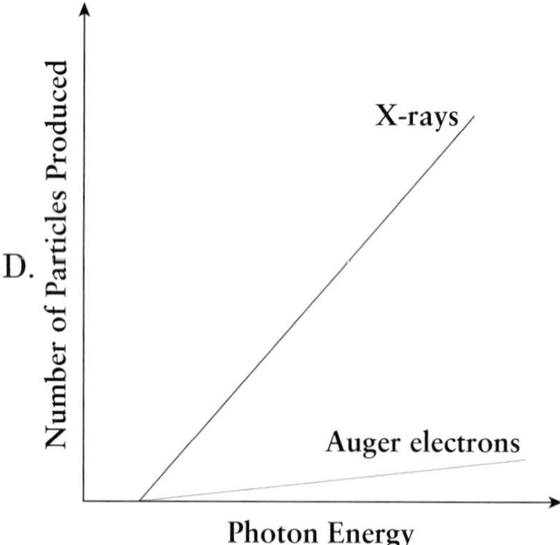

9. When a certain γ-ray causes an electron to drop from energy level *a* to energy level *b*, the resultant x-ray produces an Auger electron in energy level *c* if

A. $E_a + E_b - E_c \geq 0$.
B. $E_a - E_b + E_c \geq 0$.
C. $E\gamma + E_b - E_a + E_c \geq 0$.
D. $E\gamma + E_b + E_a + E_c \geq 0$.

PASSAGE II (QUESTIONS 10–17)

Many automatic temperature-monitoring systems take advantage of a device known as a thermocouple. Thermocouples measure change in temperature by taking advantage of the thermoelectric effect, a reversible phenomenon in which electric voltage is produced as a result of differences in temperature across a circuit. When the temperature changes, a certain voltage is applied to the thermocouple; this voltage can be measured and converted into a precise temperature.

Instead of a thermocouple, some monitoring systems use a resistance temperature detector (RTD), which calculates the temperature by comparing the resistance across a circuit to the expected resistance at any given temperature. The temperature and resistance exhibit a linear relationship. The RTD is based on observations that electrical conductors increase their resistance with increasing temperatures.

10. An increased voltage across a thermocouple indicates a(n)

A. increase in temperature.
B. decrease in temperature.
C. increased temperature difference across the circuit.
D. decreased temperature difference across the circuit.

11. If the voltage applied to an RTD is increased, its resistance will

A. decrease.
B. increase.
C. remain constant.
D. depend on the current.

12. The thermoelectric effect happens as a result of an energy imbalance across the circuit. What type of energy imbalance is responsible for the signal produced by a thermocouple?

A. Potential energy imbalance
B. Kinetic energy imbalance
C. Heat imbalance
D. Electric energy imbalance

13. Which type of temperature sensor is likely to require an external power source?

A. A thermocouple, because the voltage can only be measured if external power is available.
B. A thermocouple, because the voltage will only be produced if external power is available.
C. An RTD, because the resistance can only be measured if external power is available.
D. An RTD, because the resistance will only be produced if external power is available.

14. A student attempts to use four identical resistors to produce an RTD. Which of the following configurations is likely to detect temperature changes most accurately?

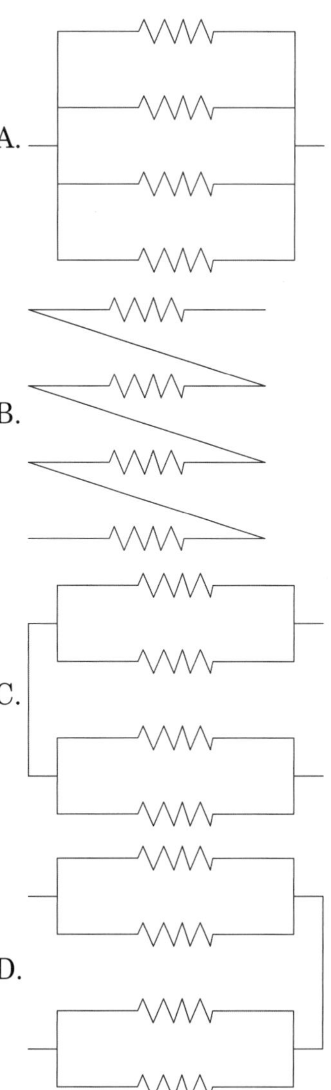

15. Which of the following diagrams best represents the optimal location within a circuit to measure voltage in a thermocouple? "V" is the device used to measure voltage, while T_1 and T_2 are the two individual temperatures.

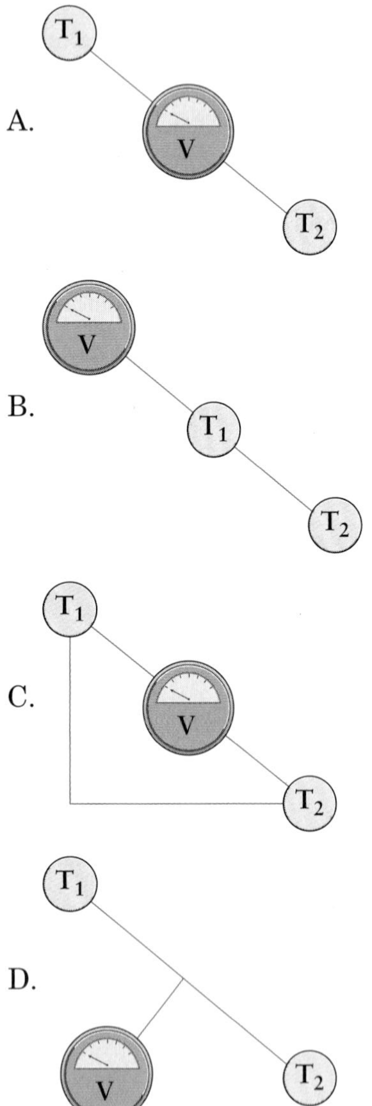

16. The thermoelectric effect CANNOT be used to

A. store electricity.
B. generate electricity.
C. heat an object by applying a voltage.
D. cool an object by applying a voltage.

17. The resistivity of a good RTD will most likely be

A. highly stable with respect to temperature.
B. highly variable with respect to temperature.
C. greater than 1.
D. less than 1.

QUESTIONS 18–21 ARE NOT BASED ON A DESCRIPTIVE PASSAGE.

18. What phenomenon can occur with light but not with sound?

A. Polarization
B. Refraction
C. Doppler effect
D. Interference

19. What is the critical angle in air for a substance whose index of refraction is 2?

A. 30°
B. 60°
C. 45°
D. 90°

20. Completely destructive interference has been used by the military in the construction of stealth planes. Suppose a new military project was launched to coat all stealth planes with a material that would function as a cloaking device and render them invisible to people. Assuming that white light has an average wavelength of 600 nm, what should the thickness of the cloaking coat be?

A. 300 nm
B. 600 nm
C. 1,200 nm
D. 1,800 nm

21. When an 8 eV photon strikes a photoemissive surface, the surface can eject electrons that have at most a maximum kinetic energy of 6 eV. What is the maximum frequency of the photons being emitted? (h = 4e-15 eV × s)

A. 5e-14 Hz
B. 5e14 Hz
C. 5e15 Hz
D. 2e14 Hz

PASSAGE III (QUESTIONS 22–30)

In the figure below, a plate sits on the edge of a table. As it sits motionless, the plate possesses gravitational potential energy due to its position above the ground. This energy is given by U = mgh. Suddenly the plate falls from the table, traveling down to the ground. When it hits the ground, it breaks into three pieces of masses: 1 m, 2 m, and 3 m. Assume that gravitational acceleration is 10 m/s^2.

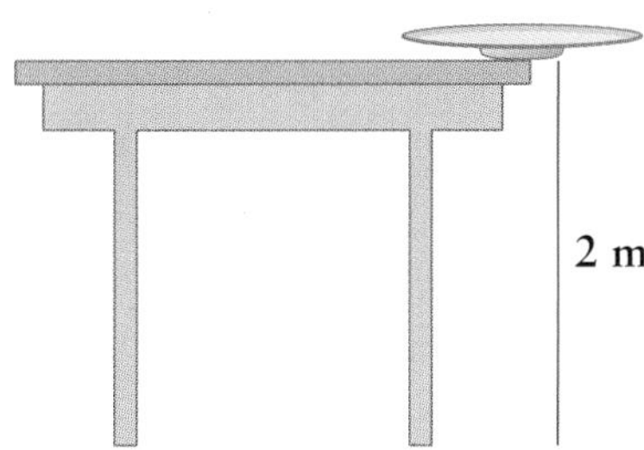

22. The plate was initially placed on the ground. If the plate has a mass of 2 kg and force is applied directly upward, how much work is done to move the plate to the table?

A. 4 J
B. 10 J
C. 40 J
D. 0.1 J

23. How much potential energy does the plate possess as it sits on the table's edge if it has a mass of 40 g and the table's height is 150 cm?

A. 60 J
B. 0.06 J
C. 60,000 J
D. 0.6 J

24. At the point when the plate has traveled 1/3 of the distance between the table and the ground

A. its total energy is 2/3 of its original energy.
B. its total energy is equal to its original energy.
C. its total energy is 4/3 of its original energy.
D. it has more potential energy, but less kinetic energy.

25. At what point in its path from the table to the ground does the plate have the greatest kinetic energy?

A. At the instant after it leaves the table
B. Halfway to the ground
C. At the instant before it hits the ground
D. The kinetic energy is the same throughout the path

26. After the plate breaks, what is the total momentum of all the pieces?

A. 720 M m/s
B. 720 M^2 kg × m/s
C. 120 M m/s
D. 120 M^2 kg × m/s

27. The piece with a mass of 3M is traveling at a speed of 5 m/s when it hits a stationary block of mass M. The piece comes to a complete stop and sends the block flying. Assuming that friction is negligible, what is the velocity of the block?

A. 15 m/s
B. (15 M) m/s
C. (75 M) m's
D. 75 m/s

28. Assume that the piece with a mass of 1M kg is moving at 4 m/s. How much force is required to bring the piece to a complete stop in 3 seconds?

A. (4/3 M) N
B. (3/4 M) N
C. (−4/3 M) N
D. (−3/4 M) N

29. If the plate was thrown into the air and then allowed to fall back down to its original position, at what point is its energy the greatest?

A. At the highest point, because the potential energy is greatest
B. At the lowest point, because kinetic energy is the greatest
C. It is the same at all points because energy is conserved
D. At the halfway point between the highest and lowest points of its path

30. If the plate moves one meter to the left while experiencing a downward force of 2 N that makes an angle of 90 degrees with the horizontal, how much work is done on the plate by the force?

A. 180 J
B. 4 J
C. 0 J
D. 1 J

PASSAGE IV (QUESTIONS 31–37)

A guitar produces its sound through the vibrations of a string that is fixed at both ends. When a force is applied to this string, it oscillates at its fundamental frequency, which determines the pitch observed by a listener. To adjust the pitch of the sound emitted by the guitar, a guitarist will usually change the effective length of a string by applying his finger to the point where he wants the new "fixed end" of the string to be:

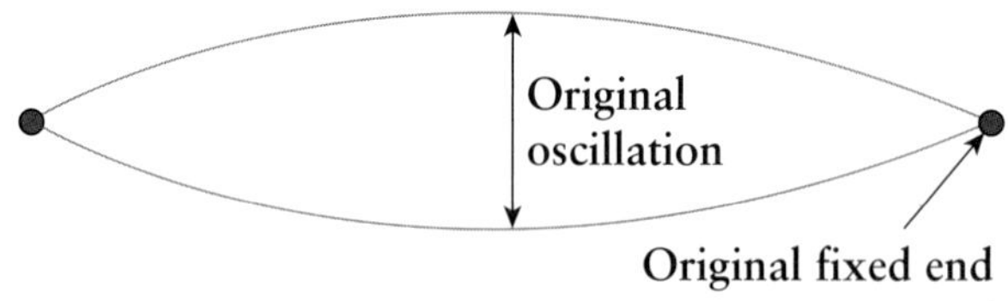

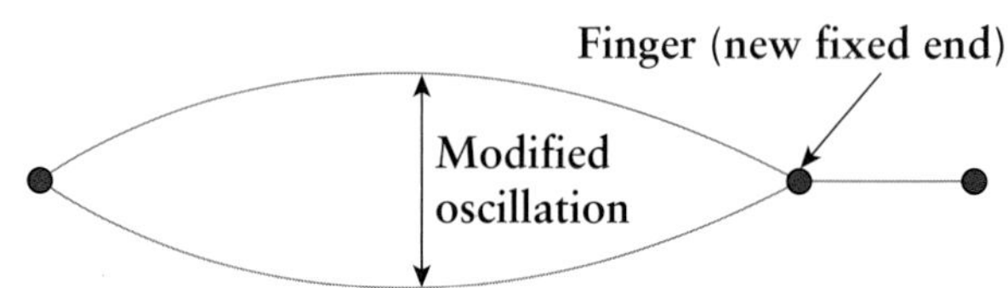

There are two common types of guitars: acoustic guitars and electric guitars. In an acoustic guitar, the waves created on the string move into an empty wooden compartment, where they build up and cause vibrations in the wood. The oscillations in the wood create sound waves in the surrounding air. These sound waves maintain the same frequency as the waves produced by the string, but they have significantly greater amplitude.

An electric guitar uses the same types of strings, but the sound waves are absorbed by a special type of magnetic microphone known as a "pickup." The waves are transmitted through a wire to an amplifier, where electrical energy is used to increase their amplitude. The amplified waves are then converted back into a sound wave by a speaker, which converts the electrical energy back into a sound wave. The best amplifiers are usually capable of applying more power to the wave thereby further increasing its amplitude.

31. A beat is produced as a result of the vibrations of two specific guitar strings. If one string is vibrating at 430 Hz and the other is vibrating at 440 Hz, how many beats will an observer hear every minute?

A. 6
B. 10
C. 600
D. 870

32. In order to increase the pitch of a sound emitted by a certain string, a guitarist must

A. move his finger down the string to decrease its effective length.
B. move his finger up the string to increase its effective length.
C. wiggle his finger on the string to increase the number of vibrations.
D. hold his finger steady in order to decrease the number of vibrations.

33. The wooden compartment in the acoustic guitar serves to

A. increase the frequency of the individual sound waves.
B. increase the intensity of the emitted sound.
C. reduce the variation between the frequencies of different sound waves.
D. reduce the background noise in the emitted sound.

34. A certain electric guitar amplifier contains a speaker that is constantly rotating, thereby emitting sounds in different directions at different times. What will happen to the pitch of the sound as the speaker rotates towards a listener?

A. It will increase because of the increased intensity.
B. It will increase because of the Doppler effect.
C. It will decrease because of the increased intensity.
D. It will decrease because of the Doppler effect.

35. Which of the following graphs best describes the relationship between the effective length of a string and the pitch of the tone that it produces?

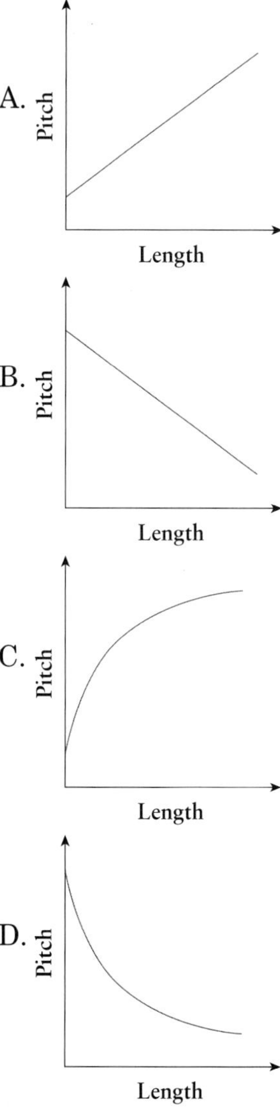

36. One of the two sound waves below represents the sound waves going from an acoustic guitar string to the environment, while the other represents the sound waves going from an electric guitar string to its pickups. The electric guitar is represented by which of the following?

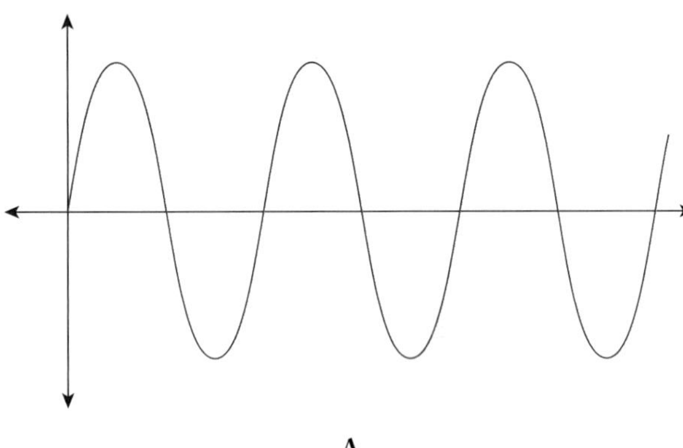

A

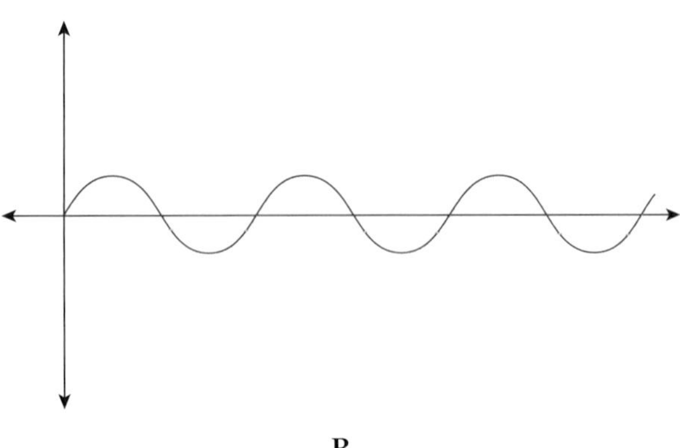

B

A. Graph A, because the sound wave from an electric guitar can be amplified.
B. Graph A, because the pickup is in close proximity to the string.
C. Graph B, because the acoustic guitar emits a sound wave with greater amplitude than the electric guitar string.
D. Graph B, because the acoustic guitar emits a sound wave over a larger area.

37. An acoustic guitarist strikes a note with a frequency of 1,000 Hz. If she applies enough force to displace the wood by 1 cm, what is the intensity of the sound observed at a distance of 1 meter from the string? Assume that the spring constant of the wood is 500 N/m and there is no loss due to friction.

A. 200 W/m^2
B. 100 W/m^2
C. 50 W/m^2
D. 25 W/m^2

QUESTIONS 38–45 ARE NOT BASED ON A DESCRIPTIVE PASSAGE.

38. For a projectile thrown with an initial speed of 40 m/s at an angle of 30°, the horizontal component of velocity is closest to

A. 50 m/s.
B. 40 m/s.
C. 30 m/s.
D. 20 m/s.

39. If two different pure substances are placed in an isolated system and a net flow of heat occurs between them, which of the following thermodynamic quantities MUST be different between the two objects?

A. Initial temperatures
B. Specific heats
C. Masses
D. Heat capacities

40. Which of the following statements is part of the kinetic theory of ideal gases?

A. Molecules transfer energy via collisions.
B. Molecules are always stationary.
C. Intermolecular forces of attraction are significant in guiding a molecule's path.
D. The size of the molecules is large compared to the distance that separates them.

41. A strong resistor in parallel with a voltage source is the essential component of which of the following?

A. Ammeter
B. Dynamo
C. Generator
D. Voltmeter

42. A perfectly spherical mirror that forms only virtual images has a radius of curvature of 1 meter. What is the focal length of this mirror?

A. 2 m
B. 1 m
C. 0.5 m
D. Infinity

43. A student is supplied with four one-ohm resistors. How many functionally different resistors can be made if all resistors must be used in each configuration?

A. 2
B. 3
C. 4
D. 5

44. If a dielectric is inserted into a parallel plate capacitor, which of the following MUST happen to the potential difference and charge on each plate, respectively?

A. Nothing, increase
B. Nothing, decrease
C. Nothing, nothing
D. Increase, increase

45. If the mass of a pendulum is doubled, the frequency of its oscillations

A. doubles.
B. quadruples.
C. halves.
D. stays the same.

PASSAGE V (QUESTIONS 46–52)

A 100 kg man decided to ride his 400 kg motorcycle around a circular track of radius R = 100 m. As his speed increased, his motorcycle tilted toward the center of the circle, making an angle alpha with the ground. When he reached a speed of 50 m/s, he felt that his body was too close to the ground and he decided to stop accelerating. Figure 1 shows some of the forces acting on the motorcycle. It does not show the force of the motor, which accelerates the motorcycle out of the page, or the force of friction which resists that motion. Note that F2 is the centripetal force. The centrifugal force opposing the centripetal force is not shown.

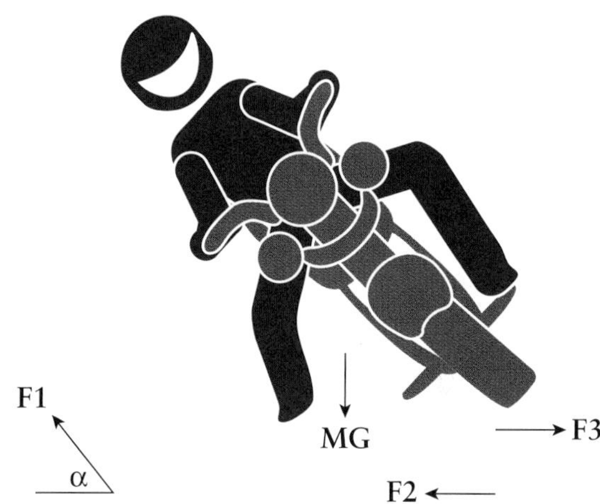

He then conducted another trial during which he accelerated to 50 m/s on a flat surface and then rode inside a cylindrical track of radius R in which he seemed to defy gravity. The schematic diagram in figure 2 shows the motorcyclist in a counterclockwise movement, being upside down at point A:

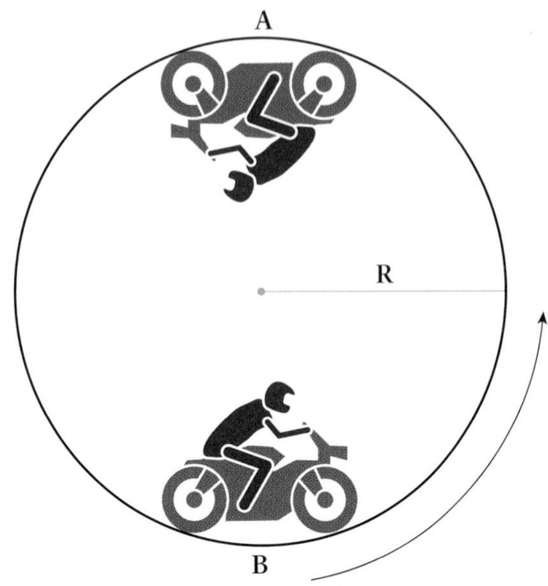

At the end of the second experiment, he observed that his tires were burnt. These observations led him to make conclusions about motorcycle safety.

46. The man believes that when on a flat surface, the tires can withstand speeds in excess of 100 m/s, because the force of friction would still be smaller than in trial 2. Is he correct?

A. Although the forces of friction increase as the speed increases, the centrifugal forces on the rotating tires might offset this effect and keep the tires from burning.
B. Although the force of friction would still be smaller than in trial 2, increasing centrifugal forces on the rotating tires might cause the tires to burst.
C. The force of friction would be smaller than in trial 2 and his prediction is absolutely correct.
D. The force of friction would be smaller than in trial 2 but this would cause him to lose control at higher speeds.

47. What is the net force acting on the motorcycle in trial 1 at any given moment, when he maintains a constant speed of 50 m/s?

A. 0 N
B. 1,000 N
C. 10,000 N
D. 100,000 N

48. What are the directions of forces F1 and F2 from trial 1, if they are measured at point B during trial 2?

A. F1 points into the ground and F2 points toward the center.
B. F1 points toward the center and F2 points in the direction behind the motorcycle.
C. Both F1 and F2 point into the ground.
D. Both F1 and F2 point toward the center.

49. What is the maximum height of track 2 that would allow a motorcyclist to execute the gravity-defying stunt while maintaining a minimum speed of 50 m/s?

A. 10 m
B. 50 m
C. 250 m
D. 500 m

50. During trial 2, the engine must supply increasing amounts of power between points A and B in order to maintain constant speed. As the motorcyclist goes up from point A to point B, the

A. force of friction on the tires increases.
B. force of friction on the tires decreases.
C. net force on the motorcycle decreases.
D. net force on the motorcycle increases.

51. If the motorcyclist wishes to increase the safety of trial 1, which of the following are effective strategies for that goal?

I. Increase the coefficient of friction of the track surface
II. Increase the radius of the track
III. Increase the mass of the motorcycle

A. I only
B. II only
C. I and II only
D. II and III only

52. What are the average net forces acting on the motorcyclist during a single round trip around tracks 1 and 2, respectively?

A. 0 N in both cases
B. 0 N and 10,000 N, respectively
C. 10,000 N in both cases
D. More information is needed

PRACTICE SECTION 2

Time—70 minutes

QUESTIONS 1–52

Directions: Most of the questions in the following Physics Practice Section are organized into groups, with a descriptive passage preceding each group of questions. Study the passage, then select the single-best answer to the question in each group. Some of the questions are not based on a descriptive passage; you must also select the best answer to these questions. If you are unsure of the best answer, eliminate the choices that you know are incorrect, then select an answer from the choices that remain.

PASSAGE I (QUESTIONS 1–9)

An experiment is conducted to test the quality of newly manufactured springs. One spring is attached to the back of a car and another one is attached to the front. The car is driven inside a specialized track (shown below):

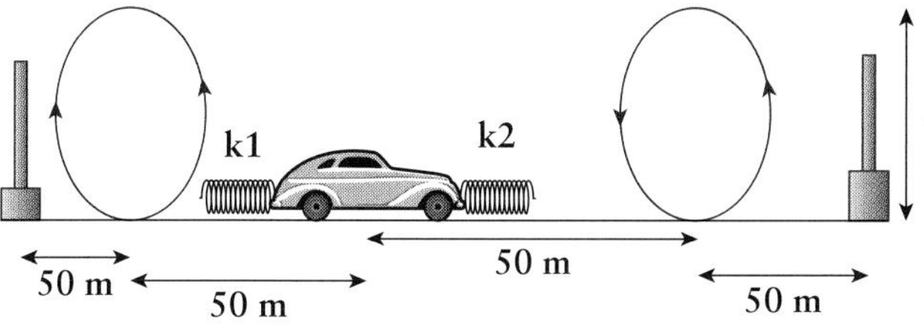

Initially, the car accelerates to the right, travels through a circular loop (with diameter of 5 m), and hits a brick, rectangular wall. If the spring causes it to rebound, it goes backward, passes through the two identical circles, and hits the other wall. A device on each wall records the maximum force of impact. This cycle may continue indefinitely.

Each wall is equipped with a transformer that converts mechanical energy into heat. Heat energy is transferred from the wall to the cylinder on top of it according to the formula $Q/t = kA\Delta T/L$, where Q is heat, t is time, A is cross-sectional area, k is the coefficient of conductivity for the cylinder, L is the length of the boundary between the wall and the inner part of the cylinder, and ΔT is the nonzero temperature difference between the surfaces.

The liquid inside the cylinder will accept heat according to the formula $Q = mC\Delta T$, where C is specific heat capacity ($c = 4.184$ J g^{-1} K^{-1} for water) and m is the liquid's mass in grams.

The car weighs 100 kg. Some of the results of the experiment are shown in Table 1:

Trial	K_1	K_2	Speed	Force R	Force L
1	2,000	3,000	50	25×10^6	23×10^6
2	3,000	3,000	20	11×10^6	11×10^6
3	4,000	3,000	7	n/a	n/a
4	10,000	2,000	12	5×10^6	n/a

During each trial the car accelerates to a certain speed in the first 50 m and then the engine is turned off for the duration. Force R and Force L represent the maximal recorded forces upon the impact with the right or left wall, respectively. K_1 and K_2 are the spring constants of the two springs. All measurements are in standard metric units.

1. What was the change in momentum of the car in trial 1 after it hit the right wall?

A. 0 kg × m/s
B. 500 kg × m/s
C. 5,000 kg × m/s
D. 10,000 kg × m/s

2. Which of the following best explains the results of trial 4?

A. The car broke down after hitting the first brick wall.
B. The spring constant K_1 was so high that the measuring device on the left wall malfunctioned.
C. The car lost some kinetic energy due to friction, thereby preventing it from reaching the top of a circle on the way back.
D. All of the above

3. In trial 1, what is the difference between the time when the car passes the first circle and the time when it comes to a stop at the right wall?

A. 1 s
B. 2.3 s
C. 3.6 s
D. 4 s

4. What graph best describes the magnitude of the car's acceleration with respect to time as it hits the wall and rebounds?

A.
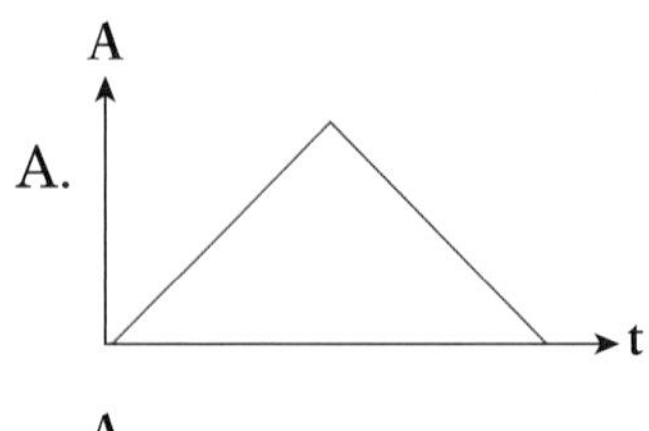

B.
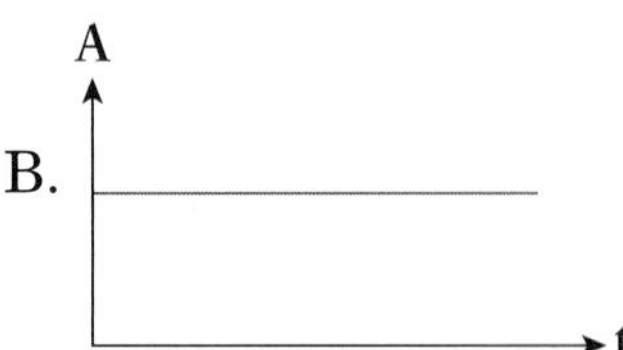

C.
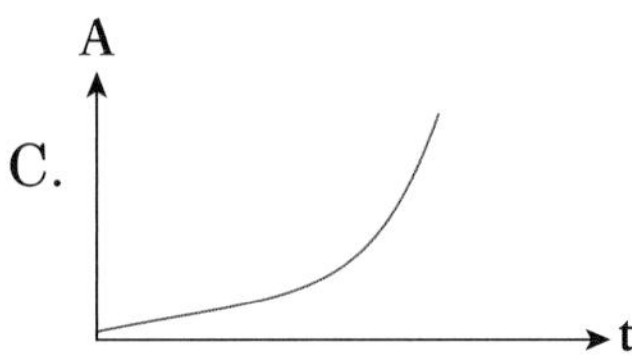

D.
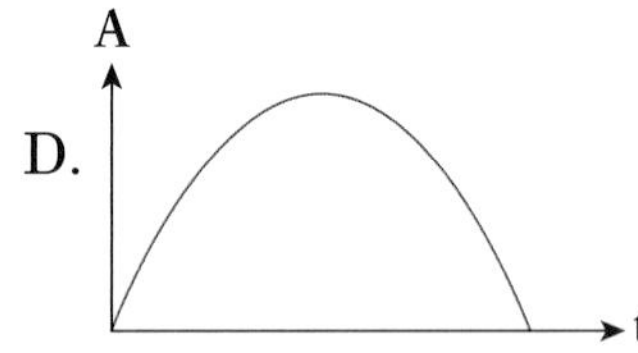

5. If 50 percent of the energy from the spring is converted into heat, how much power is delivered to each liquid cylinder in trial 2?

A. 90 W
B. 116 W
C. 180 W
D. 232 W

6. If the cylinder contains 1 kg of water and has a cross-sectional area of 1 m^2, a length of 1 cm, a coefficient of conductivity of 400 W/(m × K), how much heat will be added to the water after 5 cycles of trial 2? Assume that 50 percent of energy from the spring is converted into heat.

A. 100 J
B. 1,000 J
C. 12 kJ
D. 25 kJ

7. Which of the following would NOT affect the temperature change of a liquid inside the cylinder?

A. The number of times that the cycle is conducted
B. The magnitude of the spring constant
C. The speed of the car
D. The type of liquid inside the cylinder

8. If 50 percent of spring energy is converted into heat, then how many cycles will trial 1 last?

A. 1
B. 2
C. 4
D. Indefinitely

9. Which of the following graphs best represents the increase in temperature of a cylinder of water with respect to time if trial 1 is conducted indefinitely?

A.
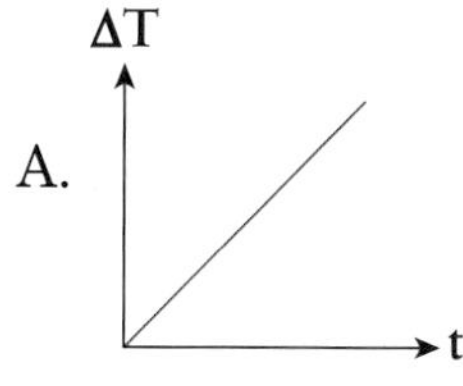

B.
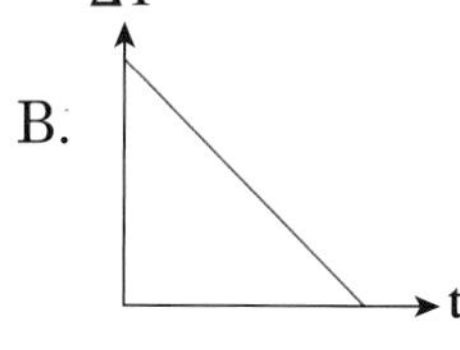

C.
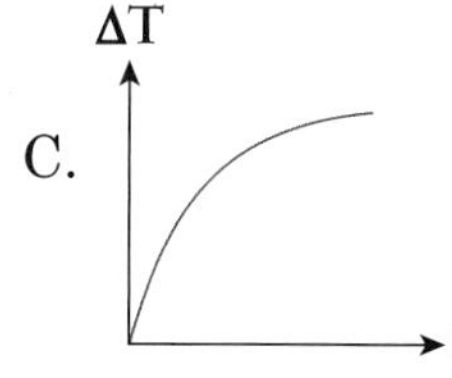

D.
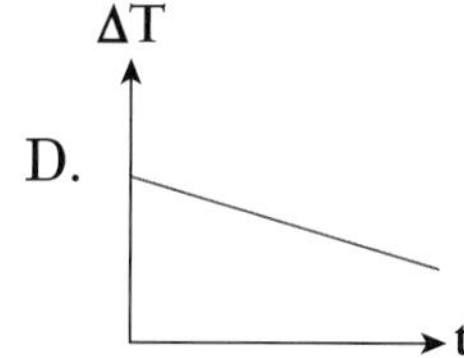

PASSAGE II (QUESTIONS 10–17)

A material's ability to conduct heat is measured by its *thermal conductivity*, k. Based on the thermal conductivity of an object, we can determine the rate of heat conduction by using the following formula:

$$\frac{\Delta Q}{\Delta t} = \frac{k \times A \times \Delta T}{x}$$

Where $\Delta Q/\Delta t$ is the change in heat per unit time, A is the cross-sectional area of the conductor, x is the width of the conductor, and ΔT is the difference in temperature between the warmer side of the conductor and the colder side.

To learn more about thermal conductivity, a student divides two compartments containing 100 mL of water (specific heat = 1 cal/[g × K]) with a plate made of copper (see figure), whose thermal conductivity is about 400 J/msK. The container is made of glass, which has a thermal conductivity of about 1 J/msK. The student uses a thermometer to measure the change in temperature of the water with respect to time. In order to compare different situations, he uses various thicknesses of copper and various temperatures of water. The total area of contact between the water and the container is 100 cm^2, while the area of contact between the water and the copper is 50 cm^2.

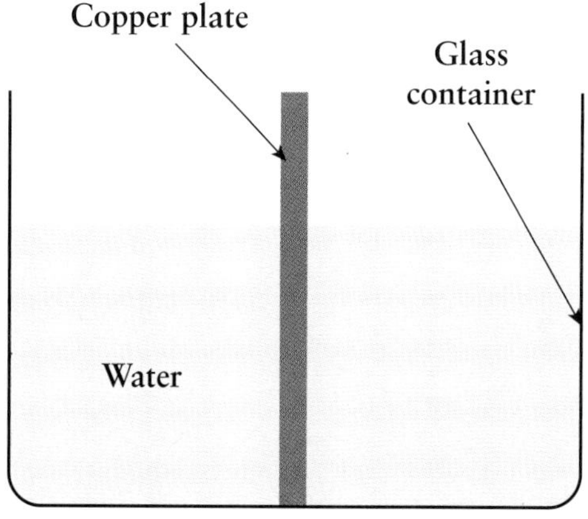

After recording the results of the experiment, the student compares them with the results that would be expected for each setup based on the thermal conductivity formula. In each calculation, the actual value of ΔQ is somewhat lower than the expected value. He notices that increases in this experimental error are almost directly proportional to the thickness of the copper plate. There is also some error present in the rest of the system.

10. The experimental error is proportional to the thickness of the plate because the student did not subtract the

A. specific heat capacity of the plate, which is directly proportional to its mass.
B. specific heat capacity of the plate, which is directly proportional to its thickness.
C. amount of heat stored by the plate, which is directly proportional to its mass.
D. amount of heat stored by the plate, which is directly proportional to its thickness.

11. None of the errors in the calculation comes from the fact that the student failed to account for

A. heat transferred by radiation from the warm water to the cold water.
B. heat transferred by conduction from the warm water to the copper plate.
C. heat transferred by conduction from the water to the environment.
D. heat transferred by conduction from the water to the glass.

12. If the environmental temperature is equal to the temperature of the cold water compartment, how much heat is conducted from through the copper plate for every 1 J that is conducted through the glass container?

A. 0.5 J
B. 2 J
C. 0.2 Kj
D. 0.5 kJ

13. If one water compartment is at a temperature of 350 K and the other compartment is at 300 K, how much heat is transferred between the two compartments when the copper divider is removed?

A. 5 Kj
B. 2.5 Kj
C. 5 Cal
D. 2.5 Cal

14. What would be the primary mode of heat transfer if the copper divider were removed?

A. Convection
B. Conduction
C. Radiation
D. Dissolution

15. The entropy change is

A. positive for the warmer compartment and zero for the cooler compartment.
B. positive for the cooler compartment and zero for the warmer compartment.
C. positive for both compartments.
D. negative for both compartments.

16. Which of the following graphs best represents the rate of heat transfer with respect to time?

A.

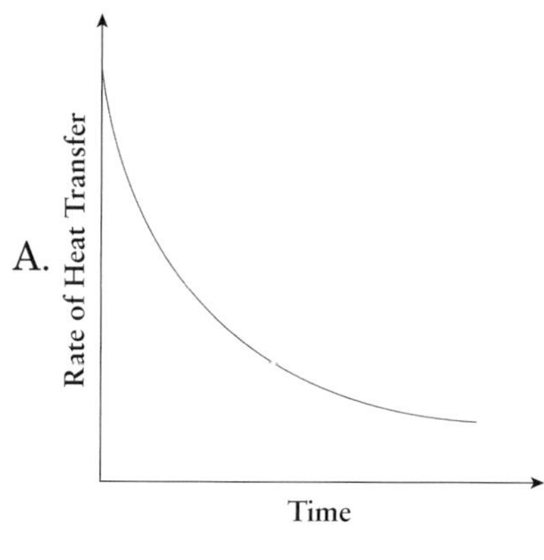

B.

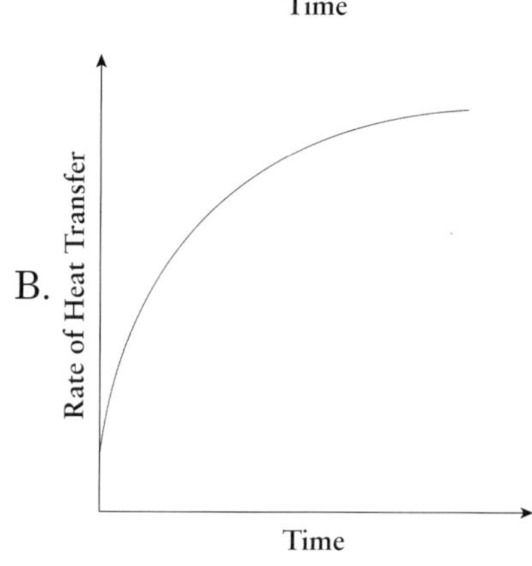

C.

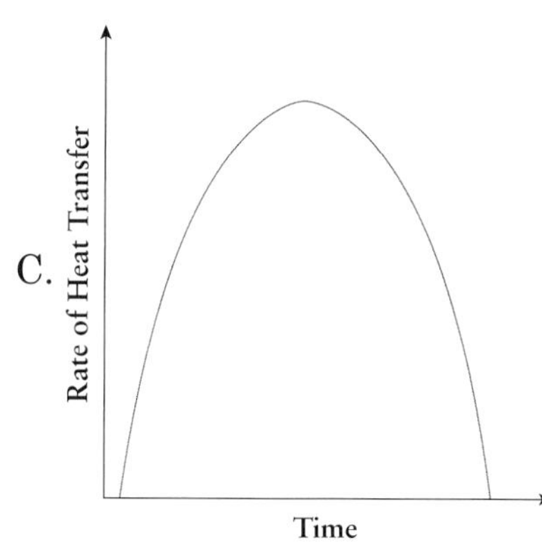

D.

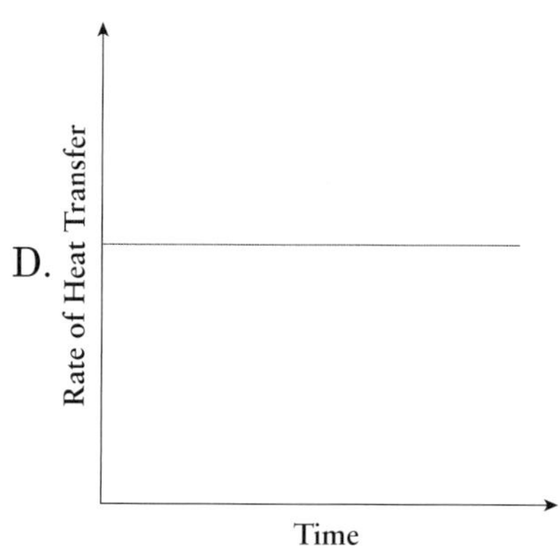

17. The kinetic energy of the molecules most likely decreases in

A. the copper plate.
B. the glass of the container.
C. the warm water compartment.
D. the cold water compartment.

QUESTIONS 18–21 ARE NOT BASED ON A DESCRIPTIVE PASSAGE.

18. A police car speeds toward you at 50 m/s. Its siren wails at 400 Hz. You are driving toward the police car at 20 m/s. What is the frequency of the sound you hear (velocity of sound in air is 330 m/s)?

A. 350 Hz
B. 370 Hz
C. 490 Hz
D. 500 Hz

19. A car moving 10 km/hr skids 15 m while stopping. How far will the car skid if it were moving originally at 100 km/hr?

A. 150 m
B. 300 m
C. 1,500 m
D. 3,000 m

20. Two identical speakers driven by an identical signal each produce 680 Hz waves. If the speakers are different distances from you, what must the difference in their distances be to completely destructively interfere? Assume that the speed of sound in air is 340 m/s.

A. 0.25 m
B. 0.5 m
C. 0.68 m
D. 1 m

21. A hydraulic lift has a small platform with a surface area of 1 m^2 and a large platform with a surface area of 100 m^2, both of which are connected by an enclosed fluid. Approximately how much force must be applied to the small platform in order to lift a 1,000 kg car that sits on the large platform?

A. 1 N
B. 5 N
C. 10 N
D. 100 N

PASSAGE III (QUESTIONS 22–30)

When operating a flight, pilots need to take into account tailwinds and headwinds. These components will affect their path and speed of flight. "Headwinds" will decrease the amount of time required for takeoff and landing, while "tailwinds" will affect the ground speed of the plane, which must be taken into account during takeoff and landing.

Headwind refers to wind at 180° of the direction of travel that opposes the forward motion of the plane. For example, if a plane is headed west at 850 m/s and the headwind is 150 m/s, then the net speed is calculated by subtracting vectors. The net resultant speed of the plane will be 700 m/s. Conversely, tailwind refers to wind at 180° of the direction of travel that adds to the forward motion of the plane. Tailwind will, hence, increase the plane's ground speed. In the above example, the net speed of the plane would be 900 m/s. Both headwinds and tailwinds occur at all altitudes. When the incident angle of the headwind or tailwind varies from 180°, vector analysis is required to isolate the component in the direction of travel.

A plane takes off from an airport at 8:00 A.M. and makes a flight path that is 30° north of east. It travels 1,500 meters in 2 hours before it is met by a tailwind blowing at 400 m/s at an angle of 45° south of east. (cos 30° = $\sqrt{3}/2$; sin 30° = 0.5; sin 45° = $\sqrt{2}/2$; cos 45° = $\sqrt{2}/2$)

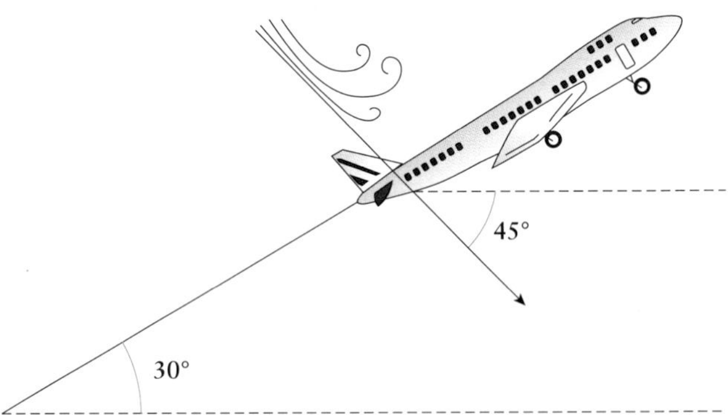

22. Which of the following is an example of a vector?

A. The speed at which the airplane is flying
B. The distance that the airplane travels
C. The velocity at which the airplane is traveling
D. The angle that the airplane makes with respect to the horizon

23. What is the average velocity of the airplane before it meets the tail wind?

A. 750 m/s
B. 750 m/s at 30° north of east
C. 3,000 m/s
D. 3,000 m/s at 30° north of east

24. What is the horizontal component of the airplane's velocity vector before it meets the tailwind?

A. 650 m/s east
B. 375 m/s east
C. 650 m/s west
D. 750 m/s east

25. What is the vertical component of the velocity after the plane meets the tailwind?

A. 92 m/s S
B. 92 m/s N
C. 658 m/s N
D. 658 m/s S

26. What is the resultant velocity of the airplane after it is met by the tailwind?

A. 938 m/s at 84° N of E
B. 1,142 m/s at 35° N of E
C. 1,142 m/s at 55° N of E
D. 938 m/s at 6° N of E

27. If there were no tailwind, how long would it take the plane to travel another 1,000 meters?

A. 1.33 minutes
B. 1.33 hours
C. 0.75 hours
D. 0.75 minutes

28. Imagine the plane at rest. If the plane traveled at 500 m/s east for 3 hours and then 175 meters west for 0.5 hours, what would be its total displacement?

A. 1,325 meters
B. 675 meters
C. 325 meters
D. 1,675 meters

29. If the tailwind were 300 m/s east, what would be the plane's total displacement at 11:30 A.M.?

A. 1,500 meters
B. 3,032 meters
C. 1,532 meters
D. 2,625 meters

30. What wind velocity would be required to change the plane's velocity to 500 m/s east?

A. 404 m/s W
B. 250 m/s at 22° S of W
C. 250 m/s W
D. 404 m/s at 68° S of W

PASSAGE IV (QUESTIONS 31–38)

The gas-filled radiation detector was one of the first instruments used to measure radiation. Particles of sufficient energy will ionize the gas molecules, causing a polarization of the gas as the positive ions migrate towards the cathode and the negative ions migrate towards the cathode. The cathode and anode are connected to a device that measures current and the readings are interpreted in order to determine the activity of the radioactive sample.

More recently, semiconductor detectors have become widespread. The basic principle of these detectors is similar to that of the gas-filled detectors, but the gas is replaced by a sample of solid silicon or germanium, both of which allow the creation of a hole in the valence shell upon contact with radiation of sufficient energy. Instead of measuring the number of gas ions produced (like the gas-filled detector), the semiconductor then measures the number of holes.

The readings from most radiation detectors are given in terms of the number of "counts." Each individual detector must be calibrated in order to relate the number of counts with the exact activity of the radioactive sample. In a certain experiment, a student tests different radionuclides with both types of radiation detectors. Each sample is counted several times in order to account for the error in the detection system; the average readings are reported here.

Sample ID	Activity	Decay Mode	Reading from Detector 1	Reading from Detector 2
None	0	?	12 counts	18 counts
A	1 mCi	α	53 counts	138 counts
B	2 mCi	α	95 counts	257 counts
C	4 mCi	α	?	?
D	0.5 mCi	?	12 counts	26 counts

31. Which of the following types of radiation is LEAST likely to be detected by a gas-filled detector?

A. α
B. β
C. γ
D. x-rays

32. Which of the following is true regarding the capabilities of both types of detectors?

A. Gas-filled detectors can measure the activity of a sample, while semiconductor detectors can measure the activity and identify the mode of decay.
B. Gas-filled detectors can identify the mode of a sample's decay, while semiconductor detectors can measure the activity and identify the mode of decay.
C. Both detectors can measure the activity of a sample and identify the mode of decay.
D. Both detectors can measure the activity of a sample, but neither can accurately identify the mode of decay.

33. Why is the semiconductor detector more sensitive than the gas-filled detector?

A. Semiconductors have a higher atomic mass than gases, making it more likely for any individual atom to interact with radiation.
B. Semiconductors are denser than gases, making it more likely for any individual atom to interact with radiation.
C. Semiconductors are more likely than gases to lose an electron.
D. Semiconductors are more likely than gases to undergo radioactive decay.

34. Why does the student notice a nonzero reading from the detectors when no sample is present?

A. Erroneous readings are caused by the inherent error in the detection system.
B. Even identical amounts of radiation may or may not interact with the particles in the detector.
C. A small number of ionization occurs even when no radiation source is present.
D. Small amounts of radiation remain in the detector from the last time that it was used.

35. Which of the following curves is most likely to be produced during the calibration of a radiation detector?

A.

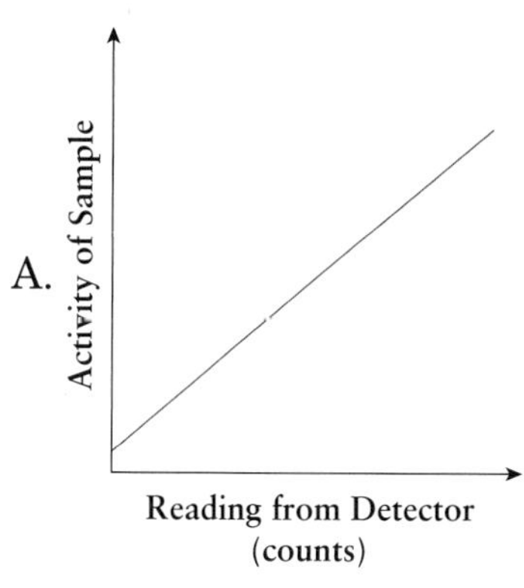

B.

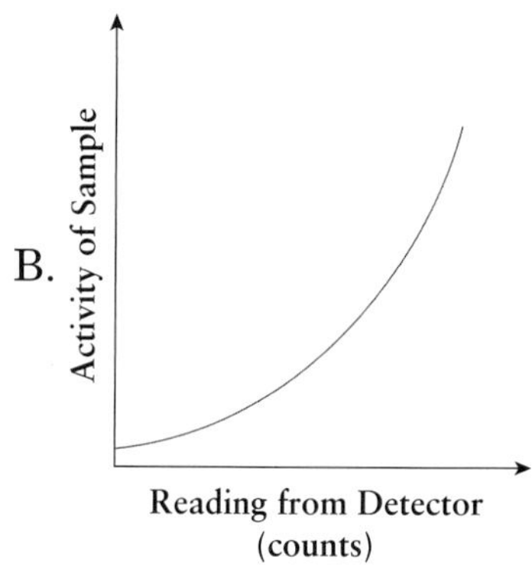

C.

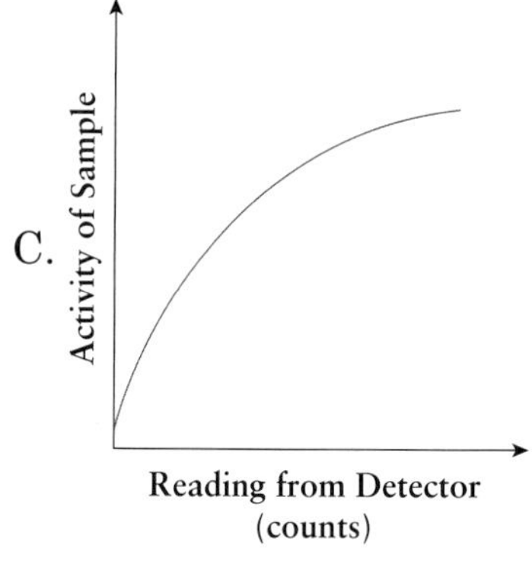

D.

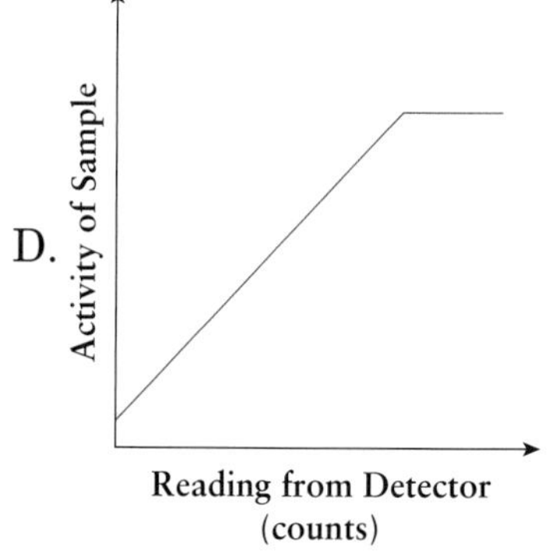

36. If sample C is tested with detector 1, the reading will probably be approximately

A. 135 counts.
B. 160 counts.
C. 175 counts.
D. 190 counts.

37. When sample A is measured again after 3 days, detector 1 reads 16 counts and detector 2 reads 32 counts. Which of the following is closest to the half-life of sample A?

A. 1 day
B. 2 days
C. 3 days
D. 4 days

38. If the activity of sample D is doubled, then

A. the readings from both detectors will definitely increase.
B. the reading from detector 2 will definitely increase, but the reading from detector 1 might not change.
C. the reading from detector 1 will definitely increase, but the reading from detector 2 might not change.
D. neither reading will definitely increase.

PASSAGE V (QUESTIONS 39–46)

Whether objects are in motion or stationary, there are always forces acting upon them. Newton's second law states that a force exerted on an object of mass m will cause it to accelerate in the direction of the force with a magnitude that is proportional to that of the force: F = ma. The concept of force is most commonly thought of as an interaction between two objects in direct contact with each other, resulting in some motion. However, one object can exert a force upon another, even across large distances and forces can be acting upon an object even if it is perfectly still. Below are two examples of such situations.

In the diagram below, a clock of mass 2M is placed on a 45° incline. The coefficient of static friction between the two surfaces is 1.2 and the coefficient of kinetic friction is 0.50.

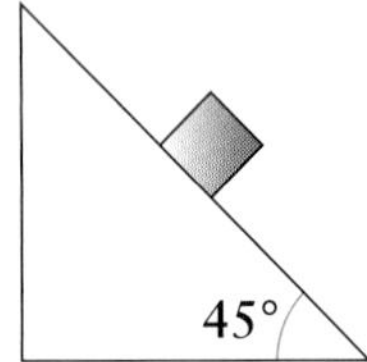

The diagram below shows two spheres. Sphere 1 has a mass of 4M and sphere 2 has a mass of M. The spheres are separated by a distance of D.

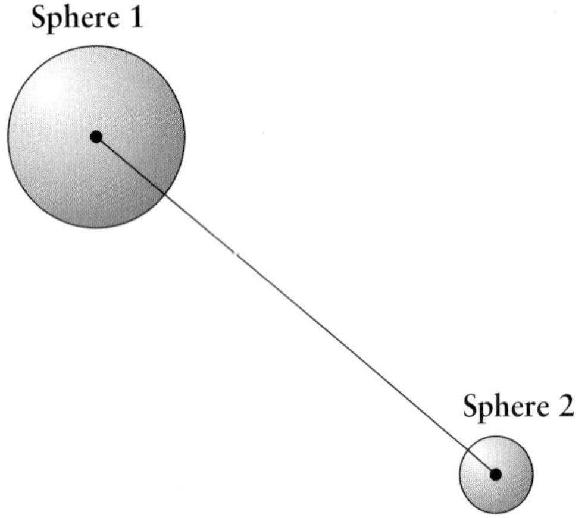

39. Which of the following correctly depicts the direction of the normal force acting upon the block in Figure 1?

A.

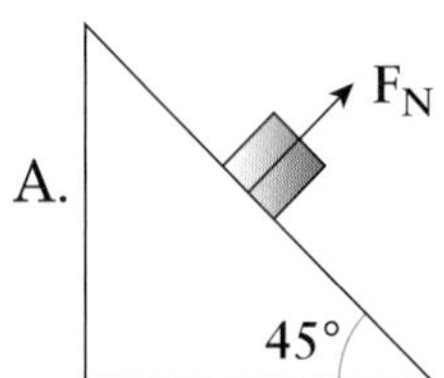

B.

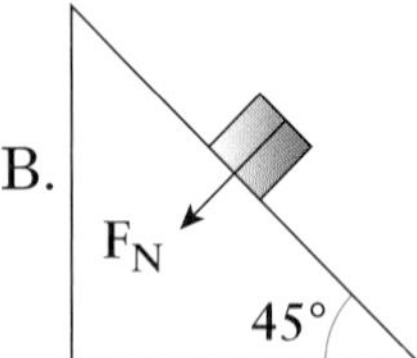

C.

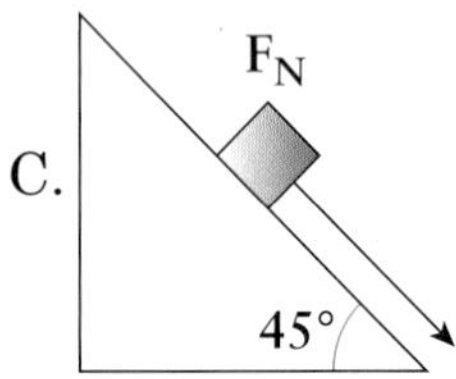

D.

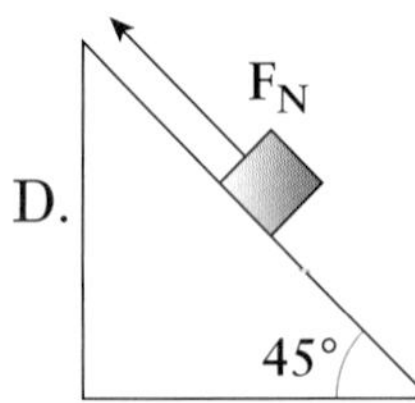

40. What is the magnitude of the force of weight exerted on the incline by the block in the y-direction?

A. sin(45°) × 2m
B. cos(45°) × 2M
C. sin(45°) × 2M × g
D. cos(45°) × 2M × g

41. If the block had a mass of 2 kg and was sitting on a flat surface, what would be the minimum force required to move it from its resting position?

A. 2.4 N
B. 1.2 N
C. 24 N
D. 20 N

42. What is the gravitational force between the two spheres in figure 2?

A. $(4GM^2)/D^2$
B. $G(m_1m_2)/d^2$
C. $(4GM)/D^2$
D. $(4GM^2)/D$

43. If the distance D in figure 2 is increased by a factor of 4, the gravitational force between the spheres will

A. increase by a factor of 4.
B. decrease by a factor of 4.
C. increase by a factor of 8.
D. decrease by a factor of 16.

44. After a certain process, the density of sphere 1 increased while its diameter decreased. The final mass of the sphere is 4 M and the position of the sphere's center is unchanged. What has happened to the gravitational force between the two spheres?

A. The force increased because the density of sphere 1 has increased.
B. The force decreased because the diameter of sphere 1 has decreased.
C. The force would be multiplied by a factor of 4.
D. The force remained the same because neither mass nor distance was altered.

45. If the block from figure 1 was placed between the two spheres such that an upward force of 75 N was applied to the block while a downward force of 33 was also applied, what would be the net force on the block?

A. 42 N upward
B. 108 N upward
C. 42 N downward
D. 108 N downward

46. If an object of mass 1 kg is sitting on the surface of a planet of mass 8 M and diameter 4 D, what is the force of gravity on the object?

A. $\frac{(8GM)}{16D^2}$

B. $\frac{(8GM)}{4D^2}$

C. $\frac{GMm}{d^2}$

D. $\frac{GM^2}{D^2}$

PASSAGE VI (QUESTIONS 47–52)

It is often invaluable to determine the blood flow rate in different vessels of the circulatory system so that information about tissue oxygen supply and possible vessel blockage can be obtained. One device commonly used for this purpose is an electromagnetic blood flow meter, which utilizes the movement of charged particles (ions) in the magnetic field. Blood plasma concentrations of different ions are presented in table 1 below, even though generally only two ions of the highest concentrations are considered when measuring the flow.

Plasma Electrolytes	Concentration
Na^+	140 mmol/L
Cl^-	100 mmol/L
K^+	4.5 mmol/L
Carbonate ion	25 mmol/L
Ca^{++}	2.5 mmol/L

During the measurement, as ions move within the artery with the velocity v = 25cm/s, magnetic poles are placed on both sides of the artery creating the magnetic field. Under the influence of magnetic forces, ions gather at opposite sides of the artery. Polarized plasma electrolytes produce electric fields across the artery which is considered uniform for the calculations. The voltage across the artery is measured with a voltmeter and $V = Ed$ ($d = 2$ cm is the diameter of the artery). The electric forces $F = qE$ produced by the electric field acting on the ions are in opposite direction to the magnetic forces $F = qvB$. The ions will continue to separate accumulating on different sides of the artery until the equilibrium is reached and magnetic force equals the electric force.

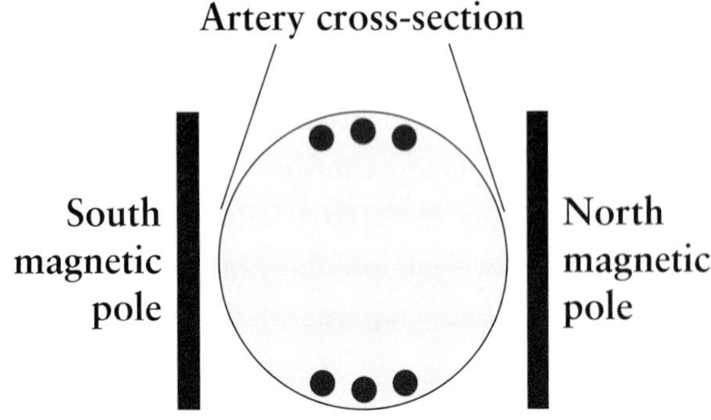

Direction of blood flow is into the page

47. What is the direction of the magnetic force on negatively charged ions in the artery?

A. Left
B. Right
C. Up
D. Down

48. Upon the application of a vasoconstricting agent, the radius of the artery decreases by 2. What will happen to the flow rate of blood and voltage, respectively?

A. Decrease by 4 and decrease by 2
B. Decrease by 2 and increase by 2
C. Both decrease by 2
D. Decrease by 2 and decrease by 8

49. Assume that calcium ion movement is considered by the flow meter. If a researcher is interested in keeping magnetic force constant for all positive ions, which of the following would need to be adjusted when considering calcium?

A. Increasing particle velocity
B. Decreasing the diameter of the artery
C. Decreasing magnetic field
D. Increasing voltage

50. As sodium and chloride are moving through the artery, what can be concluded about the magnetic force acting on the ions?

A. It is perpendicular to the ions' velocity and parallel to magnetic field.
B. It is parallel to both the ions' velocity and magnetic field.
C. It is perpendicular to the magnetic field and parallel to ions' velocity.
D. It is perpendicular to both the ions' velocity and the magnetic field.

51. If plasma electrolytes were to move from left to right in the cross-section of the artery, which of the following could be inferred?

A. There is no net magnetic force or torque on the particles.
B. There is no net magnetic force on the particles.
C. There is no torque on the particles.
D. Torque and net magnetic force are acting on the particles.

52. Calculate the current passing through the artery due to the anions' movement if the arterial resistance is 3Ω and the magnetic field of 1T is applied across the walls of the artery

A. 17×10^{-2}A
B. 1.7×10^{-5}A
C. 3.4×10^{-5}A
D. 34×10^{-2}A

PRACTICE SECTION 3

Time—70 minutes

QUESTIONS 1–52

Directions: Most of the questions in the following Physics Practice Section are organized into groups, with a descriptive passage preceding each group of questions. Study the passage, then select the single-best answer to the question in each group. Some of the questions are not based on a descriptive passage; you must also select the best answer to these questions. If you are unsure of the best answer, eliminate the choices that you know are incorrect, then select an answer from the choices that remain.

PASSAGE I (QUESTIONS 1–9)

Automotive audio systems often contain a complex wiring network, which must be optimized in order to maximize their cost-effectiveness. Typically, these systems are based around a 12 V battery, several speakers, and an amplifier, which increases the power delivered to the speakers. More elaborate customized systems often include large capacitors, multiple amplifiers, more speakers, and, occasionally, extra batteries. The best designs also consider the nature of the wire and the connectors that carry the signal between the various circuit components.

The wiring in a home audio system can be equally elaborate, but there are some clear differences. These systems extract their power from normal electrical outlets, which supply 110 V of RMS potential to most American homes. This eliminates the need for a battery and reduces the need for a capacitor while still permitting the amplifier to produce adequate amounts of power. The remaining circuit components are similar in home systems and automotive systems.

1. Which of the following are changed by the amplifier in order to increase the power delivered to the speakers?

I. Current
II. EMF
III. Resistance

A. I only
B. I and II only
C. I and III only
D. II and III only

2. A capacitor is added to an automotive system in order to provide an extra 2 A of current for up to 12 seconds at a time. What is the capacitance?

A. 2 F
B. 6 F
C. 12 F
D. 24 F

3. Assuming identical length, what type of wire should be used in order to optimize power delivery?

A. Silver wire (resistivity of 16 nΩ • m) with radius of 1 cm
B. Aluminum wire (resistivity of 28 nΩ • m) with radius of 2 cm
C. Copper wire (resistivity of 17 nΩ • m) with radius of 1.5 cm
D. Gold wire (resistivity of 24 nΩ • m) with radius of 1 cm

4. A system includes six speakers, each of which carries a resistance of 4 Ω. Assuming the speakers are the only source of resistance, what is the resistance of the circuit that would minimize overall power dissipation?

A. 2/3 Ω
B. 3/2 Ω
C. 4 Ω
D. 24 Ω

5. In a circuit containing a battery, an amplifier, a group of speakers, and a capacitor, the best place to put the capacitor is

A. between the amplifier and the speakers.
B. between the battery and the amplifier.
C. wired in parallel along with the speakers.
D. wired in series along with the speakers.

6. A car amplifier and a home amplifier are found to produce exactly the same amount of power. Which of the following statements is true?

A. Both amplifiers draw the same amount of current.
B. Both amplifiers produce the same amount of resistance.
C. The home amplifier draws more current.
D. The car amplifier draws more current.

7. Capacitors are less useful for home systems than for automotive systems because

A. the components of a home system are more likely to act as natural capacitors than the components of an automotive system.
B. the electrical outlet stores charge and, therefore, acts as a capacitor.
C. home amplifiers can extract the necessary current without the help of a capacitor.
D. car amplifiers cannot extract the necessary current without the help of a capacitor.

8. Although the published potential of most car batteries is 12 V, a typical battery will produce approximately 14 V under normal conditions. Which of the following best explains this phenomenon?

A. Fluctuations in the DC current typically lead to a higher potential.
B. Fluctuations in the AC current occasionally lead to a higher potential.
C. The RMS potential is 12 V, while the peak potential is higher.
D. The RMS potential is 14 V, while the average potential is 12 V.

9. A home amplifier and a car amplifier both have identical resistances. Which amplifier will consume more electrical energy?

A. A home amplifier, because a higher potential will draw more current
B. A car amplifier, because more energy is needed to compensate for the decreased potential
C. Both (identically), because power is directly proportional to resistance
D. Neither can be determined unless the current is known

PASSAGE II (QUESTIONS 10–17)

Early scientists measured electric charge by using an electroscope, which provides approximate measurements based on the movement of a standard charge with respect to the test object. The two most common types of such devices were the pith-ball electroscope and the gold-leaf electroscope, both of which function through electrostatic induction.

Pith-ball electroscope

The pith-ball electroscope is based on a ball suspended from a hook via a silk thread.

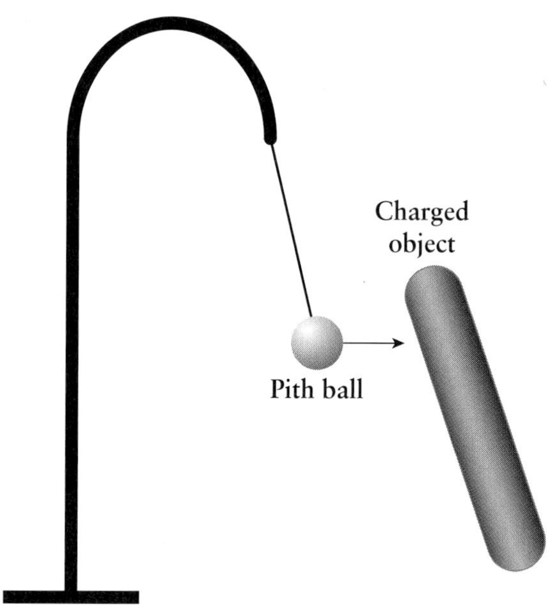

The ball is typically made of pith, which is a lightweight electrical insulator. When the electroscope is placed in the vicinity of a positively charged object, the electrons in the ball move slightly toward the object and the protons move slightly away from it. Because the electrons are now closer to the charge than the protons, the ball is attracted to the test object.

If the test object touches the pith ball, the ball will become charged. This gives the electroscope the ability to distinguish between a positive and a negative charge.

Gold-leaf electroscope

The gold-leaf electroscope consists of a metal ball (or plate) that is attached to two ultra-thin pieces of gold (also known as gold "leaves") via a brass rod.

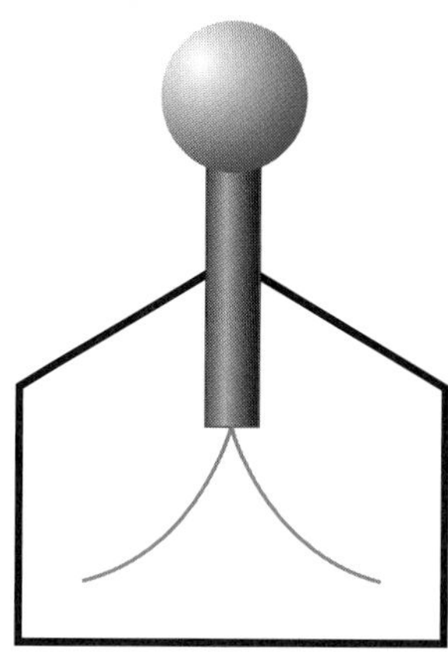

If a charged object is brought near the electroscope, the two gold leaves repel one another through a mechanism similar to the one in the pith-ball electroscope. When the object touches the ball, charge is conducted through the rod, also causing the gold leaves to repel one another.

The instrument was invented a few years after the pith-ball electroscope; it maintains several advantages because the gold leaf is much lighter than the pith ball, but still exerts a similar amount of force.

10. According to the passage, what is the definition of *electrostatic induction*?

A. The transfer of electric charge through an electrical insulator
B. The transfer of electric charge through an electrical conductor
C. A change in the distribution of electric charge in a certain object due to the influence of an outside object
D. A change in the net electric charge in a certain object due to the influence of an outside object

11. How would the pith ball interact with a negatively charged test object?

A. It would repel, because the effect should be opposite that of a positively charged object.
B. It would repel, because the electrons move slightly toward the object and the protons move slightly away from it.
C. It would attract, because metals form positively charged ions.
D. It would attract, because the electrons would move slightly away from the object and the protons would move slightly toward it.

12. Some electroscopes contain two suspended pith balls that touch each other when they are uncharged. What would be the effect of touching one of these pith balls with a negatively charged object?

A. The balls would repel each other and repel the test object.
B. The balls would repel each other and attract the test object.
C. The balls would attract each other and repel the test object.
D. The balls would attract each other and attract the test object.

13. Which of the following can be partially responsible for the movement of the pith ball or the gold leaf?

I. Electrostatic force
II. Electric conduction
III. Electric field

A. I only
B. I and II only
C. II and III only
D. I, II, and III

14. Why is it important for the pith ball to be lightweight?

A. Heavier objects will contain more atoms, which will make it more difficult for electrons and protons to migrate.
B. Heavier objects will require more force to move, which will reduce the sensitivity of the instrument.
C. Lighter objects are more likely to conduct a charge than heavier objects.
D. Lighter objects are less likely to conduct a charge than heavier objects.

15. Which of the following would be the least effective replacement for gold leaf in a gold-leaf electroscope?

A. Silver leaf
B. Copper wire
C. Gold foil
D. Pith

16. A negatively charged object is placed to the right of a pith ball. What is the direction of the electric field?

A. Left
B. Right
C. Up
D. Down

17. Which of the following does NOT describe the interaction between the two gold leaves?

A. Electrostatic repulsion
B. Charge redistribution
C. Production of an electric dipole
D. Production of an electric field

QUESTIONS 18–22 ARE NOT BASED ON A DESCRIPTIVE PASSAGE.

18. The total energy (kinetic plus potential) of a falling object is conserved. If a 5 kg object is dropped from a height of 5 m, approximately how fast is it traveling just before it touches the ground?

A. 1 m/s
B. 10 m/s
C. 25 m/s
D. 100 m/s

19. The distance a car travels relates to its initial velocity and acceleration. Suppose a car traveling at 10 m/s notices a road block which is 30 m away. The driver instantly presses the brakes, and the car decelerates at 2 m/s^2. The car will

A. crash into the roadblock.
B. just barely touch the roadblock.
C. safely miss the roadblock by 5 m.
D. safely miss the roadblock by 10 m.

20. The total resistance of a circuit is related to the resistances of individual resistors, and the orientation of those resistors. If a circuit consists of two 6 ohm resistors in parallel, and those resistors are placed in series instead, the total resistance of the circuit will do which of the following?

A. Increase four-fold
B. Increase two-fold
C. Decrease four-fold
D. Decrease two-fold

21. In a perfectly elastic collision, two objects can be considered one larger object after the collision. If a 150 kg football played traveling south at 3 m/s has a perfectly inelastic collision with a 100 kg player travelling north at 5 m/s, what is the velocity of the two players after the collision?

A. 2 m/s North
B. 0.2 m/s North
C. 0.2 m/s South
D. 2 m/s South

22. The result of two waves interfering with each other can be determined using the principal of linear superimposition. If two waves of equal amplitude A_1 interfere in phase, what will be the amplitude of the resultant wave?

A. $2 \cdot A_1$
B. $4 \cdot A_1$
C. A_1
D. $\frac{1}{2} \cdot A_1$

PASSAGE III (QUESTIONS 23–30)

The pentathlon has changed much during the years of its existence. One of the original Olympic games, it comes from the Greek for "five competitions." Among these were wrestling, long jump, javelin throw, discus throw, and a short foot race. The foot race, or *stadion*, was 180 m long. Though wrestling and the discus throw were similar to their modern forms, the javelin throw was quite different, with the athlete using a leather strap rather than gripping the javelin itself. One of the most remarkable Olympic records in this sport is held by Osleidys Menendez of Cuba, with a throw of 71.53 m, obtained in Athens at the start of this century.

The modern Olympics has changed these sports around. Starting in 1912 for men, they included 110/100 m hurdles, shot put, high jump, long jump, and 1,500/800 meter run. Today, in addition to this athletic pentathlon is a modern pentathlon, which features five completely different sports. In the shooting competition, participants must use an air pistol to shoot 20 50 g bullets at a 17 cm square target from 10 m away, all in 40 seconds. These bullets typically travel at 500 m/s! Fencing is next and is in the form of a round-robin tournament. Following that is swimming, a freestyle race spanning 200 m. Next is probably one of the most unusual parts, a riding competition featuring an obstacle course about 400 m long, with 12 obstacles and 15 jumps. Finally comes the 3 km run. Athletes are assigned handicaps based on their points total from the last four events. This allows the athlete who crosses the finish line first to be given the gold medal.

23. Consider the discus throw from the original Olympics. Which of the following describes the inward pull of the athlete's arm on the discus?

A. It is known as centrifugal force.
B. It is inversely proportional to the speed of the object.
C. It is inversely proportional to the square of the speed.
D. It is proportional to the square of the speed.

24. Imagine that a representative from Chile practices his shot put. As a conditioning exercise, he throws from the top of a peak in the Andes and launches the ball horizontally from 1,000 m above sea level. A microchip in the ball records that it has an initial speed of 30 m/s and hits something (not necessarily at sea level) within 7 seconds of its release. What is its release during the sixth second?

A. 4.2 m/s^2
B. 5.0 m/s^2
C. 10.0 m/s^2
D. 32.2 m/s^2

25. If the record-breaking javelin throw was made at an angle of 45° with the horizontal and at an initial speed of 45 m/s, how far had it traveled in its first 2 seconds in flight?

A. 2.25 m
B. 45.0 m
C. 63.6 m
D. 78.0 m

26. Imagine that an air pistol operates by spring motion. If the spring is compressed 1 cm while cocked, what is the theoretical spring constant?

A. 1.25 N/m
B. 1.25×10^7 N/m
C. 1.25×10^8 N/m
D. More information is required

27. Two fencers training on ice stand face-to-face, with their sabers crossed and pressed on each other at a single point. If fencers 1 and 2 have a mass of 67 kg and 45 kg, respectively, what is the ratio of fencer 1's speed to fencer 2's speed as they push off in opposite directions?

A. 1:1
B. 1:2
C. 45:67
D. 67:54

28. A rider pushes his horse to the break point, traveling an average of 10 m/s through the first 40 percent of the riding portion of the pentathlon. The horse becomes exhausted and finishes the second 60 percent of the race at half the original rate. What is its average speed for the race?

A. 5.00 m/s
B. 6.25 m/s
C. 7.00 m/s
D. 7.14 m/s

29. A record-holder from Cuba jumped about 2.5 m in 1989. Imagining he fell straight to the ground on his way back down, what was his speed just before he hit the ground?

A. 0.7 m/s
B. 7 m/s
C. 50 m/s
D. 20 m/s

30. An athlete training for the swimming portion of the modern pentathlon spends 30 minutes swimming at a constant rate of 2 m/s. After pushing herself to the limit and surpassing her personal record for round-trip laps swum, she determines that her displacement during this period has been

A. 0 m.
B. 1,800 m.
C. 3,600 m.
D. dependant on her acceleration.

PASSAGE IV (QUESTIONS 31–37)

A student conducts an experiment to study the rules of simple harmonic motion. To do this, he attaches a block to a spring (K = 100 N/m) on a horizontal table as shown in the figure below.

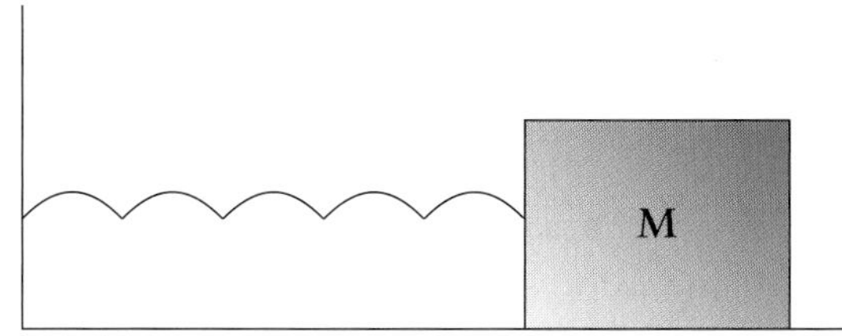

He stretches the block to the right, releases it, and watches it oscillate. After the block comes to rest, he attaches another block of a different mass and records the new findings. He repeats this experiment with varying forces and block masses. He used formulas from his physics book to compute the measurements. Some of his measurements are shown below.

$E = \frac{1}{2}mv^2 + \frac{1}{2}kx^2 = \frac{1}{2}kA^2$, where A is the maximum amplitude of the system

$\omega = 2\pi f$

	Force Applied (F)	Amplitude (A)	Period (T)	Mass (m)
Block A	50 N	0.5 m		1 kg
Block B	150 N		7 s	2 kg
Block C	200 N		1 s	5 kg

31. How many cycles does block A complete in a quarter of a second?

A. $1/(2\pi) \times \sqrt{(100/1)}$
B. $\pi \times \sqrt{(1/100)}$
C. $\pi/8 \times \sqrt{(1/100)}$
D. $1/(8\pi) \times \sqrt{(100/1)}$

32. What is the maximum velocity of block C?

A. $2A \times \sqrt{(k/m)}$
B. $A \times \sqrt{(m/k)}$
C. $A \times \sqrt{(k/m)}$
D. $2A \times \sqrt{(m/k)}$

33. Which of the following would increase the maximum amplitude of block B?

I. Increasing the mass of block B
II. Increasing the spring constant, K
III. Performing the experiment where the gravity constant is 19.6 m/s^2

A. I only
B. II only
C. I and II only
D. I, II, and III

34. Which of the following would increase the amplitude of the system?

I. Reducing the coefficient of friction between the table and the block

II. Introducing an external force (i.e., hitting the block) at the right moment during its motion

III. Increasing the length of the spring without changing the spring constant

A. II only
B. I and III only
C. II and III only
D. I, II, and III

35. How does the maximum acceleration and amplitude compare between blocks B and C?

A. B's maximum acceleration and amplitude are both greater than C's.
B. B's maximum acceleration is greater and amplitude is less than C's.
C. B's maximum acceleration is less and amplitude is greater than C's.
D. B's maximum acceleration and amplitude are both less than C's.

36. The figure below is a graph of velocity versus time for block D. Which of the following statements best describe block D?

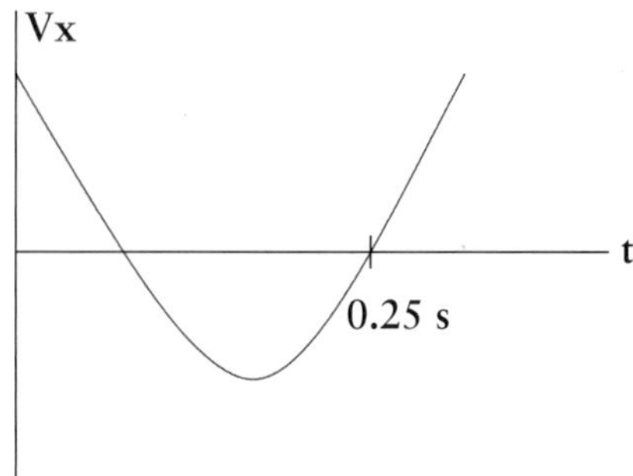

A. The spring is initially compressed and passes the equilibrium point at 0.25 seconds.
B. The block is passing the equilibrium position at t = 0 and the spring is extended at 0.25 seconds.
C. The block is passing the equilibrium position at t = 0 and the spring is compressed at 0.25 seconds.
D. The spring is initially extended and is going through the equilibrium position at 0.25 seconds.

37. When the velocity of a block A is zero and the spring is extended, which of the following is true?

A. The acceleration is at its maximum and points to the left.
B. The acceleration is at its maximum and points to the right.
C. The acceleration is zero and points to the left.
D. The acceleration is zero and points to the right.

PASSAGE V (QUESTIONS 38–44)

Nuclear energy is having a resurgence in potential popularity as a cost-effective way to meet the enormous energy demands in the United States. Together with how radiation and particles affect living organisms, an understanding of basic nuclear processes such as radioactive decay and nuclear fission will influence future energy policy and medical technology. In general, nuclear phenomena involve relatively large quantities of energy for a given amount of material; they also lead to relatively large biological effects.

Figure 1a shows a nuclear fission reaction in which weapons-grade uranium breaks up to form two fission fragments plus some neutrons. Together with protons, protons and neutrons are collectively known as nucleons. The fission reaction shown in Figure 1a involves neutron-induced fission of ${}_{92}U^{235}$, which temporarily produces a compound nucleus (${}_{92}U^{236}$) and then breaks up to form many combinations of nuclei. A typical fission reaction with one possible combination of fission fragments is given in the second reaction shown in Figure 1b. ${}_{92}U^{235}$ has a half-life of 7.1 x 10^8 years.

$${}_0n^1 + {}_{92}U^{235} \quad {}_{92}U^{236} \quad N_1 + N_2 + \text{neutrons} \qquad (1a)$$

$${}_0n^1 + {}_{92}U^{235} \quad {}_{92}U^{236} \quad {}_{36}Kr^{92} + {}_{56}Ba^{141} + 3\ {}_0n^1 \qquad (1b)$$

Radioactive carbon dating is extremely useful for dating events because human and other living organisms ingest radioactive carbon produced by cosmic rays in our atmosphere. The radioactive carbon mixes with the normal carbon in the environment and is ingested by all living organisms. Once an organism dies, the radioactive carbon in the organism begins to decay, and the ratio of radioactive carbon to ordinary carbon decreases with time. The amount of radioactive carbon can be used to determine approximately when the death occurred.

Three naturally occurring isotopes of carbon are currently known to exist on Earth. The most common, making up about 99 percent of the earth's carbon, is carbon-12. Carbon-13, a stable isotope, makes up about 1 percent. Finally, carbon-14, a radioactive isotope, makes up trace amounts, but is this form that is of most interest in radiocarbon dating. This form has a half-life of 5,630 years and a decay rate of 2000 counts/second. Figure 2 describes this decay.

$${}_0n^1 + {}_{92}U^{235} \quad {}_{92}U^{236} \quad {}_{36}Kr^{92} + {}_{56}Ba^{141} + 3\ {}_0n^1$$

38. How many neutrons exist in an atom of the uranium intermediary produced during nuclear fission?

A. 92
B. 143
C. 144
D. 236

39. Considering the half-life of ${}_{92}U^{235}$, the amount of untouched naturally occurring weapons-grade uranium embedded in the earth has

A. increased since Earth's formation 4.6 x 10^9 years ago.
B. remained constant since Earth's formation 4.6 x 10^9 years ago.
C. decreased by more than a factor of 2 since Earth's formation 4.6 x 10^9 years ago.
D. decreased by less than a factor of 2 since Earth's formation 4.6 x 10^9 years ago.

40. Approximately how much of a 200 g sample of ${}_6C^{14}$ remains after 11,460 years?

A. 200 g
B. 100 g
C. 50 g
D. 25 g

41. What will be the decay rate of ${}_6C^{14}$ in 5,730 years?

A. 2,000 count/sec
B. 1,000 count/sec
C. 500 count/sec
D. 250 count/sec

42. ${}_6C^{14}$ decay, shown below, is best described as

$${}_6C^{14} \quad {}_7N^{14} + {}_{-1}e^0$$

A. α decay.
B. β decay.
C. γ decay.
D. All of the above.

43. Which of the following is true concerning the ${}_6C^{14}$ decay (shown above)?

A. A proton and an electron are destroyed, while a neutron is created.
B. A proton and a neutron are destroyed, while an electron is created.
C. A proton and a neutron are created, while an electron is destroyed.
D. A proton and an electron are created, while a neutron is destroyed.

44. Assuming 15 decays per minute per gram of carbon in a living organism, how old is a bone containing 100 gram of carbon having a decay rate of 187.5 decays per minute?

A. 5,730 years
B. 11,460 years
C. 17,190 years
D. 22,920 years

PASSAGE VI (QUESTIONS 45–52)

The Hubble space telescope first went up into orbit in April 1990 and is scheduled to be retrieved around 2013. Remarkable for the quality of its images, Hubble is also known as one of the largest telescopes in the world. Weighing in at 11,110 kg, it orbits quite close to the Earth, about 600 km away from the surface. It orbits the Earth about every 1½ hours, going at a speed of 7,500 m/s.

Many observatories exist around the world with lenses even larger than that of Hubble. However, one of the things that sets it apart from earth-bound telescopes is actually its position relative to the Earth. The near absence of background light allows it to produce exceptionally clear and distinct images. Another unique feature is its ultra deep field abilities, which allows the scope to take images of especially far away objects using only visible light.

The inner-workings of the scope are itself remarkable. Hubble is capable of observing visible, ultraviolet, and near-infrared wavelengths and has a focal length of 57.6 m. One of the most important aspects of the telescope system is its concave mirror.

However, there have been several servicing missions since the telescope was launched. The first was scheduled to repair a flawed mirror. Though the mirror had been ground very precisely, the issue was that it had been produced with an incorrect shape. Because it was too flat at the edges, although the length of the imperfection was only a few micrometers, the mirror caused light reflecting off the edge and the light reflecting off the center to focus on different points. Although this flaw did not disrupt all kinds of observations, it was largely catastrophic for some of them.

45. At one point in the construction of Hubble, a company built a blank copy mirror from ultra-low expansion glass, with an index of refraction of 2. Imagine that a thick block of this material had been brought up in space while astronauts were on a service mission. If a laser beam had been pointed at the block, what would the astronaut determine its critical angle to be?

A. 30°
B. 45°
C. 60°
D. None of the above

46. A student builds a scale model of the telescope for a class project. However, his teacher notices that there are several inconsistencies with the actual telescope. In terms of size, everything is accurately 10 percent the size of the original. However, the optical portion consists of converging lenses rather than a single convex mirror. The lenses touch and there are two of them. If the student were to use the model for optical experiments, what would be its total focal length?

A. –2.9 m
B. 0.3 m
C. 2.9 m
D. 5.8 m

47. Rank the following by their wavelength, from highest frequency to lowest frequency.

I. Visible light
II. Ultraviolet
III. Infrared
IV. X-rays

A. III, I, IV, II
B. IV, II, I, III
C. I, II, IV, III
D. II, IV, III, I

48. Imagine that Hubble somehow hits a momentarily stationary spacecraft on the plane of its orbit. Hubble falls to Earth, starting from rest and moving with constant acceleration along a straight line as it falls. You are asked to sketch two graphs of Hubble's fall. Graph A represents speed, while Graph B represents distance. Which of the following would describe these graphs?

I. A is a flat line with 0 slope.
II. A is a straight line with a nonzero slope.
III. B is parabolic, sloping away from the x-axis.
IV. B is parabolic, sloping toward the x-axis.

A. I only
B. IV only
C. II and III only
D. II and IV only

49. Suppose that during a maintenance mission, an astronaut drops a hammer (n = 10 N) and washer (n = 0.01 N) from his hands. Instead of remaining in orbit with the satellite, space station, and astronaut, the objects drop straight down, falling freely. Neglecting air resistance, which of the following statements would be true about the subsequent motion of the two objects?

I. The two fall with the same acceleration.
II. The two have the same speed before hitting the earth.
III. The hammer has more potential energy before falling.
IV. The two have the same potential energy before falling.

A. III only
B. I and IV only
C. I, II, and III
D. I, II, and IV

50. A scientist monitoring Hubble's speed as it rounds the earth in orbit notices that the speed has become quite erratic. She looks at a chart of the motion and realizes that over the course of five seconds, Hubble's speed has decreased by 10 percent. As this speed reduction is treacherous when maintaining orbit, the scientist needs to get the telescope on track. Among the values she needs is the distance that Hubble has traveled since its speed began to decline. Assuming smooth deceleration, what is this distance?

A. 1,425 m
B. 7,125 m
C. 33,750 m
D. 35,625 m

51. A foil-covered instrument attached to the side of the telescope falls off while Hubble is steadily in orbit. How much time is required for this instrument to reach the earth's surface? Assume that the acceleration due to gravity is approximately 10 m/s^2.

A. 11 sec
B. 1 min
C. 1 min, 16 sec
D. 5 min, 46 sec

52. Imagine that a ray of light travels parallel to the principal axis of the most important aspect of the telescope. After reflecting off, the light ray will travel

A. normal to the mirror's principal axis.
B. parallel to the mirror's principal axis.
C. to a point 57.6 m in front of its initial position.
D. to a point 115.2 m in front of its initial position.

Answers and Explanations

Another way to do this problem is to use $v^2 = v_0^2 + 2a(x - x_0)$ for the vertical component. This method is quicker, as v_y and y_0 are zero and the equation reduces to $y = \frac{v_{0y}^{\ 2}}{2g}$.

7. A

Though this question may seem straightforward, it does require familiarity with scalars and vectors. Displacement is a vector made up of magnitude and direction, the magnitude being distance. Distance is composed only of magnitude and so it is considered a scalar. (B) is incorrect; we might often say that weight is the "force of gravity" on an object, but in fact it is the magnitude of the force of gravity on an object. So we can give the weight of an object in newtons and not have to indicate a direction for the force of gravity. (C) includes speed and so might peak our interest, but unless velocity is the other choice, this is incorrect. In (D), acceleration is incorrectly paired with velocity.

8. D

Two methods are possible here. The quickest and easiest method is $v^2 = v_0^2 + 2a(x - x_0)$. If we know our values, this substitution is quick: $(3 \text{ m/s})^2 = (1 \text{ m/s})^2 + 2(0.5 \text{ m/s}^2)(x - 50 \text{ m})$, so $x = 58$ m. A second method is to use $v = v_0 + at$, where $v = 3$. After we obtain t, we can use $x - x_0 = v_0t + (1/2)at^2$.

9. C

Stick to the basic principles in projectile motion and one-dimensional motion, and this question shouldn't be too difficult. The rock, A, has to rise higher than the ball, B. At the apex of its movement, it will be falling freely. We can think of B as doing so, at least in its horizontal sense. However, at the point where A starts falling freely, B has already begun doing so. It will reach the ground before the rock. (A) would be correct if the rock were dropped straight down at the same time that the ball was projected. (B) would be tempting if you allowed yourself to be swayed by the inclusion of masses. (A) and (B) are included as distractors—mass has nothing to do with the time these would take to reach the ground.

10. D

To find the maximum resultant of two concurrent forces, we add their magnitudes. Then, to find the minimum resultant, we subtract their magnitudes. This leads us only to (D).

11. C

Again, we must remember our basics or easily fall prey to traps. The horizontal velocity of the ball has nothing to do with vertical velocity. Acceleration in the horizontal component is always zero and its velocity therefore remains constant at 35 m/s. One might hastily choose A because it is familiar as g or might be tempting when compared to B. Furthermore, we might use $v^2 = v_0^2 + 2a(x - x_0)$. After doing some time-consuming calculations and estimating, we would obtain something close to (D). This would be incorrect and would have certainly wasted time. Remember, distractors are often included to accommodate flawed calculations and logic/reasoning in equation use.

12. D

Vectors are quantities that are composed of magnitude and direction. An electron's charge will be the same no matter its motion (A). It may change as a function of some variable, but that is not indicated to have a direct relationship to the direction provided. The same goes for (B), because the mass will remain the same no matter where it is thrown (even into the far reaches of the atmosphere). Here, weight would have been a tempting answer as well, but it is indeed a vector. (C) is also tempting, as potential energy is energy as a function of distance. However, it is reported in joules and the magnitude itself changes based on that distance. Direction is not a component of potential energy. Finally, (D) is correct; gravitational field strength is a ratio of the gravitational force on an object (a vector quantity) to its mass. Therefore, gravitational field strength is itself a vector quantity.

13. A

When the ball is thrown horizontally, its vertical velocity is 0 m/s and changes as per the vertical acceleration, g. The rock is dropped from *rest* and as it has no horizontal velocity component, its vertical velocity and velocity overall, is initially 0 m/s. (B) is incorrect because the rock has no horizontal velocity; it simply moves vertically. (D) can be ruled out right away because of the discrepancy in the heights of the buildings. Even if the objects were released at the same height, though, (D) would not be true because of the nature of the path of each.

14. D

Drawing a diagram here will help. Looking at our equations, we choose:

$$x - x_0 = v_0t + (1/2)at^2$$
$$20\text{ m} = (0\text{ m/s})(t) + (1/2)(10\text{ m/s}^2)t^2$$
$$t = 2$$

We use 20 m for $x - x_0$ because we add the 19 m height of the bleachers and the 1 m height to the boy's arm. This is the height at which the projectile is launched. Furthermore, we use 0 m/s for v_0 because we are concerned with vertical motion, and the initial vertical speed in a projectile question is 0 m/s. If we stop here, we might choose (B). Furthermore, if we had used 25 m/s for v_0 and in our haste dropped the t in that term, we might have chosen (A). Our next step is simple:

$$v = x/t$$
$$(25\text{ m/s}) = x/2\text{ s}$$
$$x = 50\text{ m}$$

Use 25 m/s for v because we're now concerned with horizontal distance. Using 1 s here might lead us to choice (C).

15. D

The key here is to remember that the horizontal component of the velocity has nothing to do with the vertical component. When the projectile reaches its highest point, the vertical component of the object's velocity is 0 m/s. Simply using $v = v_0 + at$, we get $0\text{ m/s} = 100\text{ m/s} + (-10\text{ m/s}^2)(t)$. Therefore, $t = 10$ s.

Remember your sign conventions. V will be 0 m/s because we're concerned with the apex, where vertical velocity is as such. Furthermore, don't forget that acceleration here is g and is negative. Otherwise, you'll get a negative time and likely be at a loss for an answer.

16. C

Because we're concerned with horizontal distance, we need to find the horizontal component of the velo-city. $v_x = v \cos\theta = (40\text{ m/s}) \cos 30° =$ appx 35 m/s. Then simply use the following:

$$v = x/t$$
$$35\text{ m/s} = x/(2.5\text{ s})$$
$$x = 87.5\text{ m}$$

Using 40 m/s during this step would lead you to (D), and confusing cos 30° with sin 30° or cos 45° would lead you to (A) and (B), respectively.

17. B

Draw a diagram here to keep all the information straight. First, because the question has to do with height, we will have to use $y - y_0 = v_0t + (1/2)at^2$. We can figure out v_0 easily, but it's more pressing to find t. We know that the post is 25 m away and need to find out how long it took to get there. We can use the following:

$$v = x/t \quad \text{but need the proper value for v. This is the horizontal component.}$$

$$v_x = (20 \text{ m/s})(\cos 45°)$$
$$= \text{appx } 14 \text{ m/s}$$
$$14 \text{ m/s} = (28 \text{ m})(t)$$
$$t = 0.5 \text{ s}$$

Looking at our original equation, we need v_0, in the vertical dimension.

$$V_{0y} = 20 \sin 45°$$
$$= \text{appx } 14 \text{ m/s}$$

Substituting into our original equation, we get:

$$y = 0 + (14 \text{ m/s})(0.5 \text{ s}) - (1/2)(10 \text{ m/s}^2)(0.5)^2$$
$$= 5.75\text{m}$$

Finally, we have to remember the last part of the question. The low post is 2.5 m high and the ball reaches 5.75 m, so the ball goes 3.25 m over. The answer is (B).

18. B

Though there's a lot to consider here, the ideas are very basic. There are two methods we could use. The fastest method is as follows:

$$v^2 = v_0^2 + 2a(x - x_0)$$
$$= (0 \text{ m/s})^2 + 2(10 \text{ m/s}^2)(30 \text{ m})$$
$$= 600 \text{ m/s}$$
$$v = \text{appx } 24 \text{ m/s}$$

Remember that $x - x_0$ is only 30 m. If you use 350, you'll have a lot of calculating to do and will most likely fall into a trap. (Coming to a point where the math leads you to $v^2 = 77{,}000$, you might well choose (D) 277 m/s, but that is incorrect.)

For the second method, you would use $x - x_0 = v_0t + (1/2)at^2$. This would give you t, which you could plug into $v = v_0 + at$. (B) is the correct answer.

19. B

Sketch a graph to make the visualization easier. The table provides information about velocity versus time, so the area under such a graph would represent change in distance traveled. It would be difficult to get the area of the shape all at once, but you can easily break up the area into two shapes: the rectangle has an area of 21 m and the triangle has an area of 4.5 m. Forgetting that the area of the triangle involves dividing by 2 would get you to (C). Knowing what the slope and area of a graph indicate is an especially important skill for kinematics. It's also possible to answer this question without sketching a graph. Calculate the average speed over the time interval and multiply it by the time interval itself. The answer is (B); the child had wobbled 25.5 m after the first 7 minutes.

CHAPTER 2: NEWTONIAN MECHANICS

1. A

The expulsion of fuel has an equal and opposite reaction from the rocket (Newton's third law). As this expulsion is at a constant flow rate, the force pushing the rocket is constant. Had this question asked about acceleration of the rocket, it would have increased with time, because the mass of the rocket is steadily decreasing and $F = m \times a$. (D) describes acceleration versus time. (A) is the correct answer.

2. C

It may help to draw a force diagram. The forces due to acceleration and those due to gravity are perpendicular. This means that the tension on the lamp is equal to m × (vector addition of a and g) = $5 \times \sqrt{4^2 + 10^2}$, which is closest to 55 N, choice (C).

3. D

To start the movement, F_A must overcome the force of static friction. So $F_A = Ks \times mg = 0.8 \times 5 \times 10 = 40$ N. Coefficient of kinetic friction only applies to the object when it is already in motion.

4. A

To continue movement, Fa must only overcome the force of kinetic friction. But the pulley system decreases the force required to move the object in half. Because the pulleys are connected by two ropes, both of which move an equal distance, the back pulley (and the box) accelerates twice as slowly as the front pulley, to which the force is applied. So if $\bar{a}$ is the acceleration of the box, then Fa = 2 × m × a. Force × distance is always conserved in such systems, and Fa has to cover twice as much distance as the box. Therefore:

$$Fa = 0.5 \times 5 \times \frac{10}{2} = 12.5 \text{ N}$$

5. D

Normally, acceleration of a box down a ramp is equal to g × sin(alpha), which is equal to g if the incline is perpendicular to the ground and to 0 if the ramp is flat. So if the ramp is not accelerating, the box will accelerate down at a rate $0 < a < g$. But when the ramp accelerates, additional forces act on the box. Writing the equations of motion for such a system is beyond the scope of the MCAT. But intuitively, you may notice than when your car accelerates forward, raindrops may move up your front window. If the box in this example were frozen in space for a moment, it would stay behind, relative to the accelerating cart. This is why the cart pushes it backward and up. In the same way, if the cart accelerated in the opposite direction, the box would accelerate down. The answer is (D), because the question doesn't indicate whether the acceleration of the cart is great enough to actually move the box up the incline.

6. C

You may imagine that the fish is attached to a string, and the tension in the string is given by ma = mg – T (because a and g point in the same direction). Then T = m × (g – a) =10 × (10 – 4) = 60 N. A quicker way to solve this is to notice that when the elevator accelerates down with magnitude g, the fish is in free fall and weighs 0 N. Alternatively, when the elevator goes up, one usually feels heavier.

7. B

The swordsman must supply both vertical and horizontal components of force with his hands. It is useful to draw a diagram.

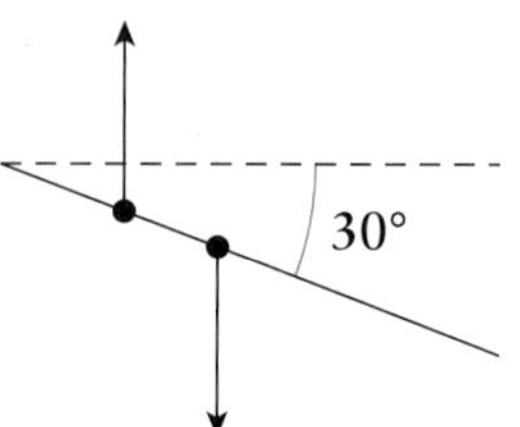

The question asks only about the vertical component. To maintain equilibrium, the knight must balance the force on the center of mass due to gravity. Therefore:

$$F_{up} \times d1 \times \cos 30 = mg \times d2 \times \cos 30$$

$$F_{up} = 10 \text{ k} \times g \times \frac{50 \text{ cm}}{10 \text{ cm}} = 500 \text{ N}$$

This vertical component of force is the same at any angle, but it is harder to hold the sword in a position close to horizontal; in that case, only a small percentage of the applied force contributes to the vertical component.

8. C

Deceleration, a, of 50 m/s divided by 10 s must be added to the force required to overcome gravity. Hence, the total force is as follows:

$$F = m \times \left(\frac{50}{10} + 10\right) = m \times (a + g) = 70 \times 15 = 1{,}050 \text{ N}$$

9. C

This question is tricky. It offers a lot of irrelevant information, some of which might have been useful had we been asked about the work done on the arrow. As written, the question can be answered with the simple equation Fa = ma. That is, with the force applied, the arrow is in equilibrium, but once let go, it starts to accelerate. So Fa = 1 × 10 = 10 N, choice (C). If the question asked about the tension of the bow, then the solution would have been 2 T × cos 30 = Fa. That means the tension in the string is 8.7 N, but that's not what is being asked.

10. B

When you pull in opposite directions, the tension in a rope is always equal throughout and is equal to the lesser of the two forces. The answer is (B) 100 N.

11. A

In one second, the ball passes 8 m. One revolution is $2\pi \times R = 1.3$ m, so 8/1.3 is 6 revs/s.

12. B

Because the ball is not slipping, the force of friction is static. If the ball were to slip, it would rotate in the movement opposite to its translational motion. The force of friction opposes this movement.

13. B

Friction takes away some of the energy of the ball by turning it into rotational motion. If the ramp were frictionless, the ball would slip but it would develop greater speed. Because the present force of static friction is enough to keep the ball from slipping, any further increases in Ks will not affect the movement of the ball.

14. B

Because these are the opposing forces acting on the satellite, the equation to solve this is:

$$G \times Me \times Ms/R^2 = Ms \times v^2/R$$

Beyond this, the question is straightforward: $GMe/R = v^2$ implies that the velocity is inversely proportional to the square of the radius.

15. A

This is an annoying question because it mixes symbols with numbers. The best way is to solve it, and then look at the answers:

$$ma = F - mg \text{ implies } F = m(a + g).$$

$$x = 1/2a \times t^2$$

Now you can find that $F = 100 \times (10 + 2x/t^2) = 1{,}000 + 2x$.

16. B

Because the train moves at constant velocity, it moves by inertia and there is no net force. Because the runner moves east by pushing off the train floor, he supplies the force in the opposite direction (west). Therefore, item III is correct for the same reason that item II is wrong.

17. D

Here you must equate gravitational force against centripetal force:

$$G \times Ms \times \frac{Me}{R^2} = Me \times \frac{v^2}{R}$$

$$\text{Period } T = 2\pi \times R/V$$

Combining these equations, you get:

$$T^2 = 4\pi^2 \times R^2/v^2 = 4\pi^2 \times R^3/(G \times Ms)$$

This indicates that if the period increases, the radius of the orbit must also increase. Therefore, (D) is impossible. The other choices satisfy the expression $T = 2\pi \times R/V$.

CHAPTER 3: WORK, ENERGY, AND MOMENTUM

1. D

As Tom moves, the center of mass of the boat + Tom + Becky system changes. Momentum is equal to the product of the mass and the velocity of the system's center of mass. Because the position of the center of mass moved toward the bow, so did the velocity of the center of mass and the momentum of the system. If you take the center of the boat to be 0 m, the bow to be +1 m, and the stern to be −1 m, then initially the center of mass was at the following:

$$\frac{(+50 \text{ kg} \times \text{m} + 0 \text{ kg} \times \text{m} - 80 \text{ kg} \times \text{m})}{(50 \text{ kg} + 50 \text{ kg} + 80 \text{ kg})} = -\frac{30}{180} \text{ m}$$

But the final position of the center of mass is:

$$\frac{(+50 \text{ kg} \times \text{m} + 0 \text{ kg} \times \text{m} + 80 \text{ kg} \times \text{m})}{(50 \text{ kg} + 50 \text{ kg} + 80 \text{ kg})} = \frac{130}{180} \text{ m}$$

To calculate the change in momentum or velocity, one needs to know the rate of change of the position of the center of mass. It is important to understand that as the boat moves in the same direction as Tom, it pushes water in the opposite direction, so that the momentum of the universe is conserved. (C) is incorrect because if a boat starts moving, it will stop only when some force acts on it, such as the resistance of water. You might have suspected (B) had you thought that, as Tom jumps and gains positive momentum, the boat would move in the opposite direction to compensate. That would be true only if Tom jumped overboard. In fact, he stays inside the Tom+Becky+boat system, and it is the water underneath the boat that must move in the opposite direction.

2. C

When Tom lands and jumps back up, the change in velocity is $v_i - (-v_i)$ or twice his original speed. The force required to produce this effect is derived from the equation:

$$F \times t = \Delta P = m \times v_i - (-v_i)$$

At the same time, the force of gravity (mg) is always acting on Tom. Therefore, the total force is $2 \text{ m} \times v_i/t + mg$. To find v_i, his velocity when he first touches the ground, use the kinematics equation: $v^2 = 2ax$, where v is the velocity at the time of contact if he drops from height x. So,

$$v^2 = 2 \times 10 \frac{\text{m}}{\text{s}^2} \times 1 \text{m} = 20 \frac{\text{m}^2}{\text{s}^2}$$

Substituting this gives:

$$F = \frac{(2 \times 80 \text{ kg} \times 4.5 \text{ m/s})}{(0.2 \text{ s} + 80 \times 10)} = 4{,}400 \text{ N}$$

Since both feet contribute equally to the effort of the jump, the force from one foot is 2,200 N.

3. C

The most direct way to do this is to set up equations of motion:

$$m_4 \times a = m_4 \times g - T$$
$$m_2 \times a = T - m_2 \times g$$

Adding these equations gives"

$a \times (m_4 + m_2) = g \times (m_4 - m_2)$, which can be rewritten to give the acceleration in the rope as he following:

$$a = g \times \frac{(m_4 - m_2)}{(m_4 + m_2)}$$

It's also possible to solve by looking at the changes in energy when the rope moves a certain distance. The gain in kinetic energy is $\frac{1}{2} m_2 \times v^2 + \frac{1}{2} m_4 \times v^2$. Potential energy is gained by the lighter block and lost by the heavier block, so loss in potential energy is as follows:

$m_4 \times gh - m_2 \times gh$ and $\frac{1}{2} \times v^2 \times (m_2 + m_4) = gh(m_4 - m_2)$

After substituting $v_2 = 2 \times a \times h$ into this equation, you'll arrive at the same answer:

$$a = 10 \times (4 - 2)/(4 + 2) = 10/3 \text{ m/s}^2$$

It is important to know both approaches for solving such problems.

4. D

Power is the total change in energy divided by time, so it can also be expressed as the change in (potential energy + kinetic energy)/(time). Potential energy is decreasing because the elevator is descending, while kinetic energy is increasing along with increasing velocity.

$$P = -\frac{(mgh)}{t} + \frac{\left(\frac{1}{2}mv^2\right)}{t}$$

After 5 seconds, the change in displacement, h, is $\frac{1}{2}at^2$, and v^2 is $2\,ah = 2\,a \times \frac{1}{2}at^2$, so:

$P = mg \times \frac{1}{2}at - \frac{1}{2}ma^2t = 100 \times 10 \times \frac{1}{2} \times 4 \times 5 - \frac{1}{2} \times 100 \times 4^2 \times 5 = 6{,}000$ W

You could also set up the equations of motion as $m \times a = F + mg$ and $P = F \times V$ or $F \times \frac{1}{2}a \times t$.

5. C

Because the skydiver has reached his terminal velocity, he is no longer accelerating. The net force from the gravity and the air resistance is equal to 0. The parachute must cause him to decelerate such that his speed drops by 50 m/s in 10 s. So the parachute must exert a force of 50/10 m/s² × 60 kg = 300 N over 10 s to cause this deceleration. Had the parachutist been accelerating with a magnitude of g at this point, then he would have had to act with a force of $m \times (a + g) = m \times (5 + 10) = 900$ N. When the parachutist's speed has decreased to 10 m/s, the net force acting on him would be close to his weight if there had been no parachute, that is $m \times g$; the force of air resistance on the parachutist is almost nonexistent at low speeds. Therefore, the net force of (gravity – air resistance on the parachutist) uniformly increases from 0 N to 600 N. As a result, the parachute will have to exert an additional force of 300 N to overcome the force of gravity, which amounts to 600 N. The distance covered over 10 s is as follows:

$$[(v_f + v_i)/2] \times t = (60 + 10)/2 \times 10 = 350 \text{ m}$$

So the work done by the parachute is:

$$F \times d = 600\text{N} \times 350 \text{ m} = 210 \text{ kJ}$$

6. A

The total change in potential energy for the pilot is 0, because his total displacement is 0 m. The change in kinetic energy is negative for the lower portion of the hook:

$$(\tfrac{1}{2} \times m \times 200^2) - (\tfrac{1}{2} \times m \times 100^2)$$

By the same token, the change over the upper portion of the hook is positive, and the total change in kinetic energy is 0. This is always the case when the initial speed (before the hook) and the final speed are the same. Note that the radius of the circle allows you to calculate the forces acting on the pilot, but since the movement of the plane is always perpendicular to the centripetal forces acting on it, centripetal work is always equal to 0; definition of work is $F \times d \times \cos$ (angle between F and d). If the pilot's final speed had been different from the initial of 200 m/s, then total kinetic work would be nonzero, and if his final altitude were different from the initial, then there would also be a nonzero change in potential energy.

7. C

Gravitational potential energy is equal to $-G \times m_1 \times m_2/d$ at distances far enough from the planet where $m \times g \times h$ is no longer accurate. Because the asteroid is initially 4R away from the center of the planet, where R is the radius of the planet, and it is converted to heat when it is 3R away, it means that $-G \times m_1 \times m_2/3R - (-G \times m_1 \times m_2/4R)$ is the fraction of the original gravitational potential energy converted into heat. To simplify, let $-G \times m_1 \times m_2 = x$. Then $(x/3 - x/4)/(x/4) = 1/3$ is the fraction converted into heat.

8. B

Only item II is correct. Elastic collisions occur when both momentum and kinetic energy are conserved. When a planet breaks into several pieces, each of them gains kinetic energy; their sum, of course, is greater than the kinetic energy of the initial object. When two balls collide and move way from each other at the same speeds, kinetic energy is conserved. All collisions must conserve momentum. The volleyball lost kinetic energy to the collision, so it is partly inelastic.

9. D

The molecule alternates between states where all of the energy is potential (elastic) and where all of the energy is kinetic. When it is completely kinetic, it is at its maximum velocity and has no elastic energy. When it is completely stretched or compressed, its velocity is 0. When its speed is halfway between the two extremes, its elastic potential energy equals its kinetic energy. Energy is conserved in the process, so the sum is always the same. The top speed of the molecules is twice the average speed, so the total energy is $2 \times ½ mv^2 = 10^{-26} \times 100^2 = 10^{-22}$.

10. C

The law of conservation of momentum states that both the vertical and horizontal components of m × v for the system must stay constant. If you take the initial movement of the cart as horizontal and the 2 balls move in perpendicular directions to the horizontal, it means that the cart must maintain its horizontal component of velocity. Therefore, (A) and (B) are wrong. If the billiard balls move as described, then kinetic energy is not conserved; the system gains energy in this inelastic collision. (C) correctly describes how this is possible.

11. A

Mary will not bounce higher than Tom. Because Tom and Mary land on the net at the same time, the net does the same amount of work on both of them. The work done by the net is equal to $½ kx^2$. For either person, this is converted into kinetic energy ($½ m_1v^2$ and $½ m_2v^2$), which is in turn converted into potential energy as m_1gh and m_2gh, respectively. The end result is that weight does not affect the height of the rebound. If the spring is perfectly efficient at converting its energy into kinetic energy, then they would both rebound back to the point from which they jumped. The change in momentum for Tom is 80 kg × $(v_i - (-v_i))$. v_i^2, the square of his speed at impact, is $2 \times g \times h = 2 \times 10 \times 20$; therefore, his momentum is 80 kg × 2 × 20 = 3,200 kg/m/s. The force upon impact is equal to the change in momentum divided by the time of contact (which is the same for both individuals). Tom weighs more, which explains his greater momentum.

12. B

The bow is initially stretched to its maximum capacity, so all of the elastic potential energy will be converted into kinetic energy. At equilibrium, the length of each part of the string is 80 cm; after it is stretched, the length is 100 cm. Therefore, each part of the string contributes $½ kx^2 = ½ k (1 - 0.8)^2$ of energy. Because they work together, $½ \times 2 \times (k \times 0.2^2) = ½ mv^2$. So, $v^2 = 100 \times 0.2^2 \times 2/1 = 8$ and mv = 2.8 kg × m/s. Notice that the arrow will leave the bow when the string passes its equilibrium point; that is, when it is perpendicular to the arrow. If the value of k were not given, it would still be possible to find it. In that case, F = ma = 2 × k × x. Unlike energy, force is a vector and we are interested in the force pointing parallel to the direction of the arrow. Therefore, x in this case would be 0.2 × 60/100, which would yield F = 1 × 24 = 2 × k × x; k = 24/2 × 100/(0.2 × 60) = 100 N/m.

13. D

If the initial speed is v = 100 m/s, then the power of the engine is proportional to the power of the torpedo. The work done by the torpedo is equal to F_e × v × t, where F_e is the average force generated by the torpedo. Because the torpedo travels at a constant speed, the force of resistance by the water is equal to the force generated from the engine and it is proportional to v, so we can set it equal to b × v (where b is some constant). Therefore, the work of resistance by the water is equal to b × v × v × t. If fuel consumption per second (F_e × v) is doubled, then 2 × F_e × v = b × v × v. For the right side of this equation to increase by a factor of 2, the speed must have increased by a factor of √2. Kinetic energy is proportional to the square of the speed, and it would have increased by a factor of 2.

14. D

If you imagine that each rope above the lower pulley moves a distance x when the lower rope is pulled a distance x, then the applied force actually moves the box a distance 2x. Because the work is the same for both parts of the system, this divides the necessary applied force by a factor of 2. Therefore, a force of 100 N applied through this pulley system is the same as a force of 200 N being applied to pull the block directly up the ramp. Now you can set up equations of motion: The forces acting on the block are 200 N up the ramp and m × g × sin 30° down the ramp. So ma = 200 N – mg × sin 30° implies that a = 200 N/20 kg – g × sin 30° = 5 m/s² upward.

15. D

The question does not specify any specific velocities, so we can assign any number that we'd like. If both molecules initially have horizontal components of +5 m/s and vertical components of +3 m/s and –3 m/s, then possible values after collision could be horizontal components of +8 m/s and +2 m/s and vertical components of +10 m/s and –10 m/s. This would conserve the momentum, but not the kinetic energies of the molecules. Kinetic energy does not have to be conserved we're not told that this is an elastic collision. While the magnitude of the vertical components must remain the same for it to add up to 0, the magnitude of the horizontal components can vary as long as their sum adds up to +10. This implies that either molecules A or B may have a greater horizontal component, and therefore greater overall speed and momentum, so (B) could be true. (D) is not true, because it would violate the law of conservation of momentum.

HIGH-YIELD SIMILAR QUESTIONS

Power and Energy

1. 213,840 J
2. 750 J
3. 37 W

Circular Loops

1. 88.2 N
2. 28 m/s
3. 35.9 m/s

Conservation of Momentum

1. 300%; no
2. 1 m/s
3. 965 m/s

Elastic Collisions

1. Kinetic energy is conserved in an elastic collision. If one nucleus is moving faster than the other, it loses some kinetic energy (as velocity) and the other gains some. If the nuclei are moving at the same speed, there should be no transfer of energy.

2. 97.4 kJ
3. 5.2 kJ; 41.5%

Collisions and Energy

1. The 10 kg block reaches a height of 0.051 m. The 50 kg block reaches a height of 0.883 m.
2. The momentum of the system immediately after the throw is 0.
3. The speed of ball 2 after impact = 1.6 v_1 = 2 v_2.

CHAPTER 4: THERMODYNAMICS

1. A

A particle's kinetic energy increases along with its velocity. The best measure of a particle's velocity is its temperature; an increase in temperature always leads to an increase in particle velocity. An increase in pressure or volume will only lead to an increase in kinetic energy if it also causes an increase in temperature. Isothermal systems (C) and (D) always remain at a constant temperature. An isobaric volume increase (B) could cause an increase in temperature, but that will not occur if the volume increase is caused by an increase in the number of moles of gas.

2. D

Temperature is essentially a measure of the kinetic energy of the molecules in an object. Because a particle's kinetic energy increases along with its velocity, an object with zero temperature will be made up of molecules with zero velocity. The phase of an object is related to its pressure as well as its temperature, and you should have no reason to believe that a liquid couldn't be produced at absolute zero (A). The molecules can still have potential energy (B). The molecule will still react if another molecule collides with it (C).

3. D

All of the items are correct. The expansion of solids and liquids due to increases in temperature can be determined by their thermal expansion coefficients. The change in the volume of a gas in different temperatures is one of the most basic principles of ideal gases.

4. C

In an adiabatic process, no heat enters or leaves the system, so (D) is out right away. The internal energy will increase if either kinetic or potential energy is increased, so (A) and (B) are incorrect. The first law of thermodynamics tells us that $\Delta U = Q - W$ (where ΔU is change in internal energy, Q is heat transferred into the system, and W is work done by the system); because the process is adiabatic, we can simplify this into $\Delta U = -W$. Because ΔU is positive, we know that W must be negative, which means that work is done on the system. This question can also be answered with simple logic. Because the total energy of a system must always be constant, the only way to increase the energy of an adiabatic system is to make the system do a negative amount of work; in other words, work must be done on the system.

5. D

Entropy is the measure of the disorder in a system. A system with more entropy is one in which the molecules are spread far apart and are in no particular arrangement. The molecules in Option D are spread randomly throughout the diagram. In options A, B, and C, they are clustered together in an uncharacteristic order.

6. C

Radiation is the type of heat transfer in which energy is transported in the form of electromagnetic radiation, which travels in discrete waves. Each of these waves has a specific direction, as in the figure. Conduction (A) is heat transfer through direct contact between objects. Convection (B) is the heat transfer that happens when a warmer substance mixes with a colder substance. Work (D) is done in a specific direction, not in random directions as in the figure. (C) is correct.

7. A

To find the amount of heat needed to bring the substance to its melting point, you can use the specific heat; the product of the specific heat, the amount of the substance, and the change in temperature. This means that the heat is equal to (1 J/mol × K) (1 mol)(1 K) = 1 J. After the substance reaches its melting point, additional heat (which can be determined by the formula $Q = m\Delta H_f$) is needed to actually induce the phase change. Therefore, the total amount of heat required is greater than 1 J.

8. B

(C) can be ruled out immediately because temperature is always constant in isothermal reactions. Because of an object's heat of fusion, energy is always released when something freezes. When a reaction releases energy, its net change in enthalpy is negative. Although the process is usually caused by a change in temperature or pressure, this is not necessary if the object was already at its freezing point before the start of the process.

9. C

According to the first law of thermodynamics, the total energy of a system is always conserved. The movement of the lid was a result of the conversion of thermal energy to work. Because this work was equal to a total of 100 J, the thermal energy of the pot must have decreased by 100 J (so the answer is –100 J). If work had been done *on* the pot instead of being done *by* the pot, then the change in energy would have been positive.

10. A

The energy of the universe will always remain constant, while the entropy will always stay constant or increase. If the energy and entropy decrease in the object but remain unchanged inside the rest of the refrigerator, then the refrigerator must be somehow releasing this energy and entropy.

11. A

When a gas is expanding or contracting at constant pressure, we can determine the work done in the process by finding the area under the pressure-volume curve by using the formula $W = P\Delta V$ (where P is pressure and ΔV is change in volume). In (A), ΔV is positive, meaning that the amount of work must also be positive and that work was done *by* the system. In (D), the amount of work is negative, so work was done *on* the system. In (B) and (C), ΔV is equal to zero. You can also answer this question with simple logic; if the volume of a gas is decreasing while the pressure stays constant, something must be doing work on the gas in order to overcome the pressure, which will push in the opposite direction to prevent the volume from changing. If the volume is increasing while the pressure stays constant, the gas must be doing work on the environment for the same reason.

12. C

In this situation, heat will transfer from the warm gas to the metal and then to the cold gas. Convection (B) is the transfer of heat when two substances are mixed together; this cannot happen here because the gas will not naturally mix with the metal. Heat transfer through radiation (A) is also implausible, not only because gases are unlikely to emit heat in the form of waves, but also because the radiation would be unlikely to penetrate the thick metal container. Enthalpy (D) is not a form of heat transfer. Conduction (C) is the most likely option; that happens when two substances make direct contact with one another. Here, gas A makes contact with the lead container, which makes contact with bas B.

13. D

Saying that substance B has a higher internal energy (D) could not explain the phenomenon because the internal energy is irrelevant; the heat involved in the process is related only to the specific heat, the heat of fusion, and the heat of vaporization. All the other choices could explain the phenomenon. The heat required to melt the solid is determined by the heat of fusion (C). The heat required to bring the liquid to its boiling point is determined by the specific heat (A). The heat required to boil the liquid is determined by the heat of vaporization (B).

14. B

When the ink randomly intersperses throughout the water, the final state is more disordered than the initial state, so the entropy change of the system is positive. When the oil separates from the water, the final state is just as ordered as the initial state (because the oil and the water are still completely separate), so the entropy change is zero. You can also answer this question by noticing the reversibility of the two experiments: experiment A has a positive entropy change because it is irreversible, while experiment B has no entropy change because the reaction is reversible. According to the second law of thermodynamics, the entropy change can never be negative in a thermodynamic process which moves from one equilibrium state to another.

15. B

The pressure on an object is equal to the force applied to the object divided by the area across which the force is distributed. In this example, the force is applied by object B, so it is distributed across the surface of object B. That means that the pressure on object C will be equal to the force (F) divided by the area of object B (b). To visualize this situation more easily, think of a person who steps on your foot: object A is the person, object B is the person's shoe, and object C is your foot. If object B is a sneaker, then it won't hurt too much; if it's a high-heeled shoe, then the pain will be excruciating. The pressure increases as the area of object B decreases.

16. C

The containers experience the same amount of pressure because their contents are identical. (A) and (B) might be tempting because the pressure is equal to force per unit area. However, the exact same force is applied to every part of a container. While container B has a larger surface area than container A, it also experiences more force from the gas particles. The pressure can be changed only by modifying the quantity of the gas, the temperature of the gas, or the volume of the container.

17. B

In thermal expansion, the change in the length of a solid is directly proportional to the change in its temperature. Because a 200 K temperature increase causes a 2 cm length change, a 400 K temperature increase will cause a 4 cm length change. The answer is (B) 304 cm.

18. A

Only item II is correct: because the entropy of a process can never be negative, a process with a positive entropy can never be reversed. Item I is incorrect because, although entropy is related to spontaneity, the spontaneity of a reaction is determined by its Gibbs Free Energy. Item III is incorrect because many exothermic systems can be reversed to produce endothermic systems.

19. A

In a closed system, the change in internal energy is zero. According to the first law of thermodynamics ($\Delta U = Q - W$), this means that the work done on the gas is equal to the heat released by the system. (B) is incorrect because a change in temperature would cause a change in kinetic energy, which is part of the internal energy. (C) and (D) are incorrect because the question stem provides no evidence which would expect us to believe that a change in pressure or volume would occur in all cases.

20. C

If a substance is undergoing a phase change, any added heat will be used toward overcoming the heat of transformation of the phase change. During the phase change, the temperature will remain constant. Temperature is a measure of the kinetic energy of the molecules in a sample, so a change in kinetic energy (A) is essentially the same thing as a change in temperature. The heat transfer by radiation described in (B) will definitely change the temperature of the solid as long as it is not in the process of melting. (D) describes heat transfer by convection, in which the warm gas will transfer heat to the cold gas until they both reach a moderate temperature.

21. C

The total amount of heat required to raise the temperature of the object can be determined by $Q = mc\Delta T$, while the total amount of heat required to melt the object can be determined by $Q = m\Delta H_f$. If we plug the individual values into the equations, we get $Q = (10\text{ g})(1\text{ J/g} \times \text{K})(100\text{ K}) + (10\text{ g})(120\text{ J/g}) = 2{,}200\text{ J}$.

22. B

Adding heat will increase the temperature until the solid starts to melt. When the phase starts to change, the temperature will remain constant until all of the solid is converted to liquid, at which point the temperature will start increasing again. It will then go through the same process again when the liquid starts to boil. (A), (C), and (D) fail to consider the constant temperature during phase changes. Additionally, (C) and (D) incorrectly represent the linear relationship between heat and temperature.

23. A

In a piston system such as this, the pressure (which is equal to F/A, where F is the force and A is the cross-sectional area) is always constant. In this particular case, the force applied by piston A is doubled, which means that the force applied to piston B is doubled. Because the cross-sectional diameter of piston B is doubled, the cross-sectional area must increase by a factor of $2^2 = 4$. Therefore, we know that the final pressure is twice the initial pressure and the final area is four times the initial area; because the pressure is always constant, we can plug this into $P_1 = P_2 = F_1/A_1 = F_2/A_2$. When the pressure is doubled and the area increases by a factor of four, the force is cut in half.

24. D

A material's heat of vaporization is unrelated to its current temperature or phase; it is a constant value that tells us how much energy is involved in the phase change that the material undergoes at its boiling point. The thermal expansion coefficient of a material (A) is not only clearly different between the solid and liquid phases, but would also be expected to change slightly as the molecules in the substance gain and lose kinetic energy along with any temperature changes. Specific heat capacity (B) is constant within any given phase, but changes between the solid, liquid, and gas phases. The internal energy of a system (C) changes whenever work is done or heat is transferred.

CHAPTER 5: FLUIDS AND SOLIDS

1. B

This question requires an understanding of specific gravity, pressure, and Young's modulus. Under water, pressure is defined as P = Po + pgh, where Po is the pressure at the surface, p is the density of the fluid, g is acceleration due to gravity, and h is the depth of interest. In this case, the density of seawater will be greater than fresh water, so the pressure experienced at increased depth will be greater. Pressure is equal to force/area, and bulk modulus, a measure of change in pressure and the resulting change in volume, will depend on the pressure of the fluid. Because the density of seawater is greater due to the presence of salt in the water, the pressure of seawater will be greater, and therefore the bulk modulus will be greater. Material shows a larger modulus because the pressure is greater, and Young's modulus = (force/area)/dL/L. (A) is incorrect because strain is directly related to pressure in Young's modulus. Young's modulus is independent of bulk modulus, and applies only to solids. You know that the polymer does not absorb anything, so (C) is incorrect.

2. B

Pressure is equal to force over area. If the second woman is only using half as much force, but we would like for the pressure to be equal for both women, she must apply the smaller force over a proportionately smaller area for the pressures to be equal.

3. C

Surface tension is defined as the tendency of similar molecules to feel an attractive force for each other. When water enters the lung, it becomes difficult for alveoli to remain open and to exchange air. Surfactant acts as a detergent to break up the bonding of the water molecules and prevent surface tension from collapsing alveoli and blocking air exchange.

4. B

Turbulent flow can be envisioned as a scatter bundle of molecules continuing to bump into each other, contrasted with orderly laminar fluid that files in orderly fashion down its course. Resistance will be increased if molecules are all bumping into each other.

5. A

This question requires an understanding of the relationship between density and weight. If density equals mass over volume (d = m/v), and weight equals mass time acceleration due to gravity (W = mg), then W = density × volume × acceleration due to gravity, or W= dvg. As such, gold unit volume is 50 percent as dense as iron, so:

$$W\text{ gold, Earth} = \frac{1}{2}d\,(v)\,(g) = \frac{1}{2}\text{dvg on Earth}$$

On Mars, the density of iron will remain d relative to gold on Earth. The g, however, will be ¾ of g on Earth because the gravitation pull is 75 percent less. So:

$$W\text{ iron, Mars} = (d)\,(v)\left(\frac{3}{4}g\right) = \frac{3}{4}\text{dvg}$$

The weight of gold on Earth is 25 percent less than weight of iron on Mars.

6. B

This is a basic restatement of Pascal's principle that a force applied to an area will be transmitted through a fluid. This will result in changing fluid levels through the system. The relationship is stated as $F_2 = F_1A_2/A_1$. Plugging in the numbers clearly shows the answer is (B) 16 N.

7. B

The key concept here is colligative properties. Boiling, as well as freezing, is considered a colligative property, where the behavior of the fluid depends on the number of particles involved. For a given tank of water, there will be more molecules of water in fresh water versus salt water because room must be made for the salt molecules. The boiling point of salt water will be elevated because of the presence of a solute in the solvent. This phenomenon is known as boiling point elevation. The converse is true for freezing; there will be freezing point depression when solutes are present, which is why we put salt on icy sidewalks—it will have to be colder to freeze! Remember, cold weather is depressing: freezing point depression.

8. D

The mass of these two objects is the same, but their volumes are different. As such, their density will be different; ball B is much denser than ball A. The force of buoyancy will be equal to the weight of the water displaced by the object. The weight of the displaced water is equal to the density of the ball multiple by the volume of the ball and the acceleration due to gravity. We know that B is more dense, but we do not know how much greater the volume of A is than B. It is possible these two terms could cancel each other out. As such, (D) is the correct answer.

9. C

This question requires an understanding of the relationship between kinetic and potential energy. Total energy is the sum of potential and kinetic energy. PE = mgh, with m as mass of fluid, g as acceleration due to gravity, and h as the height above the ground. As height = 10 m, all the energy is potential; no movement is taking place. At height 0, all the energy will be kinetic, so the speed at h = 0 can be calculated as:

$$PE = KE$$

$$mgh = \frac{1}{2}mv^2$$

Plugging in the numbers, v will equal the square root of 50, or approximately 7, choice (C).

10. B

A disruption of laminar flow is the key concept in this question. Blood flow does not like to be disturbed; it likes a nice easy path. Any angular changes are vulnerable points to disrupt the integrity of the tissue. The abrupt change in diameter of the path will intermittently increase the turbulence of flow at the branch points. Cohesion is a concept related to surface tension that describes the tendency of like molecules to be attracted to each other in fluids. Surface tension is the result of cohesive forces. Agglutination makes no sense in this situation.

11. B

Bernoulli's principle states that airflow over a curved surface will be faster than airflow over a flat surface. This is why wings have a curved upper surface and a flat lower surface. The fluid, in this case, air, will move more quickly over the curved surface because it has further to travel to the end of the wing than the air at the flat bottom surface. Increased air speed will mean lower pressure within the fluid. This will result in higher pressure below the wing, and an upward force. (D) is an incorrect restatement of the principle of buoyancy that applies to fluids.

12. D

This question relies on an understanding of which factors impact viscosity. By definition, viscosity is a measure of resistance to flow. Increased temperature will result in increased movement of water molecules as they gain energy from the heat. This will cause viscosity to decrease as temperature increases. As the temperature increases toward 100, the equilibrium will shift toward more molecules being present as gas/steam, and that will decrease the resistance to flow. Viscosity is not a colligative property; resistance to flow is a characteristic of the substance, not of the number of molecules in the substance.

13. D

It does not make sense for bulk modulus to be an inverse of Young's modulus when both are measuring deformity in response to stress, so (A) is wrong. Both Bulk and Young's modulus relate to solids (B). If the two measured the same thing (C), there would be no need to have two different moduli. Young's is a measure of stress over strain in one direction, while Bulk's measures the overall changes in volume, which is in three dimensions. (D) is the correct answer; you can think of bulk modulus as a more developed version of a Young's modulus.

14. A

This question is a simple application of the following formula: pressure = force/area. The area is 18 square meters per window, and there are two windows. The thickness of the glass has no bearing on the pressure. If pressure decreases 1 percent and area does not change, and pressure is directly proportional to force, the force will be decreased 1 percent if the atmospheric pressure decreases 1 percent. (B) is included to throw you off on an easy decimal issue. (C) and (D) are included to tempt you into considering the thickness of the glass, but it will not impact the pressure calculation.

15. B

The transition from laminar to turbulent flow is determined by a dimensionless constant known as the Reynolds constant. It is a reflection of the balance between inertial and turbulent forces. A Reynolds number below 2,000 suggests flow will be laminar; above 4,000 suggests turbulance, and a number between the two suggests transitional flow. Bernoulli's constant relates to thermodynamics and flow, not laminar-turbulent transitions. Magentic constant is related to electromagentic forces that are not relevant here. There is no such thing as a Pascal constant.

16. C

The chart is distracting. If you know the equation for absolute pressure, this will be fairly easy to figure out. $P = Po + pgh$, where p = density. Po, pressure at the surface, is always 2. Acceleration due to gravity, g, will be 10, and p will be x or 2x. As such, the only variable to consider is h. The pressures below the surface will be equal where the depth of fluid A is two times that of fluid B. In this case, the 2 times greater depth will cancel out the 2 contributed from the 2x of greater density.

17. C

Think about phase transition questions in terms of equilibrium. Vapor pressure is a measure of the number of particles of the solid that have transitioned to a liquid or gas form and are present in close proximity to the solid. Consider ice as the example. As the temperature increases, the solid will melt, and some ice will transition to water. Some of the water will be held in the gas above the solid. The greater the increases in temperature, the more molecules are activated to leave the solid as vapor, so the vapor pressure increases.

18. B

This is a basic interpretation of Bernoulli's equation that states, at equal heights, velocity and pressure of a fluid are inversely related. Decreasing the speed (B) of the water will increase its pressure.

An increase in pressure over a given area will result in increased force being transmitted to the piston. Releasing water intermittently against the pipe (D) may produce greater force at that instant, but this is unsustainable and we have no information in (D) as to the speed of the water to be released.

19. C

This question may seem confusing, but you need only focus on the pressure in pipes A and B at any given initial pressure. Because pipe A is wider, there will be less pressure; this is the continuity principle. Pipe B is narrower, and will have more pressure. This relationship holds no matter what the initial pressure is.

20. C

Pressure increases linearly based on the density of the fluid, not on the density of the object in the liquid. The pressure will be equal on both objects.

HIGH-YIELD SIMILAR QUESTIONS

Specific Gravity

1. 1,020
2. 4/3
3. 3.5 N

Hydraulic Lift

1. 15.8 cm
2. 0.5 cm
3. 0.4 m^3

Gauge Pressure

1. 20,612 kg/m^3
2. 591 kPa
3. Gauge pressure increases by a factor of 4/3.

Hydrostatics

1. $32\frac{2}{3}$ N
2. $\frac{2}{3}$ g/cm^3
3. 49 m/s^2

Hydrodynamics

1. $v_1 = \sqrt{\dfrac{\rho v_0^2 - 4P_0}{\rho}}$, where ρ is the density of the fluid, v_o is the fluid speed at a point in the pipe where pressure = P_o, and v_1 is the fluid speed at a point in the pipe where pressure = $3P_o$.
2. v_B:v_A = 4:1
3. 3.13 m/s

CHAPTER 6: ELECTROSTATICS

1. C

The MCAT places a great deal on emphasis on the fact that, according to the equation $F = kq_1q_2/r_2$, the force between two charges is inversely proportional to the square of the distance between the charges. This means that when the distance is cut in half, the force increases by a factor of 4. (C) is correct.

2. B

Electric potential energy (in joules) is equal to the product between the charge of the particle (in coulombs) and the electric potential (in volts); this relationship is represented by the equation U = qV. Because *V* is always positive, *U* can only be greater than zero if *q* is positive. Because the question specifies that *U* is greater than zero, it is impossible for the particle to have a negative charge; therefore, (B) is definitely not true.

3. B

This question can be answered either through direct knowledge of dipole moments or process of elimination. A charged particle at the midpoint of an electric dipole will move in a random direction whenever no external field is present. If the dipole is in a uniform outside field, then the particle will move according to the field's force. (A) is incorrect because the electric field in a dipole is never zero (the field can be predicted by an equation, but the equation is unnecessary for this question). (C) and (D) are incorrect because all points along the perpendicular bisector of the dipole will be subject to the same electric potential.

4. A

When an electric dipole is subjected to an external field, both particles move with equal force in opposite directions in order to produce a net force of zero. The overall movement of the dipole will be rotational. Because both particles are moving with equal velocity and acceleration, the bisecting point (point *a*) does not move.

5. D

The electric potential (V) is equal to the amount of work done (W) divided by the test charge (q_0), according to the equation $V = W/q_0$. This means that the potential is directly proportional to the amount of work done, which is equal to the amount of energy exerted by the particle; therefore, the overall amount of energy increases by a factor of 4. Because energy is directly proportional to the square of the velocity (according to $E = \frac{1}{2} mv^2$), the velocity must increase by a factor of 2.

6. D

You should know that the field lines for a positively charged particle will always point away from the particle in a radial pattern, regardless of the direction in which the particle is moving. (A) represents the field lines of a negatively charged particle. (B) and (C) do not represent any particular scheme.

7. B

For a positively charged particle, the electrostatic force has the same direction as the movement of the particle; a negatively charged particle moves in the direction opposite to the force.

8. C

Electric potential (V) is equal to the quotient of the amount of work done (W) divided by the charge of the particle on which the work is done (q_0), according to the equation $V = W/q_0$. Because the potential equals 9 V and the charge equals 2C, the work done must equal 9V × 2C = 18 J.

9. C

An equipotential line, as the name suggests, is a line along which the electric potential remains constant. In other words, $V_1 = V_2 = V_3$ and $V_4 = V_5 = V_6$. (B) and (D) are true statements because the difference between two equal values is zero. Meanwhile, the potential decreases as the distance from the original charge (q) increases (according to the equation $V = kq/r$), so V_1, V_2, and V_3 are lower than V_4, V_5, and V_6. This means that $V_1 - V_6$ is less than zero and that (A) is true. Meanwhile, $V_5 - V_2$ is greater than zero, so (C) is the one answer choice that is not a true statement.

10. B

The electric potential is constant along an equipotential line. Because potential is directly proportional to work, the work is also constant along this line. This means that no work is required to transport electron C from point 6 to point 4. For electrons A and B, the change in potential is negative (potential decreases as distance from the charge increases) and the charge is negative, so the work is positive (according to the equation $V = W/q_0$). Because A and B experience positive work and C experiences negative work, (B) is the only correct option.

11. C

The electrostatic force can be calculated by the equation $F = kq_1q_2/r$. This means that the force is related to the charges on each particle and the distance between the particles. Coulomb's constant (k) does not change for different systems, so it cannot affect the overall force, so (C) is the correct answer. An increased number of particles will indeed create additional forces, so (D) is not the answer.

12. A

The total electric potential at any given point is equal to the scalar sum of the potentials due to each charge. Each potential can be determined by the equation V = kq/r, where q is the charge and r is the distance to the charge (2 meters). Based on the equation, the individual potentials for q_1, q_2, q_3, and q_4 are equal to $k/2$, k, $3k/2$, and $2k$, respectively. The sum of these potentials is equal to $5k$.

13. C

The electrostatic force is given by the equation F = kq_1q_2/r. Because the distance does not change during the interaction in the question, the value of r is irrelevant to the answer. Currently, q_1 and q_2 are equal to +1e and +2e, respectively; the addition of three electrons (each of which carries a charge of $-e$) will change the charges to $-2e$ and $-1e$. Therefore, the product q_1q_2 before the interaction is equal to the product q_1q_2 after the interaction ($q_1q_2 = +2e^2$). Because k and r remain constant in this system, the value of kq_1q_2/r does not change.

14. D

A field line shows the direction of the electrostatic force that would act on a positively charged test particle. The field lines in this diagram are pointed toward q_1 and q_2, meaning that a positive particle would be accelerated in the direction of q_1 and q_2. This can only happen if both charges are negative, choice (D). The lines from q_1 can never intersect with the lines from q_2, because a positively charged test particle at any given point will always move in one specific direction; if the lines intersected, then a test particle at the intersection point would have to move in both directions at once.

15. A

In the horizontal direction, particle p is repelled toward the right by a charge of 10 C and repelled to the left by a charge of 15 C, so the net charge is equal to 5 C toward the left (according to the rules of vector addition). In the vertical direction, the particle is repelled toward the bottom by a charge of 5 C and attracted toward the bottom by a charge of 7 C, so the net charge is equal to 12 C toward the bottom. (A) is the only choice which considers the fact that the 12 C charge will exert a stronger force (downward) than the 5 C charge will exert (toward the left).

16. D

The net charge is equal to 5 C toward the left and 12 C toward the bottom. Because electrostatic force is a vector quantity, the rules of vector addition can be used to determine the magnitude of the overall net charge. This magnitude is equal to $5^2 + 12^2 = 169 = 13^2$.

17. B

The net force is equal to the product of mass and net acceleration. Because mass is 10 kg and net acceleration is 5 m/s^2, the net force is equal to 50 N in the upward direction. The downward force due to gravity, meanwhile, is always equal to the product of the mass and the acceleration due to gravity, which is −100 N in this case. Therefore, the electric field must supply 150 N ([upward force] − [downward force]) of force in order to provide the observed acceleration. The strength of the electric field is equal to (force)/(charge), which amounts to −30 V, so the magnitude is 30 V (because magnitudes are always positive). The field is pointed downward because negatively charged particles always move in the direction opposite to the field.

18. B

Item II is correct because an electric dipole always exists between two identical charges of opposite magnitude. Item I is incorrect because there is always an electric field at every point in an electric dipole; though the potential may be equal to zero at certain points, the field can always be calculated. Item III is incorrect because the electrostatic force (and, consequently, the acceleration) increases as the distance between the particles decreases.

HIGH-YIELD SIMILAR QUESTIONS

Net Electric Field with Multiple Sources

1. By symmetry, the electric field is zero.
2. No.
3. $5.0 \times 10^{-4} \frac{N}{C}$

Charge Distribution and Work

1. 1.2 J
2. 1.22 J
3. +126 J

Voltage and Energy

1. $V_f = 14.1$ m/s
2. 1.4×10^5 m/s
3. 3.8×10^3 m/s

Electrostatics and Velocity

1. 1.38×10^5 m/s
2. 2.07×10^{-19} J
3. 0.52 V

Electric Force

1. 1.36 N
2. 0.4012 m
3. 6.796×10^{-9} C

Electron Between Charged Plates

1. 4.4×10^{10} F (a humongous capacitance!)
2. 1.9×10^7 m/s
3. 1.6×10^{-16} m

Electrostatic Impulse

1. 4.38×10^{-25} J
2. 4.8×10^{-14} N
3. V_a

Photoelectric Effect

1. 4.8×10^{14} Hz
2. 1.9×10^{-18} J
3. frequency = 1.5×10^{15} Hz; power = 10^{-14} W

CHAPTER 7: MAGNETISM

1. A

Using the right-hand rule for the positive charge: Let the thumb point to the right-charge movement direction, with fingers pointing into the page (direction of magnetic field lines); then the palm is up and is showing the direction of magnetic force (up). However, as the charge in question is negative, the direction of the magnetic force is reversed (down).

2. B

A motionless charge cannot generate a magnetic field, and a field is required to generate a force. No magnetic force can be experienced by the charge.

3. B

Charge A is experiencing a stronger magnetic field than charge B as it is located closer to the wire and according to the formula $B = \mu_0 i/2\pi r$ the strength of the magnetic field is inversely proportional to the distance from a current carrying wire. While charges are motionless and don't produce magnetic field on their own they still experience the one produced by the wire.

4. A

Applying the right-hand rule for the current: Let the thumb of the right hand point to the left-direction of the current. Wrap the fingers of the right hand as if around the wire; the magnetic field experienced by the negative charge is coming into the page, indicating the direction of the field lines.

5. C

The magnetic force experienced by both charges is zero, as one charge is traveling parallel and another charge antiparallel to the direction of magnetic field. That makes the angle between v and B 0° and $\sin 0 = 0$, thus $F = qvB \sin 0 = 0$.

6. A

Using the right-hand rule, find the direction of the magnetic force (responsible for changing the trajectory) acting on the electron. Thumb pointing up (for the direction of electron movement), fingers pointing at you (for the direction of magnetic field lines), then the palm of the right hand (magnetic force) is pointing to the right, curving the path of the positive particle to the right. However, as an electron's charge is negative, the direction of the magnetic force is opposite (to the left); thus, the trajectory will curve to the left.

7. D

In the current-carrying wire, the magnitude of the magnetic force due to an external magnetic field can be determined by the following formula:

$$F = LBI\sin\theta$$

(L = length of the wire, B = magnetic field, I-current through the wire portion, θ = angle between magnetic field lines and current)

B is perpendicular to I so $\sin 90 = 1$. Current can be determined by the formula $I = V/R$. V is known, and R can be calculated as $R_{total} = (R1 \times R2)/(R1 + R2)$ for resistors in parallel. As a result, $R_{total} = (6 \times 3)/(6 + 3) = 2$, $I = 6/2 = 3$ A, $F = 2 \times 5 \times 3 \times 1 = 30$ N.

8. C

A charged particle moving perpendicular to the direction of a uniform magnetic field is rotating. A centripetal force associated with circular motion is the magnetic force acting on the particle. Thus, $mv^2/r = qvB$. Eliminating v on both sides, we get $mv/r = qB$, and from there, $v = qBr/m$. For the question we must convert mass to kg: $0.005g = 5 \times 10^{-6}$ kg, and circle radius to meters: 8 cm = 8×10^{-2} m. Plugging the numbers into the equation, we have $v = 2 \times 5 \times 8 \times 10^{-2}/5 \times 10^{-6} = 16 \times 10^4$ m/s.

9. A

The magnetic force does no work, as it is perpendicular to the movement of the charged particle and magnetic field lines, and as $W = Fd\cos\theta = 0$ as $\cos 90 = 0$. (A) is correct.

10. A

The magnetic forces on the different sides of a loop of wire of any shape point in opposite directions and have the same magnitude. Thus, they cancel each other out and there is no net magnetic force.

11. B

This is a case of diamagnetism. Paramagnetic (A) elements have an uneven number of electrons and would be weakly attracted to the pole of a strong magnet. Ferromagnetic (C) elements (generally metals and alloys) have great numbers of unpaired electrons, are strongly attracted to the magnet, and can themselves be magnetized. Torque (D) has no relationship to the described situation.

12. A

The magnetic field produced by the current at particular distance away from the wire can be calculated by applying the formula $B = \mu_0 i/2\pi r$, where μ_0– is the permeability of free space and r is a distance away from the wire, in this case 8 m. Plugging values into the formula, we calculate 1.26×10^{-6} T as the answer, choice (A).

13. B

A charged particle moving perpendicular to the direction of a uniform magnetic field is rotating. A centripetal force associated with circular motion is the magnetic force acting on the particle. Thus, $mv^2/r = qvB$, and eliminating v on both sides we have $mv/r = qB$. From there we get $v = qBr/m$. From this formula, to receive the highest v B-magnetic field strength, the charge of the particle (D) and orbital radius (C) can be increased, yet increasing the mass of the particles (B) would decrease the speed of rotation.

14. D

The portion BC of the wire carrying current is parallel to the direction of the magnetic field lines. If direction of the current or single moving charge is parallel/anti-parallel to the magnetic field, $\sin 0 = 0$ and $F = qvB \sin 0 = 0\,N$. There is no magnetic force on the portion BC of the wire.

15. D

All of the statements are false. The magnetic force on both particles is not zero as the particles move perpendicular to the magnetic field lines and not parallel. Acceleration of the proton would be less than that of an electron as the net force $F = ma$, according to Newton's second law, and F_{net} is the same for both proton and electron. Thus, as the proton's mass is greater, its acceleration would be less. The magnetic force does not do work, so it cannot change the kinetic energy of either particle.

16. B

As the question mentions, the velocity filter detects charged particles. The neutron is the only particle mentioned without charge and is therefore correct.

17. D

According to the formula given in the question $F = \mu_0 I^2/2\pi r$. When the researcher increases the current by two, he would need to increase the distance between wires by four (as I value is squared). (D) is correct. Decreasing the permeability of the free space (A) would help to balance the equation but the specific value of decrease is not given and μ_0 is a proportionality constant whose value is not changed.

18. A

According to the question, the speed of the particle detected occurs when $F_{electric}$ equals $F_{magnetic}$ or $Eq = qvB$; from here, $v = E/B$. In order to increase the velocity of a charge, one would need to increase the electric field strength (A) or decrease the magnetic field strength. As the particle charge (B) is not in the equation, increasing it would not bring the result needed. Increasing both electric and magnetic fields (D) would cause the effects to oppose each other, resulting in no change in velocity.

19. C

Draw a diagram of the square wire loop with the current and magnetic field. Use the right-hand rule to determine the direction of magnetic forces on the horizontal sides on the square. (Vertical sides of the square have no magnetic forces as they're parallel/antiparallel to the magnetic field.) For the top side of the square, the magnetic force is pointing out of the page; for the bottom side of the square, it's pointing into the page. Therefore, the loop would rotate top over bottom (C). The loop would not remain still (A) as torque causes it to rotate and there are magnetic forces on the loop even though the net force is zero.

HIGH-YIELD SIMILAR QUESTIONS

Magnetic Field

1. For a set of points outside the loop the magnetic field is zero.
2. $B = 0$
3. 2.1×10^{-7} into the page

Magnetic Force

1. For the angle of 90°, force = 2.4×10^{-12} N; for the angle of 45°, force = 1.7×10^{-12} N
2. 6×10^{-16} N
3. 2.4×10^{-15} N up the page

CHAPTER 8: DC AND AC CIRCUITS

1. B

Items I and III are correct. Resistance increases with length, because longer wires make it more difficult for current to travel from one end of the wire to another. Increased temperature causes increased thermal oscillations of the atoms in the conductor, which inhibits electron flow. Item II is incorrect because a larger cross-sectional area gives the current more room to travel.

2. D

Materials with high resistivity are usually good insulators, while materials with low resistivity are usually good conductors. Because metals are usually good conductors, we can assume that they have low resistivity; therefore, glass is likely to have a higher resistivity than the other options.

3. B

This question can be answered by applying the relation P = iV (power equals the product of current and voltage). The current is 4 C/s and the potential is 6 J/C, so the power is 24 J/s. Because 24 J is delivered every second, 240 J will be delivered in 10 seconds.

4. A

Kirchhoff's current law states that the sum of all currents directed into a point is always equal to the sum of all currents directed out of the point. The currents directed into point P are equal to 8 A, 2 A, and 3 A, so the sum is 13 A. The currents directed out of point P are equal to 5 A and 6 A, so the total is 11 A. Because the two numbers must always be equal, an additional current of 2 A must be directed away from point P.

5. C

Kirchhoff's voltage law states that the sum of all potential changes is equal to zero; in other words, the potential supplied by the battery (the EMF) is equal to the sum of all of the potential drops in the circuit. We can find the voltage drop across each resistor by V = iR, which is equal to 2 V. Because each resistor dissipates 2 V, the other 5 V must be dissipated by object X. Power is equal to the product of current (1 A) and potential (5 V), so the total power used by object X is 5 W.

6. C

Because the current is equal to 1 A and the total EMF is equal to 9 V, the total resistance must be equal to V/i = 9 Ω. According to the given information, the resistance due to the resistors (R_1 and R_2) and Object X is equal to 2 Ω + 2 Ω + 3 Ω = 7 Ω. This means that the remaining 2 Ω must come from the wire. Because 2 Ω is a very high resistance, the wire must have a very high resistivity. (A) is incorrect because the current remains constant throughout a circuit. (B) is incorrect because, while there may be a potential difference across object X, the overall potential of the circuit will not change. (D) is incorrect because a large cross-sectional area will give the wire a lower resistance, not a higher one.

7. A

Increasing the cross-sectional area will lead to a decrease in resistance. Adding more resistors in parallel will also decrease the resistance of the circuit. Adding more resistors in series (B) would increase the overall resistance. (C) and (D) would have no effect on the resistance.

8. D

Capacitance is given by the formula C = Q/V (capacitance = charge/voltage difference). Keep in mind that the SI unit for capacitance is F; because the question gives capacitance in µF, the answer will be in µC rather than C. Based on the formula, the capacitor stores 320 µC (3.2×10^{-4} C) of charge.

9. D

The electric field between two plates of a parallel plate capacitor is related to the potential difference between the plates of the capacitor and the distance between the plates (according to the formula E = V/d). The addition of another battery will increase the total voltage applied to the circuit, which is likely to consequently increase the electric field. (D) is correct. The addition of a resistor (A) and (B), whether in series or parallel, will increase the resistance and decrease the voltage applied to the capacitor. Increasing the distance between the plates would not work because electric field is inversely proportional to the distance between the plates.

10. A

A dielectric material acts by reducing the voltage between the plates of a capacitor, thereby increasing the capacitance (because the definition of capacitance, C = Q/V, tells us that capacitance is inversely proportional to voltage). You should know that the dielectric constant is directly proportional to capacitance.

11. A

Stored charge increases and decreases gradually along with current. As the charge begins to saturate the capacitor, the rate of charging decreases. Similarly, the rate of discharging decreases as the capacitor loses charge. (B) suggests a sharp change when the capacitor switches between its charging and discharging states. (C) and (D) both suggest a linear change.

12. B

The ability of a parallel plate system to store charge at a given potential difference (capacitance) is given by the equation $C = \varepsilon_0 A/d$, where C represents capacitance, ε_0 is a constant, A is the overlapping area of the two plates, and d is the distance between the plates. (B) is the best choice because the plates are closer together than in any of the other options. (A) is incorrect because, although the overlapping area is the highest, the distance between the plates is much greater than the distance in (B).

13. C

The rms current of an AC signal is equal to $(I_{max})/(\sqrt{2})$, where I_{max} is the maximum current. Because the maximum value of $\sin(4\pi t)$ is equal to 1, the maximum value of I is equal to 14 A. This means that the rms current is approximately 10 A.

14. B

When an atom loses an electron, the charge from the electron is transferred to another part of the material. This causes the charge to be conduced across the sample in question, as in copper, silver, gold, and some other metals. The other answer choice describe electrical insulators which are unlikely to lose an electron.

15. D

The resistance of the three resistors wired in series is equal to the sum of the individual resistances (12 Ω). This means that the circuit essentially contains a 12 Ω resistor and a 4 Ω resistor. To determine the overall resistance of this system, we can use the formula $1/R = 1/R_1 + 1/R_2 + \ldots$, where R is equal to the overall resistance when R_1 and R_2 are wired in parallel. Based on the formula, the resistance is equal to 3 Ω.

16. A

Because an AC current is described by a sin curve, it fluctuates evenly between positive and negative values. Therefore, the average current of an AC circuit is always equal to zero.

17. C

Unlike the average current, the average power of an AC circuit is not equal to zero. This is because power is proportional to the square of the current, so it carries a positive sign even when the current is negative. The power of an AC circuit is given by the formula $P = i_{RMS}^2R$; since i_{RMS} is equal to 20 A and R is equal to 2 Ω, the total power is 800 W.

18. D

A dielectric material increases capacitance by decreasing the voltage between the plates of a parallel plate capacitor. For this reason, better insulators are more likely to be more dielectric and, consequently, have a higher dielectric constant. The best insulators are atoms and molecules that are unlikely to lose an electron; of the options given, Iodine is the only choice that has a much stronger tendency to gain an electron than to lose one.

19. D

The capacitance of a series circuit is given by the formula $1/C = 1/C_1 + 1/C_2 + 1/C_3 + \ldots$, where C is equal to the overall capacitance of C_1, C_2, and C_3. Based on this formula, the capacitance of the series portion of the circuit is equal to 1 F. For a parallel circuit, the capacitance is equal to the sum of the individual values; this means that the overall system has a capacitance of 1 F + 3 F = 4 F. Based on the formula C = Q/V, we can use the voltage (4 V) to determine that the system can store 4 F × 4 V = 16 C of charge.

20. B

Charge per second is equal to current, which is always fluctuating in an AC circuit, so item I is incorrect. Charge per volt is equal to capacitance, which remains constant as long as the capacitors are not changed, so item II is correct. Charge per joule is the inverse of electric potential (J/C = V), which changes along with the fluctuations in current, so item III is incorrect. Only item II is correct so (B) is correct.

CHAPTER 9: PERIODIC MOTION, WAVES, AND SOUND

1. B

The only thing that you need to remember for this question is the formula for angular frequency, ω. By definition, ω = 2πf, but in simple harmonic motion it can be rewritten as ω = √(k/m). Therefore, the angular frequency is √(2/3) its original value.

2. B

Recall the formula for the period of a pendulum, T = 2π × √(L/g). It is a common misconception that mass has an effect on frequency of a pendulum. Remember that this is a pendulum and not a spring! In a pendulum system, the only factors that can affect the motion are the ones in that formula: the length of the string and the gravitational acceleration (usually 9.8 m/s^2, unless the pendulum is on a different planet or under some special conditions). Only item III is correct.

3. C

First ask yourself what is going on in this question. The student wants to convert the potential energy stored in a spring into gravitational energy. From here you realize that $E_{spring} = E_{gravitational}$, or ½ kx^2 = mgh. The question asks how all of the variables will affect the height, so solve for the "h" to get h = (kx^2)/(2mg). Reducing the value of the variables in the denominator and increasing the values of the variables in the numerator will increase "h." From here, just plug in the numbers. Doubling the mass and halving the compression (A) will give you 1/8 of the initial height. Doubling the mass of the ball and halving the spring constant (B) will give you ¼ of the initial height. Halving the mass of the ball and doubling the spring constant (D) will give you four times the initial height.

4. A

Depending on which formula you remember, you'll have to do some rearranging before you can plug in any numbers. You should know that $f = 1/T$, and that $T = 2\pi \times \sqrt{(L/g)}$; we can substitute the second equation into the first equation to get $f = 1/(2\pi) \times \sqrt{(g/L)}$. g/L is roughly 5, so the frequency is equal to approximately $1/6 \times \sqrt{(5)}$, where $\sqrt{(5)}$ is a little over $2.2/6 = 1/3$, or (A).

5. A

Here, an observer is moving closer to a stationary source. The formula needed is $f_L = [(v + v_L)/v] \times f_s$, where v is the velocity of the sound and the subscripts L and S stand for listener and source, respectively. Because the numerator is greater than the denominator, f_L will be greater than f_s; therefore, item I is correct. Item II will produce a similar, but not identical, effect. The frequency formula here will be $f_L = [v/(v - v_s)] \times f_s$. The listener's frequency will also increase, but the increase will not be exactly the same; that means item II is incorrect. Because the medium through which the wave travels does not change, the velocity of the wave does not change either. That means item III is incorrect.

6. A

We're being asked for the wavelength behind the car at a stationary point as the car is moving forward. This means the "listener" is stationary and the "source" is moving away. $f_L = [(v + v_L)/v] \times f_s$ is the formula needed. Plugging in the numbers, the frequency is 70 Hz. $\lambda = v/f = 300/70$, which is roughly 4.3 m (A). You might arrive at (B) and (C) had you used the incorrect version of the Doppler effect formula.

7. B

In transverse waves, the oscillation of the particles is perpendicular to the direction of the wave's motion. This eliminates (C) and (D). All you have to realize now is that the string moves up and down, and because string movement is perpendicular to the direction in which the wave travels, (B) is correct.

8. A

The frequency for standing waves on strings is given as $f = (nv)/(2L)$, where n is the principal number, v is the velocity of sound, and L is the length of the string. Even though the speed of sound is not given in this question, it is unnecessary because "v" is constant, so it cancels out when you take the ratio of two frequencies. We can rearrange the formula to see that the string's length is $L = (3 \times v)/(2 \times 600)$, or ¾$v$ m. In the second case, we get $(1 \times v)/(2 \times 600)$, or ¼$v$ m.

9. C

If you visualize a transverse wave, you know that the higher the harmonic, the more crests and troughs are generated. Thus, with higher harmonics, the wavelength should be decreased (more nodes and antinodes). A decrease in wavelength results in higher energy and velocity. I and III are true and (C) is the correct answer.

10. A

In simple harmonic motion, displacement versus time is given as $x = A \times \cos(\omega t + \varphi)$, where A is the amplitude, ω is the angular frequency and φ is the phase angle. We are told that $x = -2$ and A is 2, so solving for $\cos(\omega t + \varphi) = -1$; because cosine is -1 when the angle equals π, we can say that $\omega t + \varphi = \pi$. Also notice that the phase angle is zero because we're starting from the origin. This means that $\omega t = \pi$. If we substitute the equation $\omega = 2\pi f$, we get $t = \pi/(2\pi f) =$ 0.1 seconds.

This question can also be solved logically if you understand the definition of frequency. Because the frequency is 5 Hz, we know that the seesaw traverses the amplitude 5 times every second. The distance between 0 m and –2 m is half the amplitude, so the seesaw can travel this distance 10 times every second. This means that it can travel the distance once every 1/10 second.

11. A

Because all the units presented in the question stem are the same in the answers, there is no need to convert anything. Some students get stumped when they see surface area of the detector and try to figure out how to incorporate that number into the answer. Remember, Intensity = Power/Area, where area is the square of the distance between the listener and the source; you can disregard the 5 meters. Just do $10^{-4}/4$ which is easier if you think about it as $10/4 \times 10^{-5}$. This gives you (A).

12. B

Let's look at the possible answer choices and see if we can deduce anything first. (C) states that the two tuning forks have the same frequency. This implies that they are in sync and that you shouldn't have any wavering sounds. Because this is false, so (C) is incorrect. (A) and (D) contradict themselves: if a tuning fork has a higher frequency, it must have a higher pitch. Since high-pitched sounds are produced from high frequencies, (A) and (D) are wrong. (B) is correct because higher frequency and higher pitch mean the same thing. You can also find the y-intercept by letting $t = 0$ to verify the second half of the answer choice.

13. C

Constructive interference occurs when the two waves arrive at a particular point and there is no difference in their phases, or in other words, the distances from the two speakers differ by either λ, 2λ, 3λ, and so forth. Destructive interferences happens at all other instances. This eliminates (A) and (D). Even though the waves from the speakers are in phase, the question says that at point "P" the wavelengths differ by $\lambda/2$. This is the definition of destructive interference, so (C) is the answer.

14. B

Look out for absolute statements as in (C) and (D). There are usually exceptions to most rules, and while you shouldn't automatically eliminate these, be suspicious. If a pulse is sent down a rope and the end is fixed, it will be inverted. Visualize holding a rope where the other end is attached to a free ring that can move up and down. As you flick the rope, the wave will propagate to the other end. You can imagine that once wave gets to the ring, it will want to flick the ring up. The wave that comes back will be inverted if the end is fixed, but (B) has it backward. (C) and (D) are just inaccurate.

15. D

From the generic formula, $x(t) = A \times \text{Cos}(\omega t + \varphi)$, there are three numbers given here: the amplitude, angular frequency, and the initial displacement. You should realize that a greater period means the same thing as a *smaller frequency*; (A), (B), and (C) are saying the same thing. Because all three answers cannot be correct, we can eliminate them and immediately choose (D). From $\omega = 2\pi f$, we see that the first wave has a greater frequency than the second wave, which confirms our decision to eliminate (A), (B), and (C). (D) is the answer.

16. B

This question tries to confuse you with useless information. If a transverse wave hits a fixed end, it will always be reflected in a way opposite to the way in which it entered. If it hits a free end, it will be reflected the same way in which it entered. This leaves (B) as the answer.

17. A

The frequency of a pendulum is defined as $f = 2\pi \times \sqrt{(g/L)}$. Because "g" is under a square root, the gravitational constant has to be f^2 as big, or 16 in this case. (B) and (C) assume you think that the relationship between frequency and the gravitational acceleration is 1:1. (C) assumes that you mistakenly wrote "g" in the denominator when trying to solve.

18. C

The displacement for a harmonic oscillator is given as $x = A \times \cos(\omega t + \varphi)$, Remember that A has to be in meters (0.03 m) and that $\omega = \sqrt{(k/m)}$, or $\sqrt{(10/0.1)} = 10$. If you're wondering about the phase angle, remember that the question stem asks which of the following it *could* be. It cannot be (A) because the angular velocity is wrong; it cannot be (B) because that contains a sine; and it can't be (D) because the angular velocity is wrong. All the values that are given in the question correspond to the values in (C).

HIGH-YIELD SIMILAR QUESTIONS

Energy and Springs

1. 0.0051 m
2. 1200 J
3. The ratio is 5:2, where the numerator refers to the spring with the 5 kg mass and the denominator refers to the spring with the 2 kg mass.

Acceleration of a Pendulum

1. Magnitude: 144 $m\backslash s^2$, Direction: points to the center of the motion
2. $\theta = 151.9°$ measured counterclockwise from east
3. $\theta = 68.5°$ east of north; $a = 17.3 \text{ m/s}^2$

Dampened Harmonic Motion

1. 0.0125%
2. Please disregard this problem
3. Period = 0.51 s; 98.9%

Doppler Effect

1. 18 bullets/minute
2. Perceived frequency by the observers on the bridge: 330.7 Hz
3. Perceived frequency by the observers on the boat: 371.7 Hz

CHAPTER 10: LIGHT AND OPTICS

1. A

We simply have to weed out the important information here to get some quick points and move on. Remember our important equations in this chapter. We know that for the position of maxima, we should be looking at $d \sin \theta = m\lambda$ ($m = 0, 1, 2 \ldots$). Notice that this equation doesn't contain a term for intensity. The distance between maxima in a diffraction pattern is unrelated to the intensity of the light used. (B) is tempting, because one might assume that the spacing would increase with intensity. So is (D), but we see that frequency is not a term in the equation either. Wavelength would have been a more tempting answer. (C) exists as a foil to (B).

2. B

Electromagnetic waves are transverse waves. Simply put, the vectors for electric field and magnetic field oscillate and are perpendicular to the direction of propagation and to each other. Simply refer to figure 10.1. Knowing this image and understanding what it means would lead you to choice B. Included in the spectrum of electromagnetic waves is visible light. Longitudinal vibrations come into question when considering sound and a few other types of motion, so (A) is incorrect.

3. B

Draw a diagram of the described system and sketch some rays coming from it. First, we have to find the placement of the first image. We first use (1/o) + (1/i) = (1/f). So (1/6 m) + (1/i) = (1/4 m), and i = 12 m. Stopping here would give us either (C) or (D). Based on our drawing, we know that the image is upside-down and beyond the focal point on the other side of the lens. This can be confirmed by determining the magnification and then the height of the first image. To find the distance of the first image from the second lens, we see that 18 m – 12 m = 6 m. We must now use the same equation for the second lens, using the first image as the object in this equation. Thus, (1/6 m) + (1/i) = (1/3 m), and i = 3 m. Our diagram confirms that the image is to the right of the second lens and upright.

4. D

All images produced by plane mirrors will be virtual. The same goes for mirrors that are convex. Lenses are a bit different; all concave lenses will produce virtual images, but this is not necessarily true for convex lenses. Virtual images will not typically be produced unless an object is placed between the center and the focal point of the lens, but it is still possible.

5. A

If you're rusty on the concept of total internal reflection, refer to the text. For light to undergo this phenomenon, it has to go from a substance of high index of refraction to a substance of low index. Furthermore, it has to have an angle of incidence greater than the critical angle for the original medium. The second medium is n_2, the first is n_1, and the second must have a higher index than the second. Therefore, the relative index of refraction, which we can think of as the ratio of the two indices, must be less than 1.0. (B) is certainly not correct because if this were the case, then the two media will be the same and so the light will simply pass through. With (C), total internal reflection cannot occur when the ratio is greater than 1.0, signaling that the second medium is of higher index than the second.

6. C

Mirrors do not transmit light and one will not be able to see anything while looking through one, so items I and II are incorrect. If the object were a concave lens (item IV), one would see a virtual image of the teddy bear. Though this specific example might come to mind, it is not the only possibility; this is also possible with a convex lens (item III). The teddy bear is 10 m from the lens, which is twice its focal length (5 m). The student will observe a real image on the other side of the lens, 10 m from the lens. However, if there is nothing there to stop the light, nothing will be seen. This is because the light actually continues to travel and diverges as though an object was there. The eye will observe an object 12.5 m from it (22.5 m – 10 m). An image of the teddy bear will be observed. Because items III and IV are correct, (C) is the answer.

7. B

White light is the type of light that we usually deal with in scenarios such as these. White light produces a central white band and the spectrum of colors is produced on either side. With blue light, however, one sees alternating bands of light (whichever color of light is involved) alternating with black regions (B). Blue light consists of only a single wavelength, which is not the case with white light. Light composed of only a single wavelength does not disperse and so all bands will be composed of the color light in question. (C) and (D) would not exhibit this phenomena, and (A) suggests there is no perceptible difference between white and blue light.

8. A

First, the color of the light is irrelevant here; the ratio would be the same even if the specific color were not mentioned. Second, recall two handy equations: $n_1 \sin\theta_1 = n_2 \sin\theta_2$. Though we don't know the value of *n* for either medium, we do know the simple relationship: $n = c/v$. Replacing n in the first equation, canceling out c and rearranging, we can ultimately get $\sin\theta_2/\sin\theta_1 = v_2/v_1$. We're asked for the ratio between 2 and 1 so let's rearrange accordingly: $v_2/v_1 = \sin 45°/\sin 30°$ = approx. 0.7/0.5. Thus, $v_2 = 1.4v_1$. Having the relationship the other way around would give us (B). Using approximately 0.86 for sin 45° will give us (C) or (D).

9. C

First consider that the fringe under consideration is bright. Therefore, the kind of interference involved is constructive. The equation $d \sin\theta = m\lambda$ should come to mind. This equation is specific to maxima and we know that it is only valid with m = 0, 1, 2... We know that the difference in path length must be a whole number times the wavelength, so (B) and (D) are incorrect. Because the central maximum is equidistant from the two slits, $d \sin\theta = 0$ there and (A) is incorrect. At the first bright fringe above the central maximum, we know that $d \sin\theta = \lambda$.

10. D

A basic optics principle is tested here, but you need to know how to discern between and assign values to variables, as well as choose the correct equation. Here, our choice of equation should not be very difficult. The question points to $1/o + 1/i = 1/f = 2/r$. We know that the goal of the lens is to create a virtual image of your friend's face at the near point of your eye. Consider this when assigning amounts to variables: 1/50 cm + 1/–100 cm = 2/r, and r = 200 cm. If we fail to realize that the question asks about r rather than f, we might get (A) or (C). (B) would be your result had you used a positive value, getting a value of 67 cm for r. Pay attention to signs! Finally, to get power, we know that $P = 1/f$ and $1/f = 2/r$. This means that P = 1.0 diopters. Remember, this equation works only if *f* and *r* are measured in meters.

11. D

Drawing a diagram is best here. Because the angle given is with respect to the horizontal, we know that our angle in question, θ_1, must equal 30°. So we know that the reflected beam will produce a mirror image of the incident beam angles on the other side of the plane of symmetry. Therefore, the reflected beam will make an angle of 60° with the horizontal. Since we're given that the reflected and refracted beams are perpendicular to each other, the refracted beam will make a 30° angle with the horizontal. However, because our θ_2 must be with respect to the plane of symmetry, it equals 60°. Be careful in this analysis: confusing 30° and 60° throughout will lead you to an incorrect n_2 = 1.7. Using $n_1 \sin\theta_1 = n_2 \sin\theta_2$, we have $(1)(\sin 30°) = n_2(\sin 60°)$, and $n_2 = 0.58$. (A) would demonstrate a lack of understanding of index of refraction, which can never be smaller than 1.

12. A

We may not have the actual angles of incidence and refraction, but having relative values will do just fine. First, we refer to $n_1 \sin\theta_1 = n_2 \sin\theta_2$. As the angle in medium A ($\theta - 10°$) is smaller than the angle in glycerol ($\theta°$), we know that the index of refraction of medium A must be larger that the index of refraction of glycerol. Therefore, (B) and (C) are incorrect. Next, we see that as light travels from medium A to B, the angle changes from $\theta - 10°$ to θ. We can therefore conclude that medium B must have an index of refraction equal to the index of refraction of glycerol. Though only (B) includes this scenario for medium B, it has already been eliminated. Instead, realize that corn oil can also work, since it has the same index of refraction as glycerol. (A) is correct.

13. C

Though we may not be given the index of refraction for the glass of a greenhouse, we know that its index will be higher than that of air. Whenever light passes from low to high index, $n = c/v$ shows us that an increase in n leads to a decrease of v. This eliminates (A) and (B). Knowing $c = f\lambda$ and replacing c with v, we must note that the frequency of a specific wave doesn't change as it passes from one medium to another. This allows wavelength to become shorter. However, if that simple fact were unknown, one could easily choose (D).

14. B

It would be difficult to answer this question correctly without knowing that frequency remains the same through different media; (A) and (B), especially, would have been hard to distinguish. While you cannot use a calculator during the test, this math can be done easily through estimation. First we realize that we can use $c = f\lambda$ and v instead, so $v = f\lambda$. Next, we need $n = c/v$ rearranged to $v = c/n$. Substituting, we get $c/n = f\lambda$. Separately, we can use $v = f\lambda$ again, specifically to obtain $\lambda_{\text{in diamond}}$, so we would have $\lambda_{\text{diamond}} = v_{\text{diamond}}/f$. So now we have $n_{\text{diamond}} = c/v_{\text{dia}}$. After rearranging and substituting from above, we get $\lambda_{\text{dia}} = c/f\, n_{\text{dia}}$. After rearranging and substituting again, we have something more useful: $\lambda_{\text{dia}} = \lambda_{\text{air}}/n_{\text{dia}}$. Substituting our values, 620 nm/1.92 = 322 nm, choice (B). Had we switched these two amounts around, we might have gotten (A). Multiplying rather than dividing would have produced (D), and simply assuming that the wavelength would remain unchanged would have produced (C).

15. D

At the point where the ray hits one of the legs, we know that the angle of incidence is 0° and thus that the angle of refraction will also be 0°. Therefore, the ray will enter the prism without bending and will hit the hypotenuse at an angle of 30° with the axis of symmetry. Right away, we know that (A) is incorrect. Next, we need to know if the critical angle of the surface between the prism and the air will be reached. Regarding the critical angle, we know that:

$$\sin\theta_c = n_{\text{air}}/n_{\text{prism}}$$
$$= 1/1.4$$
$$= \text{appx } 0.71$$
$$\theta_c = 45°$$

Because we know that the angle of the ray is 30° and that the critical angle is 45°, we know that the ray will not continue through the prism. Total internal reflection will not happen and the ray must immediately exit the prism into the air. (D) is correct.

16. A

Don't be put off by the lack of information. This question sets out to test a very basic idea which, even if you don't remember, can be deduced by knowing the correct formula. For maximums in the pattern that will be produced on this screen, $d \sin\theta = m\lambda$ (m = 0, 1, 2...). Using the small angle approximation will lead us to y, the linear distance between maxima. Ultimately, $\Delta y = (\Delta m\ \lambda\ D)/d$.

HIGH-YIELD SIMILAR QUESTIONS

Snell's Law

1. 51.1°
2. 42.2 mm
3. 13.8°; 17.6°

Refraction

1. 19.2°
2. 24.4°
3. 1.62

Total Internal Reflection

1. 2.79
2. 1.22
3. 35°

Converging Lens

1. 14 cm
2. The image is located $6\frac{2}{3}$ cm in front of the lens. It is $1\frac{1}{3}$ cm tall.
3. A coverging lens with f = 10 cm.

CHAPTER 11: ATOMIC PHENOMENA

1. B

The most common use of Planck's constant is in the formula $E = hf$ (the energy of a photon equals the product of Planck's constant and the frequency of the photon). This means that Planck's constant is equal to the ratio of a photon's energy to its frequency. Items I and II are not true.

2. A

In this system, heat energy is being added to the system; this means that the total energy of the system increases. According to the formula $E = hc/\lambda$, the wavelength of light decreases as the energy increases; a decrease in wavelength means that the color of the light approaches violet and ultraviolet.

3. D

A window in a furnace is an approximate replica of a black body system. In such a system, the total emitted energy is proportional to the fourth power of the temperature (according to the equation $E_T = \sigma T_4$). If the temperature is doubled, then the total energy must increase by a factor of 16.

4. A

At every temperature, a black body has a different wavelength at which the energy of its radiation is at its peak. When the temperature is higher, this peak can be achieved at a lower wavelength. Wien's displacement law summarizes this idea by stating that λ_{peak} is inversely proportional to temperature, where λ_{peak} is equal to the wavelength at which the radiation's energy is at its peak.

5. C

In the photoelectric effect, an electron escapes from a metal if it is struck by a photon whose energy is at least as high as the metal's work function. After it is ejected, its kinetic energy is equal to the difference between the photon's energy and the work function. Because the photon in this question has an energy that is equal to the work function, the kinetic energy is equal to zero. This means that the energy of the photon is just enough to let the electron escape; afterward, its velocity will be approximately zero.

6. B

The electron moves from a higher energy level to a lower energy level; this can only occur if the extra energy is dissipated through the emission of a photon. (A) suggests the opposite of that. (C) is incorrect because the work function is equal to the amount of energy necessary to eject the electron, which increases as the electron becomes more difficult to separate from the nucleus. (D) is incorrect because the energy of the atom will decrease when it emits a photon.

7. C

The energy of an electron is inversely proportional to the principal quantum number. If we say that the energy in the first energy level is equal to x, then the energy in the second energy level (which is given as –40 eV) is equal to $x/4$. This means that $x = -40$ eV, so the difference between the energies is –10 eV – –40 eV = 30 eV.

8. D

An electron in its excited state is in a higher energy level than before, so it is at a greater physical distance from the nucleus. This will decrease the attractive force between the negatively-charged electron and the positively-charged protons. The other answer choices are all true in this scenario.

9. A

The Bohr energy of an electron is positive when the electron is free from an atom and negative when the electron is in orbit. The energy decreases as the electron moves into orbit and decreases further as it moves toward a lower energy orbit. This energy change occurs instantaneously through the release (or absorption) of a photon, as depicted in all four answer choices.

10. D

An electron can absorb a photon only if the energy of the photon (i) is not precisely equal to the amount of energy needed for the electron to move up an energy level (according to Bohr's atomic theory postulates) or (ii) is greater than the work function of the atom (according to Einstein's explanation of the photoelectric effect). In this case, the principal energy level contains electrons with an energy of –20 eV; because an electron's energy is inversely proportional to the square of the principal quantum number, the second energy level must contain electrons with an energy of $-20/2^2 = -5$ eV. This means that a photon must contain at least 15 eV of energy in order to be absorbed by the electron and, consequently, move the electron from the –20 eV energy level to the –5 eV energy level.

11. B

Fluorescent light is produced when excited electrons return to their ground state. Colored light (D) appears when electrons jump up to a higher energy level and absorb photons.

12. A

The maximum frequency of light will be emitted if the electron drops to the lowest energy level. Because the energy is inversely proportional to the square of the principal quantum number, the energy in the lowest energy level is equal to $3^2 = 9$ times the energy in the third energy level. Therefore, the electron can achieve an energy as low as –18 eV, which is 16 eV lower than its initial energy. This means that the emitted radiation will carry 16 eV of energy and will exhibit a frequency of $16/h$ Hz.

13. C

Our current atomic model suggests the presence of various atomic orbitals of different shapes; although some of these orbitals are spherical, most of them are not.

14. D

The photoelectric effect occurs when a photon of sufficiently high energy strikes an atom with a sufficiently low work function. This means that a photon with higher energy is more likely to produce the effect. Because ultraviolet light has a higher frequency and lower wavelength than visible light, it also carries more energy according to the formula E = hf.

15. C

If the atom has two excited states, then it has three total energy levels including the ground state. For a photon to be emitted, an electron must drop to a lower energy level from one of these excited states. This means that the electron can drop from level 3 to level 2, level 3 to level 1, or level 2 to level 1; therefore, there are three total possibilities.

16. A

A photon with a longer wavelength will have a shorter frequency and, consequently, the least energy. The transition between two outer energy levels requires less energy than the transition between inner energy levels, because there is significantly less attraction to the nucleus. Therefore, the transition between the third and fourth energy levels will emit a photon with the lowest energy and the longest wavelength.

17. D

If a metal has a high work function, it requires a relatively large amount of energy in order to eject an electron. Because infrared light carries less energy than most other types of radiation, it is unlikely to eject an electron. The intensity of the light and the time of exposure would both increase the number of photons, but would not change the energy of each photon; because a photon is only absorbed if it carries the right amount of energy, the quantity of photons is irrelevant in this case.

18. A

The capability of hydrogen to accept an electron does not change the typical structure of a hydrogen atom, which is the basis for most atomic theories. Moreover, hydrogen is indeed capable of accepting an electron in rare circumstances.

19. C

Photons always travel at the speed of light and cannot be accelerated. The other answer choices are incorrect because energy is directly proportional to frequency and inversely proportional to wavelength, which directly determines color.

20. B

An electron is ejected from its atom if the sum of its Bohr energy and its absorbed energy (the energy of the photon) is greater than zero. When this sum is less than zero, the electron will absorb the photon only if the photon carries precisely enough energy to move the electron to one of its excited states.

HIGH-YIELD SIMILAR QUESTIONS

Energy Emission from Electrons

1. This is now a free electron which has been completely ejected from the hydrogen atom, so it does not occupy any of the atom's energy levels.
2. -4×10^{-19} J
3. 91 nm

CHAPTER 12: NUCLEAR PHENOMENA

1. A

The mass of the protons and the neutrons is (1.007 amu/proton)(2 protons) + (1.009 amu/neutron)(2 neutrons) = 4.032 amu. Some of this mass is converted to energy in order to overcome the binding energy of the nucleus, so the overall mass must be less than 4.032 amu.

2. B

The change in energy is determined by the equation $E = \Delta mc^2$, so it is directly proportional to the change in mass. This is equal to the mass of the final state ($m_p + m_n$) minus the mass of the initial state (m). c^2, meanwhile, is clearly equal to the ratio of E/m (based on $E = mc^2$), so its units must be in terms of energy/mass. (B) is the only one that correctly represents both m and c^2.

3. C

The reaction in (C) is an example of α decay. This means that any extra energy is stored in the alpha particle, so free energy is not necessarily released. (A) is a fusion reaction and (B) is a fission reaction, both of which involve the release of energy. (D) is an atom that goes from its excited state to its ground state, which is always accompanied by the emission of energy in the form of a photon.

4. C

A typical carbon nucleus contains 6 protons and 6 neutrons. An α particle contains 2 protons and 2 neutrons. Therefore, one carbon nucleus can dissociate into 6/2 = 3 α particles.

5. B

β decay occurs when an electron or a positron is released by the nucleus. This means that a proton is converted to a neutron or vice versa. Therefore, a β particle is emitted in any reaction in which the atomic number of the parent atom increases or decreases by 1 while the mass number stays the same.

6. D

In a fission process, the parent nuclide is split into two or more daughter nuclides, each of which has a significantly lower mass. (A) and (B) are incorrect because the mass number does not change in β decay and γ decay. (C) is incorrect because a fusion process involves the combination of two nuclei into one heavier nucleus.

7. B

When mass is converted completely into energy, the total energy is equal to mc^2. In this case, two particles with mass m_e are converted completely into energy, so the total energy is equal to $2\ m_e c^2$. The kinetic energy of the individual particles is irrelevant to the calculation of the total energy.

8. A

Because the half-life of ^{12}C is essentially infinite, a 25 percent decrease in the ratio of ^{14}C to ^{12}C means the same thing as a 25 percent decrease in the amount of ^{14}C. If less than half of the ^{14}C has deteriorated, then less than one half-life has elapsed; therefore, the sample is less than 5,730 years old.

9. D

The activity of a nuclide is cut in half after every half-life ("$t_{1/2}$" is shorthand for "half-life"). (D) is the only graph which suggests such a trend, in which the rate of decline decreases as time goes on.

10. D

In an alpha decay, an element loses two protons. In a positron decay, a proton is converted to a neutron. Gamma decay, meanwhile, has no impact on the atomic number of the nuclide. Therefore, two alpha decays and two positron decays will yield a daughter nuclide with six less protons than the parent.

11. B

Over the course of the first 6 hours, the concentration decreases eight-fold. During the last 6 hours, the concentration also decreases eight-fold. An eight-fold decrease suggests that 3 half-lives have elapsed; because 6 hours have passed, the total half-life must be equal to (6 hours)/(3 half-lives) = 2 hours/half-life.

12. C

After the stable nucleus fuses with three hydrogen atoms, it has a plethora of protons. In order to balance the size of the nucleus, it will either lose some protons (via α decay), convert some protons into neutrons (via β^+ decay), or gain additional neutrons. It is unlikely for it to acquire another proton through β^- decay.

13. D

The instantaneous decay rate at any given time is equal to $-\lambda n$, where λ is equal to approximately $0.7/t_{1/2}$. Therefore, λ is equal to $-(7/10) \times (1/14 \text{ days}^{-1}) = -1/20 \text{ days}^{-1}$. Because the quantity is 1 mol, the decay rate must be equal to $(-1/20 \text{ days}^{-1})(1 \text{ mol}) = -1/20$ mol/day. This question can also be solved without knowing the equation if you are familiar with basic calculus; if you take the derivative of the equation $n = n_0e^{-\lambda t}$ with respect to time, you get $dn/dt = -\lambda n$.

14. C

If a neutron combines with a positron, a proton is formed. Because protons have a lower mass than neutrons, the extra mass must be converted to energy and released from the system.

15. A

The fusion of a hydrogen nucleus (one proton) and a helium nucleus (two protons, two neutrons) will produce ^{5}Li. If the ^{5}Li nucleus captures an electron, a proton will be converted to a neutron, producing ^{5}He. Although the atom will initially carry a positive charge in most cases, the positive charge is a property of the atom and not of the nuclide.

16. A

A particle is likely to be deflected if it interacts with an atom in the lead sheet. Because an α particle is larger in size and carries a larger charge than the other types of radiation, it is also more likely to be attracted to an atom or to randomly collide with an atom.

HIGH-YIELD SIMILAR QUESTIONS

Mass Defect

1. 0.76206 amu
2. 1.68398 amu
3. 1.08484 amu

PRACTICE SECTIONS

PRACTICE SECTION 1

ANSWER KEY

1. D	19. A	37. B
2. D	20. A	38. B
3. B	21. B	39. A
4. C	22. C	40. A
5. A	23. D	41. D
6. D	24. B	42. C
7. A	25. C	43. D
8. C	26. B	44. A
9. B	27. A	45. D
10. C	28. A	46. B
11. C	29. C	47. C
12. A	30. C	48. D
13. C	31. C	49. D
14. B	32. A	50. B
15. C	33. B	51. C
16. A	34. B	52. A
17. B	35. D	
18. A	36. C	

PASSAGE I

1. D

The Bohr energy is negative for an atomic electron and positive for a free electron. The largest negative energy values are found in the first energy level; the energy increases for electrons closer to the outer energy levels, but never reaches zero. The electron is only ejected when it is struck by a photon carrying enough energy to bring the electron's energy above zero. For this reason, it is easier for a photon to eject a high-energy outer electron than a lower-energy inner electron.

2. D

Electrons always occupy the lowest possible energy level. If one of the inner shells has a vacancy, an electron from an outer shell will immediately occupy it in order to minimize its own energy. The energy level drop causes the emission of the x-ray, not vice versa as in (A). The charge on the atom doesn't change when an electron moves from one energy level to another, so (B) is incorrect. The gravitational force between the nucleus and the electron (C) is insignificant compared to the electrostatic force; also, the gravitational force does not change when an empty shell is created.

3. B

Because the x-ray moves in a random direction, only the energy of the photon will impact the likelihood of the production of an Auger electron. A photon carrying more energy, meanwhile, is more likely to carry enough energy to eject a second electron. We can tell by looking at the figures that (A) and (B) involve the largest energy change. A more precise value can be determined by considering the fact that the total energy is inversely proportional to the square of the principal quantum number. If we set the energy of the first level as x, the energy of the drop from level 2 to level 1 (B) is equal to x/1 − x/4 = 3x/4. The energy of the trop from level 4 to level 2 (A), meanwhile, is x/4 − x/16 = 3x/16. Therefore, (B) carries far more energy than (A).

4. C

The passage states that the emission of the x-ray photon is caused by the decrease in energy of the electron, so the photon will carry all of the energy lost by the electron. Because energy is inversely proportional to the square of the principal quantum number, we can say that the energy of an electron in level 3 is equal to $x/9$ and the energy of an electron in level 2 is equal to $x/4$, where x is the energy of an electron in level 1. Since $x/9$ is equal to 10 eV, x must be equal to 90 eV; this means that $x/4$, the energy of level 2, is equal to 2.5 eV. Therefore, the change in energy from level 3 to level 2 is 7.5 eV.

5. A

As the passage suggests, the energy from Auger electrons will slightly distort the measurements of an x-ray's energy. If the Auger electrons are eliminated, this error in the measurements will be decreased. A fairly constant number of Auger electrons is produced (on average) along with an x-ray, so this is not a significant source of variability (B). Auger electrons are unrelated to the sensitivity and resolution of the equipment (C) and (D). Also, no details are provided about the equipment used to measure the energy of x-rays.

6. D

The number of electrons will change the likelihood of the production of an Auger electron, but will not affect the energy of the electron. If a negatively-charged ion is produced through the addition of an extra electron, each of the electrons in orbit will feel a decreased net electrostatic force with the nucleus; this means that it will take less energy to remove the electron from orbit. Therefore, an Auger electron released from substance A will have a higher kinetic energy because it used up less of its energy when being ejected from orbit.

7. A

Hydrogen and helium have only one energy level, so they do not produce Auger electrons. All the other elements have the potential to produce Auger electrons because they all have multiple energy levels from which an outer electron can drop to fill a hole.

8. C

An increase in photon energy will not directly cause an increase in the number of x-rays unless the increase is significant enough to eject an electron in a lower energy level. Once the energy of the photon reaches this point, the number of x-rays will suddenly increase. The energy of these x-rays, however, will increase continuously. When this energy becomes adequate to start ejecting Auger electrons, it will begin to do so. The number of steps in the Auger electron curve is greater than the number of steps in the x-ray curve because every x-ray has the potential to produce several different Auger electrons.

9. B

When an electron drops from level a to level b, the excess energy will, according to the passage, take the form of an x-ray. This x-ray, whose energy is now equal to $E_a - E_b$, sometimes collides with the potential Auger electron. This electron will be ejected if its new energy (the sum of its energy, E_c, and the x-ray's energy, $E_a - E_b$) is greater than zero. This sum will be equal to the kinetic energy of the electron after it is ejected.

PASSAGE II

10. C

According to the passage, the thermocouple measures voltage changes that occur as a result of the temperature difference across the circuit. As this temperature difference increases, the energy difference between the two sides will also increase; this will lead to the production of a larger voltage.

11. C

The resistance does not change when more voltage is applied. According to Ohm's law (V = IR), an increase in electric potential (V) will cause an increase in current (I). The amount of current depends on the total resistance in a circuit, but the amount of resistance does not depend on the current (D). The resistance of a material is an innate property of that material and based on $R = (\rho L)/A$, where ρ is the resistivity of the material, L is the length of the resistor, and A is the cross-sectional area of the resistor.

12. A

According to the passage, a thermocouple determines temperature differences based on differences in voltage; you should know that voltage is produced as a result of differences in potential energy.

13. C

The voltage in a thermocouple is produced as a result of the temperature difference across the circuit; therefore, it can function without an external source of electric current. That means (A) and (B) are incorrect. Resistance, however, cannot be easily measured without applying a current across the circuit. (D) is incorrect because resistance always exists, whether or not external power is present. Because an RTD functions by measuring changes in resistance, a small amount of external power is always necessary in order to accurately determine these changes.

14. B

The passage states that the temperature is directly proportional to the resistance. This means that the temperature changes will be greater for circuits with larger resistances. The resistance in a circuit is maximized when the resistors are wired in series, as in (B); in this case, the total resistance is equal to the sum of the individual resistances. In (A), the resistors are wired in parallel, so the total resistance is equal to one-fourth of each individual resistance. (C) and (D) represent a circuit that contains both a series and a parallel connection; no matter how this is organized, the total resistance will be lower than the resistance in a series wiring scheme.

15. C

A complete circuit is always organized in a loop; (C) is the only one that includes such a loop. (B) and (D) disregard the fact that a voltage is always created between two points, so a voltmeter must measure voltage through two different wires. (A) does not feature a loop.

16. A

A thermoelectric system can store thermal energy and convert it to electrical energy, but it cannot store electrical energy unless a capacitor is added. The passage mentions that the thermoelectric effect is reversible, meaning that it can also produce heat from voltage (instead of just producing voltage from heat). Because voltage can be either positive or negative, it can be used for either heating or cooling.

17. B

If the resistivity changes easily with respect to temperature, changes in temperature will lead to significant changes in the readings from the RTD. This will make it more likely for the RTD to detect relatively small changes in temperature.

QUESTIONS 18–21

18. A

How do light and sound waves differ? Polarization requires that the direction of propagation of the wave be perpendicular to the direction of propagation of energy. Electromagnetic waves like light can accomplish this because they are transverse waves. Sound cannot produce this phenomenon because it is a longitudinal wave and so the direction of its propagation is parallel to the direction in which it carries energy.

19. A

The question assumes you know that the index of refraction of air is, by definition, 1. This assumption is also made on the actual MCAT. For any material with an index of refraction n, the critical angle is arcsin(1/n). The angle whose sine is 1/2 is 30. For Test Day, be familiar with the sines and cosines of 0, 30, 45, 60, and 90 because they occur so commonly in calculations.

20. A

When light reflects off any object, its phase is shifted by pi radians causing constructive interference. If a material is made that is half the thickness of the wavelength, then as the light passes through the film (once incoming and once outgoing), it will be shifted by another wavelength causing completely destructive interference.

21. B

Think: What formula relates the work function to an emitted photon's frequency? $hf = \phi$. The work function, ϕ, is the difference in kinetic energy between incoming and outgoing electrons. This difference is an energy and so is related to frequency as $E = hf$, with h being Planck's constant. Be careful with the units.

PASSAGE III

22. C

This problem asks that you calculate work: $W = Fd(\cos\theta)$, where F is the force, d is the distance, and θ is the angle between the work and the displacement. Because the force being applied is in the exact same direction as the displacement, θ is equal to 0. $\cos(0) = 1$, so we have $W = Fd$. The force required to lift the plate is equal to the weight of the plate. Weight = mg = 2 kg × 10 m/s^2 = 20 N and the displacement is 2 m, so the work is equal to 20 N × 2 m = 40 J. (C) is correct. (A) confuses the mass of the plate with its weight. (B) uses the incorrect formula $W = F/d$, and (D) uses $W = d/F$.

23. D

The formula for potential energy is $U = mgh$, where m is the mass of the object, g is the acceleration due to gravity, and h is the height of the object off the ground. First, make sure that all of the variables are converted into standard units: 40 g = 0.04 kg and 150 cm = 1.5 m. Then plug in the variables to find the answer. (0.04 kg)(1.5 m)(10 m/s^2) = 0.6 J. (A) and (C) omit one or more conversions.

24. B

It is important to remember the concept of conservation of energy. Although the energy of the plate may change forms throughout its path, its total energy will remain constant. The plate does not simply lose or gain energy by simply falling (A) and (C). The potential energy of the plate will decrease as its height decreases, while its kinetic energy will increase as its velocity increases (D).

25. C

When the plate sits on the table, all of its energy is potential energy. As it falls, the potential energy is converted to kinetic energy. The further it falls to the ground, the more the potential energy is converted to kinetic. Thus, although the total energy stays the same, the kinetic energy is greatest right before the plate hits the ground (C).

26. B

Utilizing the concept of conservation of momentum, we know that the individual pieces will have a total momentum equal to the momentum of the plate right before it breaks. Momentum is given by p = mv. If the plate is falling at 10 m/s^2 for 2 m, its velocity as it reaches the ground is given by $v^2 = 2\ ax$. The mass of the plate before it breaks into pieces is 6M. Thus, v = 2(10 m/s^2)(6M); v = 120M m/s. Now we calculate the momentum. We have 120M (6M) = 720M^2 kg × m/s, so (B) is correct. If you stop after the first step, you end up with the velocity instead of the momentum, as in (A) and (C). (D) calculates a momentum, but incorrectly calculates velocity as the product of the distance and acceleration.

27. A

Because friction is negligible, momentum will be conserved in this interaction. The piece of the plate has a momentum of p = (3M)(5 m/s) = 15M kg × m/s. Because it comes to a complete stop, all of its momentum is transferred to the block. Thus, 15M m/s = M(v); v = 15 m/s. (A) is correct. (B) is the total momentum, not velocity. (C) and (D) are derived incorrectly using the kinetic energy formula, not the momentum formula.

28. A

Here you must apply the concept of impulse. Impulse is given by $J = Ft = mv_f - mv_0$. If we want to find how much for is required to stop the 1M kg piece in 3 seconds, we must plug in our variables (m = 1M kg, v_0 = 4 m/s, v_f = 0 m/s, t = 3s, F = ?). Thus, (F)(3s) = (M)(4 m/s) – (M)(0 m/s) = 4/3MN. (A) is correct. (C) and (D) confuse the initial velocity with the final velocity.

29. C

Due to conservation of energy, the position of the plate does not matter. As it reaches its highest point, its kinetic energy is decreasing because its velocity is decreasing. However, its potential energy is increasing due to an increase in height from the original position. As it falls, the opposite happens. Overall, the total energy stays constant even if the potential and kinetic energies change. (C) is correct.

30. C

Work is done only by the force that is responsible for an object's movement. Because the force points downward and the plate moves to the left, this particular force does no work on the plate. (C) is correct. (A) multiplies the force by the value of the angle. (B) correctly multiplies force by distance but doesn't consider the fact that the force is not in the same direction as the displacement. (D) also ignores the angle of the force and uses the incorrect formula by dividing the force by the distance.

PASSAGE IV

31. C

Two nearby sound waves will typically emit a beat whose frequency is equal to the difference between the frequencies of the individual waves. In this case, the frequency of the beat is equal to 440 Hz – 430 Hz = 10 Hz, or 10 beats per second. There will be a total of (10 Hz)(60 seconds/minute) = 600 beats per minute.

32. A

The pitch of a sound is determined by its frequency, which is inversely proportional to the length of the string. Therefore, if the length of the string is decreased, the frequency will increase.

33. B

The passage mentions that the sound waves emerging from the compartment have a greater amplitude than those entering the compartment. This means that the waves carry more energy and that the individual sounds are louder. Either of these two observations should lead you to the conclusion that the sound has a greater intensity, because the intensity of the wave increases with increasing energy and determines how loud the sound is.

34. B

As the sound wave approaches the listener, its relative velocity is greater than the typical velocity of sound in air. According to the Doppler effect, this increased velocity will cause the apparent frequency of the sound to increase, since frequency is directly proportional to velocity.

35. D

The length of a fixed string is inversely proportional to its frequency. This means that the pitch of the string will decrease as the length increases. The curve will demonstrate a y = 1/x curve, which is represented approximately by the graph in (D). (A) represents a curve with the formula y = x, (B) represents a curve with the formula y = –x, and (C) represents a curve with the formula y = –1/x.

36. C

The passage states that a pickup absorbs a sound wave directly from the electric guitar strings. The acoustic guitar strings, on the other hand, are amplified in the wooden compartment. Therefore, the acoustic guitar produces a louder sound wave than the electric guitar strings; this means that the sine curve will have a larger amplitude.

37. B

Assuming no loss due to friction, the energy transmitted by the string is equal to ½ kx^2, where *k* is the spring constant (500 N/m) and *x* is the total displacement (0.02 m). So ½ kx^2 is equal to 0.1 J. Power is equal to energy per unit time, which can be determined by multiplying the energy by the frequency (1,000 s^{-1}), so the total power equals 100 W. The intensity of a sound is equal to the power divided by the square of the distance (1 m), so the total intensity is 100 W/m^2.

QUESTIONS 38–45

38. B

A combined approach of test-taking skills and physical reasoning makes this question easier than it seems. First, the horizontal component is always less than the total velocity vector unless the object is moving only in the horizontal direction. Furthermore, it is never greater than the total velocity vector of which it is a component. This eliminates (A), but be careful when reviewing (B), because the form of the question means that a velocity of 35 m/s or greater would indicate (B) as correct. In fact, the horizontal component of velocity is equal to the total velocity vector multiplied by the cosine angle made with the horizontal. Estimating cos 30 to be 0.9, the horizontal component is closest to 40 m/s (B).

39. A

Heat flow is directly proportional to temperature change according to the laws of thermodynamics. For heat exchange to have occurred, there must have been an initial difference in temperature. To disprove the other answer choices, reason by counterexample: heat can flow from one object to an object of identical composition at a lower temperature, so (B) and (D) are incorrect. The mass (C) will influence the amount of heat transferred but not the fact that heat is transferred.

40. A

(B) is too extreme. (C) and (D) directly contradict the postulates of the kinetic theory of gases.

41. D

Whereas high resistance would increase the error associated with measuring a current because of the creation of a non-negligible current drop across any resistor, it would decrease the error associated with measuring any voltage in parallel because of the very same effect. Both dynamos and generators rely on electromagnetic induction, as can some ammeters.

42. C

How is the focal length related to the radius of curvature? It is one-half the radius of curvature. This is a straightforward application of the formula stating that the focal length of a perfectly spherical mirror is equal to one-half the length of the radius of curvature.

43. D

While this question may seem daunting because these are one-ohm resistors, the key lies in discovering the symmetry. They can be arranged as follows: all in series; all in parallel; in a train of two groups of resistors (three then one or two then two); or in a train of three groups of resistors. That makes a total of five combinations.

44. A

A dieletric allows more charge to be stored on each plate in a parallel plate capacitor as it decreases the effective electric field between the plates. Because $F = qE$, at a constant force, the charge stored must go up. The potential difference is unchanged because the addition of additional charge is proportional on both plates.

45. D

The angular frequency (which is directly proportional to the frequency of oscillation) of a pendulum is directly proportional to the square root of acceleration due to gravity, and inversely proportional to the square root of the length of the pendulum's stem. The mass has no effect, eliminating all answer choices but (D).

PASSAGE V

46. B

Centrifugal forces on the tires are proportional to the speed of the vehicle. This may lead them to expand and burst, even if the force of friction is smaller than in trial 2.

47. C

The net force is not 0 N; it is the centripetal force which causes the constant change in direction, measured by mv^2/R. (C) is the answer, 10,000 N.

48. D

F1 and F2 are normal and centripetal forces, respectively. At point B in figure 2, they point toward the center. At point A, they also point toward the center.

49. D

It's important to set the equation up correctly. Fn at point A must be greater than 0 N. $m \times v^2/R = Fn + mg$. So $m \times v^2/R - mg >= 0$. Or $v^2/R = g$. Therefore, $R = v^2/g = 25$ and the maximum height is 500 m. Of course, the motorcyclist is burning up his engine by going against gravity, but that is not of concern here.

50. B

As the motorcycle moves away from the lowest point, the normal force decreases. The force of friction is proportional to the normal force. The net force is always of the same magnitude and points toward the center of the circle.

51. C

Item I is correct: The radial force of friction is responsible for keeping the motorcycle from wiping out. (This is what may happen if the road is slick.)

This force is equal in magnitude and direction to the horizontal component of the normal force. If it didn't exist, the wheels would slip radially outward. Item II is correct: A greater radius means that a smaller radial force of friction is required to sustain the smaller centripetal force (m × v^2/R). Item III is wrong; the mass of the motorcycle is proportional to both the centripetal and the frictional forces, creating no net effect. Items I and II are correct so (C) is the answer.

52. A

In both scenarios the forces are nonzero in magnitude at any given moment, but the summation of force vectors for a circle happens to be 0 N. This indicates that centripetal forces do not do any work over a circular trip.

PRACTICE SECTION 2

ANSWER KEY

1. D	19. C	37. A
2. C	20. A	38. B
3. B	21. D	39. A
4. A	22. C	40. D
5. B	23. B	41. C
6. D	24. A	42. A
7. B	25. B	43. D
8. C	26. D	44. D
9. C	27. B	45. A
10. C	28. A	46. B
11. B	29. B	47. D
12. C	30. D	48. A
13. D	31. D	49. C
14. A	32. D	50. D
15. C	33. B	51. B
16. A	34. C	52. B
17. C	35. A	
18. D	36. C	

PASSAGE I

1. D

The car maintains its speed when it goes through the circle (change of kinetic energy to potential and back to kinetic) and it also maintains its speed when it hits the wall and rebounds, assuming there is no energy loss to heat. The change in momentum is m × $(v_i - (-v_i))$ = 2 × 100 kg × 50 m/s = 10,000 kg × m/s.

2. C

(A) and (B) are unlikely to happen because trial 1 used more kinetic energy and, therefore, subjected the car and the wall to greater stress. (C) is reasonable because most collisions are not perfectly elastic.

3. B

If friction is negligible, then the speed of the car after coming out of the circle is the same as the speed when it went in, because no work was done on it. The distance to travel toward the wall is 50 m, which can be traversed in 1 second. But the car will have to convert all of its kinetic energy into elastic potential energy before it stops.

$\frac{1}{4}\sqrt{k/m}$ = 1.3 s. Therefore, the total time is 2.3 s.

4. A

At first, the spring on the car is relaxed (x = 0), but as it hits the wall, a force proportional to the length of compression is applied to it: F = –kx = ma. Therefore, deceleration grows in magnitude as the spring compresses until it comes to a stop. After that, the reverse happens, as the car accelerates and rebounds.

5. B

With 50 percent efficiency, half of the kinetic energy will be delivered to the cylinders. The rest will cause the car to rebound with half of its original kinetic energy. So the heat delivered is 50% × ½ × mv^2 = ¼ ×

$100 \times 20^2 = 10{,}000$ J. To find power, one must find the time it takes the car to complete one cycle—to go from one wall to another and back. The length of the track is 200 m and the circumference of the circle is 5π, so the time can be found by computing the distance: $x = 2 \times (200 + 5\pi)$ and $t = x/v = (400 + 10\pi)/20 = 21$ s. Power is energy divided by time, which is equal to 10,000 J/21 s = 116 W.

6. D

The heat delivered to the cylinder is equal to the product of power and time. With 10,000 J per cycle, that means 10,000 J × 5 = 25 kJ. If you used the heat transfer formula, $Q/t = k \times A \times \Delta T/L$ to calculate ΔT, you would end up with a small value, which tells you only that the wall of the cylinder quickly transfers heat from the outside to the inside of the cylinder. It does not tell you how much heat will be added to the water inside the cylinder system, only how quickly the temperature is equilibrated. The question asked how much heat was added, and the best way to answer it was to compute how much kinetic energy was delivered to the system.

7. B

The more the car hits the spring, the more energy (and, therefore, more heat) will be delivered to the water cylinder. Unless the water cylinder quickly loses this heat to the environment (which is not mentioned in the passage), its temperature will increase. The speed of the car determines how much energy is delivered. According to the formula $Q = mC\ \Delta T$ and as explained in the passage, specific heat is different for every liquid and affects the propensity of the liquid to change temperature. The magnitude of the spring constant does not affect the amount of energy generated in the collision. There is no indication in the passage that greater or smaller spring constants increase the efficiency of transfer from elastic to heat energy.

8. C

In order for the car to continue moving from wall to wall, it must overcome the circular track with diameter 5 m centripetal forces help the car to keep moving along the ceiling of the circle. According to the equation $mv^2/r = mg + F_N$, the car always needs a velocity which would provide a normal force greater than 0. This means that $mv^2/r = mg$, so $v^2 > g \times r$, which means that $v^2 > 25\ m^2/s^2$ at the top of the track. The car also needs to overcome the gravitational potential energy, while maintaining a speed of at least 5 m/s. The law of conservation of energy is PE final + KE initial = KE initial, which translates into $gh + \frac{1}{2} v^2$ final = $\frac{1}{2} v^2$ initial. Solving this equation yields $v^2 = 2 \times 10 \times 5 + 25\ m^2/s^2 = 125\ m^2/s^2$ at the bottom of the track, or v must be > 11 m/s. If the car loses energy and slows down with each collision, eventually it will get stuck between the circles (or fall off the track) if it cannot generate a speed of greater than 11 m/s. If half of its kinetic energy is lost, then its speed declines by a factor of $\sqrt{2}$ with each cycle. After 4 cycles, its speed will be $50/(\sqrt{2}^4)$, or 12.5 m/s.

9. C

According to the equation $Q/t = k \times A \times \Delta T/L$, the rate of heat transfer is proportional to the temperature difference between the hot and cold surfaces. If the cylinder becomes almost as hot as the heated engine, the rate of heat transfer decreases. This means that while water still keeps accepting heat, it will eventually reach a plateau and its rate of cooling will approach its rate of heating.

PASSAGE II

10. C

The amount of heat stored by the copper plate can be calculated by the equation $Q = mc\Delta T$, where m is the mass of the plate, c is its specific heat capacity, and ΔT is the change in its temperature. According to this equation, the plate will absorb some of the heat emitted by the warm water, and this absorption will be directly proportional to both the mass and the heat capacity. In his calculations, the student did not subtract this heat from the total amount of heat that is transferred from the warm water to the cold water.

11. B

The main purpose of the student's calculation is to determine the amount of heat transferred by conduction from the warm water to the copper plate and from the copper plate to the cold water. Although this is not specifically mentioned in the passage, it is something you should be able to infer. (A), (C), and (D) all mention potential types of heat transfer that the student did not consider in his calculations.

12. C

The passage states that the thermal conductivity of copper is about 400 times the thermal conductivity of glass. Therefore, according to the equation in the passage, the copper plate will conduct 400 times as much heat per unit area. Because the area of the copper is half the area of the glass, then it will conduct 400/2 = 200 times as much heat as the glass. The total amount of heat conducted by the copper is equal to 200 J, or 0.2 kJ.

13. D

The amount of heat transferred can be determined by the formula $Q = mc\Delta T$. In this case, the system reaches equilibrium when the temperature of the warm tank decreases by 25 K and the temperature of the cold tank increases by 25 K, so ΔT is equal to 25 K. Because the mass of 100 mL of water is 100 g and the heat capacity is given as 1 cal/(g × K), the total heat transfer equals (100 g)(1 cal/[g × K])(25 K) = 2500 cal. One Cal (with a capital "C") is equal to 1,000 cal (with a lowercase "c"), so the correct answer is 2.5 Cal.

14. A

When the divider is removed, the water will mix together. In cases where heat is transferred as a result of substances that are mixing together, the process is known as convection.

15. C

The entropy change is always positive for an irreversible process. When heat is transferred from one side of the system to the other, the process cannot be reversed without artificially heating or cooling either side; therefore, the entropy change is positive.

16. A

The heat transfer, $\Delta Q/\Delta t$, is directly proportional to the difference in temperature between the two sides of the copper plate (ΔT). As heat is transferred from one side of the plate to the other, the temperature of the warm water decreases and the temperature of the cold water increases. This means that ΔT is constantly decreasing, which also causes a decrease in $\Delta Q/\Delta t$. (A) is the only answer choice in which $\Delta Q/\Delta t$ continuously decreases.

17. C

The kinetic energy of the molecules in an object is measured by its temperature; if the kinetic energy is decreasing, then the temperature must also be decreasing. The temperature of the warm water tank will always decrease in the system, because this is the entire purpose of the experimental setup. Conversely, the temperature of the cold water tank will always increase (D). The passage suggests that the copper and the glass are conducting heat, so their temperatures are likely to increase (A) and (B).

QUESTIONS 18–21

18. D

Because both the source and the receiver are heading toward one another, the frequency will be increased, removing (A) and (B). Because (C) and (D) are so close together one should be careful in his calculation; the change in apparent frequency will be 380/310 as per the Doppler equation.

19. C

Because the change in velocity in the second case is 10 times that in the first case, the increase distance needed in multiplied by a factor equal to 10 squared since the square difference in velocities is directly proportional to the distance skidded. If you just multiplied by 10 and forget to square, you would get (A).

20. A

Completely destructive interference occurs when two waves are one wavelength or 180° out of phase. With the wave equation v = fλ, the wavelength is 0.25 m and is the distance that would ensure no net wave reached your ears. One could eliminate (B) and (D) because they are both even integer multiples of the wavelength and thus both cannot be correct.

21. D

According to Pascal's principle, $F_1/A_1 = F_2/A_2$. The force due to the car, F_2, is mg = 10,000 N. The surface area of the larger platform is 100 m^2, and so F_2/A_2 = 100 N/m^2. Because A_1 = 1 m^2, then the force which must be applied to the small platform, F_1, is 100 N.

PASSAGE III

22. C

The velocity gives both the speed of the plane and the direction in which the plane is traveling, so (C) is correct. A vector is a quantity that has both a magnitude and a direction. The speed of the plane (A) tells us how fast it is going but nothing about its direction. The distance the plane travels (B) also tells us nothing about its direction. The angle that the airplane makes with the horizon (D) tells us the direction of the plane's velocity but not the magnitude.

23. B

Average velocity is given by the formula v = d/t. We know that the plane traveled 1,500 meters in 2 hours. Thus, 1,500/2 = 750 m/s. The question asks for velocity and not speed; velocity considers the direction in addition to the magnitude. To have a complete answer, you must write 750 m/s at 30° north of east (the angle is given in the passage), so (B) is correct. (A) correctly specifies the magnitude of the velocity but fails to give a direction. (C) and (D) miscalculate the magnitude by multiplying distance by time.

24. A

First set up a right triangle with the velocity of the airplane as the hypotenuse.

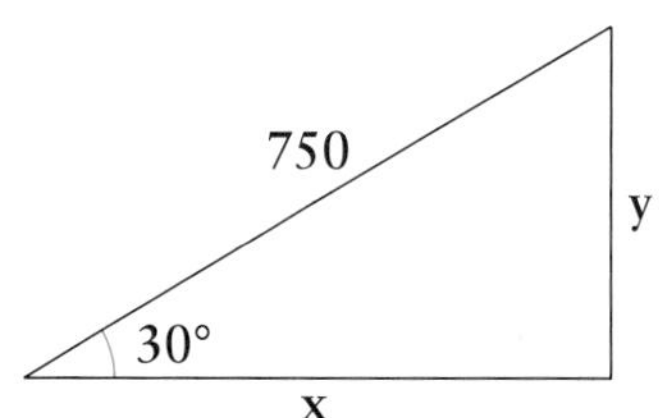

Here you can see that the x- and y-components are the legs of the right triangle. To solve for the x-component, you will utilize your trigonometric formulas: Soh Cah Toa.

Sin = opp/hyp
Cos = adj/hyp
Tan = opp/adj

Here we're looking for the x-component, which is the side adjacent to the 30° angle, so we use the equation cos(30°) = x/750 m/s. Thus, x = 750[cos(30)] which gives us 650 m/s. Because the airplane is traveling in the northeast direction, the x-component is directed east, and (A) is correct. If you had mistakenly used sin(30) = x/750 you would have gotten (B) 375 m/s, which is the y-component. (D) pairs the magnitude of the resultant velocity vector with the direction of the x-component.

25. B

To find the sum of the two y-components, you must first break down each velocity vector. Draw a right triangle to represent each vector and its x- and y-components. Then use your trigonometric identities to determine the components that you need.

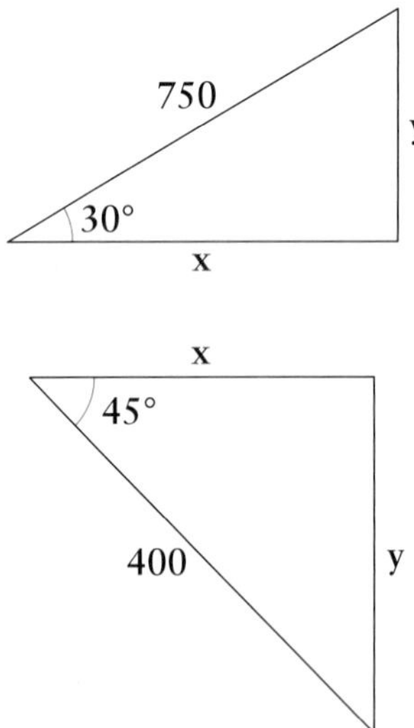

Now you can easily see that the y-component of the plane's velocity will be y_1 = sin(30) × 750 = 375 m/s heading north. The y-component for the tailwind's velocity is given by y_2= sin(45) × 400 = 283 m/s heading south. It is important to note the direction of each vector before you take their sum. To prevent adding together velocities that actually oppose one another, first designate one direction as "positive" and let the opposite direction be "negative." It is most common to indicate north as the positive direction. Thus, we have 375 m/s – 283 m/s = 92 m/s heading north. (B) is correct.

26. D

To find the resultant velocity of two separate vectors, you must add the vectors together. Draw the two vectors in a tip-to-tail manner, then draw a final line which connects the two to form a triangle.

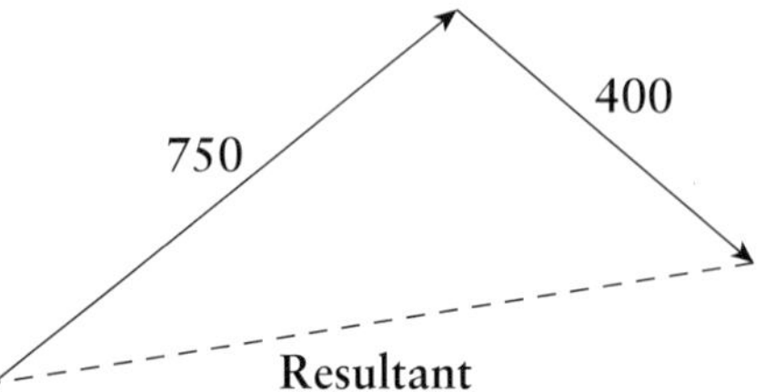

To find the magnitude of this resultant vector you'll need to break down the velocities into their x- and y-components. The x- and y-components are given by:

$$X_1 = \cos(30) \times 750 = 650 \text{ m/s E}$$
$$y_1 = \sin(30) \times 750 = 375 \text{ m/s N}$$

$$X_2 = \cos(45) \times 400 = 283 \text{ m/s E}$$
$$y_2 = \sin(45) \times 400 = 283 \text{ m/s S}$$

Now add up the x- and y-components to get a total for each.

$$X_{total} = 933 \text{ m/s E}$$
$$y_{total} = 92 \text{ m/s N}$$

These sums will be the vectors used to find the resultant velocity of the airplane after it meets the wind.

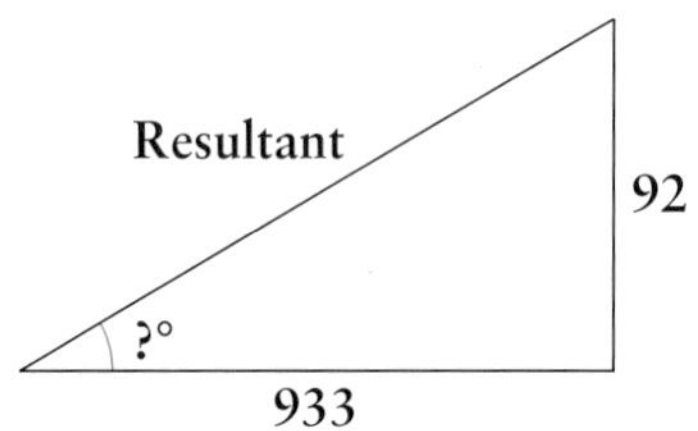

To obtain the magnitude of the velocity, use the Pythagorean theorem ($a^2 + b^2 = c^2$) to determine the hypotenuse of this right triangle. We get a result of 938 m/s. To obtain the direction of the velocity, you will use tan(θ)=opp/adj.

$$\theta = \tan^{-1}(92/933)$$
$$\theta = 6^{\circ}\text{N of E}$$

Our full answer will be 938 m/s at 6° N of E, choice (D). You might have gotten (A) if you had used the formula tan = adj/opp.

27. B

Because the plane traveled 1,500 meters in the 2 hours before it met the tailwind, we know that its average speed was 1,500/2 = 750 m/s. The question asks how long it takes the plane to travel another 1,000 meters at this speed. Because speed = d/t, we can solve for time as t = d/v. Thus, 1,000 meters/750 m/s = 1.33 hours. (B) is correct.

28. A

You're asked for displacement, not distance. That means it doesn't matter how far the plane travels, but rather how far it is from its original position. The plane traveled at 500 m/s for 3 hours, yielding a total of 1,500 meters east. Then it travels 175 meters west, so we can subtract the 175 from the 1,500 meters and end up with a total displacement of 1,325 meters. You might have gotten (C) had you forgotten to multiply the velocity by the time and simply taken the velocity as the meters traveled.

29. B

This question asks for total displacement. When the tailwind meets the plane, it has already traveled 1,500 meters. Once the wind and plane meet, a new velocity must be calculated for the next 1.5 hours. Break the velocities down into their components and add them up to get the totals. The x-component of the plane's velocity is cos(30) × 750 = 650 m/s east. Add the x-component of the wind, 300 m/s east, and the total x-velocity is 950 m/s east. Because there is no y-component for the wind, we just have sin(30) × 750 = 375 m/s north which we obtain for the plane's velocity. Using these two vectors, 950 m/s E and 375 m/s N, we get a resultant vector of 1,021 m/s. If the plane travels at this speed for another 1.5 hours, we get a displacement of 1,021 × 1.5 = 1,532 meters. Add this to the original 1,500 meters traveled and we have a total of 3,032 meters, choice (B). (D) assumes that the plane is traveling at 750 m/s for the entire 3.5 hours.

30. D

Here you need to break up the velocity into its components and then cancel out the parts until you're left with only 500 m/s east. Once you find the x- and y-components that will do this, you can add them to find the resultant vector, which is equal to the velocity of the wind. The x-component of the plane's velocity is 650 m/s east and the y-component is 375 m/s north. Because we want the resultant velocity to be in the east direction, we need to completely cancel out the y-component. This means the wind should have a y-component of 375 m/s south. To reduce the x-component to 500 m/s, we must subtract 150 m/s from the plane's x-component. Therefore, we have the following for the wind vectors:

x-component = 150 m/s west
y-component = 375 m/s south

Using the Pythagorean theorem, we can find a resultant with magnitude 404 m/s and a direction of 68° S of W. (D) is correct. (A) and (C) assume that a wind directed west will cancel out the velocity of the plane and do not give the proper angle. (B) gives the correct angle but assumes you can directly cancel out the speed by subtracting 250 m/s from the original speed.

PASSAGE IV

31. D

According to the passage, a gas-filled detector functions by allowing its particles to be ionized by radiation. You should know that radiation is more likely to ionize a particle if it carries more energy. Also, photons are less likely to interact with atoms because they are infinitely small and they carry no charge. X-rays and γ-rays are the only options that are photons. Because x-rays typically carry much less energy than γ-rays, they are also the least likely to induce ionization.

32. D

Both types of detectors function by ionizing a particle and measuring the extent of the ionization. Radiation with higher energy will produce more ions; however, different modes of decay are capable of carrying the same amount of energy and, consequently, producing the same number of ions. This makes the mode of decay indistinguishable by either of the means mentioned in the passage.

33. B

Because semiconductors are solid, they contain more molecules in the same volume. Therefore, radiation is more likely to interact with an atom in a semiconductor detector. (A) is incorrect because there are several gases that are heavier than silicon and germanium; also, the mass has very little effect on the likelihood of an interaction. (C) is a true statement, but is incorrect because the difference in ionization potential is minimal when compared with the effect of (B). (D) is irrelevant.

34. C

The passage states that ionization occurs as a result of the energy of the radiation; any other form of energy, including the ultraviolet light in the room, can also cause an ionization. For this reason, radiation detectors typically report a small amount of background noise; this noise must be subtracted from any counts in order to get an accurate reading.

35. A

A sample with higher activity simply produces more radiation particles than a sample with lower activity. Every additional radiation particle will produce a constant number of additional ions, so the readings from the detector should be directly proportional to the activity. This is clear based on the data in the table, which suggest a linear trend.

36. C

After the impact of the background radiation is subtracted (12 counts), the ratio of counts to activity for detector 1 is approximately 41 counts/curie. Because the sample in question has a known activity of 4 Ci, it will directly produce $41 \times 4 = 164$ counts. After the background radiation (12 counts) is added, the reading should be close to 175 counts.

37. A

After the background is subtracted, the reading from detector 1 is 4 counts ($16 - 12 = 4$) and the reading from detector 2 is 14 counts ($32 - 18 = 14$). On the first day, the reading from detector 1 was 41 counts ($53 - 12 = 41$) and the reading from detector 2 was 120 counts ($138 - 18 = 120$). Both of the values recorded after 3 days are slightly less than 1/8 of the value from the first day. The number of half-lives elapsed can be determined by finding n in the equation $1/8 = (\frac{1}{2})^n$; because n is 3, we know that approximately three half-lives have passed over the course of the 3 days. Therefore, one half-life is equal to approximately one day.

38. B

Detector 1 is unable to detect Sample D at its current activity, so there is no indication that the radiation from the sample will be adequate to ionize the particles in detector 1 if the activity is increased. Detector 2, however, can effectively detect Sample D at its current activity; therefore, an increase in activity will clearly lead to an increase in the reading.

PASSAGE V

39. A

The normal force is to the surface and opposes the force of the object on the surface. Thus, the normal force should be drawn perpendicular to the surface of the incline and directed outward. (B) indicates a force perpendicular to the surface, but it is facing into the incline, suggesting that this is the force exerted on the incline by the block. (C) and (D) indicate the force of gravity acting on the block and force of friction, respectively.

40. D

Because of the orientation of the force vectors for an object on an incline, the cosine function should be used to determine the y-component of this force instead of the typical sine function. We want to use cos(45) × 2M × g to obtain the y-component of force weight, and (D) is correct. (C) assumes that a sin function is used to determine the force in the y-direction.

41. C

The force due to friction is equal to the normal force multiplied by the coefficient of friction (static in this case). Thus, to obtain the force of friction we must first calculate the normal force. Because the surface is flat, $F_N = mg = 2\text{ kg} \times 10\text{ m/s}^2 = 20\text{N}$. This normal force is then multiplied by the coefficient of static friction: 20 N × 1.2 = 24 N. This is the force of friction that must be overcome in order to move the object. (A) ignores gravity and units by using the mass of the block instead of its weight. (B) is simply the coefficient of static friction.

42. A

For this question you simply need to remember the formula for gravitational force: $F_g = G(m_1m_2)/d^2$. Now just plug in the variables you are given to derive the formula $(4\ GM^2)/D^2$. (C) neglects the mass of the second sphere and (D) does not square the distance between the two spheres.

43. D

Looking at the formula again, $F_g = G(m_1m_2)/d^2$,we see that the force is inversely proportional to the square of the distance. Therefore, if we alter the distance from D to 4D, we will change the value of the denominator from D^2 to $16D^2$. That means the force will be decreased by a factor of 16.

44. D

The equation for force gravitational does not include diameter or density $F_g = G(m_1m_2)/d^2$. If the changes made did not affect the mass of the sphere or the position of its center, then the gravitational force will remain the same between the two spheres.

45. A

Here you simply need to add the two force vectors to get a net result. Because the forces are acting in opposite directions, you must subtract the smaller quantity from the larger one to obtain 42 N. Since the force in the upward direction is greater than that in the downward direction, the overall direction of the force is up and (A) is correct. (B) and (D) both feature the sum of the two vectors without accounting for the direction. (C) correctly states the magnitude but gives the opposite direction.

46. B

To find the gravitational acceleration of a planet on an object that is on its surface, you can use: $g = Gm/r^2$ where m is the mass of the planet and r is the radius of the planet. If we plug in 8 M for mass and 2D for radius, we get $(8\ GM)/4D^2$. (A) uses the diameter instead of the radius.

PASSAGE VI

47. D

From the diagram of the flow meter, the direction of the magnetic field is determined to be from right to left (leaving north pole, entering south). Knowing the direction of blood/electrolyte flow and applying the right-hand rule for the negative charge, we determine the direction of magnetic force to be down, perpendicular to both the magnetic field and electrolytes' velocity.

48. A

Volume flow rate equal $Q = Av = \pi r^2 v$. Thus, decreasing the radius by 2 will decrease volume flow rate by 4. As for voltage, $V = Ed$, so decreasing the radius by 2 will decrease both diameter and voltage by 2.

49. C

Remember that $F = qvB$. The ions in the passage that are being measured are univalent. However, calcium is bivalent with a 2+ positive charge. Thus, when the charge goes up, the magnetic field must decrease to maintain a constant magnetic force. In other words, the charge and magnetic field are inversely related. The correct answer is (C).

50. D

Applying the right-hand rule for both ions, we can determine that for both positive and negative electrolytes, magnetic force is perpendicular to both the magnetic field and velocity. The most important thing to remember when assessing the direction of current is that it is opposite the direction of electron flow. Using this, and knowing the direction of the magnetic field, you can determine the direction of force. It will always be perpendicular to both magnetic field and current.

51. B

There is no net magnetic force on the particles moving from left to right as they move parallel/antiparallel to magnetic field lines. The torque is indeed present (C), as the particles would be rotating in the uniform magnetic field at the given direction of magnetic field and particle movement.

52. B

According to Ohm's law $I = V/R$. We know from the passage that, at equilibrium, $E = vB$ and $V = Ed = vBd$. Thus, $I = vBd/R = (25 \times 10^{-2} \times 2 \times 10^{-2} \times 1)/3 = 17 \times 10^{-4} = 1.7 \times 10^{-5}$A.

PRACTICE SECTION 3

ANSWER KEY

1. A	19. C	37. A
2. A	20. A	38. C
3. B	21. B	39. C
4. A	22. A	40. C
5. B	23. D	41. B
6. D	24. C	42. B
7. C	25. C	43. D
8. A	26. C	44. C
9. A	27. C	45. D
10. C	28. B	46. C
11. D	29. B	47. B
12. A	30. A	48. D
13. D	31. D	49. D
14. B	32. C	50. D
15. D	33. A	51. D
16. A	34. A	52. C
17. C	35. B	
18. B	36. C	

PASSAGE I

1. A

Based on the equations P = IV and P = I^2R, we can tell that power is related to current, voltage, and resistance. The passage states that the battery supplies a constant 12 V of potential, which cannot be increased without the addition of another battery, so item II is incorrect. Item III is incorrect because, although increased resistance would cause the amplifier to *dissipate* more power, the question asks how the amplifier *produces* more power. Therefore, only the current (item I) can be increased by the amplifier.

2. A

The capacitance can be determined by using the formula C = Q/V, where Q is charge and V is voltage. We also know that Q = It, where I is current and t is time, so we can conclude that C = It/V. The question states that *I* equals 2 A and *t* equals 12 seconds, while the passage states that *V* equals 12 V; therefore, *C* equals (2 A × 12 s)/(12 V) = 2 F.

3. B

A wire will be more effective if it minimizes resistance, which is directly proportional to resistivity and inversely proportional to the square of the radius. Of the four options, the aluminum wire has the smallest ratio of the resistivity to the square of the radius.

4. A

Power dissipation can be determined by the formula P = I^2R, so it will be decreased if resistance is decreased. This can be accomplished if the speakers are wired in parallel, in which case the reciprocal of the circuit's resistance (1/R) is equal to the sum of the reciprocals of the individual resistances. In this case, this means that 1/R = ¼ + ¼ + ¼ + ¼ + ¼ + ¼ = 3/2 Ω, so R = 2/3 Ω.

5. B

The purpose of a capacitor is to store charge. It is placed after the battery so that it can provide an extra burst of current whenever the amplifier needs it. If it was placed after the amplifier, the current from the capacitor would not take advantage of the amplifier's ability to increase the power delivered.

6. D

According to the passage, the voltage source is much higher in magnitude for home systems than for automotive systems. This means that, to produce the same amount of power, the automotive system would need to draw more current in order to make up for its lack of potential.

7. C

Home amplifiers extract their power from a 110 V EMF, while automotive amplifiers can use only a 12 V EMF. Because current is directly proportional to electric potential (voltage), the home amplifier can easily acquire all of the necessary current. Capacitance is inversely proportional to electric potential, so the components in a home system (which has more electric potential) are actually less likely to function as a capacitor (A). There is no indication that the power outlet stores charge (B); in fact, it acquires its charge from the power lines outside. Not all car systems include capacitors as per the passage (D), so it is clear that an amplifier can function without a capacitor.

8. A

The easiest way to answer this question is by eliminating the incorrect options. (B) and (C) are incorrect because the ratio of the peak current to the rms current in an AC circuit is equal to approximately 1.41, which is far from the ratio of 14 V to 12 V. (D) is incorrect because an rms current only applies to AC circuits, whose average potential is always equal to zero. DC circuits can, however, experience fluctuations that will affect the exact value of the voltage.

9. A

The current of a circuit can be determined by the formula V = IR. Because the resistances are identical, the current must be higher for the system with a higher voltage (the home system). Power is directly proportional to current and voltage, so the home amplifier will consume much more power and, consequently, much more energy.

PASSAGE II

10. C

The passage states that both types of electroscopes function primarily through electrostatic induction. It also mentions that the mechanism of action of the instruments involves the movement of protons and electrons to different parts of any given atom. This is an example of a redistribution of charge.

11. D

According to the passage, a positively charged object pushes protons toward the opposite side of the pith ball, causing the electrons to propel the ball toward the object. A negatively charged object, therefore, will push electrons to the opposite side of the ball. This would mean that the protons are near the test object, which would cause an attractive force.

12. A

A pith ball becomes charged when it is touched by a charged object. When this object is negatively charged, the ball will also gain a negative charge and will be repelled from the object. The second ball will then receive some of the charge from the first ball, causing a repulsive force between the two balls.

13. D

All three items are correct. An object will always move at a constant velocity unless it is acted upon by an external force. In this case, the attraction of the pith ball and the repulsion of the gold leaves are causes by an electrostatic force. In addition, the gold-leaf electroscope requires electric conduction from the ball to the leaves. Finally, electrostatic force is produced by an electric field.

14. B

The pith ball moves as a result of an electrostatic force. Because force is directly proportional to mass and acceleration, a decrease in mass will lead to an increase in acceleration. A heavier pith ball may be too heavy to move as a result of the electrostatic force. The protons and electrons move within an atom, so the number of atoms (A) is irrelevant. (C) and (D) are simply false; there is no trend relating conductivity to weight.

15. D

Pith is an electrical insulator. Gold, silver, and copper are all electrical conductors. An insulator would be unable to absorb the charge conducted through the brass rod.

16. A

For a negatively charged object, the electric field points in the direction opposite that of the electrostatic force. Because the charged object will attract the pith ball, the force must be pointing to the right; that means the electric field points to the left.

17. C

Choice (C) is the only item that does not accurately describe the gold leaf interaction. A dipole moment is defined as a pair of charges with opposite sign and equal magnitude. The two gold leaves in the electroscope have charges with the same sign, so they do not form a dipole moment. Electrostatic repulsion (A) is the reason why the leaves spread apart. The charge is conducted from the metal ball through the brass rod and distributed around the gold leaf; this redistribution (B) is the reason for the electrostatic force. An electrostatic force is produced by an electric field (D).

QUESTIONS 18–22

18. B

The total energy of the object is conserved. When the object is dropped, it only has potential energy, which is mgh. Right before the object hits the ground, it has only kinetic energy, which is $\frac{1}{2} \cdot (mv^2)$. Thus, $mgh = \frac{1}{2} \cdot mv^2$, and so $v^2 = 2gh = 100 m^2/s^2$, and $v = 10$ m/s.

19. C

The time it takes for the car to decelerate can be calculated using $V_f = V_i + a \cdot t$, where $V_f = 0$ m/s, $V_i =$ 10 m/s, and $a = -2$ m/s^2. Thus, it takes the car 5 s to decelerate. The distance traveled during that time can be calculated by $d = t \cdot (V_i + V_f)/2 = 25$ m. The road block is 30 m away when the car starts braking, and so the car misses the road block by 5 m.

20. A

For circuits in parallel, the equation is $1/R_T = 1/R_1 + 1/R_2$, so for two 6 ohm circuits, the total resistance is 3 ohms. For circuits in series, the equation is $R_T = R_1 + R_2$, so the total resistance is 12 ohms. Overall then, the total resistance increases by a factor of 4.

21. B

The linear momentum is conserved. Before the collision, assuming north is positive, is $m_1v_1 + m_2v_2 =$ 100 kg · 5 m/s – 150 kg · 3 m/s = 50 kg · m/s north. Because this is a perfectly inelastic collision, the total momentum after the collision is $(m_1 + m_2)v$, and this equals 50 kg · m/s north. Thus, (100 kg + 150 kg)v = 50 kg · m/s, and so v = 0.2 m/s north.

22. A

If two waves are in phase, constructive interference takes place, and the amplitude of the resultant wave is the sum of the amplitudes of the interfering waves,. In this case, that is $A_1 + A_1 = 2 \cdot A_1$.

PASSAGE III

23. D

First, we must know that (A) can't be correct: the pull of the string on the stone is centripetal, not centrifugal force. The expression for centripetal force is $F_c = mv^2/R$, leading us to (D).

24. C

There is a lot of unnecessary information here, included just to annoy and confuse you. If you stick to basics though, you'll realize that horizontal motion has nothing to do with vertical motion. This is basically a projectile motion question. (Though it mentions the shot put, which would be projectile motion but with an angle for the initial velocity, the ball is projected horizontally and no arc-like motion is observed.) Remembering our basic principles of projectile motion, acceleration is 0 m/s^2 in the horizontal direction and constant in the vertical direction. It will always be g, for our purposes, 10 m/s^2. (A) might be your selection had you used a = v/t, where $v_i = 30$ m/s, $v_f = 0$ m/s, and t = 7 s. (B) is half of g and included to make the question more challenging. (D) might be your selection had you used a one-dimensional motion equation, $x - x_0 = v_0t + (at^2)/2$. Here, $x - x_0$ is 1,000, v_0 is 30 m/s, and t = 7.

25. C

Gathering our facts for this situation, we see that all the required information is provided from the question stem and from the passage. However, the information in the passage might not be necessary. The question only has to do with horizontal motion, as it asks for a distance. We know, then, that we need to find the horizontal component of the given speed. Using the cos function, we find the following:

$$v_x = v_i \cos\theta$$
$$= (45 \text{ m/s}) (\cos 45°)$$
$$= 31.82 \text{ m/s (approx.)}$$

The more complicated kinematics equations aren't necessary here; we can simply work with v = x/t. Substituting our values, we get the distance traveled to be 63.64, choice (C).

26. C

More firearms work by way of creating explosions, not by using springs. However, this question is theoretical. You might first think you haven't been given enough information, but the passage provided a great deal. You're being asked about spring constants, and there are only a few things required to figure that out. We know here that the loss of potential energy of the spring is equal to the gain in kinetic energy of the bullet. The bullet itself is released from the spring when it is at its equilibrium point. So we have the following:

$$PE = KE$$
$$\tfrac{1}{2} kx^2 = \tfrac{1}{2} mv^2$$
$$k(0.01 \text{ m})^2 = (0.050 \text{ kg})(500 \text{ m/s})^2$$
$$k = 1.25 \times 10^8 \text{ N/m}$$

Notice that we use only variables x, m, and v, and we need to convert m and x to the necessary units.

27. C

In this situation, momentum must be conserved. We know that p = mv and that initially, total momentum is 0. For this reason, we know that the final momenta of each skater must be equal in magnitude and opposite in direction. In other words, they must add up to zero. Using variables, we have $m_1v_1 = m_2v_2$. Rearranging, we have $V_1/v_2 = m_2/m_1 = 45/67$.

28. B

To get average speed, we use v = total distance/total time. We know from the passage that the length of the race is 400 m. To get the total time, we calculate in parts: v = x/t. For the first part of the race (the first 200 m), we have 10 m/s = 160 m/t, so t = 16 s. For the remaining 240 m, we have 5 m/s = 240 m/t, so t = 48 s. So our original equation becomes v = 400 m/(16 + 48) = 6.25 m/s. Had you averaged 10 m/s and 5 m/s, you would have gotten (A). Had you switched around the percentages, you would have gotten (D).

29. B

We are not provided with much information here, but we can still determine our answer. All we need is the following equation: $v_f^2 = v_i^2 + 2ax$. So (0) + 2 (-10 m/s^2)(-2.5 m) = 50. You'll need to know the square root of 50. Thus, v_f is appx 7 m/s. Another strategy would be to use $x - x_0 = v_0t + (at^2)/2$. Considering vertical motion, x's should be changed to y's. Using this will give us t, and again, we'll need to know a square root. We use that value of t in $v^2 = v_0^2 + 2a(x - x_0)$.

30. A

This is a trick question that can yield easy points. You're given a lot of information and might be tempted to look back at the passage for details, but all you need to consider is the word *displacement*, a net change in position for the object in question. The athlete has completed round-trips, so you can assume she ends her exercise where she began it. This would mean that she hasn't changed her position at all, and the answer is (A). (D) is definitely incorrect because she is swimming at constant speed. Acceleration in that case would be 0 m/s^2.

PASSAGE IV

31. D

Know the formula for frequency in simple harmonic motion. Frequency is the number of cycles per second, whereas the period is the number of seconds needed to complete one cycle. This question asks for the frequency, so we need to use $f = 1/(2\pi) \times \sqrt{(k/m)}$. Because we're asked about one-quarter of the cycle, we have to divide our answer by 4, which is (D). (A) is the frequency for one full cycle. (B) and (C) are wrong because initial inspection shows that the locations of k and m are inverted.

32. C

Maximum velocity will be achieved when the kinetic energy of the system is greatest. Because the sum of kinetic and potential energy is always constant, the potential energy is zero. Looking at the given formula, this reduces to $\frac{1}{2}kA^2 = \frac{1}{2}mv_{max}^2$. If you rearrange the terms to isolate v, you end up with the expression in (C). (A) and (D) are incorrect because there is no "2" term in the equation.

33. A

Only item I is correct. The question asks you to clarify the relationship of amplitude, mass, spring constant, and gravity. v_{max} = amplitude $\times \sqrt{(k/m)}$, so if we rearrange, we get $A = v_{max} \times \sqrt{(m/k)}$. Now we have an equation which shows the relationship between amplitude, mass, and spring constant. Notice that gravity has no effect, because we are conducting this experiment on a horizontal table. Because m is in the numerator, amplitude and mass are directly related. Because k is in the denominator, amplitude and the spring constant are inversely related, and increasing "k" would decrease amplitude.

34. A

Only item II is correct. Amplitude is just the maximum displacement of a system. If you stretched a block to 2 meters and let it oscillate, the block's amplitude would be 2 meters. If the friction is decreased, that will affect only the duration of the oscillation and not the amplitude. (Item I is incorrect.) If the spring is oscillating and you push it as it is compressing, you can see that the energy introduced will be incorporated by the spring and will oscillate with a greater amplitude. (Item II is correct.) The length of the spring has no impact on amplitude; all measurements are taken from the equilibrium position of the block and the displacement of the block from that position. (Item III is incorrect.)

35. B

This is the perfect equation for using Hooke's law because it incorporates all of the variables into one simple equation, $F_b = kx$, where x is the maximum displacement. In this case, the maximum displacement is equal to the amplitude because the block cannot oscillate at a greater displacement than the initial displacement unless an external force is applied. So we get $x_b = F_b/k$, which is equal to 1.5 m. Repeating the calculation for block C, we get $x_c = 2$ m. This leaves only (B) and (D). If we equate $F = ma$ and $F = kx$, we get $a = kx/m$. The best place to use the x value is at the ends, because we just found out what their maximum displacement is at those points and we are given the k and m values. Plugging in the numbers, we get $a_b = 75$ m/s^2 and $a_c = 40$ m/s^2. (B) is correct.

36. C

The graph shows that block has its greatest velocity at the beginning. This occurs when it is at the equilibrium position, so we can eliminate (A) and (D). At the ends, the block comes to a rest and the restoring force pulls/pushes it back. Notice from the graph that the block's velocity is going to be positive. This implies that after the block passes 0.25 seconds, it will be moving toward the positive direction (the right side). We know the block is moving to the right because $v_x = 0$ when it is compressed, just as the spring is just beginning to extend again. This leaves (C).

37. A
The block has a velocity of zero only when the spring is fully compressed or extended, or at the ends. You can visualize that at this point, the spring wants to jerk the block back toward the equilibrium position, so it is at its maximum acceleration. If the spring is extended, the acceleration will point to the left (check Figure 1), leaving choice (A).

PASSAGE V

38. C
The number of neutrons in a given isotope is determined by subtracting the number of protons in the nucleus from the number of nucleons, N = A – Z = 236 – 92 = 144 neutrons for a ${}_{92}U^{235}$. Not knowing that the question refers to the intermediate product would lead us to the other answer choices.

39. C
The amount of untouched naturally occurring weapons-grade uranium, ${}_{92}U^{235}$, has decreased due to radioactivity by more than a factor of two, because the age of the earth is more than the half-life of this isotope. Half-life is defined as the time it takes for half of the original amount a given radioactive isotope to decay.

40. C
The amount of a radioactive sample decreases exponentially. Here, 11,460 years happens to be equal to two times 5,730 years, which is the half-life for ${}_6C^{14}$. This means that one quarter of the original sample will remain after two half-lives. One must refer to the passage for specific values.

41. B
The radioactive decay rate, also called the activity, decreases exponentially, just like the amount of a radioactive sample. After one half-life, 5,730 years, the decay rate will be half of the initial value. Refer to the passage for the values needed to carry out this problem.

42. B
ß decay is defined as the emission of an electron by a nucleus. The figure shows this sort of emission, so it clearly represents a ß decay. An anti-neutrino is also emitted in the decay, but is not shown in the figure.

43. D
A neutron is converted into a proton, an electron and an electron/anti-neutrino.

44. C
Assuming 15 decays per minute per gram of carbon, a 100-gram sample would initially have a decay rate of 1,500 decays per minute when the organism dies. If the decay rate is currently 187.5 decays per minute, that means that the organism died three half-lives ago.

PASSAGE VI

45. D
Critical angles are only a consideration when light moves from a medium of high index of refraction into a medium of low index, relative to the first. In outer space, the originating medium is a vacuum for which the index of refraction is infinity. Had we used the equation for critical angles, $\sin\theta_c = n_2/n_1 = n_{glass}/n_{vacuum}$, we would have gotten a number greater than 1 (and the sine of an angle can never be greater than 1). This might have tempted us to choose (A) over (D). Had we flipped this, however, we would have seen that $\sin\theta_c$ was 0.5 and that

θ_c was 30°. (D) is indeed the answer, as no critical angle would exist. Total internal reflection cannot occur.

46. C

Although the lenses touched, this should be considered a multiple-lens system. For such a system, there is one very helpful equation from our arsenal of optics equations: $1/f = 1/f_1 + 1/f_2 \ldots$ The question is mathematically quite simple after we realize these few points. Our objective is f, because we have f_1 and f_2. We have the focal length of the original, 57.5 m. 10 percent of this is 5.75, or 23/4. The inverse of that is 4/23 and we double this to get 8/23. Setting this equal to 1/f, we find that f is about 2.9 m. Mathematical errors along the way would produce or assuming the focal length of one lens to be sufficient would produce (D). Using 8/23 instead would produce (B) 0.3 m. Using negative focal lengths would give us the negative of our correct answer, and this is incorrect when using converging lenses.

47. B

The relationship between wavelength and frequency is inverse; a wave with high frequency must have small wavelength and vice versa. Though we might not know the entire order of the visible spectrum, we can still make some headway with these options. If we know that wavelength decreases in the order of ROYGBIV, we know that red has the longest wavelength of the visible spectrum. Also recall that infrared light falls right next to red visible light and that it has higher wavelength. On the other side, ultraviolet light lays next to violet light, which has a smaller wavelength. You should be familiar with the general fact that x-rays are very high-energy waves. The relationship between energy and frequency is direct ($E = hf$) and thus between energy and wavelength, it is indirect. We can then say that the order of these waves, from smallest wavelength, is x-rays, UV, visible, and infrared.

48. D

This question is a bit time-consuming because it requires you to sketch some graphs. Items II and IV are correct. We know that for an object starting from rest and moving with constant acceleration, $a = v/t$. Because Graph A reflects speed versus time, we know that the slope of the line is acceleration. We're told that acceleration is constant, so the line representing it will be straight. However, we know that acceleration is not zero and so item I is incorrect. Next, for distance, we can look to one of our one-dimensional motion equations: $x - x_0 = v_0t + \frac{1}{2}at^2$. The equation shows us that the relationship between distance and time is parabolic and symmetrical about the x-axis. Distance is constantly decreasing. We know, then, that item IV is correct.

49. D

Only item III is incorrect. Acceleration is the same for all falling objects. Even though acceleration may be different at this height above the Earth's surface, it will affect the two objects identically (as long as we can neglect air resistance). Item I is correct. Next, $v = at$ tells us that the speed of a falling object starting from rest is proportional to the acceleration and the time of fall. These values have nothing to do with the mass of the object. Therefore, item II is incorrect. Items III and IV differentiate potential energy. Recalling the formula $PE = mgh$, in this case g and h are identical for the two objects, though mass is of some consequence. Because potential energy and mass are proportional, the hammer—with greater mass—will have greater potential energy. Though we're given weight, both objects are at the same height above the Earth and therefore both experience the same force of gravity.

50. D

There are several ways to go about this problem. One is to make a graph of the known values. With a graph indicating velocity versus time, we could find the area under the graph. Another way is to use the average speed (we can only do this because acceleration is constant). We simply multiply the average speed by the time traveled. To get the average speed, we add the initial speed to the final speed and divide by 2. We're told the speed has decreased by 10 percent, but what was the speed to begin with? Such a speed was provided in the passage and we can quickly refer back for this number: 7,500 m/s. When this decreases by 10 percent, we have a new speed of 6,750 m/s. This would give us that the average speed is 7,125 m/s, or simply a reduction of 5 percent overall. Stopping here would produce (B). Multiplying this by 5 seconds, we get that the distance covered is 35,625 m. Dividing would produce (A). Using 6,750 m/s here instead would produce (C).

51. D

While we might be relieved that the passage provides the speed of the telescope, this is not the speed with which we're concerned. In fact, this is only the initial horizontal velocity. Rather, an object falls under the influence of gravity and its descent is not affected by this value. We use the equation $x - x_0 = v_0t + \frac{1}{2}at^2$. We do not completely dismiss the passage, because we need Hubble's height, 600 km. Plugging this in, we get 600,000 m = (0 m/s)(t) + $\frac{1}{2}$(10 m/s^2)(t^2), and t^2 = 1,200,000. Though it would be difficult to know the value of *t* right off the bat, it is safe at this point to choose from the given answer choices. The only value which comes close is 346 s, or 5 minutes and 46 seconds. Failing to convert km to m would have given you (A) about 11 seconds. Of course, carrying units would prevent that mistake. Using a = v/t would have given you 60 s (1 min), choice (B).

52. C

The concave spherical mirror identified in the passage will be of most help here. Though the equation 1/o + 1/i = 1/f might guide you here, you should also be able to visualize the actual rays that produce the images whose distances and heights we calculate. This question tests that ability. First, we must realize that incident rays parallel to the axis of a concave mirror will converge to the focal point. This will be the case for all rays that travel parallel. If we imagined that a certain source of light was producing these rays, a ray which goes through the focal point would reflect back through the focal point. A ray which travels straight to the center of curvature will return back at the same angle that the original ray had made, with the horizontal *above* the horizontal and do that *below* the horizontal. A ray would not travel normal, or perpendicular, to the axis, so (A) is out. Due to the curvature of the mirror, it would not travel parallel. This would happen with a plane mirror. (B) is out as well. (C) is the focal length of 57.6 m, from the passage, and (D) uses 2f as a value. Knowing that all parallel rays will converge at the focus, we choose (C) over (D).

INDEX

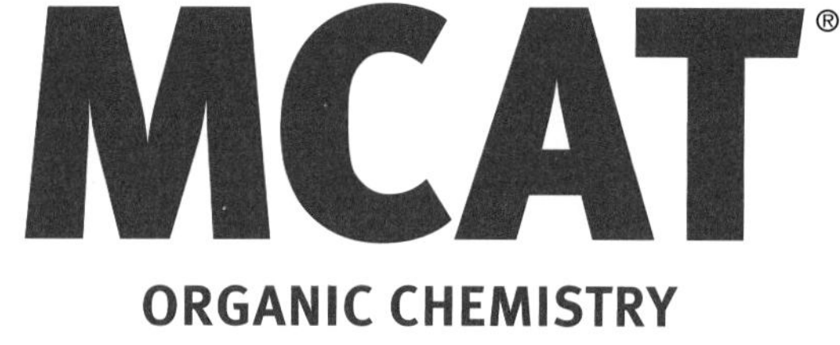

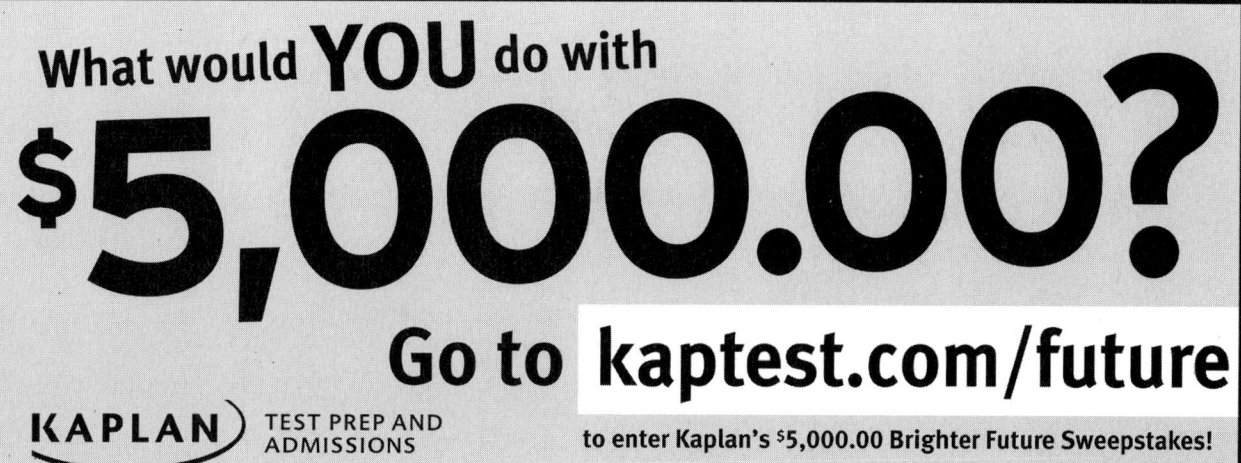

ORGANIC CHEMISTRY

2009–2010 EDITION

Related Titles

Kaplan MCAT Biology 2009–2010
Kaplan MCAT General Chemistry 2009–2010
Kaplan MCAT Physics 2009–2010
Kaplan MCAT Verbal Reasoning 2009-2010

MCAT®

ORGANIC CHEMISTRY

2009–2010 EDITION

The Staff of Kaplan

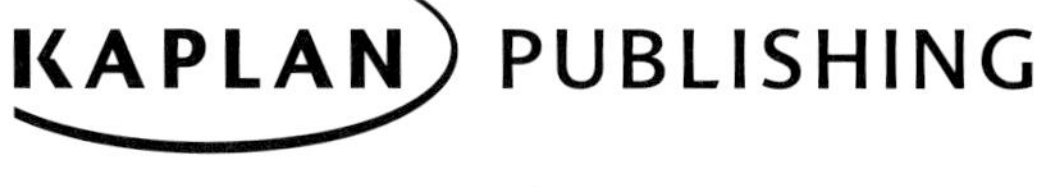

New York

Published by Kaplan Publishing, a division of Kaplan, Inc.
1 Liberty Plaza, 24th Floor
New York, NY 10006

Printed in the United States of America

10 9 8 7 6 5 4 3 2 1

ISBN: 978-1-4277-9874-9

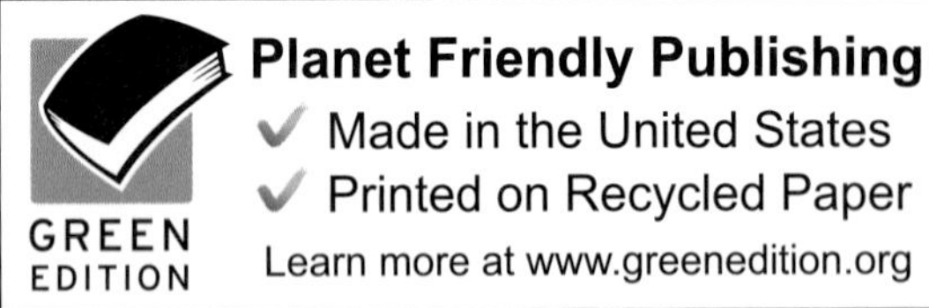

- Manufacturing books in the United States ensures compliance with strict environmental laws and eliminates the need for international freight shipping, a major contributor to global air pollution. Printing on recycled paper helps minimize our consumption of trees, water and fossil fuels.
- Trees Saved: 52 • Air Emissions Eliminated: 4,629 pounds
- Water Saved: 20,179 gallons • Solid Waste Eliminated: 2,095 pounds

Contents

How to Use this Book

Kaplan MCAT Organic Chemistry, along with the other four books in our MCAT subject review series, brings the Kaplan classroom experience right into your home!

Kaplan has been preparing premeds for the MCAT for more than 40 years in our comprehensive courses. In the past 15 years alone, we've helped over 400,000 students prepare for this important exam and improve their chances of medical school admission.

TEACHER TIPS

Think of Kaplan's five MCAT subject books as having a private Kaplan teacher right by your side! We've created a team of the **top MCAT teachers in the country,** who have read through these comprehensive guides. On every page, they offer the same tips, advice, and test day insight as in their Kaplan classroom.

Pay close attention to **Teacher Tip** sidebars like this:

> **TEACHER TIP**
>
> The MCAT is not a "picky" exam. You probably won't have two answers that will differ only in their alphabetization, though the rule about the prefixes may come in handy.

When you see these, you know what you're getting the same insight and knowledge that students in Kaplan MCAT classrooms across the country receive.

HIGH-YIELD MCAT REVIEW

At the end of several chapters, you'll find a special **High-Yield Questions** spread. These questions tackle the most frequently tested topics found on the MCAT. For each type of problem, you will be provided with a stepwise technique for solving the question and key directional points on how to solve for the MCAT specifically.

Included on each spread are two icons: the first, a sideways hand pointing toward equations, notes equations that you should memorize for the MCAT. The second, an open hand, indicates where in a problem you can stop without doing further calculation.

At the end of each topic you will find a "Takeaways" box, which gives a concise summary of the problem-solving approach; and a "Things to watch out for" box, which points out any caveats to the approach discussed above that usually lead to wrong answer choices. Finally, there is a "Similar Questions" box at the end so you can test your ability to apply the stepwise technique to analogous questions. You can find the answers in the Answers and Explanations section of this book.

We're confident that this guide, and our award-wining Kaplan teachers, can help you achieve your goals of MCAT success and admission into medical school!

Good luck!

EXPERT KAPLAN MCAT TEAM

Marilyn Engle

MCAT Master Teacher; Teacher Trainer; Kaplan National Teacher of the Year, 2006; Westwood Teacher of the Year, 2007; Westwood Trainer of the Year, 2007; Encino Trainer of the Tear, 2005

John Michael Linick

MCAT Teacher; Boulder Teacher of the Year, 2007; Summer Intensive Program Faculty Member

Dr. Glen Pearlstein

MCAT Master Teacher; Teacher Trainer; Westwood Teacher of the Year, 2006

Matthew B. Wilkinson

MCAT Teacher; Teacher Trainer; Lone Star Trainer of the Year, 2007

INTRODUCTION TO THE MCAT

THE MCAT

The Medical College Admission Test, affectionately known as the MCAT, is different from any other test you've encountered in your academic career. It's not like the knowledge-based exams from high school and college, whose emphasis was on memorizing and regurgitating information. Medical schools can assess your academic prowess by looking at your transcript. The MCAT isn't even like other standardized tests you may have taken, where the focus was on proving your general skills.

Test Tip

The MCAT places more weight on your thought process. However you must have a strong hold of the required core knowledge. The MCAT may not be a perfect gauge of your abilities, but it is a relatively objective way to compare you with students from different backgrounds and undergraduate institutions.

Medical schools use MCAT scores to assess whether you possess the foundation upon which to build a successful medical career. Though you certainly need to know the content to do well, the stress is on thought process, because the MCAT is above all else a thinking test. That's why it emphasizes reasoning, critical and analytical thinking, reading comprehension, data analysis, writing, and problem-solving skills.

The MCAT's power comes from its use as an indicator of your abilities. Good scores can open doors. Your power comes from preparation and mindset, because the key to MCAT success is knowing what you're up against. That's where this section of this book comes in. We'll explain the philosophy behind the test, review the sections one by one, show you sample questions, share some of Kaplan's proven methods, and clue you in to what the test makers are really after. You'll get a handle on the process, find a confident new perspective, and achieve your highest possible scores.

ABOUT THE MCAT

Information about the MCAT CBT is included below. For the latest information about the MCAT, visit www.kaptest.com/mcat.

MCAT CBT

Format	U.S.—All administrations on computer International—Most on computer with limited paper and pencil in a few isolated areas
Essay Grading	One human and one computer grader
Breaks	Optional break between each section
Length of MCAT Day	Approximately 5.5 hours
Test Dates	Multiple dates in January, April, May, June, July, August, and September Total of 24 administrations each year.
Delivery of Results	Within 30 days. If scores are delayed notification will be posted online at www.aamc.org/mcat Electronic and paper
Security	Government-issued ID Electronic thumbprint Electronic signature verification
Testing Centers	Small computer testing sites

PLANNING FOR THE TEST

As you look toward your preparation for the MCAT consider the following advice:

Complete your core course requirements as soon as possible. Take a strategic eye to your schedule and get core requirements out of the way now.

Take the MCAT once. The MCAT is a notoriously grueling standardized exam that requires extensive preparation. It is longer than the graduate admissions exams for business school (GMAT, 3½ hours), law school (LSAT, 3¼ hours) and graduate school (GRE, 2½ hours). You do not want to take it twice. Plan and prepare accordingly.

KAPLAN EXCLUSIVE

Go online and sign up for a local Kaplan Pre-Med Edge event to get the latest information on the test.

THE ROLE OF THE MCAT IN ADMISSIONS

More and more people are applying to medical school and more and more people are taking the MCAT. It's important for you to recognize that while a high MCAT score is a critical component in getting admitted to top med schools, it's not the only factor. Medical school admissions officers weigh grades, interviews, MCAT scores, level of involvement in extracurricular activities, as well as personal essays.

In a Kaplan survey of 130 pre-med advisors, 84 percent called the interview a "very important" part of the admissions process, followed closely by college grades (83%) and MCAT scores (76%). Kaplan's college admissions consulting practice works with students on all these issues so they can position themselves as strongly as possible. In addition, the AAMC has made it clear that scores will continue to be valid for three years, and that the scoring of the computer-based MCAT will not differ from that of the paper and pencil version.

REGISTRATION

The only way to register for the MCAT is online. The registration site is: www.aamc.org/mcat.

You will be able to access the site approximately six months before your test date. Payment must be made by MasterCard or Visa.

Go to www.aamc.org/mcat/registration.htm and download *MCAT Essentials* for information about registration, fees, test administration, and preparation. For other questions, contact:

MCAT Care Team
Association of American Medical Colleges
Section for Applicant Assessment Services
2450 N. St., NW
Washington, DC 20037
www.aamc.org/mcat
Email: mcat@aamc.org

You will want to take the MCAT in the year prior to your planned start date. For example, if you want to start medical school in Fall 2010, you will need to take the MCAT and apply in 2009. Don't drag your feet gathering information. You'll need time not only to prepare and practice for the test, but also to get all your registration work done.

ANATOMY OF THE MCAT

TEST TIP

The MCAT should be viewed just like any other part of your application: as an opportunity to show the medical schools who you are and what you can do. Take control of your MCAT experience.

Before mastering strategies, you need to know exactly what you're dealing with on the MCAT. Let's start with the basics: The MCAT is, among other things, an endurance test.

If you can't approach it with confidence and stamina, you'll quickly lose your composure. That's why it's so important that you take control of the test.

The MCAT consists of four timed sections: Physical Sciences, Verbal Reasoning, Writing Sample, and Biological Sciences. Later in this section we'll take an in-depth look at each MCAT section, including sample question types and specific test-smart hints, but here's a general overview, reflecting the order of the test sections and number of questions in each.

Physical Sciences

Time	70 minutes
Format	• 52 multiple-choice questions: approximately 7–9 passages with 4–8 questions each • approximately 10 stand-alone questions (not passage-based)
What it tests	basic general chemistry concepts, basic physics concepts, analytical reasoning, data interpretation

Verbal Reasoning

Time	60 minutes
Format	• 40 multiple-choice questions: approximately 7 passages with 5–7 questions each
What it tests	critical reading

Writing Sample

Time	60 minutes
Format	• 2 essay questions (30 minutes per essay)
What it tests	critical thinking, intellectual organization, written communication skills

Biological Sciences

Time	70 minutes
Format	• 52 multiple-choice questions: approximately 7–9 passages with 4–8 questions each • approximately 10 stand-alone questions (not passage-based)
What it tests	basic biology concepts, basic organic chemistry concepts, analytical reasoning, data interpretation

TEST TIP

There's no penalty for a wrong answer on the MCAT, so NEVER LEAVE ANY QUESTION BLANK, even if you only have time for a wild guess.

The sections of the test always appear in the same order:

Physical Sciences

[optional 10-minute break]

Verbal Reasoning

[optional 10-minute break]

Writing Sample

[optional 10-minute break]

Biological Sciences

SCORING

Each MCAT section receives its own score. Physical Sciences, Verbal Reasoning, and Biological Sciences are each scored on a scale ranging from 1–15, with 15 as the highest. The Writing Sample essays are scored alphabetically on a scale ranging from J to T, with T as the highest. The two essays are each evaluated by two official readers, so four critiques combine to make the alphabetical score.

TEST TIP

The percentile figure tells you how many other test takers scored at or below your level. In other words, a percentile figure of 80 means that 80 percent did as well or worse than you did, and that only 20 percent did better.

The number of multiple-choice questions that you answer correctly per section is your "raw score." Your raw score will then be converted to yield the "scaled score"—the one that will fall somewhere in that 1–15 range. These scaled scores are what are reported to medical schools as your MCAT scores. All multiple-choice questions are worth the same amount—one raw point—and *there's no penalty for guessing*. That means that *you should always select an answer for every question, whether you get to that question or not!* This is an important piece of advice, so pay it heed. Never let time run out on any section without selecting an answer for every question.

Your score report will tell you—and your potential medical schools—not only your scaled scores, but also the national mean score for each section, standard deviation, national scoring profile for each section, and your percentile ranking.

WHAT'S A GOOD SCORE?

There's no such thing as a cut-and-dry "good score." Much depends on the strength of the rest of your application (if your transcript is first rate, the pressure to strut your stuff on the MCAT isn't as intense) and on where you want to go to school (different schools have different score expectations). Here are a few interesting statistics:

For each MCAT administration, the average scaled scores are approximately 8s for Physical Sciences, Verbal Reasoning, and Biological Sciences, and N for the Writing Sample. You need scores of at least 10–11s to be considered competitive by most medical schools, and if you're aiming for the top you've got to do even better, and score 12s and above.

You don't have to be perfect to do well. For instance, on the AAMC's Practice Test 5R, you could get as many as 10 questions wrong in Verbal Reasoning, 17 in Physical Sciences, and 16 in Biological Sciences and still score in the 80th percentile. To score in the 90th percentile, you could get as many as 7 wrong in Verbal Reasoning, 12 in Physical Sciences, and 12 in Biological Sciences. Even students who receive perfect scaled scores usually get a handful of questions wrong.

It's important to maximize your performance on every question. Just a few questions one way or the other can make a big difference in your scaled score. Here's a look at recent score profiles so you can get an idea of the shape of a typical score distribution.

Physical Sciences		
Scaled Score	Percent Achieving Score	Percentile Rank Range
15	0.1	99.9–99.9
14	1.2	98.7–99.8
13	2.5	96.2–98.6
12	5.1	91.1–96.1
11	7.2	83.9–91.0
10	12.1	71.8–83.8
9	12.9	58.9–71.1
8	16.5	42.4–58.5
7	16.7	25.7–42.3
6	13.0	12.7–25.6
5	7.9	04.8–12.6
4	3.3	01.5–04.7
3	1.3	00.2–01.4
2	0.1	00.1–00.1
1	0.0	00.0–00.0
Scaled Score Mean = 8.1 Standard Deviation = 2.32		

Verbal Reasoning		
Scaled Score	Percent Achieving Score	Percentile Rank Range
15	0.1	99.9–99.9
14	0.2	99.7–99.8
13	1.8	97.9–99.6
12	3.6	94.3–97.8
11	10.5	83.8–94.2
10	15.6	68.2–83.7
9	17.2	51.0–68.1
8	15.4	35.6–50.9
7	10.3	25.3–35.5
6	10.9	14.4–25.2
5	6.9	07.5–14.3
4	3.9	03.6–07.4
3	2.0	01.6–03.5
2	0.5	00.1–01.5
1	0.0	00.0–00.0
Scaled Score Mean = 8.0 Standard Deviation = 2.43		

TEST TIP

The raw score of each administration is converted to a scaled score. The conversion varies with administrations. Hence, the same raw score will not always give you the same scaled score.

Writing Sample		
Scaled Score	Percent Achieving Score	Percentile Rank Range
T	0.5	99.9–99.9
S	2.8	94.7–99.8
R	7.2	96.0–99.3
Q	14.2	91.0–95.9
P	9.7	81.2–90.9
O	17.9	64.0–81.1
N	14.7	47.1–63.9
M	18.8	30.4–47.0
L	9.5	21.2–30.3
K	3.6	13.5–21.1
J	1.2	06.8–13.4
		02.9–06.7
		00.9–02.8
		00.2–00.8
		00.0–00.1
75th Percentile = Q 50th Percentile = O 25th Percentile = M		

Biological Sciences		
Scaled Score	Percent Achieving Score	Percentile Rank Range
15	0.1	99.9–99.9
14	1.2	98.7–99.8
13	2.5	96.2–98.6
12	5.1	91.1–96.1
11	7.2	83.9–91.0
10	12.1	71.8–83.8
9	12.9	58.9–71.1
8	16.5	42.4–58.5
7	16.7	25.7–42.3
6	13.0	12.7–25.6
5	7.9	04.8–12.6
4	3.3	01.5–04.7
3	1.3	00.2–01.4
2	0.1	00.1–00.1
1	0.0	00.0–00.0
Scaled Score Mean = 8.2 Standard Deviation = 2.39		

WHAT THE MCAT REALLY TESTS

It's important to grasp not only the nuts and bolts of the MCAT, so you'll know *what* to do on test day, but also the underlying principles of the test so you'll know *why* you're doing what you're doing on test day. We'll cover the straightforward MCAT facts later. Now it's time to examine the heart and soul of the MCAT, to see what it's really about.

THE MYTH

Most people preparing for the MCAT fall prey to the myth that the MCAT is a straightforward science test. They think something like this:

> *"It covers the four years of science I had to take in school: biology, chemistry, physics, and organic chemistry. It even has equations. OK, so it has Verbal Reasoning and Writing, but those sections are just to see if we're literate, right? The important stuff is the science. After all, we're going to be doctors."*

Well, here's the little secret no one seems to want you to know: The MCAT is not just a science test; it's also a thinking test. This means that the test is designed to let you demonstrate your thought process, not only your thought content.

The implications are vast. Once you shift your test-taking paradigm to match the MCAT modus operandi, you'll find a new level of confidence and control over the test. You'll begin to work with the nature of the MCAT rather than against it. You'll be more efficient and insightful as you prepare for the test, and you'll be more relaxed on Test Day. In fact, you'll be able to see the MCAT for what it is rather than for what it's dressed up to be. We want your Test Day to feel like a visit with a familiar friend instead of an awkward blind date.

THE ZEN OF MCAT

Medical schools do not need to rely on the MCAT to see what you already know. Admission committees can measure your subject-area proficiency using your undergraduate coursework and grades. Schools are most interested in the potential of your mind.

In recent years, many medical schools have shifted pedagogic focus away from an information-heavy curriculum to a concept-based curriculum. There is currently more emphasis placed on problem solving, holistic thinking, and cross-disciplinary study. Be careful not to dismiss this important point, figuring you'll wait to worry about academic trends until you're actually in medical school. This trend affects you right now, because it's reflected in the MCAT. Every good tool matches its task. In this case the tool is the test, used to measure you and other candidates, and the task is to quantify how likely it is that you'll succeed in medical school.

Your intellectual potential—how skillfully you annex new territory into your mental boundaries, how quickly you build "thought highways" between ideas, how confidently and creatively you solve problems—is far more important to admission committees than your ability to recite Young's modulus for every material known to man. The schools assume they can expand your knowledge base. They choose applicants carefully because expansive knowledge is not enough to succeed in medical school or in the profession. There's something more. It's this "something more" that the MCAT is trying to measure.

Every section on the MCAT tests essentially the same higher-order thinking skills: analytical reasoning, abstract thinking, and problem solving.

Most test takers get trapped into thinking they are being tested strictly about biology, chemistry, and so on. Thus, they approach each section with a new outlook on what's expected. This constant mental gear-shifting can be exhausting, not to mention counterproductive. Instead of perceiving the test as parsed into radically different sections, you need to maintain your focus on the underlying nature of the test: It's designed to test your thinking skills, not your information-recall skills. Each test section thus presents a variation on the same theme.

WHAT ABOUT THE SCIENCE?

With this perspective, you may be left asking these questions: "What about the science? What about the content? Don't I need to know the basics?" The answer is a resounding "Yes!" You must be fluent in the different languages of the test. You cannot do well on the MCAT if you don't know the basics of physics, general chemistry, biology, and organic chemistry. We recommend that you take one year each of biology, general chemistry, organic chemistry, and physics before taking the MCAT, and that you review the content in this book thoroughly. Knowing these basics is just the beginning of doing well on the MCAT. That's a shock to most test takers. They presume that once they recall or relearn their undergraduate science, they are ready to do battle against the MCAT. Wrong! They merely have directions to the battlefield. They lack what they need to beat the test: a copy of the test maker's battle plan!

> **TEST TIP**
>
> Don't think of the sections of the MCAT as unrelated timed pieces. Each is a variation on the same theme, because the underlying purpose of each section and of the test as a whole is to evaluate your thinking skills. Memorizing formulas won't boost your score. Understanding fundamental scientific principles will.

You won't be drilled on facts and formulas on the MCAT. You'll need to demonstrate ability to reason based on ideas and concepts. The science questions are painted with a broad brush, testing your general understanding.

TAKE CONTROL: THE MCAT MINDSET

In addition to being a thinking test, as we've stressed, the MCAT is a standardized test. As such, it has its own consistent patterns and idiosyncrasies that can actually work in your favor. This is the key to why test preparation works. You have the opportunity to familiarize yourself with those consistent peculiarities, to adopt the proper test-taking mindset.

> **TEST TIP**
>
> Those perfectionist tendencies that make you a good student and a good medical school candidate may work against you in MCAT Land. If you get stuck on a question or passage, move on. Perfectionism is for medical school—not the MCAT, and you don't need to understand every word of a passage before you go on to the questions—what's tripping you up may not even be relevant to what you'll be asked.

The following are some overriding principles of the MCAT mindset that will be covered in depth in the chapters to come:

- Read actively and critically.
- Translate prose into your own words.

- Save the toughest questions for last.
- Know the test and its components inside and out.
- Do MCAT-style problems in each topic area after you've reviewed it.
- Allow your confidence to build on itself.
- Take full-length practice tests a week or two before the test to break down the mystique of the real experience.
- Learn from your mistakes—get the most out of your practice tests.
- Look at the MCAT as a challenge, the first step in your medical career, rather than as an arbitrary obstacle.

That's what the MCAT mindset boils down to: Taking control. Being proactive. Being on top of the testing experience so that you can get as many points as you can as quickly and as easily as possible. Keep this in mind as you read and work through the material in this book and, of course, as you face the challenge on Test Day.

Now that you have a better idea of what the MCAT is all about, let's take a tour of the individual test sections. Although the underlying skills being tested are similar, each MCAT section requires that you call into play a different domain of knowledge. So, though we encourage you to think of the MCAT as a holistic and unified test, we also recognize that the test is segmented by discipline and that there are characteristics unique to each section. In the overviews, we'll review sample questions and answers and discuss section-specific strategies. For each of the sections—Verbal Reasoning, Physical/Biological Sciences, and the Writing Sample—we'll present you with the following:

- **The Big Picture**
  You'll get a clear view of the section and familiarize yourself with what it's really evaluating.
- **A Closer Look**
  You'll explore the types of questions that will appear and master the strategies you'll need to deal with them successfully.
- **Highlights**
  The key approaches to each section are outlined, for reinforcement and quick review.

TEST EXPERTISE

The first year of medical school is a frenzied experience for most students. In order to meet the requirements of a rigorous work schedule, students either learn to prioritize and budget their time or else fall hopelessly behind. It's no surprise, then, that the MCAT, the test specifically designed to predict success in the first year of medical school, is a high-speed, time-intensive test. It demands excellent time-management skills as well as that sine qua non of the successful physician—grace under pressure.

It's one thing to answer a Verbal Reasoning question correctly; it's quite another to answer several correctly in a limited time frame. The same goes for Physical and Biological Sciences—it's a whole new ballgame once you move from doing an individual passage at your leisure to handling a full section under actual timed conditions. You also need to budget your time for the Writing Sample, but this section isn't as time sensitive. However, when it comes to the multiple-choice sections, time pressure is a factor that affects virtually every test taker.

TEST TIP

For complete MCAT success, you've got to get as many correct answers as possible in the time you're allotted. Knowing the strategies is not enough. You have to perfect your time-management skills so that you get a chance to use those strategies on as many questions as possible.

So when you're comfortable with the content of the test, your next challenge will be to take it to the next level—test expertise—which will enable you to manage the all-important time element of the test.

THE FIVE BASIC PRINCIPLES OF TEST EXPERTISE

On some tests, if a question seems particularly difficult you'll spend significantly more time on it, as you'll probably be given more points for correctly answering a hard question. Not so on the MCAT. Remember, every MCAT question, no matter how hard, is worth a single point. There's no partial credit or "A" for effort, and because there are so many questions to do in so little time, you'd be a fool to spend 10 minutes getting a point for a hard question and then not have time to get a couple of quick points from three easy questions later in the section.

TEST TIP

In order to meet the stringent time requirements of the MCAT, you have to cultivate the following elements of test expertise:

- Feel free to skip questions.
- Learn to recognize and seek out questions you can do.
- Use a process of answer elimination.
- Remain calm.
- Keep track of time.

Given this combination—limited time, all questions equal in weight—you've got to develop a way of handling the test sections to make sure you get as many points as you can as quickly and easily as you can. Here are the principles that will help you do that:

1. FEEL FREE TO SKIP AROUND

One of the most valuable strategies to help you finish the sections in time is to learn to recognize and deal first with the questions that are easier and more familiar to you. That means you must temporarily skip those that promise to be difficult and time-consuming, if you feel comfortable doing so. You can always come back to these at the end, and if you run out of time, you're much better off not getting to questions you may have had difficulty with, rather than not getting to potentially feasible material. Of course, because there's no guessing penalty, always put an answer to every question on the test, whether you get to it or not. (It's not practical to skip passages, so do those in order.)

This strategy is difficult for most test takers; we're conditioned to do things in order. Nevertheless, give it a try when you practice. Remember, if you do the test in the exact order given, you're letting the test makers control you. You control how you take this test. On the other hand, if skipping around goes against your moral fiber and makes you a nervous wreck—don't do it. Just be mindful of the clock, and don't get bogged down with the tough questions.

2. LEARN TO RECOGNIZE AND SEEK OUT QUESTIONS YOU CAN DO

Another thing to remember about managing the test sections is that MCAT questions and passages, unlike items on the SAT and other standardized tests, are not presented in order of difficulty. There's no rule that says you have to work through the sections in any particular order; in fact, the test makers scatter the easy and difficult questions throughout the section, in effect rewarding those who actually get to the end. Don't lose sight of what you're being tested for along with your reading and thinking skills: efficiency and cleverness.

Don't waste time on questions you can't do. We know that skipping a possibly tough question is easier said than done; we all have the natural instinct to plow through test sections in their given order, but it just doesn't pay off on the MCAT. The computer won't be impressed if you get the toughest question right. If you dig in your heels on a tough question, refusing to move on until you've cracked it, well, you're letting your ego get in the way of your test score. A test section (not to mention life itself) is too short to waste on lost causes.

TEST TIP

Every question is worth exactly one point, but questions vary dramatically in difficulty level. Given a shortage of time, work on easy questions and then move on to the hard ones.

TEST TIP

Don't let your ego sabotage your score. It isn't easy for some of us to give up on a tough, time-consuming question, but sometimes it's better to say "uncle." Remember, there's no point of honor at stake here, but there are MCAT points at stake.

3. USE A PROCESS OF ANSWER ELIMINATION

Using a process of elimination is another way to answer questions both quickly and effectively. There are two ways to get all the answers right on the MCAT. You either know all the right answers, or you know all the wrong answers. Because there are three times as many wrong answers, you should be able to eliminate some if not all of them. By doing so you either get to the correct response or increase your chances of guessing the correct response. You start out with a 25 percent chance of picking the right answer, and with each eliminated answer your odds go up. Eliminate one, and you'll have a $33\frac{1}{3}$ percent chance of picking the right one, eliminate two, and you'll have a 50 percent chance, and, of course, eliminate three, and you'll have a 100 percent chance. Increase your efficiency by actually crossing out the wrong choices on the screen using the strike-through feature. Remember to look for wrong-answer traps when you're eliminating. Some answers are designed to seduce you by distorting the correct answer.

4. REMAIN CALM

It's imperative that you remain calm and composed while working through a section. You can't allow yourself to become so rattled by one hard reading passage that it throws off your performance on the rest of the section. Expect to find at least one killer passage in every section, but remember, you won't be the only one to have trouble with it. The test is curved to take the tough material into account. Having trouble with a difficult question isn't going to ruin your score—but getting upset about it and letting it throw you off track will. When you understand that part of the test maker's goal is to reward those who keep their composure, you'll recognize the importance of not panicking when you run into challenging material.

5. KEEP TRACK OF TIME

Of course, the last thing you want to happen is to have time called on a particular section before you've gotten to half the questions. Therefore, it's essential that you pace yourself, keeping in mind the general guidelines for how long to spend on any individual question or passage. Have a sense of how long you have to do each question, so you know when you're exceeding the limit and should start to move faster.

So, when working on a section, always remember to keep track of time. Don't spend a wildly disproportionate amount of time on any one question or group of questions. Also, give yourself 30 seconds or so at the end of each section to fill in answers for any questions you haven't gotten to.

SECTION-SPECIFIC PACING

Let's now look at the section-specific timing requirements and some tips for meeting them. Keep in mind that the times per question or passage are only averages; there are bound to be some that take less time and some that take more. Try to stay balanced. Remember, too, that every question is of equal worth, so don't get hung up on any one. Think about it: If a question is so hard that it takes you a long time to answer it, chances are you may get it wrong anyway. In that case, you'd have nothing to show for your extra time but a lower score.

VERBAL REASONING

Allow yourself approximately eight to ten minutes per passage and respective questions. It may sound like a lot of time, but it goes quickly. Keep in mind that some passages are longer than others. On average, give yourself about three or four minutes to read and then four to six minutes for the questions.

> **TEST TIP**
>
> For Verbal Reasoning, here are some of the important time techniques to remember:
>
> - Spend eight to ten minutes per passage
> - Allow about three to four minutes to read and four to six minutes for the questions

PHYSICAL AND BIOLOGICAL SCIENCES

Averaging over each section, you'll have about one minute and 20 seconds per question. Some questions, of course, will take more time, some less. A science passage plus accompanying questions should take about eight to nine minutes, depending on how many questions there are. Standalone questions can take anywhere from a few seconds to a minute or more. Again, the rule is to do your best work first. Also, don't feel that you have to understand everything in a passage before you go on to the questions. You may not need that deep an understanding to answer questions, because a lot of information may be extraneous. You should overcome your perfectionism and use your time wisely.

> **TEST TIP**
>
> Some suggestions for maximizing your time on the science sections:
>
> - Spend about eight to nine minutes per passage
> - Maximize points by doing the questions you can do first
> - Don't waste valuable time trying to understand extraneous material

WRITING SAMPLE

You have exactly 30 minutes for each essay. As mentioned in discussion of the seven-step approach to this section, you should allow approximately five minutes to prewrite the essay, 23 minutes to write the essay, and two minutes to proofread. It's important that you budget your time, so you don't get cut off.

COMPUTER-BASED TESTING STRATEGIES

ARRIVE AT THE TESTING CENTER EARLY

Get to the testing center early to jump-start your brain. However, if they allow you to begin your test early, decline.

USE THE MOUSE TO YOUR ADVANTAGE

If you are right-handed, practice using the mouse with your left hand for Test Day. This way, you'll increase speed by keeping the pencil in your right hand to write on your scratch paper. If you are left-handed, use your right hand for the mouse.

KNOW THE TUTORIAL BEFORE TEST DAY

You will save time on Test Day by knowing exactly how the test will work. Click through any tutorial pages and save time.

PRACTICE WITH SCRATCH PAPER

Going forward, always practice using scratch paper when solving questions because this is how you will do it on Test Day. Never write directly on a written test.

GET NEW SCRATCH PAPER

Between sections, get a new piece of scratch paper even if you only used part of the old one. This will maximize the available space for each section and minimize the likelihood of you running out of paper to write on.

REMEMBER YOU CAN ALWAYS GO BACK

Just because you finish a passage or move on, remember you can come back to questions about which you are uncertain. You have the "marking" option to your advantage. However, as a general rule minimize the amount of questions you mark or skip.

MARK INCOMPLETE WORK

If you need to go back to a question, clearly mark the work you've done on the scratch paper with the question number. This way, you will be able to find your work easily when you come back to tackle the question.

LOOK AWAY AT TIMES

Taking the test on computer leads to faster eye-muscle fatigue. Use the Kaplan strategy of looking at a distant object at regular intervals. This will keep you fresher at the end of the test.

PRACTICE ON THE COMPUTER

This is the most critical aspect of adapting to computer-based testing. Like anything else, in order to perform well on computer-based tests you must practice. Spend time reading passages and answering questions on the computer. You often will have to scroll when reading passages.

Part I
Subject Review

PERIODIC TABLE OF THE ELEMENTS

Period	1 IA 1A	2 IIA 2A	3 IIIB 3B	4 IVB 4B	5 VB 5B	6 VIB 6B	7 VIIB 7B	8 -------	9 VIII -- (------- 8 -------)	10 -----	11 IB 1B	12 IIB 2B	13 IIIA 3A	14 IVA 4A	15 VA 5A	16 VIA 6A	17 VIIA 7A	18 vIIIA 8A
1	1 H 1.008																	2 He 4.003
2	3 Li 6.941	4 Be 9.012											5 B 10.81	6 C 12.01	7 N 14.01	8 O 16.00	9 F 19.00	10 Ne 20.18
3	11 Na 22.99	12 Mg 24.31											13 Al 26.98	14 Si 28.09	15 P 30.97	16 S 32.07	17 Cl 35.45	18 Ar 39.95
4	19 K 39.10	20 Ca 40.08	21 Sc 44.96	22 Ti 47.88	23 V 50.94	24 Cr 52.00	25 Mn 54.94	26 Fe 55.85	27 Co 58.47	28 Ni 58.69	29 Cu 63.55	30 Zn 65.39	31 Ga 69.72	32 Ge 72.59	33 As 74.92	34 Se 78.96	35 Br 79.90	36 Kr 83.80
5	37 Rb 85.47	38 Sr 87.62	39 Y 88.91	40 Zr 91.22	41 Nb 92.91	42 Mo 95.94	43 Tc (98)	44 Ru 101.1	45 Rh 102.9	46 Pd 106.4	47 Ag 107.9	48 Cd 112.4	49 In 114.8	50 Sn 118.7	51 Sb 121.8	52 Te 127.6	53 I 126.9	54 Xe 131.3
6	55 Cs 132.9	56 Ba 137.3	57 La* 138.9	72 Hf 178.5	73 Ta 180.9	74 W 183.9	75 Re 186.2	76 Os 190.2	77 Ir 190.2	78 Pt 195.1	79 Au 197.0	80 Hg 200.5	81 Tl 204.4	82 Pb 207.2	83 Bi 209.0	84 Po (210)	85 At (210)	86 Rn (222)
7	87 Fr (223)	88 Ra (226)	89 Ac~ (227)	104 Rf (257)	105 Db (260)	106 Sg (263)	107 Bh (262)	108 Hs (265)	109 Mt (266)	110 --- ()	111 --- ()	112 --- ()		114 --- ()		116 --- ()		118 --- ()

Lanthanide Series*	58 Ce 140.1	59 Pr 140.9	60 Nd 144.2	61 Pm (147)	62 Sm 150.4	63 Eu 152.0	64 Gd 157.3	65 Tb 158.9	66 Dy 162.5	67 Ho 164.9	68 Er 167.3	69 Tm 168.9	70 Yb 173.0	71 Lu 175.0
Actinide Series~	90 Th 232.0	91 Pa (231)	92 U (238)	93 Np (237)	94 Pu (242)	95 Am (243)	96 Cm (247)	97 Bk (247)	98 Cf (249)	99 Es (254)	100 Fm (253)	101 Md (256)	102 No (254)	103 Lr (257)

CHAPTER 1

NOMENCLATURE

Nomenclature, the set of accepted conventions for naming compounds, is crucial to a discussion of organic chemistry. The rules of nomenclature presented in this chapter are for general cases only. More specific examples will be discussed in the chapters dealing with particular types of compounds.

You may see specific nomenclature questions on the MCAT, such as "Name the following compound," or "Which structure represents the following named compound?" But more importantly, nomenclature represents the basic language of organic chemistry. If you don't know it, you may feel like you're taking a test in a foreign language—which, in a way, you would be!

TEACHER TIP

How is nomenclature usually tested on the MCAT? A reactant is written out in IUPAC in the question stem and only structures are given as answer choices, leaving you to figure out both the structure of the reactant and the reaction taking place.

ALKANES

Alkanes are the simplest organic molecules, consisting only of carbon and hydrogen atoms held together by single bonds.

A. STRAIGHT-CHAIN ALKANES

The names of the four simplest alkanes are:

CH_4	CH_3CH_3	$CH_3CH_2CH_3$	$CH_3CH_2CH_2CH_3$
methane	ethane	propane	butane

MCAT SYNOPSIS

All straight-chain alkanes have the general formula $C_nH_{2n} + 2$ (n is an integer).

The names of the longer-chain alkanes consist of prefixes derived from the Greek root for the number of carbon atoms, with the ending **-ane.**

C_5H_{12} = **pent**ane C_9H_{20} = **non**ane
C_6H_{14} = **hex**ane $C_{10}H_{22}$ = **dec**ane
C_7H_{16} = **hept**ane $C_{11}H_{24}$ = **undec**ane
C_8H_{18} = **oct**ane $C_{12}H_{26}$ = **dodec**ane

TEACHER TIP

Be careful about the number of carbons in the compounds when evaluating a question and answer. Often, a wrong answer choice will have the correct functional groups but will differ by the amount of carbons.

These prefixes are applicable to more complex organic molecules and should be memorized.

B. BRANCHED-CHAIN ALKANES

The International Union of Pure and Applied Chemistry (IUPAC) has proposed a set of simple rules for naming complex molecules. This basic system can be used to name all classes of organic compounds. Throughout these notes, the IUPAC names will be listed as the primary name, and common names will appear in parentheses.

TEACHER TIP

While this is an important rule, the MCAT is not looking to trick you. Most often, you will have smaller chains and not have to work too hard to find the longest carbon chain.

1. Find the longest chain in the compound.

The longest continuous carbon chain within the compound is taken as the backbone. If there are two or more chains of equal length, the most highly substituted chain takes precedence. The longest chain may not be obvious from the structural formula as it is drawn. For example, the backbone shown below is an octane (it contains eight carbon atoms).

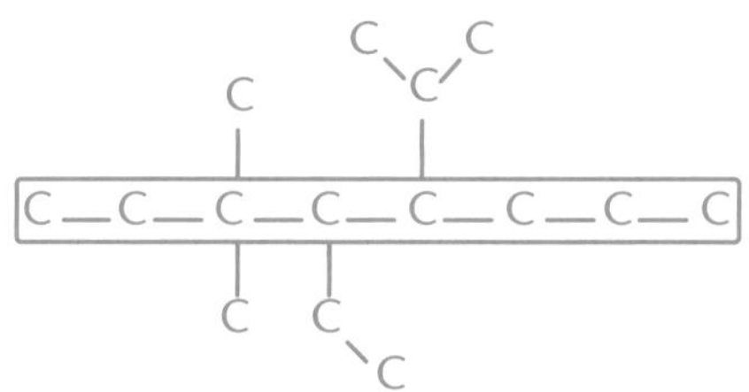

Figure 1.1

MCAT SYNOPSIS

1. Identify the longest backbone.
2. Number it, keeping numbers for the substituents as low as possible.
3. Name substituents.
4. Assign numbers.
5. Put the whole name together, remembering to alphabetize substituents.

2. Number the chain.

Number the chain from one end in such a way that the lowest set of numbers is obtained for the substituents.

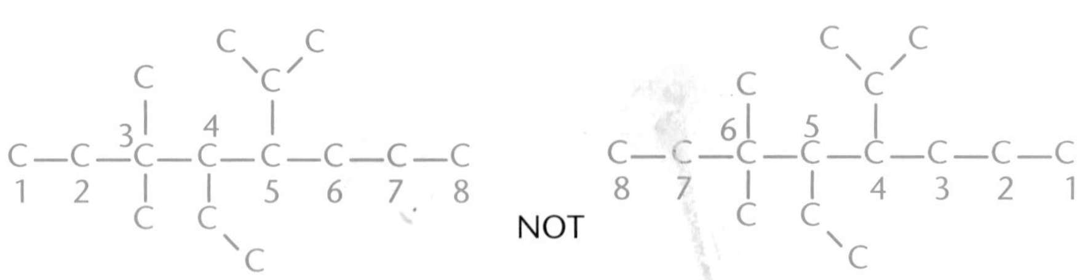

Figure 1.2

3. Name the substituents.

Substituents are named according to their appropriate prefix with the ending **-yl.** More complex substituents are named as derivatives of the longest chain in the group.

CH_3–	CH_3CH_2–	$CH_3CH_2CH_2$–
methyl	ethyl	*n*-propyl

The prefix *n*- in the previous example indicates an unbranched ("normal") compound. There are special names for some common branched alkanes, and these are usually used in the naming of substituents.

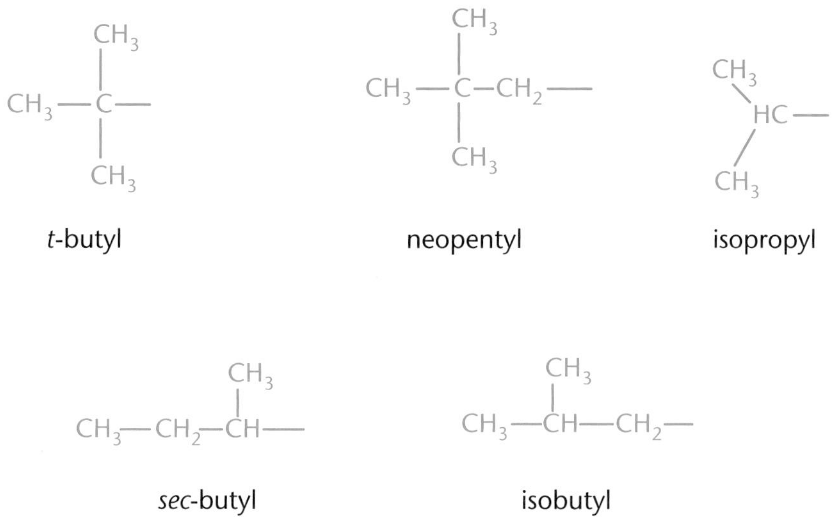

t-butyl   neopentyl   isopropyl

sec-butyl   isobutyl

Figure 1.3

If there are two or more equivalent groups, the prefixes **di-, tri-, tetra-,** and so on are used.

4. Assign a number to each substituent.

Each substituent is assigned a number to identify its point of attachment to the principal chain. If the prefixes **di-, tri-, tetra-,** and so on are used, a number is still necessary for each individual group.

5. Complete the name.

List the substituents in alphabetical order with their corresponding numbers. Prefixes such as di-, tri-, and so on as well as the hyphenated prefixes (tert- [or t-], sec-, n-) are ignored in alphabetizing. In contrast, **cyclo-, iso-,** and **neo-** are considered part of the group name, and are alphabetized. Commas should be placed between numbers, and dashes should be placed between numbers and words. For example:

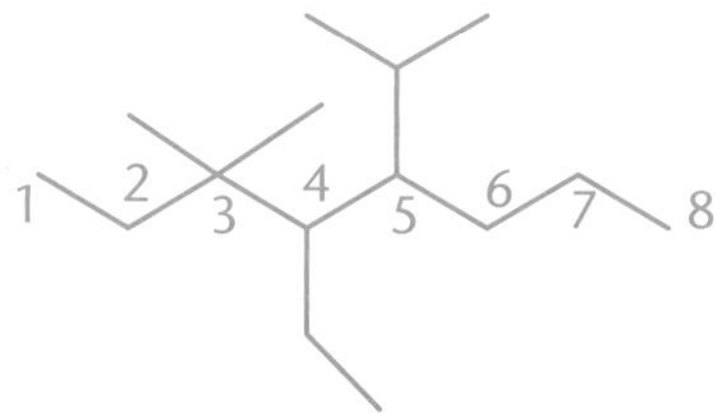

4-ethyl-5-isopropyl-3,3-dimethyl octane

Figure 1.4

TEACHER TIP

While the MCAT will most likely give IUPAC names, knowing the "common" names will prepare you for all possibilities.

TEACHER TIP

The MCAT is not a "picky" exam. You probably won't have two answers that will differ only in their alphabetization, though the rule about the prefixes may come in handy.

You may also need to indicate the isomer you are describing, e.g., *cis* or *trans, R* or *S,* and so on. Isomers will be discussed in detail in chapter 2.

Teacher Tip

Cycloalkanes will have the same general formula (C_nH_{2n}) as the alkenes that will be discussed below. They are both said to have "one degree of unsaturation" (i.e., missing two hydrogens from a straight chain alkane).

C. CYCLOALKANES

Alkanes can form rings. These are named according to the number of carbon atoms in the ring with the prefix **cyclo-.**

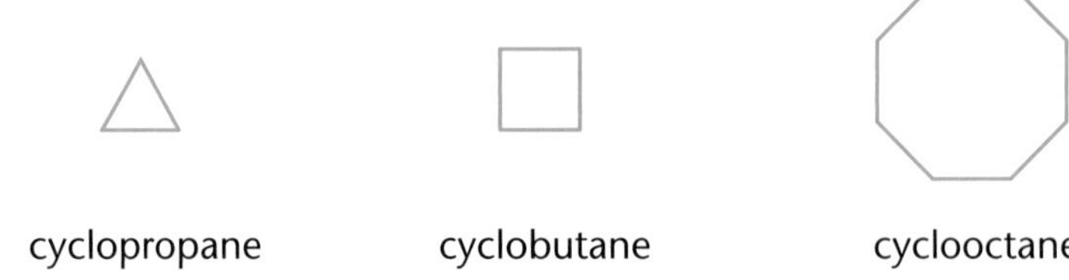

cyclopropane cyclobutane cyclooctane

Figure 1.5

Substituted cycloalkanes are named as derivatives of the parent cycloalkane. The substituents are named, and the carbon atoms are numbered around the ring *starting from the point of greatest substitution.* Again, the goal is to provide the lowest series of numbers as in rule 2 mentioned previously.

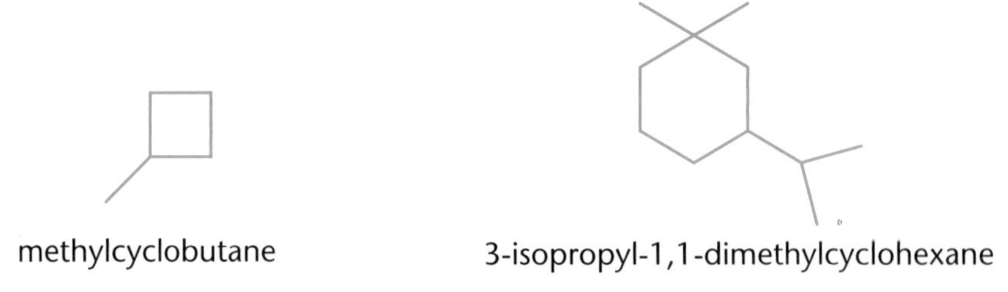

methylcyclobutane 3-isopropyl-1,1-dimethylcyclohexane

Figure 1.6

Teacher Tip

Straight chain alkanes and cycloalkanes both have the general formula C_nH_{2n} (*n* is an integer).

MORE COMPLICATED MOLECULES

Organic molecules that are more complicated than simple alkanes can also be named using this five-step process, with a few additional considerations.

MULTIPLE BONDS

Teacher Tip

While alkenes will not be tested directly, the nomenclature is important. Alkenes are products in the elimination reactions.

A. ALKENES

Alkenes (or **olefins**) are compounds containing carbon-carbon double bonds. The nomenclature rules are essentially the same as for alkanes, except that the ending **-ene** is used rather than **-ane.** (Exceptions: The common names *ethylene* and *propylene,* which are used preferentially over the IUPAC names *ethene* and *propene*).

When identifying the carbon backbone, select the longest chain that contains the double bond (or the greatest number of double bonds, if more than one is present).

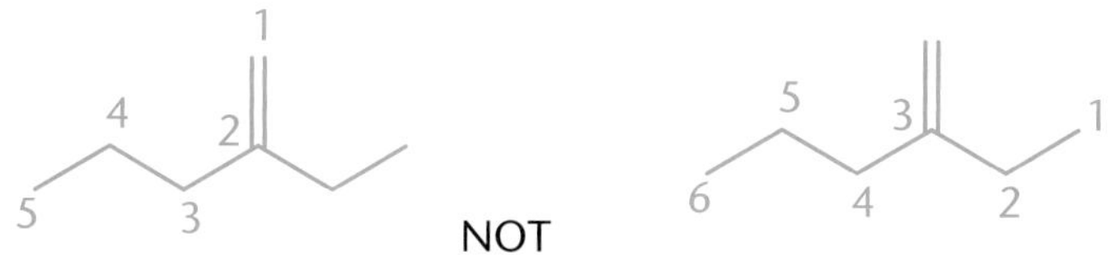

NOT

Figure 1.7

Number the backbone so that the double bond receives the lowest number possible. Remember that multiple double bonds must be named using the prefixes di-, tri-, and so on and that each must receive a number. Also, you may need to name the configurational isomer *(cis/trans, Z/E)*. This topic will be discussed further in chapter 2.

Substituents are named as they are for alkanes, and their positions are specified by the number of the backbone carbon atom to which they are attached.

Frequently, an alkene group must be named as a substituent. In these cases, the systematic names may be used, but common names are more popular. **Vinyl-** derivatives are monosubstituted ethylenes **(ethenyl-),** and **allyl-**derivatives are propylenes substituted at the C–3 position **(2-propenyl-). Methylene-** refers to the $-CH_2$ group.

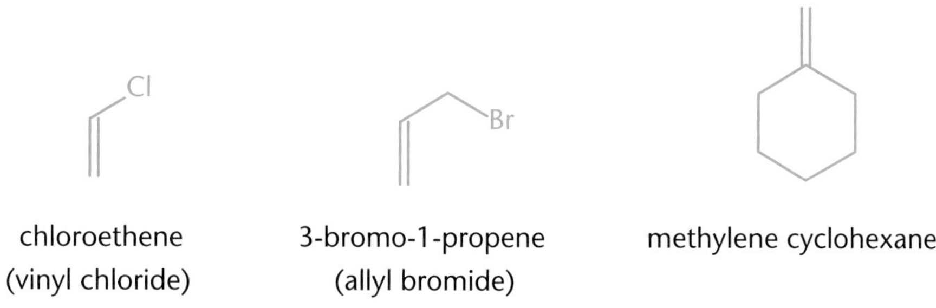

chloroethene (vinyl chloride) | 3-bromo-1-propene (allyl bromide) | methylene cyclohexane

Figure 1.8

B. CYCLOALKENES

Cycloalkenes are named like cycloalkanes but with the suffix **-ene** rather than **-ane.** If there is only one double bond and no other substituents, a number is not necessary.

TEACHER TIP

Because we have a ring and a double bond, we have "two degrees of unsaturation," or four "missing" hydrogens. These will also have the same general formula as the alkynes.

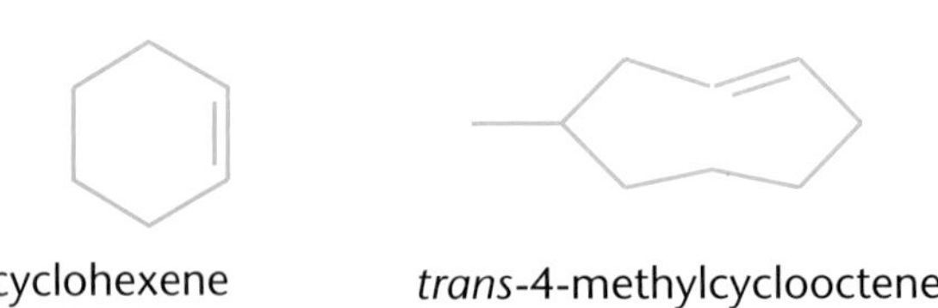

cyclohexene *trans*-4-methylcyclooctene

Figure 1.9

C. ALKYNES

MCAT SYNOPSIS

Straight chain alkynes have the general formula C_nH_{2n-2} (*n* is an integer).

Alkynes are compounds that possess carbon-carbon triple bonds. The suffix **-yne** replaces -ane in the parent alkane. The position of the triple bond is indicated by a number when necessary. The common name for ethyne is **acetylene,** and this name is used almost exclusively.

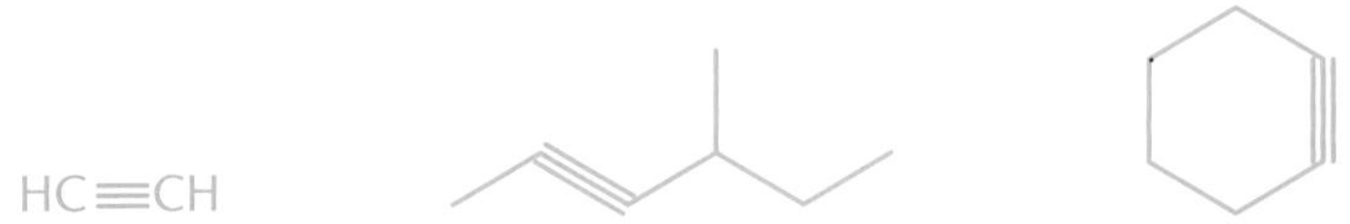

$HC\equiv CH$

ethyne (acetylene) **4-methyl-2-hexyne** **cyclohexyne**

Figure 1.10

SUBSTITUTED ALKANES

A. HALOALKANES

TEACHER TIP

Halogens are often good leaving groups and, as such, are likely to be seen on the MCAT as part of the many reactions.

Compounds that contain a halogen substituent are named as **haloalkanes.** The appendages are numbered and alphabetized as alkyl groups are treated. Notice that the presence of the halide does not dramatically affect the numbering of the chain—you should still proceed so that substituents receive the lowest possible numbers. For example:

Cl Cl I

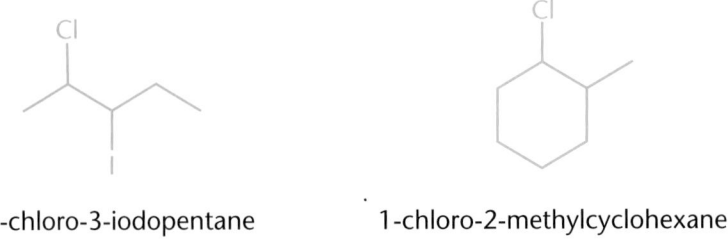

2-chloro-3-iodopentane 1-chloro-2-methylcyclohexane

Figure 1.11

Alternatively, the haloalkane may be named as an **alkyl halide.** In this system, chloroethane is called **ethyl chloride.** Other examples are:

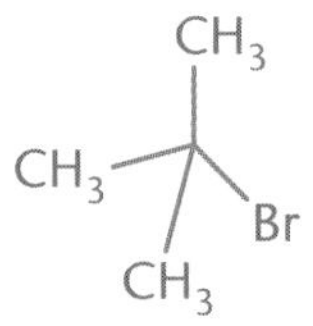

CH_3 / CH_3 / Br / CH_3

2-bromo-2-methylpropane
(*t*-butyl bromide)

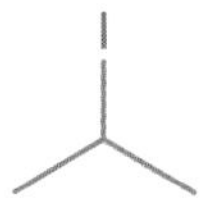

I

2-iodopropane
(isopropyl iodide)

Figure 1.12

B. ALCOHOLS

In the IUPAC system, **alcohols** are named by replacing the **-e** of the corresponding alkane with **-ol.** The chain is numbered in such a way that the carbon attached to the hydroxyl group (–OH) receives the lowest number possible.

In compounds that possess a multiple bond and a hydroxyl group, numerical priority is given to the carbon attached to the –OH.

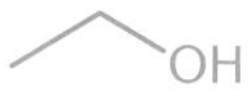

TEACHER TIP

Because the alcohol will be important in determining the reactions and properties of the compound, it becomes an integral part of the name. The more important the functional group is to the compounds properties, the higher priority it takes in the naming.

OH

ethanol

OH

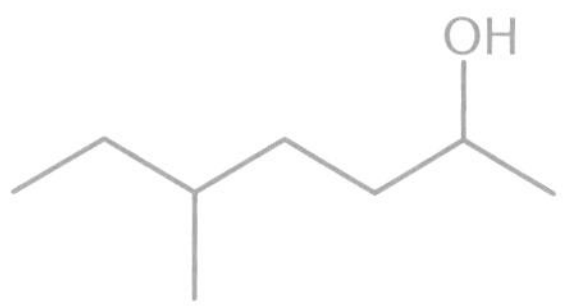

5-methyl-2-heptanol

OH

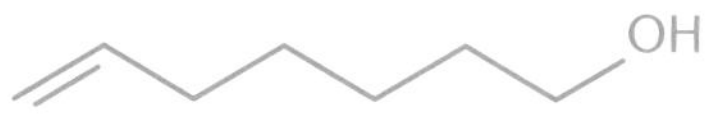

hept-6-en-1-ol

Figure 1.13

A common system of nomenclature exists for alcohols in which the name of the alkyl group is combined with the word *alcohol*. These common names are used for simple alcohols. For example, methanol may be named "methyl alcohol," while 2-propanol may also be named "isopropyl alcohol."

Molecules with two hydroxyl groups are called **diols** (or **glycols**) and are named with the suffix **-diol.** Two numbers are necessary to locate the two functional groups. Diols with hydroxyl groups on adjacent carbons are referred to as **vicinal,** and diols with hydroxyl groups on the same carbon are **geminal.** Geminal diols (also called **hydrates**) are not commonly observed because they spontaneously lose water **(dehydrate)** to produce carbonyl compounds (containing C=O; see chapter 8).

TEACHER TIP

Ethers are just as often given in IUPAC and common names. Be aware of both naming methods.

C. ETHERS

In the IUPAC system, **ethers** are named as derivatives of alkanes, and the larger alkyl group is chosen as the backbone. The ether functionality is specified as an **alkoxy-** prefix, indicating the presence of an ether (-oxy-), and the corresponding smaller alkyl group (alk-). The chain is numbered to give the ether the lowest position. Common names for ethers are frequently used. They are derived by naming the two alkyl groups in alphabetical order and adding the word *ether*. The generic term *ether* refers to diethyl ether, a commonly used solvent.

For **cyclic ethers,** numbering of the ring begins at the oxygen and proceeds to provide the lowest numbers for the substituents. Three-membered rings are termed **oxiranes** by IUPAC, although they are commonly called **epoxides.**

MCAT SYNOPSIS

Cyclic ethers with three members are *epoxides*.

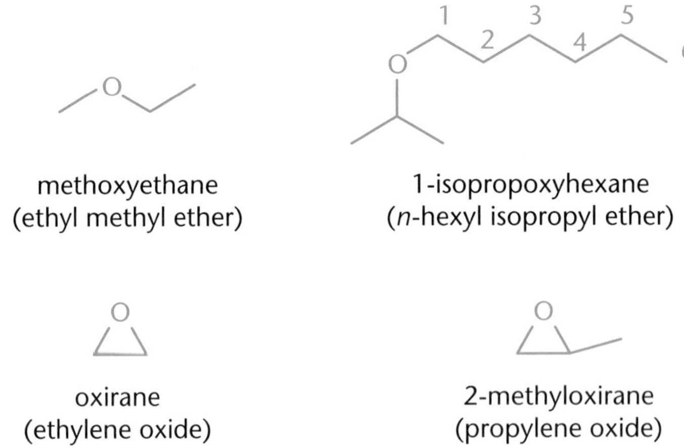

Figure 1.14

O

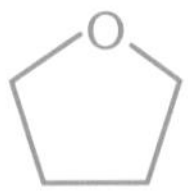

tetrahydrofuran
(THF)

Figure 1.15

TEACHER TIP

An aldehyde is always at the end of a carbon chain and, because it is often the highest priority functional group, it is reflected in the suffix of the name (-al) and is C–1 of the compound.

D. ALDEHYDES AND KETONES

Aldehydes are named according to the longest chain containing the aldehyde functional group. The suffix **-al** replaces the **-e** of the corresponding alkane. The carbonyl carbon receives the lowest number, although numbers are not always necessary because by definition an aldehyde is terminal and receives the number 1.

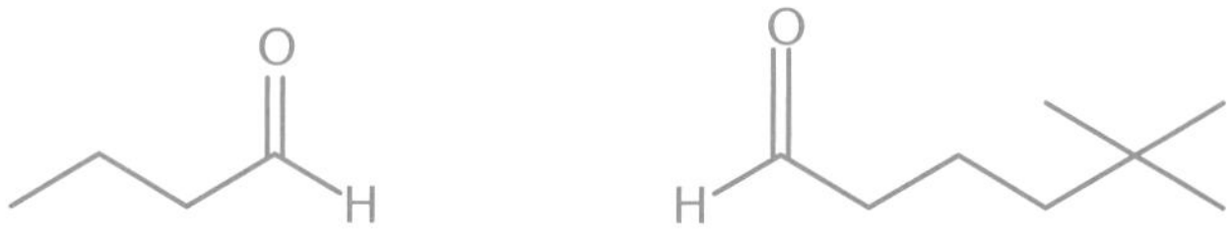

n-butanal   5,5-dimethylhexanal

Figure 1.16

The common names *formaldehyde, acetaldehyde,* and *propionaldehyde* are used almost exclusively instead of the IUPAC names *methanal, ethanal,* and *propanal,* respectively.

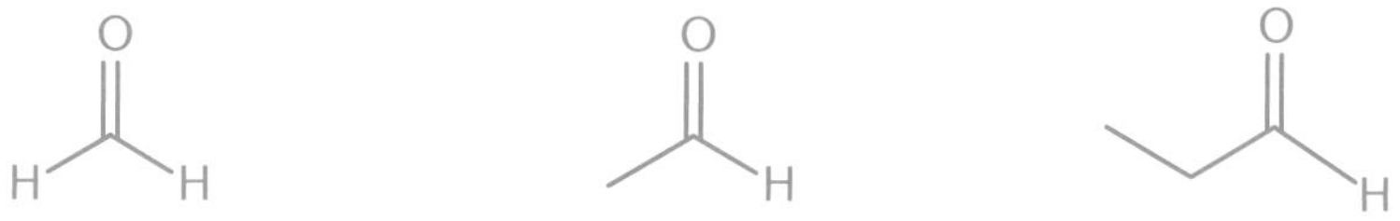

MCAT SYNOPSIS

The carbonyl in a ketone should receive the lowest number possible unless there is a higher priority group.

methanal (formaldehyde)   ethanal (acetaldehyde)   propanal (propionaldehyde)

Figure 1.17

Ketones are named analogously, with **-one** as a suffix. The carbonyl group has to be assigned the lowest possible number. In complex molecules, the carbonyl group can be named as a prefix with the term **oxo-.** Alternatively, the individual alkyl groups may be listed in alphabetical order, followed by the word **ketone.**

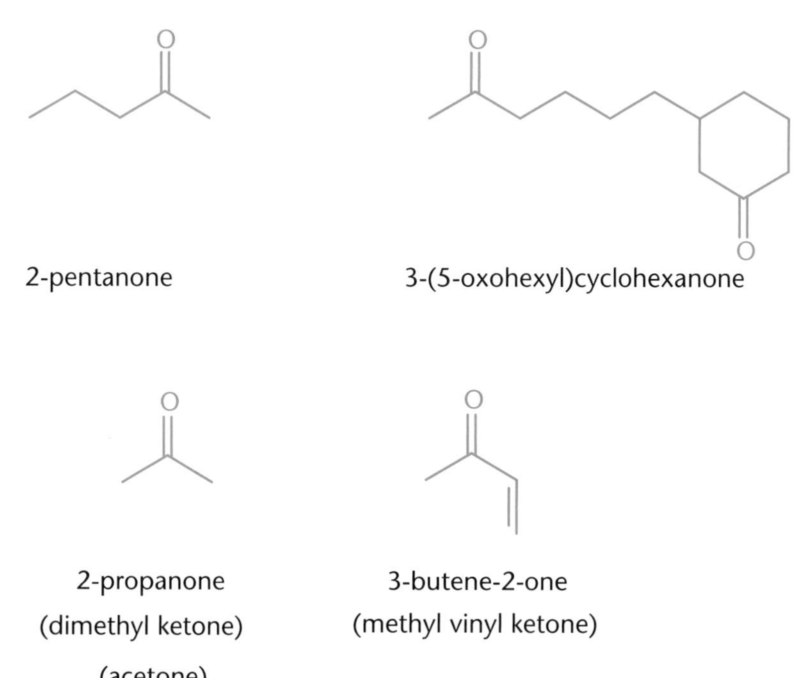

Figure 1.18

TEACHER TIP

When the ketone is not the main functional group, or when there are two ketones, you need to use the prefix oxo- to denote the group.

TEACHER TIP

In biological molecules, we often use the Greek letter designations rather than numbers (*i.e.* β-ketoacids). This will be seen later when we discuss α-hydrogen acidity in the Carboxylic Acids chapter.

A commonly used alternative to the numerical designation of substituents is to term the carbon atom adjacent to the carbonyl carbon as α and the carbon atoms successively along the chain as β, γ, δ, and so on. This system is encountered with dicarbonyl compounds and halocarbonyl compounds.

E. CARBOXYLIC ACIDS

TEACHER TIP

Rule of Thumb: The more oxidized the group the higher the priority! So, carboxylic acids are always the highest priority because they are the most oxidized a carbon can be without turning into CO_2.

Carboxylic acids are named with the ending **-oic** and the word **acid** replacing the **-e** ending of the corresponding alkane. Carboxylic acids are terminal functional groups and, like aldehydes, are numbered one (1). The common names formic acid (methanoic acid), acetic acid (ethanoic acid), and propionic acid (propanoic acid) are used almost exclusively.

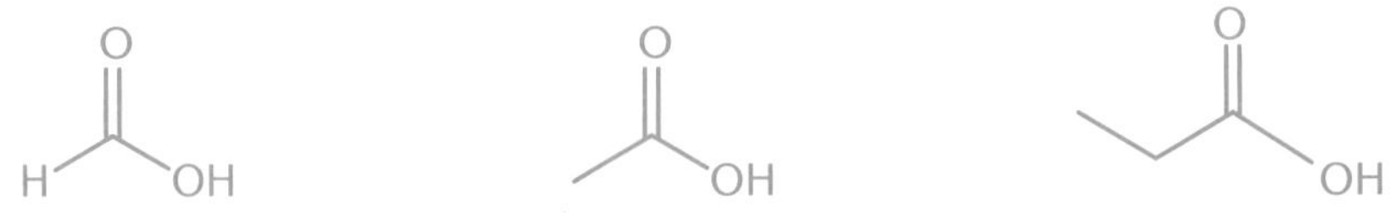

methanoic acid (formic acid) | ethanoic acid (acetic acid) | propanoic acid (propionic acid)

Figure 1.19

F. AMINES

The longest chain attached to the nitrogen atom is taken as the backbone. For simple compounds, name the alkane and replace the final "e" with "amine."

MCAT SYNOPSIS

When additional alkyl groups are attached to the nitrogen, use the prefix N–.

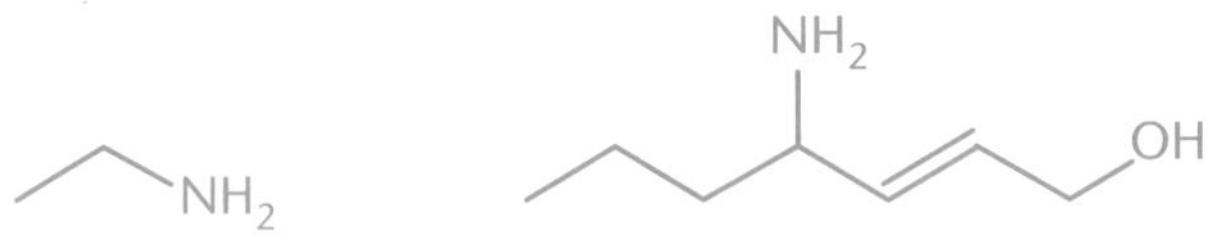

ethanamine | 4-aminohept-2-en-1-ol

Figure 1.20

To specify the location of an additional alkyl group that is attached to the nitrogen, the prefix N- is used:

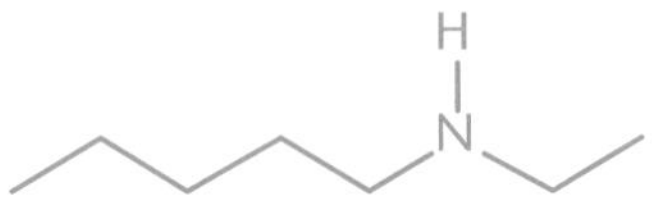

N-ethylpentanamine
(ethylpentylamine)

Figure 1.21

SUMMARY OF FUNCTIONAL GROUPS

Table 1.1 lists the major functional groups you need to known for the MCAT.

Table 1.1.

Functional Group	Structure	IUPAC Prefix	IUPAC Suffix
Carboxylic acid	R–C(=O)–OH	carboxy-	-oic acid
Ester	R–C(=O)–OR	alkoxycarbonyl-	-oate
Acyl halide	R–C(=O)–X	halocarbonyl-	-oyl halide
Amide	R–C(=O)–NH_2	amido-	-amide
Nitrile/Cyanide	RC≡N	cyano-	-nitrile
Aldehyde	R–C(=O)–H	oxo-	-al
Ketone	R–C(=O)–R	oxo-	-one
Alcohol	ROH	hydroxy-	-ol
Thiol	RSH	sulfhydryl-	-thiol
Amine	RNH_2	amino-	-amine
Imine	R_2C=NR’	imino-	-imine
Ether	ROR	alkoxy-	-ether
Sulfide	R_2S	alkylthio-	
Halide	-I, -Br, -Cl, -F	halo-	
Nitro	RNO_2	nitro-	
Azide	RN_3	azido-	
Diazo	RN_2	diazo-	

MCAT SYNOPSIS

More complex molecules can also be named with the same five steps, with a few additional considerations:

1. Multiple bonds should be on the main carbon backbone whenever possible.
2. –OH is a high priority functional group, placed above multiple bonds in numbering.
3. Haloalkanes, ethers, and ketones are often given common names (*e.g.*, methyl chloride, ethyl methyl ether, diethyl ketone).
4. Aldehydes and carboxylic acids are terminal functional groups. If present, they define C–1 of the carbon chain (taking precedence over hydroxy, –OH, or multiple bonds).
5. Remember to specify the isomer, if relevant (such as *cis* or *trans*, *R* or *S*, etc.).

PRACTICE QUESTIONS

1. What is the most appropriate IUPAC name for the structure shown below?

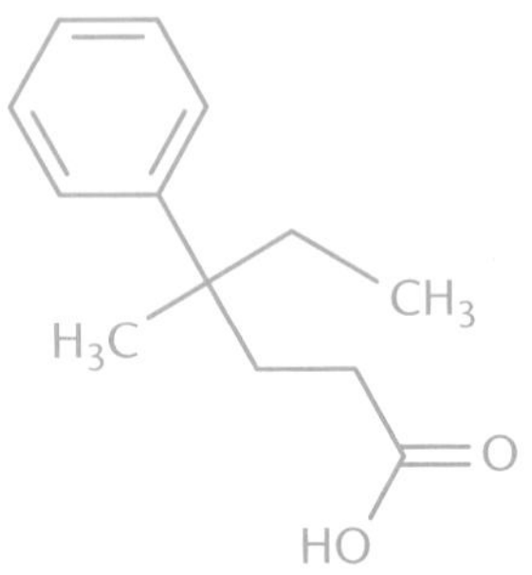

A. 4-methyl-4-phenylhexanoic acid
B. 4-ethyl-4-phenylpentanoic acid
C. 4-methyl-4-phenylhexanal
D. 4-carboxy-1-ethyl-1-methylbenzene

2. Name the compound below according to IUPAC convention.

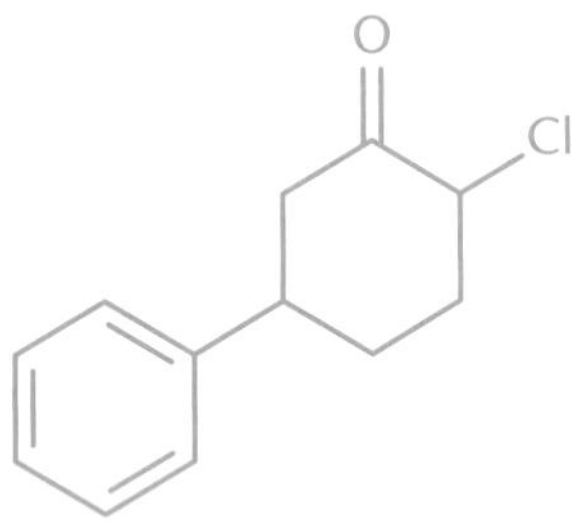

A. 4-chloro-3-oxo-1-phenylcyclohexane
B. Para-chlorophenylcyclohexan-1-one
C. 2-chloro-5-phenylcyclohexanone
D. 6-chloro-3-phenylcyclohexanone

3. In the figure below, what is the correct name for the molecule shown in the Haworth projection?

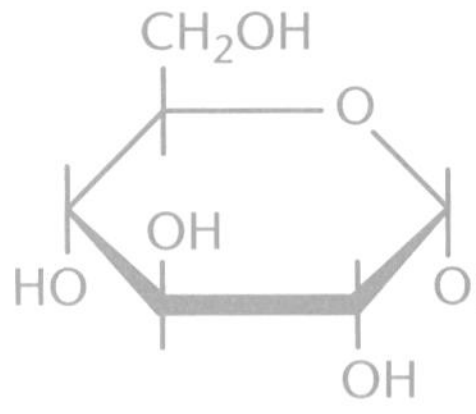

A. α-L-glucose
B. α-glucose
C. β-L-glucose
D. β-D-glucose

4. Which of the following is the most appropriate IUPAC name for the structure shown below?

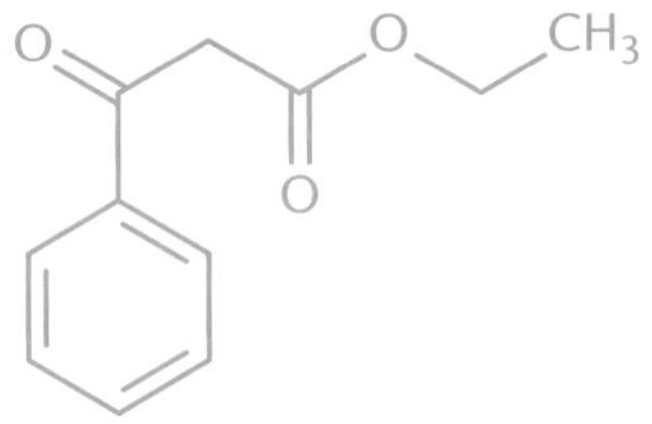

A. 1,3-dioxo-3-phenylethyl ether
B. 1,3-dioxo-3-phenyl-1-ethoxypropane
C. 3-oxo-3-phenylpropanoic acid
D. Ethyl 3-oxo-3-phenylpropanoate

5. The IUPAC name for the structure below ends with what suffix?

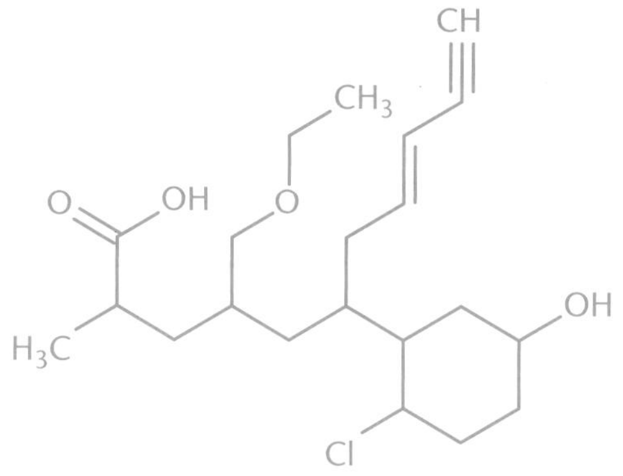

A. –ol
B. –ide
C. –oic acid
D. -yne

KEY CONCEPTS

Nomenclature

Functional group priority

TAKEAWAYS

The key to the nomenclature problems is to be as systematic as possible. Don't try to do everything at once, or you risk confusing yourself.

THINGS TO WATCH OUT FOR

Don't forget to include parentheses if a substituent is further substituted, so that you don't confuse the two numbering systems.

NOMENCLATURE

What is the IUPAC name for the following compound?

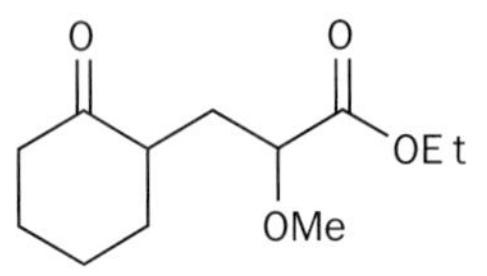

---

1) Identify the highest priority functional group.

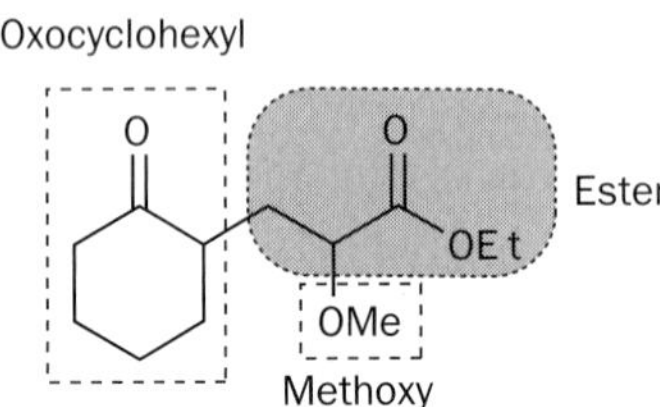

In this case, the highest priority functional group is the ester. Therefore, we will name everything attached to the ester as a substituent, including the cyclohexyl ring on the left.

---

2) Determine the longest continuous carbon chain attached to the highest priority functional group, and number them accordingly.

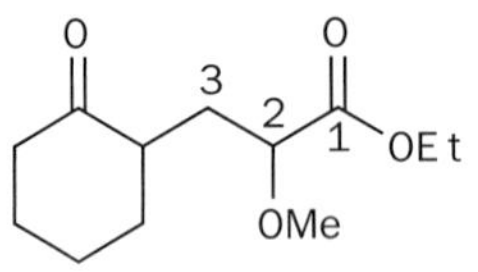

In this case, the longest continuous chain is three carbons, with carbon 1 being the carbonyl carbon (because the ester is the highest priority functional group). Because the ester has three carbons, it will be a propanoate ester.

---

3) Locate the substituents on the carbon chain identified in step 2, and name and number them.

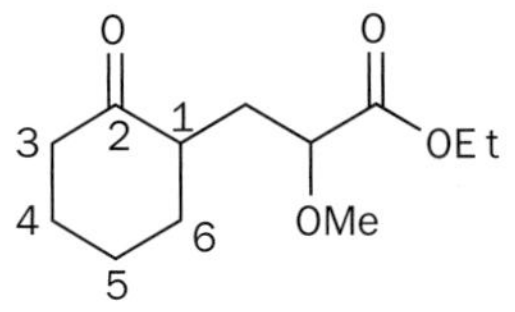

The first substituent is the ethyl group on the ester, which we will name by placing the word "ethyl" in front of the ester name.

Next, there is a methyl group attached to an oxygen at carbon 2, which will be named as a methoxy group.

Finally, how do we handle the ring attached to carbon 3? If there were nothing attached to the ring, we would name the ring as a cyclohexyl substituent. However, there is a ketone on the ring. When there are aldehydes or ketones that are named as substituents, recall that they are named as "oxo" groups. The numbering works by assigning the carbon attached to the ester carbon chain as carbon 1 as shown.

Therefore, the ketone on the ring will be at carbon 2. We'll name the whole ring as a (2-oxocyclohexyl) substituent, and put it in parentheses so that we don't confuse the two numbering systems.

---

4) Put it all together.
The name of our compound will therefore be:

Ethyl 2–methoxy–3–(2–oxocyclohexyl)propanoate

SIMILAR QUESTIONS

1) How would the name be altered if the alkyl group attached to the ester oxygen contained substituents?
2) Upon reduction with sodium borohydride, followed by dilute acid workup, the molecule below gave two products in unequal yield. Draw them and provide the correct IUPAC name for each.

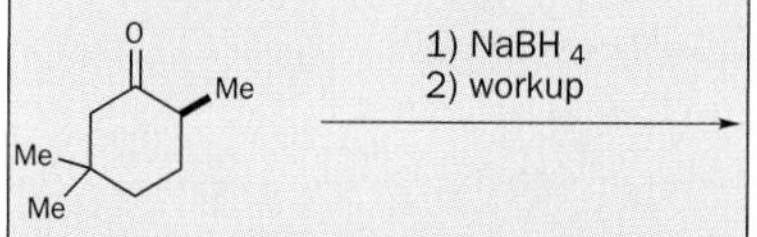

O, Me, Me, Me — 1) $NaBH_4$ 2) workup →

3) What are the two possible products of the reaction shown below? Draw and provide IUPAC names for both.

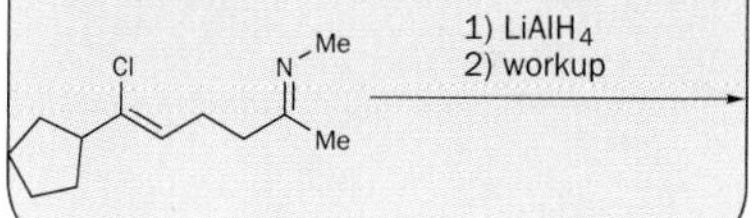

Cl, N, Me, Me — 1) $LiAlH_4$ 2) workup →

CHAPTER 2

ISOMERS

Isomers are chemical compounds that have the same molecular formula but differ in structure—that is, in their atomic connectivity, rotational orientation, or the three-dimensional position of their atoms. Isomers may be extremely similar, sharing most or all of their physical and chemical properties, or they may be very different.

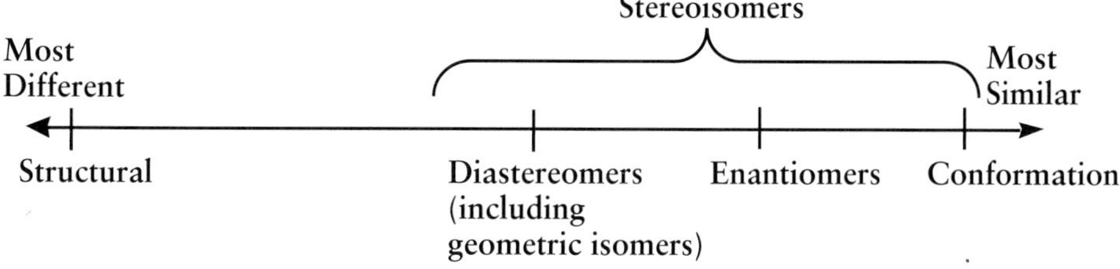

Structural isomers are the most unlike each other, while conformational isomers are the most similar.

STRUCTURAL ISOMERISM

Structural isomers are compounds that share only their molecular formula. Because their atomic connections may be completely different, they often have very different chemical and physical properties (such as melting point, boiling point, solubility, etc.). For example, five different structures exist for compounds with the formula C_6H_{14}.

TEACHER TIP

Structural isomers all have the same molecular formula but different atomic connectivity. The various shapes and functional groups cause different physical and chemical properties, respectively.

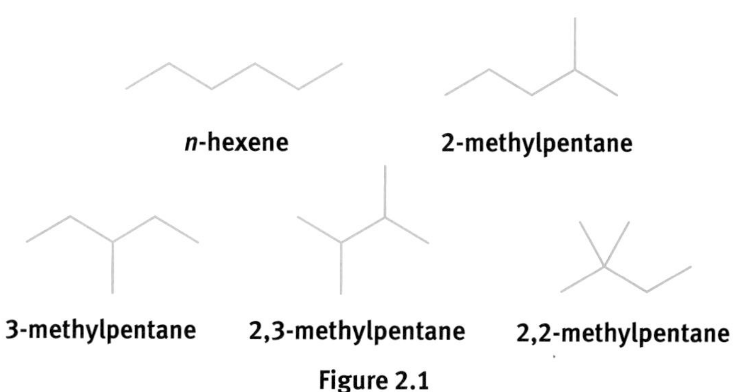

Figure 2.1

All have the same formula, but they differ in their carbon framework and in the number and type of atoms bonded to each other.

TEACHER TIP

Stereoisomers have the same connectivity but different orientations in three-dimensional space. Because they have the same functional groups (due to the same connectivity), then they'll have the same chemical properties, but with different shapes they may have different physical properties.

STEREOISOMERISM

Stereoisomers are compounds that differ from each other only in the way that their atoms are oriented in space. Geometric isomers; enantiomers, diastereomers, and *meso* compounds; and conformational isomers all fall under this heading.

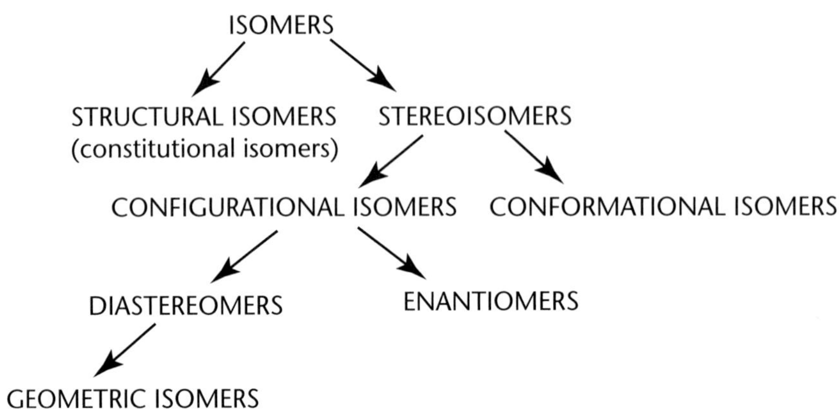

Figure 2.2

TEACHER TIP

Geometric isomers are a subset of diastereomers that differ only in their placement of groups around the double bond. This difference may affect their polarity and thereby their physical properties.

A. GEOMETRIC ISOMERS

Geometric isomers are compounds that differ in the position of substituents attached to a double bond. If two substituents are on the same side, the double bond is called ***cis.*** If they are on opposite sides, it is a ***trans*** double bond.

For compounds with polysubstituted double bonds, the situation can be confusing, and an alternative method of naming is employed. The highest priority substituent attached to each double-bonded carbon has to be determined: The higher the atomic number, the higher the priority, and if the atomic numbers are equal, priority is determined by the substituents of these atoms. The alkene is called **(*Z*)** (from the German *zusammen*, meaning "together") if the two highest priority substituents on each carbon lie on the same side of the double bond, and (*E*) (from the German *entgegen*, meaning opposite) if they are on opposite sides.

KAPLAN EXCLUSIVE

Z = zame zide (same side)
E = epposite (opposite sides)

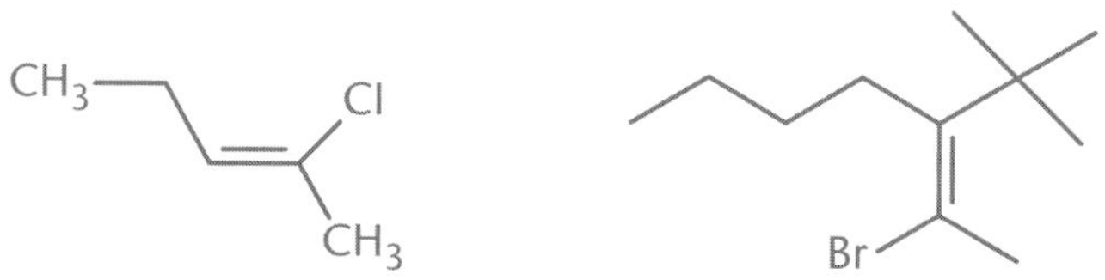

(*Z*)-2-chloro-2-pentene (*E*)-2-bromo-3-*t*-butyl-2-heptene

Figure 2.3

B. CHIRALITY

An object that is not superimposable upon its mirror image is called **chiral.** Familiar chiral objects are your right and left hands. Although essentially identical, they differ in their ability to fit into a right-handed glove. They are mirror images of each other, yet cannot be superimposed. **Achiral** objects are mirror images that can be superimposed; for example, the letter A is identical to its mirror image and therefore achiral.

> **MCAT SYNOPSIS**
> Chirality = handedness
> Nonsuperimposable mirror images exist—like your right and left hands.

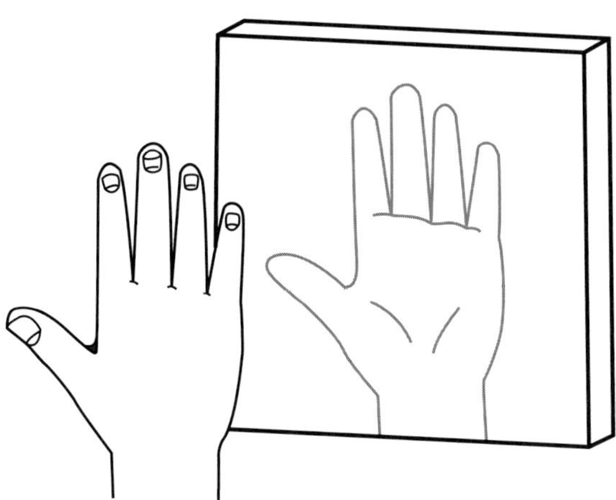

Figure 2.4

In organic chemistry, chirality is most frequently encountered when carbon atoms have four different substituents. Such a carbon atom is called *asymmetric* because it lacks a plane or point of symmetry. For example, the C–1 carbon atom in 1-bromo-1-chloroethane has four different substituents. The molecule is chiral because it is not superimposable on its mirror image. Chiral objects that are nonsuperimposable mirror images are called **enantiomers** and are a specific type of stereoisomer.

MCAT SYNOPSIS

Rotating a molecule in space does not change its chirality.

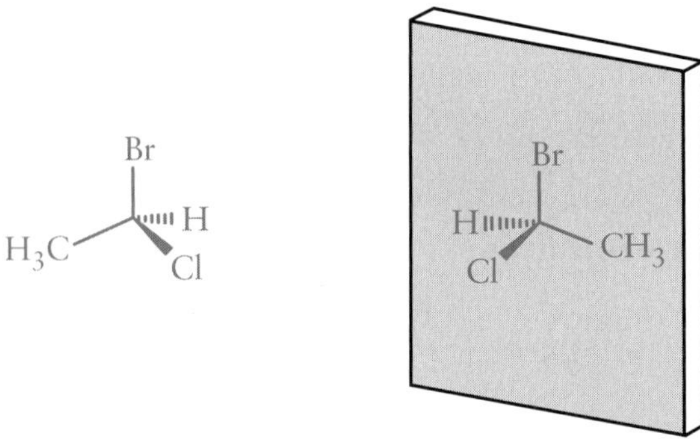

Figure 2.5

TEACHER TIP

On the exam, you may see a compound drawn to show three-dimensional orientation, but it is only chiral if four different groups are attached to the carbon.

A carbon atom with only three different substituents, such as 1, 1-dibromoethane, has a plane of symmetry and is therefore achiral. A simple 180° rotation along the *y*-axis allows the compound to be superimposed upon its mirror image.

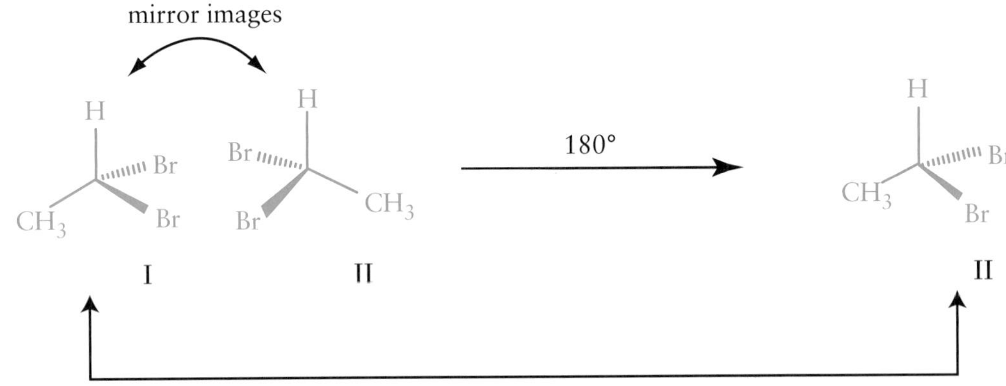

Figure 2.6

TEACHER TIP

Absolute configuration is similar to a state function in that they're both path independent. When dealing on the exam with chiral compounds in a reaction, don't assume the chirality is based on a "relative" relationship.

1. Relative and Absolute Configuration

The **configuration** is the spatial arrangement of the atoms or groups of a stereoisomer. The **relative configuration** of a chiral molecule is its configuration in relation to another chiral molecule. The **absolute configuration** of a chiral molecule describes the spatial arrangement of these atoms or groups. There is a set sequence to determine the absolute configuration of a molecule at a single chiral center:

Step 1:

Assign priority to the four substituents, looking only at the first atom that is directly attached to the chiral center. Higher atomic number takes precedence over lower atomic number. If the atomic numbers are equal, then priority is determined by the substituents attached to these atoms. For example:

Figure 2.7

Step 2:

Orient the molecule in space so that the line of sight proceeds down the bond from the asymmetric carbon atom (the chiral center) to the substituent with lowest priority. The three substituents with highest priority should radiate from the asymmetric atom like the spokes of a wheel.

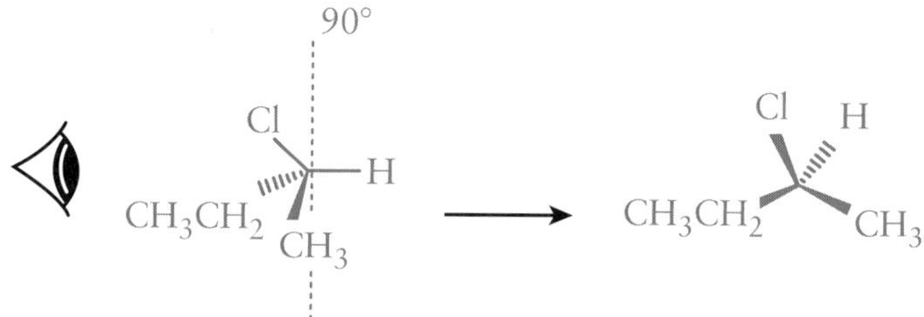

Figure 2.8

Step 3:

Proceeding from highest priority (#1) on down, determine the order of substituents around the wheel as either clockwise or counterclockwise. If the order is clockwise, the asymmetric atom is called ***R*** (from the Latin *rectus*, meaning "right"). If it is counterclockwise, it is called ***S*** (from the Latin *sinister*, meaning "left").

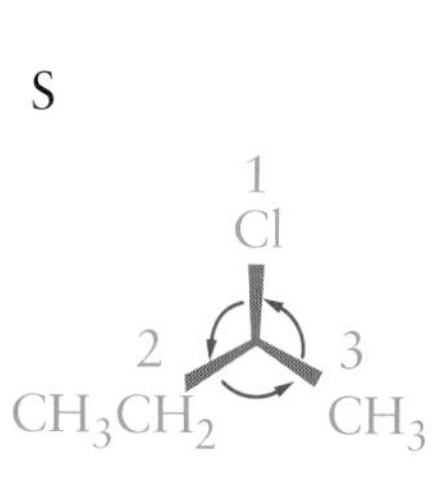

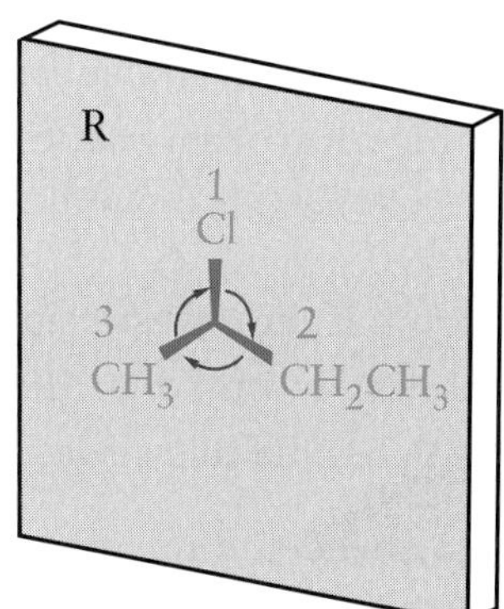

Figure 2.9

Teacher Tip

When assigning priority for chirality or to determine E and Z designations, look only at the first atom of the group that is attached to the carbon (which will be sufficient for most compounds on the MCAT) and move out one bond at a time, if necessary. Do not look at the whole group, and remember—the higher the atomic number, the higher the priority!

Teacher Tip

Before Test Day, practice manipulating molecules in your head to move the lowest priority in the back. If you have trouble doing that, there's also a different trick: If the lowest priority is pointing at you (the opposite of where you want it), then the configuration will be opposite of what it seems.

MCAT Synopsis

To determine the absolute configuration at a single chiral center:

1. Assign priority by atomic number.
2. Orient the molecule with the lowest priority substituent in the back.
3. Move around the molecule from highest to lowest priority ($1 \rightarrow 2 \rightarrow 3$).
4. Clockwise = *R*
   Counterclockwise = *S*.

Step 4:
Provide a full name for the compound. The terms *R* and *S* are put in parentheses and separated from the rest of the name by a dash. If there is more than one asymmetric carbon, location is specified by a number preceding the *R* or *S* within the parentheses, without a dash.

2. Fischer Projections
A three-dimensional molecule can be conveniently represented in two dimensions in a **Fischer projection.** In this system, horizontal lines indicate bonds that project out from the plane of the page, while vertical lines indicate bonds behind the plane of the page. The point of intersection of the lines represents a carbon atom. They can be interconverted by interchanging any two pairs of substituents, or by rotating the projection in the plane of the page by 180°. If only one pair of substituents is interchanged, or if the molecule is rotated by 90°, the mirror image of the original compound is obtained.

Teacher Tip

Chiral centers are present in different types of compounds. Enantiomers are a pair of compounds that are nonsuperimposable mirror images of one another. Diastereomers (except geometric isomers) have more than one chiral center and won't be mirror images of one another. Meso compounds will contain chiral centers, but because they have an internal plane of symmetry, the molecule itself will not be chiral or optically active.

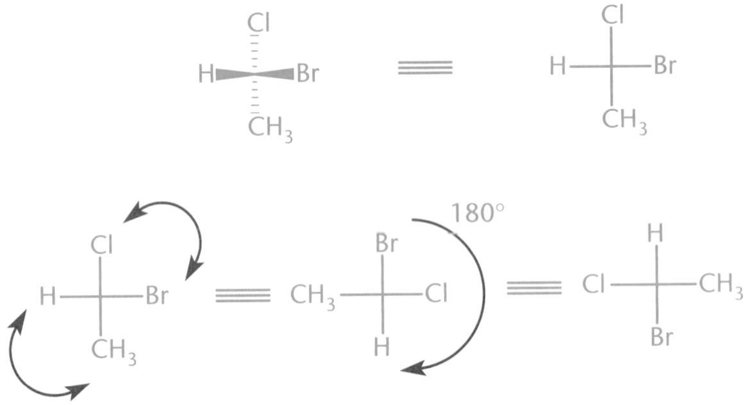

Figure 2.10

This provides another way to determine the chirality at a chiral center. If the lowest priority substituent is on the vertical axis, it is already pointing away from you. Simply picture moving from $\#1 \rightarrow \#2 \rightarrow \#3$, and you'll be able to name the center.

However, if the lowest priority substituent is on the horizontal axis, it is pointing toward you, and so the situation is trickier. Here are some ways to handle this situation:

1. Go ahead and imagine rotating from $\#1 \rightarrow \#2 \rightarrow \#3$. Obtain a designation (*R* or *S*). The *true* designation will be the opposite of what you have just obtained.

2. Alternatively, make a single switch—move the low priority substituent so that it is on the vertical axis. Obtain the designation (*R* or *S*). Again, the *true* designation will be the opposite of what you have just obtained.
3. Another approach is to make two switches or interconversions—that is, move the low-priority atom to the vertical axis and "trade" some other pair of atoms at the same time. This new molecule has the same configuration as the molecule you started with. So you can go ahead and determine the correct designation right away.

3. Optical Activity

Enantiomers have identical chemical and physical properties with one exception: **optical activity.** A compound is optically active if it has the ability to rotate plane-polarized light. Ordinary light is unpolarized. It consists of waves vibrating in all possible planes perpendicular to its direction of motion. A polarizer allows light waves oscillating only in a particular direction to pass, producing plane-polarized light.

TEACHER TIP

Optical activity is when plane-polarized light is shifted in one direction by a chiral molecule. It's like handedness in people: If we throw a tennis ball at a right-handed person, we can predict that he'd hit the ball in a different direction than a left-handed person. This is the same as a molecule where one enantiomer will rotate plane-polarized light in the opposite direction of its mirror image.

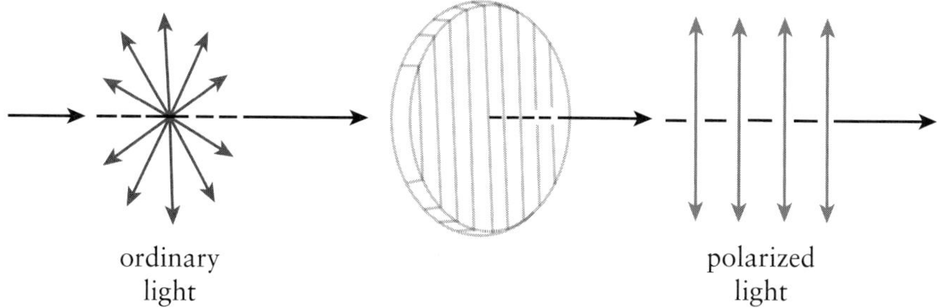

Figure 2.11

If plane-polarized light is passed through an optically active compound, the orientation of the plane is rotated by an angle α. The enantiomer of this compound will rotate light by the same amount, but in the opposite direction. A compound that rotates the plane of polarized light to the right, or clockwise (from the point of view of an observer seeing the light approach), is **dextrorotatory** and is indicated by (+). A compound that rotates light toward the left, or counterclockwise, is **levorotatory** and is labeled (–). The direction of rotation cannot be determined from the structure of a molecule and must be determined experimentally.

TEACHER TIP

The only thing we know about the relation of optical activity and the absolute configurations, *R* and *S*, is that they will be opposite one another. The direction of rotation is a relative property and must be experimentally determined.

The amount of rotation depends on the number of molecules that a light wave encounters. This depends on two factors: the concentration of the optically active compound and the length of the tube through which the light passes. Chemists have set standard conditions of

1 g/mL for concentration and 1 dm for length in order to compare the optical activities of different compounds. Rotations measured at different concentrations and tube lengths can be converted to a standardized **specific rotation** (α) using the following equation:

$$\text{specific rotation } ([\alpha]) = \frac{\text{observed rotation } (\alpha)}{\text{concentration (g/mL)} \times \text{length (dm)}}$$

MCAT SYNOPSIS

A racemic mixture displays no optical activity and is analogous to a person that is ambidextrous.

A **racemic mixture,** or **racemic modification,** is a mixture of equal concentrations of both the (+) and (–) enantiomers. The rotations cancel each other and no optical activity is observed.

C. OTHER CHIRAL COMPOUNDS

1. Diastereomers

For any molecule with n chiral centers, there are 2^n possible stereoisomers. Thus, if a compound has two chiral carbon atoms, it has four possible stereoisomers (see Figure 2.12).

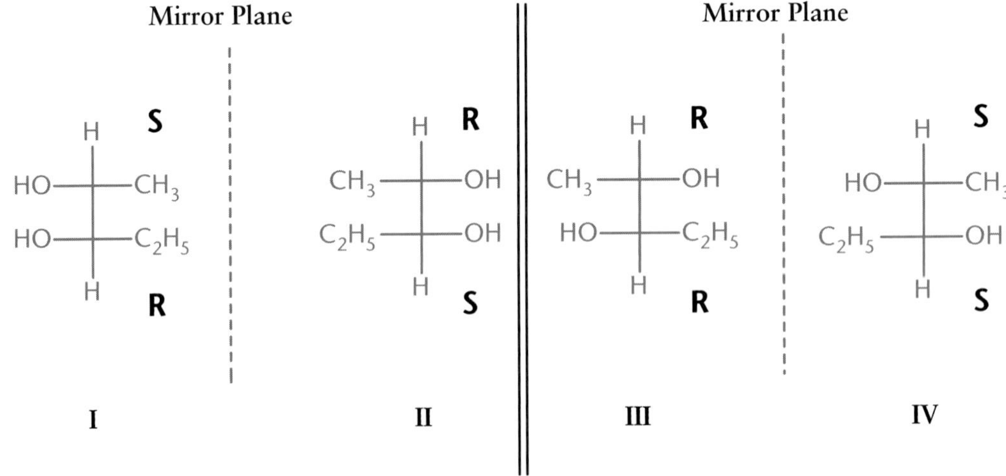

Figure 2.12

TEACHER TIP

Diastereomers will have the same functional group, meaning they'll have the same chemical reactivity. But because they have different arrangements in space, they'll have different physical properties.

I and II are mirror images of each other and are therefore enantiomers. Similarly, III and IV are enantiomers. However, I and III are not. They are stereoisomers that are not mirror images, and so they are called **diastereomers.** Notice that other combinations of nonmirror image stereoisomers are also diastereomeric. Hence I and IV, II and III, I and III, and II and IV are all pairs of diastereomers.

2. Meso Compounds

The criterion for optical activity of a molecule containing a single chiral center is that it has no plane of symmetry. The same criterion applies to a molecule with two or more chiral centers. If a plane of symmetry exists, the molecule is not optically active, even though it possesses chiral centers. Such a molecule is called a *meso* compound. For example:

COOH	COOH	COOH
H—OH	H—OH	HO—H
	- - - Line of Symmetry	
HO—H	H—OH	H—OH
COOH	COOH	COOH
L-tartaric acid	***Meso* -tartaric acid**	**D-tartaric acid**

Figure 2.13

> **KAPLAN EXCLUSIVE**
>
> MeSo compounds have a Mirror plane of Symmetry

D- and L-tartaric acid are both optically active, but *meso*-tartaric acid has a plane of symmetry and is not optically active. Although *meso*-tartaric acid has two chiral carbon atoms, the lack of optical activity is a function of the molecule as a whole.

D. CONFORMATIONAL ISOMERISM

Conformational isomers are compounds that differ only by rotation about one or more single bonds. Essentially, these isomers represent the same compound in a slightly different position—analogous to a person who may be either standing up or sitting down. These different conformations can be seen when the molecule is depicted in a **Newman projection,** in which the line of sight extends along a carbon-carbon bond axis. The conformations are encountered as the molecule is rotated about this axis. The classic example for demonstrating conformational isomerism in a straight chain is *n*-butane. In a Newman projection, the line of sight extends through the C–2—C–3 bond axis.

> **MCAT SYNOPSIS**
>
> Think of conformational isomers as being different positions (conformations) of a compound—like a person who may be standing up or sitting down. Thus, they are often easily interconverted.

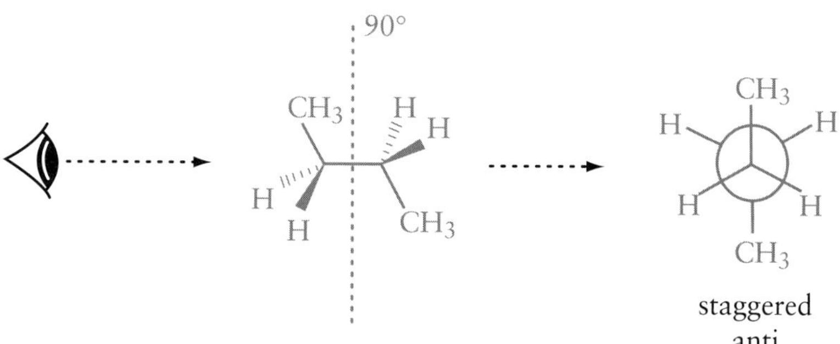

Figure 2.14

1. Straight-Chain Conformations

The most stable conformation is when the two methyl groups (C–1 and C–4) are oriented 180° from each other. There is no overlap of atoms along the line of sight (besides C–2 and C–3), so the molecule is said to be in a

staggered conformation. Specifically, it is called the ***anti*** conformation, because the two methyl groups are antiperiplanar to each other. This particular orientation is very stable and thus represents an energy minimum because all atoms are far apart, minimizing repulsive steric interactions.

Kaplan Exclusive

It's "gauche" (or inappropriate) for one methyl group to stand too close to another group!

The other type of staggered conformation, called ***(gauche),*** occurs when the two methyl groups are 60° apart. In order to convert from the *anti* to the *gauche* conformation, the molecule must pass through an **eclipsed** conformation, in which the two methyl groups are 120° apart and overlap with the H atoms on the adjacent carbon. When the two methyl groups overlap with each other, the molecule is said to be **totally eclipsed** and is in its highest energy state.

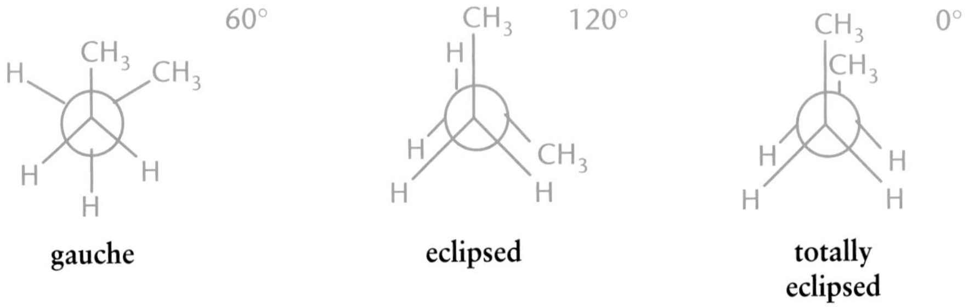

60° 120° 0°

gauche **eclipsed** **totally eclipsed**

Figure 2.15

A plot of potential energy versus the degree of rotation about the C–2—C–3 bond shows the relative minima and maxima the molecule encounters throughout its various conformations.

Teacher Tip

Notice that the *anti* isomer (A and G) has the lowest energy, while the totally eclipsed (D) has the highest energy.

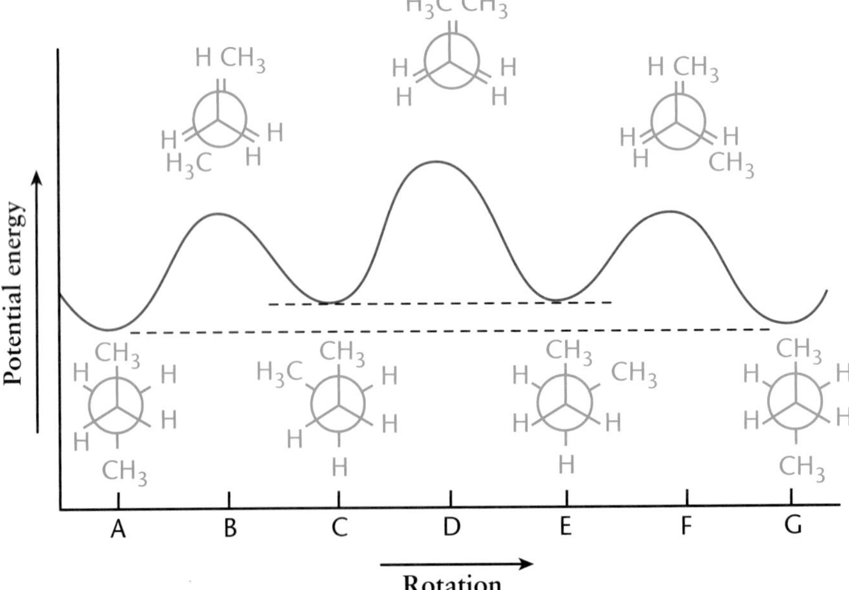

Figure 2.16

It is important to note that these barriers are rather small (3–4 kcal/ mol) and are easily overcome at room temperature. Very low temperatures will slow conformational interconversion. If the molecules do not possess sufficient energy to cross the energy barrier, they may not rotate at all.

2. Cyclic Conformations

a. Strain Energies

In cycloalkanes, ring strain arises from three factors: angle strain, torsional strain, and nonbonded strain. Angle strain results when bond angles deviate from their ideal values; torsional strain results when cyclic molecules must assume conformations that have eclipsed interactions; and nonbonded strain (van der Waals repulsion) results when atoms or groups compete for the same space. In order to alleviate these three types of strain, cycloalkanes attempt to adopt nonplanar conformations. Cyclobutane puckers into a slight V shape, cyclopentane adopts what is called the **envelope** conformation, and cyclohexane exists mainly in three conformations called the **chair,** the **boat,** and the **twist** or **skew-boat.**

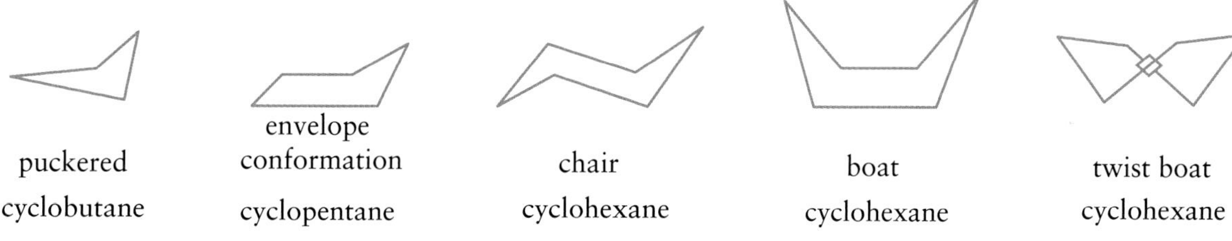

Conformations of cyclic hydrocarbons

Figure 2.17

b. Cyclohexane

i. Unsubstituted

The most stable conformation of cyclohexane is the chair conformation. In this conformation, all three types of strain are eliminated. The hydrogen atoms that are perpendicular to the plane of the ring are called **axial,** and those parallel are called **equatorial.** The axial-equatorial orientations alternate around the ring.

The boat conformation is adopted when the chair "flips" and converts to another chair. In such a process, hydrogen atoms that were equatorial become axial, and vice versa, in the new chair. In the boat conformation, all of the atoms are eclipsed, creating a high-energy state. To avoid this strain, the boat can twist into a slightly more stable form called the twist or skew-boat conformation.

KAPLAN EXCLUSIVE

- When you have low energy, you sit down in a chair to rest. Boats can be tippy, so they are less stable.
- Axial substituents are on a vertical axis, like your axial skeleton (skull and spine).
- Equatorial substituents go around the middle, like the earth's equator.

ii. Monosubstituted

The interconversion between the two chairs can be slowed or even prevented if a sterically bulky group is attached to the ring. The equatorial position is favored over the axial position because of steric repulsion with other axial substituents. Hence, a large group such as *t*-butyl can lock the molecule in one conformation.

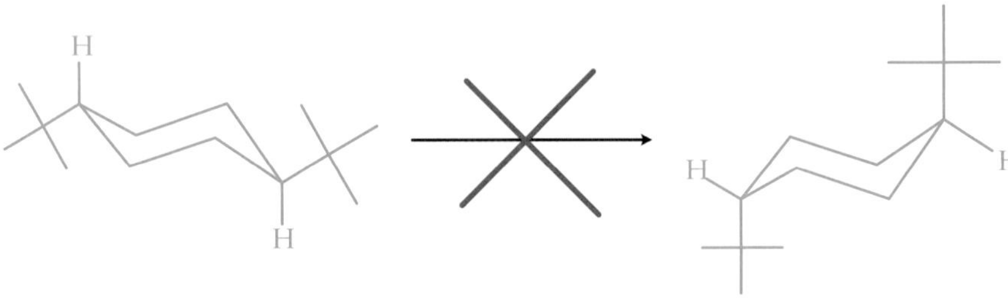

Bulky groups prefer equatorial positions

Figure 2.18

TEACHER TIP

A bulky substituent will favor one of the chair confirmations. The bulky groups will prefer to be equatorial so that they'll minimize the steric repulsion.

iii. Disubstituted

Different isomers can exist for disubstituted cycloalkanes. If both substituents are located on the same side of the ring, the molecule is called ***cis***; if the two groups are on opposite sides of the ring, it is called ***(trans)***.

TEACHER TIP

(Cis) and *(trans)* are used not only for simple alkenes, but also for multi-substituted cycloalkanes. On the exam, keep stereochemistry in mind because many a wrong answer will include an incorrect stereochemical designation (or will lack one that is needed).

cis-1,2-dimethylcyclohexane

trans-1,2-dimethylcyclohexane

Figure 2.19

In *trans*-1,4-dimethylcyclohexane, both of the methyl groups are equatorial in one chair conformation and axial in the other, but in either case they point in opposite directions relative to the plane of the ring.

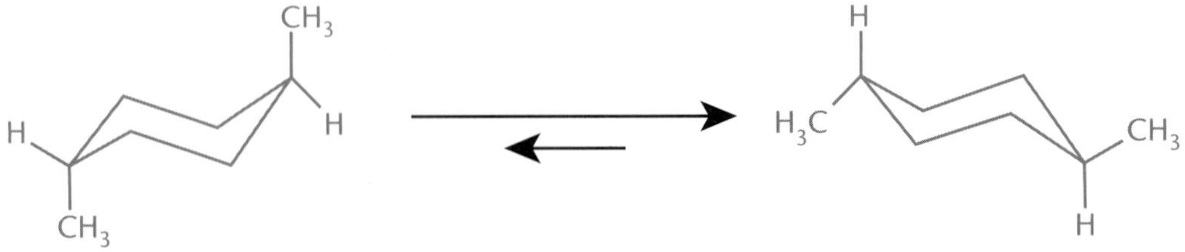

trans-1,4-dimethylcyclohexane

Figure 2.20

PRACTICE QUESTIONS

1. How many chiral centers are in the molecule shown below?

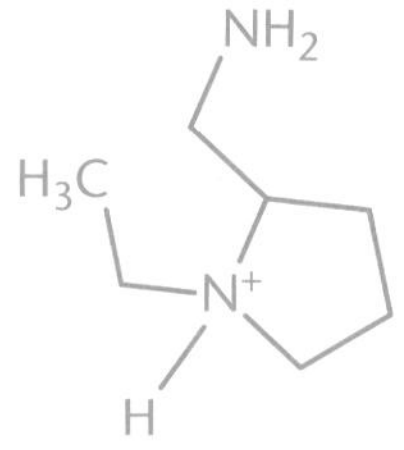

A. 0
B. 1
C. 2
D. 3

2. What is the most appropriate R-/S-naming prefix for the compound shown below?

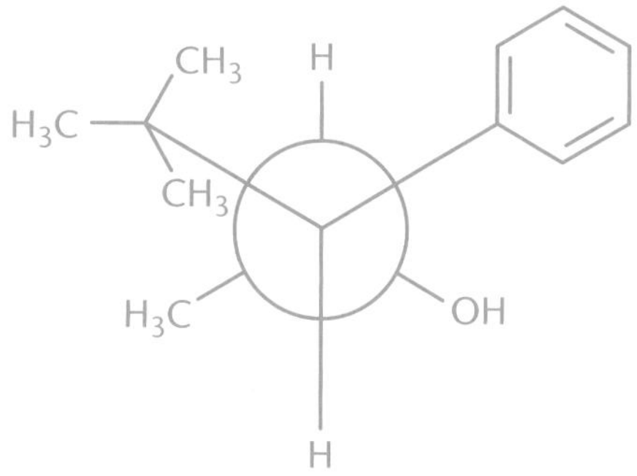

A. (3S,4S)-
B. (2R,3S)-
C. (3S,4R)-
D. (2R,3R)-

3. Which of the following statements is NOT true of the molecule shown below?

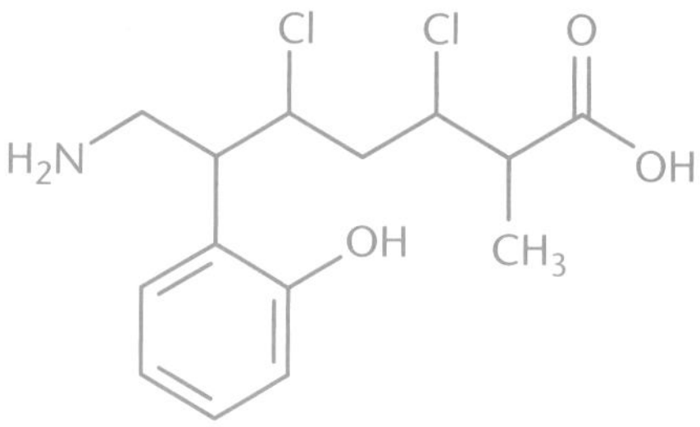

A. The compound is an amino acid.
B. The compound contains a primary amine and a phenol group.
C. The IUPAC name for the compound ends with the suffix -oic acid.
D. The compound has 32 possible stereoisomers.

4. The compound shown below is reacted with Br_2. Which of the following is the most likely major product?

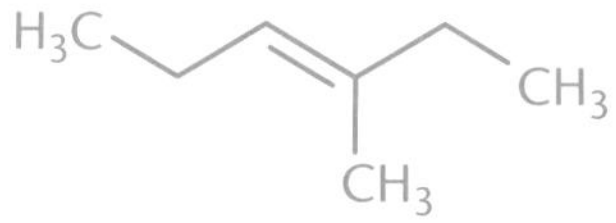

A. *Cis-* and *trans*-3,4-dibromo-3-methylhexane
B. *Trans*-3,4-dibromo-3-methylhexane
C. *Cis*-3,4-dibromo-3-methylhexane
D. 3-Bromo-3-methylhexane

KEY CONCEPTS

Isomers

Enantiomers

Diastereomers

TAKEAWAYS

Be as systematic as possible in assigning isomeric relationships in order to avoid making mistakes and missing easy points on Test Day! Follow the flowchart provided in the Lesson Book to accomplish this goal.

THINGS TO WATCH OUT FOR

Avoid confusing *enantiomers* and *diastereomers*. This is where a great many mistakes are made on MCAT questions. Remember that if two molecules are nonsuperimposable mirror images, they are enantiomers. Provided that you have determined that the molecules are configurational isomers without a plane of symmetry, *any other molecules are diastereomers.*

ISOMERS

The reagent *meta*–chloroperoxybenzoic acid (mCPBA) is often used to convert alkenes to epoxides. If the alkene shown below is treated with mCPBA, two products result. Draw these products and determine their isomeric relationship.

Me, OH, Me, mCPBA, $CHCl_3$, ?

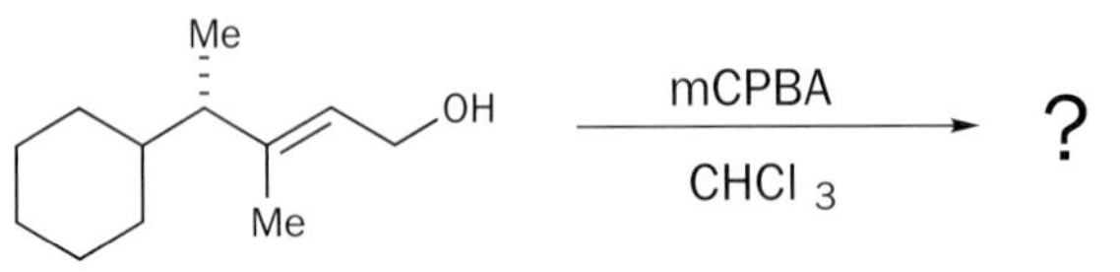

1) Draw the product(s) and note the major differences between them.

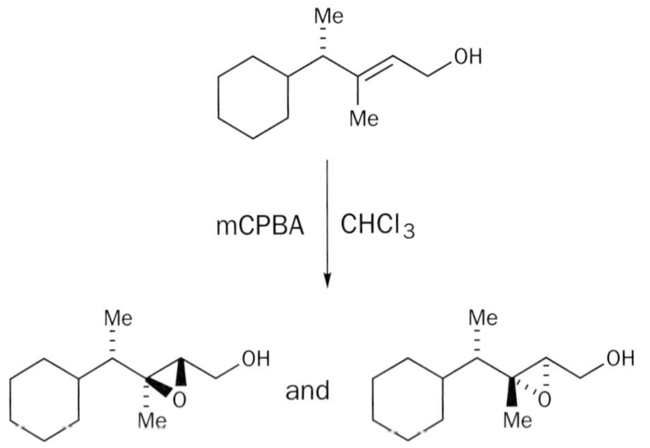

Me, OH, Me, mCPBA, $CHCl_3$

Me, OH, O, Me and Me, OH, O, Me

Recall that alkenes are flat due to both carbons being sp^2 hybridized. Therefore, the epoxide can form on either face of the alkene, giving rise to two possible products.

Notice that each isomer differs only in the stereochemical sense.

---

2) Determine the isomeric relationship.

The first question you should ask yourself is whether or not the molecules have the same connectivity. Here, they do because they differ only in the orientation of two stereocenters, so they are not structural isomers.

Next, you need to figure out whether bond breaking would be required to interconvert them. Here, that is definitely true because to convert the top isomer to the bottom one, you would have to break both epoxide carbon–oxygen bonds and reassemble them on the opposite face of the molecule. Therefore, our molecules are configurational isomers.

Then, you will want to see if the molecules are nonsuperimposable mirror images of one another.

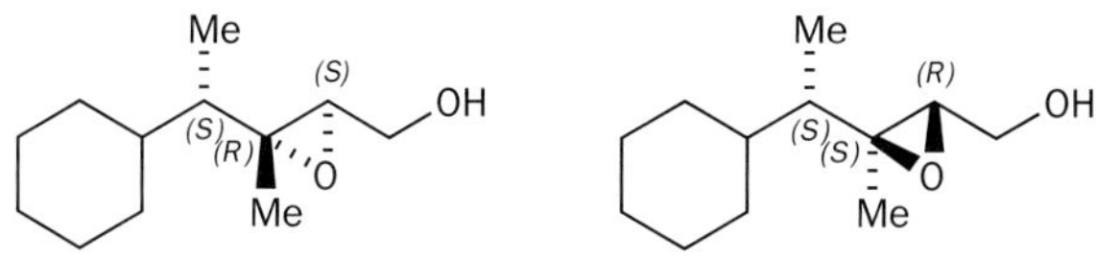

The molecules are not nonsuperimposable mirror images of one another because the stereocenter adjacent to the cyclohexyl ring has the same orientation in both products. (Note that the carbon where the ring is joined to the acyclic portion of the molecule is *not* a stereocenter. Why?) Therefore, our two molecules are *diastereomers*.

You can confirm this by assigning *R/S* designations to each stereocenter and then seeing that some of the stereocenters have the same orientation and some are different. For our two molecules to be *enantiomers,* each stereocenter would have to have the opposite orientation in each product.

SIMILAR QUESTIONS

1) Alkynes can be reduced to alkenes selectively by manipulating the reaction conditions. Examine the reaction scheme below and determine the relationship between the two products.

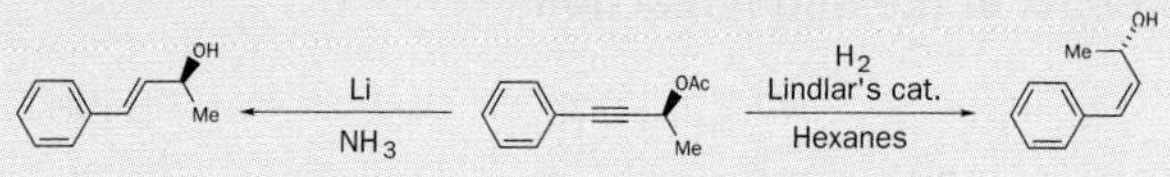

2) If the alkenes in question 1 were reduced with Pd/H_2, would the isomeric relationship change?

3) Would the physical properties of the alkenes in question 1 be the same or different? What about when the alkenes were reduced?

KEY CONCEPTS

- Stereochemistry
- Fischer projections
- Oxidation/reduction
- *Meso* compounds

TAKEAWAYS

Anytime a molecule with stereocenters behaves as an achiral molecule, that must mean there is a plane of symmetry somewhere in the molecule.

THINGS TO WATCH OUT FOR

With molecules with multiple stereocenters, be sure to draw them as Fischer projections to be able to spot the symmetry planes easily.

MESO COMPOUNDS

A student wanted to prepare chiral polyols by taking sugars and reacting them with sodium borohydride. She took D-xylose, shown below, and treated it with sodium borohydride, followed by a dilute aqueous acid workup. On purifying and isolating the product, she found that it did not rotate plane-polarized light. What was the structure of the product and why did it not rotate light?

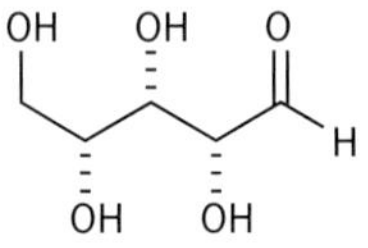

D-xylose

1) Convert the molecule from standard projection to Fischer projection.

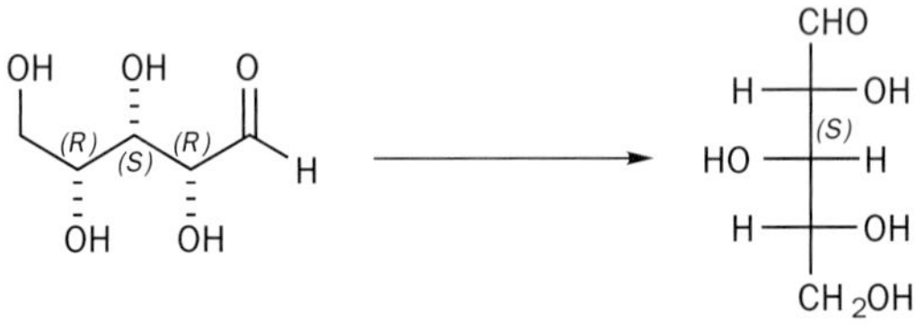

This will enable you to see stereochemical relationships much more clearly.

---

2) Draw the product of the initial reaction.

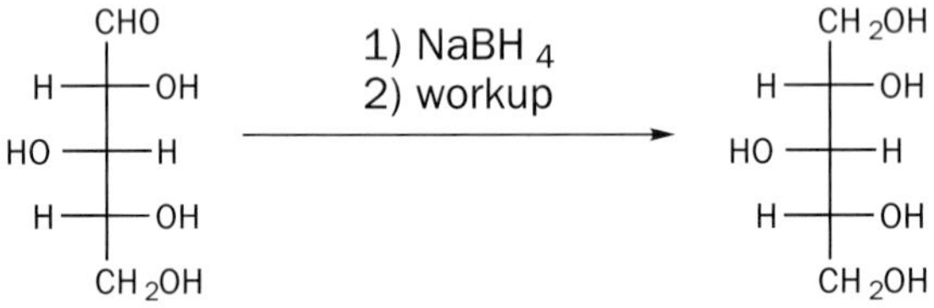

1) $NaBH_4$
2) workup

In this case, sodium borohydride reduces the aldehyde to an alcohol.

---

3) Look for planes of symmetry in the product.

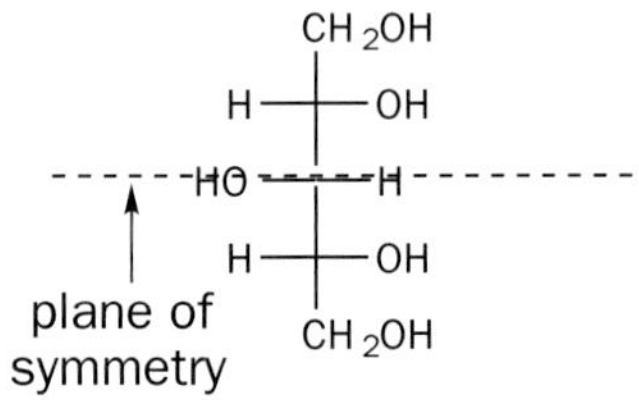

plane of symmetry

The fact that a molecule possesses stereocenters but is achiral is a dead giveaway that the molecule must be a *meso* compound. This would be caused by a plane of symmetry in the molecule. The plane of symmetry runs right through C3 in this case.

SIMILAR QUESTIONS

1) Which of the remaining three D–aldopentoses (shown below) would result in achiral polyols when subjected to borohydride reduction?

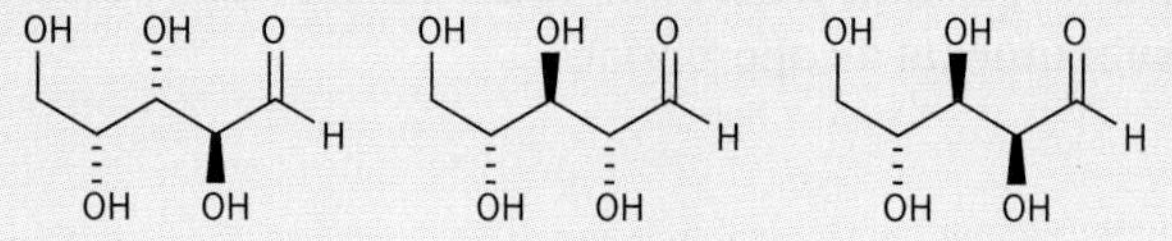

Key Concepts

Stereochemistry

Fischer projections

Stereocenter

Takeaways

Assigning priorities is based on atomic number and is done one atom at a time. When you "turn" from the highest priority to the lowest priority substituent, think about the three highest priority substituents as being on a steering wheel in a car, with the lowest priority substituent as the steering column.

Things to Watch Out For

Don't forget that if a substituent is attached to a horizontal bond in a Fischer projection, that means that it is *coming out of the page at you.* If it is attached to a vertical bond, it is *going into the page away from you.*

FISCHER PROJECTIONS

Redraw the following molecule in a Fischer projection:

HO OH O H OH

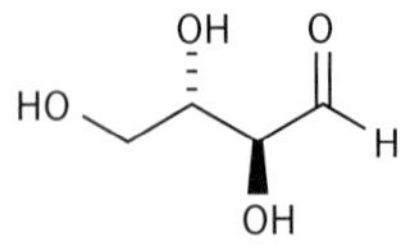

1) Begin by drawing a flat vertical line to account for all of the stereocenters. Draw in end substituents as appropriate.

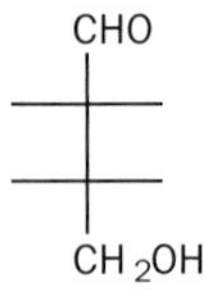

CHO

CH_2OH

2) Determine the stereochemical orientation of the stereocenters in the original molecule by assigning *R*/*S* to each.

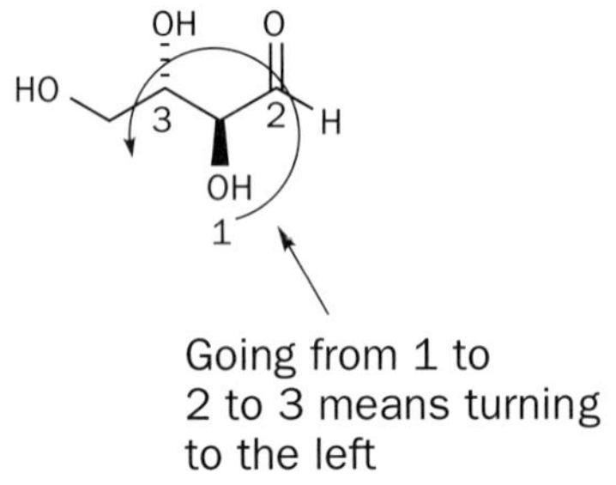

HO OH O 3 2 H OH 1

Going from 1 to 2 to 3 means turning to the left

For the stereocenter adjacent to the aldehyde, the alcohol is the highest priority substituent, followed by the aldehyde, then the carbon with the other stereocenter, and finally the hydrogen. Because the hydrogen is already oriented away from us, we can go ahead and assign the stereocenter to be *S*, because we "turn the wheel" to the left.

Applying the same methodology to the other stereocenter gives an *S* stereocenter as well.

MCAT Pitfall: *Be careful with assigning the second stereocenter because the hydrogen is coming out of the page at you.*

3) Draw in the substituents in the Fischer projection and make sure that they match the original molecule.

CHO
HO—+—H
H—+—OH
CH_2OH

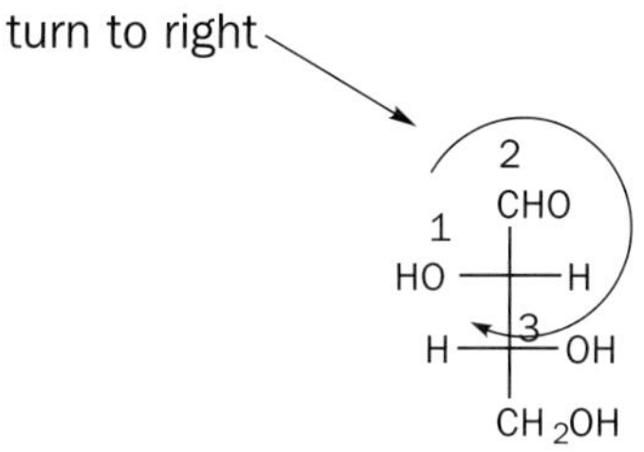

turn to right

2
CHO
1
HO—+—H
H—+—OH 3
CH_2OH

S CHO
HO—+—H
H—+—OH
CH_2OH
R

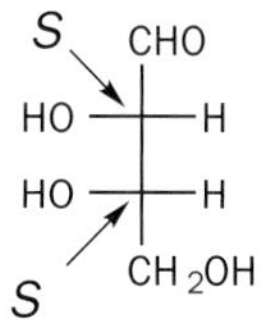

S CHO
HO—+—H
HO—+—H
CH_2OH
S

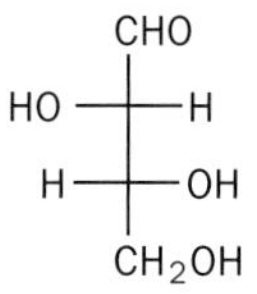

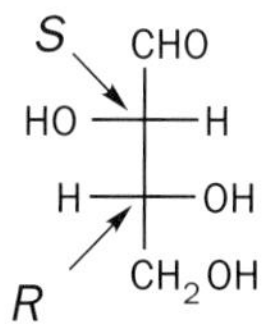

At this point, you can randomly insert the substituents and check to make sure that they match the original molecule. Assigning priorities as before.

For the first stereocenter, we would turn to the right, meaning that you would think it would be *R*. However, note that the lowest priority substituent, the hydrogen, is coming *out of the page* because it is attached to a horizontal line; we want the hydrogen to be going into the page. So, we would flip the assignment from *R* to *S*. The first stereocenter then matches. Applying the same idea to the second stereocenter would give an *R* assignment.

However, we need the *S*, *S* compound. So, we can do that by just exchanging the alcohol and the proton in the second stereocenter.

SIMILAR QUESTIONS

1) Draw the Fischer projection of the enantiomer compound.
2) Draw the Fischer projection of all the diastereomers for the compound and the compound's enantiomer, diagramming the relationships between each.
3) Fumaric acid (trans-2-butenedioic acid) can undergo *syn* addition with D_2. Draw the Fischer projection of the product(s). If multiple products are produced, what is the relationship between them?

CHAPTER 3

BONDING

As discussed in General Chemistry, there are two types of chemical bonds: **ionic,** in which an electron is transferred from one atom to another, and **covalent,** in which pairs of electrons are shared between two atoms. In organic chemistry, it is important to understand the details of covalent bonding, as these play a crucial role in determining the properties and reactions of organic compounds.

> **TEACHER TIP**
>
> In Organic Chemistry, we're primarily concerned with polar and nonpolar covalent bonds. These will have effects on the physical properties, which will be discussed in the chapter on Purification and Separation Techniques.

ATOMIC ORBITALS

The first three quantum numbers, n, l, and m, describe the size, shape, and number of the atomic orbitals that an element possesses. The number n, which can equal 1, 2, 3, . . , corresponds to the energy levels in an atom and is essentially a measure of size. Within each electron shell, there can be several types of orbitals (s, p, d, f, g, . . . , corresponding to the quantum numbers $l = 0, 1, 2, 3, 4, \ldots$). Each type of atomic orbital has a specific shape. An s orbital is spherical and symmetrical, and it is centered around the nucleus. A p orbital is composed of two lobes located symmetrically about the nucleus and contains a **node** (an area in which the probability of finding an electron is zero). A d orbital is composed of four symmetrical lobes and contains two nodes. Both d and f orbitals are complex in shape and are rarely encountered in organic chemistry.

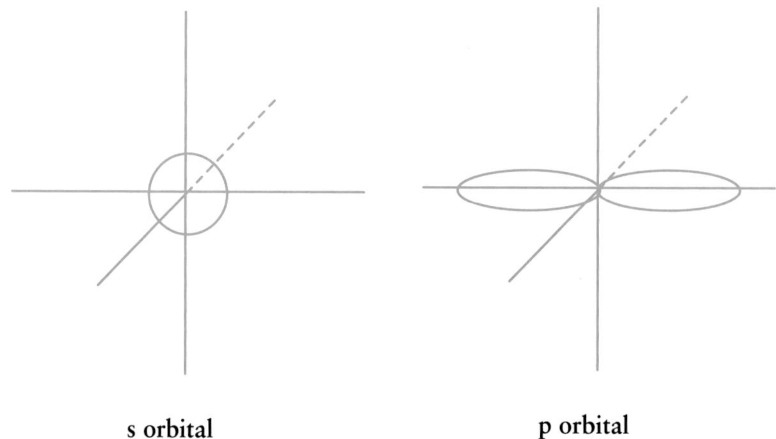

Figure 3.1

MOLECULAR ORBITALS

Teacher Tip

Orbitals might also be tested in the Physical Sciences section as part of the General Chemistry subject matter.

A. SINGLE BONDS

Two atomic orbitals can be combined to form what is called a **molecular orbital (MO).** Molecular orbitals are obtained mathematically by adding the wave functions of the atomic orbitals. If the signs of the wave functions are the same, a lower-energy **bonding orbital** is produced. If the signs are different, a higher-energy **antibonding orbital** is produced. This is represented schematically by the addition of two s orbitals. Two p orbitals or one p and one s orbital can be combined in a similar fashion.

Teacher Tip

Sigma bonds are the most common and will be a big part of the organic compounds seen on the MCAT.

When a molecular orbital is formed by head-to-head overlap as in Figure 3.2, the resulting bond is called a **sigma (σ) bond**. All single bonds are sigma bonds, accommodating two electrons. Shorter single bonds are stronger than longer single bonds.

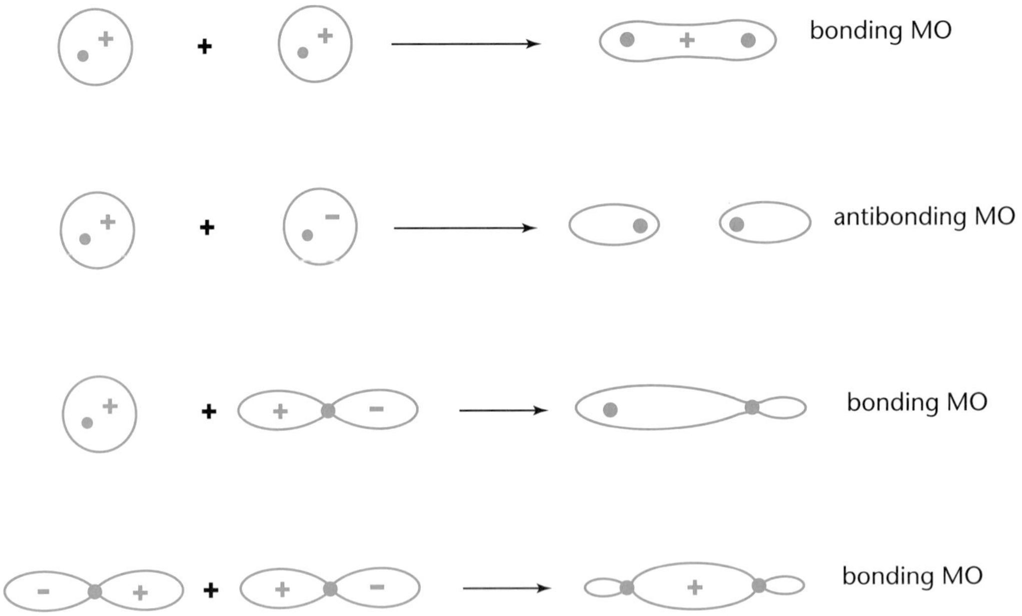

Figure 3.2

B. DOUBLE AND TRIPLE BONDS

When two p orbitals overlap in a parallel fashion, a bonding MO is formed, called a **pi (π) bond.** When both a sigma and a pi bond exist between two atoms, a **double bond** is formed. When a sigma bond and two pi bonds exist, a **triple bond** is formed. As can be seen in Figure 3.3, the overlap of the p orbitals involved in a p bond hinder rotation about double and triple bonds.

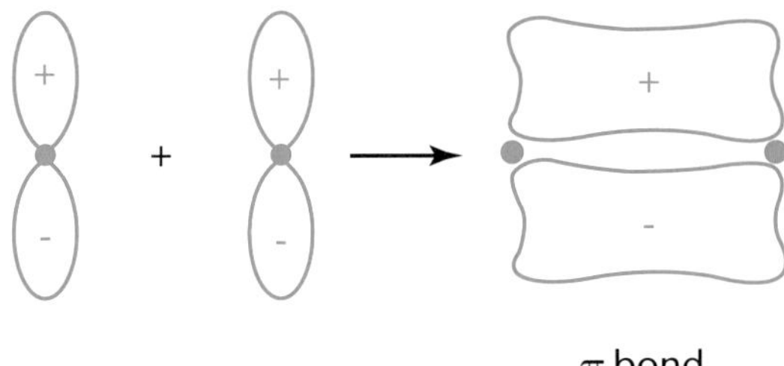

Figure 3.3

> **TEACHER TIP**
>
> A double bond consists of both a σ bond and a π bond (and a triple bond consists of a σ bond and 2π bonds). π bonds are weaker than σ bonds in isolation, but the strength is additive when it comes to double and triple bonds, making those stronger.

A pi bond cannot exist independently of a sigma bond. Only after the formation of a sigma bond will the p orbitals of adjacent carbons be parallel, because without the bond the three p orbitals are orthogonal to one another.

In general, pi bonds are weaker than sigma bonds; it is possible to break one bond of a double bond, leaving a single bond intact.

HYBRIDIZATION

The carbon atom has the electron configuration $1s^2 2s^2 2p^2$ and therefore needs four electrons to complete its octet. A typical molecule formed by carbon is methane, CH_4. Experimentation shows that the four sigma bonds in methane are equal. This is inconsistent with the unsymmetrical distribution of valence electrons: two electrons in the 2s orbital, one in the p_x orbital, one in the p_y orbital, and none in the p_z orbital.

A. SP³

The theory of **orbital hybridization** was developed to account for this discrepancy. Hybrid orbitals are formed by mixing different types of atomic orbitals. If one s orbital and three p orbitals are mathematically combined, the result is four sp^3 hybrid orbitals that have a new shape.

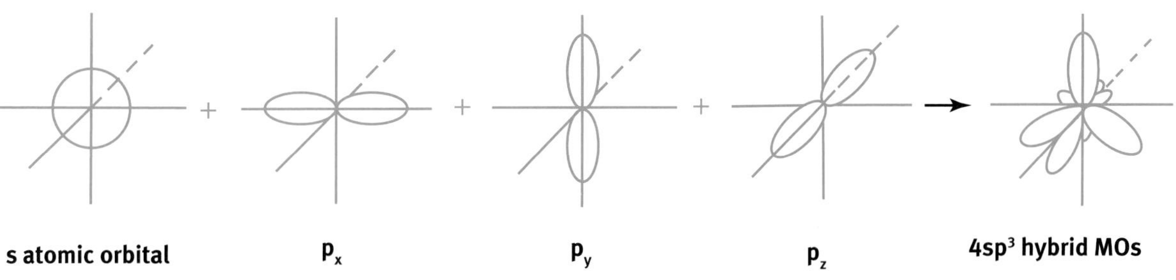

Figure 3.4

These four orbitals will point toward the vertices of a tetrahedron, minimizing repulsion. This explains the preferred tetrahedral geometry adopted by carbon.

The hybridization is accomplished by promoting one of the 2s electrons into the $2p_z$ orbital (see Figure 3.5). This produces four valence orbitals, each with one electron, which can be mathematically mixed to provide the hybrids.

TEACHER TIP

Hybridization is a way of making all of the bonds to a central atom equivalent to one another. The sp^3 orbitals are the reason for the tetrahedral shape which is a hallmark of carbon-containing compounds.

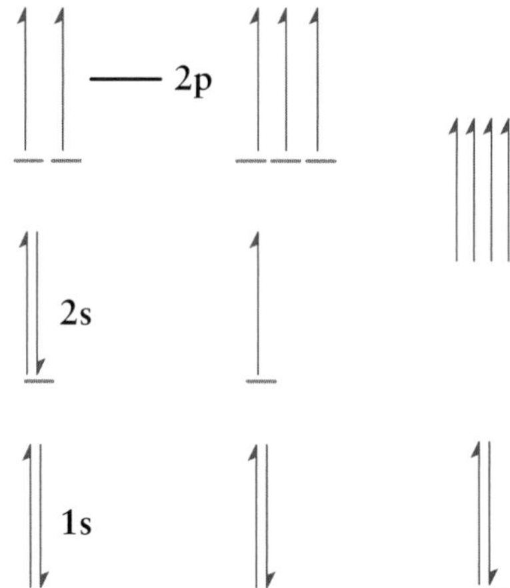

Figure 3.5

B. SP^2

Although carbon is most often found with sp^3 hybridization, there are other possibilities. If one s orbital and two p orbitals are mixed, three sp^2 hybrid orbitals are obtained.

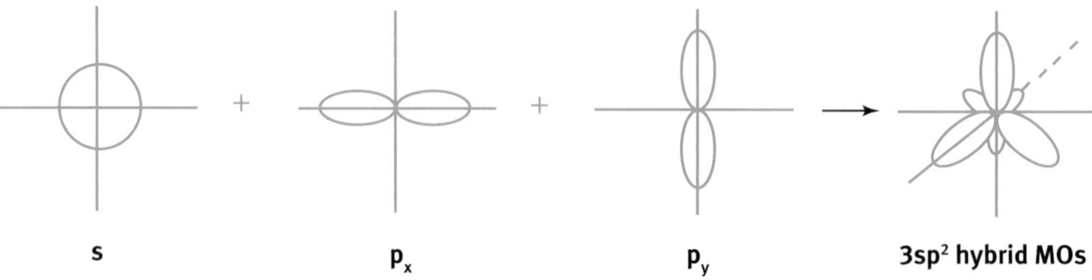

Figure 3.6

This occurs, for example, in ethylene. The third p orbital of each carbon atom is left unhybridized and participates in the pi bond. The three sp^2 orbitals are 120° apart, allowing maximum separation. These orbitals participate in the formation of the C–C and C–H single bonds.

C. SP

If two p orbitals are used to form a triple bond, and the remaining p orbital is mixed with an s orbital, two sp hybrid orbitals are obtained. They are oriented 180° apart, explaining the linear structure of molecules like acetylene.

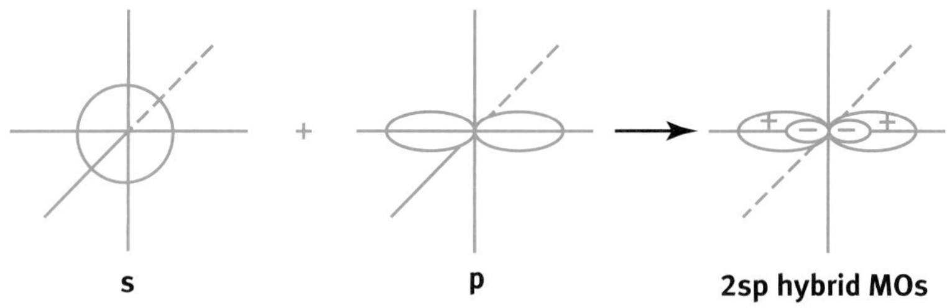

Figure 3.7

BONDING SUMMARY

The following table summarizes the major features of bonding in organic molecules.

Bond Order	Component Bonds	Hybridization	Angles	Examples
single	sigma	sp^3	109.5°	C–C; C–H
double	sigma pi	sp^2	120°	C=C; C=O
triple	sigma pi pi	sp	180°	C≡C; C≡N

PRACTICE QUESTIONS

1. Which of the following is true about carbon-carbon single bonds?

   A. They are comprised of one sigma and one pi bond.
   B. They are sp^2 hydridized.
   C. They have a bond angle of 109.5°.
   D. All of the above

2. Which of the following statements in NOT correct?

   A. SO_2 has no dipole moment.
   B. CO_2 has no dipole moment.
   C. The dipole moment of NH^3 is greater than NF^3.
   D. $BeCl_2$ has no dipole moment.

3. Which of the following is NOT a result of hydrogen bonding?

   A. The boiling point for H_2O is higher than HF.
   B. NH_3 is more soluble in water than CH_4.
   C. DMSO dissolves NaCl.
   D. The boiling point of 1-butanol is higher than its isomer diethyl ether.

4. Which of the following statements is correct?

   A. Benzene exhibits both sp^2 and sp^3 hybridized orbitals.
   B. 1-butyne exhibits both sp^2 and sp^3 hybridized orbitals.
   C. Propene exhibits both sp and sp^2 hybridized orbitals.
   D. 2,3-hexadiene exhibits sp, sp^2 and sp^3 hybridized orbitals.

CHAPTER 4

ALKANES

Alkanes are fully saturated hydrocarbons, compounds consisting only of hydrogen and carbon atoms joined by single bonds. Their general formula is C_nH_{2n+2}, which means they have the maximum possible number of hydrogen atoms attached to each carbon atom.

NOMENCLATURE

Once again, be sure that you are familiar with the common, frequently encountered names. These include:

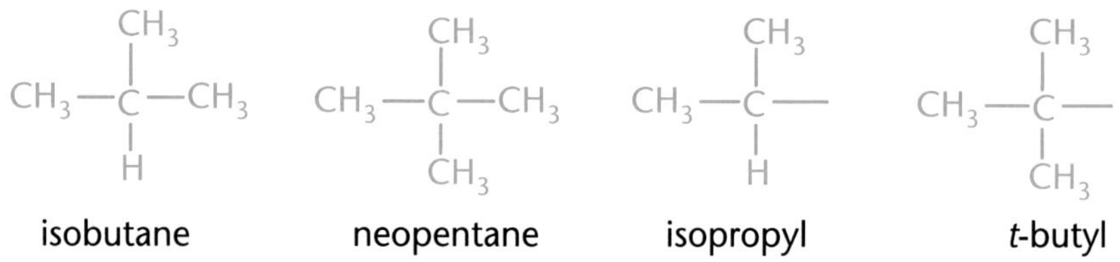

isobutane neopentane isopropyl *t*-butyl

Figure 4.1

Carbon atoms can be characterized by the number of other carbon atoms to which they are directly bonded. A **primary** carbon atom (written as **1°**) is bonded to only one other carbon atom. A **secondary (2°)** carbon is bonded to two; a **tertiary (3°)** to three, and a **quaternary (4°)** to four other carbon atoms. In addition, hydrogen atoms attached to 1°, 2°, or 3° carbon atoms are referred to as 1°, 2°, or 3°, respectively.

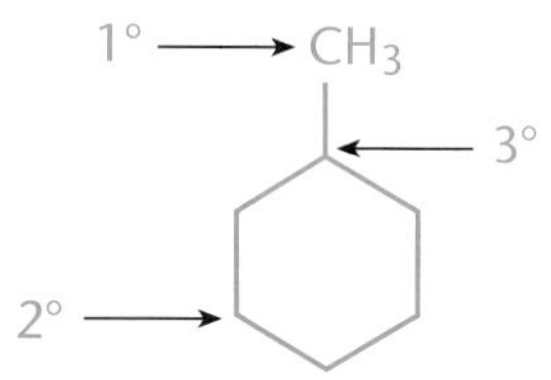

MCAT Favorite

The ability to identify 1°, 2°, and 3° carbons is crucial to determining the products of many chemical reactions and to understanding NMR spectroscopy.

Figure 4.2

IN A NUTSHELL

↑ chain length	↑ b.p. ↑ m.p. ↑ density
↑ branching	↓ b.p. ↓ m.p. ↓ density

PHYSICAL PROPERTIES

The physical properties of alkanes vary in a regular manner. In general, as the molecular weight increases, the melting point, boiling point, and density also increase. At room temperature, the straight-chain compounds C_1 through C_4 are gases, C_5 through C_{16} are liquids, and the longer-chain compounds are waxes and harder solids. Branched molecules have slightly lower boiling and melting points than their straight-chain isomers. Greater branching reduces the surface area of a molecule, decreasing the weak intermolecular attractive forces (van der Waals forces). Hence, the molecules are held together less tightly, effectively lowering the boiling point. In addition, branched molecules are more difficult to pack into a tight, three-dimensional structure. This difficulty is reflected in the lower melting points of branched alkanes.

REACTIONS

A. FREE RADICAL HALOGENATION

One frequently encountered reaction of alkanes are **halogenations,** in which one or more hydrogen atoms are replaced by halogen atoms (Cl, Br, or I) via a **free-radical substitution** mechanism. These reactions involve three steps:

1. **Initiation**—Diatomic halogens are homolytically cleaved by either heat or light (hν), resulting in the formation of free radicals. Free radicals are neutral species with unpaired electrons (such as Cl• or R_3C•). They are extremely reactive and readily attack alkanes.

$$\text{Initiation: } X_2 \xrightarrow[\text{or } \Delta]{h\nu} 2X\bullet$$

2. **Propagation**—A propagation step is one in which a radical produces another radical that can continue the reaction. A free radical reacts with an alkane, removing a hydrogen atom to form HX, and creating an alkyl radical. The alkyl radical can then react with X_2 to form an alkyl halide, generating X•.

Propagation:
$$X\bullet + RH \rightarrow HX + R\bullet$$
$$R\bullet + X_2 \rightarrow RX + X\bullet$$

3. **Termination**—Two free radicals combine with one another to form a stable molecule.

Termination: $2X\bullet \rightarrow X_2$

$X\bullet + R\bullet \rightarrow RX$

$2R\bullet \rightarrow R_2$

A single free radical can initiate many reactions before the reaction chain is terminated.

Larger alkanes have many hydrogens that the free radical can attack. Bromine radicals react fairly slowly, and primarily attack the hydrogens on the carbon atom that can form the most stable free radical, i.e., the most substituted carbon atom.

$$\bullet CR_3 > \bullet CR_2H > \bullet CRH_2 > \bullet CH_3$$
$$3° > 2° > 1° > \text{methyl}$$

Thus, a tertiary radical is the most likely to be formed in a free-radical bromination reaction.

TEACHER TIP

Think of carbocations and free radicals as "electron-deficient" because both species have fewer than the eight electrons needed to be complete. In this way, we can remember the trends of stability of both of these species: 3° > 2° > 1° > methyl.

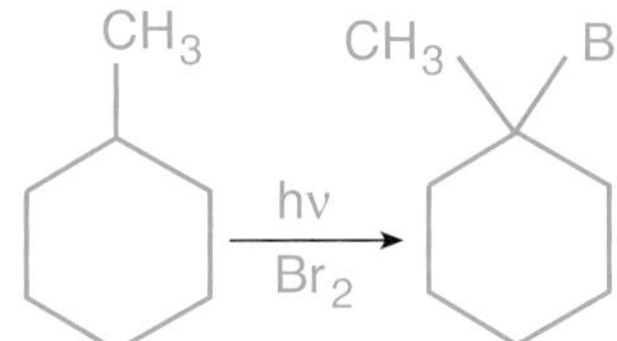

Figure 4.3

Free-radical chlorination is a more rapid process and thus depends not only on the stability of the intermediate, but on the number of hydrogens present. Free-radical chlorination reactions are likely to replace primary hydrogens because of their abundance, despite the relative instability of primary radicals. Unfortunately, free-radical chlorination reactions produce mixtures of products, and are preparatively useful only when just one type of hydrogen is present.

B. COMBUSTION

The reaction of alkanes with molecular oxygen, to form carbon dioxide, water, and heat, is a process of great practical importance. It is an unusual reaction because heat, not a chemical species, is generally the desired product. The reaction mechanism is very complex and is believed to proceed through a radical process. The equation for the complete **combustion** of propane is:

$$C_3H_8 + 5O_2 \rightarrow 3CO_2 + 4H_2O + \text{heat}$$

REAL-WORLD ANALOGY

Nitrogen in the air is also often oxidized in the internal combustion engine. Various nitrogen oxides are major contributors to air pollution.

Combustion is often incomplete, producing significant quantities of carbon monoxide instead of carbon dioxide. This frequently occurs, for example, in the burning of gasoline in an internal combustion engine.

C. PYROLYSIS

Pyrolysis occurs when a molecule is broken down by heat. Pyrolysis, also called **cracking,** is most commonly used to reduce the average molecular weight of heavy oils and to increase the production of the more desirable volatile compounds. In the pyrolysis of alkanes, the C–C bonds are cleaved, producing smaller-chain alkyl radicals. These radicals can recombine to form a variety of alkanes:

TEACHER TIP

When a reaction involves UV light, you'll almost always see a free radical. When a reaction involves heat, consider the possibility of free radicals and elimination reactions (which do not involve radicals and will be discussed in later chapters).

$$CH_3CH_2CH_3 \xrightarrow[\Delta]{} CH_3\bullet + \bullet CH_2CH_3$$

$$2\ CH_3\bullet \longrightarrow CH_3CH_3$$

$$2\ \bullet CH_2CH_3 \longrightarrow CH_3CH_2CH_2CH_3$$

Figure 4.4

Alternatively, in a process called **disproportionation,** a radical transfers a hydrogen atom to another radical, producing an alkane and an alkene:

$$CH_3\bullet + \bullet CH_2CH_3 \rightarrow CH_4 + CH_2 = CH_2$$

Figure 4.5

SUBSTITUTION REACTIONS OF ALKYL HALIDES

Alkyl halides and indeed other substituted carbon atoms can take part in reactions known as *nucleophilic substitutions*. **Nucleophiles** ("nucleus lovers") are electron-rich species that are attracted to positively polarized atoms.

A. NUCLEOPHILES

1. Basicity

If the nucleophiles have the same attacking atom (for example, oxygen) then nucleophilicity is roughly correlated to basicity. In other words, the stronger the base, the stronger the nucleophile. For example, nucleophilic strength decreases in the order:

$$RO^- > HO^- > RCO_2^- > ROH > H_2O$$

2. Size and Polarizability

If the attacking atoms differ, nucleophilic ability doesn't necessarily correlate to basicity. In a protic solvent, large atoms tend to be better nucleophiles as they can shed their solvent molecules and are more polarizable. Hence, nucleophilic strength decreases in the order:

$$CN^- > I^- > RO^- > HO^- > Br^- > Cl^- > F^- > H_2O$$

In aprotic solvents however, the nucleophiles are "naked"; they are not solvated. In this situation, nucleophilic strength is related to basicity. For example in DMSO, the order of nucleophilic strength is the same as base strength:

$$F^- > Cl^- > Br^- > I^-$$

Note that this is the opposite of what happens in polar solvents.

TEACHER TIP

When it comes to nucleophilicity, *size matters* in protic solvents (those capable of hydrogen bonding). The smaller atoms can be surrounded easily by the solvent to decrease its ability to act as a nucleophile. A larger atom, then, becomes more nucleophilic in comparison.

TEACHER TIP

Because aprotic solvents do not have a positive pole, they're unable to stabilize the negative charges of a nucleophile; thus, they're said to be "naked" and are able to act as expected—the more basic, the more nucleophilic.

B. LEAVING GROUPS

The ease with which nucleophilic substitution takes place is also dependent on the leaving group. The best leaving groups are those that are weak bases, as these can accept an electron pair and dissociate to form a stable species. In the case of the halogens, therefore, this is the opposite of base strength:

$$I^- > Br^- > Cl^- > F^-$$

MCAT SYNOPSIS

Weak bases make good leaving groups.

C. S_N1 REACTIONS

S_N1 is the designation for **unimolecular nucleophilic substitution** reaction. It is called unimolecular because the rate of the reaction is dependent upon only one species. Generally, the rate-determining step is the dissociation of this species to form a stable, positively charged ion called a **carbocation** or **carbonium ion.**

TEACHER TIP

The carbocation intermediate is the hallmark of the S_N1 reaction and our understanding of the intermediate will be essential in determining all of the facts surrounding the reaction, including the rate and the products.

1. Mechanism of S_N1 Reactions

S_N1 reactions involve two steps: the dissociation of a molecule into a carbocation and a good leaving group, followed by the combination of the carbocation with a strong nucleophile.

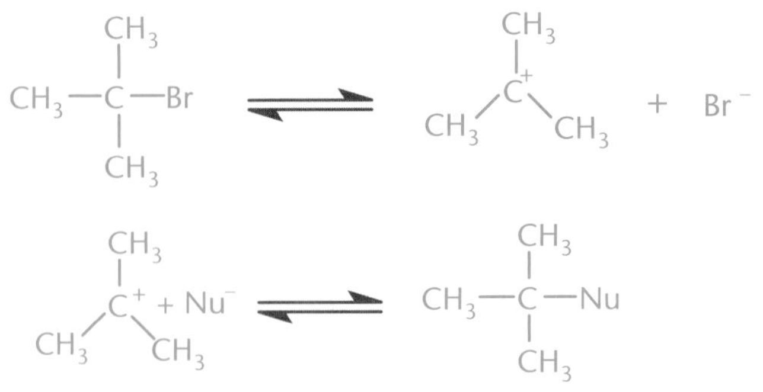

$$(CH_3)_3C{-}Br \rightleftharpoons (CH_3)_3C^+ + Br^-$$

$$(CH_3)_3C^+ + Nu^- \rightleftharpoons (CH_3)_3C{-}Nu$$

Figure 4.6

In the first step, a carbocation is formed. Carbocations are stabilized by polar solvents that have lone electron pairs to donate (*e.g.*, water, acetone). Carbocations are also stabilized by charge delocalization. More highly substituted cations are therefore more stable. The order of stability for carbocations is:

tertiary > secondary > primary > methyl

To get the desired product, the original substituent should be a better leaving group than the nucleophile, so that at equilibrium, RNu is the main product. Conditions are usually chosen so that the second step of the reaction is essentially irreversible.

2. Rate of S_N1 Reactions

The rate at which a reaction occurs can never be greater than the rate of its slowest step. Such a step is termed the **rate-limiting** or **rate-determining step** of the reaction, because it limits the speed of the reaction. In an S_N1 reaction, the slowest step is the dissociation of the molecule to form a carbocation, a step that is energetically unfavorable. The formation of a carbocation is therefore the rate-limiting step of an S_N1 reaction. The only reactant in this step is the original molecule, and so the rate of the entire reaction, under a given set of conditions, depends only on the concentration of this original molecule (a so-called *first-order reaction*). The rate is *not* dependent on the concentration or the nature of the nucleophile, because it plays no part in the rate-limiting step.

The rate of an S_N1 reaction can be increased by anything that accelerates the formation of the carbocation. The most important factors are as follows:

a. Structural factors: Highly substituted alkyl halides allow for distribution of the positive charge over a greater number of carbon atoms, and thus form the most stable carbocations.

b. Solvent effects: Highly polar solvents are better at surrounding and isolating ions than are less polar solvents. Polar protic solvents such as water work best because solvation stabilizes the intermediate state.

c. Nature of the leaving group: Weak bases dissociate more easily from the alkyl chain and thus make better leaving groups, increasing the rate of carbocation formation.

D. S_N2 REACTIONS

The formation of a carbocation is not always favorable. Under certain conditions, substitution can proceed by a different mechanism, which does not involve a carbocation. An S_N2 **(bimolecular nucleophilic substitution)** reaction involves a nucleophile pushing its way into a compound while simultaneously displacing the leaving group. Its rate-determining, and only, step involves two molecules: the **substrate** and the nucleophile.

TEACHER TIP

The pentavalent transition state (where there are five bonds to the carbon atom) is the hallmark of the S_N2 reaction. The increased crowding around that central atom will guide the rate and products of the reaction.

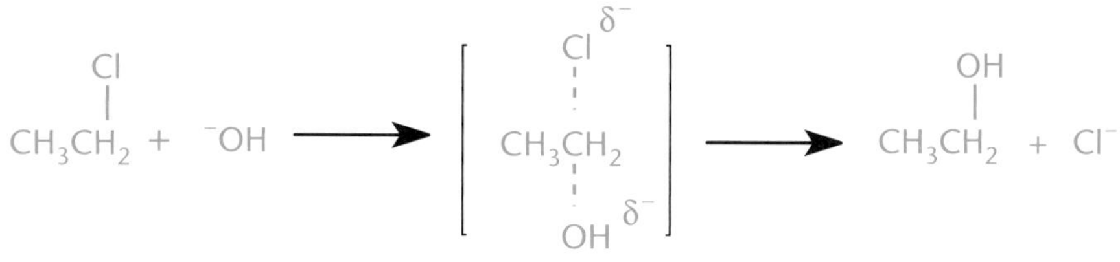

$$CH_3CH_2Cl + {}^-OH \longrightarrow \left[CH_3CH_2 (Cl^{\delta-})(OH^{\delta-}) \right] \longrightarrow CH_3CH_2OH + Cl^-$$

Figure 4.7

1. Mechanism of S_N2 reactions

In S_N2 reactions, the nucleophile actively displaces the leaving group. For this to occur, the nucleophile must be strong, and the reactant cannot be sterically hindered. The nucleophile attacks the reactant from the backside of the leaving group, forming a trigonal bipyramidal **transition state.** As the reaction progresses, the bond to the nucleophile strengthens while the bond to the leaving group weakens. The leaving group is displaced as the bond to the nucleophile becomes complete.

MCAT SYNOPSIS

An intermediate is distinct from a transition state. An intermediate is a well-defined species with a finite lifetime. On the other hand, a transition state is a theoretical structure used to define a mechanism.

2. Rate of S_N2 Reactions

The single step of an S_N2 reaction involves *two* reacting species: the substrate (the molecule with a leaving group, usually an alkyl halide), and the nucleophile. The concentrations of both therefore play a role in determining the rate of an S_N2 reaction; the two species must "meet" in solution, and raising the concentration of either will make such a meeting more likely. Because the rate of the S_N2 reaction depends on the concentration of two reactants, it follows **second-order kinetics.**

TEACHER TIP

The comparison of molecules and which mechanism is favored by particular reactants under specific conditions is a common topic on the MCAT.

S_N1 VERSUS S_N2

Certain reaction conditions favor one substitution mechanism over the other. It is also possible for both to occur in the same flask. Sterics, nucleophilic strength, leaving group ability, reaction conditions, and solvent effects are all important in determining which reaction will occur.

TEACHER TIP

S_N1 leads to loss of stereochemistry; S_N2 leads to a relative inversion due to backside attack. Be careful though, because the *absolute* configuration is independent of the path.

STEREOCHEMISTRY OF SUBSTITUTION REACTIONS

A. S_N1 STEREOCHEMISTRY

S_N1 reactions involve carbocation intermediates, which are approximately planar and therefore achiral.

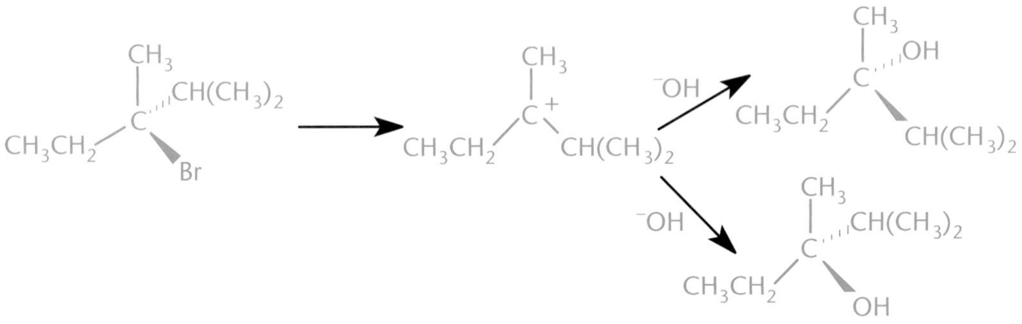

Figure 4.8

If the original compound is optically active because of the reacting chiral center, then a racemic mixture will be produced. S_N1 reactions result in a loss of optical activity.

MCAT SYNOPSIS

S_N1	S_N2
• 2 steps	• 1 step
• favored in polar protic solvents	• favored in polar aprotic solvents
• 3° > 2° > 1° > methyl	• 1° > 2° > 3°
• rate = k[RX]	• rate = k[Nu] [RX]
• racemic products	• optically active/inverted products
• favored with the use of bulky nucleophiles	

B. S_N2 STEREOCHEMISTRY

The single step of an S_N2 reaction involves a chiral transition state. Since the nucleophile attacks from one side of the central carbon and the leaving group departs from the opposite side, the reaction "flips" the bonds attached to the carbon.

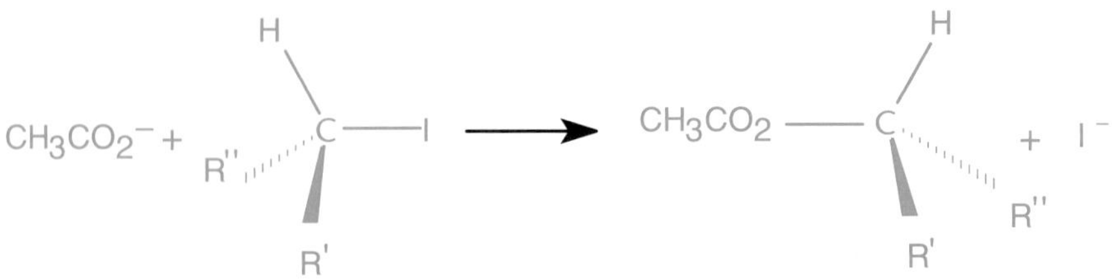

Figure 4.9

If the reactant is chiral, optical activity is usually retained; however, in the case of S_N2 reactions, an inversion of configuration occurs.

PRACTICE QUESTIONS

1. Two structures for C_8H_{18} are shown below. Which one has a higher boiling point and why?

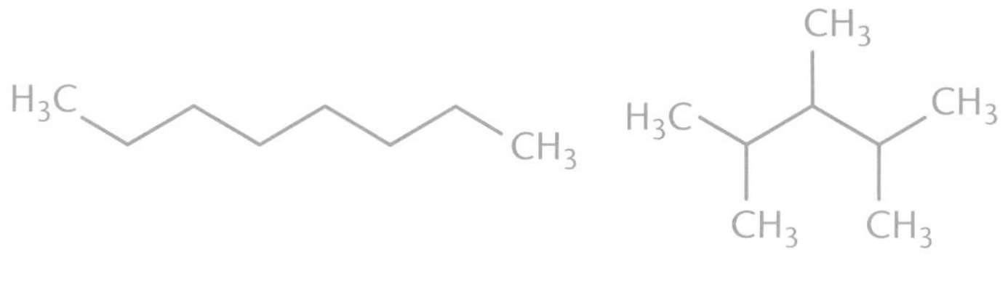

A. N-octane: Linear, unbranched alkanes have greater surface area and greater Van der Waals forces acting on them.

B. N-octane: The atom pairs in octane have a smaller electronegativity difference than in 2,3,4-trimethylpentane.

C. 2,3,4-trimethylpentane: The boiling point of alkanes increases proportionally to the chain length and number of substituents.

D. 2,3,4-trimethylpentane: The increased branching increases the polarity of the molecule.

2. Which of the circled protons below can destroy Grignard reagents?

A.

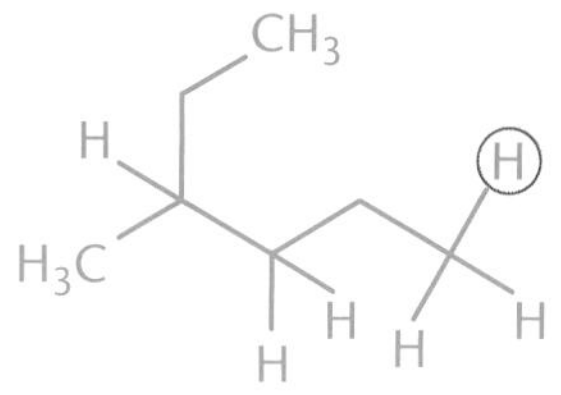

B.

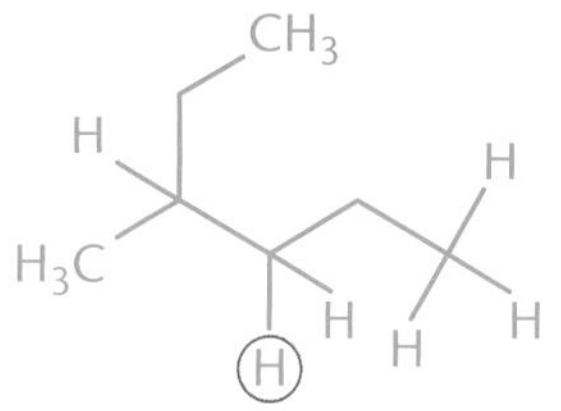

C.

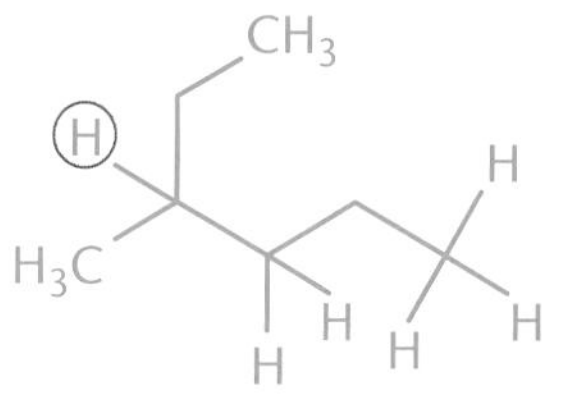

D. None of the above

3. A Wurtz reaction is performed on 1,3-dichlorocyclobutane. What is the major product?

A.

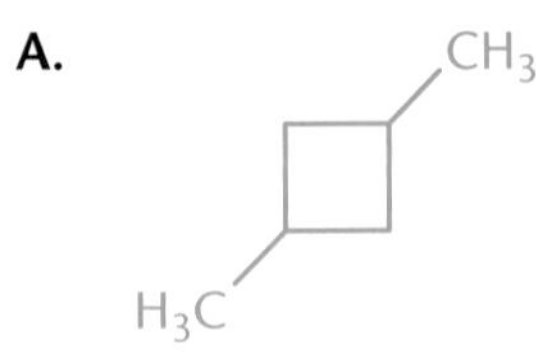

B.

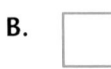

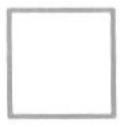

C.

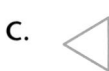

D.

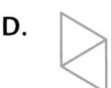

4. Which of the following alkanes is the best candidate to synthesize using a Wurtz synthesis?

A. 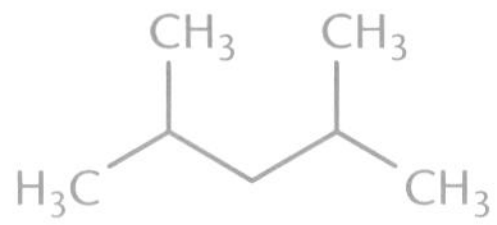 This molecule is symmetrical.

B. 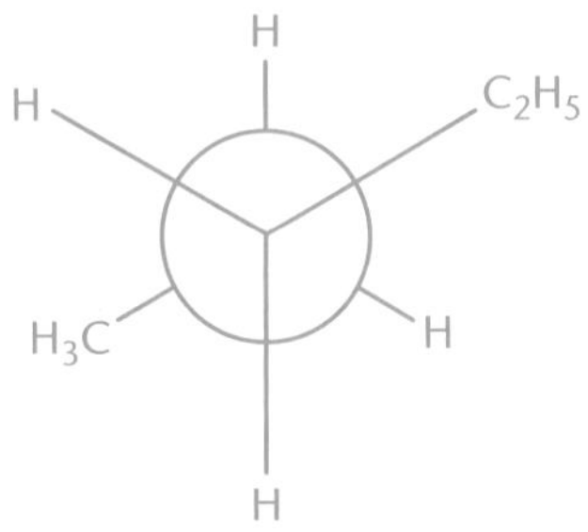 This molecule is the simplest alkane.

C. 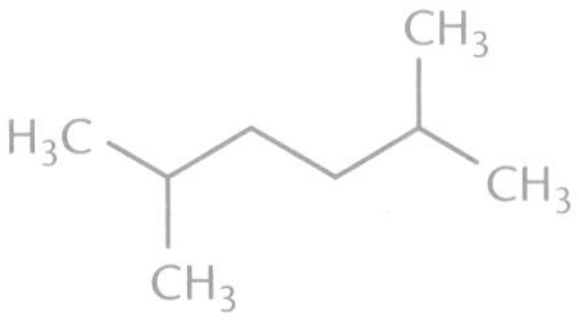 This molecule is symmetrical.

D. 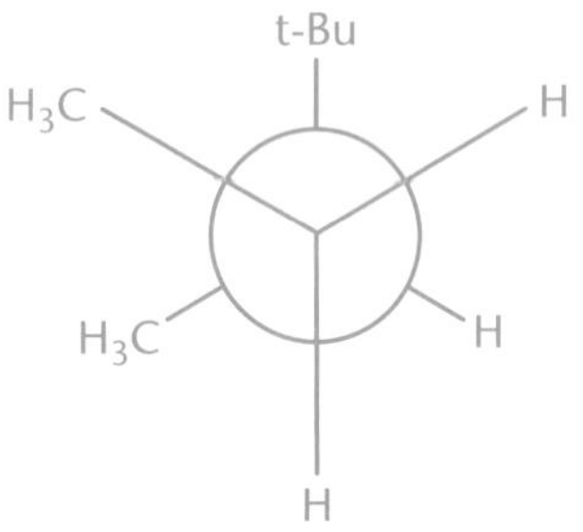 This alkane is too complex to form without using a Wurtz reaction.

5. Which of the following could be used to reduce an alkyl halide to an alkane?

A. $LiAlH_4$
B. Zn, H^+
C. Mg in anhydrous ether, then water
D. All of the above

NUCLEOPHILICITY TRENDS

Rank the following compounds in order of *increasing nucleophilicity* toward the same electrophile in a *polar, protic* solvent:

CH_3OH Et_3N $H_3C(C{=}O)O^{\ominus}$ Et_3P $CH_3O^{\ominus}$

1) Separate out nucleophiles with the same attacking atom and rank them first.

Look at the oxygen nucleophiles first. Here the methoxide anion is more basic than the acetate anion ($CH_3CO_2^-$), which in turn is more basic than methanol. Therefore, the methoxide anion will be the most nucleophilic of the three oxygen-containing molecules.

With the methoxide anion, the lone pair on oxygen is "stuck" on the oxygen atom, whereas with acetate, the negative charge can be delocalized through resonance; this makes methoxide more basic. Both molecules are more basic than methanol, because methanol lacks a negative charge.

Remember: *When the attacking atom of different nucleophiles is the same, nucleophilicity and basicity are* ***directly proportional****. Recall that* ***basicity*** *is proportional to how* ***localized a lone pair*** *is.*

---

2) Look next for nucleophiles where the attacking atom is in the same group.

Because phosphorus is directly below nitrogen in the periodic table, triethylphosphine is more nucleophilic. This is where the nature of the solvent makes a big difference. The more basic molecules are better hydrogen bond *acceptors,* meaning that they will be surrounded by solvent molecules and therefore less available to attack the substrate. The differences in basicity are *less pronounced* when molecules are in the same period, so this effect is only noticeable when the attacking atoms are in the same group.

If the solvent were *polar, aprotic,* then the trend would be *exactly the opposite.* Here, the hydrogen bonding effect is removed, so the molecules with the most localized charge density—the most basic—will also be the most nucleophilic.

Comparing the basicity of triethylphosphine and triethylamine is a bit more complicated. The key to determining basicity is remembering that in triethylphosphine, the lone pair on phosphorus is contained in an sp^3 hybrid orbital that is made up of one s and three 3p orbitals. Contrast this with triethylamine, where the nitrogen lone pair is in an sp^3 hybrid composed of one s and three 2p orbitals. This means that the electrons in the phosphorus lone pair are in a larger hybrid orbital, as 3p orbitals are larger than 2p orbitals.

KEY CONCEPTS

Acids and bases

Nucleophilicity

Polar solvent

Protic solvent

TAKEAWAYS

Sort out differences in nucleophilicity two molecules at a time. Don't try to order all the molecules at once, or you risk confusing yourself.

THINGS TO WATCH OUT FOR

Remember that basicity *sometimes* parallels nucleophilicity, but *sometimes* opposes it.

This, in turn, means that the electrons in the phosphorus lone pair are more stable, because they probably have more volume to exist in. If the phosphorus lone pair is *more stable,* then the lone pair is *less reactive* and *less basic* (less likely to want to reach out and grab a proton).

---

3) Look for relationships between nucleophiles in the same period.

$CH_3OH < CH_3CO_2^- < CH_3O^- < Et_3N < Et_3P$ (polar, protic solvent)

Nucleophile	Relative Rate
CH_3OH	1
$CH_3CO_2^-$	20,000
CH_3O^-	1,900,000
Et_3N	4,600,000
Et_3P	520,000,000

Now the question is between the two groups we have ordered separately, which one is more nucleophilic? In most cases, this question is answered by realizing that for different nucleophiles where the attacking atoms are in the *same period, nucleophilicity roughly parallels basicity.* That being the case, triethylamine is more basic than the acetate anion.

This trend is borne out experimentally. The relative reactivities of each nucleophile toward CH_3I in CH_3OH as solvent are as follows:

In a *polar, aprotic* solvent, the order of nucleophilicity would parallel basicity:

$CH_3OH < Et_3P < CH_3CO_2^- < Et_3N < CH_3O^-$ (polar, aprotic solvent)

SIMILAR QUESTIONS

1) Place the following molecules in order of increasing nucleophilicity: pyridine (benzene with one of the carbons in the ring replaced by a nitrogen), triethylamine, acetonitrile (CH_3CN), and DMAP (4–dimethylaminopyridine)? (Note that the solvent doesn't impact nucleophilicity here, because the same atom is nucleophilic in all four compounds.) Which of the two nitrogens in DMAP is more nucleophilic, and why?
2) How would the nucleophlicity of fluoride, chloride, bromide, and iodide rank in an S_N2 reaction with methyl iodide in methanol? In dimethyl sulfoxide?
3) How would you order the nucleophilicity of the following molecules in methanol: Et_3N, Ph_3P, Et_3P, Ph_3N, and Et_3As? Provide a rationale for your ordering. (*Hint*: What about their structures makes all of the molecules above both basic *and* nucleophilic?)

SUBSTRATE REACTIVITY: S_N1 REACTIONS

Place the following molecules in order of *increasing* reactivity towards methanol under solvolytic conditions:

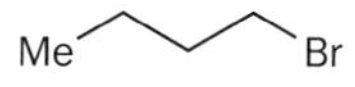

1 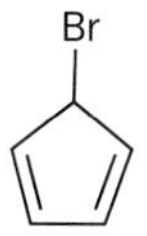 2 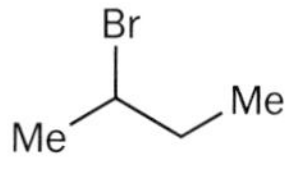 3

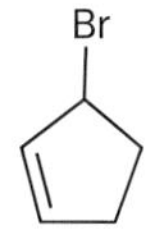

4 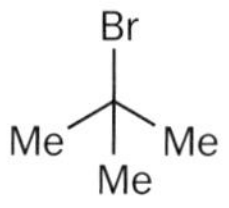 5

1) Determine the potential stabilizing effects on each molecule.
"Solvolytic conditions" is code for an S_N1 reaction. With that in mind, the question is essentially asking you to place the molecules in order of increasing carbocation stability.

Molecules 2 and 4 would benefit from resonance stabilization, so at first glance they will be more stable carbocations than the others.

Remember: *When it comes to charge stabilization,* ***resonance stabilization*** *is* ***always*** *more powerful than* ***inductive stabilization.***

---

2) Look for resonance stabilization first.
Molecule four clearly would have a resonance structure were the bromide to leave and form a cation:

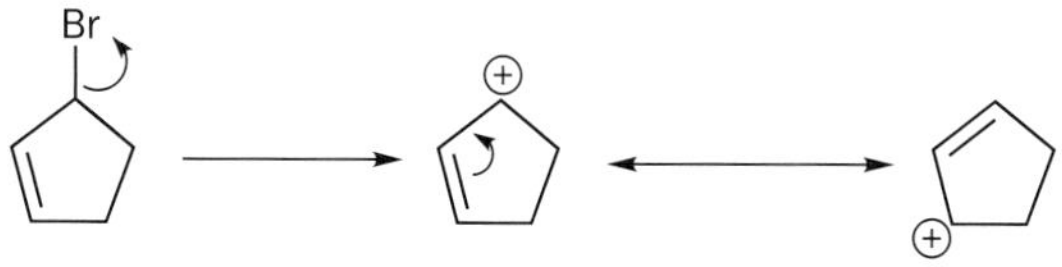

You might think that if one alkene helps stabilize the carbocation, then *two* alkenes would do it better. Be careful with this, though: take a look at the carbocation generated from 2:

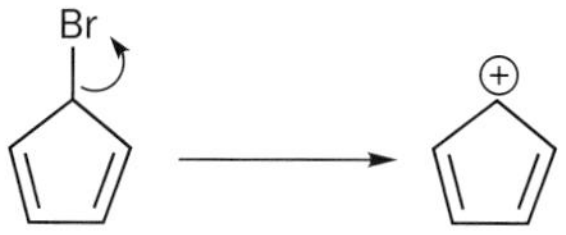

KEY CONCEPTS

Reaction mechanisms

Carbocation stability

Aromaticity

Solvolytic conditions

Hückel's rule

TAKEAWAYS

Reactivity in the S_N1 reaction is determined by carbocation stability because carbocation formation is the rate-limiting step.

THINGS TO WATCH OUT FOR

Don't forget that charged molecules can be aromatic as well!

SIMILAR QUESTIONS

1) 1-Cromocycloheptatriene is dramatically more reactive in S_N1 reactions than is 1-bromocyclohexadiene. Why is this the case?
2) If 1-bromobutane (molecule 1) were forced to become a carbocation, what product(s) would be isolated from the solvolytic reaction with methanol?
3) Compare the reactivity of 1-iodocyclopropene to 1-iodocyclopropane in a solvolysis reaction with ethanol, and provide an explanation for your comparison.

Even though the carbocation at the left could have five resonance structures, notice that it is *antiaromatic*: it is cyclic, planar, and with conjugated alkenes, but it does not fit Hückel's rule. Therefore, this carbocation will be the *least stable* of all five molecules.

---

3) Look for inductive stabilization next.

Now we will look at the remaining molecules to determine their carbocation stability. If you draw the carbocations resulting from each bromide, you get the following:

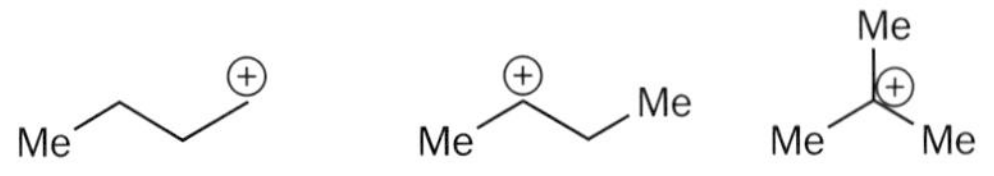

1 **3** **5**

Because the stability of a carbocation is proportional to its substitution, 5 (tertiary) will be more stable than 3 (secondary), and finally 1 (primary).

---

4) Place all of the molecules in order of their reactivity.

The final order in increasing reactivity is thus:

2 < 1 < 3 < 5 < 4

CHAPTER 5

ALKENES AND ALKYNES

ALKENES

Alkenes are hydrocarbons that contain carbon-carbon double bonds. The general formula for a straight-chain alkene with one double bond is C_nH_{2n}. The degree of unsaturation (the number N of double bonds or rings) of a compound of molecular formula C_nH_m can be determined according to the equation:

$$N = \frac{1}{2}(2n + 2 - m)$$

Double bonds are considered functional groups, and alkenes are more reactive than the corresponding alkanes.

TEACHER TIP

Alkenes and Alkynes will not be tested directly on the MCAT and, if they appear, much of the relevant information will be included in the passage and/or question stem. Elimination reactions, however, are indeed tested because they relate to the substitution reactions discussed in the previous chapter.

NOMENCLATURE

Alkenes, also called **olefins,** may be described by the terms *cis, trans, E,* and *Z*. The common names *ethylene, propylene,* and *isobutylene* are often used over the IUPAC names.

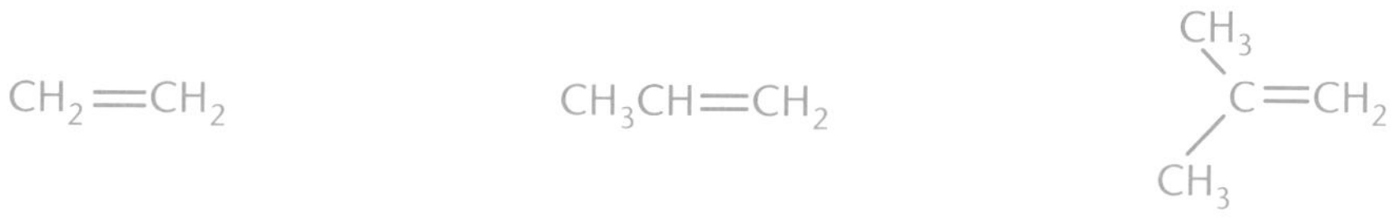

$CH_2{=}CH_2$

ethene (ethylene)

$CH_3CH{=}CH_2$

propene (propylene)

$(CH_3)_2C{=}CH_2$

2-methyl-1-propene (isobutylene)

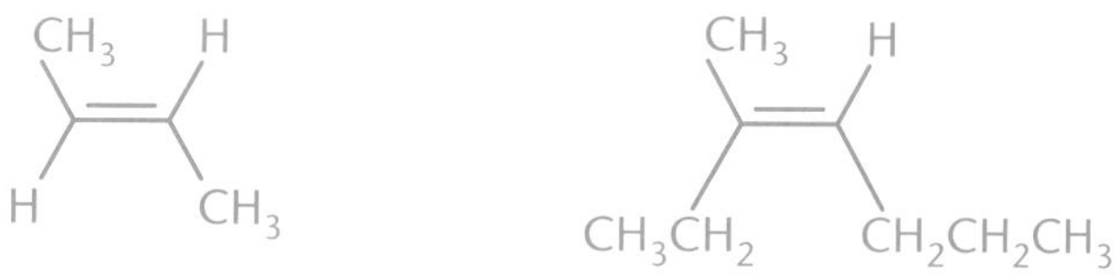

CH$_3$, H / H, CH$_3$

***trans*-2-butene**

CH$_3$, H / CH$_3$CH$_2$, CH$_2$CH$_2$CH$_3$

(*Z*)-3-methyl-3-heptene

Figure 5.1

TEACHER TIP

Trans-alkenes have higher melting points than *cis*-alkenes do due to higher symmetry, allowing them to have more efficient packing in the solid state. *Cis*-alkenes have higher boiling points than *trans*-alkenes because they are polar (as we see in Figure 5.2).

PHYSICAL PROPERTIES

The physical properties of alkenes are similar to those of alkanes. For example, the melting and boiling points increase with increasing molecular weight and are similar in value to those of the corresponding alkanes. Terminal alkenes do (or 1-alkenes) usually boil at a lower temperature than internal alkenes do, and can be separated by fractional distillation (see chapter 12). *Trans*-alkenes generally have higher melting points than *cis*-alkenes do because their higher symmetry allows better packing in the solid state. They also tend to have lower boiling points than *cis*-alkenes do because they are less **polar.**

Polarity is a property that results from the asymmetrical distribution of electrons in a particular molecule. In alkenes, this distribution creates dipole moments that are oriented from the electropositive alkyl groups toward the electronegative alkene. In *trans*-2-butene, the two dipole moments are oriented in opposite directions and cancel each other. The compound possesses no net dipole moment and is not polar. On the other hand, *cis*-2-butene has a net dipole moment, resulting from addition of the two smaller dipoles. The compound is polar, and the additional intermolecular forces tend to raise the boiling point.

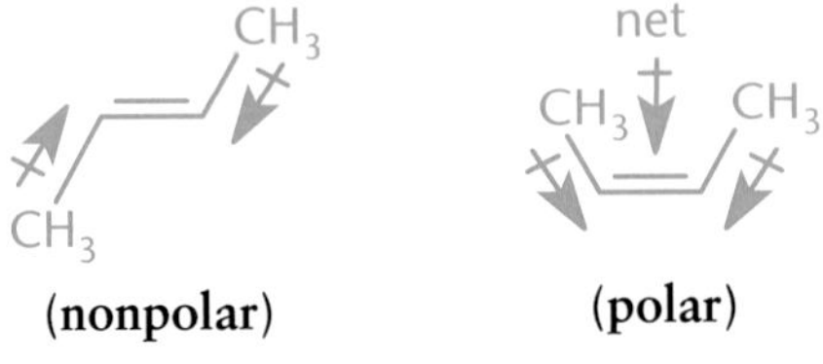

Figure 5.2

SYNTHESIS

Alkenes can be synthesized in a number of different ways. The most common method involves **elimination reactions** of either alcohols or alkyl halides. In these reactions the carbon skeleton loses HX (where X is a halide), or a molecule of water, to form a double bond (see Figure 5.3).

Elimination occurs by two distinct mechanisms, unimolecular and bimolecular, which are referred to as **E1** and **E2,** respectively.

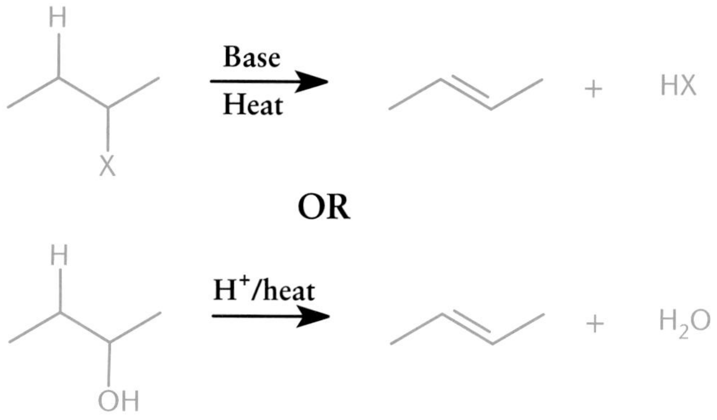

H / X; Base / Heat → + HX

OR

H / OH; H^+/heat → + H_2O

Figure 5.3

> **TEACHER TIP**
> When a reaction involves heat, consider the possibility of elimination reactions and free radicals.

A. UNIMOLECULAR ELIMINATION

Unimolecular elimination, which is abbreviated E1, is a two-step process proceeding through a carbocation intermediate. The rate of reaction is dependent on the concentration of only one species, namely the substrate. The elimination of a leaving group and a proton results in the production of a double bond. In the first step, the leaving group departs, producing a carbocation. In the second step, a proton is removed by a base.

> **TEACHER TIP**
> The carbocation intermediate is the hallmark of the E1 reaction, just like the S_N1 reaction, and our understanding of the intermediate will be essential in determining all of the facts surrounding the reaction, including the rate and the products. E1 and S_N1 reactions both occur because the formation of the intermediate, which is the slow step in both, is the same.

E1 is favored by the same factors that favor S_N1: highly polar solvents, highly branched carbon chains, good leaving groups, and weak nucleophiles in low concentration. These mechanisms are therefore competitive, and directing a reaction toward either E1 or S_N1 alone is difficult, although high temperatures tend to favor E1.

B. BIMOLECULAR ELIMINATION

Bimolecular elimination, termed E2, occurs in one step. Its rate is dependent on the concentration of two species, the substrate and the base. A strong base such as the ethoxide ion ($C_2H_5O^-$) removes a proton, while a halide ion *anti* to the proton leaves, resulting in the formation of a double bond.

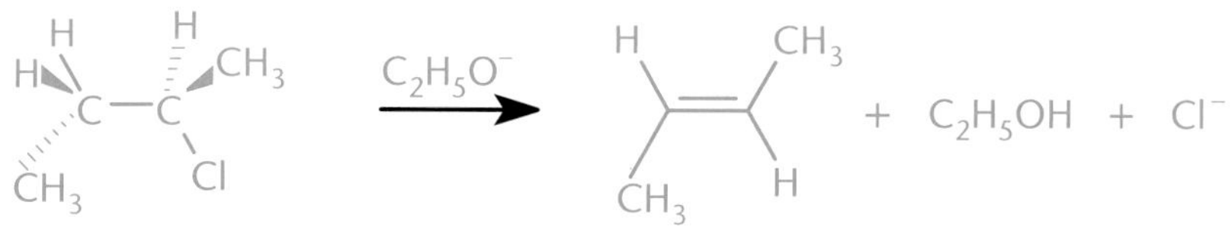

H, H, CH_3, CH_3, Cl; $C_2H_5O^-$ → H, CH_3, CH_3, H + C_2H_5OH + Cl^-

Figure 5.4

Often there are two possible products. In such cases, the more substituted double bond is formed preferentially.

Controlling E2 versus S_N2 is easier than controlling E1 versus S_N1.

1. Steric hindrance does not greatly affect E2 reactions. Therefore, highly substituted carbon chains, which form the most stable alkenes, undergo E2 most easily and S_N2 rarely.
2. A strong base favors E2 over S_N2. S_N2 is favored over E2 by weak Lewis bases (strong nucleophiles).

Teacher Tip

E2 and S_N2 are not in direct competition like the unimolecular reactions.

Other factors, such as the polarity of the solvent and branching of the carbon chain, can be modified in order to reduce the competition between E1 and S_N1 reactions.

REACTIONS

A. REDUCTION

Catalytic hydrogenation is the reductive process of adding molecular hydrogen to a double bond with the aid of a metal catalyst. Typical catalysts are platinum, palladium, and nickel (usually Raney nickel, a special powdered form), but occasionally rhodium, iridium, or ruthenium are used.

MCAT Synopsis

Reactions where one stereoisomer is favored are termed stereospecific reactions.

The reaction takes place on the surface of the metal. One face of the double bond is coordinated to the metal surface, and thus the two hydrogen atoms are added to the same face of the double bond. This type of addition is called *syn* addition.

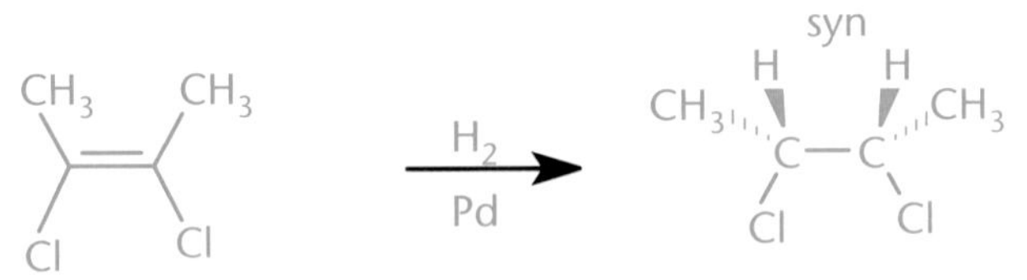

Figure 5.5

Teacher Tip

Markovnikov's rule refers to the addition of a group to the more substituted carbon of the double bond. It does so because the more stable carbocation intermediate will form in the slow first step, and the nucleophile will then attack that positive charge in the fast step.

B. ELECTROPHILIC ADDITIONS

The π bond is somewhat weaker than the σ bond, and can therefore be broken without breaking the σ bond. As a result, one can *add* compounds to double bonds while leaving the carbon skeleton intact. Though many different **addition reactions** exist, most operate via the same essential mechanism.

The electrons of the π bond are particularly exposed and are thus easily attacked by molecules that seek to accept an electron pair (Lewis acids). Because these groups are electron-seeking, they are more often termed **electrophiles** (literally, "lovers of electrons").

1. Addition of HX

The electrons of the double bond act as a Lewis base and react with electrophilic HX molecules. The first step yields a carbocation intermediate after the double bond reacts with a proton. In the second step, the halide ion combines with the carbocation to give an alkyl halide. In cases where the alkene is asymmetrical, the initial protonation proceeds to produce the *most stable carbocation*. The proton will add to the less substituted carbon atom (the carbon atom with the most protons), because alkyl substituents stabilize carbocations. This phenomenon is called **Markovnikov's rule.** An example is:

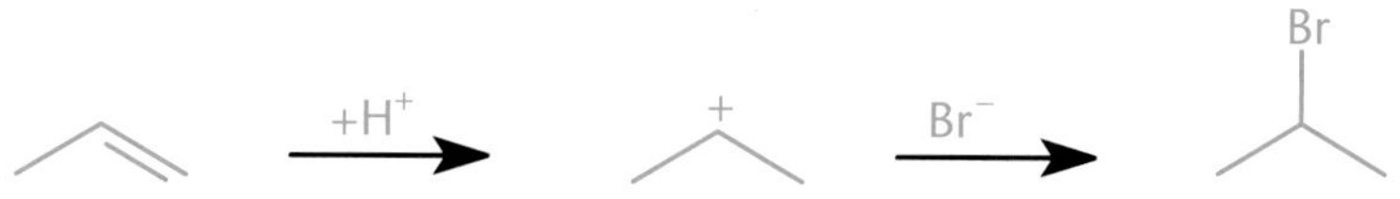

+H⁺ → + Br⁻ → Br

Figure 5.6

2. Addition of X_2

The addition of halogens to a double bond is a rapid process. It is frequently used as a diagnostic tool to test for the presence of double bonds. The double bond acts as a nucleophile and attacks an X_2 molecule, displacing X^-. The intermediate carbocation forms a **cyclic halonium ion,** which is then attacked by X^-, giving the dihalo compound. Note that this addition is *anti*, because the X^- attacks the cyclic halonium ion in a standard S_N2 displacement.

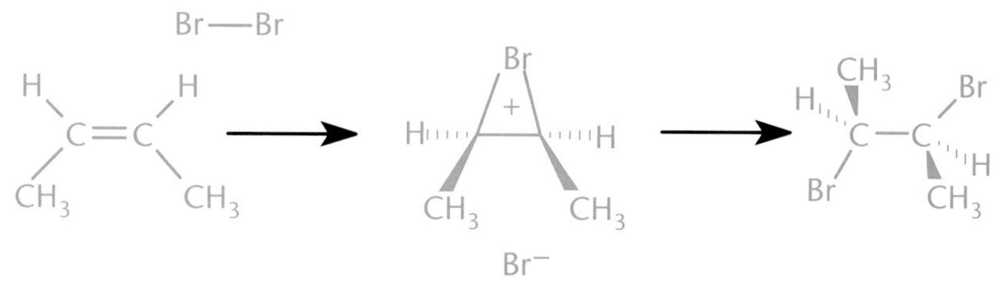

Br—Br; H, H, C=C, CH_3, CH_3 → Br, +, H, H, CH_3, CH_3, Br^- → CH_3, Br, H, C—C, H, Br, CH_3

Anti-addition

Figure 5.7

TEACHER TIP

While the halonium ion may seem odd from your knowledge of the "rules" of chemistry, realize that the products were found experimentally to be anti-addition, and the halonium ion is a good explanation of these findings. On the MCAT, don't question what is given to you as fact in the text; just use those facts to find the correct answer.

If the reaction is carried out in a nucleophilic solvent, the solvent molecules can compete in the displacement step, producing, for example, a **halo alcohol** (rather than the **dihalo** compound).

3. Addition of H_2O

Water can be added to alkenes under acidic conditions. The double bond is protonated according to Markovnikov's rule, forming the most stable carbocation. This carbocation reacts with water, forming a protonated alcohol, which then loses a proton to yield the alcohol. The reaction is performed at low temperature because the reverse reaction is an acid-catalyzed **dehydration** that is favored by high temperatures.

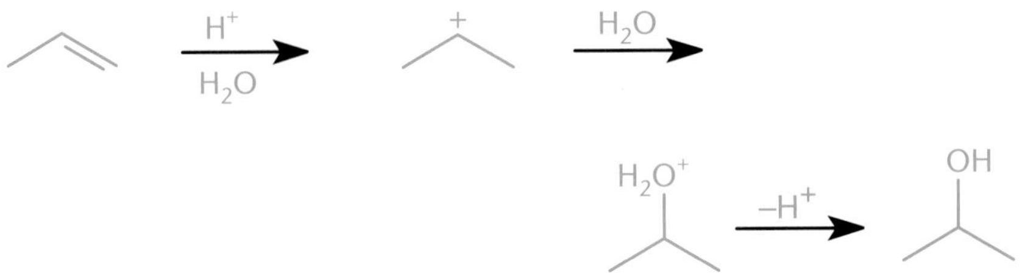

Figure 5.8

Direct addition of water is generally not useful in the laboratory because yields vary greatly with reaction conditions; therefore, this reaction is generally carried out indirectly using mercuric acetate, $Hg(CH_3COO)_2$.

C. FREE RADICAL ADDITIONS

An alternate mechanism exists for the addition of HX to alkenes, which proceeds through **free-radical intermediates**, and occurs when peroxides, oxygen, or other impurities are present. Free-radical additions disobey the Markovnikov rule because X• adds first to the double bond, producing the most stable free radical, whereas H^+ adds first in standard electrophilic additions, producing the most stable carbocation. The reaction is useful for HBr, but is not practical for HCl or HI, because the energetics are unfavorable.

TEACHER TIP

In "anti-Markovnikov" reactions we can see that the most stable radical forms on the most substituted carbon (just like the most stable carbocation formed earlier), but since the halogen adds first, then it ends up on the least substituted carbon. Remember, the most stable intermediate and least energetic transition state will *always* determine the favored products, so on the ecam, identify those species in a particular reaction.

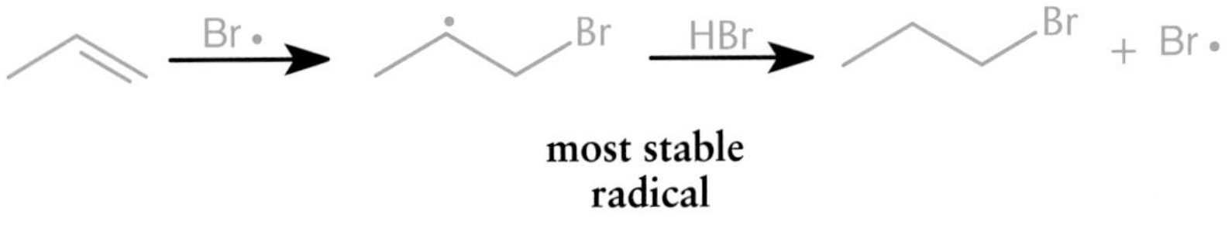

Figure 5.9

D. HYDROBORATION

Diborane (B_2H_6) adds readily to double bonds. The boron atom is a Lewis acid and attaches to the less sterically hindered carbon atom. The second step is an oxidation-hydrolysis with peroxide and aqueous base, producing the alcohol with overall anti-Markovnikov, *syn* orientation.

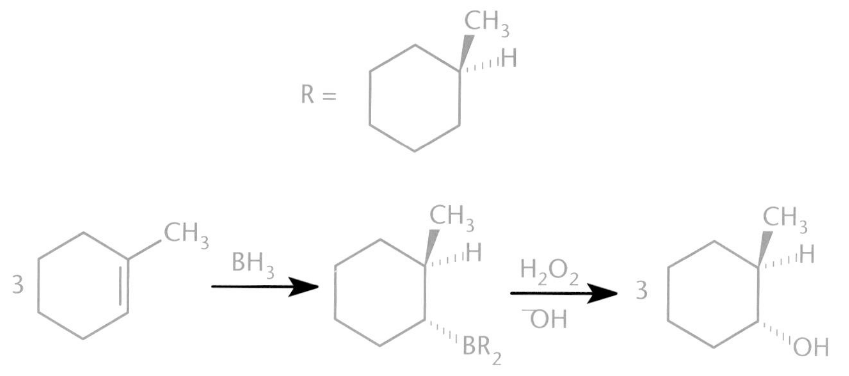

Figure 5.10

E. OXIDATION

1. Potassium Permanganate

Alkenes can be oxidized with $KMnO_4$ to provide different types of products, depending upon the reaction conditions. Cold, dilute, aqueous $KMnO_4$ reacts to produce 1,2 diols (vicinal diols), which are also called glycols, with *syn* orientation:

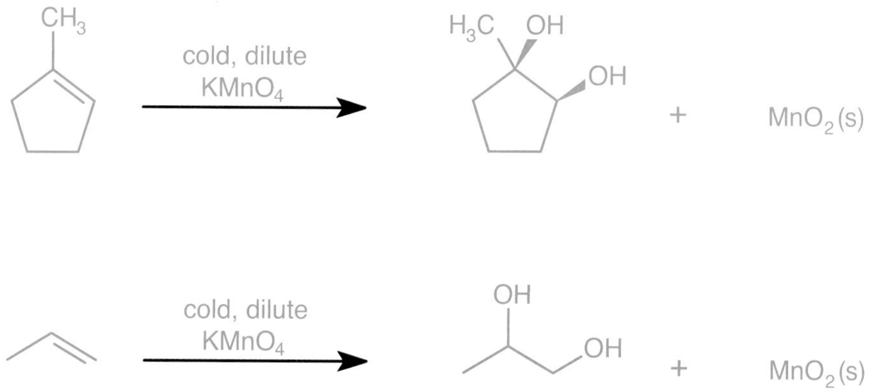

Figure 5.11

TEACHER TIP

Cold and *dilute* conditions should always make you think mild or weak reaction (adding alcohols to a double bond). *Hot* should make you think of rigorous or strong reactions (breaking the double bond altogether and forming carboxylic acids).

If a hot, basic solution of potassium permangenate is added to the alkene and then acidified, nonterminal alkenes are cleaved to form two molar equivalents of carboxylic acid, and terminal alkenes are cleaved to form a carboxylic acid and carbon dioxide. If the nonterminal double-bonded carbon is disubstituted, however, a ketone will be formed:

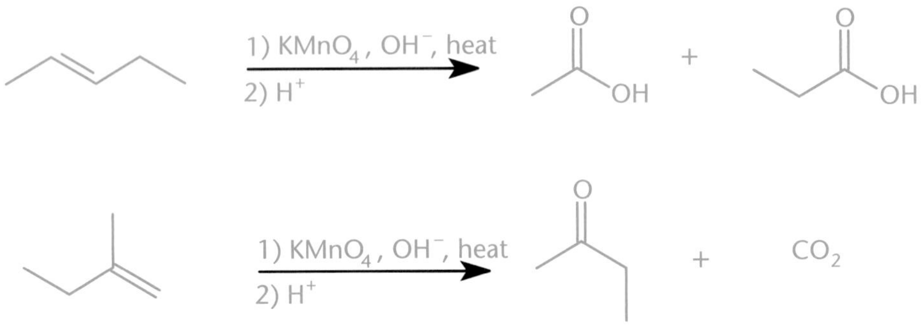

1) $KMnO_4$, OH^-, heat
2) H^+
OH + OH

1) $KMnO_4$, OH^-, heat
2) H^+
+ CO_2

Figure 5.12

2. Ozonolysis

Treatment of alkenes with ozone followed by reduction with zinc and water results in cleavage of the double bond in the following manner:

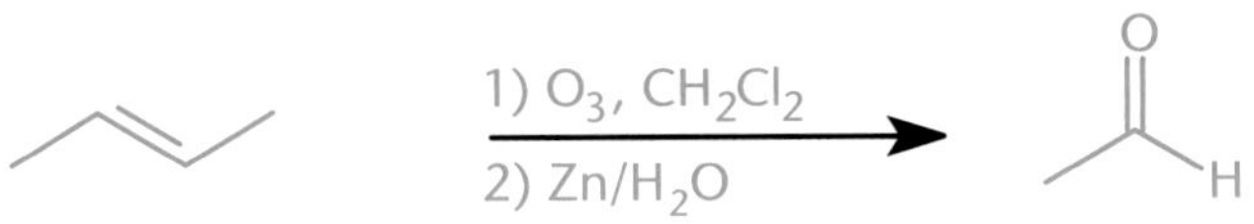

1) O_3, CH_2Cl_2
2) Zn/H_2O
H

Figure 5.13

If the reaction mixture is reduced with sodium borohydride, $NaBH_4$, the corresponding alcohols are produced:

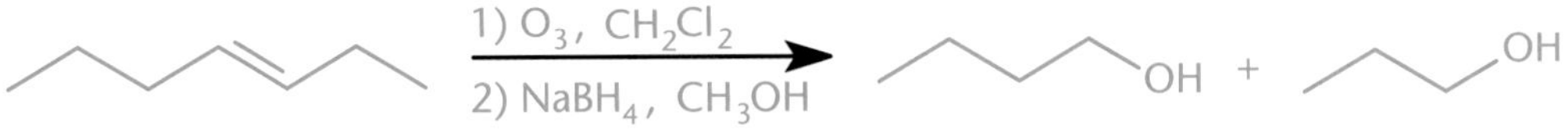

1) O_3, CH_2Cl_2
2) $NaBH_4$, CH_3OH
OH + OH

Figure 5.14

3. Peroxycarboxylic Acids

Alkenes can be oxidized with peroxycarboxylic acids. Peroxyacetic acid (CH_3CO_3H) and *m*-chloroperoxybenzoic acid (mcpba) are commonly used. The products formed are **oxiranes** (also called **epoxides**):

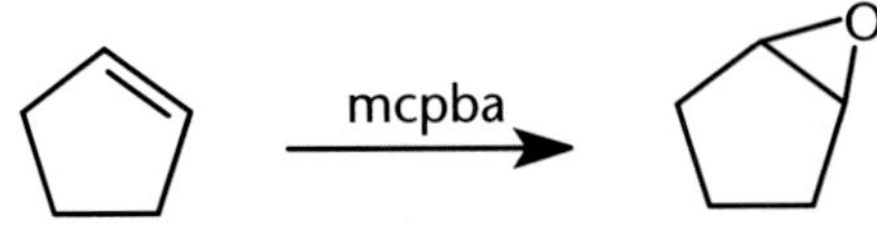

Figure 5.15

F. POLYMERIZATION

Polymerization is the creation of long, high molecular weight chains **(polymers),** composed of repeating subunits (called **monomers**). Polymerization usually occurs through a radical mechanism, although anionic and even cationic polymerizations are commonly observed. A typical example is the formation of polyethylene from ethylene (ethene) that requires high temperatures and pressures:

$$CH_2{=}CH_2 \xrightarrow[\text{high pressure}]{R\cdot,\ \text{heat}} RCH_2CH_2(CH_2CH_2)_nCH_2CH_2R$$

Figure 5.16

TEACHER TIP

When heat is present, consider the possibility of a radical mechanism.

ALKYNES

Alkynes are hydrocarbon compounds that possess one or more carbon-carbon triple bonds.

TEACHER TIP

Alkynes will not be directly tested and will therefore show up even more infrequently than alkenes on the exam. However we'll see similar reactions to those with alkenes because the π-bond is the impetus for most reactions in these two types of compounds.

NOMENCLATURE

The suffix **-yne** is used, and the position of the triple bond is specified when necessary. A common exception to the IUPAC rules is ethyne, which is called *acetylene*. Frequently, compounds are named as derivatives of acetylene.

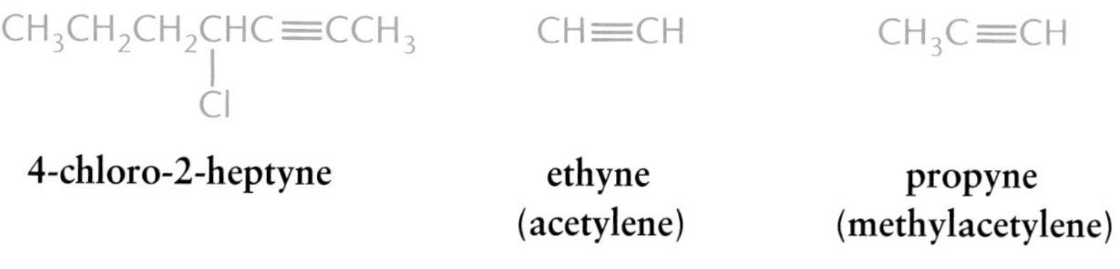

4-chloro-2-heptyne **ethyne (acetylene)** **propyne (methylacetylene)**

Figure 5.17

PHYSICAL PROPERTIES

The physical properties of the alkynes are similar to the properties of the analogous alkenes and alkanes. In general, the shorter-chain compounds are gases, boiling at somewhat higher temperatures than the corresponding alkenes. Internal alkynes, like alkenes, boil at higher temperatures than terminal alkynes.

TEACHER TIP

The acidity of the hydrogen on a terminal alkyne is the one major difference with all other hydrocarbon molecules. If anything about alkynes shows up on the MCAT, it may be in a question about acidity or in a synthesis passage involving the reactions seen in Figure 5.19.

Asymmetrical distribution of electron density causes alkynes to have dipole moments which are larger than those of alkenes, but still small in magnitude. Thus, solutions of alkynes can be slightly polar.

Terminal alkynes are fairly acidic, with a pKa of approximately 25. This property is exploited in some of the reactions of alkynes, which will be discussed later.

SYNTHESIS

Triple bonds can be made by the elimination of two molecules of HX from a geminal or vicinal dihalide:

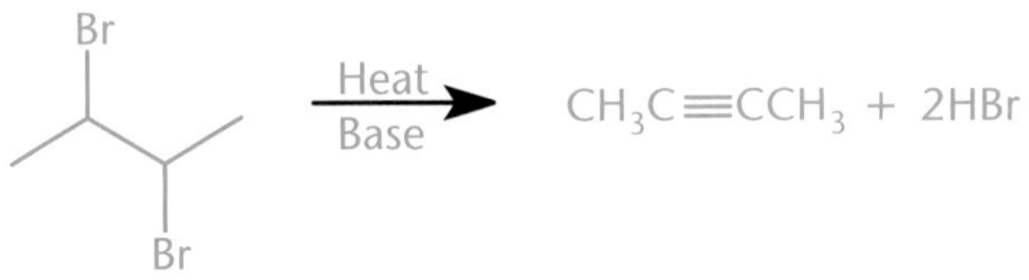

$$\text{(2,3-dibromobutane)} \xrightarrow[\text{Base}]{\text{Heat}} CH_3C{\equiv}CCH_3 + 2HBr$$

Figure 5.18

This reaction is not always practical and requires high temperatures and a strong base. A more useful method adds an already existing triple bond into a particular carbon skeleton. A terminal triple bond is converted to a nucleophile by removing the acidic proton with strong base, producing an *acetylide ion*. This ion will perform nucleophilic displacements on alkyl halides at room temperature:

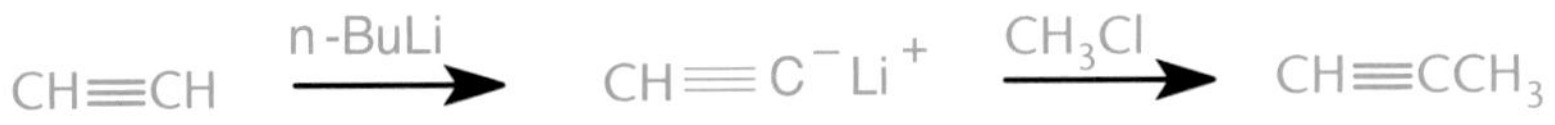

$$CH{\equiv}CH \xrightarrow{\text{n-BuLi}} CH{\equiv}C^-\,Li^+ \xrightarrow{CH_3Cl} CH{\equiv}CCH_3$$

Figure 5.19

REACTIONS

TEACHER TIP

Reduction can be seen as adding electrons in a General Chemistry sense or adding bonds to hydrogen in Organic Chemistry, just as oxidation can be seen as removing electrons or adding bonds to oxygen.

A. REDUCTION

Alkynes, just like alkenes, can be hydrogenated with a catalyst to produce alkanes. A more useful reaction stops the reduction after addition of just one equivalent of H_2, producing alkenes. This partial hydrogenation can take place in two different ways. The first uses **Lindlar's catalyst,** that is palladium on barium sulfate ($BaSO_4$) with quinoline, a poison that stops the reaction at the alkene stage. Because the reaction occurs on a metal surface, the product alkene is the *cis* isomer. The other method uses sodium in liquid ammonia below –33°C (the boiling point of ammonia), and produces the *trans* isomer of the alkene via a free radical mechanism:

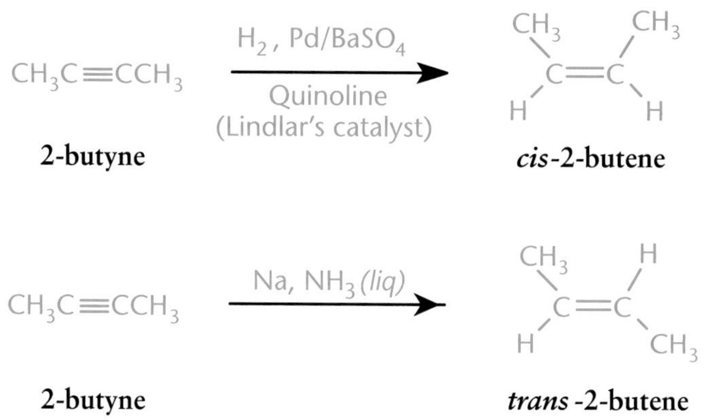

$CH_3C{\equiv}CCH_3$ (**2-butyne**) $\xrightarrow[\text{Quinoline (Lindlar's catalyst)}]{H_2,\ Pd/BaSO_4}$ **cis-2-butene** (CH_3 and CH_3 on the same side of C=C, H and H on the same side)

$CH_3C{\equiv}CCH_3$ (**2-butyne**) $\xrightarrow{Na,\ NH_3\,(liq)}$ ***trans*-2-butene** (CH_3 and H on each carbon, CH_3 groups on opposite sides of C=C)

Figure 5.20

B. ADDITION

1. Electrophilic

Electrophilic addition to alkynes occurs in the same manner as it does to alkenes. The reaction occurs according to Markovnikov's rule. The addition can generally be stopped at the intermediate alkene stage, or carried further. The following examples are illustrative:

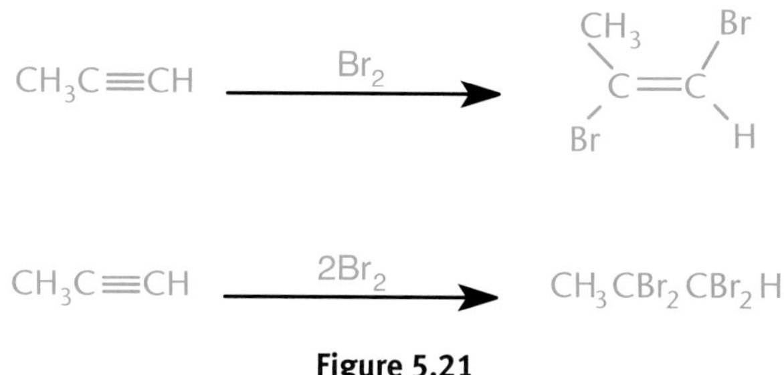

Figure 5.21

TEACHER TIP

As expected, we see anti-addition here just as we did in halogenation of alkenes.

2. Free Radical

Radicals add to triple bonds as they do to double bonds—with anti-Markovnikov orientation. The reaction product is usually the *trans* isomer, because the intermediate vinyl radical can isomerize to its more stable form.

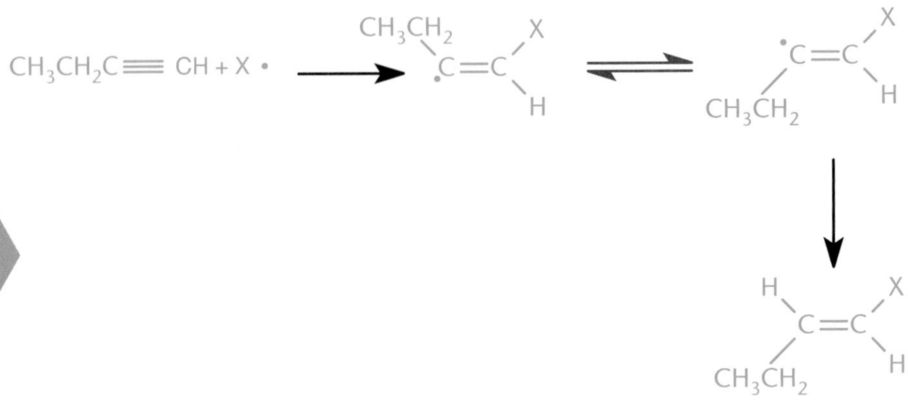

$CH_3CH_2C \equiv CH + X\cdot \longrightarrow$ (CH3CH2)(•)C=C(X)(H) $\rightleftharpoons$ (•)C=C(X)(H) with CH_3CH_2 → (H)(CH3CH2)C=C(X)(H)

Figure 5.22

TEACHER TIP

As always, the most stable "electron-deficient" species forms in this reaction, giving us an anti-Markovnikov product.

C. HYDROBORATION

Addition of boron to triple bonds occurs by the same method as addition of boron to double bonds. Addition is *syn,* and the boron atom adds first. The boron atom can be replaced with a proton from acetic acid, to produce a *cis* alkene:

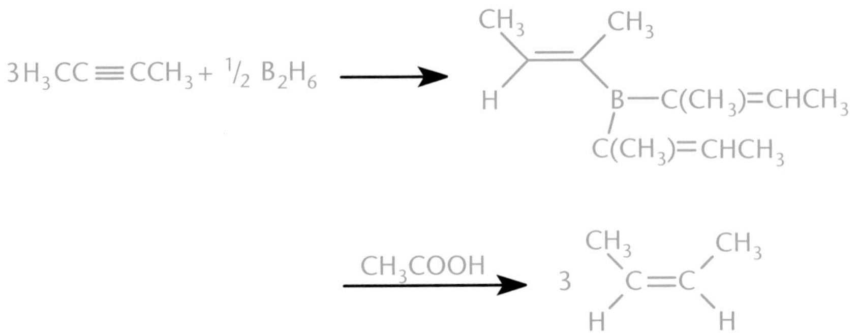

$3H_3CC \equiv CCH_3 + \frac{1}{2} B_2H_6 \longrightarrow$ (CH3)(H)C=C(CH3)(B—C(CH3)=CHCH3 / C(CH3)=CHCH3)

$\xrightarrow{CH_3COOH}$ 3 (CH3)(H)C=C(CH3)(H)

Figure 5.23

MCAT SYNOPSIS

Keto-enol tautomerisms will be discussed in chapter 8.

With terminal alkynes, a disubstituted borane is used to prevent further boration of the vinylic intermediate to an alkane. The vinylic borane intermediate can be oxidatively cleaved with hydrogen peroxide (H_2O_2), creating an intermediate vinyl alcohol, which rearranges to the more stable carbonyl compound (via **keto-enol tautomerism**).

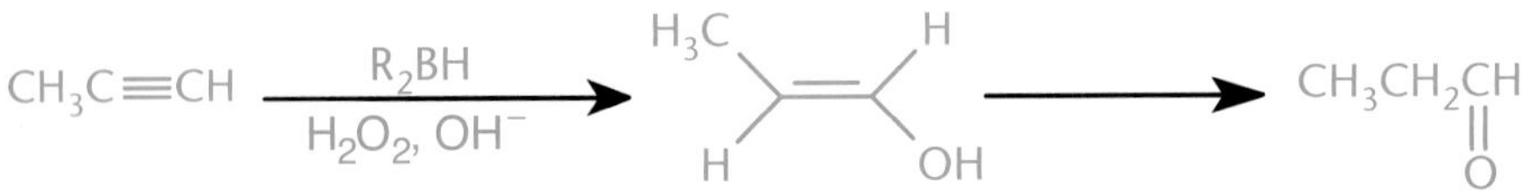

$CH_3C \equiv CH \xrightarrow[H_2O_2,\ OH^-]{R_2BH}$ (H3C)(H)C=C(H)(OH) $\longrightarrow CH_3CH_2CH(=O)$

Figure 5.24

D. OXIDATION

Alkynes can be oxidatively cleaved with either basic potassium permanganate (followed by acidification) or ozone.

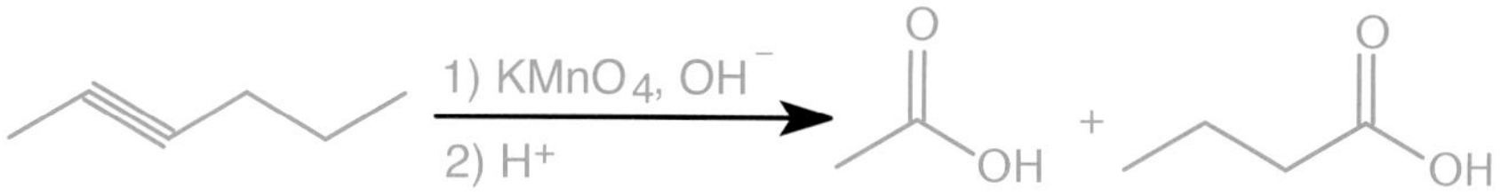

1) $KMnO_4$, OH^-
2) H^+

Figure 5.25

1) O_3, CCl_4
2) H_2O

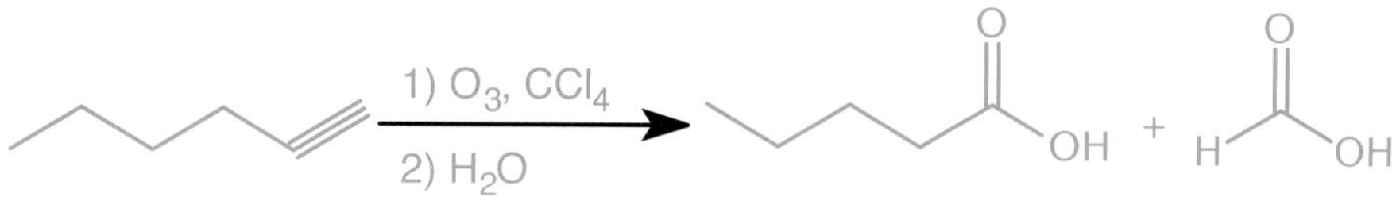

Figure 5.26

PRACTICE QUESTIONS

1. What is the IUPAC name for the compound shown below?

CH$_3$

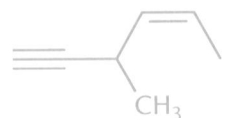

A. (4E)-4-Methylhex-2-en-4-yne
B. (4Z)-4-Methylpent-4-yn-2-ene
C. (4E)-3-Methylhept-1-yn-4-ene
D. (4Z)-3-Methylhex-4-en-1-yne

2. What is the major product of the reaction shown below?

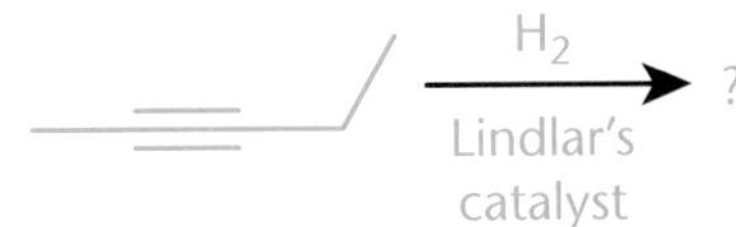

A. (Z)-2-pentene
B. Pentane
C. (E)-2-pentene
D. There is no reaction.

3. Given the reaction shown below, what is the major product, not counting stereoisomers?

Br$_2$, –78°C → ?

A. Br, Br

B. Br, Br

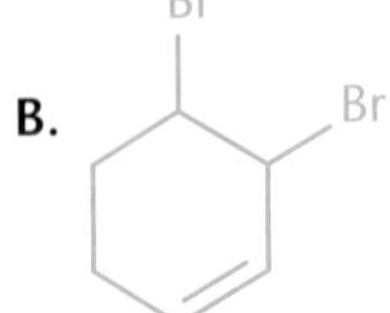

C. Br, Br

D. Br, Br

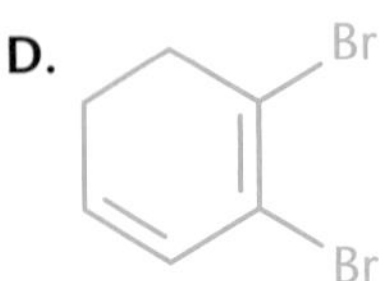

4. Which of the reagents shown below will furnish 2-butanone starting with either 2-butyne or 1-butyne?

A. H_3O^+/H_2O
B. BH_3/THF, followed by H_2O_2/NaOH
C. Acidic $KMnO_4$, heat
D. H_2SO_4, $HgSO_4$, and H_2O

5. What modification must be made to the reaction shown below for it to yield the product indicated?

HBr, ? → Br

A. No modification needed
B. Addition of a peroxide, RO-OR
C. Addition of heat
D. Addition of Br_2

CHAPTER 6

AROMATIC COMPOUNDS

The terms **aromatic** and **aliphatic,** meaning "fragrant" and "fatty," respectively, were used originally to distinguish types of organic compounds. The terms persist with new definitions. "Aromatic" now describes any unusually stable ring system. These compounds are cyclic, conjugated polyenes that possess $4n + 2$ pi electrons and adopt planar conformations to allow maximum overlap of the conjugated pi orbitals. "Aliphatic" describes all compounds that are not aromatic.

The criterion of $4n + 2$ pi electrons is known as **Hückel's rule,** and is an important indicator of aromaticity. In general, if a cyclic conjugated polyene follows Hückel's rule, then it is an aromatic compound. Neutral compounds, anions, and cations may all be aromatic. Some typical aromatic compounds and ions are:

Teacher Tip

Because the MCAT won't provide the formula for a 100 carbon fullerene molecule and ask you to determine if it's aromatic, just remember the smaller numbers 2, 6, 10, 14, and 18 and you won't even need to use the formula.

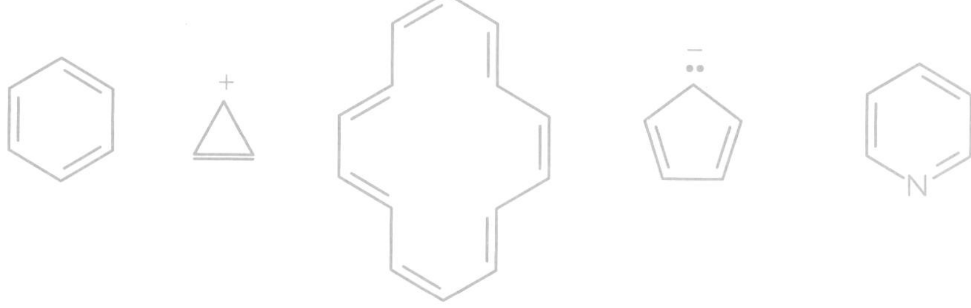

Figure 6.1

A cyclic, conjugated polyene that possesses $4n$ electrons is said to be **antiaromatic** (a cyclic, conjugated polyene that is destabilized). Some typical antiaromatic compounds are:

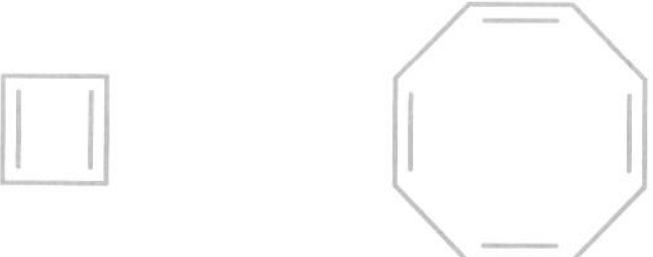

Figure 6.2

NOMENCLATURE

TEACHER TIP

It helps to be familiar with the most common of the common names so they don't cause unnecessary stress on Test Day.

Aromatic compounds are referred to as **aryl** compounds, or **arenes,** and are represented by the symbol **Ar.** Aliphatic compounds are called **alkyl** and are represented by the symbol **R.** Common names exist for many mono- and disubstituted aromatic compounds.

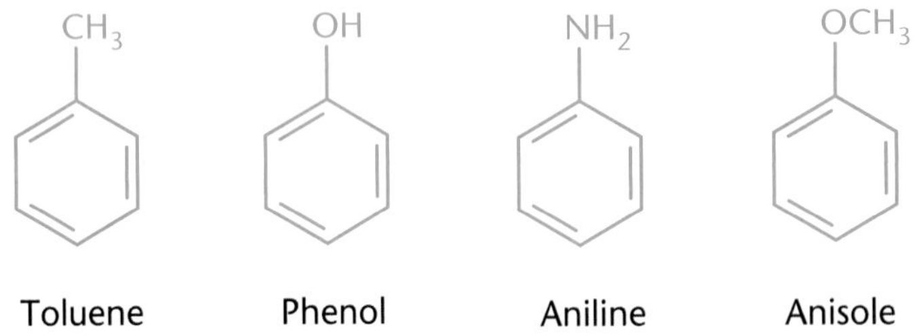

CH_3 OH NH_2 OCH_3

Toluene Phenol Aniline Anisole

Figure 6.3

The benzene group is called a **phenyl** group **(Ph)** when named as a substituent. The term **benzyl** refers to a toluene molecule substituted at the methyl position.

TEACHER TIP

Because many wrong answer choices will be missing a carbon or have an extra carbon, pay attention to the names used in the questions and answers and how they relate to the structures. Knowing the substituent names seen here can earn you points.

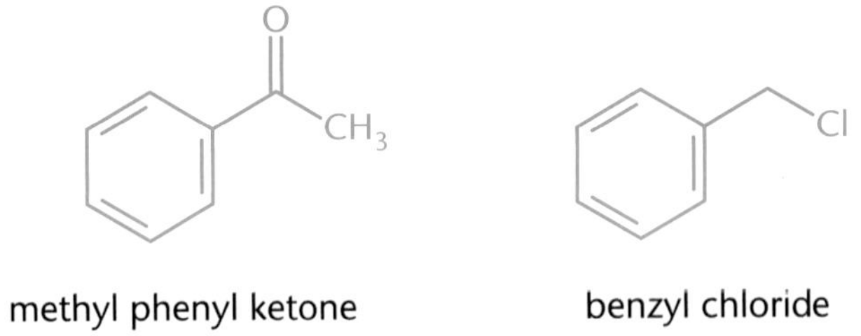

O CH_3 Cl

methyl phenyl ketone benzyl chloride

Figure 6.4

Substituted benzene rings are named as alkyl benzenes, with the substituents numbered to produce the lowest sequence. A 1,2-disubstituted compound is called ***ortho-*** or ***o-***; a 1,3 disubstituted compound is called ***meta-*** or ***m-***; and a 1,4 disubstituted compound is called ***para-*** or ***p-***.

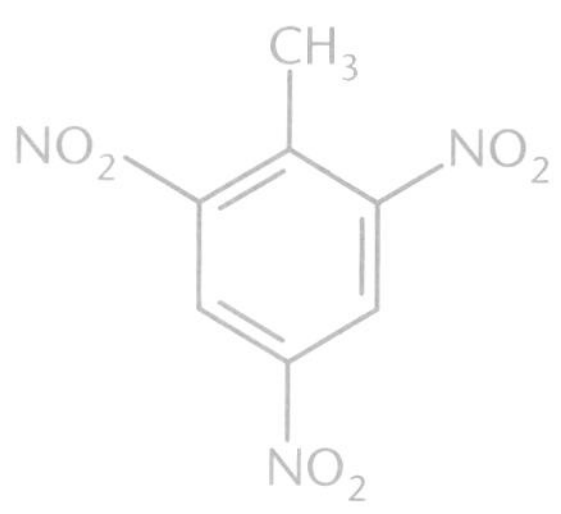

2,4,6-trinitrotoluene (TNT)

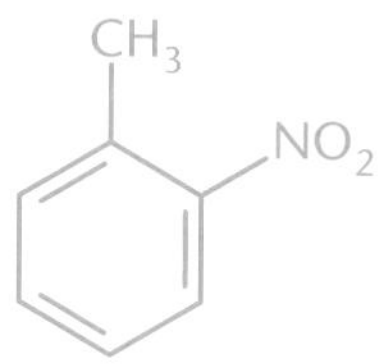

o-nitrotoluene

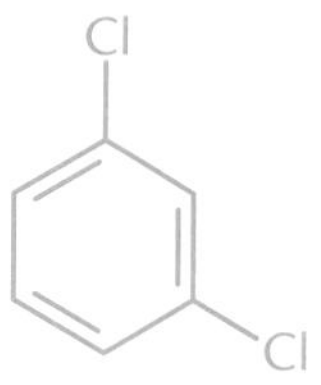

m-dichlorobenzene

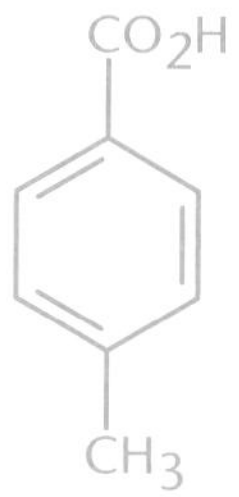

p-methylbenzoic acid

Figure 6.5

> **TEACHER TIP**
>
> *Ortho* (*o*-), *meta* (*m*-) and *para* (*p*-) are designations that you should know and will play an essential role in your understanding of electrophilic aromatic substitution.

There are many polycyclic and heterocyclic aromatic compounds.

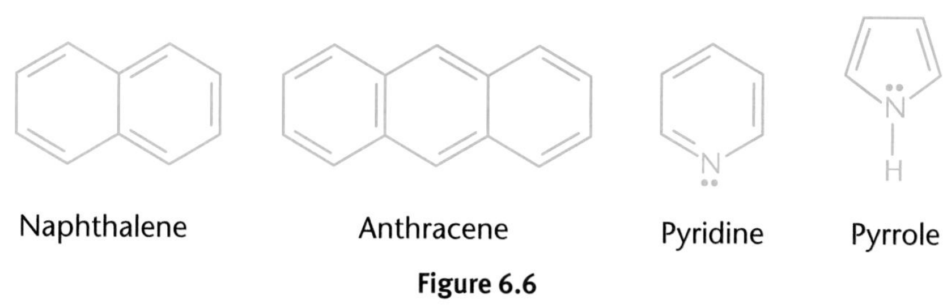

Figure 6.6

> **MCAT SYNOPSIS**
>
> The nonbonding electron pair in pyridine is in a nitrogen sp^2 orbital. This orbital is perpendicular to the p orbitals around the ring and therefore is not involved in the conjugated pi system. On the other hand, the nonbonding pair in pyrrole is in a nitrogen sp^3 orbital parallel to the ring p orbitals and therefore can participate in the delocalized pi system.

PROPERTIES

The physical properties of aromatic compounds are generally similar to those of other hydrocarbons. By contrast, chemical properties are significantly affected by aromaticity. The characteristic planar shape of benzene permits the ring's six pi orbitals to overlap, delocalizing the electron density. All six carbon atoms are sp^2 hybridized, and each of the six orbitals overlaps equally with its two neighbors. As a result, the delocalized electrons form two "pi electron clouds," one above and one below the plane of the ring. This delocalization stabilizes the molecule, making it fairly unreactive: In particular, benzene does not undergo addition reactions as do alkenes. The same holds true for other aromatic compounds, because the definition of an aromatic compound includes the condition that it have a delocalized pi electron system.

REACTIONS

A. ELECTROPHILIC AROMATIC SUBSTITUTION

TEACHER TIP

Because the aromaticity of benzene provides a significant amount of stability, almost all of the reactions with benzene will involve "keeping" the aromaticity. In other words, we see here an overall substitution, not an addition to the molecule.

The most important reaction of aromatic compounds is electrophilic aromatic substitution. In this reaction an electrophile replaces a proton on an aromatic ring, producing a substituted aromatic compound. The most common examples are halogenation, sulfonation, nitration, and acylation.

1. Halogenation

Aromatic rings react with bromine or chlorine in the presence of a Lewis acid, such as $FeCl_3$, $FeBr_3$, or $AlCl_3$, to produce monosubstituted products in good yield. Reaction of fluorine and iodine with aromatic rings is less useful, as fluorine tends to produce multisubstituted products, and iodine's lack of reactivity requires special conditions for the reaction to proceed.

TEACHER TIP

Because our reactant, benzene, is so stable, we need some kind of catalyst and/or extreme conditions to drive these reactions.

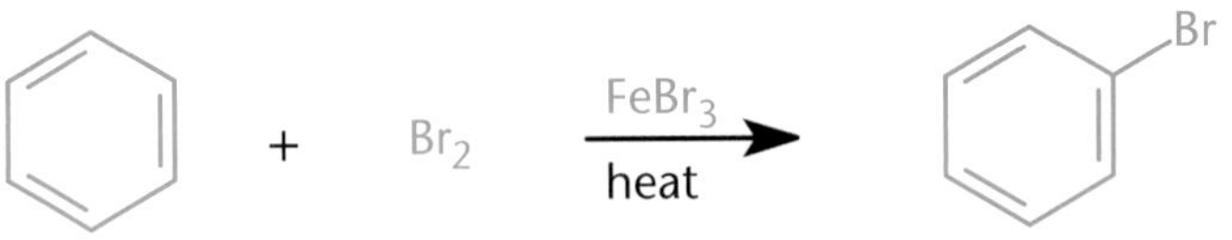

$$C_6H_6 + Br_2 \xrightarrow[\text{heat}]{FeBr_3} C_6H_5Br$$

Figure 6.7

2. Sulfonation

Aromatic rings react with fuming sulfuric acid (a mixture of sulfuric acid and sulfur trioxide) to form sulfonic acids.

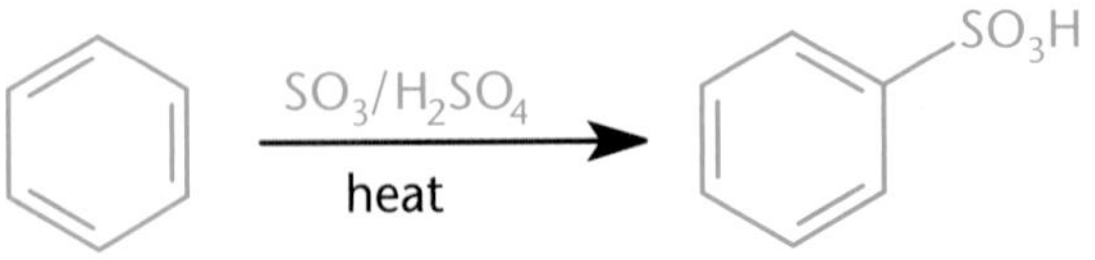

$$C_6H_6 \xrightarrow[\text{heat}]{SO_3/H_2SO_4} C_6H_5SO_3H$$

Figure 6.8

3. Nitration

The nitration of aromatic rings is another synthetically useful reaction. A mixture of nitric and sulfuric acids is used to create the nitronium ion, NO_2^+, a strong electrophile. This reacts with aromatic rings to produce nitro compounds.

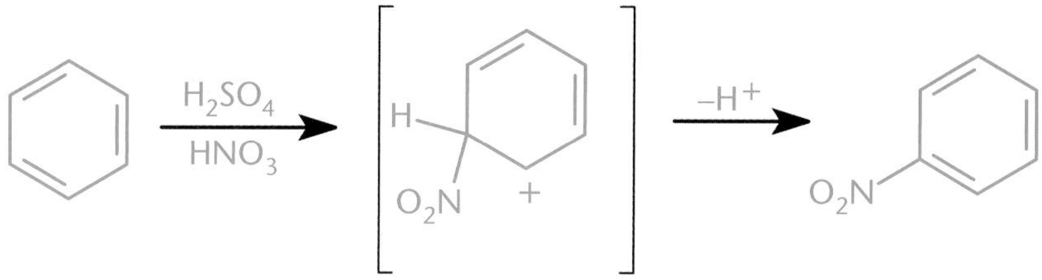

Figure 6.9

4. Acylation (Friedel-Crafts Reactions)

In Friedel-Crafts acylation reaction, a carbocation electrophile, usually an acyl group, is incorporated into the aromatic ring. These reactions are usually catalyzed by Lewis acids such as $AlCl_3$.

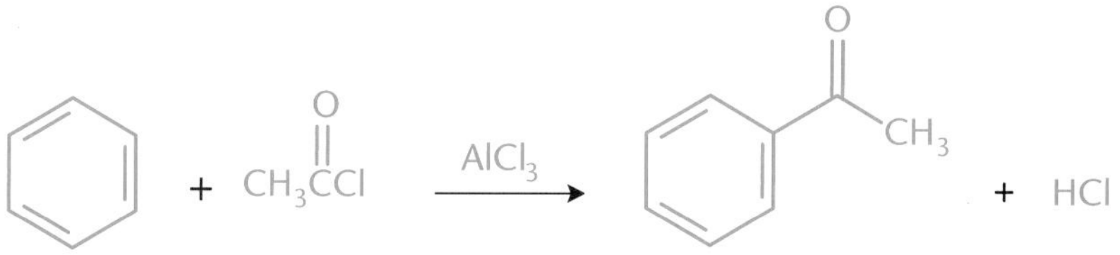

Figure 6.10

MCAT FAVORITE

Be sure to understand substituent effects:

- activating = *ortho/para* directing = e^- donating
- deactivating = *meta* directing = e^- withdrawing

(Halogens are exceptions: although they are e^- withdrawing and deactivators, they are *ortho/para* directors.)

5. Substituent Effects

Substituents on an aromatic ring strongly influence the susceptibility of the ring to electrophilic aromatic substitution, and also strongly affect what position on the ring an incoming electrophile is most likely to attack. Substituents can be grouped into three different classes according to whether substitution is enhanced (activating) or inhibited (deactivating), and where the reaction is likely to take place with respect to the group already present. These effects depend on whether the group tends to donate or withdraw electron density, and how it does so; the specifics of these mechanisms will not be discussed here. Arranged in order of decreasing strength of the substituent effect, the three classes are listed below:

a. Activating, *ortho/para*-directing substituents (electron-donating): NH_2, NR_2, OH, NHCOR, OR, OCOR, and R.
b. Deactivating, *ortho/para*-directing substituents (weakly electron-withdrawing): F, Cl, Br, and I.
c. Deactivating, *meta*-directing substituents (electron-withdrawing): NO_2, SO_3H, and carbonyl compounds, including COOH, COOR, COR, and CHO.

For example, when toluene undergoes electrophilic aromatic substitution, the methyl group directs substitution to occur at the *ortho* and *para* positions:

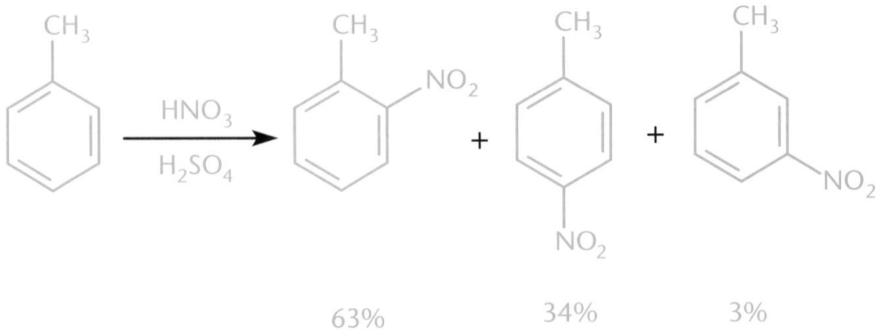

CH_3 HNO_3 H_2SO_4 CH_3 NO_2 + CH_3 NO_2 + CH_3 NO_2

63% 34% 3%

Figure 6.11

B. REDUCTION

1. Catalytic Reduction

Benzene rings can be reduced by catalytic hydrogenation under vigorous conditions (elevated temperature and pressure) to yield cyclohexane. Ruthenium or rhodium on carbon are the most common catalysts; platinum or palladium may also be used.

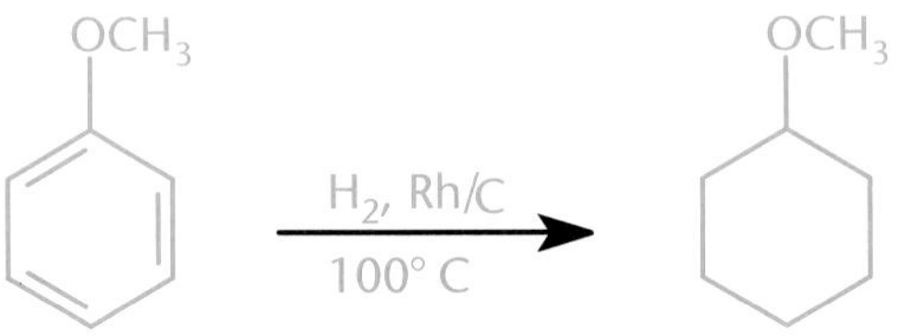

OCH_3 H_2, Rh/C 100° C OCH_3

Figure 6.12

PRACTICE QUESTIONS

1. Starting with phenol, what is the major product of the reaction sequence shown below?

Phenol $\xrightarrow[AlCl_3]{CH_3COCl}$ $\xrightarrow[AlCl_3]{CH_3Cl}$ $\xrightarrow[CH_3I]{NaOH}$ $\xrightarrow[HCl]{Zn}$?

A. Aceto(4-methoxy-3-methyl)phenone
B. 4-Ethyl-2,6-dimethylphenol
C. 4-Ethyl-2-methylanisole
D. 3-Chloro-4-ethyl-2-methylanisole

2. How would an ammonium group affect a benzene ring for subsequent reactions?

A. Deactivate the ring; *m*-directing
B. Activate the ring, *o*/*p*-directing
C. Deactivate the ring; *o*/*p*-directing
D. Activate the ring; *m*-directing

3. Which of the molecules shown below are aromatic?

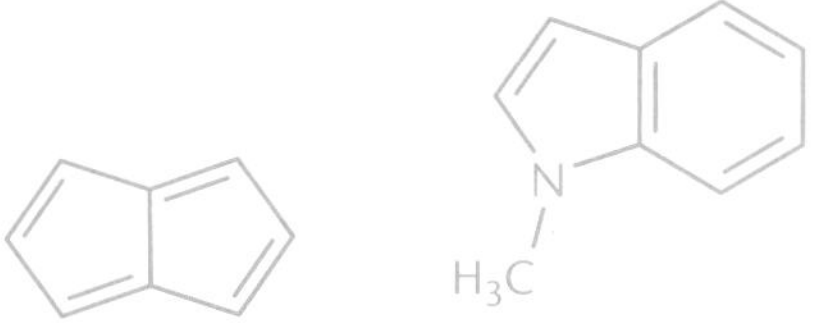

Compound I   Compound II

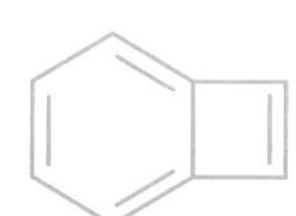
Compound III

A. I only
B. II only
C. I and III
D. I, II, and III

4. What is the major product for the following reaction shown between ethylbenzene and N-bromosuccinimide (NBS)?

Ethylbenzene $\xrightarrow{NBS}$?

A.   B.

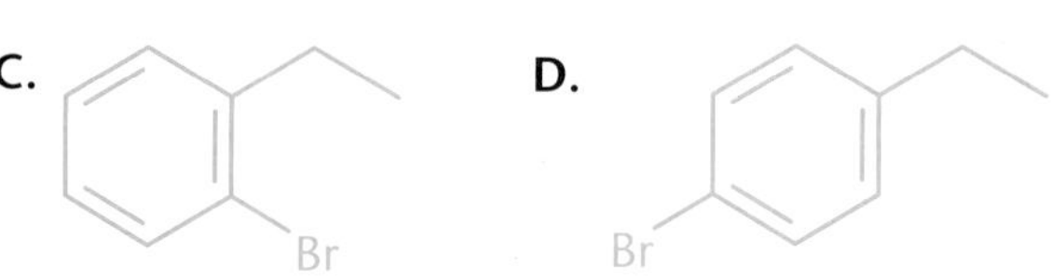

5. ^1H NMR data for compound X, with general formula $C_{10}H_{12}O$, is given below. What is the most likely structure of compound X?

δ 0.95 (triplet, 3H); δ 3.53 (quartet, 2H); δ 3.60 (singlet, 2H); δ 7.20 (multiplet, 5H)

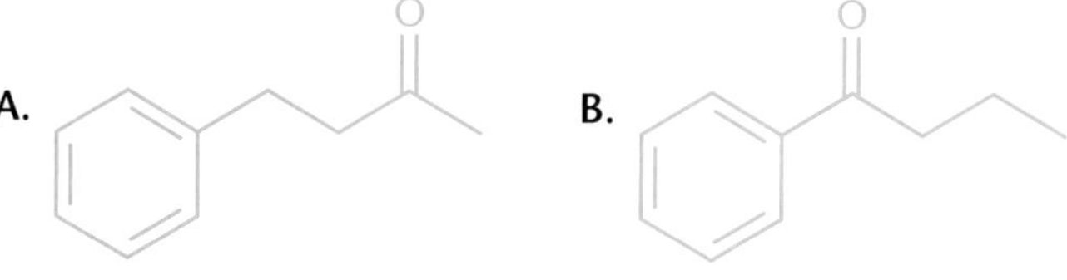

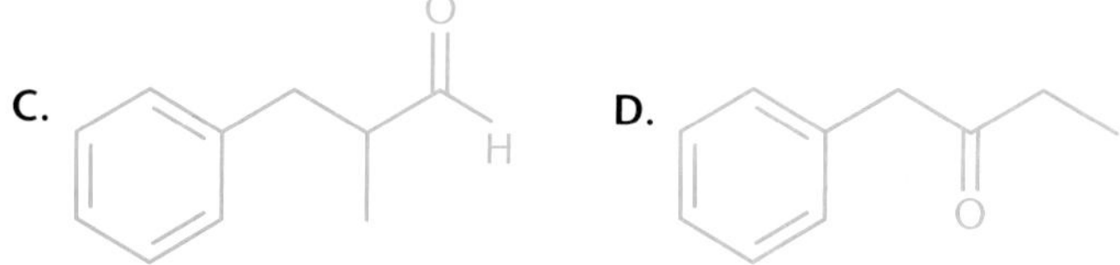

KEY CONCEPTS

Aromaticity

Electrophilic aromatic substitution

ELECTROPHILIC AROMATIC SUBSTITUTION

Show how you might prepare *p*–bromobenzoic acid starting from benzene.

1) Identify the substituents on the ring and their regiochemical preferences. Work backwards, if necessary.

$E^{\oplus}$

CO_2H E CO_2H

$E^{\oplus}$

Br Br E + E Br

TAKEAWAYS

Identify the regiochemical preferences of each substituent on an aromatic ring before thinking about specific reactions.

Clearly, we can't put both substituents on the ring at the same time. So, we'll have to put one substituent on at a time.

If the intermediate before the last step is the carboxylic acid, when this molecule is substituted the electrophile will go to the *meta* position, giving the incorrect regiochemistry.

If bromobenzene is substituted, the electrophile will go to the *ortho* and *para* positions. We can then separate the isomers to give the desired para isomer.

Remember: *The carboxylic acid is a* meta *director because it is resonance electron withdrawing. The bromo group is an* ortho/para *director because it is resonance electron donating.*

---

2) Establish reaction conditions to get to the desired product.

Me $KMnO_4$ CO_2H

Br Br

THINGS TO WATCH OUT FOR

Be sure to arrange the synthetic steps in the correct order!

Now that we've decided to brominate first, we have to figure out which electrophile we will place on bromobenzene to get to the carboxylic acid.

The most straightforward way to do this is to place a methyl group on bromobenzene, and then oxidize the methyl group to the carboxylic acid.

---

3) Write down the complete synthetic scheme in the forward direction.

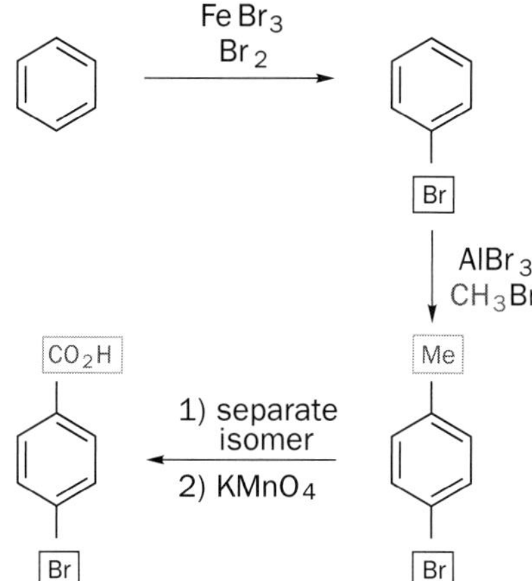

SIMILAR QUESTIONS

1) How might *para*–bromobenzoic acid be prepared from *para*–dibromobenzene?
2) If 3–bromomethoxybenzene were nitrated once, where do you expect that the nitro group would appear in the product?
3) Show how triphenylmethane could be prepared from excess benzene and chloroform.

KEY CONCEPTS

Electrophilic aromatic substitution

Nucleophilic acyl substitution

Spectroscopy

1H NMR

TAKEAWAYS

Be sure to move one step at a time with these problems and to use the spectroscopic data together, rather than in separate pieces, if possible.

THINGS TO WATCH OUT FOR

Make sure you know the IR stretches that are diagnostic for given functional groups. There aren't that many to learn—perhaps six at the most.

IDENTIFYING STRUCTURE OF UNKNOWN AROMATIC

Given the diagram and the 1H NMR spectra shown below, determine the structures of molecules **A** through **H.**

D (C_6H_7N) —(Cl(C=O)CH₂Me, $AlCl_3$)→ **E** ($C_9H_{11}NO$) —(Cl(C=O)CH₂Me, $AlCl_3$)→ **F + G + H** ($C_{12}H_{15}NO_2$)

%-Yield:
F = 38%
G = 5%
H = 47%

Benzene —(1) HNO_3, H_2SO_4; 2) H_2, Pt/C)→ **D**

Benzene —(Cl(C=O)CH₂Me, $AlCl_3$)→ **B** ($C_9H_{10}O$) —(Zn(Hg), HCl)→ **C** (C_9H_{12})

IR Stretch:
1690 cm^{-1}
2950 cm^{-1}
3010 cm^{-1}

Benzene —(n–PrCl, $AlCl_3$)→ **A** (C_9H_{12})

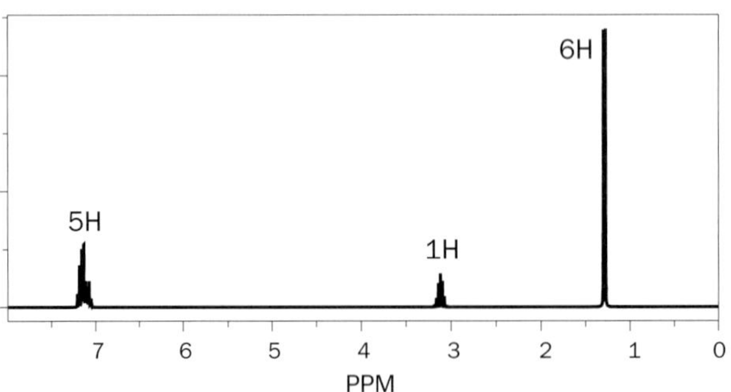

1H NMR of compound **A**

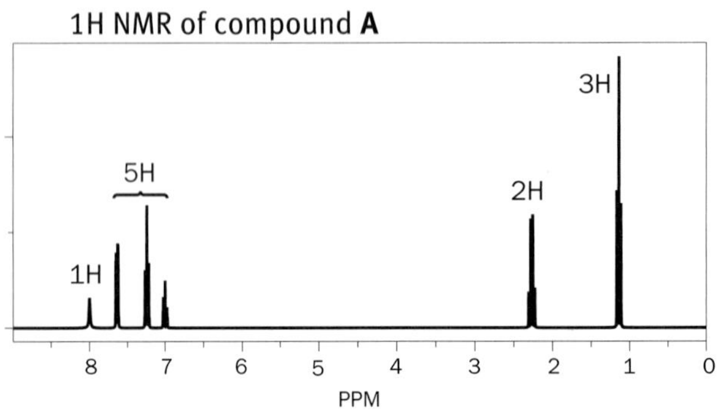

1H NMR of compound **E**

1) Determine the type of reaction.

Me Cl AlCl 3 → Me H (+) hydride shift Me Me (+) – H+ Me Me A

For the reaction to form product A, you should immediately recognize these conditions as that of a Friedel–Crafts alkylation. However, note from the NMR that the product is not simply propylbenzene because there are only two aliphatic signals in the NMR, not three. Therefore, the product must be isopropylbenzene.

---

2) Identify product B.
Product B is the product of a Friedel–Crafts *acylation*, giving a carbonyl.

O Me Zn(Hg) HCl → Me

$C_9H_{10}O$ C_9H_{12}

B **C**

Even if you didn't remember this, you should know that B contains a ketone from the stretch in the IR [the other stretches are for sp^3 C–H's (just to the *right* of 3,000 cm^{-1}) and the aromatic sp^2 C–H's (just to the *left* of 3,000 cm^{-1})]. In the next step, the carbonyl is removed and replaced with a methylene in the *Clemmensen reduction*.

---

3) Identify product D.

NH_2 O Cl Me AlCl 3 → O HN Me

C_6H_7N $C_9H_{11}NO$

D **E**

SIMILAR QUESTIONS

1) How might compound E be converted back into D?
2) Why is the IR stretch for the ketone in B slightly less than 1700 cm^{-1}?
3) What is the driving force for the rearrangement of the cation derived from propyl chloride (in the reaction to give A)?

In the reaction to give molecule D, note that benzene is first *nitrated,* then the nitro group is reduced to an *amine*. Remember that if you see a nitrogen-bearing functional group followed by reductive conditions, an amine is almost certainly being generated. You should recognize the conditions to give E as another Friedel–Crafts acylation; however, note that in the NMR, there are still five aromatic protons. Therefore, the only other place that the acyl group can go is on the amine.

Remember: *The amino group is much more nucleophilic than the benzene ring, so with a Lewis acid in the reaction, the amine adds to the acid chloride carbonyl and then eliminates chloride to give the amide E.*

---

4) Rerun the reaction with molecule E.

$C_9H_{11}NO$

E

$AlCl_3$

$C_{12}H_{15}NO_2$

F G H

The third time seems to be the charm for this grad student. When he repeats the acylation reaction on E, this time the reaction works. You should suspect this not only from the molecular formula, but from the fact that three products are formed in unequal yield—one of the telltale signs of electrophilic aromatic substitution. Because the nitrogen in E is still an *ortho/para* director, even with the adjacent carbonyl, the major products F and G will be the *ortho* and *para* isomers and H will be the *meta* isomer.

CHAPTER 7

ALCOHOLS AND ETHERS

ALCOHOLS

Alcohols are compounds with the general formula **ROH.** The functional group −**OH** is called the **hydroxyl** group. An alcohol can be thought of as a substituted water molecule, with an alkyl group R replacing one H atom.

TEACHER TIP

Alcohols are an important group of compounds and will be seen on the MCAT as protic solvents, reactants, products, and a prime example of hydrogen bonding.

NOMENCLATURE

Alcohols are named in the IUPAC system by replacing the **-e** ending of the root alkane with the ending **-ol.** The carbon atom attached to the hydroxyl group must be included in the longest chain and receives the lowest possible number. Some examples are:

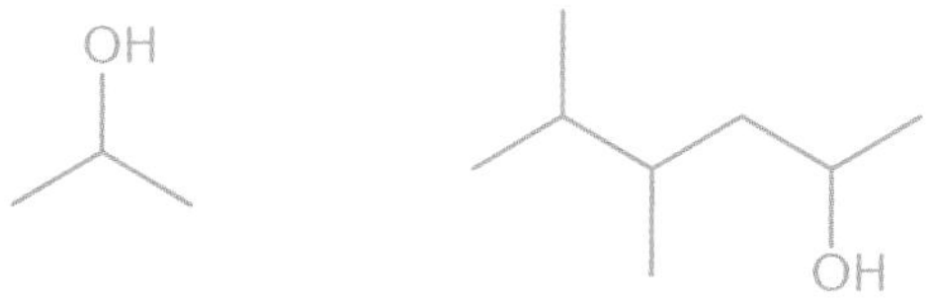

OH

OH

2-propanol　　4,5-dimethyl-2-hexanol

Figure 7.1

Alternatively, the alkyl group can be named as a derivative, followed by the word *alcohol*.

OH

OH

ethyl alcohol　　isobutyl alcohol

Figure 7.2

TEACHER TIP

Don't be thrown by these two naming systems; they both follow IUPAC rules!

Compounds of the general formula ArOH, with a hydroxyl group attached to an aromatic ring, are called **phenols** (see chapter 6).

TEACHER TIP

Aromatic alcohols (ArOH) are called phenols. The possible resonance between the ring and the lone pairs of the oxygen atom makes the hydrogen of the alcohol more acidic than other alcohols.

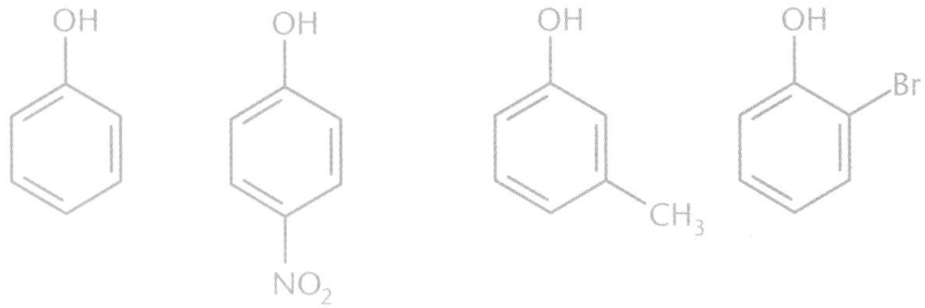

phenol   *p*-nitrophenol   *m*-cresol (*m*-methylphenol)   *o*-bromophenol

Figure 7.3

PHYSICAL PROPERTIES

The boiling points of alcohols are significantly higher than those of the analogous hydrocarbons, due to **hydrogen bonding.**

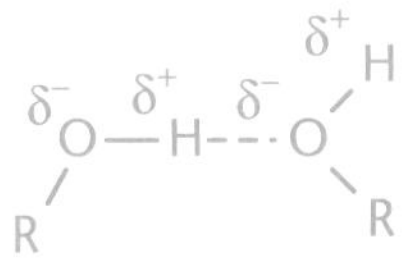

Figure 7.4

Molecules with more than one hydroxyl group show greater degrees of hydrogen bonding, as is evident from the following boiling points.

TEACHER TIP

Hydrogen bonding causes a great increase in boiling points!

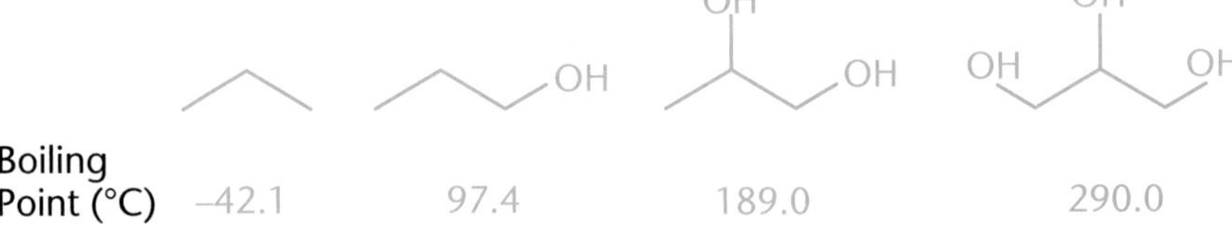

Figure 7.5

KAPLAN EXCLUSIVE

Hydrogen bonds form on the "phone"—the "FON"!

(Fluorine, Oxygen, Nitrogen)

Hydrogen bonding can also occur when hydrogen atoms are attached to other highly electronegative atoms, such as nitrogen and fluorine. HF has particularly strong hydrogen bonds because the high electronegativity of fluorine causes the HF bond to be highly polarized.

The hydroxyl hydrogen atom is weakly acidic, and alcohols can dissociate into protons and alkoxy ions just as water dissociates into protons and hydroxide ions. pK_a values of several compounds are listed in Table 7.1.

Table 7.1.

Dissociation			pK$_a$
H_2O	$\rightleftharpoons$	$HO^- + H^+$	15.7
CH_3OH	$\rightleftharpoons$	$CH_3O^- + H^+$	15.5
C_2H_5OH	$\rightleftharpoons$	$C_2H_5O^- + H^+$	15.9
i-PrOH	$\rightleftharpoons$	*i*-PrO$^-$ + H$^+$	17.1
t-BuOH	$\rightleftharpoons$	*t*-BuO$^-$ + H$^+$	18.0
CF_3CH_2OH	$\rightleftharpoons$	$CF_3CH_2O^- + H^+$	12.4
PhOH	$\rightleftharpoons$	PhO$^-$ + H$^+$	≈10.0

TEACHER TIP

$pK_a = -\log K_a$

Strong acids have high Ka's and small pKa's. Thus, phenol, which has the smallest pKa, is the most acidic.

The hydroxyl hydrogens of phenols are more acidic than those of alcohols, due to resonance stuctures that distribute the negative charge throughout the ring, thus stabilizing the anion. As a result, these compounds form intermolecular hydrogen bonds and have relatively high melting and boiling points. Phenol is slightly soluble in water (presumably due to hydrogen bonding), as are some of its derivatives. Phenols are much more acidic than aliphatic alcohols and can form salts with inorganic bases such as NaOH.

MCAT SYNOPSIS

Acidity decreases as more alkyl groups are attached because the electron-donating alkyl groups *destabilize* the alkoxide anion. Electron-withdrawing groups stabilize the alkoxy anion, making the alcohol more acidic.

The presence of other substituents on the ring has significant effects on the acidity, boiling points, and melting points of phenols. As with other aromatic compounds, electron-withdrawing substituents increase acidity, and electron-donating groups decrease acidity.

REVIEW

A. KEY REACTION MECHANISMS FOR ALCOHOLS AND ETHERS

As you read about synthesis of (and from) alcohols and ethers, you'll see the same basic reaction mechanisms recurring over and over. Rather than memorizing each reaction individually, try to think of them in broad categories. Focus on how the basic mechanism works and on how this particular reaction exemplifies it. The "Big Three" mechanisms for alcohols and ethers are:

TEACHER TIP

The first two reactions here are the ones discussed earlier in our chapters on Alkanes and Alkenes. The third mechanism is one that will get more attention in the upcoming chapters.

1) S_N1, S_N2: nucleophilic substitution

   e.g., $CH_3Br + OH^- \longrightarrow CH_3OH + Br^-$

   See chapter 4 for review.

2) Electrophilic addition to a double bond,

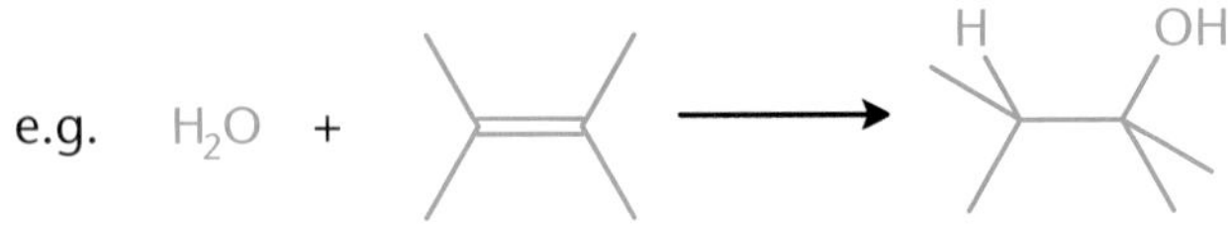

e.g. H_2O + (alkene) → (alcohol with H and OH)

This and other reactions adding H_2O to double bonds are covered in chapter 4.

3) Nucleophilic addition to a carbonyl,

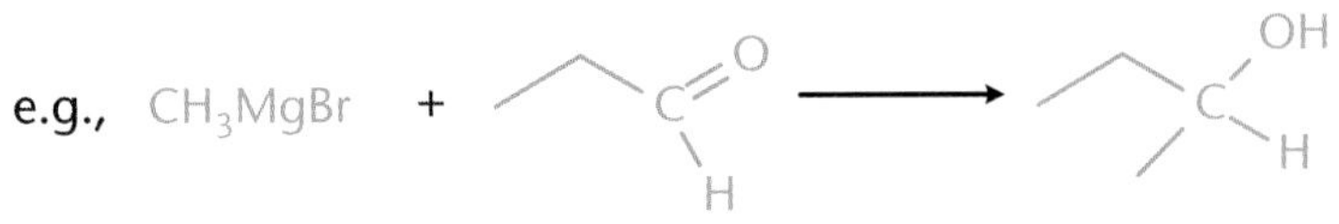

e.g., CH_3MgBr + (aldehyde) → (secondary alcohol)

This mechanism is discussed further in chapters 8–10.

Also, when thinking about alcohols, you should keep in mind their place on the oxidation-reduction continuum:

KAPLAN EXCLUSIVE

More bonds to oxygen means more oxidized.

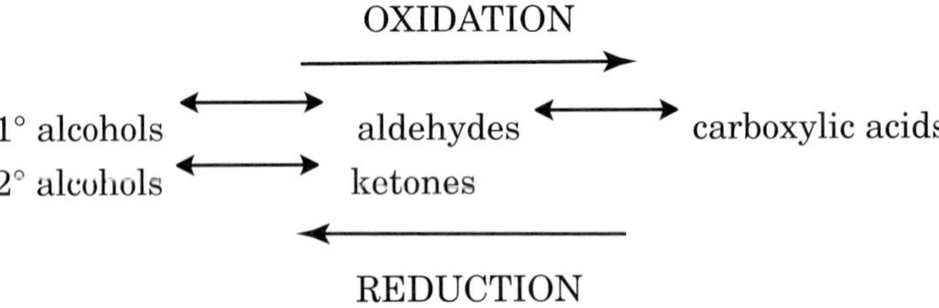

As you read about the individual reactions in which alcohols participate, try to fit them into this framework (possible for most reactions, though not all).

SYNTHESIS

Alcohols can be prepared from a variety of different types of compounds. Methanol, also called wood alcohol, is obtained from the destructive distillation of wood. It is toxic and can cause blindness if ingested. Ethanol, or grain alcohol, is produced from the fermentation of sugars and can be metabolized by the body; however, in large enough quantities, it too is toxic.

A. ADDITION REACTIONS

Alcohols can be prepared via several reactions which involve addition of water to double bonds (discussed in chapter 5). Alcohols can also be prepared from the addition of organometallic compounds to carbonyl groups (discussed in chapter 10).

B. SUBSTITUTION REACTIONS

Both S_N1 and S_N2 reactions can be used to produce alcohols under the proper conditions (discussed in chapter 4).

C. REDUCTION REACTIONS

Alcohols can be prepared from the reduction of aldehydes, ketones, carboxylic acids, or esters. Lithium aluminum hydride ($LiAlH_4$, or LAH) and sodium borohydride ($NaBH_4$) are the two most frequently used reducing reagents. LAH is more powerful and more difficult to work with, whereas $NaBH_4$ is more selective and easier to handle. For example, LAH will reduce carboxylic acids and esters, while $NaBH_4$ will not.

Teacher Tip

Oxidation and reduction reactions are important tools to the organic chemist and will be important for you to know on the MCAT. Remember, reducing agents have a lot of H's ($NaBH_4$ and $LiAlH_4$), and oxidizing agents have a lot of O's ($KMnO_4$).

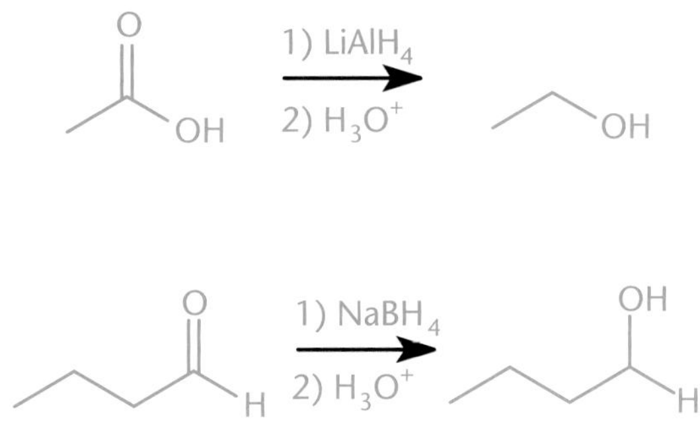

Figure 7.6

D. PHENOL SYNTHESIS

Phenols may be synthesized from arylsulfonic acids with hot NaOH, as described in chapter 6. However, this reaction is useful only for phenol or its alkylated derivatives, as most functional groups are destroyed by the harsh reaction conditions.

A more versatile method of synthesizing phenols is via hydrolysis of diazonium salts.

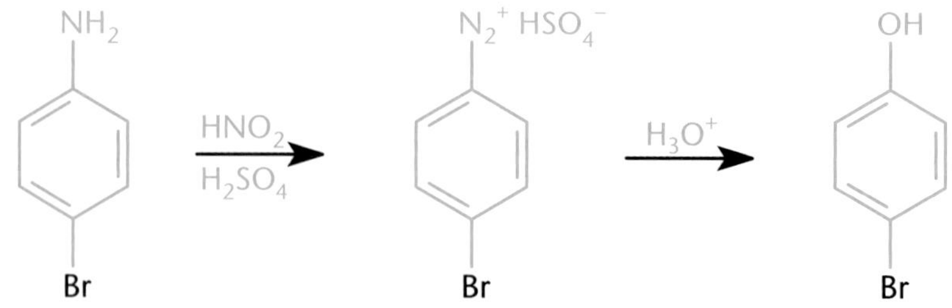

Figure 7.7

REACTIONS

A. ELIMINATION REACTIONS

Alcohols can be **dehydrated** in a strongly acidic solution (usually H_2SO_4) to produce alkenes. The mechanism of this dehydration reaction is E1, and proceeds via the protonated alcohol.

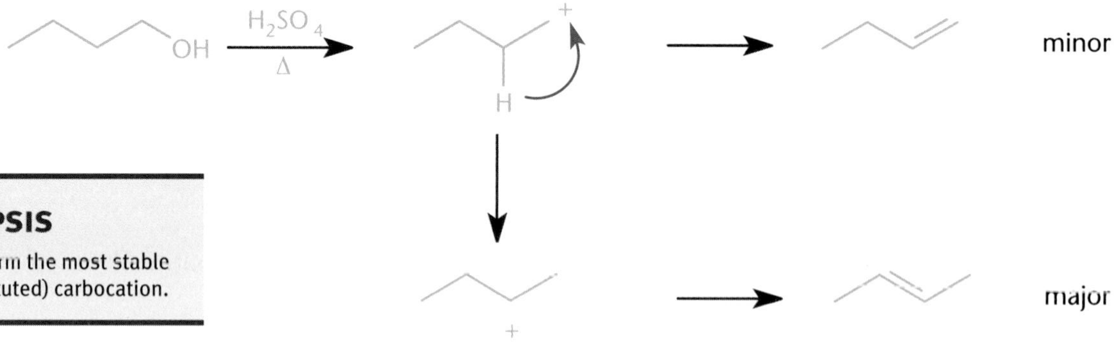

Figure 7.8

MCAT SYNOPSIS

In E1, you want to form the most stable (that is, most substituted) carbocation.

Notice that two products are obtained, with the more stable alkene being the major product. This occurs via movement of a proton to produce the more stable 2° carbocation. This type of rearrangement is commonly encountered with carbocations.

B. SUBSTITUTION REACTIONS

The displacement of hydroxyl groups in substitution reactions is rare because the hydroxide ion is a poor leaving group. If such a transformation is desired, the hydroxyl group must be made into a good leaving group. Protonating the alcohol makes water the leaving group, which is good for S_N1 reactions; even better, the alcohol can be converted into a tosylate (*p*-toluenesulfonate) group, which is an excellent leaving group for S_N2 reactions (see Figures 7.9a and 7.9b).

MCAT SYNOPSIS

Alcohols can participate in S_N1 or S_N2 reactions, but only if you turn the –OH into a better leaving group by one of the following methods:

- —protonate it;
- —convert to a tosylate;
- —form an inorganic ester.

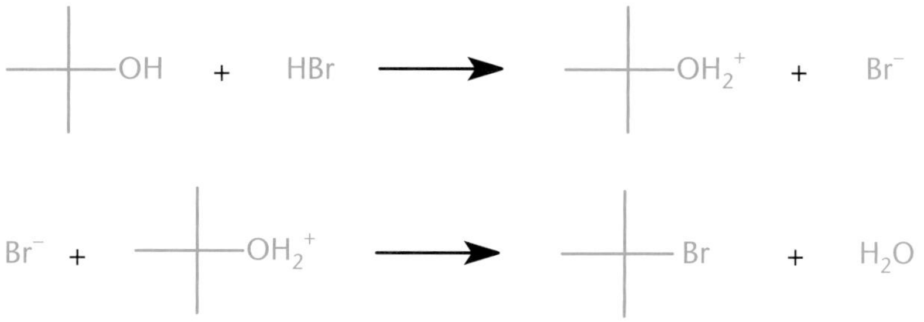
OH
HBr
OH_2^+
Br^-
Br^-
OH_2^+
Br
H_2O

Figure 7.9a

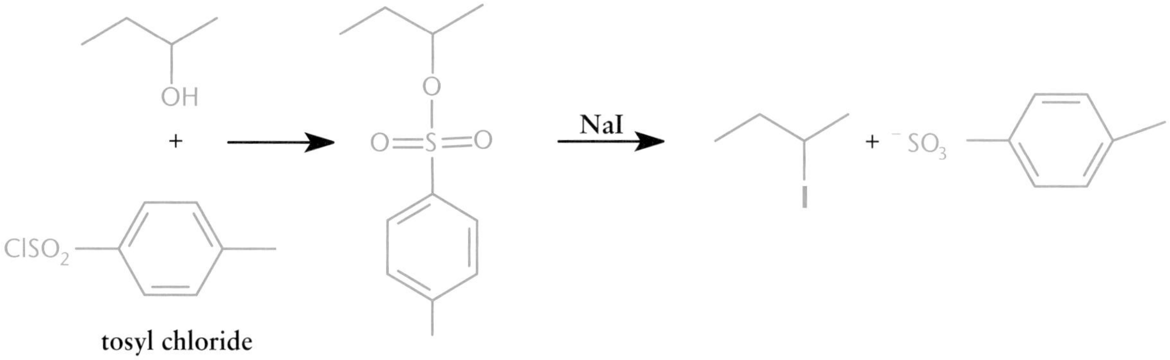
OH
O
O=S=O
NaI
$^-SO_3$
$ClSO_2$
I
tosyl chloride

Figure 7.9b

A common method of converting alcohols into alkyl halides involves the formation of inorganic esters, which readily undergo S_N2 reactions. Alcohols react with thionyl chloride to produce an intermediate inorganic ester (a chlorosulfite) and HCl. The chloride ion of HCl displaces SO_2 and regenerates Cl^-, forming the desired alkyl chloride.

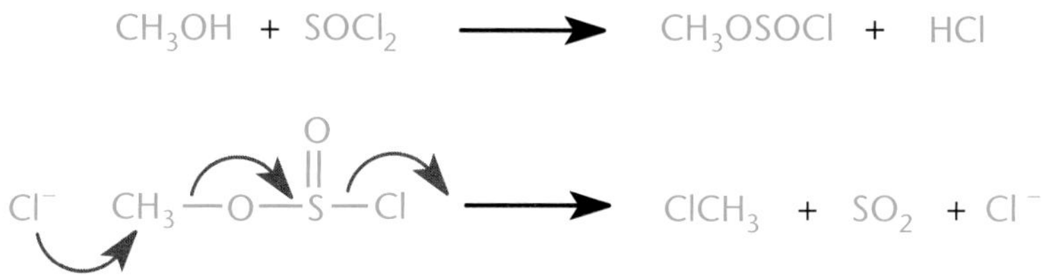
CH_3OH + $SOCl_2$
CH_3OSOCl + HCl
Cl^-
CH_3—O—S—Cl
O
$ClCH_3$ + SO_2 + Cl^-

Figure 7.10

An analogous reaction, where the alcohol is treated with PBr_3 instead of thionyl chloride, produces alkyl bromides.

Phenols readily undergo electrophilic aromatic substitution reactions; because it has lone pairs that it can donate to the ring, the –OH group is a strongly activating, *ortho/para*-directing ring substituent (see chapter 6).

Teacher Tip

Phenols are good substrates for the EAS reactions from chapter 6. Remember that the lone pair from the oxygen makes it an electron donating substituent. Therefore, the -OH will be activating and *ortho/para* directing.

C. OXIDATION REACTIONS

The oxidation of alcohols generally involves some form of chromium (VI) as the oxidizing agent, which is reduced to chromium (III) during the reaction. PCC (pyridinium chlorochromate, $C_5H_6NCrO_3Cl$) is commonly used as a mild oxidant. It converts primary alcohols to aldehydes without overoxidation to the acid. (In contrast, $KMnO_4$ is a very strong oxidizing agent that will take the alcohol all the way to the carboxylic acid.) It can also be used to form ketones from 2° alcohols. Tertiary alcohols cannot be oxidized for valence reasons.

PAVLOV'S DOG

When you see a transition metal (such as Cr or Mn) with lots of oxygen (Cr_2O_7, CrO_3, MnO_4), think OXIDATION.

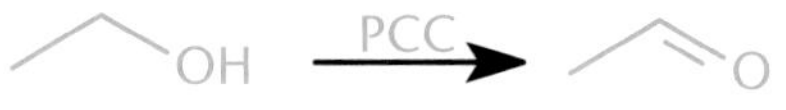

OH —PCC→ O

Figure 7.11

Another reagent used to oxidize secondary alcohols is alkali (either sodium or potassium) dichromate salt. This will also oxidize 1° alcohols to carboxylic acids.

OH —$Na_2Cr_2O_7$ / H_2SO_4→ O

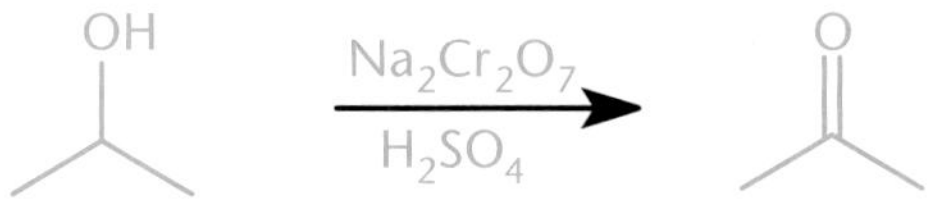

Figure 7.12

A stronger oxidant is chromium trioxide, CrO_3. This is often dissolved with dilute sulfuric acid in acetone; the mixture is called Jones' reagent. It oxidizes primary alcohols to carboxylic acids and secondary alcohols to ketones.

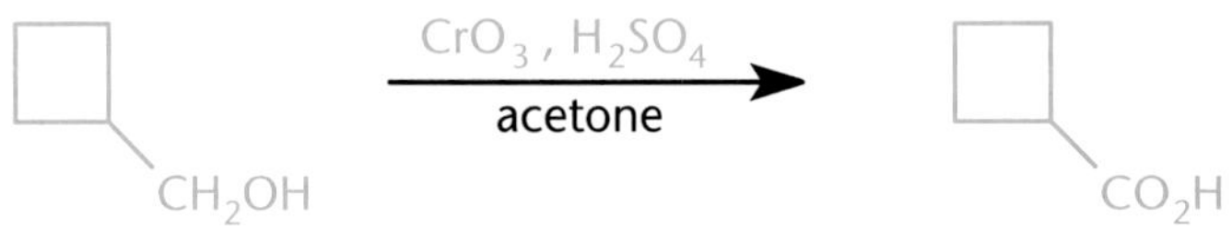

CH_2OH —CrO_3, H_2SO_4 / acetone→ CO_2H

Figure 7.13

Treatment of phenols with oxidizing reagents produces compounds called quinones (2,5-cyclohexadiene-1,4-diones).

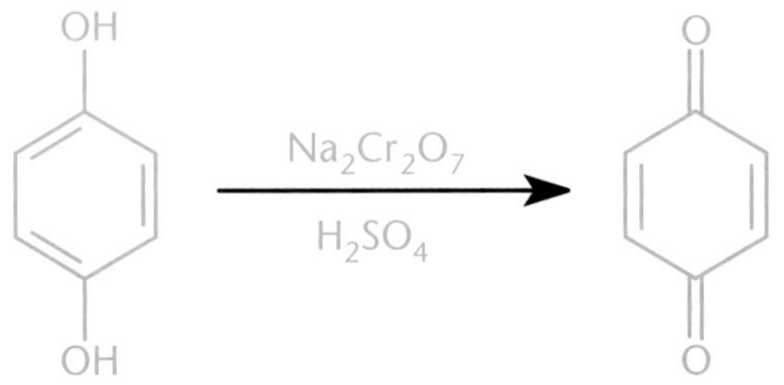

OH, OH —$Na_2Cr_2O_7$ / H_2SO_4→ O, O

1,4-Benzenediol p-Benzoquinone

Figure 7.14

ETHERS

An ether is a compound with two alkyl (or aryl) groups bonded to an oxygen atom. The general formula for an ether is **ROR.** Ethers can be thought of as disubstituted water molecules. The most familiar ether is diethyl ether, once used as a medical anesthetic, and still often used that way in the laboratory.

TEACHER TIP

Ethers, like alcohols, are important solvents, though ethers are *aprotic*.

NOMENCLATURE

Ethers are named according to IUPAC rules as **alkoxyalkanes,** with the smaller chain as the prefix and the larger chain as the suffix. There is a common system of nomenclature in which ethers are named as alkyl alkyl ethers. In this system, methoxyethane would be named ethyl methyl ether. The alkyl substituents are alphabetized.

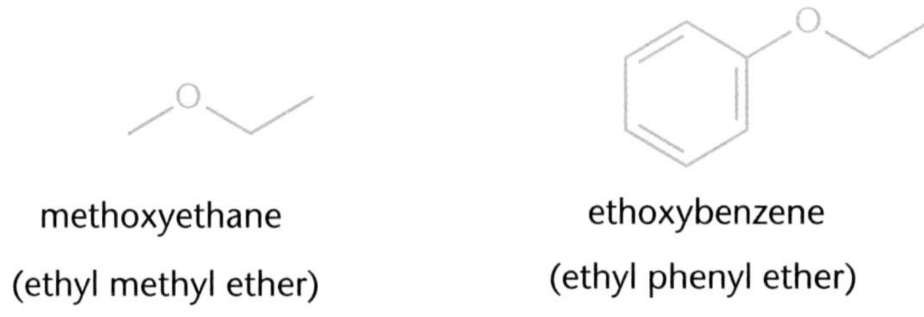

Figure 7.15

Exceptions to these rules occur for cyclic ethers, for which many common names also exist.

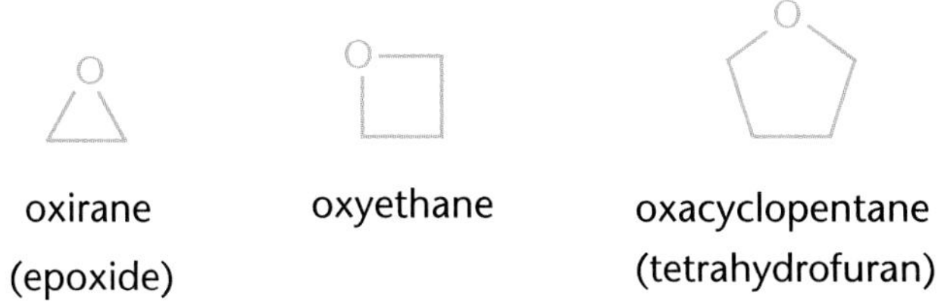

Figure 7.16

MCAT SYNOPSIS

Remember that smaller rings have more angle strain, making them less stable.

PHYSICAL PROPERTIES

Ethers do not undergo hydrogen bonding because they have no hydrogen atoms bonded to the oxygen atoms. Ethers therefore boil at relatively low temperatures compared to alcohols; in fact, they boil at approximately the same temperatures as alkanes of comparable molecular weight.

TEACHER TIP

The *lack* of hydrogen bonds is significant when determining the physical properties of ethers.

Ethers are only slightly polar and therefore only slightly soluble in water. They are rather inert to most organic reagents and are frequently used as solvents.

SYNTHESIS

The Williamson ether synthesis produces ethers from the reaction of metal alkoxides with primary alkyl halides or tosylates. The alkoxides behave as nucleophiles, and displace the halide or tosylate via an S_N2 reaction, producing an ether.

MCAT SYNOPSIS

Look! It's S_N2 again! Therefore, you need a strong nucleophile (alkoxides are good) and an unhindered substrate (*not* bulky or highly substituted).

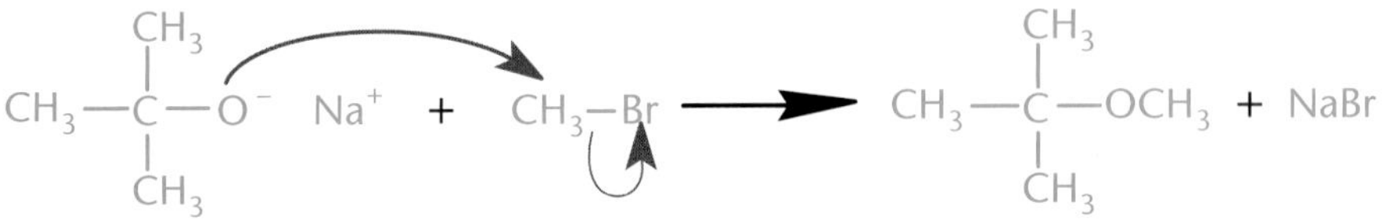

$$(CH_3)_3C{-}O^- \; Na^+ + CH_3{-}Br \longrightarrow (CH_3)_3C{-}OCH_3 + NaBr$$

Figure 7.17

It is important to remember that alkoxides will attack only nonhindered halides. Thus, to synthesize a methyl ether, an alkoxide must attack a methyl halide; the reaction cannot be accomplished with methoxide ion attacking a hindered alkyl halide substrate.

The Williamson ether synthesis can also be applied to phenols. Relatively mild reaction conditions are sufficient, due to the phenols' acidity.

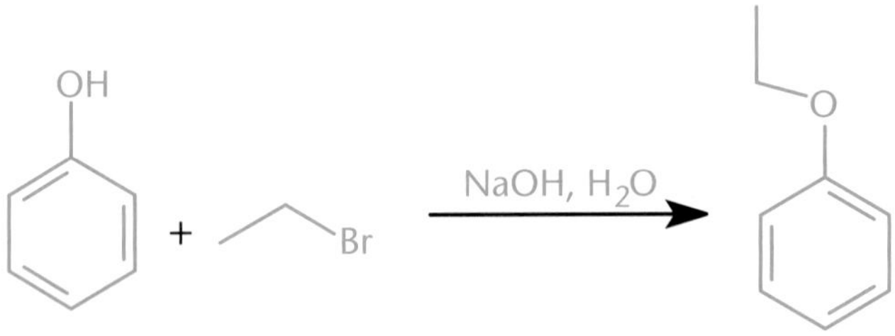

OH (phenol) + Br (ethyl bromide) —NaOH, H_2O→ O (ethoxybenzene)

Figure 7.18

Cyclic ethers are prepared in a number of ways. Oxiranes can be synthesized by means of an internal S_N2 displacement.

MCAT SYNOPSIS

More S_N2! This time, however, it's intramolecular—the nucleophile and leaving group are part of the same molecule.

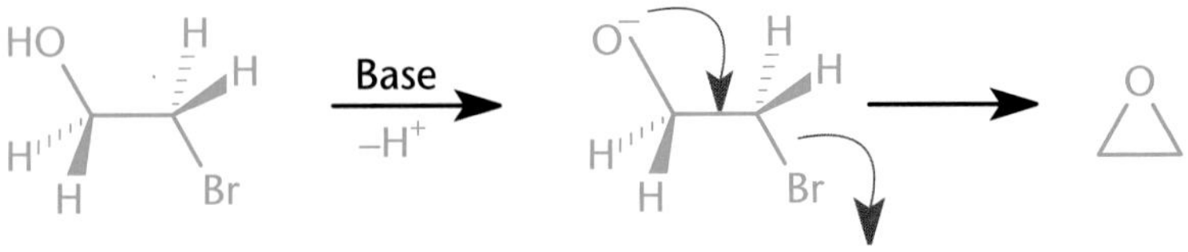

HO, H, H, H, H, Br —Base, $-H^+$→ O^-, H, H, H, H, Br → O

Figure 7.19

Oxidation of an alkene with a **peroxy acid** (general formula RCOOOH) such as mcpba (*m*-chloroperoxybenzoic acid) will also produce an oxirane.

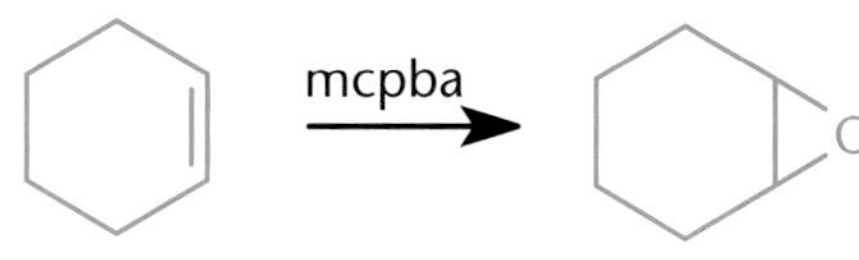

Figure 7.20

TEACHER TIP

Intramolecular reactions are often seen on the MCAT because they can be confusing to test takers. With every reaction on the exam, identify an electrophile (positive) and a nucleophile (negative) first and you know that they will then come together—even if they are part of the same molecule.

REACTIONS

A. PEROXIDE FORMATION

Ethers react with the oxygen in air to form highly explosive compounds called **peroxides** (general formula ROOR).

MCAT SYNOPSIS

Remember, strong bases are poor leaving groups. Without protonation, the leaving group would be an alkoxide (strongly basic), and the reaction would be unlikely to proceed.

B. CLEAVAGE

Cleavage of straight-chain ethers will take place only under vigorous conditions: usually at high temperatures in the presence of HBr or HI. Cleavage is initiated by protonation of the ether oxygen. The reaction then proceeds by an S_N1 or S_N2 mechanism, depending on the conditions and the structure of the ether (Figure 7.20). Although not shown below, the alcohol products usually react with a second molecule of hydrogen halide to produce an alkyl halide.

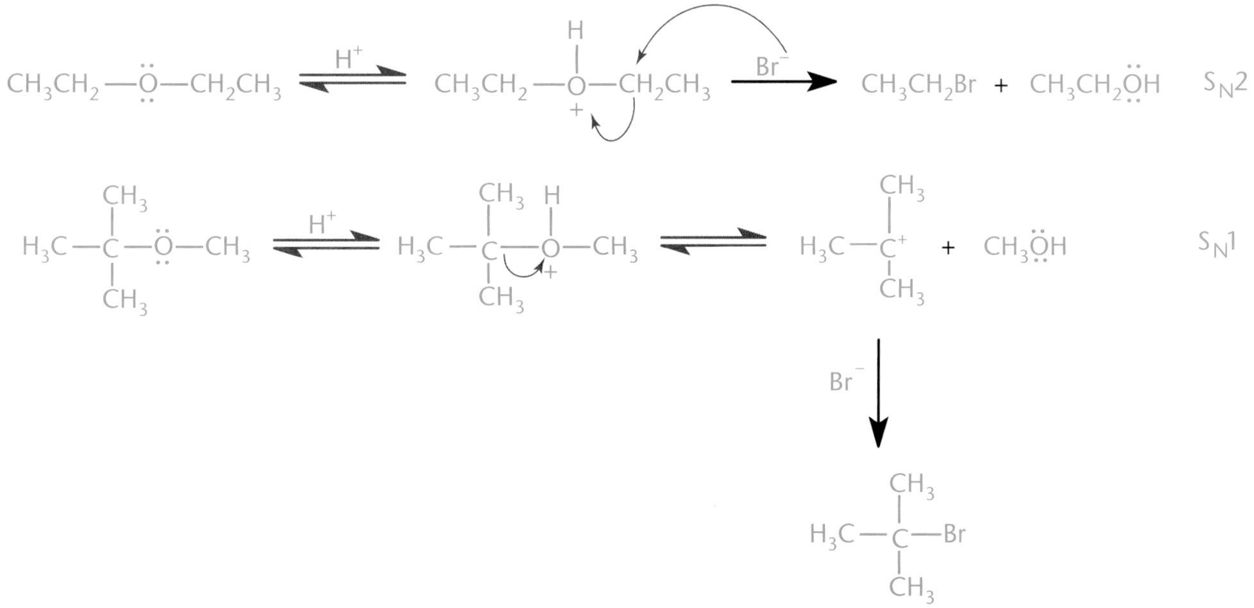

$$CH_3CH_2-\ddot{O}-CH_2CH_3 \overset{H^+}{\rightleftharpoons} CH_3CH_2-\overset{+}{O}(H)-CH_2CH_3 \xrightarrow{Br^-} CH_3CH_2Br + CH_3CH_2\ddot{O}H \quad S_N2$$

$$(CH_3)_3C-\ddot{O}-CH_3 \overset{H^+}{\rightleftharpoons} (CH_3)_3C-\overset{+}{O}(H)-CH_3 \rightleftharpoons (CH_3)_3C^+ + CH_3\ddot{O}H \quad S_N1$$

$$(CH_3)_3C^+ \xrightarrow{Br^-} (CH_3)_3C-Br$$

Figure 7.21

MCAT SYNOPSIS

Cleavage of straight chain ethers is acid-catalyzed. Cleavage of cyclic ethers can be acid- or base-catalyzed.

Because epoxides are highly strained cyclic ethers, they are susceptible to S_N2 reactions. Unlike straight-chain ethers, these reactions can be catalyzed by acid or base. In symmetrical epoxides, either carbon can be nucleophilically attacked; but in asymmetrical epoxides, the most substituted carbon is nucleophilically attacked in the presence of acid, and the least substituted carbon is attacked in the presence of base:

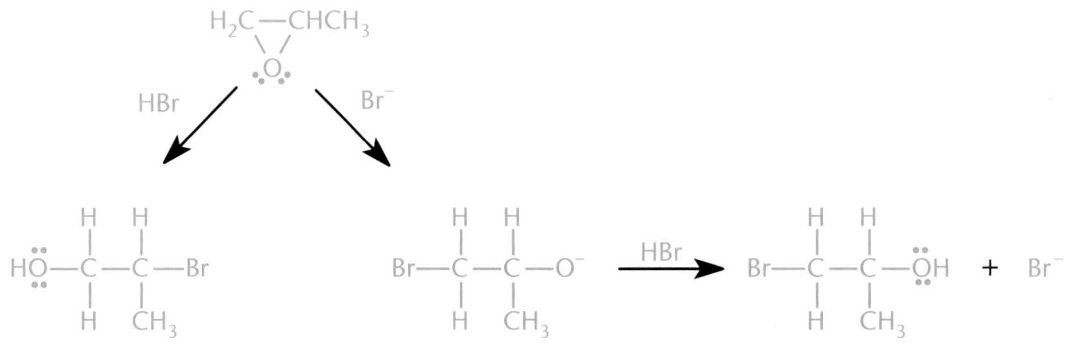

Figure 7.22

MCAT SYNOPSIS

Base-catalyzed cleavage has the most S_N2 character, while acid-catalyzed cleavage seems to have some S_N1 character.

Base-catalyzed cleavage has the most S_N2 character, so it occurs at the least hindered (least substituted) carbon. The basic environment provides the best nucleophile.

In contrast, acid-catalyzed cleavage is thought to have some S_N1 character as well as some S_N2 character. The epoxide O can be protonated, making it a better leaving group. This gives the carbons a bit of positive charge. Because substitution stabilizes this charge (remember, 3° carbons make the best carbocations), the more substituted C becomes a good target for nucleophilic attack.

Don't let epoxides intimidate you; the same basic principles and reaction mechanisms apply, just as we've seen with more simple compounds.

PRACTICE QUESTIONS

1. Given the reaction shown below with *m*-chloroperoxybenzoic acid, which could be the stereochemistry of the product?

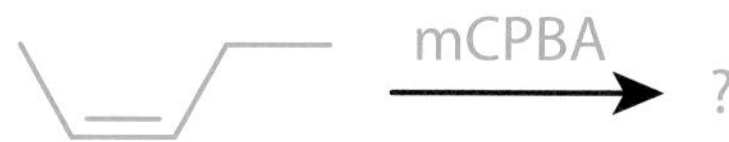

I. 2(R), 3(R)
II. 2(R), 3(S)
III. 2(S), 3(R)
IV. 2(S), 3(S)

A. I and II
B. II and IV
C. II and III
D. I and IV

2. What are the major products of the reaction shown below?

O HBr ?

A. Phenol and bromopropane
B. Bromobenzene and propanol
C. Bromobenzene and propane
D. Benzene and propane

3. Which of the compounds below can undergo oxidation?

A. OH

B. O

C. O OH

D. OH

4. How many different products (excluding water) can be obtained from the dehydration reaction shown below?

OH CH_3 H^+, heat

A. 1
B. 2
C. 3
D. 4

5. What reagents most effectively produce the following transformation shown below?

O ? OH OCH_3

A. CH_3OH, H^+
B. CH_3Br
C. H_3O^+, CH_3Cl
D. CH_3OH, CH_3O–Na^+

CHAPTER 8

ALDEHYDES AND KETONES

Aldehydes and **ketones** are compounds that contain the **carbonyl group, C=O,** a double bond between a carbon atom and an oxygen atom. A ketone has two alkyl or aryl groups bonded to the carbonyl, whereas an aldehyde has one alkyl group and one hydrogen (or, in the case of formaldehyde, two hydrogens) bonded to the carbonyl. The carbonyl group is one of the most important functional groups in organic chemistry. In addition to aldehydes and ketones, it is also found in carboxylic acids, esters, amides, and more complicated compounds.

NOMENCLATURE

In the IUPAC system, aldehydes are named with the suffix **-al.** The position of the aldehyde group does not need to be specified: it must occupy the terminal (C–1) position. Common names exist for the first five aldehydes: formaldehyde, acetaldehyde, propionaldehyde, butyraldehyde, and valeraldehyde.

TEACHER TIP

These common names actually do have a pattern: *form-* will be seen also in formic acid (a one carbon carboxylic acid), and *acet-* is seen in many two-carbon compounds (acetic acid, acetyl CoA).

TEACHER TIP

Aldehydes and ketones are important functional groups because they can be reduced to form alcohols and oxidized to form carboxylic acids.

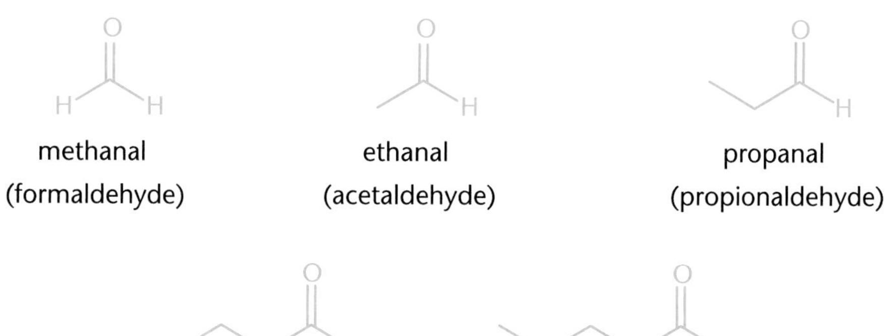

Figure 8.1

In more complicated molecules, the suffix **-carbaldehyde** can be used. In addition, the aldehyde can be named as a functional group with the prefix **formyl-.**

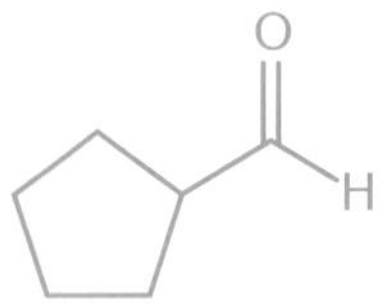

cyclopentanecarbaldehyde

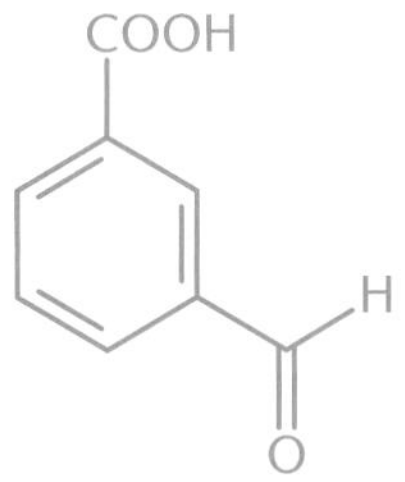

m-formylbenzoic acid

Figure 8.2

Ketones are named with the suffix **-one.** The location of the carbonyl group must be specified with a number, except in cyclic ketones, where it is assumed to occupy the number 1 position. The common system of naming **ketones** lists the two alkyl groups followed by the word *ketone*. When it is necessary to name the carbonyl as a substituent, the prefix **oxo-** is used.

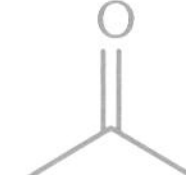

2-propanone
(dimethyl ketone)
(acetone)

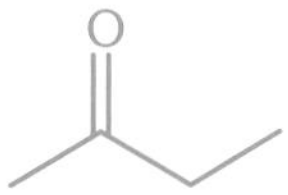

2-butanone
(ethyl methyl ketone)

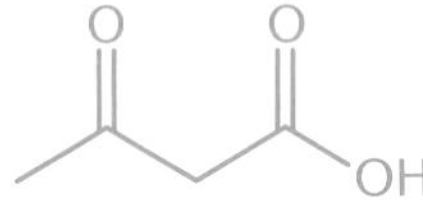

3-oxobutanoic acid

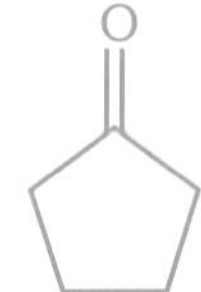

cyclopentanone

Figure 8.3

TEACHER TIP

The carbonyl group (in aldehydes and ketones) has a dipole moment. Oxygen is more electronegative—it is an "electron hog,"—pulling the electrons away from the carbon, making the carbon electrophilic.

PHYSICAL PROPERTIES

The physical properties of aldehydes and ketones are governed by the presence of the carbonyl group. The dipole moments that are associated with the polar carbonyl groups align, causing an elevation in boiling point relative to the alkanes. This elevation is less than that in alcohols, as no hydrogen bonding is involved.

TEACHER TIP

While the dipole moments in the carbonyl do increase their intermolecular forces and therefore their boiling points, it is not as significant as the hydrogen bonds seen in alcohols.

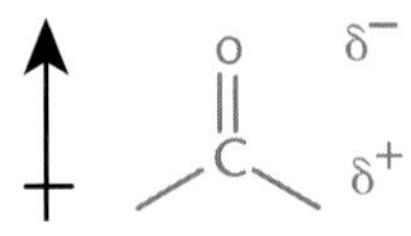

Figure 8.4

SYNTHESIS

There are numerous methods of preparing aldehydes and ketones; three of the most common are described below.

A. OXIDATION OF ALCOHOLS

An aldehyde can be obtained from the oxidation of a primary alcohol; a ketone can be obtained from a secondary alcohol. As mentioned in chapter 7, these reactions are usually performed with PCC, sodium or potassium dichromate, or chromium trioxide (Jones's reagent).

> **MCAT SYNOPSIS**
> Primary alcohols can be oxidized to aldehydes. Secondary alcohols can be oxidized to ketones.

Primary alcohols (1) $\longrightarrow$ aldehydes (2) $\longrightarrow$ carboxylic acids (3)
secondary alcohols (1) $\longrightarrow$ ketone (2)

B. OZONOLYSIS OF ALKENES

Double bonds can be oxidatively cleaved to yield aldehydes and/or ketones, typically with ozone. See chapter 5 for more details.

C. FRIEDEL-CRAFTS ACYLATION

This reaction, discussed in chapter 6, produces ketones of the form R–CO–Ar.

REACTIONS

A. ENOLIZATION AND REACTIONS OF ENOLS

Protons alpha to carbonyl groups are relatively acidic ($pK_a \approx 20$), due to resonance stabilization of the conjugate base. A hydrogen atom that detaches itself from the alpha carbon has a finite probability of reattaching itself to the oxygen instead of the carbon. Therefore, aldehydes and ketones exist in solution as a mixture of two isomers, the familiar **keto** form, and the **enol** form, representing the unsaturated alcohol (**ene** = the double bond, **ol** = the alcohol, so **ene + ol = enol**). The two isomers, which differ only in the placement of a proton, are called **tautomers.** The equilibrium between the tautomers lies far to the keto side. The process of interconverting from the keto to the enol tautomer is called **enolization.**

> **MCAT SYNOPSIS**
> Aldehydes and ketones have the traditional keto form (C=O), as well as the less common enol tautomer (enol = ene + ol). The enol form can act as a nucleophile.

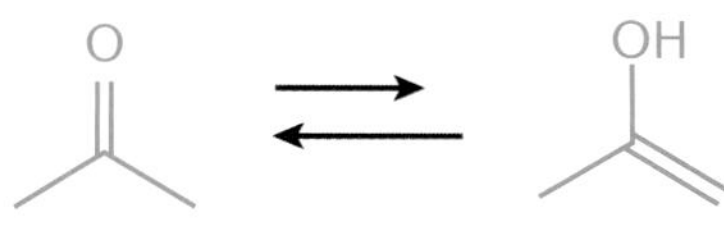

Figure 8.5

Enols are the necessary intermediates in many reactions of aldehydes and ketones. The enolate carbanion, which is nucleophilic, can be created with a strong base such as lithium diisopropyl amide (LDA) or potassium hydride, KH. This nucleophilic carbanion reacts via S_N2 with α, β-unsaturated carbonyl compounds in reactions called **Michael additions.**

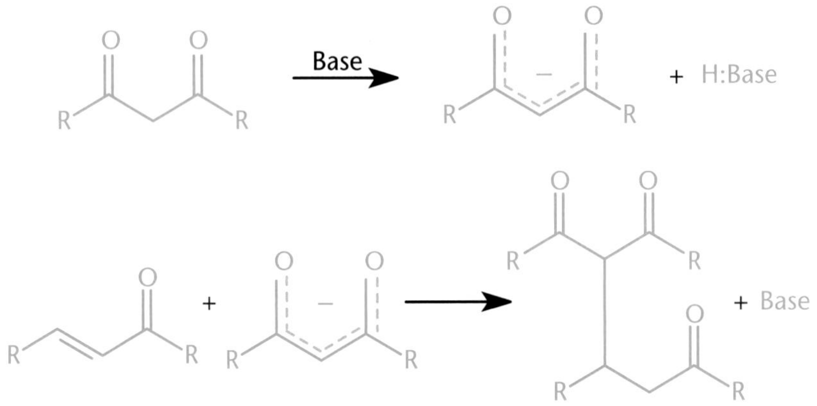

TEACHER TIP

Recall our discussion about α-hydrogen acidity. The hybrid structures in Figure 8.6 depicting resonance demonstrate why the hydrogen on the α-carbon is acidic and can then act as a nucleophile in more complex reactions such as the aldol condensation seen at the end of this chapter.

Figure 8.6

B. ADDITION REACTIONS

General Reaction Mechanism: Nucleophilic Addition to a Carbonyl

Many of the reactions of aldehydes and ketones share this general reaction mechanism. Rather than memorizing them all individually, focus on understanding the basic pattern. Then, you can learn how each reaction exemplifies it.

As shown in Figure 8.4 earlier, the C=O bond is polarized, with a partial positive charge on C and a partial negative charge on O. This makes the carbon ripe for nucleophilic attack.

The nucleophile attacks, forming a bond to the C, which causes the π bond in the C=O to break. This generates a tetrahedral intermediate. If no good leaving group is present, the double bond cannot reform, and so the final product is nearly identical to the intermediate, except that usually the O^- will accept a proton to become a hydroxyl (–OH).

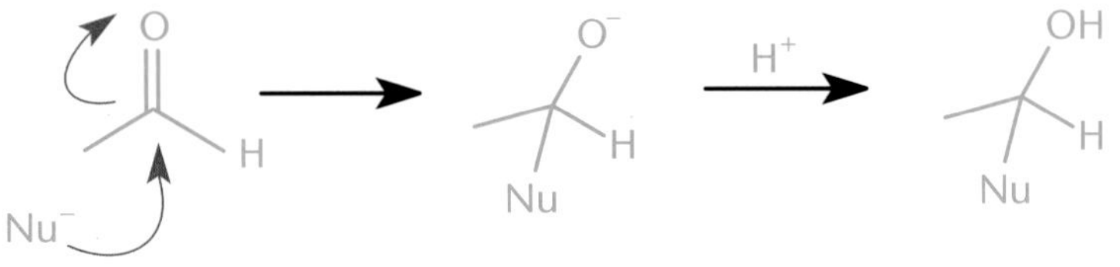

TEACHER TIP

Memorizing one reaction may get you one question correct but understanding trends and overarching concepts will get you many questions correct. The carbonyl carbon is a great target for nucleophilic attacks in many of the reactions in this chapter.

Figure 8.7

Although the figure shows only nucleophilic addition to an aldehyde, this mechanism applies to ketones as well.

1. **Hydration.** In the presence of water, aldehydes and ketones react to form *gem* diols (1,1-diols). In this case, water acts as the nucleophile attacking at the carbonyl carbon. This hydration reaction proceeds slowly; the rate may be increased by the addition of a small amount of acid or base.

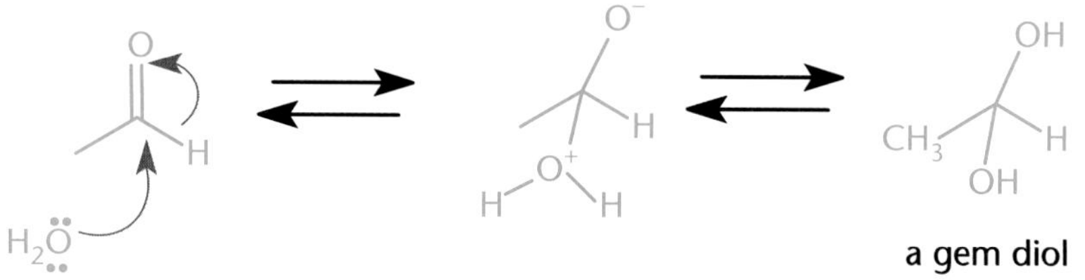

a gem diol

Figure 8.8

MCAT SYNOPSIS

Hydration is when H_2O is the nucleophile, and carbonyl carbon is the electrophile.

2. **Acetal and ketal formation.** A reaction similar to hydration occurs when aldehydes and ketones are treated with alcohols. When one equivalent of alcohol (in this reaction the nucleophile) is added to an aldehyde or ketone, the product is a **hemiacetal** or a **hemiketal,** respectively. When two equivalents of alcohol are added, the product is an **acetal** or a **ketal,** respectively. The reaction mechanism is the same as it is for hydration and is catalyzed by anhydrous acid. Acetals and ketals, comparatively inert, are frequently used as protecting groups for carbonyl functionalities. They can easily be converted back to the carbonyl with aqueous acid.

MCAT SYNOPSIS

Acetal and ketal formation is when alcohol is the nucleophile and carbonyl carbon is the electrophile.

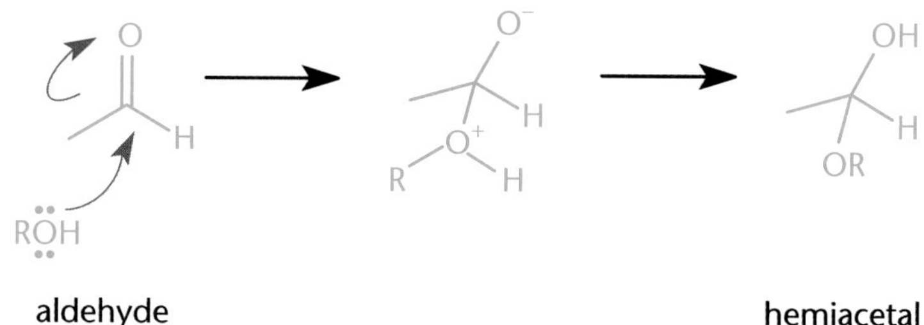

Figure 8.9

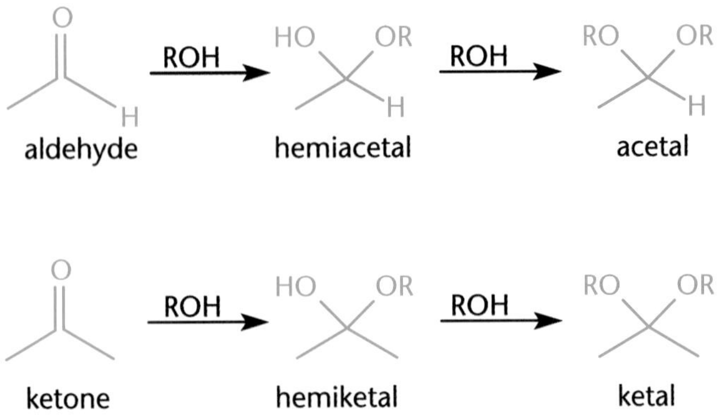

aldehyde → (ROH) hemiacetal → (ROH) acetal

ketone → (ROH) hemiketal → (ROH) ketal

Figure 8.10

MCAT SYNOPSIS

In a reaction with HCN, the CN^- is the nucleophile, and carbonyl carbon is the electrophile.

3. Reaction with HCN. Aldehydes and ketones react with HCN (hydrogen cyanide) to produce stable compounds called **cyanohydrins.** HCN dissociates and the nucleophilic cyanide anion attacks the carbonyl carbon atom. Protonation of the oxygen produces the cyanohydrin. The cyanohydrin gains its stability from the newly formed C–C bond (in contrast, when a carbonyl reacts with HCl, a weak C–Cl bond is formed, and the resulting chlorohydrin is unstable).

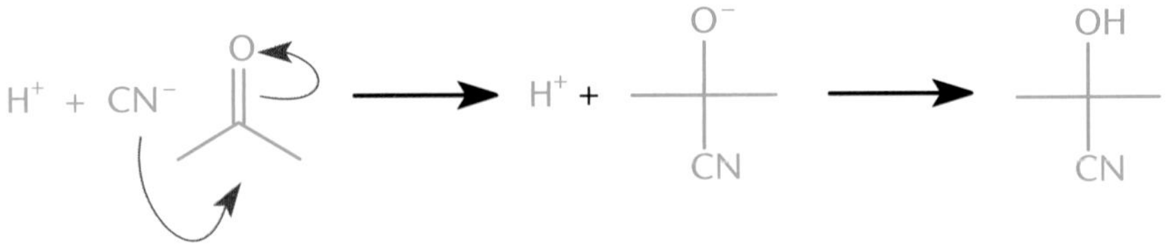

TEACHER TIP

Do you see a pattern developing? What might the carbonyl carbon do in the next reaction? Might it act as an electrophile? Most certainly! When you see a carbonyl carbon, think electrophile first.

$H^+ + CN^-$ → $H^+ +$ (O^-, CN) → (OH, CN)

Figure 8.11

4. Condensations with ammonia derivatives. Ammonia and some of its derivatives are nucleophiles and can add to carbonyl compounds. In the simplest case, ammonia adds to the carbon atom and water is lost, producing an **imine,** a compound with a nitrogen atom double-bonded to a carbon atom. (A reaction in which water is lost between two molecules is called a **condensation reaction.**)

In this case, the first part of the reaction follows the mechanism of nucleophilic addition described above. However, after formation of a tetrahedral intermediate, this reaction proceeds further: The C=O double bond reforms and a leaving group is kicked off. This mechanism is called nucleophilic *substitution* on a carbonyl and will be described in greater detail in chapter 9.

Some common ammonia derivatives that react with aldehydes and ketones are hydroxylamine (H_2NOH), hydrazine (H_2NNH_2), and semicarbazide ($H_2NNHCONH_2$); these form oximes, hydrazones, and semicarbazones, respectively.

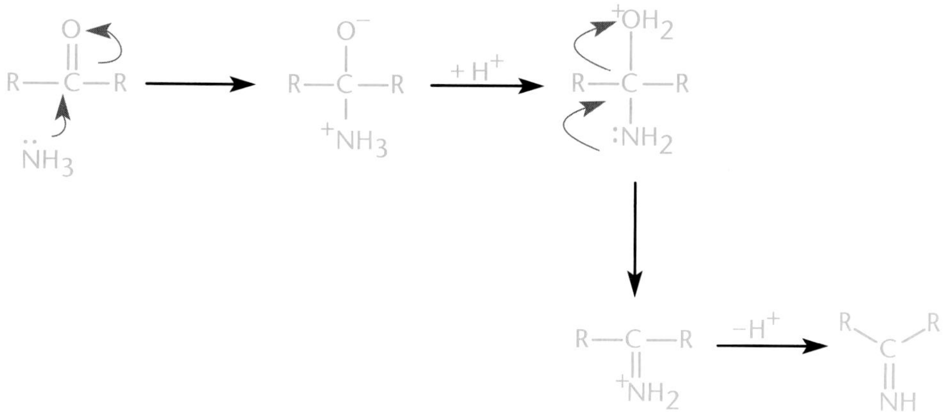

$R-C(=O)-R + :NH_3 \longrightarrow R-C(O^-)(^+NH_3)-R \xrightarrow{+H^+} R-C(^+OH_2)(:NH_2)-R \longrightarrow R-C(=^+NH_2)-R \xrightarrow{-H^+} R_2C=NH$

Figure 8.12

Don't worry too much about protons coming and going; there should be plenty in the solution, so you can transiently put them where needed to facilitate this reaction.

TEACHER TIP

There's nothing new here, just more carbonyl carbons acting as electrophiles with some other nucleophiles!

Examples of other potential nucleophiles and their respective products are shown below.

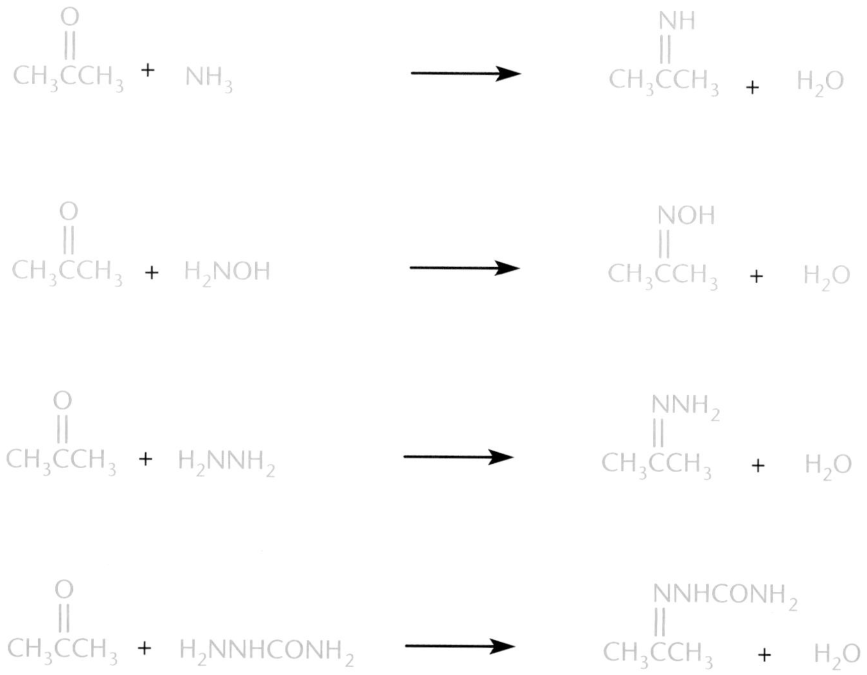

$CH_3C(=O)CH_3 + NH_3 \longrightarrow CH_3C(=NH)CH_3 + H_2O$

$CH_3C(=O)CH_3 + H_2NOH \longrightarrow CH_3C(=NOH)CH_3 + H_2O$

$CH_3C(=O)CH_3 + H_2NNH_2 \longrightarrow CH_3C(=NNH_2)CH_3 + H_2O$

$CH_3C(=O)CH_3 + H_2NNHCONH_2 \longrightarrow CH_3C(=NNHCONH_2)CH_3 + H_2O$

Figure 8.13

TEACHER TIP

In the aldol condensation it should be no surprise that the carbonyl carbon acts as an electrophile; we also have the aldehyde acting as a nucleophile as we saw in our discussion of the enol compound.

C. THE ALDOL CONDENSATION

The aldol condensation is an important reaction that basically follows the mechanism of nucleophilic addition to a carbonyl that was described above. In this case, an aldehyde acts both as nucleophile (enol form) and target (keto form). When acetaldehyde (ethanol) is treated with base, an enolate ion is produced. This enolate ion, being nucleophilic, can react with the carbonyl group of another acetaldehyde molecule. The product is 3-hydroxybutanal, which contains both an alcohol and an aldehyde functionality. This type of compound is called an **aldol,** from **alde**hyde and alcoh**ol.** With stronger base and higher temperatures, condensation occurs, producing an α, β-unsaturated aldehyde. This type of condensation reaction has become known as the **aldol condensation.**

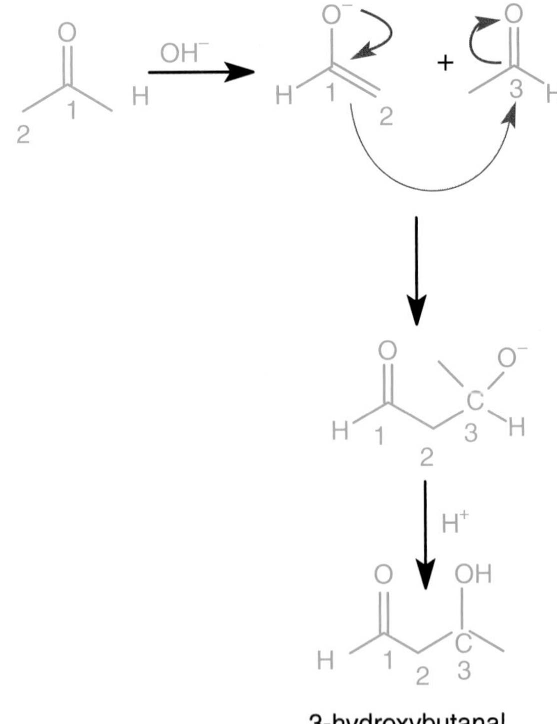

Figure 8.14a

MCAT SYNOPSIS

An aldol can lose H_2O to form a carbon–carbon double bond, in an E1 reaction.

When heated, this molecule can undergo elimination and lose H_2O to form a double bond:

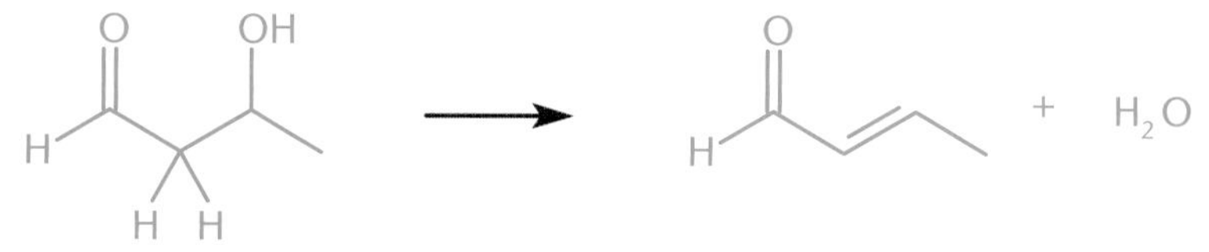

Figure 8.14b

The aldol condensation is most useful when only one type of aldehyde or ketone is present, because mixed condensations usually result in a mixture of products.

MCAT SYNOPSIS

The Wittig reaction ultimately converts C=O to C=C.

D. THE WITTIG REACTION

The **Wittig reaction** is a method of forming carbon-carbon double bonds by converting aldehydes and ketones into alkenes. The first step involves the formation of a phosphonium salt from the S_N2 reaction of an alkyl halide with the nucleophile triphenylphosphine, $(C_6H_5)_3P$. The phosphonium salt is then deprotonated (losing the proton α to the phosphorus) with a strong base, yielding a neutral compound called an **ylide** (pronounced "ill-id") or **phosphorane.** (The phosphorus atom may be drawn as pentavalent, utilizing the low-lying 3d atomic orbitals.)

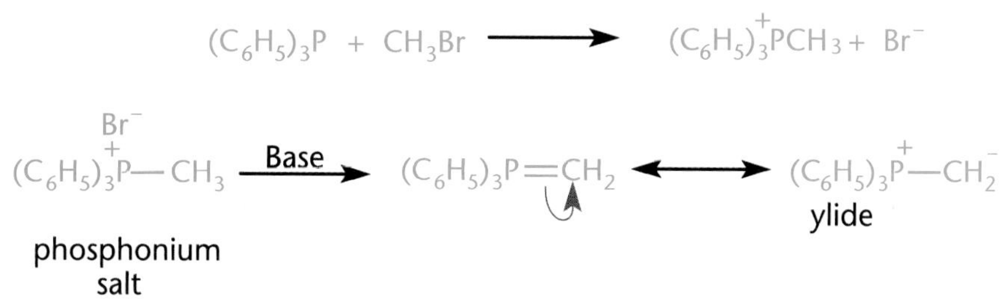

$$(C_6H_5)_3P + CH_3Br \longrightarrow (C_6H_5)_3\overset{+}{P}CH_3 + Br^-$$

$$\underset{\text{phosphonium salt}}{(C_6H_5)_3\overset{+}{P}\text{—}CH_3\ Br^-} \xrightarrow{\text{Base}} (C_6H_5)_3P\text{=}CH_2 \longleftrightarrow \underset{\text{ylide}}{(C_6H_5)_3\overset{+}{P}\text{—}\overset{-}{C}H_2}$$

Figure 8.15

Notice that an ylide is a type of carbanion and has nucleophilic properties. When combined with an aldehyde or ketone, an ylide attacks the carbonyl carbon, giving an intermediate called a *betaine,* which forms a four-membered ring intermediate called an oxaphosphetane. This decomposes to yield an alkene and triphenylphosphine oxide.

The decomposition reaction is driven by the strength of the phosphorus-oxygen bond that is formed.

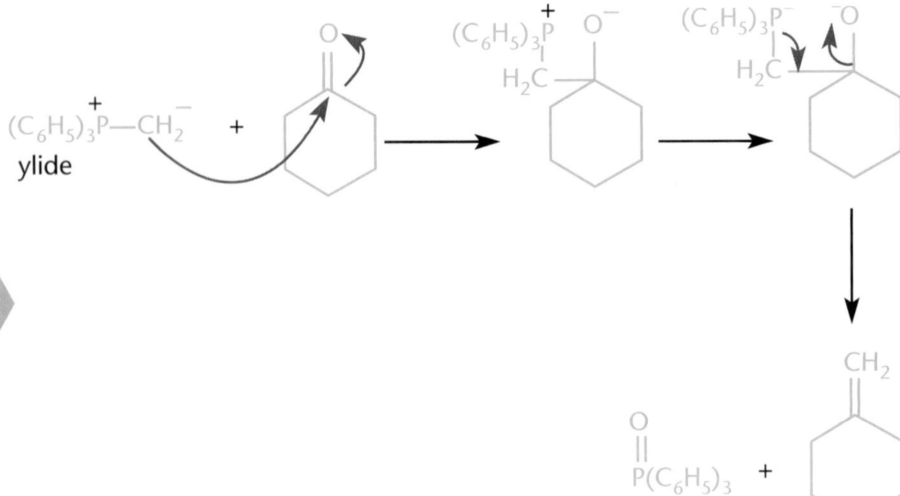

TEACHER TIP

Here's another instance where the carbonyl carbon acts as an electrophile with a random nucleophile.

Figure 8.16

E. OXIDATION AND REDUCTION

Aldehydes and ketones occupy the middle of the oxidation-reduction continuum. They are more oxidized than alcohols but less oxidized than carboxylic acids.

Aldehydes can be oxidized with a number of different reagents, such as $KMnO_4$, CrO_3, Ag_2O, or H_2O_2. The product of oxidation is a carboxylic acid.

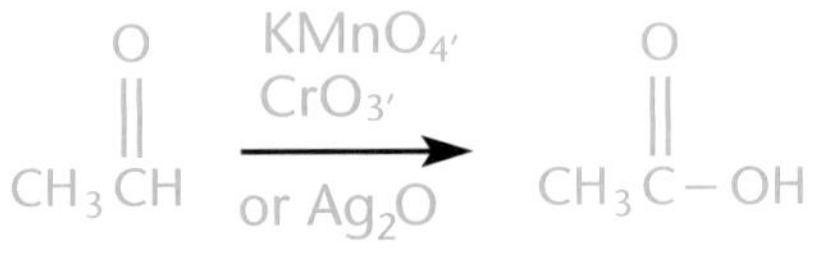

$$CH_3\overset{O}{\overset{\|}{C}}H \xrightarrow[\text{or } Ag_2O]{KMnO_4,\ CrO_3,} CH_3\overset{O}{\overset{\|}{C}}-OH$$

Figure 8.17

A number of different reagents will reduce aldehydes and ketones to alcohols. The most common is lithium aluminum hydride (LAH); sodium borohydride ($NaBH_4$) is often used when milder conditions are needed.

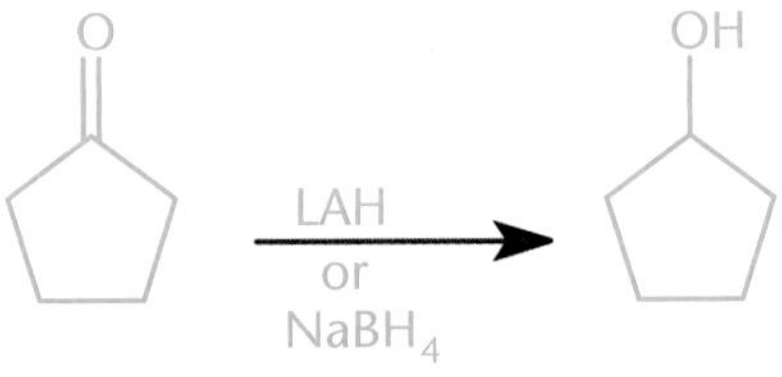

O

LAH
or
$NaBH_4$

OH

Figure 8.18

Aldehydes and ketones can be completely reduced to alkanes by two common methods. In the **Wolff-Kishner reduction,** the carbonyl is first converted to a hydrazone, which releases molecular nitrogen (N_2) when heated and forms an alkane (the protons being abstracted from the solvent). The Wolff-Kishner reaction is performed in basic solution and therefore is useful only when the product is stable under basic conditions.

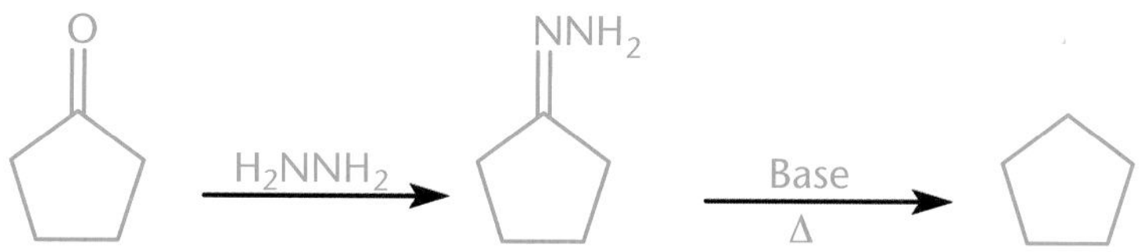

MCAT SYNOPSIS

Both aldehydes and ketones can be fully reduced to alkanes:

—Wolff-Kishner (H_2NNH_2);
—Clemmensen [Hg (Zn), HCl].

H_2NNH_2 ; NNH_2 ; Base, Δ

Figure 8.19

An alternative reduction not subject to this restriction is the **Clemmensen reduction,** in which an aldehyde or ketone is heated with amalgamated zinc in hydrochloric acid.

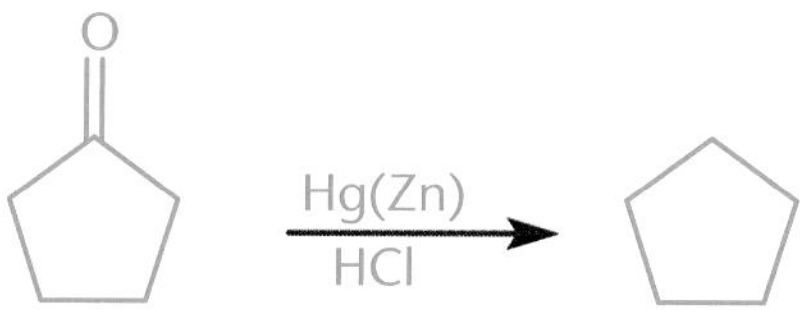

Hg(Zn) ; HCl

Figure 8.20

PRACTICE QUESTIONS

1. A student investigates the reactivity of carboxylic acid derivatives and aldehydes by reacting hydrazine ($H_2N–NH_2$) with benzaldehyde and benzoyl chloride. Which of the following statements is true about this reaction?

   A. Both compounds undergo substitution reactions but arrive at different products.
   B. Both compounds undergo elimination reactions but arrive at the same product.
   C. Unlike benzaldehyde, benzoyl chloride undergoes an elimination reaction because chlorine is a good leaving group.
   D. Unlike benzaldehyde, benzoyl chloride undergoes a substitution reaction because chlorine is a good leaving group.

2. Which of the following statements is true about the reaction below?

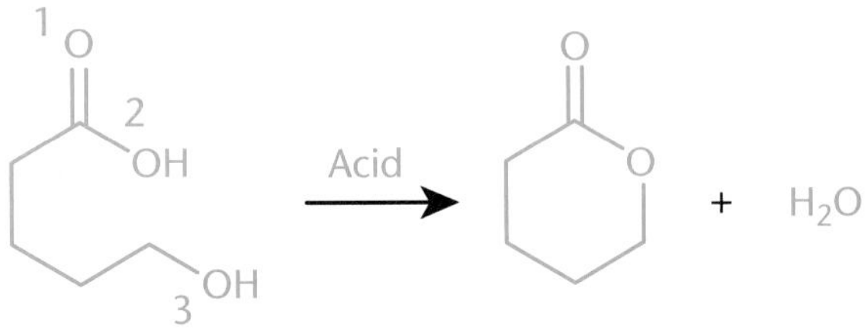

1 O, 2 OH, 3 OH — Acid → (cyclic) + H_2O

   A. The oxygen atoms labeled 1 and 3 are in the cyclic molecule and water is formed by oxygen atom number 2.
   B. The oxygen atoms labeled 1 and 2 are in the cyclic molecule and water is formed by oxygen atom number 3.
   C. The oxygen atom labeled 1 is in the cyclic molecule and water is formed by oxygen atoms 2 and 3.
   D. It is impossible to know which oxygen atom is in which position due to the stochastic nature of molecular motion.

3. Which of the following statements is NOT true about the following reaction?

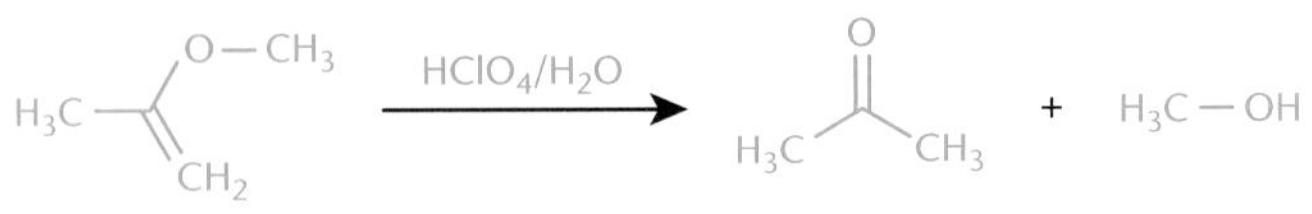

H_3C–C(O–CH_3)=CH_2 —$HClO_4/H_2O$→ H_3C–C(=O)–CH_3 + H_3C–OH

   A. The oxygen atom in the reactant is the oxygen atom in methanol after the reaction.
   B. The oxygen atom in the reactant is the carbonyl group of acetone after the reaction.
   C. The oxygen atom in water attacks the enol ether as a nucleophile.
   D. The oxygen atoms in $HClO_4$ are not transferred to acetone or methanol.

4. Assuming a meticulously anhydrous environment, which of following could be used to form 3-ethylhept-6-en-3-ol?

   A. 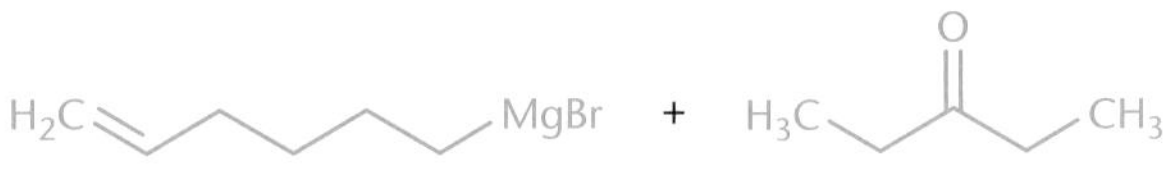 H_2C= ... MgBr + H_3C ... (C=O) ... CH_3
   B. 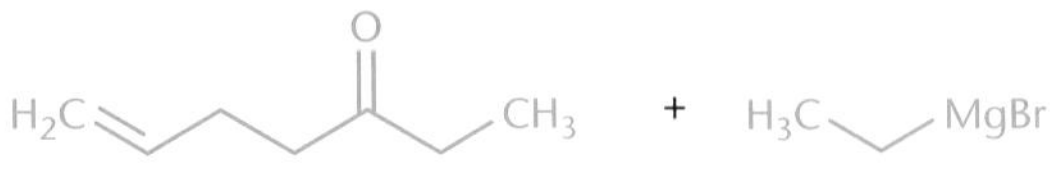 H_2C= ... (C=O) ... CH_3 + H_3C ... MgBr
   C. 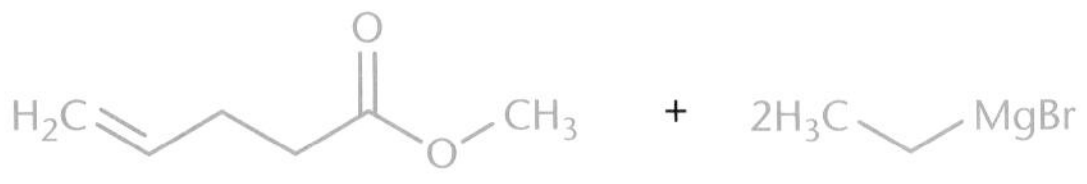 H_2C= ... (C=O)–O ... CH_3 + $2H_3C$ ... MgBr
   D. All of the above

5. A chemist wishes to form a bicyclic ring from a monocyclic compound and chooses to perform a Robinson annulation. One could best describe the set of reactions involved as a(n)

   A. intramolecular aldol condensation and a substitution.
   B. substitution, a Michael addition, and a dehydration.
   C. Michael addition and an intramolecular aldol condensation.
   D. Michael addition, a substitution, and an intramolecular aldol condensation.

CHAPTER 9

CARBOXYLIC ACIDS

Carboxylic acids are compounds that contain hydroxyl groups attached to carbonyl groups. This functionality is known as a **carboxyl group.** The hydroxyl hydrogen atoms are acidic, with pK_a values in the general range of 3 to 6. Carboxylic acids occur widely in nature and are synthesized by all living organisms.

TEACHER TIP

Carboxylic acids play an important role in biology and can also be used to flavor your food (vinegar = acetic acid). Carboxylic acids and their derivatives are sure to be on your exam.

NOMENCLATURE

In the IUPAC system of nomenclature, carboxylic acids are named by adding the suffix **-oic acid** to the alkyl root. The chain is numbered so that the carboxyl group receives the lowest possible number. Additional substituents are named in the usual fashion.

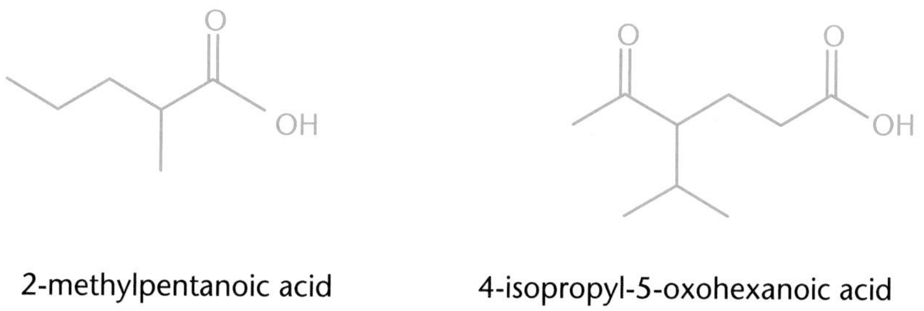

O
OH
2-methylpentanoic acid

O O
OH
4-isopropyl-5-oxohexanoic acid

Figure 9.1

TEACHER TIP

Besides being acidic, carbonyl carbon is also very electrophilic.

Carboxylic acids were among the first organic compounds discovered. Their original names continue today in the common system of nomenclature. For example, formic acid (from the Latin *formica*, meaning "ant") was found in ants and butyric acid (from the Latin *butyrum*, meaning "butter") in rancid butter. The common and IUPAC names of the first three carboxylic acids are listed in Figure 9.2.

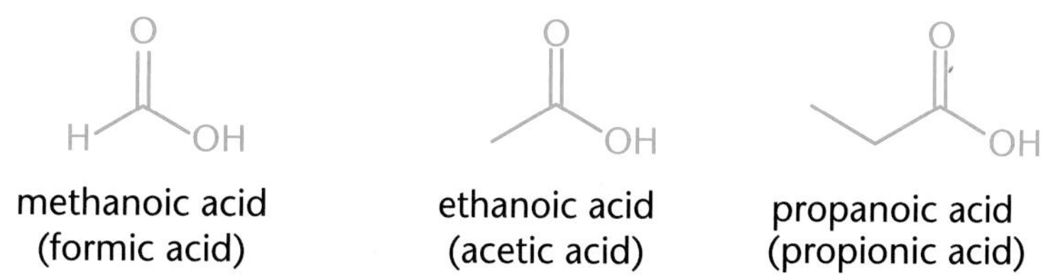

O
H OH
methanoic acid
(formic acid)

O
OH
ethanoic acid
(acetic acid)

O
OH
propanoic acid
(propionic acid)

Figure 9.2

TEACHER TIP

Here are those prefixes from before *form-* and *acet-*, including the main ingredient in salad dressing, the acetic acid.

Cyclic carboxylic acids are usually named as cycloalkane carboxylic acids. The carbon atom to which the carboxyl group is attached is numbered 1. Salts of carboxylic acids are named beginning with the cation, followed by the name of the acid with the ending **-ate** replacing **-ic acid.** Typical examples are:

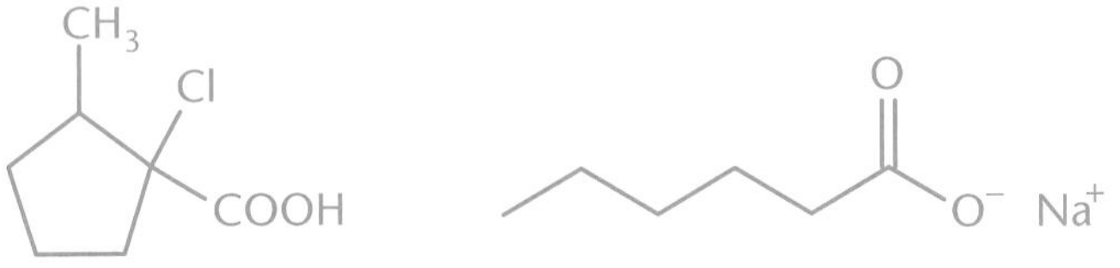

CH_3 Cl COOH O O^- Na^+

1-chloro-2-methylcyclo-pentane carboxylic acid

sodium hexanoate

Figure 9.3

Dicarboxylic acids—compounds with two carboxyl groups—are common in biological systems. The first six straight-chain terminal dicarboxylic acids are oxalic, malonic, succinic, glutaric, adipic, and pimelic acids. Their IUPAC names are ethanedioic acid, propanedioic acid, butanedioic acid, pentanedioic acid, hexanedioic acid, and heptanedioic acid.

MCAT SYNOPSIS

Carboxylic acids are polar and can form hydrogen bonds. Their acidity is due to resonance stabilization and can be enhanced by adding electronegative groups or other potential resonance structures.

PHYSICAL PROPERTIES

A. HYDROGEN BONDING

Carboxylic acids are polar and can form hydrogen bonds. As a result, carboxylic acids can form dimers: pairs of molecules connected by hydrogen bonds. The boiling points of carboxylic acids are therefore even higher than those of the corresponding alcohols. The boiling points follow the usual trend of increasing with molecular weight.

B. ACIDITY

The acidity of carboxylic acids is due to the resonance stabilization of the carboxylate anion (the conjugate base). When the hydroxyl proton dissociates from the acid, the negative charge left on the carboxylate group is delocalized between the two oxygen atoms.

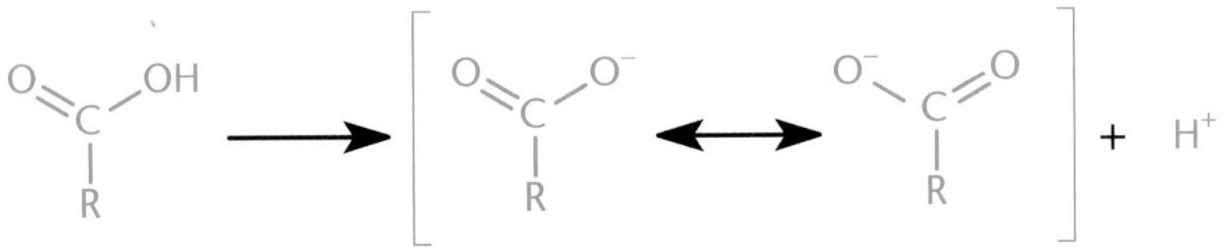

$$RCOOH \longrightarrow \left[RC(=O)O^- \longleftrightarrow RC(O^-)=O \right] + H^+$$

Figure 9.4

Substituents on carbon atoms adjacent to a carboxyl group can influence acidity. Electron-withdrawing groups such as –Cl or $-NO_2$ further delocalize the negative charge and increase acidity. Electron-donating groups such as $-NH_2$ or $-OCH_3$ destabilize the negative charge, making the compound less acidic.

In dicarboxylic acids, one –COOH group (which is electron-withdrawing) influences the other, making the compound more acidic than the analogous monocarboxylic acid. The second carboxyl group is then influenced by the carboxylate anion. Ionization of the second group will create a doubly charged species, in which the two negative charges repel each other. Because this is unfavorable, the second proton is less acidic than that of a monocarboxylic acid.

β-dicarboxylic acids are notable for the high acidity of the α-hydrogens located between the two carboxyl groups ($pK_a \sim 10$). Loss of this acidic hydrogen atom produces a carbanion that is stabilized by the electron-withdrawing effect of the two carboxyl groups (the same effect seen in β-ketoacids, $RC{=}OCH_2\,COOH$).

Figure 9.5

Similarly, the β-dicarboxylic acid also has acidic α hydrogens.

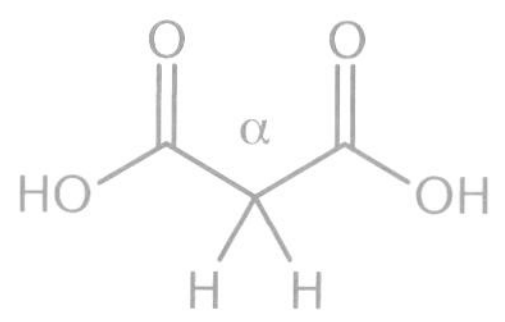

Figure 9.6

MCAT Favorite

Other ways to stabilize the negative charge (and thus increase acidity) are:

- electron-withdrawing groups (*e.g.*, halides);
- groups that allow more resonance stabilization (*e.g.*, benzyl or allyl substituents).

The more of such groups that exist, and the closer to the acid they are, the stronger the acid.

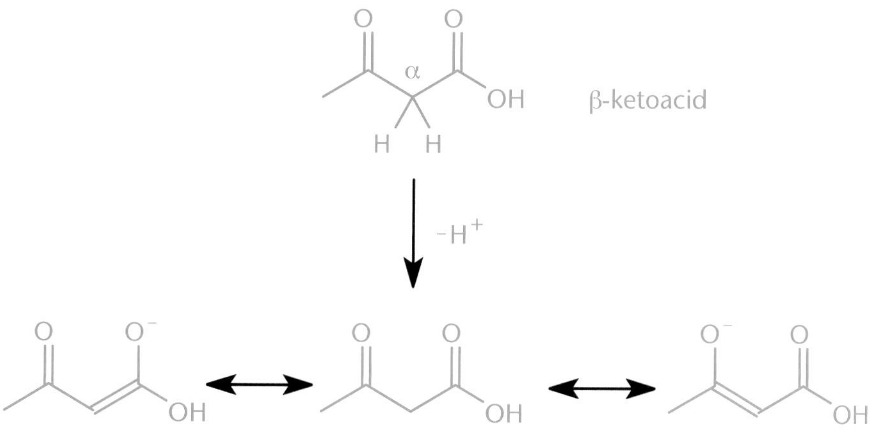

Teacher Tip

Remember β-ketoacids in our discussion about the Greek lettering convention? See them and the α-carbon in Figure 9.5. β-ketoacids will not be tested on the exam, though you should understand the significant acidity of the α-hydrogen.

SYNTHESIS

KAPLAN EXCLUSIVE

Carboxylic acids are the most oxidized.

A. OXIDATION REACTIONS

Carboxylic acids can be prepared via oxidation of aldehydes, primary alcohols, and certain alkylbenzenes. The oxidant is usually potassium permanganate, $KMnO_4$. Note that secondary and tertiary alcohols cannot be oxidized to carboxylic acids because of valence limitations.

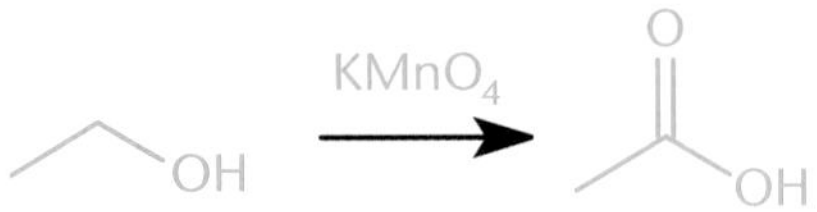

$$CH_3CH_2OH \xrightarrow{KMnO_4} CH_3COOH$$

Figure 9.7

B. CARBONATION OF ORGANOMETALLIC REAGENTS

Organometallic reagents, such as Grignard reagents, react with carbon dioxide (CO_2) to form carboxylic acids. This reaction is useful for the conversion of tertiary alkyl halides into carboxylic acids, which cannot be accomplished through other methods. Note that this reaction adds one carbon atom to the chain.

TEACHER TIP

In the second reaction, the nucleophile is essentially a carbanion that is coordinated with a positively charged magnesium, and the electrophile is the carbon of the CO_2 (which is very similar to any other carbonyl or carboxylic carbon).

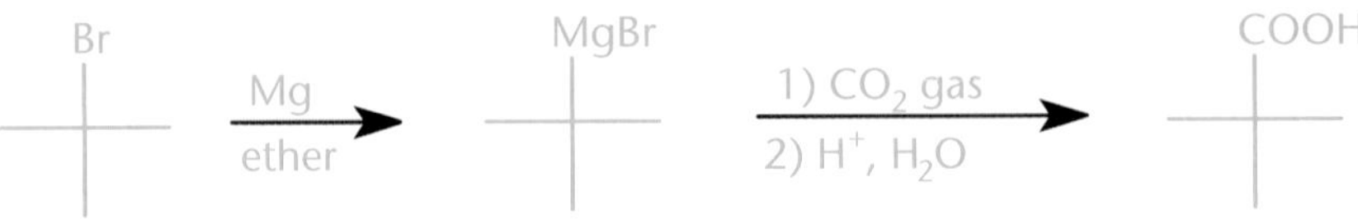

Figure 9.8

C. HYDROLYSIS OF NITRILES

Nitriles, also called cyanides, are compounds containing the functional group –CN. The cyanide anion CN^- is a good nucleophile and will displace primary and secondary halides in typical S_N2 fashion.

Nitriles can be hydrolyzed under either acidic or basic conditions. The products are carboxylic acids and ammonia (or ammonium salts).

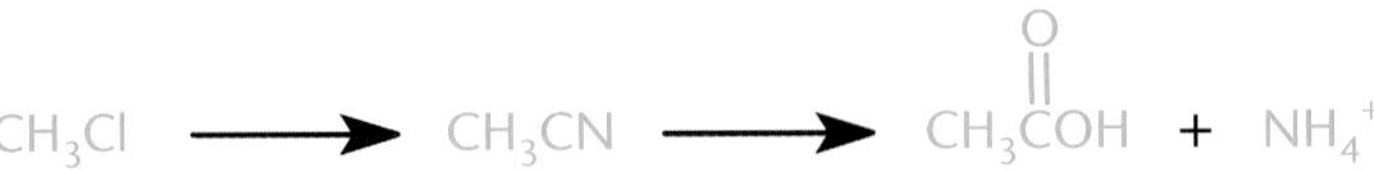

Figure 9.9

This allows for the conversion of alkyl halides into carboxylic acids. As in the carbonation reaction, an additional carbon atom is introduced. For instance, if the desired product is acetic acid, a possible starting material would be methyl iodide.

REACTIONS

A. SOAP FORMATION

When long-chain carboxylic acids react with sodium or potassium hydroxide, they form salts. These salts, called soaps, are able to solubilize nonpolar organic compounds in aqueous solutions because they possess both a nonpolar "tail" and a polar carboxylate "head."

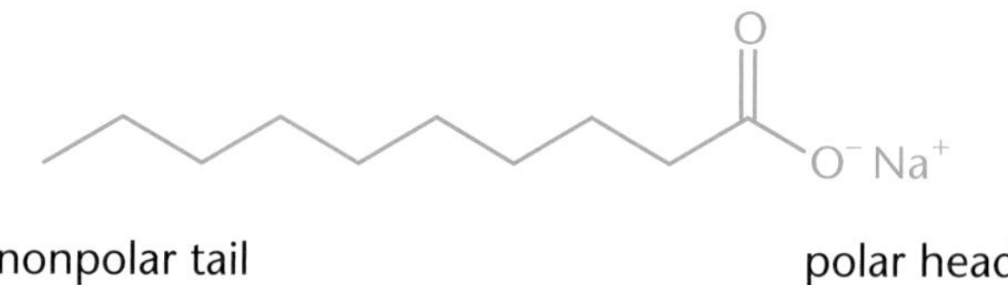

Figure 9.10

When placed in aqueous solution, soap molecules arrange themselves into spherical structures called **micelles.** The polar heads face outward, where they can be solvated by water molecules, and the nonpolar hydrocarbon chains are inside the sphere, protected from the solvent. Nonpolar molecules such as grease can dissolve in the hydrocarbon interior of the spherical micelle, while the micelle as a whole is soluble in water because of its polar shell.

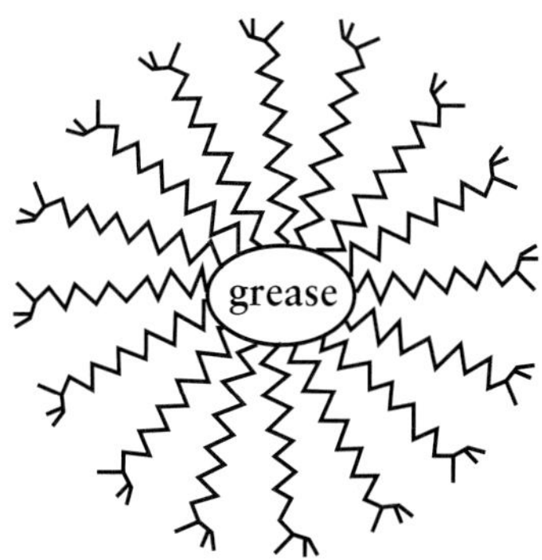

Figure 9.11

MCAT SYNOPSIS

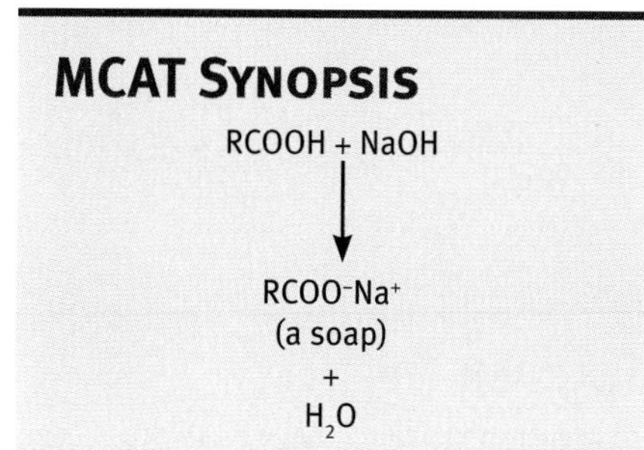

MCAT SYNOPSIS

nonpolar "tail" = hydrophobic
polar head = hydro*philic*

CLINICAL CORRELATE

In the small intestine, consumed fat is solubilized in micelles, not with detergent but with *bile salts*, which have a structure similar to soaps—hydrophobic tail and hydrophilic head!.

B. NUCLEOPHILIC SUBSTITUTION

Many of the reactions that carboxylic acids (and their derivatives) participate in can be described by a single mechanism: nucleophilic substitution. This mechanism is very similar to nucleophilic addition to a carbonyl, shown in the preceding chapter. The key difference: nucleophilic substitution concludes with reformation of the C=O double bond and elimination of a leaving group.

TEACHER TIP

Whatever the nucleophile, we can see clearly that the electrophile will still be that carbonyl carbon. For the reactions in this chapter, the first step is the same as in the last chapter, but the second step involves a leaving group rather than the oxygen as the electron acceptor.

Figure 9.12

1. Reduction

Carboxylic acids occupy the most oxidized side of the oxidation-reduction continuum (see chapter 7). Carboxylic acids are reduced with lithium aluminum hydride (LAH) to the corresponding alcohols. Aldehyde intermediates that may be formed in the course of the reaction are also reduced to the alcohol. The reaction occurs by nucleophilic addition of hydride to the carbonyl group.

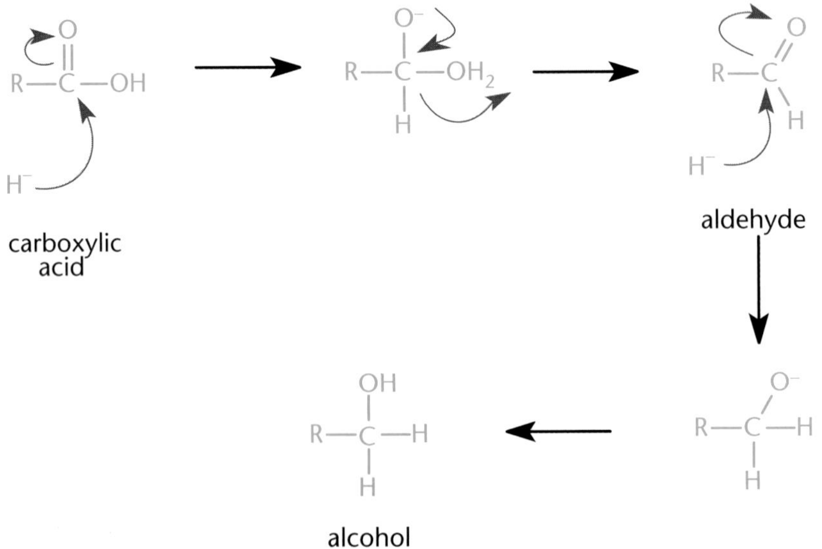

Figure 9.13

2. Ester Formation

Carboxylic acids react with alcohols under acidic conditions to form esters and water. In acidic solution, the O on the C=O can become protonated. This accentuates the polarity of the bond, putting even more positive charge on the C and making it even more susceptible to nucleophilic attack. This condensation reaction occurs most rapidly with primary alcohols.

MCAT Synopsis

Protonating the C=O makes the C even more ripe for nucleophilic attack.

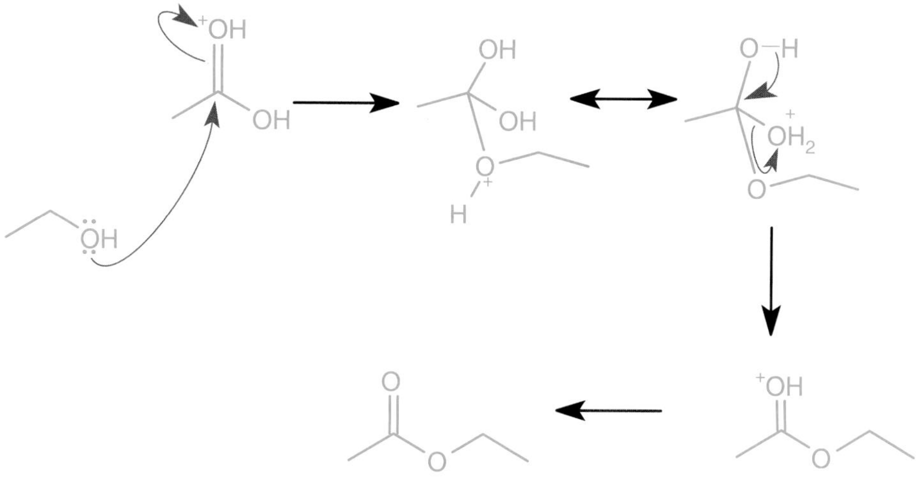

Figure 9.14

3. Acyl Halide Formation

Acyl halides, also called acid halides, are compounds with carbonyl groups bonded to halides. Several different reagents can accomplish this transformation; thionyl chloride, $SOCl_2$, is the most common.

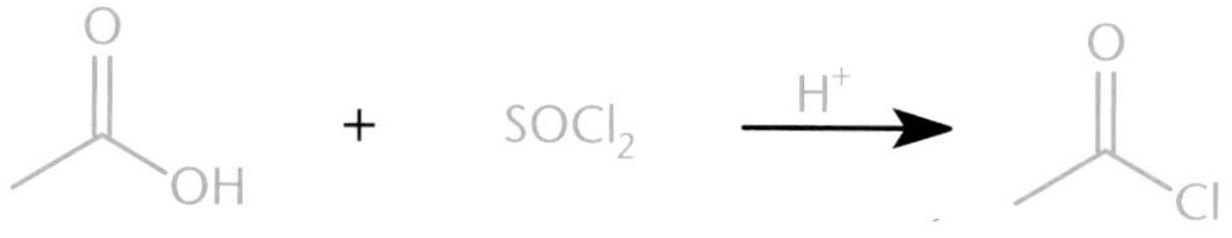

MCAT Synopsis

Acid chlorides are among the highest energy (least stable and most reactive) members of the carbonyl family.

Figure 9.15

Acid chlorides are very reactive, as the greater electron-withdrawing power of the Cl^- makes the carbonyl carbon more susceptible to nucleophilic attack than the carbonyl carbon of a carboxylic acid. Thus acid chlorides are frequently used as intermediates in the conversion of carboxylic acids to esters and amides.

MCAT Synopsis

Key reactions include:
- soap formation (*e.g.*, when neutralized by NaOH or KOH);
- nucleophilic substitution;
- decarboxylation, in which CO_2 is lost.

C. DECARBOXYLATION

Carboxylic acids can undergo decarboxylation reactions, resulting in the loss of carbon dioxide.

1,3-dicarboxylic acids and other β-keto acids may spontaneously decarboxylate when heated. The carboxyl group is lost and replaced with a hydrogen. The reaction proceeds through a six-membered ring transition state. The enol initially formed tautomerizes to the more stable keto form.

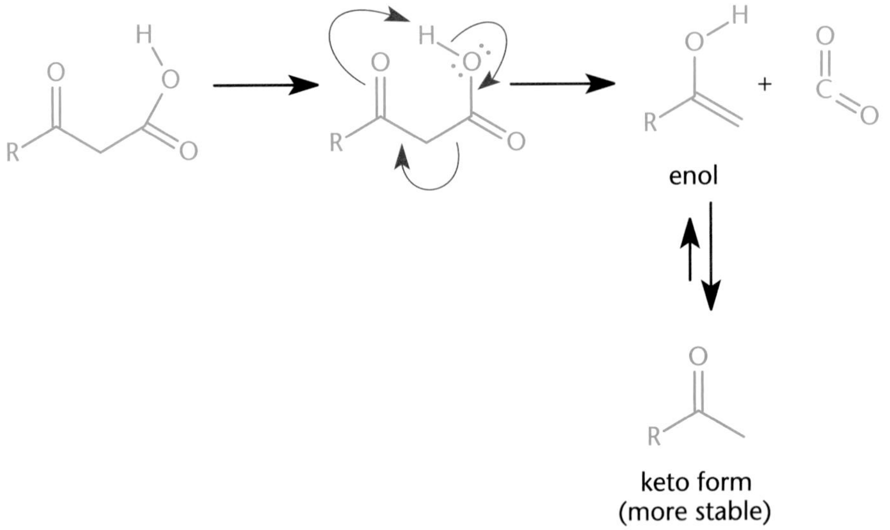

enol

keto form (more stable)

Figure 9.16

Bridge

Decarboxylation is very common in biochemical pathways in the body, such as the Krebs cycle.

PRACTICE QUESTIONS

1. Which of the following reactions does not produce hexanoic acid?

A. H_3C–(chain)–Br $\xrightarrow{Mg}$ $\xrightarrow{CO_2}$ $\xrightarrow{H^+}$

B. H_3C–(chain)–Br $\xrightarrow{CN^-}$ $\xrightarrow{H_3O^+}$

C. (cyclohexene) $\xrightarrow[H^+]{KMnO_4}$

D. H_3C–(chain)–C≡CH $\xrightarrow[H_3O^+]{KMnO_4}$

2. Which of the following cannot be used to convert butanoic acid to butanoyl chloride?

A. PCl_3
B. PCl_5
C. CCl_4
D. $SOCl_2$

3. Which of the following reagents will reduce butanoic acid to butanol?

A. $LiAlH_4$
B. $LiAlH_4$, H_2O
C. $NaBH_4$
D. All of the above

4. In the presence of an acid catalyst, the major product of ethanoic acid and ethanol is

A. acetic anhydride.
B. butene.
C. diethyl ether.
D. ethyl acetate.

5. 14C-labeled methanol is subjected to the reaction sequence shown below.

Which carbon(s) in propanoic acid will be labeled (indicated in bold)?

$CH_3OH \xrightarrow[\Delta]{Cu} \xrightarrow[2.\ H^+]{1.\ CH_3MgI} \xrightarrow{HBr} \xrightarrow[2.\ CO_2,\ 3.\ H^+]{1.\ Mg}$ propanoic acid

A. CH_3CH_2COOH
B. CH_3CH_2COOH
C. CH_3CH_2COOH
D. CH_3CH_2COOH

CHAPTER 10

CARBOXYLIC ACID DERIVATIVES

Carboxylic acids can be converted into several types of derivatives: **acyl halides, anhydrides, amides,** and **esters.** These are compounds in which the –OH of the carboxyl group has been replaced with **–X, –OCOR, –NH_2,** or **–OR,** respectively. They readily undergo nucleophilic substitution reactions, including hydrolysis (H_2O as nucleophile) which produces the original carboxylic acid. They also undergo other additions and substitutions, including various interconversions between different acid derivatives. In general, the acyl halides are the most reactive of the carboxylic acid derivatives, followed by the anhydrides, the esters, and the amides.

> **MCAT SYNOPSIS**
> Order of reactivity:
> acyl halides > anhydrides > esters > amides

ACYL HALIDES

A. NOMENCLATURE

Acyl halides are also called **acid** or **alkanoyl halides.** (The acyl group is RCO–.) They are the most reactive of the carboxylic acid derivatives. They are named in the IUPAC system by changing the *-ic acid* ending of the carboxylic acid to **-yl halide.** Some typical examples are ethanoyl chloride (also called acetyl chloride), benzoyl chloride, and *n*-butanoyl bromide.

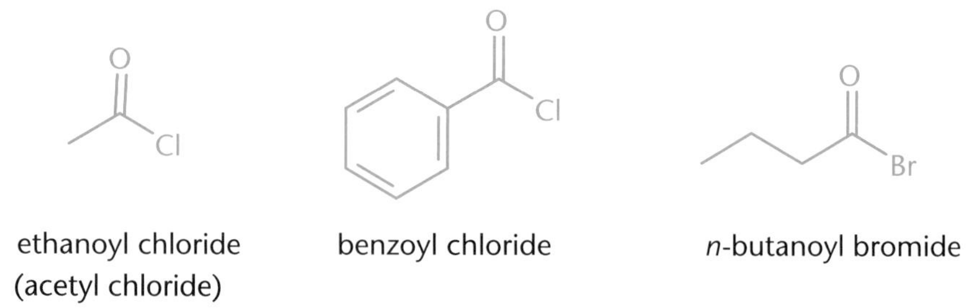

ethanoyl chloride (acetyl chloride) | benzoyl chloride | *n*-butanoyl bromide

Figure 10.1

B. SYNTHESIS

The most common acyl halides are the acid chlorides, although acid bromides and iodides are occasionally encountered. They are prepared by reaction of the carboxylic acid with thionyl chloride, $SOCl_2$, producing SO_2 and HCl as side products. Alternatively, PCl_3 or PCl_5 (or PBr_3, to make an acid bromide) will accomplish the same transformation.

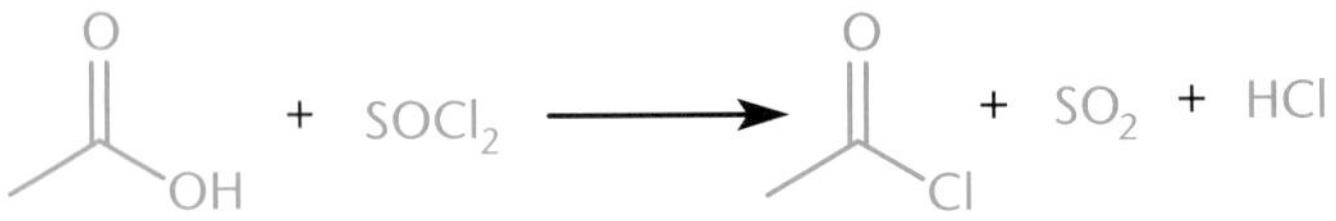

Figure 10.2

C. REACTIONS: NUCLEOPHILIC ACYL SUBSTITUTION

TEACHER TIP

The steps are the same for all of these reactions. Of course, we have the carbonyl carbon acting as an electrophile and being attacked by the nucelophile of the day. The second step involves the leaving group taking the extra electrons.

The following reactions of acyl halides proceed via the mechanism of nucleophilic substitution on a carbonyl, shown in detail in chapter 9.

1. Hydrolysis

The simplest reaction of acid halides is their reconversion to carboxylic acids. They react very rapidly with water to form the corresponding acid, along with HCl, which is responsible for their irritating odor.

KAPLAN EXCLUSIVE

Hydrolysis = hydro + lysis, or cleavage by water.

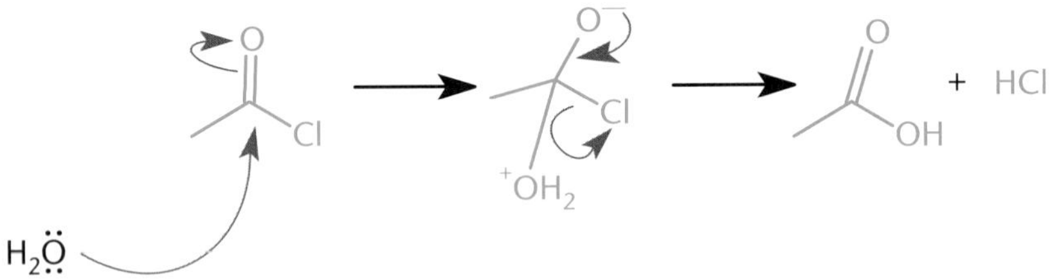

Figure 10.3

2. Conversion into Esters

Acyl halides can be converted into esters by reaction with alcohols. The same type of nucleophilic attack found in hydrolysis leads to the formation of a tetrahedral intermediate, with the hydroxyl oxygen as the nucleophile. Chloride is displaced and HCl is released as the side-product.

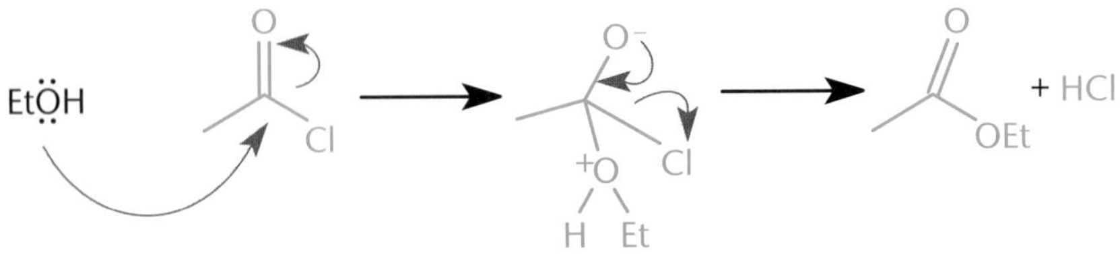

Figure 10.4

3. Conversion into Amides

Acyl halides can be converted into amides (compounds of the general formula $RCONR_2$) by an analogous reaction with amines. Nucleophilic amines, such as ammonia, attack the carbonyl group, displacing chloride. The side product is ammonium chloride, formed from excess ammonia and HCl.

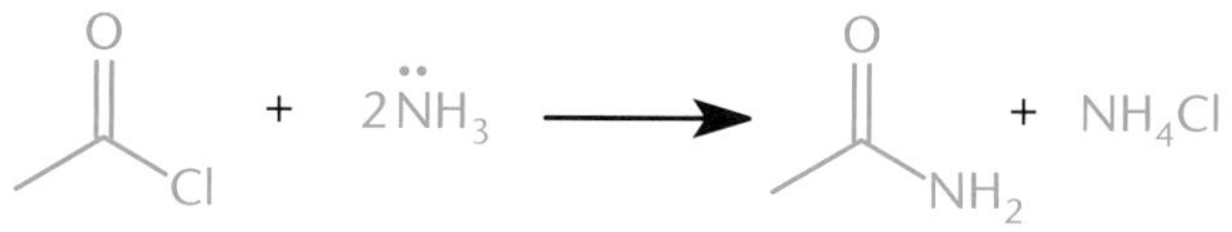

O, Cl + $2\ddot{N}H_3$ → O, NH_2 + NH_4Cl

Figure 10.5

D. OTHER REACTIONS

1. Friedel-Crafts Acylation

Aromatic rings can be acylated in a Friedel-Crafts reaction. The mechanism is electrophilic aromatic substitution, and the attacking reagent is an acylium ion, formed by reaction of an acid chloride with $AlCl_3$ or another Lewis acid. The product is an alkyl aryl ketone.

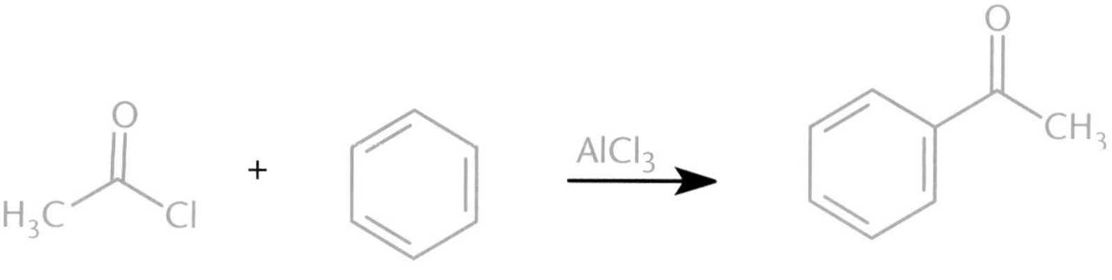

Figure 10.6

TEACHER TIP

This mechanism is a two-in-one! The electrophile is, of course, the carbonyl carbon, and the nucleophile is the benzene ring, making this a nucleophilic acyl substitution and an electrophilic aromatic substitution depending on your perspective.

2. Reduction

Acid halides can be reduced to alcohols, or selectively reduced to the intermediate aldehydes. Catalytic hydrogenation in the presence of a "poison" like quinoline accomplishes the latter transformation. (Compare with Lindlar's catalyst, chapter 5.)

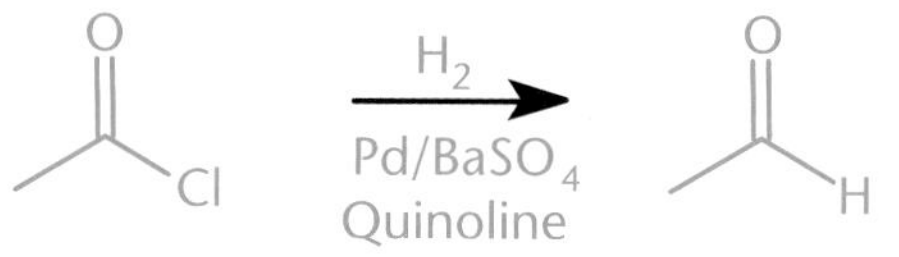

O, Cl —H_2; $Pd/BaSO_4$, Quinoline→ O, H

Figure 10.7

KAPLAN EXCLUSIVE

Anhydride means "without water." Anhydrides are formed by two acid molecules condensing (losing water).

ANHYDRIDES

A. NOMENCLATURE

Anhydrides, also called **acid anhydrides,** are the condensation dimers of carboxylic acids, with the general formula RCOOCOR. They are named by substituting the word **anhydride** for the word *acid* in an alkanoic acid. The most common and important anhydride is acetic anhydride, the dimer of acetic acid. Other common anhydrides, such as succinic, maleic, and phthalic anhydrides, are **cyclic anhydrides** arising from intramolecular condensation or dehydration of diacids (Figure 10.9).

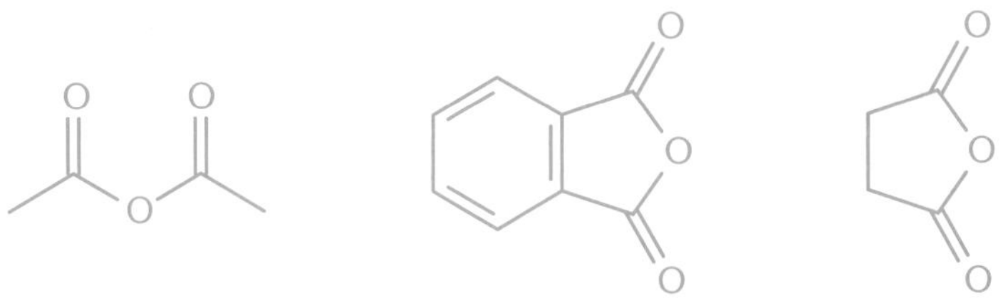

acetic anhydride (ethanoic anhydride) | phthalic anhydride | succinic anhydride

Figure 10.8

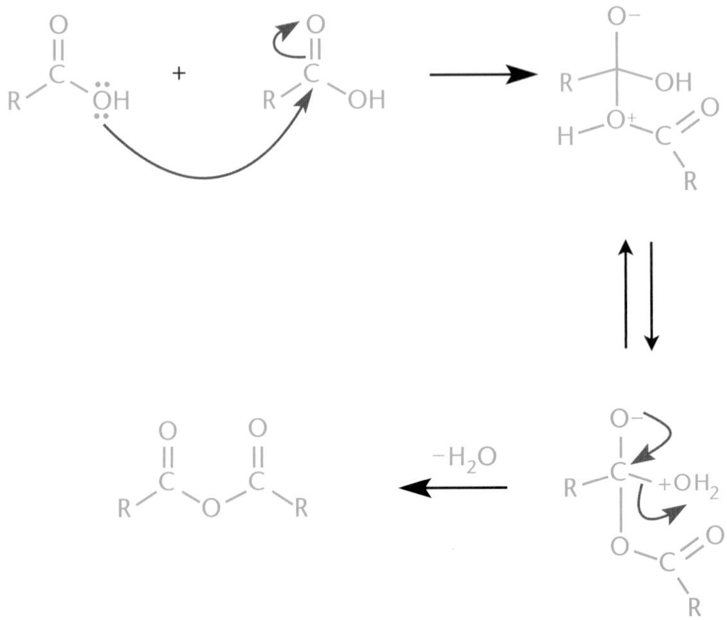

Figure 10.9

Condensation of two carboxylic acid molecules to form an anhydride.

B. SYNTHESIS

Anhydrides can be synthesized by reaction of an acid chloride with a carboxylate salt.

TEACHER TIP

Nothing new about this mechanism!

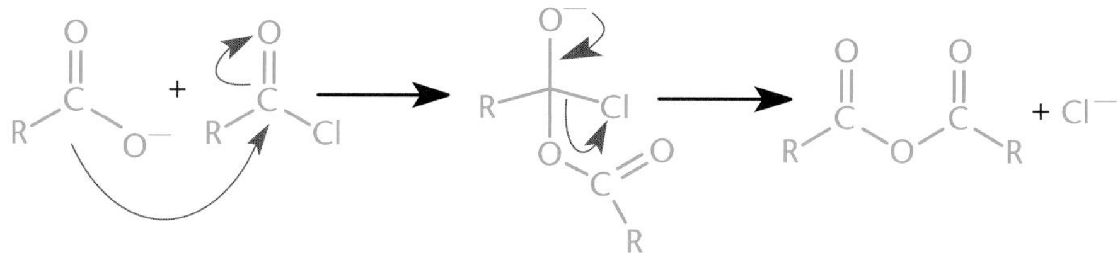

Figure 10.10

Reaction of acid chloride with carboxylate anion to form an anhydride.

Certain cyclic anhydrides can be formed simply by heating carboxylic acids. The reaction is driven by the increased stability of the newly formed ring; hence, only five- and six-membered ring anhydrides are easily made. In this case, the hydroxyl of one –COOH moiety acts as a nucleophile, attacking the carbonyl on the other –COOH moiety.

TEACHER TIP

Intramolecular reactions are more likely to occur than a reaction with two separate molecules. It's analogous to two people handcuffed together; they're much more likely to get into a fight than two random people passing on the street.

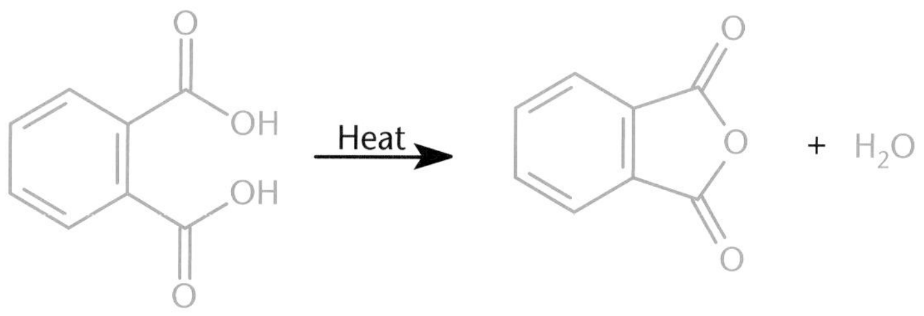

o-phtalic acid   phthalic anhydride

Figure 10.11

C. REACTIONS

Anhydrides react under the same conditions as acid chlorides, but because they are somewhat more stable, they are a bit less reactive. The reactions are slower and produce a carboxylic acid as the side product instead of HCl. Cyclic anhydrides are also subject to these reactions, which cause ring-opening at the anhydride group along with formation of the new functional groups.

1. Hydrolysis

Anhydrides are converted into carboxylic acids when exposed to water.

TEACHER TIP

Again, the carbonyl compound is the electrophile, the nucleophile is water, and the leaving group is a carboxylic acid (which is not as good of a leaving group as the halogens that took the electrons away in the acyl halide reactions).

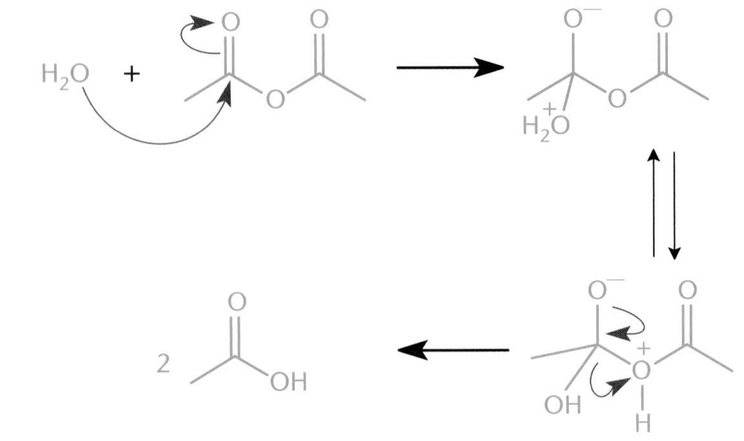

Figure 10.12

Note that in this reaction, the leaving group is actually a carboxylic acid.

2. Conversion into Amides

Anhydrides are cleaved by ammonia, producing amides and ammonium carboxylates.

TEACHER TIP

Again, these reactions differ only in the attacking nucleophile.

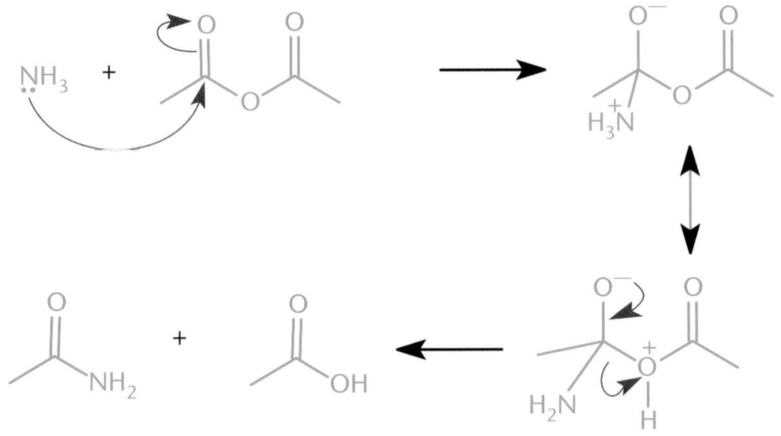

Then:

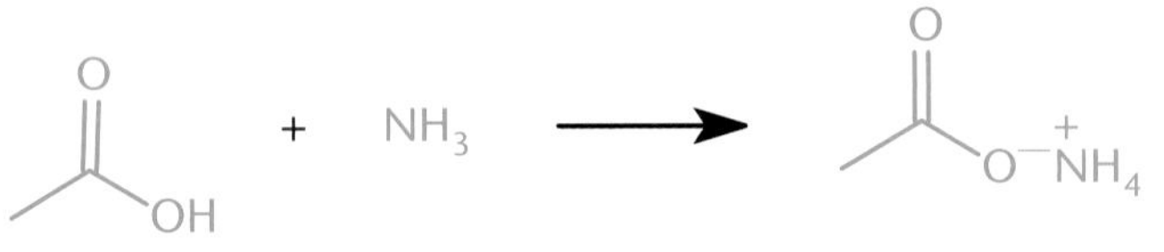

Figure 10.13

Thus, even though the leaving group is actually a carboxylic acid, the final products are an amide and the ammonium salt of a carboxylate anion.

3. Conversion into Esters and Carboxylic Acids

Anhydrides react with alcohols to form esters and carboxylic acids.

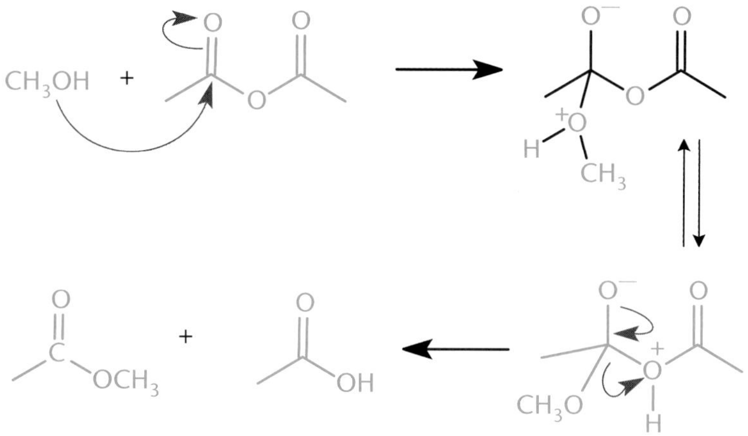

Figure 10.14

4. Acylation

Friedel-Crafts acylation occurs readily with $AlCl_3$ or other Lewis acid catalysts.

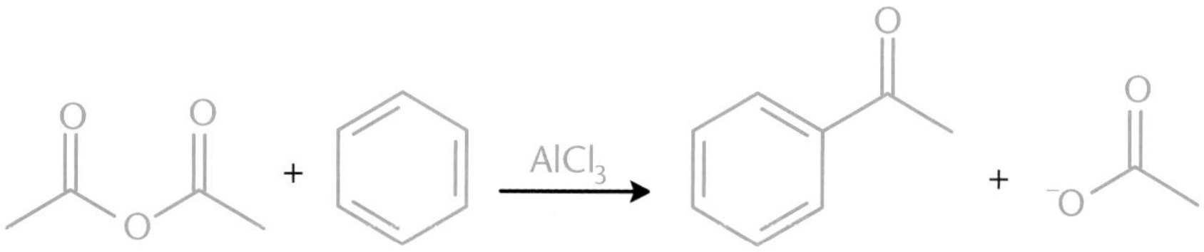

Figure 10.15

MCAT SYNOPSIS

This reaction is the same as the earlier two-in-one involving both EAS and nucleophilic acyl substitution.

AMIDES

A. NOMENCLATURE

Amides are compounds with the general formula $RCONR_2$. They are named by replacing the *-oic* acid ending with **-amide.** Alkyl substituents on the nitrogen atom are listed as prefixes, and their location is specified with the letter *N*. For example:

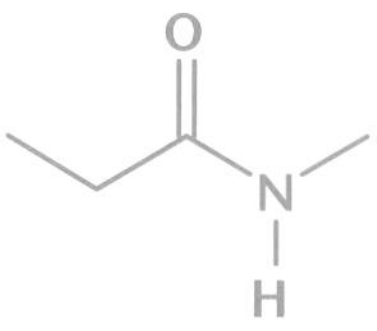

N-methylpropanamide

Figure 10.16

BRIDGE

The peptide bond is an amide linkage and is the most stable carboxylic acid derivative.

B. SYNTHESIS

Amides are generally synthesized by the reaction of acid chlorides with amines or by the reaction of acid anhydrides with ammonia (see above). Note that loss of hydrogen is required; thus, only primary and secondary amines will undergo this reaction.

C. REACTIONS

1. Hydrolysis

Amides can be hydrolyzed under acidic conditions, via nucleophilic substitution, to produce carboxylic acids or basic conditions to form carboxylates:

TEACHER TIP

We need extreme conditions—strong acid—to increase the electrophilicity to hydrolyze an amide. This is why we have stomach acid: to provide the catalysis necessary to break down proteins.

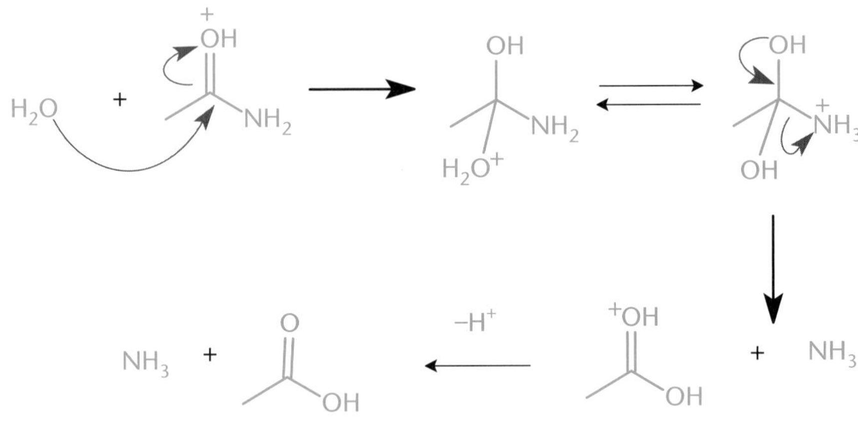

Figure 10.17

2. Hofmann Rearrangement

The **Hofmann rearrangement** converts amides to primary amines with the loss of the carbonyl carbon. The mechanism involves the formation of a **nitrene,** the nitrogen analog of a carbene. The nitrene is attached to the carbonyl group and rearranges to form an **isocyanate,** which, under the reaction condition is hydrolyzed to the amine.

MCAT SYNOPSIS

Hofmann rearrangement: amides → primary amines (with loss of a carbon)

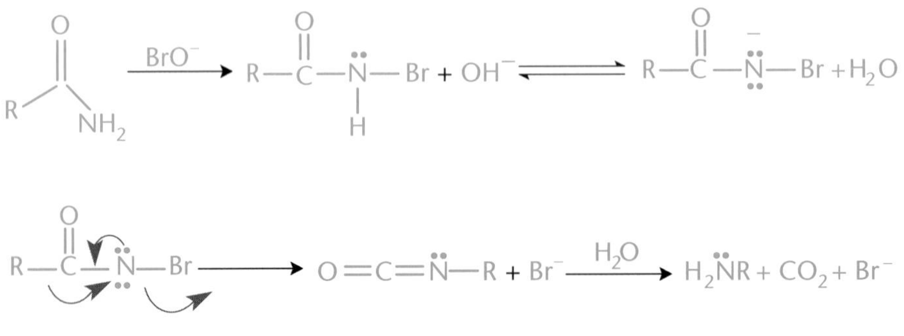

$$RC(=O)NH_2 \xrightarrow{BrO^-} R\text{—}C(=O)\text{—}\ddot{N}(H)\text{—}Br + OH^- \rightleftharpoons R\text{—}C(=O)\text{—}\ddot{N}^-\text{—}Br + H_2O$$

$$R\text{—}C(=O)\text{—}\ddot{N}\text{—}Br \longrightarrow O{=}C{=}\ddot{N}\text{—}R + Br^- \xrightarrow{H_2O} H_2\ddot{N}R + CO_2 + Br^-$$

nitrene isocyanate

Figure 10.18

3. Reduction

Amides can be reduced with LAH to the corresponding amine. Notice that this differs from the product of the Hofmann rearrangement in that no carbon atom is lost.

MCAT SYNOPSIS

Reduction also produces amines, but no carbon is lost.

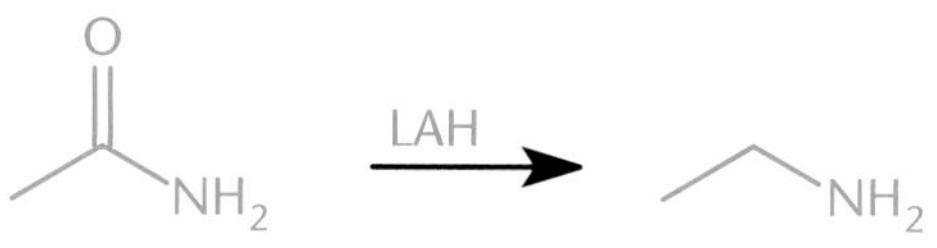

LAH

NH_2 NH_2

Figure 10.19

ESTERS

A. NOMENCLATURE

Esters are the dehydration products of carboxylic acids and alcohols. They are commonly found in many fruits and perfumes. They are named in the IUPAC system as **alkyl** or **aryl alkanoates.** For example, ethyl acetate, derived from the condensation of acetic acid and ethanol, is called ethyl ethanoate according to IUPAC nomenclature.

MCAT SYNOPSIS

An acid + an alcohol = an ester.

B. SYNTHESIS

Mixtures of carboxylic acids and alcohols will condense into esters, liberating water, under acidic conditions. Esters can also be obtained from reaction of acid chlorides or anhydrides with alcohols (see above). Phenolic (aromatic) esters are produced in the same way, although the aromatic acid chlorides are less reactive than aliphatic acid chlorides, so that base must generally be added as a catalyst.

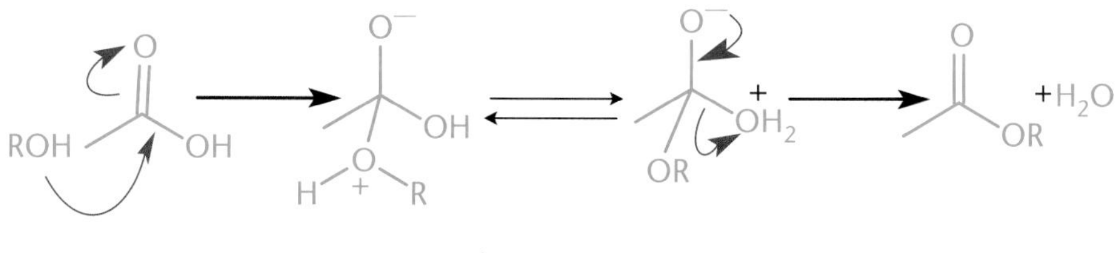

ROH O OH → O^- OH H O R + ⇌ O^- OH_2^+ OR → O OR $+H_2O$

Figure 10.20

C. REACTIONS

1. Hydrolysis

Esters, like the other derivatives of carboxylic acids, can be hydrolyzed, yielding carboxylic acids and alcohols. Hydrolysis can take place under either acidic or basic conditions.

TEACHER TIP

This mechanism keeps coming up and will surely appear on your exam.

Under acidic conditions:

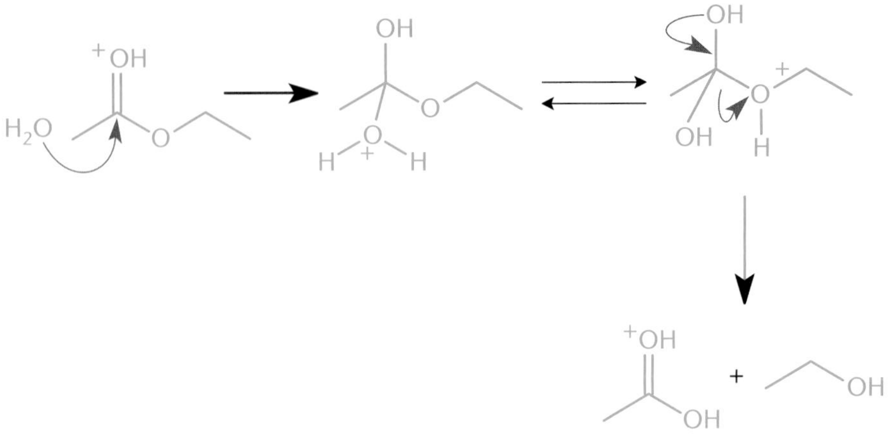

Figure 10.21

The reaction proceeds similarly under basic conditions, except that the oxygen on the C=O is not protonated, and the nucleophile is OH^-.

MCAT SYNOPSIS

Triacylglycerols are actually esters, with glycerol as the alcohol (ROH) and free fatty acids as RCOOH.

Triacylglycerols, also called fats, are esters of long-chain carboxylic acids, often called fatty acids, and glycerol (1,2,3-propanetriol). **Saponification** is the process whereby fats are hydrolyzed under basic conditions to produce soaps. (Note: Acidification of the soap retrieves triacylglycerol.)

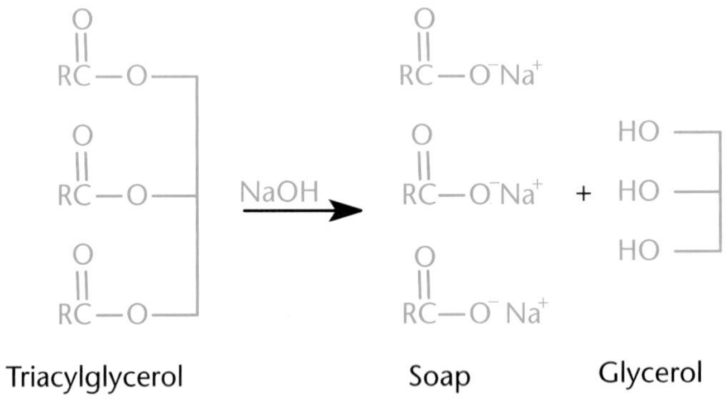

Triacylglycerol — NaOH → Soap + Glycerol

Figure 10.22

2. Conversion into Amides

Nitrogen bases such as ammonia will attack the electron-deficient carbonyl carbon atom, displacing alkoxide, to yield an amide and an alcohol side-product. Here, ammonia is the nucleophile.

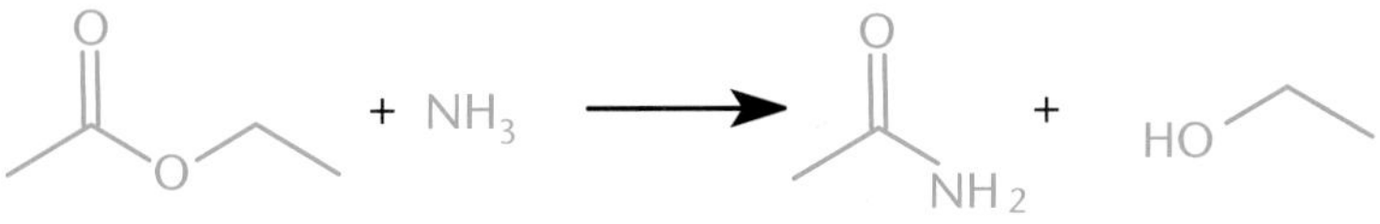

Figure 10.23

3. Transesterification

Alcohols can act as nucleophiles and displace the alkoxy groups on esters. This process, which transforms one ester into another, is called **transesterification.**

> **KAPLAN EXCLUSIVE**
>
> When a different alcohol attacks the ester, the ester is *trans*formed, and *trans*esterification results.

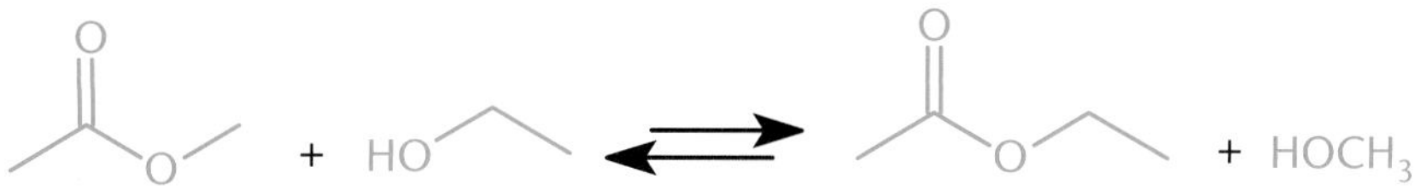

+ HO ⇌ + $HOCH_3$

Figure 10.24

4. Grignard Addition

Grignard reagents add to the carbonyl groups of esters to form ketones; however, these ketones are more reactive than the initial esters and are readily attacked by more Grignard reagent. Two equivalents of Grignard reagent can thus be used to produce tertiary alcohols with good yield. (The intermediate ketone can be isolated only if the alkyl groups are sufficiently bulky to prevent further attack.) This reaction proceeds via nucleophilic substitution followed by nucleophilic addition.

> **MCAT SYNOPSIS**
>
> Grignard reagents, RMgX, are essentially equivalent to R^- nucleophiles.

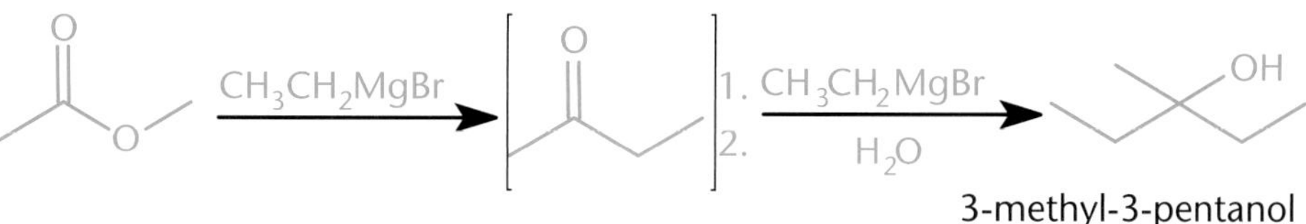

Figure 10.25

5. Condensation Reactions

An important reaction of esters is the **Claisen condensation.** In the simplest case, two moles of ethyl acetate react under basic conditions to produce a β-keto ester, ethyl 3-oxobutanoate, or acetoacetic ester by its common name. (The Claisen condensation is also called the **acetoacetic ester condensation.**) The reaction proceeds by addition of an enolate anion to the carbonyl group of another ester, followed by displacement of ethoxide ion. This mechanism is analogous to that of the aldol condensation.

> **MCAT SYNOPSIS**
>
> The Claisen condensation is similar to the aldol condensation, but instead of an aldehyde acting as an electrophile and nucleophile (in its enol form), it is an ester acting as an electrophile and a nucleophile (in its enolate form)

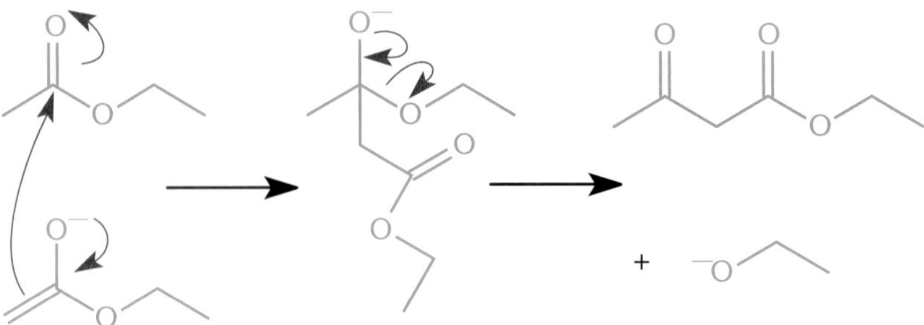

Figure 10.26

> **TEACHER TIP**
>
> The more powerful lithium aluminium hydride is necessary to reduce the ester. Remember that $NaBH_4$ is weaker and more selective than $LiAlH_4$, but both are essential equivalent to an H-nucleophile.

6. Reduction

Esters may be reduced to primary alcohols with LAH, but not with $NaBH_4$. This allows for selective reduction in molecules with multiple functional groups.

LAH

OH + OH

Figure 10.27

D. PHOSPHATE ESTERS

While phosphoric acid derivatives are not carboxylic acid derivatives they form esters similar to those above.

O=P(OH)(OH)(OH)	O=P(OR)(OR)(OR)	where R = H or hydrocarbon
phosphoric acid	phosphoric ester	

Figure 10.28

Phosphoric acid and the mono- and diesters are acidic (more so than carboxylic acids) and usually exist as anions. Like all esters, under acidic conditions they can be cleaved into the parent acid (here, H_3PO_4) and alcohols.

Phosphate esters are found in living systems in the form of **phospholipids** (phosphoglycerides), in which glycerol is attached to two carboxylic acids and one phosphoric acid.

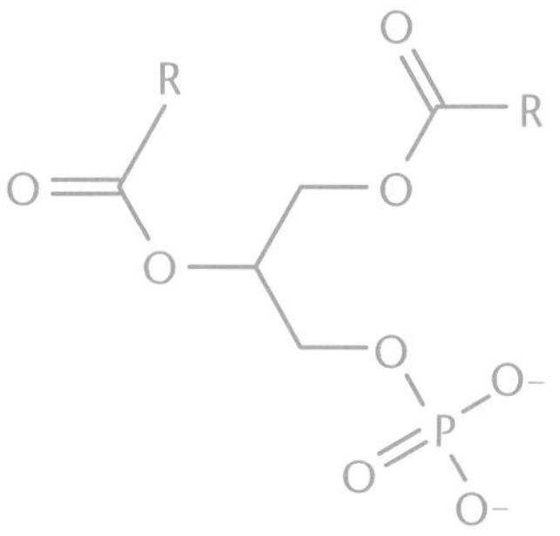

phosphatidic acid
diacylglycerol phosphate
(a phosphoglyceride)

Figure 10.29

Phospholipids are the main component of cell membranes, and phospholipid/carbohydrate polymers form the backbone of nucleic acids, the hereditary material of life (see chapter 14). The nucleic acid derivative **adenosine triphosphate (ATP)** can give up and regain one or more phosphate groups. ATP facilitates many biological reactions by releasing phosphate groups to other compounds, thereby increasing their reactivities.

Teacher Tip

These phosphate esters will act similarly to the carboxylic esters. The phosphodiester bonds should look familiar from your studies of Molecular Biology; they're responsible for holding the DNA backbone together, connecting nucleotides with covalent linkages.

SUMMARY OF REACTIONS

The most important derivatives of carboxylic acid are acyl halides, anhydrides, esters, and amides. These are listed from most reactive (least stable) to least reactive (most stable).

ACYL HALIDES

- Can be formed by adding RCOOH + $SOCl_2$, PCl_3 or PCl_5, or PBr_3
- Undergo many different nucleophilic substitutions; H_2O yields carboxylic acid, while ROH yields an ester, and NH_3 yields an amide
- Can participate in Friedel-Crafts acylation to form an alkyl aryl ketone
- Can be reduced to alcohols or, selectively, to aldehydes

ANHYDRIDES

- Can be formed by RCOOH + RCOOH (condensation) or $RCOO^-$ + RCOCl (substitution)
- Undergo many nucleophilic substitution reactions, forming products that include carboxylic acids, amides, and esters
- Can participate in Friedel-Crafts acylation

TEACHER TIP

The reactions of carboxylic acid derivatives will appear on the exam.

ESTERS

- Formed by RCOOH + ROH or, better, by acid chlorides or anhydrides + ROH
- Hydrolyze to yield acids + alcohols; adding ammonia yields an amide
- Reaction with Grignard reagent (two moles) produces a tertiary alcohol
- In Claisen condensation, analogous to the aldol, the ester acts both as nucleophile and target
- Very important in biological processes, particularly phosphate esters, which can be found in membranes, nucleic acids, and metabolic reactions

AMIDES

- Can be formed by acid chlorides + amines, or acid anhydrides + ammonia
- Hydrolysis yields carboxylic acids or carboxylate anions
- Can be transformed to primary amines via Hofmann rearrangement or reduction

PRACTICE QUESTIONS

1. Which of the following is identified by 1H NMR as having optical diastereomers?

A. 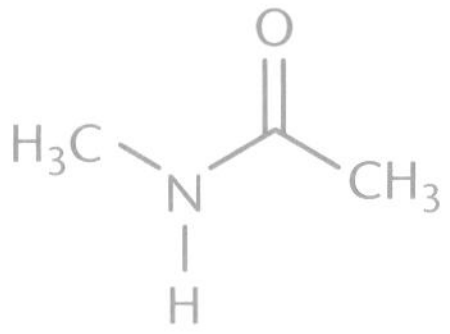 H_3C N H O CH_3

B. 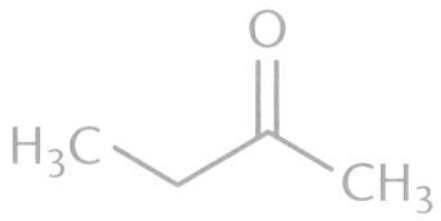 H_3C O CH_3

C. 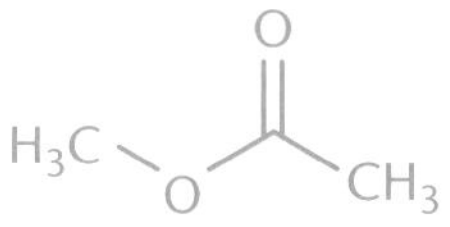 H_3C O O CH_3

D. None of the above

2. Which conversion between carboxylic acid derivatives is not possible by nucleophilic reaction?

A. Acid chloride → ester
B. Acid chloride → anhydride
C. Anhydride → amide
D. Ester → anhydride

3. Acyl halides make excellent reactants in carboxylic acid derivative synthesis becuase

A. halides are amenable to nucleophilic attack.
B. halides are amenable to electrophilic attack.
C. halide ions are good leaving groups.
D. there is a lack of rotation around the C=O bond.

4. Which of the following undergoes a Fischer esterification most rapidly?

A. 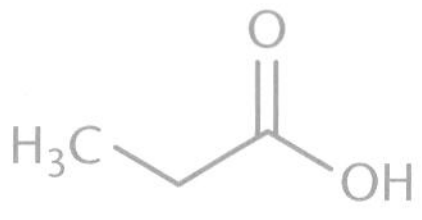 H_3C O OH

B. 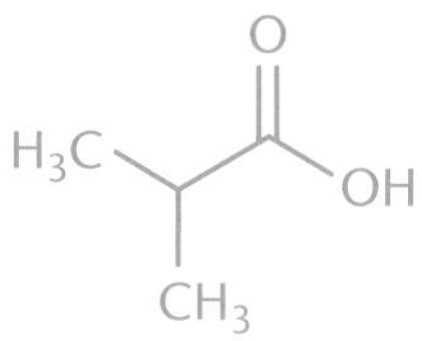 H_3C O OH CH_3

C. 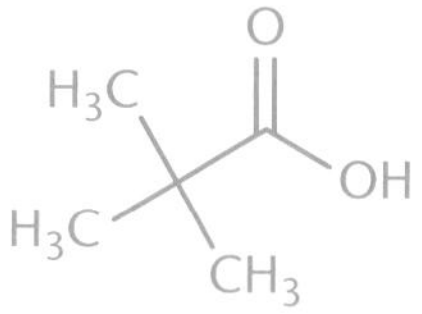 H_3C H_3C CH_3 O OH

D. 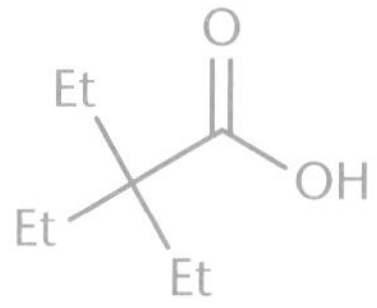 Et Et Et O OH

5. Which of the following does NOT explain why a primary acyl chloride is more susceptible to nucleophilic attack than an alkyl chloride?

A. The carbonyl carbon is more electrophilic than the chlorinated carbon of an alkane is.
B. The transition state of an alkyl halide is more sterically hindered.
C. Sigma bonds are stronger than pi bonds are.
D. The chloride in an alkyl halide is more electronegative.

KEY CONCEPTS

Acids and bases

Enolate ion

Claisen condensation

Intramolecular reactions

INTRAMOLECULAR RING CLOSURES

Provide a detailed, stepwise mechanism to account for the following transformation:

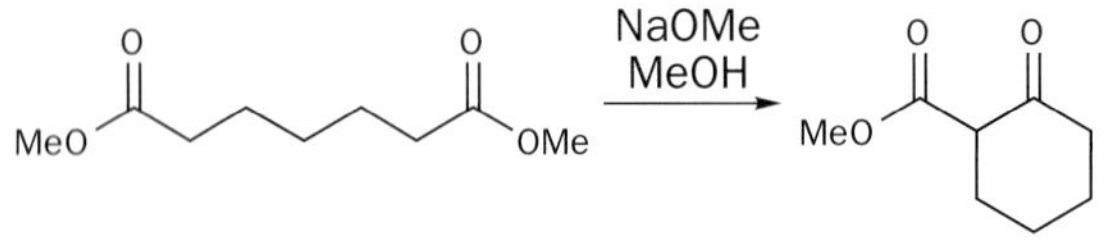

NaOMe
MeOH

1) Examine the product for clues to the connectivity.

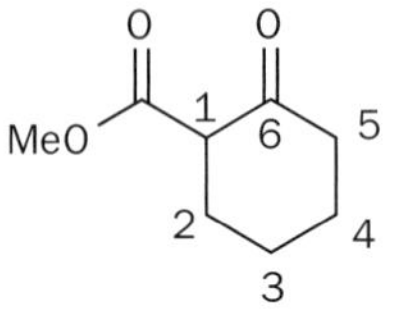

TAKEAWAYS

Remember that with mechanism problems, you always want to get toward the specified products. Don't include steps that don't get you any closer to where you want to be.

Anytime you see one molecule going to form a ring, you should suspect that there is an intramolecular reaction. Here, note that in the six-membered ring, the α–carbon of one ester is directly connected to a ketone. That, combined with the fact that there is a β–keto ester in the product, should tell you that what is going on is an intramolecular Claisen condensation.

Remember: *Intramolecular reactions are always faster than intermolecular reactions because the reactants are already close together.*

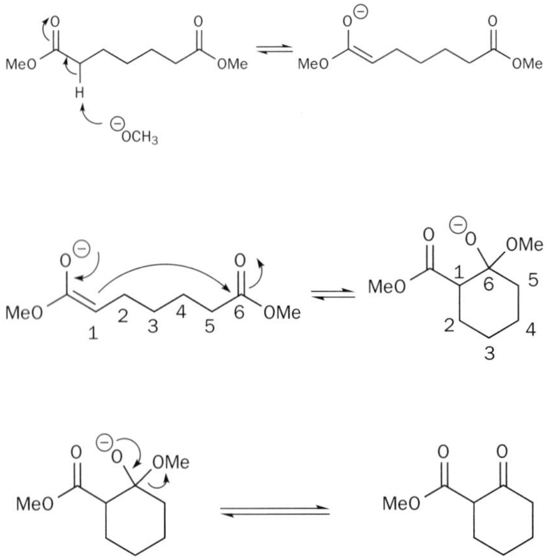

THINGS TO WATCH OUT FOR

Make sure that if charged intermediates are involved in your mechanism, they go away before you get to the product, unless the product is charged as well.

Also, be sure that your arrows are pointing in the right direction! The head of the arrow is pointing toward where the electrons are moving, not where they start from.

2) Start pushing electons.

First, generate an enolate for the Claisen condensation, which must take place next to one of the esters.

Then, the intramolecular reaction takes place. Numbering along the carbon chain and in the product is always a good idea. This will help you make sure that everything is in the right place.

Here, finish the mechanism by generating the keto ester functionality that is in the product.

SIMILAR QUESTIONS

1) Provide a detailed, step-wise mechanism for the following transformation:

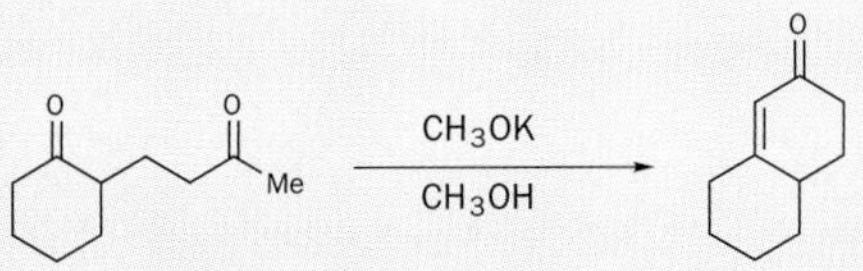

2) Provide a detailed, step-wise mechanism for the same reaction above, except run an *acid* instead of a *base*.
3) Provide a detailed, step-wise mechanism to account for the following reaction:

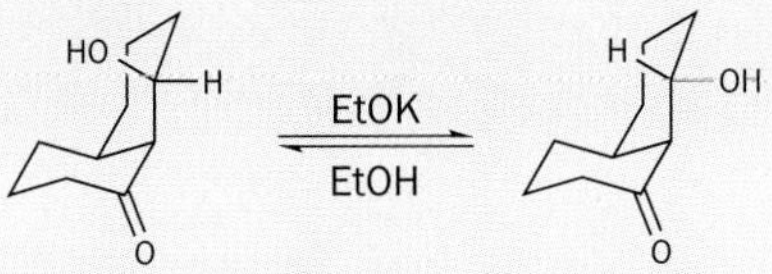

CHAPTER 11

AMINES AND NITROGEN-CONTAINING COMPOUNDS

NOMENCLATURE

Amines are compounds of the general formula NR_3. They are classified according to the number of alkyl (or aryl) groups to which they are bound. A **primary (1°)** amine is attached to one alkyl group, a **secondary (2°)** amine to two, and a **tertiary (3°)** amine to three. A nitrogen atom attached to four alkyl groups is called a **quaternary ammonium compound.** The nitrogen carries a positive charge; thus, these compounds generally exist as salts.

TEACHER TIP

Amino groups are common in biological molecules and are capable of hydrogen bonding.

In the common system, amines are generally named as alkylamines. The groups are designated individually or by using the prefixes di- or tri- if they are the same. In the IUPAC system, amines are named by substituting the suffix **-amine** for the final "e" of the name of the alkane to which the nitrogen is attached. *N* is used to label substituents attached to the nitrogen in secondary or tertiary amines. The prefix **amino-** is used for naming compounds containg an OH or a CO_2H group. Aromatic amines are named as derivatives of aniline ($C_6H_5NH_2$), the IUPAC name for which is benzenamine.

Table 11.1.

Formula:	$CH_3CH_2NH_2$	$CH_3CH_2N(CH_3)_2$	$(CH_3)_2NCH_2CH_2CH_2CH_2CH_2CH_3$
IUPAC:	ethanamine	*N,N*-dimethylethanamine	*N,N*-dimethylhexanamine
Common:	ethylamine	dimethylethylamine	dimethylhexylamine

TEACHER TIP

Don't spend time trying to figure out how to name all amines, just get a general idea. When "N" precedes the name, it means the substituent is on the nitrogen itself.

Aromatic amines are named as derivatives of **aniline** ($C_6H_5NH_2$).

There are many other nitrogen-containing organic compounds. **Amides** are the condensation products of carboxylic acids and amines, and have already been discussed in Chapter 10. **Carbamates** are compounds with the general formula RNHC(O)OR′. They are also called **urethanes,** and can form polymers called **polyurethanes**. Carbamates are derived from compounds called **isocyanates,** (general formula RNCO) by the addition of an alcohol. **Enamines** are the nitrogen analogs of enols, with an

CLINICAL CORRELATE

All amino acids, as you might guess, are amines. Peptide bonds between amino acids in proteins are amide bonds. Urea, a molecule used to store ammonia for removal from the body, is also an amide.

amine group attached to one carbon of a double bond. **Imines** are nitrogen compounds that contain nitrogen-carbon double bonds. **Nitriles,** or **cyanides,** are compounds with a triple bond between a carbon atom and a nitrogen atom. They are named with either the prefix **cyano-** or the suffix **-nitrile. Nitro** compounds contain the nitro group, NO_2. **Diazo** compounds contain an N_2 functionality. They tend to lose N_2 to form carbenes. **Azides** are compounds with an N_3 functionality. When azides lose nitrogen (N_2), they form **nitrenes,** the nitrogen analogs of carbenes. Examples of these various compounds are listed below.

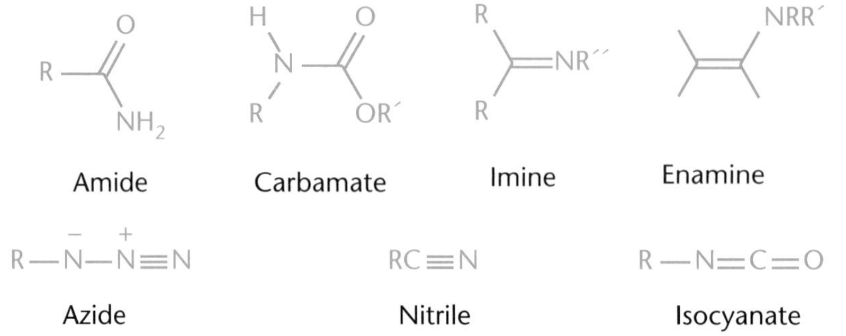

Amide — Carbamate — Imine — Enamine

$R—\overset{-}{N}—\overset{+}{N}≡N$ Azide — $RC≡N$ Nitrile — $R—N=C=O$ Isocyanate

Figure 11.1

TEACHER TIP

Hydrogen bonding will always increase boiling points. So primary and secondary amines will have hydrogens available to interact and thus will have elevated boiling points (though not as high as corresponding alcohol because the bonds will be a bit weaker). Tertiary amines will not be able to hydrogen bond.

PROPERTIES

The boiling points of amines are between those of alkanes and alcohols. For example, ammonia boils at –33°C, whereas methane boils at –161°C and methanol at 64.5°C. As molecular weight increases, so do boiling points. Primary and secondary amines can form hydrogen bonds, while tertiary amines cannot; therefore, tertiary amines have lower boiling points. Since nitrogen is not as electronegative as oxygen, the hydrogen bonds of amines are not as strong as those of alcohols.

The nitrogen atom in an amine is approximately sp^3 hybridized. Nitrogen must bond to only three substituents in order to complete its octet; a lone pair occupies the last sp^3 orbital. This lone pair is very important to the chemistry of amines; it is associated with their basic and nucleophilic properties.

Nitrogen atoms bonded to three different substituents are chiral because of the geometry of the orbitals. However, these enantiomers cannot be isolated, because they interconvert rapidly in a process called **nitrogen inversion**: an inversion of the sp^3 orbital occupied by the lone pair. The activation energy for this process is only 6 kcal/mol, and only at very low temperatures is it significantly slowed or stopped.

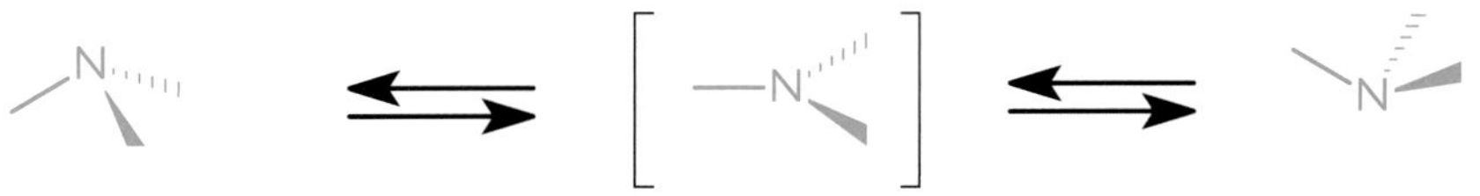

Figure 11.2

Amines are bases and readily accept protons to form ammonium ions. The pK_b values of alkyl amines are around 4, making them slightly more basic than ammonia (pK_b = 4.76), but less basic than hydroxide (pK_b = −1.7). Aromatic amines such as aniline (pK_b = 9.42) are far less basic than aliphatic amines, because the electron-withdrawing effect of the ring reduces the basicity of the amino group. The presence of other substituents on the ring alters the basicity of anilines: electron-donating groups (such as $-OH$, $-CH_3$, and $-NH_2$) increase basicity, while electron-withdrawing groups (such as NO_2) reduce basicity.

Amines also function as very weak acids. The pK_a's of amines are around 35, and a very strong base is required for deprotonation. For example, the proton of diisopropylamine may be removed with butyllithium, forming the sterically hindered base lithium diisopropylamide, LDA.

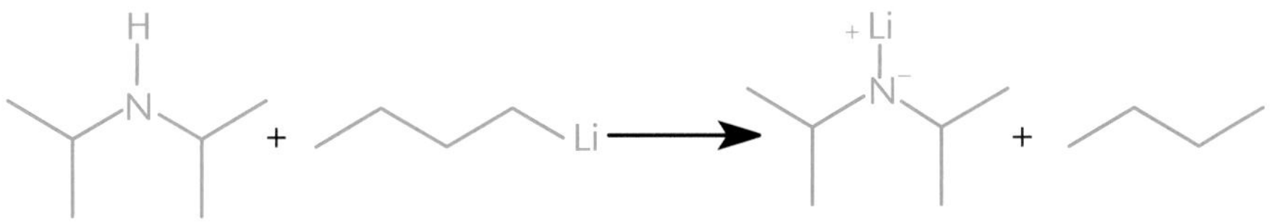

REAL-WORLD ANALOGY

An interesting property of several nitrogen-containing compounds, such as nitroglycerin and nitrous oxide, is their ability to act as relaxants. Nitroglycerine is given sublingually to relieve coronary artery spasms in people with chest pain, and nitrous oxide (laughing gas) is a common dental anesthetic. Nitroglycerine has the additional property of rapidly decomposing to form gas and is thus fairly explosive.

Figure 11.3

SYNTHESIS

A. ALKYLATION OF AMMONIA

1. Direct

Alkyl halides react with ammonia to produce alkylammonium halide salts. Ammonia functions as a nucleophile and displaces the halide atom. When the salt is treated with base, the alkylamine product is formed.

$$CH_3Br + NH_3 \longrightarrow CH_3\overset{+}{N}H_3Br^- \xrightarrow{NaOH} CH_3NH_2 + NaBr + H_2O$$

Figure 11.4

TEACHER TIP

This is an S_N2 reaction mechanism. But more important about this reaction is that the product will actually be a better product than the original nucleophile. That's because the electron-donating properties of the alkyl group causes further substitution.

This reaction often leads to side products, because the alkylamine formed is nucleophilic and can react with the alkyl halide to form more complex products.

FLASHBACK

Addition of ammonia to an alkyl halide and the Gabriel synthesis are both S_N2 reactions. With its unshared electron pair, ammonia is a very good nucleophile, while the halides are all good leaving groups (see chapter 4).

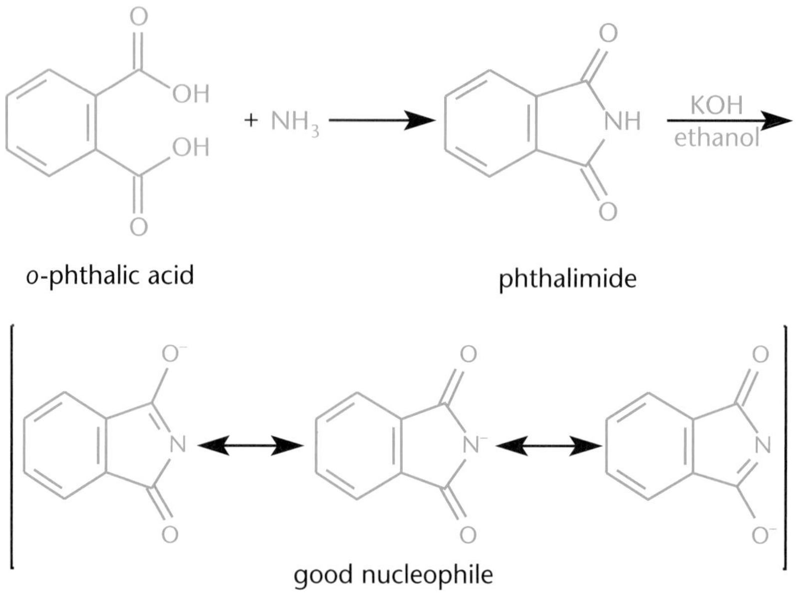

2. **Gabriel Synthesis**

The **Gabriel synthesis** converts a primary alkyl halide to a primary amine. The use of a disguised form of ammonia prevents side-product formation.

o-phthalic acid + NH_3 → phthalimide $\xrightarrow[\text{ethanol}]{\text{KOH}}$

[resonance structures of phthalimide anion] good nucleophile

Figure 11.5

Phthalimide, the condensation product of phthalic acid and ammonia, acts as a good nucleophile when deprotonated. It displaces halide ions, forming N-alkylphthalimides, which do not react with other alkyl halides. When the reaction is complete, the N-alkylphthalimide can be hydrolyzed with aqueous base to produce the alkylamine.

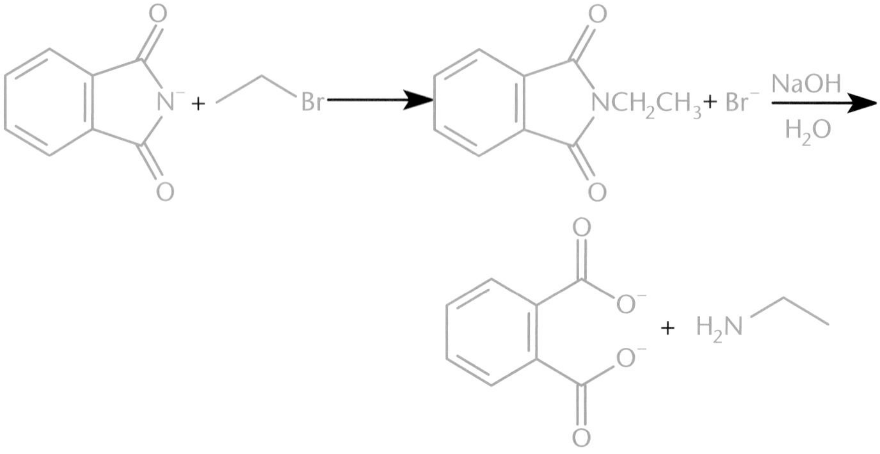

phthalimide anion (N^-) + ethyl bromide (Br) → NCH_2CH_3 + Br^- $\xrightarrow[H_2O]{\text{NaOH}}$ phthalate (O^-, O^-) + H_2N–ethyl

Figure 11.6

B. REDUCTION

Amines can be obtained from other nitrogen-containing functionalities via reduction reactions.

1. From Nitro Compounds

Nitro compounds are easily reduced to primary amines. The most common reducing agent is iron or zinc and dilute hydrochloric acid, although many other reagents can be used. This reaction is especially useful for aromatic compounds, because nitration of aromatic rings is facile.

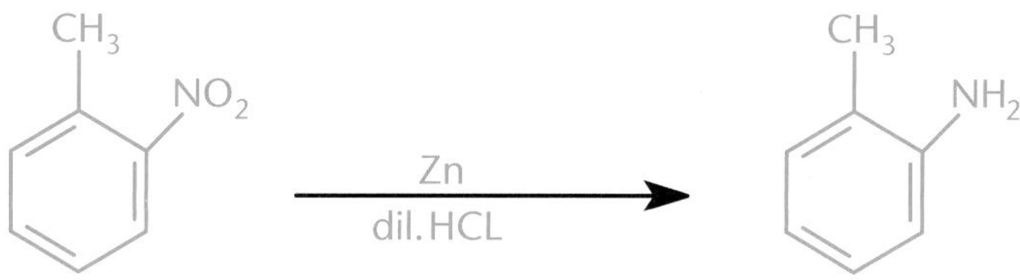

Figure 11.7

> **MCAT SYNOPSIS**
>
> Amines can be formed by:
>
> 1) S_N2 reactions
>   - ammonia reacting with alkyl halides
>   - Gabriel synthesis
> 2) Reduction of:
>   - amides
>   - aniline and its derivatives
>   - nitriles
>   - imines
>
> Amines can be destroyed (converted to alkenes) by exhaustive methylation.

2. From Nitriles

Nitriles can be reduced with hydrogen and a catalyst, or with lithium aluminum hydride (LAH), to produce primary amines.

$$CH_3CH_2C{\equiv}N \xrightarrow{LAH} CH_3CH_2CH_2NH_2$$

Figure 11.8

3. From Imines

Amines can be synthesized by **reductive amination,** a process whereby an aldehyde or ketone is reacted with ammonia, a primary amine, or a secondary amine to form a primary, secondary, or tertiary amine, respectively. When the amine reacts with the aldehyde or the ketone, an imine is produced. Consequently, it will undergo hydride reduction in much the same way that a carbonyl does. When the imine is reduced with hydrogen in the presence of a catalyst, an amine is produced.

> **MCAT SYNOPSIS**
>
> An imine is a nitrogen double bonded to a carbon atom. It looks like a carbonyl and acts like one too: Similar polarity and similar reactivity.

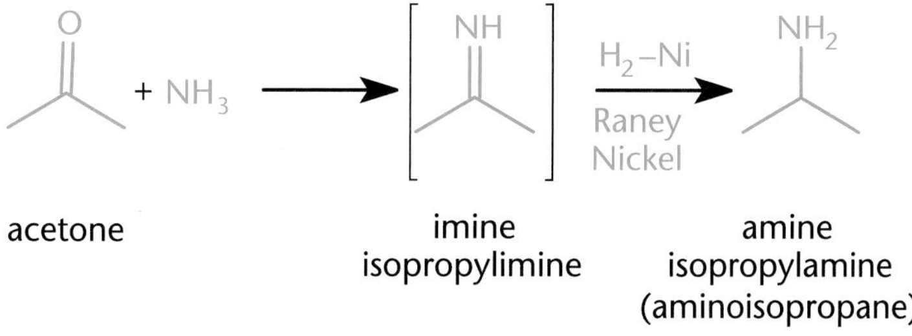

acetone | imine isopropylimine | amine isopropylamine (aminoisopropane)

Figure 11.9

4. From Amides

Amides can be reduced with LAH to form amines (see chapter 10).

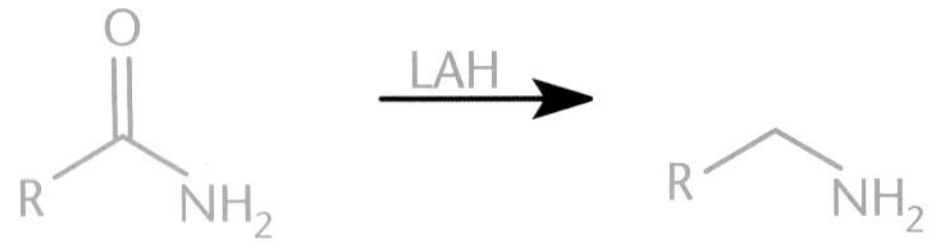

Figure 11.10

REACTIONS

A. EXHAUSTIVE METHYLATION

Exhaustive methylation is also known as **Hofmann elimination.** In this process, an amine is converted to a quaternary ammonium iodide by treatment with excess methyl iodide. Treatment with silver oxide and water converts this to the ammonium hydroxide, which, when heated, undergoes elimination to form an alkene and an amine. The predominant alkene formed is the least substituted, in contrast with normal elimination reactions, where the predominant alkene product is the most substituted.

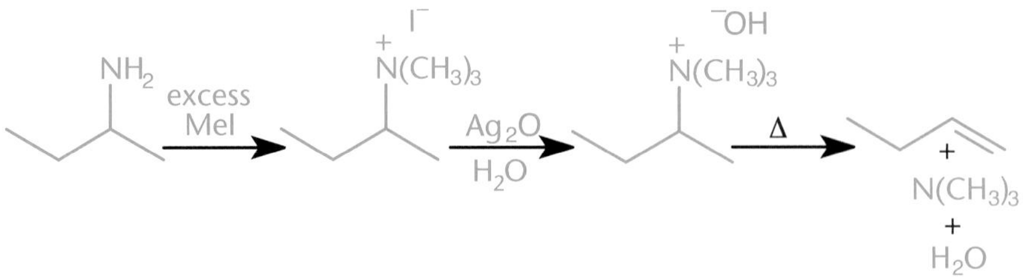

Figure 11.11

PRACTICE QUESTIONS

1. What is the IUPAC name for the compound shown below?

H_3C N H_3C N

A. 4-(N-dimethylamino)pyridine
B. Dimethylaminopyridine
C. 4-(N,N-dimethylamino)pyridine
D. N,N-dimethylaminopyridine

2. Pyrrolidine is an excellent base, with a pK_a of 11.27. In contrast, pyrrole, which has a very similar structure, is a very poor base, with a pK_a of 0.4. Why is pyrrole such a poor base compared to pyrrolidine?

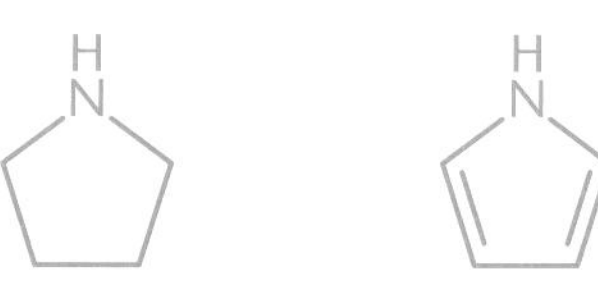

Pyrrolidine **Pyrrole**

A. Pyrrole is aromatic.
B. Pyrrolidine is anti-aromatic.
C. The nitrogen atom in pyrrole does not have any lone pairs.
D. The nitrogen in pyrrolidine contains an extra lone pair.

3. What product is formed from the following reaction?

NH → ?
1. xs CH_3I
2. Ag_2O, H_2O
3. Heat

A. NH_2
B. N—
C. + $N(CH_3)_3$
D. $N(CH_3)_2$

4. What intermediate is formed from the following reaction shown in Figure 4?

H, O, NH_2 → [?] → (H_2, Raney Nickel) Piperidine

A. $+NH_2$
B. NH
C. N
D. NH

5. What is the overall charge of the nitrogen atom in a nitrene?

A. –1
B. 0
C. +1
D. +2

CHAPTER 12

PURIFICATION AND SEPARATION

Much of organic chemistry is concerned with the isolation and purification of the desired reaction product. A reaction itself may be completed in a matter of minutes, but separating the product from the reaction mixture is often a difficult and rather time-consuming process. Many different techniques have been developed to accomplish this objective: to obtain a pure compound separated from solvents, reagents, and other products.

TEACHER TIP

Purification and separation techniques are procedures which exploit different physical properties.

BASIC TECHNIQUES

A. EXTRACTION

One way of separating a desired product is through **extraction,** the transfer of a dissolved compound (here, the desired product) from one solvent into another in which it is more soluble. Most impurities will be left behind in the first solvent. The two solvents should be immiscible (form two layers that do not mix because of mutual insolubility). The two layers are temporarily mixed together so that solute can pass from one to the other. For example, a solution of isobutyric acid in diethyl ether can be extracted with water. Isobutyric acid is more soluble in water than in ether, and so when the two solvents are placed together, isobutyric acid transfers to the water phase.

The water (aqueous) and ether (organic) phases are separated in a specialized piece of glassware called a separatory funnel. Once separated, the isobutyric acid can be isolated from the aqueous phase in pure form. Some isobutyric acid will remain dissolved in the ether phase, so the extraction should be repeated several times with fresh solvent (water). More product can be obtained with successive extractions; i.e., it is more effective to perform three successive extractions of 10 mL each than to perform one extraction of 30 mL. Once the compound has been isolated in its purified form in a solvent, it can then be obtained by evaporation of the solvent.

TEACHER TIP

Think of the organic and aqueous layers as being like oil and water, respectively, in salad dressing: you can shake the mixture to increase their interaction, but ultimately they'll separate again.

MCAT Synopsis

Extraction depends on the rules of solubility—"like dissolves like"! Remember the three intermolecular forces that affect solubility:

1. Hydrogen bonding: compounds that can do this, such as alcohols or acids, will move most easily into the aqueous layer.
2. Dipole-dipole interactions: these compounds are less likely to move into the aqueous layer.
3. van der Waals (London) forces: with only these interactions, compounds are least likely to move into the aqueous layer.

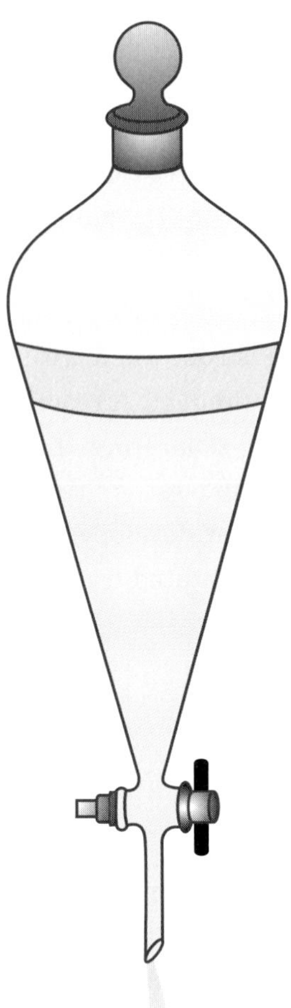

Figure 12.1 Separatory Funnel

An extraction carried out to remove unwanted impurities rather than to isolate a pure product is called a **wash.**

B. FILTRATION

Filtration is used to isolate a solid from a liquid. In this technique, a liquid/solid mixture is poured onto a paper filter that allows only the solvent to pass through. The result of this process is the separation of the solid (often referred to as the residue) from the liquid or **filtrate.** The two basic types of filtration are **gravity filtration** and **vacuum filtration.** In gravity filtration, the solvent's own weight pulls it through the filter. Frequently, however, the pores of the filter become clogged with solid, slowing the rate of filtration. For this reason, in gravity filtration it is generally desirable for the substance of interest to be in solution (dissolved in the solvent), while impurities remain undissolved and can be filtered out. This allows the desired product to flow more easily and rapidly through the apparatus. To ensure that the product remains dissolved, gravity filtration is usually carried out with hot solvent.

In vacuum filtration, the solvent is forced through the filter by a vacuum on the other side. Vacuum filtration is used to isolate relatively large quantities of solid, usually when the solid is the desired product.

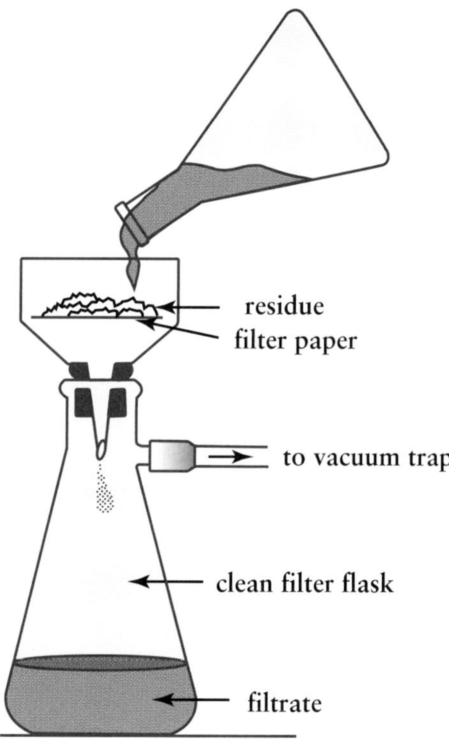

Figure 12.2 Vacuum Filtration

C. RECRYSTALLIZATION

Recrystallization is a process in which impure crystals are dissolved in a minimum amount of hot solvent. As the solvent is cooled, the crystals reform, leaving the impurities in solution. For recrystallization to be effective, the solvent must be chosen carefully. It must dissolve the solid while it is hot, but not while it is cold. In addition, it must dissolve the impurities at both temperatures, so that they remain in solution. Solvent choice is usually a matter of trial and error, although some generalizations can be made. An estimate of polarity is useful, because polar solvents dissolve polar compounds while nonpolar solvents dissolve nonpolar compounds. A solvent with intermediate polarity is generally desirable in recrystallization. In addition, the solvent should have a low enough freezing point that the solution may be sufficiently cooled.

> **MCAT SYNOPSIS**
>
> Ideally the desired product should have solubility that depends on temperature—it should be more soluble at higher temperatures, less so at low ones. In contrast, impurities should be equally soluble at various temperatures.

In some instances, a mixed solvent system may be used. Here the crude compound is dissolved in a solvent in which it is highly soluble. Another solvent, in which the compound is less soluble, is then added in drops, just until solid begins to precipitate. The solution is heated a bit more to redissolve the precipitate, and then slowly cooled to induce crystal formation.

D. SUBLIMATION

Sublimation occurs when a heated solid turns directly into a gas, without an intervening liquid stage. It is used as a method of purification because the impurities found in most reaction mixtures will not sublime easily. The vapors are made to condense on a **cold finger,** a piece of glassware packed with dry ice or with cold water running through it. Most sublimations are performed under vacuum, because at higher pressures more compounds will pass through a liquid phase rather than subliming; low pressure also reduces the temperature required for sublimation and thus the danger that the compound will decompose. The optimal conditions depend on the compound to be purified, because each compound has a different phase diagram.

MCAT Favorite

Remember the phase diagram:

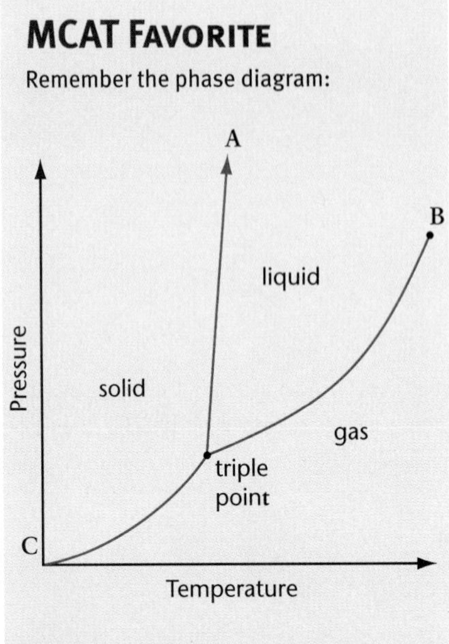

To make a solid sublime, you must either:

a) raise the temperature at a low enough pressure; or
b) lower the pressure at a very cold temperature.

Ever wonder why the ice cubes in your freezer seem to be shrinking?

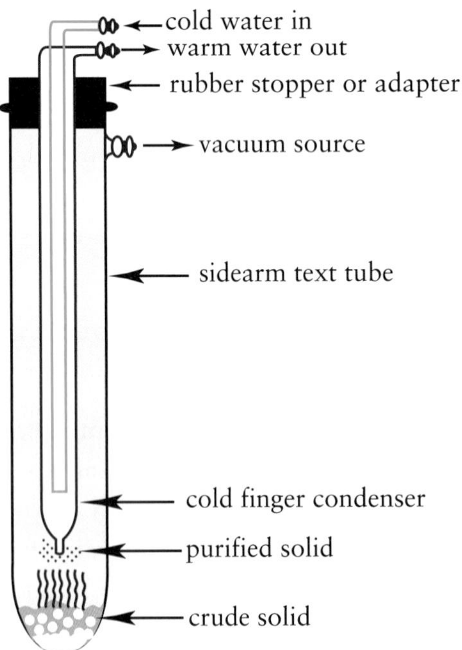

Figure 12.3 Sublimation

Clinical Correlate

Centrifugation is generally used to separate big things from each other. For example, you can:

- centrifuge blood to separate cells (RBC, WBC, platelets) from plasma;
- centrifuge cell debris to separate out organelles of interest, such as mitochondria;
- centrifuge (at ultrahigh speeds) to separate big DNA molecules, such as bacterial chromosomes, from smaller ones, such as plasmids.

E. CENTRIFUGATION

Particles in a solution settle, or **sediment,** at different rates depending upon their mass, their density, and their shape. Sedimentation can be accelerated by **centrifuging** the solution. A centrifuge is an apparatus in which test tubes containing the solution are spun at high speed, which subjects them to centrifugal force. Compounds of greater mass and density settle toward the bottom of the test tubes, while lighter compounds remain near the top. This method of separation is effective for many different types of compounds, and is frequently used in biochemistry to separate cells, organelles, and biological macromolecules.

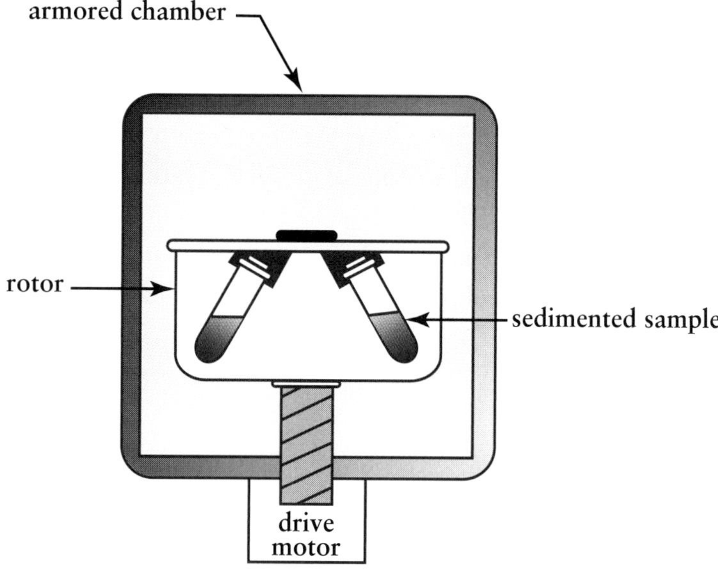

Figure 12.4 Centrifuge

KAPLAN EXCLUSIVE

SeDimentation depends on Size (mass) and Density.

DISTILLATION

Distillation is the separation of one liquid from another through vaporization and condensation. A mixture of two (or more) miscible liquids is slowly heated; the compound with the lowest boiling point is preferentially vaporized, condenses on a water-cooled distillation column, and is separated from the other, higher-boiling compound(s). (Immiscible liquids can be separated in a separatory funnel and thus do not require distillation.)

A. SIMPLE

Simple distillation is used to separate liquids that boil *below* 150°C and at least 25°C apart. The apparatus consists of a distilling flask containing the two liquids, a distillation column consisting of a thermometer and a condenser, and a receiving flask to collect the distillate.

TEACHER TIP

Remember from general chemistry that liquids boil when their vapor pressure is greater than atmospheric pressure. In vacuum filtration, lower in the atmospheric pressure means that the liquid can boil at lower temperatures.

B. VACUUM

Vacuum distillation is used to separate liquids that boil *above* 150°C and at least 25°C apart. The entire system is operated under reduced pressure, lowering the boiling points of the liquids and thus preventing their decomposition due to excessive temperature.

TEACHER TIP

Fractional distillation is like a million simple distillations in one and that is why it is highly efficient.

C. FRACTIONAL

Fractional distillation is used to separate liquids that boil less than 25°C apart. A fractionating column is used to connect the distilling flask to the distillation column. It is filled with inert objects, such as glass beads, which have a large surface area. The vapors condense on these surfaces, reevaporate, and then condense further up the column. Each time the liquid evaporates, the vapors contain a greater proportion of the lower-boiling component. Eventually, near the top of the fractionating column, the vapor is composed solely of one component, which will condense on the distillation column and collect in the receiving flask.

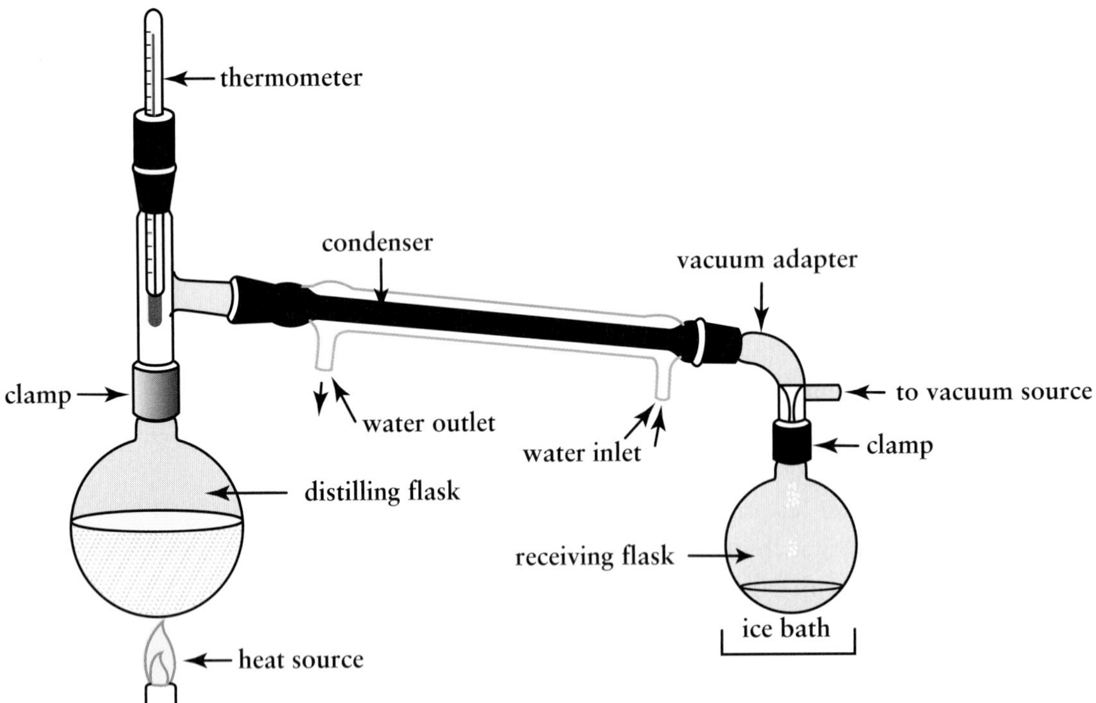

Figure 12.5: Vacuum Distillation

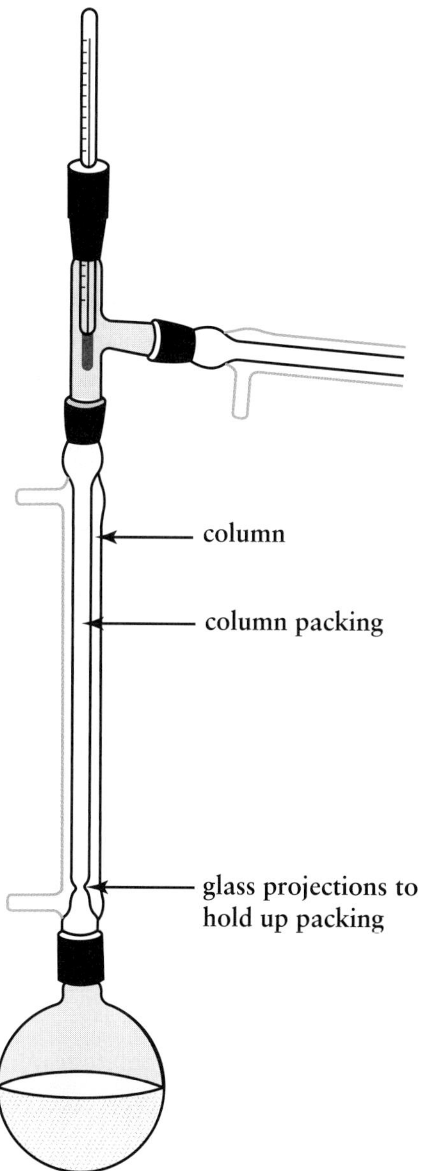

Figure 12.6: Fractional Distillation

CHROMATOGRAPHY

A. GENERAL PRINCIPLES

Chromatography is a technique that allows scientists to separate, identify, and isolate individual compounds from a complex mixture based on their differing chemical properties. First, the sample is placed, or loaded, onto a solid medium called the **stationary phase** or **adsorbant.** Then, the **mobile phase,** a liquid (or gas for gas chromatography), is run through the stationary phase, to displace (or **elute**) adhered substances. Different compounds will adhere to the stationary phase with different strengths, and therefore migrate with different speeds. This causes separation of the compounds within the stationary phase, allowing each compound to be isolated.

There are several forms of media used as the stationary phase, which separate compounds based on different chemical properties. How quickly a compound travels through the stationary phase depends on a variety of factors. Commonly, the key is polarity. For instance, thin layer chromatography often uses silica gel, which is highly polar. Thus, polar compounds bind tightly, eluting poorly into the less polar organic solvent. Size or charge may also play a role, as in column chromatography (described in detail below). Newer techniques, such as affinity chromatography, take advantage of unique properties of a substance (such as its strong binding to a specific antibody or to a known receptor or ligand) to bind it tightly to the stationary phase.

Compounds can be distinguished from each other because they travel across the stationary phase (adsorbant) at different rates. In practice, a substance can be identified based on:

- how far it travels in a given amount of time (as in TLC); or
- how rapidly it travels a given distance, *e.g.*, how quickly it elutes off the column (as in GC or column chromatography.)

The four most commonly used types of chromatography are **thin-layer chromatography, column chromatography, gas chromatography,** and **high-pressure** (or **performance**) **liquid chromatography.**

MCAT Synopsis

Key idea: Chromatography separates compounds based on how strongly they adhere to the *solid,* or *stationary,* phase (or, in other words, how easily they come off into the mobile phase).

B. THIN-LAYER CHROMATOGRAPHY

The adsorbant in thin-layer chromatography (TLC) is either a piece of paper or a thin layer of silica gel or alumina on a plastic or glass sheet. The mixture to be separated is placed on the adsorbant; this is called **spotting,** because a small, well defined spot is desirable. The TLC plate is then **developed**: placed upright in a developing chamber (usually a beaker with a lid or a wide-mouthed jar), containing **eluant** (solvent) approximately ¼-inch deep (this value depends on the size of the plate). It is imperative that the initial spots on the plate be above the level of the solvent, or they will simply elute off the plate into the solvent rather than moving neatly up the plate itself. The solvent creeps up the plate by capillary action, moving different compounds at different rates. When the **solvent front** nears the top of the plate, the plate is removed from the chamber and allowed to dry.

Chromatography is often done with silica gel, which is very polar and hydrophilic. The mobile phase, usually an organic solvent of weak to moderate polarity, is then used to "run" the sample through the gel. Nonpolar compounds move very quickly, while polar molecules are stuck tightly to the gel. The more polar the solvent, the faster the sample will migrate. Reverse-phase chromatography is just the opposite. Here the stationary phase is very nonpolar, so polar molecules run very quickly, while nonpolar molecules stick more tightly.

The spots of individual compounds (usually white) are not usually visible on the white TLC plate. They are **visualized** by placing the TLC plate under UV light, which will show any compounds that are UV-sensitive (see chapter 13, Spectroscopy); or by allowing iodine, I_2, to stain the spots. Other chemical staining agents include phosphomolybdic acid and vanillin. Note that these compounds destroy the product (usually by oxidation), so that it cannot be recovered for further study.

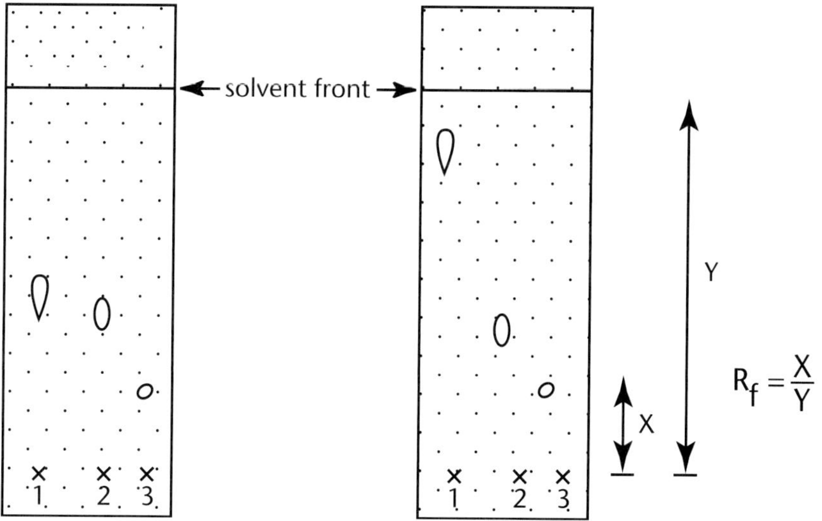

Figure 12.7 Thin-Layer Chromatograms

The distance a compound travels, divided by the distance the solvent travels, is called the **R_f value.** This value is relatively constant for a particular compound in a particular solvent, and can therefore be used for identification.

TEACHER TIP

If the sample travels further, then it is similar to the solvent.

TLC is most frequently used for qualitative identification (*i.e.*, determining the identity of a compound). It can also be used on a larger scale, as a means of purification. **Preparative** or **prep TLC** uses a large TLC plate upon which a sizeable streak of a mixture is placed. As the plate develops, the streak splits into bands of individual compounds, which can be scraped off. Rinsing with a polar solvent will recover the pure compounds from the silica.

Teacher Tip

All chromatography, except for *size-exclusion chromatography*, addresses how "like" the substance is to the mobile and stationary phases.

C. COLUMN CHROMATOGRAPHY

The principle behind column chromatography is the same as for TLC. Column chromatography, however, uses silica gel or alumina as an adsorbant (not paper), and this adsorbant is in the form of a column (not a layer), allowing much more separation. In TLC the solvent and compounds move up the plate (by capillary action), whereas in column chromatography they move down the column (by gravity). Sometimes the solvent is forced through the column with nitrogen gas; this is called **flash column chromatography.**

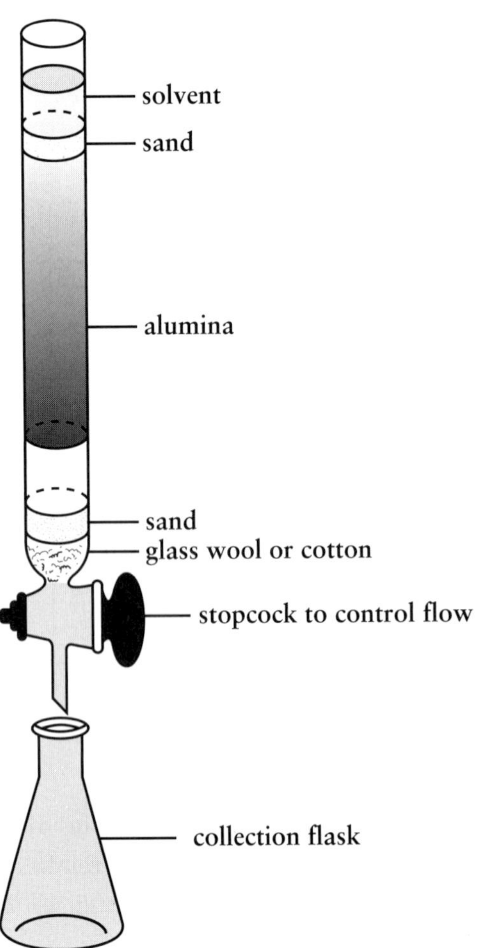

Figure 12.8: Column Chromatography

The solvent drips out the end of the column and fractions are collected in flasks or test tubes. These fractions contain bands corresponding to the different compounds, and when the solvents are evaporated, the compounds can be isolated.

Column chromatography is particularly useful in biochemistry, because it can be used to separate macromolecules such as proteins or nucleic acids. Several techniques exist:

1) In *ion exchange chromatography,* the beads in the column are coated with charged substances, and so they will attract or bind compounds with an opposing charge. For instance, a positively charged column will attract and hold negative substances while letting those with positive charge pass through.
2) In *size-exclusion chromatography,* the column contains beads with many tiny pores. Very small molecules can enter the beads, which slows down their progress, while large molecules move around or between the beads and thus travel through the column faster.
3) In *affinity chromotography,* columns can be "customized" to bind a substance of interest. For example, to purify substance A, a scientist might use a column of beads coated with something that binds A very tightly, such as a receptor for A, A's biological target, or even a specific antibody. A will bind to the column very tightly. It can later be eluted by washing with free receptor (or target or antibody), which will compete with the bead-bound receptor and ultimately free substance A from the column.

D. GAS CHROMATOGRAPHY

Gas chromatography (GC) is another method of qualitative separation. In gas chromatography, also called **vapor-phase chromatography** (VPC), the eluant that passes through the adsorbant is a gas, usually helium or nitrogen. The adsorbant is inside a 30-foot column that is coiled and kept inside an oven to control its temperature. The mixture to be separated is injected into the column and vaporized. The gaseous compounds travel through the column at different rates, because they adhere to the adsorbent to different degrees, and will separate by the time they reach the end of the column. At this point they are registered by a detector, which records the presence of a compound as a peak.

MCAT SYNOPSIS

To identify a compound or distinguish two different compounds, look at their "retention times"—that is, how *long* it took for each to travel through the column.

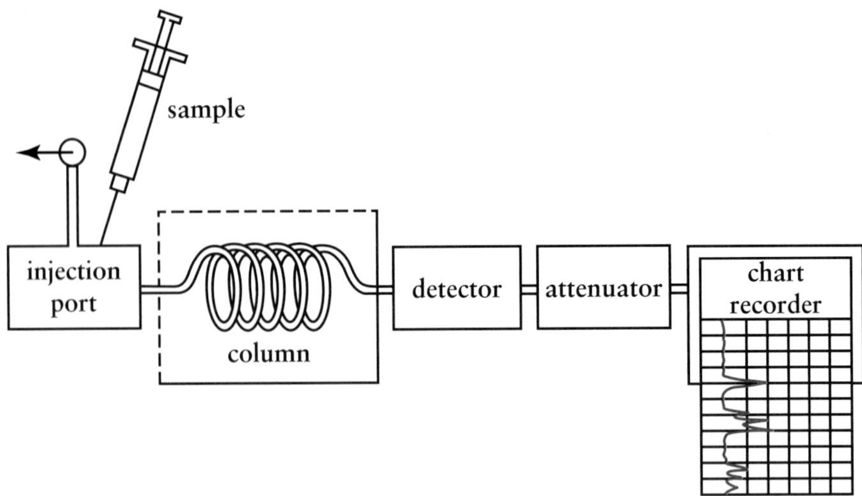

Figure 12.9: Gas Chromatography

KAPLAN EXCLUSIVE

In electrophoresis:

*An*ions are attracted to the *an*ode while

*cat*ions are attracted to the *cat*hode.

GC can be used on a larger scale for quantitative separation, and is then called preparative or prep GC. This is, however, very tedious and difficult to perform.

E. HPLC

HPLC stands for either high-pressure or high-performance liquid chromatography. The eluant is a liquid that travels through a column similar to a GC column, but under pressure. In the past, very high pressures were used; now they are much lower, hence the change from high *pressure* to high *performance*.

In HPLC, a sample is injected into the column and separation occurs as it flows through. The compounds pass through a detector and are collected as the solvent flows out the end of the apparatus. The eluant may vary, as in thin-layer or column chromatography.

MCAT SYNOPSIS

In most forms of electrophoresis, the size of a macromolecule is usually the most important factor—small molecules move faster, while large ones move more slowly and may in fact take hours to leave the well.

ELECTROPHORESIS

When a molecule is placed in an electric field, it will move towards either the cathode or the anode depending on its size and charge. **Electrophoresis** employs this phenomenon to separate macromolecules (usually biological macromolecules) such as proteins or DNA. The migration velocity, v, of a molecule is directly proportional to the electric field strength, E, and to the net charge on the molecule, z, and is inversely proportional to a frictional coefficient, f, which depends on the mass and shape of the migrating molecules.

$$v = \frac{Ez}{f}$$

Therefore, in a constant electric field, highly charged molecules will move most rapidly, as will small molecules.

A. AGAROSE GEL ELECTROPHORESIS

Agarose gel electrophoresis is used by molecular biologists to separate pieces of **nucleic acid** (usually **deoxyribonucleic acid,** DNA, but sometimes **ribonucleic acid,** RNA, as well; see chapter 15). Agarose is a plant gel, derived from seaweed, that is nontoxic and easy to manipulate (unlike SDS/polyacrylamide). Because every piece of nucleic acid is highly negatively charged, nucleic acids can be separated effectively on the basis of size even without the charge-masking provided by SDS. Agarose gels are stained with a compound called ethidium bromide, which binds to nucleic acids and is visualized by its fluorescence under ultraviolet light. Agarose gel electrophoresis can also be used preparatively, by cutting the desired band out of the gel and eluting out the nucleic acid.

KAPLAN EXCLUSIVE

SDS–PAGE and agarose gel electrophoresis separate molecules based on *size*.

B. SDS-POLYACRYLAMIDE GEL ELECTROPHORESIS

SDS-polyacrylamide gel electrophoresis separates proteins on the basis of mass, not charge. Polyacrylamide gel is the standard medium for electrophoresis. SDS is sodium dodecyl sulfate, which disrupts noncovalent interactions. It binds to proteins and creates large negative net charges, neutralizing the protein's original net charge. As proteins move through the gel, the only variable affecting their velocity is f, the frictional coefficient, which is dependent on mass. After separation, the gel is stained so that the protein bands can be visualized.

MCAT SYNOPSIS

When pH = pI, a protein stops moving.

C. ISOELECTRIC FOCUSING

A protein may be characterized by its **isoelectric point,** pI, which is the pH at which its net charge (the sum of the charges on all of its component amino acids; see chapter 15) is zero. If a mixture of proteins is placed in an electric field in a gel with a pH gradient, the proteins will move until they reach the point at which the pH is equal to their pI. At this location, the protein will be uncharged and will no longer move in the field. Molecules differing by as little as one charge can be separated in this manner, which is called **isoelectric focusing.**

BRIDGE

Because amino acids and proteins are organic molecules, the fundamental principles of acid-base chemistry apply to them as well.

- At a low pH, [H+] is relatively high. Thus, at a pH < pI, proteins will tend to be protonated and, as a result, positively charged.
- At a relatively high (basic) pH, [H+] is fairly low and proteins will tend to be depronated—thus carrying a negative charge.

SUMMARY OF PURIFICATION METHODS

Method	Use
Extraction	Separates dissolved substances based on differential solubility in aqueous versus organic solvents
Filtration	Separates solids from liquids
Recrystallization	Separates solids based on differential solubility; temperature is important here
Sublimation	Separates solids based on their ability to sublime
Centrifugation	Separates large things (like cells, organelles, and macromolecules) based on mass and density
Distillation	Separates liquids based on boiling point, which in turn depends on intermolecular forces
Chromatography	Uses a stationary phase and a mobile phase to separate compounds based on how tightly they adhere (generally due to polarity, but sometimes size as well)
Electrophoresis	Used to separate biological macromolecules (such as proteins or nucleic acids) based on size and sometimes charge

PRACTICE QUESTIONS

1. Isoelectric focusing, a process used in the isolation of proteins, is based on which of the following molecule characteristics?

   A. Mass
   B. pH
   C. Comparison to a set amino acid standard
   D. Molecule shape

2. Four compounds, I, II, III, and IV are separated by thin layer chromatography (TLC) Compound III is the most polar, II the least polar, and I and IV have intermediate polarity. The solvent system is 85:15 ethanol: methylene chloride. Which spot belongs to compound III?

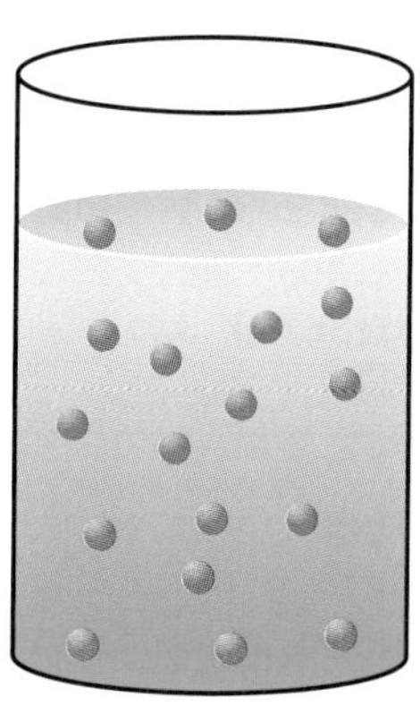

   A. Spot with the smallest R_f
   B. Spot with the second-largest R_f
   C. Spot with the largest R_f
   D. More information is needed

3. What is the function of sodium dodecyl sulfate (SDS) in SDS-PAGE?

   A. SDS stabilizes the gel matrix, improving resolution during electrophoresis.
   B. SDS solubilizes proteins to give them uniformly negative charges, so separation is based purely on size.
   C. SDS raises the pH of the gel, separating multiunit proteins into individual subunits.
   D. SDS solubilizes proteins to give them uniformly positive charges, so separation is based purely on pH.

4. Suppose an extraction with methylene chloride (d = 1.40 g/mL) is performed, with the desired compound initially in brine (d ≈ 1.00 g/mL). In a separatory funnel, which layer will be the organic layer?

   A. Bottom layer
   B. No layers are observed; methylene chloride and brine are 100 percent miscible
   C. Top layer
   D. More information is needed

KEY CONCEPTS

Isoelectric focusing

Determining isoelectric point

Electrolytic cell

TAKEAWAYS

In order to solve isoelectric focusing questions, determine the pI of the samples being separated. Then, determine the orientation of the pH gradient on the gel. The samples will migrate toward their pI, isoelectric point.

THINGS TO WATCH OUT FOR

Be careful in problems that ask you to separate proteins. Remember that the pI of a protein cannot be determined simply by averaging the pI of the individual amino acids. If the isoelectric point of a protein is not given, then another method must be used to separate the proteins.

ISOELECTRIC FOCUSING

Suppose you are trying to separate glycine, glutamic acid, and lysine given the following information:

	pKa COOH	pKa NH_3^+	pKa R group
Glycine:	2.34	9.63	—
Glutamic acid:	2.19	9.67	4.25
Lysine:	2.18	8.95	10.53

Indicate in which region of the gel each amino acid will stop migrating.

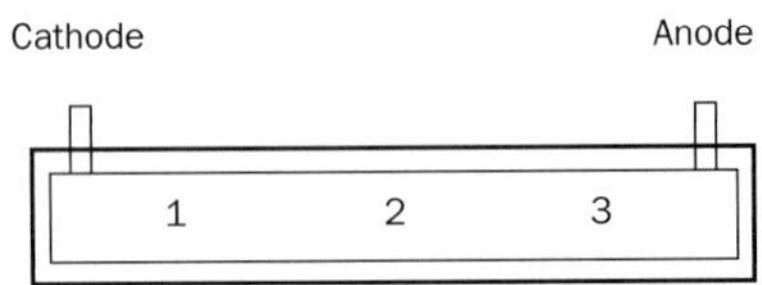

1) Identify if it is an isoelectric focusing problem.

Whenever a question gives you the pKa of the substance being purified, think ion exchange chromatography or isoelectric focusing. In the above question, we can be certain that isoelectric focusing is used because the separatory apparatus has a cathode and an anode, and because we're told that each amino acid will eventually stop migrating through the gel.

---

2) Determine the isoelectric points of the sample(s).

$$\text{pI of glycine} = \frac{(2.34 + 9.63)}{2} = 5.99$$

$$\text{pI of glutamic acid} = \frac{(2.19 + 4.25)}{2} = 3.22$$

$$\text{pI of lysine} = \frac{(8.95 + 10.53)}{2} = 9.74$$

To find the pI for an amino acid, identify the deprotonation reaction that converts the amino acid with +1 overall charge into the zwitterion with 0 overall charge; also, identify the deprotonation reaction that converts the zwitterion into a form with –1 overall charge. The pI for the amino acid is the average of the pK_a's for these two reactions.

For glycine, the sequence of deprotonation reactions is:

$$NH_3^+\text{–C(R)(H)–COOH} \xrightleftharpoons{pK_{a1} = 2.34} NH_3^+\text{–C(R)(H)–COO}^- \xrightleftharpoons{pK_{a2} = 9.63} NH_2\text{–C(R)(H)–COO}^-$$

For glycine, the pKa's for the reactions leading to and from the zwitterion are pK_{a1} and pK_{a2}. So the pI for glycine is the average of its pK_{a1} and pK_{a2}.

For glutamic acid, the sequence of deprotonation reactions is:

$$NH_3^+{-}C(RH)(H){-}COOH \underset{}{\overset{pK_{a1}=2.19}{\rightleftharpoons}} NH_3^+{-}C(RH)(H){-}COO^- \overset{pK_{a2}=4.25}{\rightleftharpoons} NH_3^+{-}C(R)(H){-}COO^- \overset{pK_{a3}=9.67}{\rightleftharpoons} NH_2{-}C(R^-)(H){-}COO^-$$

(The side chain is acidic, so we need to include a reaction for its deprotonation. The conjugate base of an acidic side chain is negatively charged.) For glutamic acid, the pKa's for the reactions leading to and from the zwitterion are pK_{a1} and pK_{a2}. So the pI for glutamic acid is the average of its pK_{a1} and pK_{a2}.

For lysine the sequence of deprotonation reactions is:

$$NH_3^+{-}C(RH^+)(H){-}COOH \overset{pK_{a1}=2.18}{\rightleftharpoons} NH_3^+{-}C(RH^+)(H){-}COO^- \overset{pK_{a2}=8.95}{\rightleftharpoons} NH_2{-}C(RH^+)(H){-}COO^- \overset{pK_{a3}=10.53}{\rightleftharpoons} NH_2{-}C(R)(H){-}COO^-$$

For lysine, the pKa's for the reactions leading to and from the zwitterion are pK_{a2} and pK_{a3}. So the pI for glycine is the average of its pK_{a2} and pK_{a3}.

---

3) Determine the relative pH gradient of the gel.
Electrophoresis is always run on electrolytic cells. Recall that electrolytic cells require an outside source of energy. The negative terminal is connected to the cathode and the positive end is connected to the anode. This means that the anode (acidic end of the gel) will attract negative anions and the cathode (basic end of the gel) will attract positive anions.

Therefore, we know that zone 1 is at a higher pH than zone 2, which is at a higher pH than zone 3.

---

4) Determine where the samples will migrate.
This means that proteins will migrate toward their pI. At the pI, the protein will not have a net charge (it will be in its zwitterion form), and thus will no longer be induced to migrate in the electric field.

In the above problem, glutamic acid will align itself in region 3, glycine will align itself in region 2, and lysine will align itself in region 1.

Remember: *Amino acids are amphoteric and thus will be positively charged at pH values below their pI and negatively charged above their pI.*

SIMILAR QUESTIONS

1) If a segment of polypeptide with a pI of 6.7 is subjected to electrophoresis at pH 5, will the segment move toward the cathode or the anode?
2) What is the isoelectric point of aspartic acid?
3) In what form is an amino acid said to be when it reaches its isoelectric point?

KEY CONCEPTS

Extraction (liquid–liquid separation)

Acid/base properties

Separation

EXTRACTION

A student wishes to separate methyl phenyl ketone, aniline, and phenol from a mixture. In order to perform the separation, the mixture is dissolved in a solution consisting of 500 ml of H_2O and 500 ml of dichloromethane. The solution is then washed with water three times and the aqueous layer (A) is extracted. The remaining solution is then washed with 20 percent Na_2CO_3 three times and the aqueous layer (B) is collected. The remaining organic layer is finally washed with 10 percent HCl and the aqueous layer (C) is once again collected, leaving behind the organic layer (D). What were the contents of samples A, B, C, and D?

TAKEAWAYS

In an extraction problem, each compound will either be dissolved in the aqueous layer or the organic layer. However, if a compound is acidic or basic, it is possible to transpose it to the aqueous layer by using basic or acidic washes, respectively.

1) Determine the difference between the molecules being separated.

Acetophenone, aniline, and phenol are all organic compounds. However, aniline is a weak base whereas phenol is a weak acid. Methyl phenyl ketone is the most hydrophobic of the three compounds because it doesn't possess any functional groups capable of making hydrogen bonds.

---

2) Determine into what phase each of the compounds will dissolve after the first set of washings.

All three compounds are uncharged organic compounds and as such will dissolve in the organic layer, in dichloromethane. Thus, the first set of washings will not aid in separating any of the three compounds.

---

3) Determine into what phase each of the compounds will dissolve after the second set of washings.

When the sample is washed with Na_2CO_3, phenol will be deprotonated to yield sodium phenoxide (the conjugate base of phenol). Because this molecule is charged, it will move into the aqueous layer. After the washing, the deprotonated phenol will move to the aqueous phase, whereas methyl phenyl ketone and aniline will remain in the organic layer.

Remember: *Washing a mixture with a base is an effective way to move acidic compounds from the organic layer into the aqueous layer.*

THINGS TO WATCH OUT FOR

Don't assume that the organic phase will be on top—this depends on the densities of the two phases. For example, dichloromethane (1.3 g mL^{-1}) is denser than water (1.0 g mL^{-1}); dichloromethane will sink to the bottom of the separatory funnel, with the water floating on top.

---

4) Determine into what phase each of the compounds will dissolve after the third set of washings.

At this point, the only remaining compounds in the organic layer are acetophenone and aniline.

When the sample is washed with HCl (a strong acid), aniline will be protonated to an anilinium ion. This positively charged molecule will move into the aqueous layer, whereas acetophenone will remain in the organic layer.

Remember: *Washing a mixture with an acid is an effective way to move basic compounds from the organic layer to the aqueous layer.*

SIMILAR QUESTIONS:

1) Design an extraction procedure to separate a mixture of phenol and benzoic acid dissolved in ether.
2) In order to extract *p*-nitrophenol from phenol in an ether solution, a student washes the organic layer with 10 ml of a 5 percent aqueous solution of NaOH. After the washing, what will be left in the organic layer?

KEY CONCEPTS

Purification

Chromatography

Ion exchange

Separation

Column chromatography

TAKEAWAYS

All forms of chromatography have two phases, a stationary phase and a mobile phase. Separations of compounds take advantage of the different affinities that compounds have for the two different phases.

THINGS TO WATCH OUT FOR

Be cautious not to assume that the desired product will attach to the stationary phase. You may be presented with a situation in which purification will be better accomplished if the desired product has a higher affinity for the mobile phase.

CHROMATOGRAPHY

In an effort to purify ATCase, a crude cell extract in a potassium phosphate buffer is run on a Q-Sepharose column (mono Q is an anion exchanger: $-CH_2-N(CH_3)_3^+$). What characteristic of ATCase allows it to be separated using an anion exchanger? Are any additives necessary to achieve a successful purification?

1) Determine the difference between the molecules being separated.

In the question stem, we are told that mono Q (the stationary phase in the column) is an anion exchanger. This means that it attracts anions and thus must have a positive charged group. Because we are trying to purify ATCase, it must bind to mono Q because if it doesn't, it will simply pass through the column along with the other positively charged proteins and thus not be purified. So we can conclude that ATCase is a negatively charged protein (an anionic protein), enabling it to be purified using an anion exchanger.

If an antibody or substrate for ATCase were available, affinity chromatography could have been used. Column chromatography could also be used to separate substances based on size.

---

2) Determine which compound has a higher affinity for the stationary phase.

When the crude cell extract is run through the column, ATCase and other anionic proteins will stick to the stationary phase, whereas the rest of the extract will pass through the column relatively easily.

---

3) Determine which compound has a higher affinity for the eluent.

Now that the anionic proteins are bound to the Q-sepharose gel, they must be eluted based on their affinities (in this case the strength of their negative charge) for the stationary phase. For this purpose, NaCl is added in an increasing concentration gradient. The least negatively charged proteins will emerge from the column before the proteins with the greatest negative charge.

SIMILAR QUESTIONS

1) Sample *A* (R_f value of 0.75) and sample *B* (R_f value of 0.50) were run on silica gel. What is the distance traveled by sample *A* if sample *B* traveled 2.0 cm?
2) If the pH of the buffer is increased from 7 to 9, how will the purification be affected?
3) If you want to separate two anionic proteins (protein *A* and protein *B*, where protein *A* is a tetramer of protein *B*) with the same anionic character, which type of chromatography will be most useful? Assume that the tetramer once formed in the cell does not dissociate and that the monomer cannot form the tetramer *in vitro*.

CHAPTER 13

SPECTROSCOPY

Once an organic compound is isolated, it must be characterized and identified. If it is a known compound, identification can often be made from elemental analysis or determination of the melting point. With new or more complex compounds, other methods must be used. **Spectroscopy** is the process of measuring the energy differences between the possible states of a molecular system by determining the frequencies of electromagnetic radiation (light) absorbed by the molecules. The possible states are quantized energy levels associated with different types of molecular motion, including molecular rotation, vibration of bonds, and electron movement. Different types of spectroscopy measure these different types of molecular motion, identifying specific functional groups and how they are connected.

Teacher Tip

You will likely be asked about IR and/or ^{1}H-NMR on the exam. Don't spend too much time on spectroscopy but don't ignore it all together.

Spectroscopy is useful because only a very small quantity of sample is needed. In addition, the sample may be reused after an IR, NMR, or UV spectrum is obtained.

INFRARED

A. BASIC THEORY

Infrared (IR) spectroscopy measures molecular vibrations, which include bond **stretching, bending,** and **rotation.** The useful absorptions of infrared light occur in the 3,000–30,000 nm region, which corresponds to 3,500–300 cm^{-1} (called **wave numbers**). When light of these wavelengths/wave numbers is absorbed, the molecules enter higher (excited) vibrational states.

Bond stretching (which can be of two types: symmetric or asymmetric) involves the largest change in energy and is observed in the region 1,500–4,000 cm^{-1}. Bending vibrations are observed in the region 400–1,500 cm^{-1}. Four different types of vibration that can occur are shown in Figure 13.1.

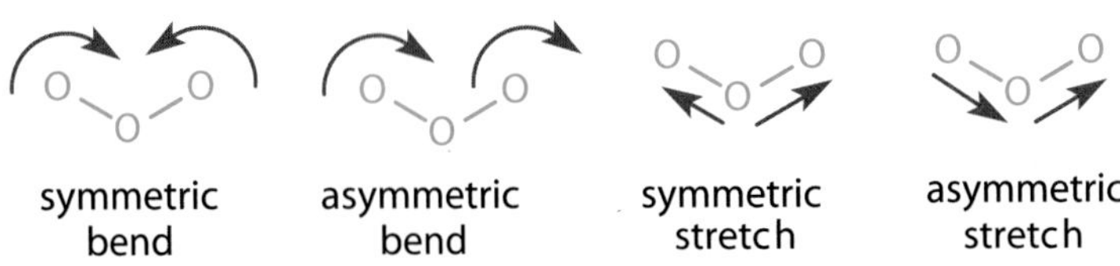

Figure 13.1

In addition to bending and stretching vibrations, more complex vibrations may occur. These can be combinations of bending, stretching, and rotation frequencies or complex frequency patterns caused by the motion of the whole molecule. Absorptions of these types are seen in the region 1,500–400 cm^{-1}. This region of the spectrum is known as the **fingerprint region** and is characteristic of a molecule; it is, therefore, frequently used to identify a substance.

MCAT SYNOPSIS

Symmetric stretches do not show up in IR spectra because they involve no net change in dipole movement.

In order for an absorption to be recorded, the motion must result in a change in a bond dipole moment. Molecules comprised of atoms with the same electronegativity, as well as symmetrical molecules, do not experience a changing dipole moment and therefore do not exhibit absorption. For example, O_2 and Br_2 do not absorb, but HCl and CO do.

A typical spectrum is obtained by passing infrared light (of frequencies from approximately 4,000–400 cm^{-1}) through a sample, and recording the absorption pattern. Percent transmittance is plotted versus frequency, where percent transmittance = absorption^{-1} ($\%T = A^{-1}$); absorptions appear as valleys on the spectrum.

MCAT SYNOPSIS

Wave numbers (cm^{-1}) are not the same as frequency.

$V = \frac{C}{\lambda}$, while wave number $= \frac{1}{\lambda}$

B. CHARACTERISTIC ABSORPTIONS

Particular functional groups absorb at localized frequencies. For example, alcohols absorb around 3,300 cm^{-1}, carbonyl groups around 1,700 cm^{-1}, and ethers around 1,100 cm^{-1}. Table 13.1 lists the specific absorptions of key functional groups and their corresponding vibrations.

Table 13.1. Common Infrared Absorption Peaks

Functional Group	Frequency (cm^{-1})	Vibration
Alkanes	2,800–3,000	C−H
	1,200	C−C
Alkenes	3,080–3,140	=C−H
	1,645	C=C
Alkynes	2,200	C≡C
	3,300	≡C−H
Aromatic	2,900–3,100	C−H
	1,475–1,625	C−C
Alcohols	3,100–3,500	O−H (broad)
Ethers	1,050–1,150	C−O
Aldehydes	2,700–2,900	(O)C−H
	1,725–1,750	C=O
Ketones	1,700–1,750	C=O
Acids	1,700–1,750	C−O
	2,900–3,300	O−H (broad)
Amines	3,100–3,500	N−H (sharp)

TEACHER TIP

IR spectroscopy is best used for identification of functional groups. The most important peaks to know are those for the –OH (BROAD peak above 2900 cm^{-1}), and the carbonyl peak (SHARP peak near 1700 cm^{-1}). If you know nothing else here, *know these!*

C. APPLICATION

A great deal of information can be obtained from an IR spectrum. Most of the useful functional group information is found between 1,400 and 4,000 cm^{-1}.

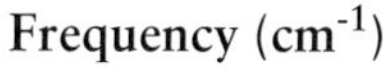

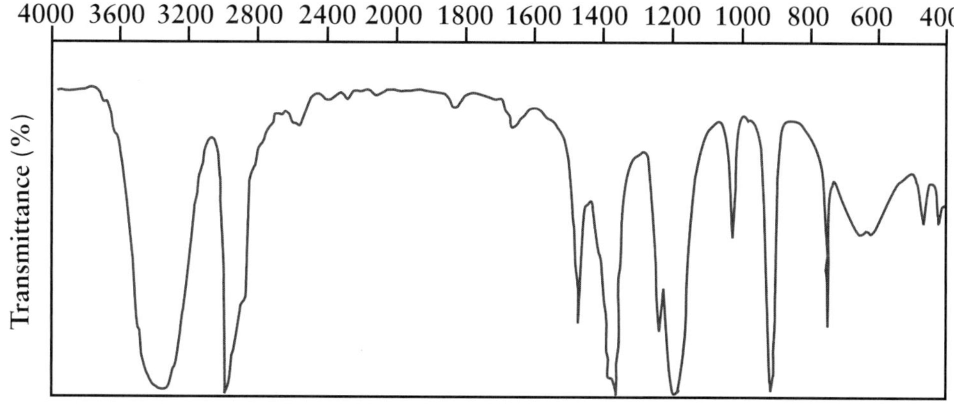

Figure 13.2

Clinical Correlate

Magnetic Resonance Imaging (MRI) is a noninvasive medical diagnostic tool which utilizes proton NMR. Multiple cross-sectional scans of the patient's body are taken, and the various chemical shifts of absorbing protons are translated into specific colors. A picture is thus produced that shows the relative density of specific types of protons; for instance, a dark blue area on the MRI output screen indicates a high concentration of the types of protons giving rise to the range of resonances which correlate to dark blue. Comparison to normal MRI then allows the diagnostician to detect abnormalities in the scanned region.

Figure 13.2 shows the IR spectrum of an aliphatic alcohol. The large peak at 3,300 cm^{-1} is due to the presence of the hydroxyl group, while the peak at 3,000 cm^{-1} can be attributed to the alkane portion of the molecule.

NUCLEAR MAGNETIC RESONANCE

A. BASIC THEORY

Nuclear magnetic resonance (NMR) spectroscopy is one of the most widely used spectroscopic tools in organic chemistry. NMR is based on the fact that certain nuclei have magnetic moments which are normally oriented at random. When such nuclei are placed in a magnetic field, their magnetic moments tend to align either with or against the direction of this applied field. Nuclei whose magnetic moments are aligned with the field are said to be in the α *state* (lower energy), while those whose moments are aligned against the field are said to be in the β *state* (higher energy). If the nuclei are then irradiated with electromagnetic radiation, some will be excited into the β state.The absorption corresponding to this excitation occurs at different frequencies depending on an atom's environment. The nuclear magnetic moments are affected by other nearby atoms that also possess magnetic moments. Hence, a compound may contain many nuclei that resonate at different frequencies, producing a very complex spectrum.

A typical NMR spectrum is a plot of frequency versus absorption of energy during resonance. Frequency *decreases* toward the right. Alternatively, varying magnetic field may be plotted on the x axis, *increasing* toward the right. Because different NMR spectrometers operate at different magnetic field strengths, a standardized method of plotting the NMR spectrum has been adopted. An arbitrary variable, called **chemical shift** (represented by the symbol δ), with units of **parts per million (ppm)** of spectrometer frequency, is plotted on the x axis.

MCAT Synopsis

TMS provides a reference peak. The signal for its H atoms is assigned a $\delta = 0$.

NMR is most commonly used to study ^{1}H nuclei (protons) and ^{13}C nuclei, although any atom possessing a nuclear spin (any nucleus with an odd atomic number or odd mass number) can be studied, such as ^{19}F, ^{17}O, ^{14}N, ^{15}N, or ^{31}P.

B. ^{1}H NMR

Most ^{1}H nuclei come into resonance between 0 and 10 δ downfield from TMS. Each distinct set of nuclei gives rise to a separate peak. The compound dichloromethyl methyl ether has two distinct sets of ^{1}H nuclei. The single proton attached to the dichloromethyl group is in a different

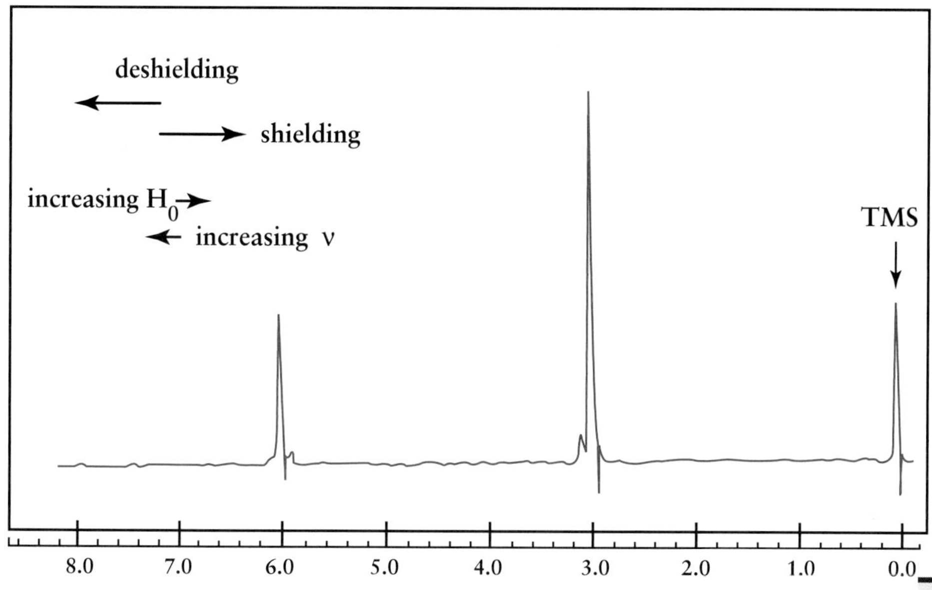

Figure 13.3

magnetic environment than are the three protons on the methyl group, and the two classes resonate at different frequencies. The three protons on the methyl group are magnetically equivalent, due to rotation about the oxygen-carbon single bond, and resonate at the same frequency. Thus, two separate peaks are expected, as shown in Figure 13.3.

The left-hand peak corresponds to the single dichloromethyl proton and the middle peak to the three methyl protons (the one on the far right is the TMS reference peak). Notice that if the areas under the peaks are integrated, the ratio between them is 3:1, corresponding to the number of protons producing each peak.

The single proton comes into resonance downfield from the methyl protons. This phenomenon is due to the electron-withdrawing effect of the chlorine atoms. The electron cloud that surrounds the ^1H nucleus ordinarily screens the nucleus somewhat from the applied magnetic field. The chlorine atoms pull away the electron cloud and **deshield** the nucleus. Thus, the nucleus resonates in a lower field than it would otherwise. By the same rationale, electron-donating atoms, such as the silicon atoms in TMS, **shield** the ^1H nuclei, causing them to come into resonance at a higher field.

If two magnetically different protons are within three bonds of each other, a phenomenon known as **coupling**, or **splitting** occurs. Consider two protons, H_a and H_b, on the molecule 1,1-dibromo-2,2-dichloroethane (Figure 13.4).

MCAT SYNOPSIS

- Each peak represents a single proton or a group of equivalent protons. (The number of peaks represents the number of groups of nonequivalent protons.)
- The relative area of each peak reflects the ratio of the protons producing each peak.
- The position of the peak (upfield or downfield) due to shielding or deshielding effects reflects the chemical environment of the protons.

KAPLAN EXCLUSIVE

When dealing with ^1H-NMR on the MCAT, think of a proton being surrounded by a shield of electrons. Therefore, as we add electronegative atoms or have double bonds, which pull electrons away from the proton, we ***D***eshield and move ***D***ownfield.

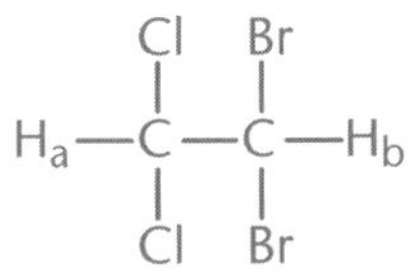

$$\begin{array}{ccccccc} & & Cl & & Br & & \\ & & | & & | & & \\ H_a & - & C & - & C & - & H_b \\ & & | & & | & & \\ & & Cl & & Br & & \end{array}$$

Figure 13.4

MCAT SYNOPSIS

The splitting of the peak represents the number of adjacent hydrogens. A peak will be split into *n* + 1 peaks where n is the number of adjacent hydrogens.

At any given time, H_a can experience two different magnetic environments, because H_b can be in either the α or the β state. These different states of H_b influence nucleus H_a (if the two H atoms are within three bonds of each other), causing slight upfield and downfield shifts. Because there is approximately a 50 percent chance that H_b will be in either state, this results in a **doublet,** two peaks of equal intensity equally spaced around the true chemical shift of H_a. H_b experiences the two different states of H_a and is likewise coupled. The magnitude of the splitting, usually denoted in Hz, is called the **coupling constant, J.**

In 1,1-dibromo-2-chloroethane (Figure 13.5), the H_a nucleus is affected by two nearby H_b nuclei, and can experience four different states: $\alpha\alpha$, $\alpha\beta$, $\beta\alpha$, or $\beta\beta$.

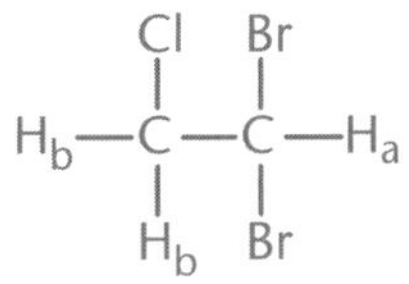

$$\begin{array}{ccccccc} & & Cl & & Br & & \\ & & | & & | & & \\ H_b & - & C & - & C & - & H_a \\ & & | & & | & & \\ & & H_b & & Br & & \end{array}$$

Figure 13.5

The $\alpha\beta$ and $\beta\alpha$ states have the same net effect on the H_a nucleus, and the resonances occur at the same frequency. The $\alpha\alpha$ and $\beta\beta$ states resonate at frequencies different from each other and from the $\alpha\beta$/$\beta\alpha$ frequency. The result is three peaks that are centered around the true chemical shift, with an area ratio of 1:2:1. In general, *n* hydrogen atoms couple to give n + 1 peaks, whose area ratios are given by Pascal's triangle, shown in Table 13.2.

MCAT SYNOPSIS

Proton NMR is good for:

1. Determining the relative number of protons and their relative chemical environments
2. Showing how many adjacent protons there are by splitting patterns
3. Showing certain functional groups

Table 13.2. Pascal's Triangle

Number of Adjacent Hydrogens	Total Number of Peaks	Area Ratios
0	1	1
1	2	1:1
2	3	1:2:1
3	4	1:3:3:1
4	5	1:4:6:4:1
5	6	1:5:10:10:5:1
6	7	1:6:15:20:15:6:1
7	8	1:7:21:35:35:21:7:1

The following table indicates the chemical shift ranges of several different types of protons:

Table 13.3. Chemical Shifts

Type of Proton	Approximate Chemical Shift δ (ppm) Downfield from TMS
RCH_3	0.9
RCH_2	1.25
R_3CH	1.5
–CH=CH	4.6–6.0
–C≡CH	2.0–3.0
Ar–H	6.0–8.5
–CHX	2.0–4.5
–CHOH/–CHOR	3.4–4.0
RCHO	9.0–10.0
RCHCO–	2.0–2.5
–CHCOOH/–CHCOOR	2.0–2.6
–CHOH–CH_2OH	1.0–5.5
ArOH	4.0–12.0
–COOH	10.5–12.0
–NH_2	1.0–5.0

TEACHER TIP

If you know nothing else about ^{1}H-NMR for the MCAT, know that the peaks for alkyl groups are upfield (1–3 ppm), peaks for alkenes are further downfield (4–7 ppm) and aldehydes are the furthest downfield (9–10 ppm). Also, just counting the number of the peaks and unique hydrogens may get you the correct answer.

C. ^{13}C NMR

^{13}C NMR *is* very similar to ^{1}H-NMR. Most ^{13}C NMR signals, however, occur 0–200 δ downfield from the carbon peak of TMS. Another significant difference is that only 1.1 percent of carbon atoms are ^{13}C atoms. This has two effects: first, a much larger sample is needed to run a ^{13}C spectrum (about 50 mg compared with 1 mg for ^{1}H-NMR), and second, coupling between carbon atoms is generally not observed.

TEACHER TIP

Don't spend too much time on ^{13}C NMR! Just know that the same principle applies to electrons in ^{1}H-NMR: the more deshielded, the further downfield.

Coupling *is* observed, however, between carbon atoms and the protons directly attached to them. This one-bond coupling is analogous to the three-bond coupling in ^{1}H-NMR. For example, if a carbon atom is attached to two protons, it can experience four different states of those protons (αα, αβ, βα, and ββ), and the carbon signal is split into a triplet with the area ratio 1:2:1.

An additional feature of ^{13}C NMR is the ability to record a spectrum *without* the coupling of adjacent protons. This is called **spin decoupling,** and produces a spectrum of **singlets,** each corresponding to a separate,

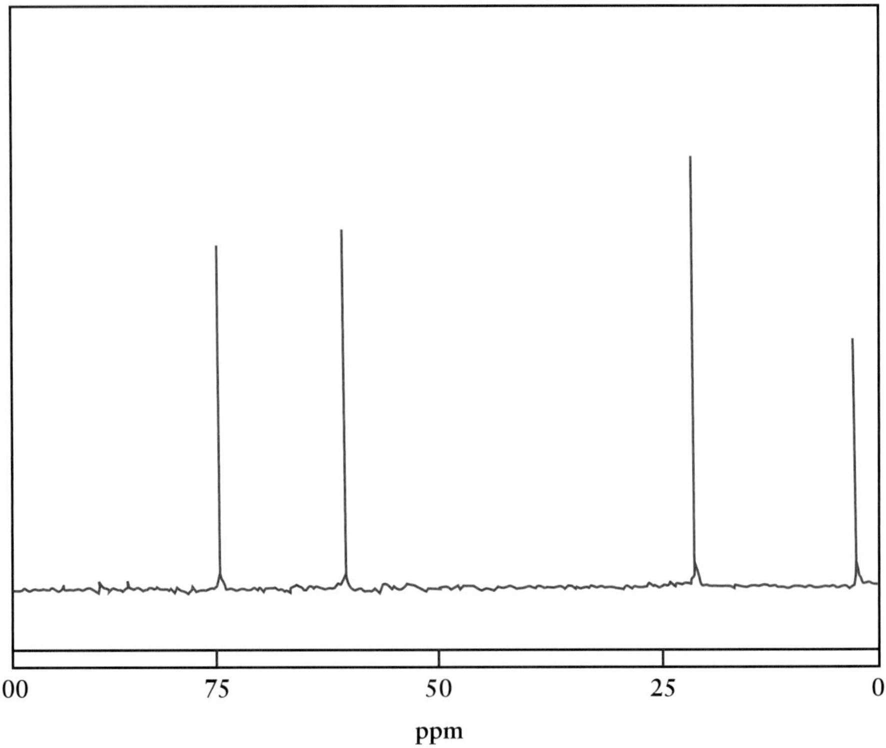

Figure 13.6. Spin-Decoupled Spectrum of 1,1,2-Trichloropropane

TEACHER TIP

Don't confuse ^{13}C NMR and ^{1}H-NMR on the MCAT! Just pay attention to the x-axis!

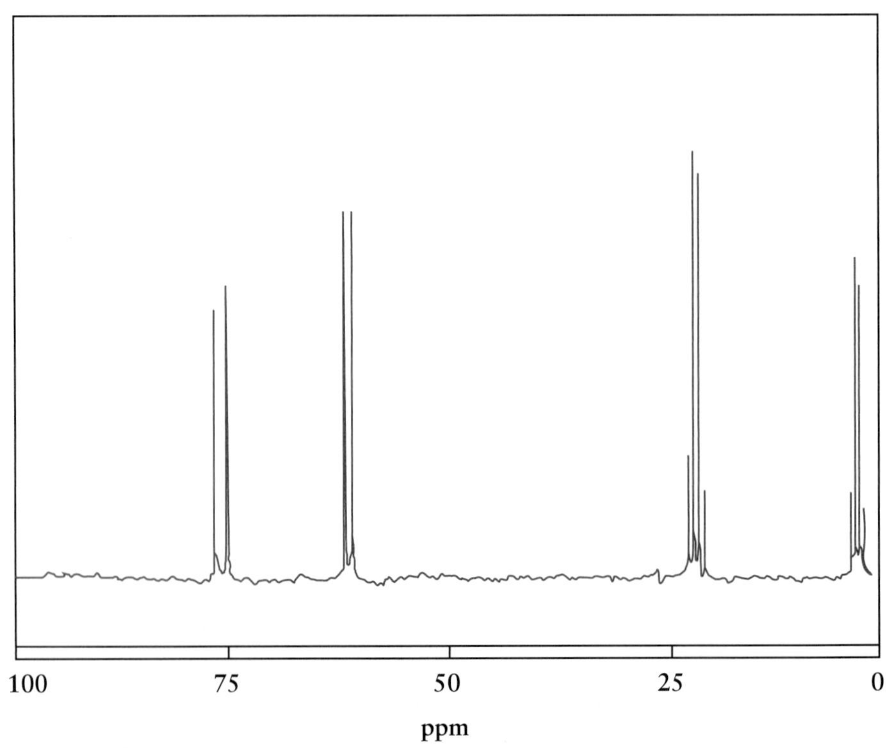

Figure 13.7. Spin-Coupled Spectrum of 1,1,2-Trichloropropane

magnetically equivalent, carbon atoms. For example, compare the following spectra of 1,1,2-trichloropropane. One (Figure 13.6) is a typical **spin-decoupled spectrum,** and the other (Figure 13.7) is spin-coupled.

In general, NMR spectroscopy provides information about the carbon skeleton of a compound, along with some suggestion of its functional groups. Specifically, NMR can provide the following types of information:

1. The number of nonequivalent nuclei, determined from the number of peaks
2. The magnetic environment of a nucleus, determined by the chemical shift
3. The relative numbers of nuclei, determined by integrating the peak areas
4. The number of neighboring nuclei, determined by the splitting pattern observed (except for ^{13}C in the spin-decoupled mode)

ULTRAVIOLET SPECTROSCOPY

A. BASIC THEORY

Ultraviolet spectra are obtained by passing ultraviolet light through a chemical sample (usually dissolved in an inert, nonabsorbing solvent) and plotting absorbance versus wavelength. The wavelength of maximum absorbance provides information on the extent of the conjugated system as well as other structural and compositional information.

TEACHER TIP

UV spectroscopy is most useful for studying compounds containing double bonds, and/or hetero atoms with lone pairs. For the MCAT, that is all you need to know!

MASS SPECTROMETRY

A. BASIC THEORY

Mass spectrometry differs from the methods thus far discussed in that it is not true spectroscopy, *i.e.,* no absorption of electromagnetic radiation is involved, and, in that it is a destructive technique, mass spectrometry, does not allow for reuse of the sample once the analysis is complete. Most commonly used mass spectrometers use a high-speed beam of electrons to ionize the sample to be analyzed, a particle accelerator to put the charged particles in flight, a magnetic field to deflect the accelerated cationic fragments, and a detector that records the number of particles of each mass exiting the deflector area. The initially formed ion is the molecular cation-radical (M^+) resulting from a single electron being removed from a molecule of the sample. This unstable species usually decomposes rapidly into a cationic fragment and a radical fragment. Because there are many molecules in the sample and (usually) more than one way for the initially formed cation-radical to decompose into fragments, a typical mass spectrum is composed of many lines, each corresponding to a specific mass/charge ratio (m/e). The spectrum itself plots mass/charge on the horizontal axis and relative abundance of the various cationic fragments on the vertical axis (see Fig. 13.8).

TEACHER TIP

Mass spectrometry is low-yield for the MCAT, but the M^+ (parent ion peak), which indicates molecular weight, can be useful.

B. CHARACTERISTICS

The tallest peak, belonging to the most common ion, is called the **base peak,** and is assigned the relative abundance value of 100 percent. The peak with the highest m/e ratio (see Figure 13.8) is generally the **molecular ion peak (parent ion peak), M^+,** from which the molecular weight, M, can be obtained. The charge value is usually 1; hence the m/e ratio can usually be read as the mass of the fragment.

C. APPLICATION

Fragmentation patterns often provide information that helps identify or distinguish certain compounds. In particular, the fragmentation pattern provides clues to the compound's structure. For example, while IR spectroscopy would be of little use in distinguishing between propionaldehyde and butyraldehyde, a mass spectrum would allow unambiguous identification.

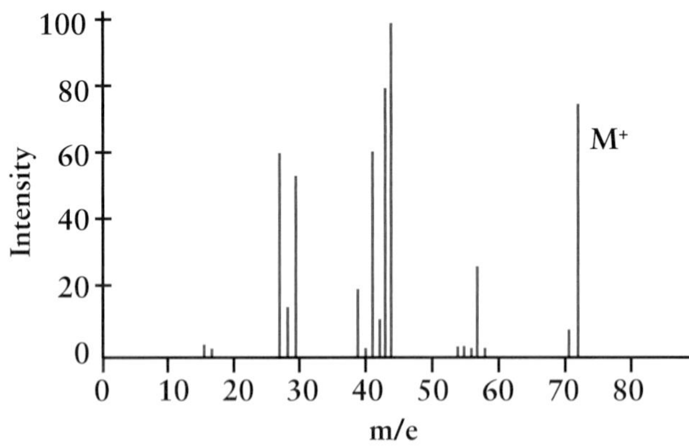

Figure 13.8

Figure 13.8 shows the mass spectrum of butyraldehyde. The peak at m/e = 72 corresponds to the molecular cation-radical, M^+, while the base peak at m/e = 44 corresponds to the cationic fragment resulting from the loss of a C_2H_4 neutral fragment (M – 28 = 44). Other peaks of note include those at 57 (M – 15, loss of CH_3 radical), 43 (M – 29, loss of C_2H_5 radical), and at 29 (M – 43, loss of C_3H_7 radical). The small peak at m/e = 15 can be attributed to the unstabled (and therefore not abundant) methyl cation.

PRACTICE QUESTIONS

1. Alkyl benzenes often provide mass spectra with a large peak at m/z 91. What aromatic fragment is responsible for the observed peak?

A.

B.

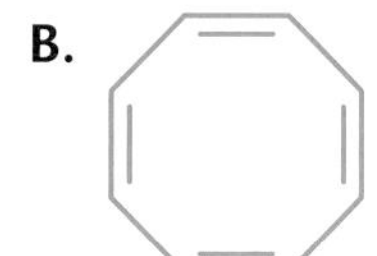

C.

D.

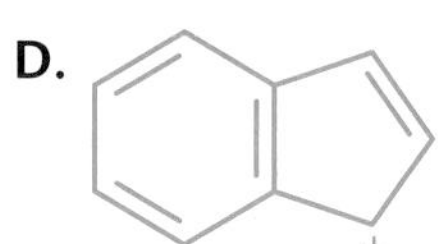

2. Using ^{1}H-NMR, and focusing on the 0–4.5 ppm region only, how is the spectrum for ethanol distinguished from the spectrum for isopropanol?

A. They cannot be distinguished from ^{1}H NMR alone.

B. A triplet and quartet are observed for ethanol, while a doublet and septet are observed for isopropanol.

C. A triplet and quartet are observed for isopropanol, while a doublet and septet are observed for ethanol.

D. The alcohol hydrogen in ethanol will appear within that region, while the alcohol hydrogen in isopropanol will not appear in that region.

3. For the compound below, how many distinct signals are observed in the ^{13}C NMR spectrum?

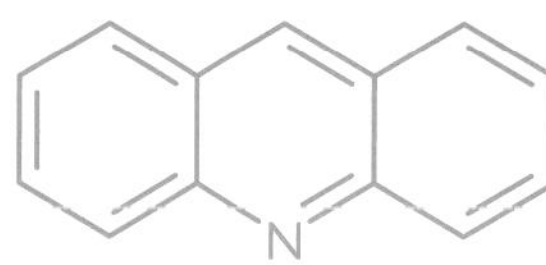

A. 13

B. 6

C. 4

D. 9

4. In an IR spectrum, how does extended conjugation of double bonds affect the absorbance band of carbonyl (C=O) stretches compared to normal absorption at 1720 cm^{-1}?

A. The absorbance band will occur at a lower wave number.

B. The absorbance band will occur at a higher wave number.

C. The absorbance band will occur at the same wave number.

D. The absorbance band will disappear.

KEY CONCEPTS

Spectroscopy

Electrophilic aromatic substitution

^{1}H-NMR

NMR SPECTROSCOPY

A grad student performed an electrophilic chlorination of phenol, as shown below.

OH — $FeCl_3$, Cl_2 → OH, Cl

The grad student obtained three products, the *ortho*, *meta*, and *para* isomers, and separated all three. Unfortunately, he forgot to label which compound was which. ^{1}H-NMRs were taken of each product and are shown below. Match each spectrum to its corresponding product.

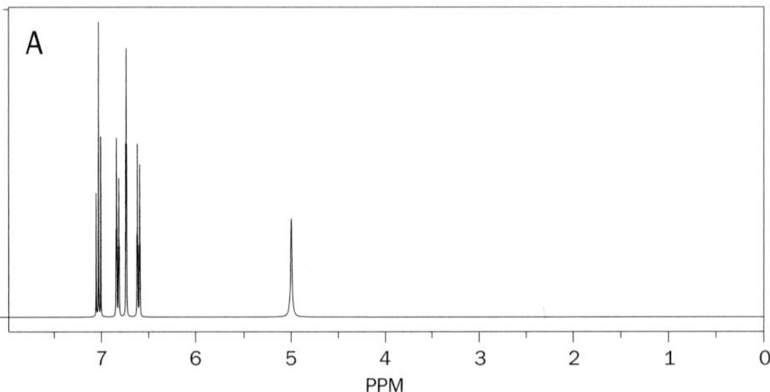

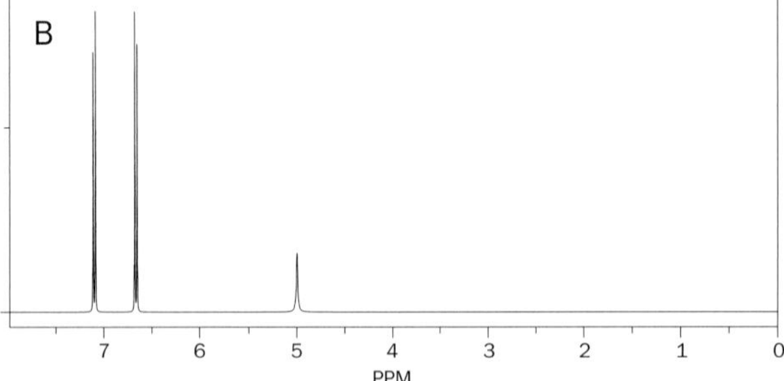

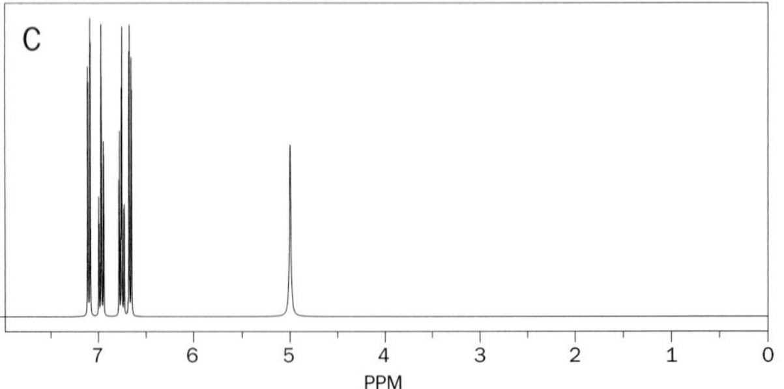

1) Examine each spectrum for the number of signals.
In this case, spectrum **B** appears to be the most symmetric molecule because it has the least number of signals (3). Spectra **A** and **C** are the least symmetric, with five signals each.

The number of signals tells you a lot about the symmetry of a molecule. The fewer signals there are, the higher symmetry the molecule possesses.

---

2) Examine the structure of each product and try to start matching spectra based on your symmetry observations.
The three possible products are:

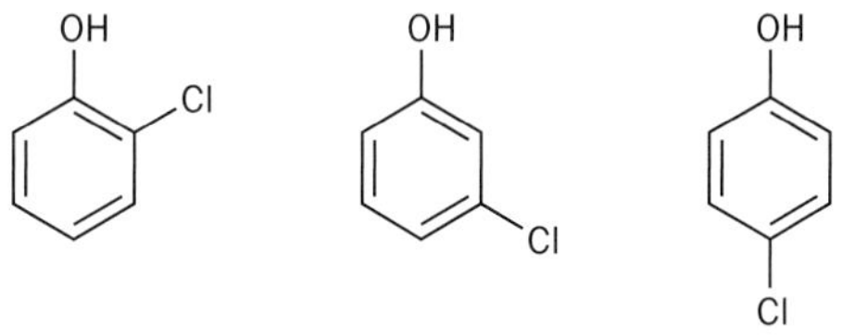

OH, Cl (ortho) — OH, Cl (meta) — OH, Cl (para)

By inspection, the *para* isomer appears to be the most symmetric. Imagine jamming a pole down the middle of the ring, through the alcohol and chlorine. If you were to rotate the molecule 180 degrees around the pole, you would get the same molecule back. The proton adjacent to the alochol will then account for one aromatic signal, and the protons adjacent to the chlorine another. Therefore, spectrum **B** must be that of the *para* isomer.

---

3) Take a closer look at each of the products to sort out the remaining spectra, if necessary.
Now we have to distinguish between the *ortho* and *meta* isomers. The main difference between them is that the *meta* isomer has one proton between the alcohol and the chlorine, whereas the *ortho* has none. In the *meta* isomer, this proton will give rise to a singlet in the NMR because there are no protons on the adjacent carbons. In the *ortho* isomer, each proton has at least one proton on the adjacent carbon, meaning no singlets.

Thus, spectrum **A** must correspond to the *meta* isomer because it is the only spectrum that has a singlet (near 6.75 ppm). By process of elimination, spectrum **C** must be the *ortho* isomer.

TAKEAWAYS

The most effective strategy in these types of problems is to try and eliminate one spectrum at a time, by looking at the most general differences between molecules and proceeding to the more specific.

THINGS TO WATCH OUT FOR

Be sure to check your assignments by ensuring that each spectrum has the correct number of proton signals.

SIMILAR QUESTIONS

1) Predict the splitting patterns resulting from all of the protons on the *ortho* and *meta* isomers.
2) Other than the chemical shift, how do you know that the signal around 5 ppm must be that of the alcohol proton? (*Hint:* Look at the *shape* of the signal.)
3) If the three isomers were of iodophenol instead of chlorophenol, how would the ^{1}H-NMR spectra be different from those displayed above?

KEY CONCEPTS

Spectroscopy

IR spectroscopy

^{1}H-NMR spectroscopy

COMBINED SPECTROSCOPY: IR AND NMR

An unknown compound was discovered in an old, unused laboratory. Its molecular formula was determined to be $C_6H_9NO_2$ by high resolution mass spectrometry. The following IR stretches were recorded: 3,300 (share), 2,890 (m), 2,220, 1,740 (s), 1,220, 984, 700, 650 cm^{-1}.

The ^{1}H-NMR spectrum of the compound is as follows:

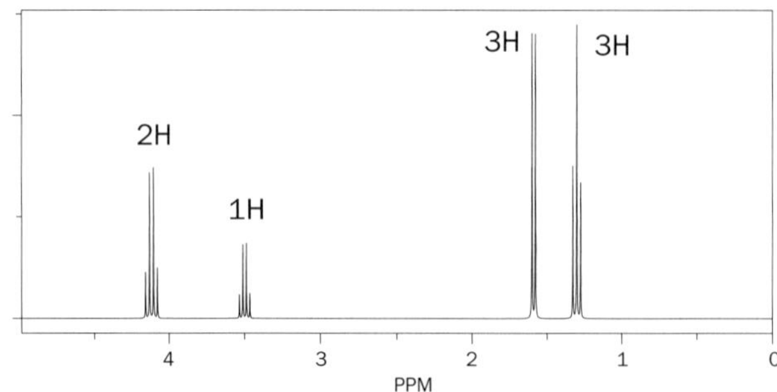

Given this information, determine the structure of the unknown compound.

TAKEAWAYS

With these combined structure problems, make sure to utilize all of the data at your disposal. The process is very much like taking the pieces of a jigsaw puzzle and putting them together.

1) Compute the number of sites of unsaturation.

$$U = \frac{(2n + 2 - m)}{2}$$

n = number of carbons; m = number of protons and/or halogens minus # of nitrogens. Ignore oxygen and sulfur.

$$\text{Thus: } U = \frac{(2 \times 6 + 2 - 8)}{2} = \frac{6}{2} = 3$$

This means that the molecule has either three double bonds, one double bond and one triple bond, or some combination of rings and double or triple bonds.

Remember: *If a molecule has four or more sites of unsaturation, you should immediately suspect that an aromatic ring is present.*

THINGS TO WATCH OUT FOR

Again, be sure not to overinterpret the IR data. There are only five or six functional groups whose presence can be conclusively indicated by the IR.

2) Look at the IR stretches to determine what functional groups are present. Here, the stretch at 1,740 cm^{-1} indicates the presence of a carbonyl, and the stretch at 2,220 cm^{-1} indicates the presence of a triple bond (either an alkyne or a nitrile).

The one thing you do *not* want to do with the IR data is to try and interpret every single stretch. The IR is not nearly as informative as the NMR. Just look for the few stretches that are indicative of functional groups.

---

3) Do a little detective work to narrow down the structural possibilities.
First let's think about the carbonyl. It can't be an aldehyde because there are no aldehyde signals in the NMR, and it can't be a carboxylic acid because there is no alcohol stretch in the IR. Because the stretch is closer to 1,740 than to 1,700, it is probably an ester rather than a ketone (you might also suspect this from the 1,220 stretch in the IR, which indicates a C–O stretch).

As for the triple-bond stretch, it is most likely a nitrile because there are no amine stretches in the IR.

---

4) Look more specifically at the information in the NMR to put the rest of the molecule together.

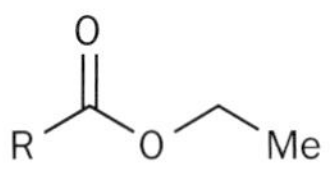

$C_6H_9NO_2 - C_4H_5NO_2 = C_2H_4$

So, we have two carbons and two hydrogens left to deal with. There can only be two possibilities, structurally:

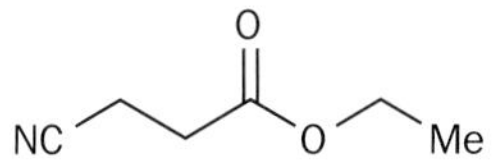

or

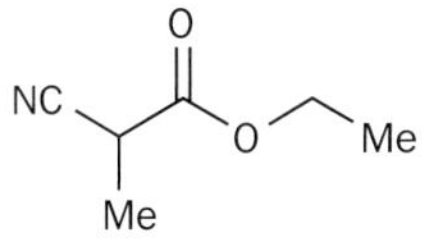

Look at the signal that's farthest downfield in the NMR. It comes from two protons that are adjacent to a methyl group (because the signal is a quartet). Because we suspect that the carbonyl is an ester, this signal must correspond to two protons that are right next to the ester oxygen. The fact that the signal is farthest downfield indicates that these protons are immediately adjacent to the oxygen, which is the most electronegative atom. We also know that this is an ethyl ester because these two protons are next to a methyl group.

We've accounted for three carbons, two oxygens, and five hydrogens in the structure above, and we also know that the nitrile accounts for an additional carbon and nitrogen.

Note that the protons in the structure on the left would have to give rise to two triplets because each is adjacent to a carbon with two protons. However, the only signals we haven't accounted for in the NMR are a doublet integrating for three protons and a quartet integrating for one. These signals exactly match the structure on the right, and so that must be the unknown.

Remember: *Once you have made a tentative structural assignment, check it against all of the data available to be sure you have the right molecule.*

SIMILAR QUESTIONS

1) Why is it unlikely that the compound in the original question is cyclic (*i.e.*, contains one or more rings)?
2) If the molecule were a methyl ketone rather than an ester (*i.e.*, replace the ethoxy group with a methyl group), where do you expect that the carbonyl IR stretch would appear, and why?
3) Where would the signal for the methyl ketone protons in the compound described in question 2 show up in the NMR relative to the signal for the protons adjacent to the oxygen in the ester?

CHAPTER 14

CARBOHYDRATES

Carbohydrates are compounds containing carbon, hydrogen, and oxygen in the form of polyhydroxylated aldehydes or ketones. They have the general formula $C_n(H_2O)_n$ and serve many functions in biological systems, most notably as the chemical energy source for most organisms. A single carbohydrate unit is a **monosaccharide** (simple sugar), and a molecule with two sugars is a **disaccharide. Oligosaccharides** are short carbohydrate chains, while **polysaccharides** are long carbohydrate chains.

TEACHER TIP

The MCAT likes to take complicated molecules and test you on the most basic information. When dealing with carbohydrates, look for the functional groups you've seen in the previous chapters and realize that they will always act the same.

MONOSACCHARIDES

Monosaccharides, the simplest carbohydrate units, are classified according to the number of carbons they possess. For example, **trioses, tetroses, pentoses,** and **hexoses** have 3, 4, 5, and 6 carbons, respectively. The basic structure of monosaccharides is exemplified by the simplest, glyceraldehyde.

MCAT SYNOPSIS

Monosaccharides are the simplest units and are classified by the number of carbons.

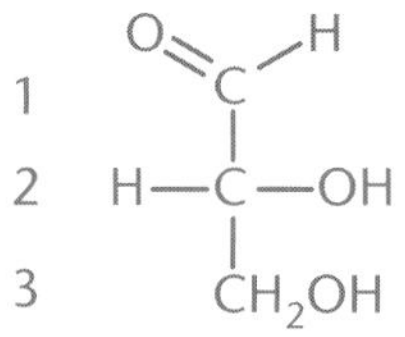

1 O=C–H (C)
2 H—C—OH
3 CH_2OH

Glyceraldehyde

Figure 14.1

Glyceraldehyde is a polyhydroxylated aldehyde or **aldose** (aldehyde sugar). A polyhydroxylated ketone is called a **ketose** (ketone sugar). The numbering of the carbon atoms in a monosaccharide begins with the end closest to the carbonyl group.

A. STEREOCHEMISTRY

The stereochemistry of monosaccharides can be understood by studying the enantiomeric configurations of glyceraldehyde.

MCAT SYNOPSIS

D and L are based on the sterochemistry of glyceraldehyde. These are not related to the + and – designations denoting optical rotation.

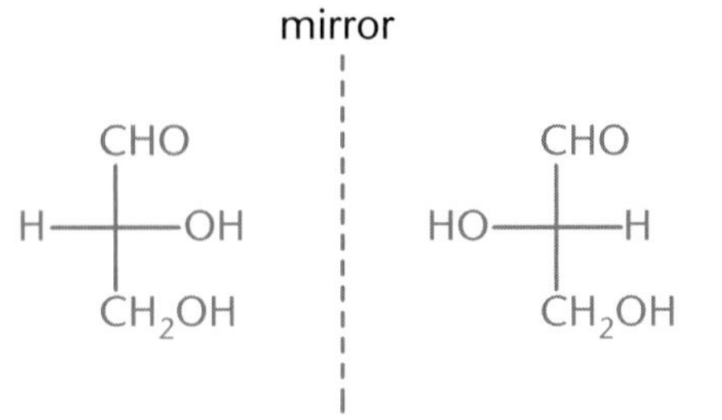

D-Glyceraldehyde *L*-Glyceraldehyde

Figure 14.2

KAPLAN EXCLUSIVE

If *L*owest –OH is on the *L*eft, the molecule is *L*. If the –OH is on the *R*ight, it's *D* (from the *L*atin root dextro, meaning "right").

The D and L configurations of glyceraldehyde were assigned early in this century (before the *R* and *S* configurations were used) to designate the optical rotation of each enantiomer. D-glyceraldehyde was later determined to exhibit a positive rotation (designated as D-(+)-glyceraldehyde) and L-glyceraldehyde a negative rotation (designated as L-(–)-glyceraldehyde. However, other monosaccharides are assigned the D or L configuration depending on their relationship to glyceraldehyde: a molecule whose highest numbered chiral center (the chiral center farthest from the carbonyl) has the same configuration as D-(+)-glyceraldehyde is classed as a D sugar. A molecule that has its highest numbered chiral center in the same configuration as L-(–)-glyceraldehyde is classed as an L sugar. This is illustrated below:

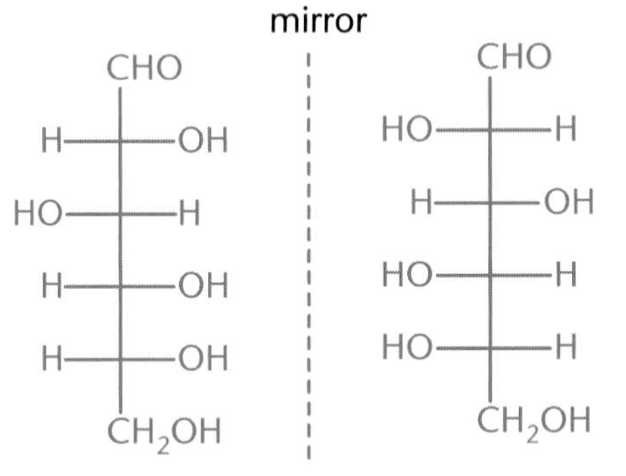

D-Glucose *L*-Glucose

Figure 14.3

MCAT SYNOPSIS

Epimers differ in configuration at only one carbon.

Monosaccharide stereoisomers are divided into two optical families, D and L; the stereoisomers within one family are known as **diastereomers.** Aldose diastereomers which differ only about the configuration of one carbon are known as **epimers.** For instance, D-ribose and D-arabinose are pentose epimers. They differ in configuration only at C–2.

Some important monosaccharides are shown in Figure 14.5.

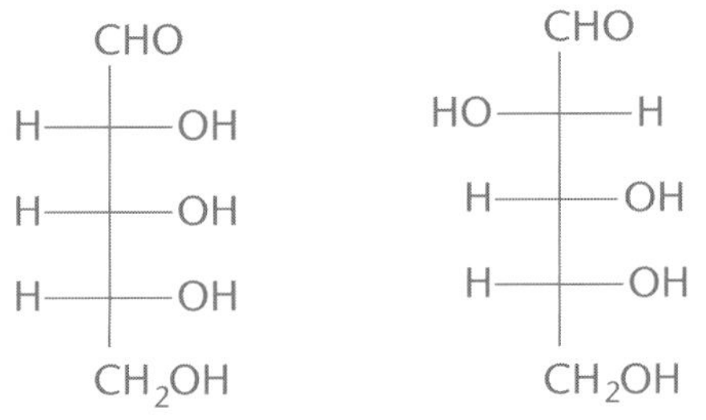

D-Ribose D-Arabinose

Figure 14.4

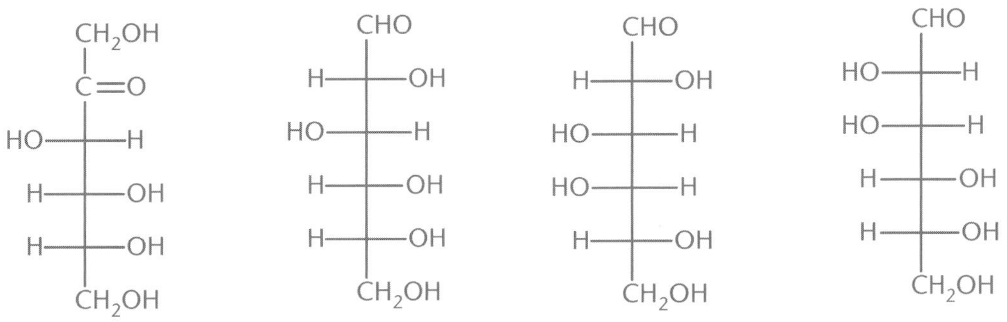

D-Fructose D-Glucose D-Galactose D-Mannose

Figure 14.5

B. RING PROPERTIES

Because monosaccharides contain both a hydroxyl group and a carbonyl group, they can undergo intramolecular reactions to form cyclic hemiacetals (or hemiketals, in the case of ketoses). These cyclic molecules are stable in solution and may exist as six-membered **pyranose** rings (as in glucose) or five-membered **furanose** rings. Like cyclohexane, the pyranose rings adopt a chairlike configuration, and the substituents assume axial or equatorial positions so as to minimize steric hindrance. When converting the monosaccharide from its straight-chain Fischer projection to the Haworth projection (shown in Figure 14.6), it is important to remember that any group on the right of the Fischer projection will be pointing down, while any group on the left side of the Fischer projection will be pointing up. The following reaction scheme depicts the formation of a cyclic hemiacetal from D-glucose.

TEACHER TIP

The carbonyl carbon is (as always) a good electrophile and the many –OH groups represent good nucleophiles. What might happen when these two groups are "handcuffed" together in the same molecule? An intramolecular nucleophilic acyl substitution.

When a straight-chain monosaccharide is converted to its cyclic form, the carbonyl carbon (C–1 for glucose) becomes chiral. Cyclic stereoisomers differing about the new chiral carbon are known as **anomers.** In glucose, the alpha anomer has the –OH group of C–1 *trans* to the CH_2OH

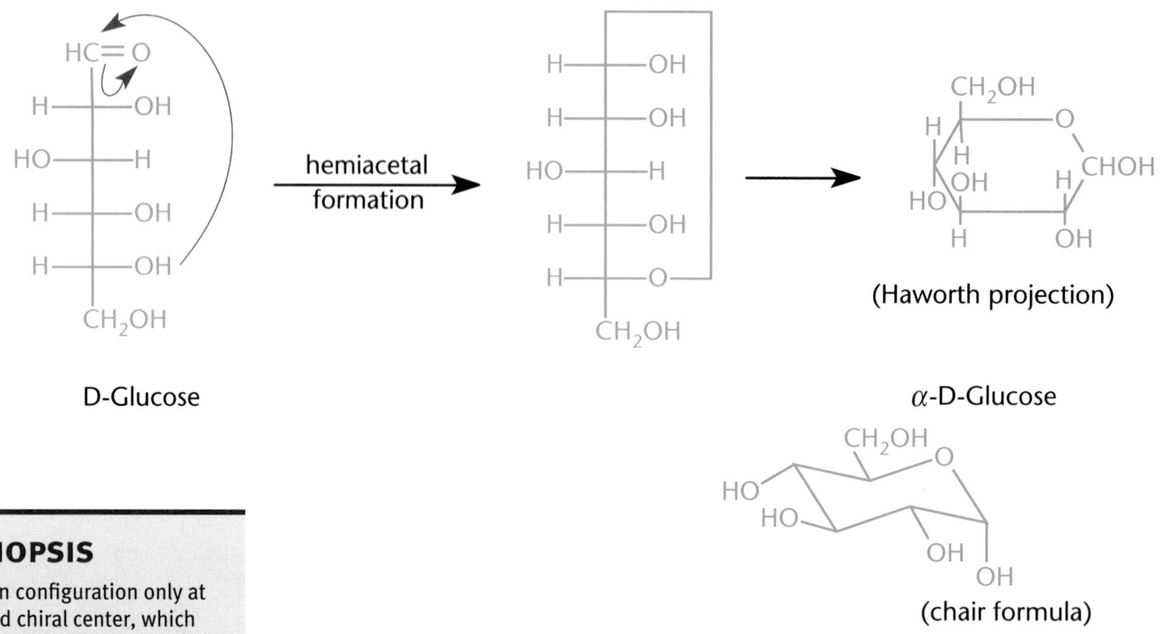

D-Glucose

hemiacetal formation

(Haworth projection)

α-D-Glucose

(chair formula)

Figure 14.6

> ### MCAT SYNOPSIS
> Anomers differ in configuration only at the newly formed chiral center, which is caused by the attack of the alcohol on two different sides of the planar carbonyl carbon. α = *trans* to the $-CH_2OH$ (down in glucose). β =*cis* to the $-CH_2OH$ (up in glucose).

substituent (down), while the beta anomer has the –OH group of C–1 *cis* to the CH_2OH substituent (up).

When exposed to water, hemiacetal rings spontaneously open and then reform. Because of bond rotation between C–1 and C–2, either the alpha or beta anomer may be formed. The reaction is more rapid when catalyzed by acid or base. The spontaneous change of configuration about C–1 is known as **mutarotation,** and results in a mixture containing both anomers in their equilibrium concentrations (for glucose, 36 percent alpha:64 percent beta). The alpha configuration is less favored because the hydroxyl group of C–1 is axial, making the molecule more sterically strained.

> ### TEACHER TIP
> Often confusing terms:
>
> *Anomerization*: the forming of one anomer or another from the straight chain sugar.
>
> *Mutarotation*: the process of one anomer changing into the other anomer by opening and reclosing.

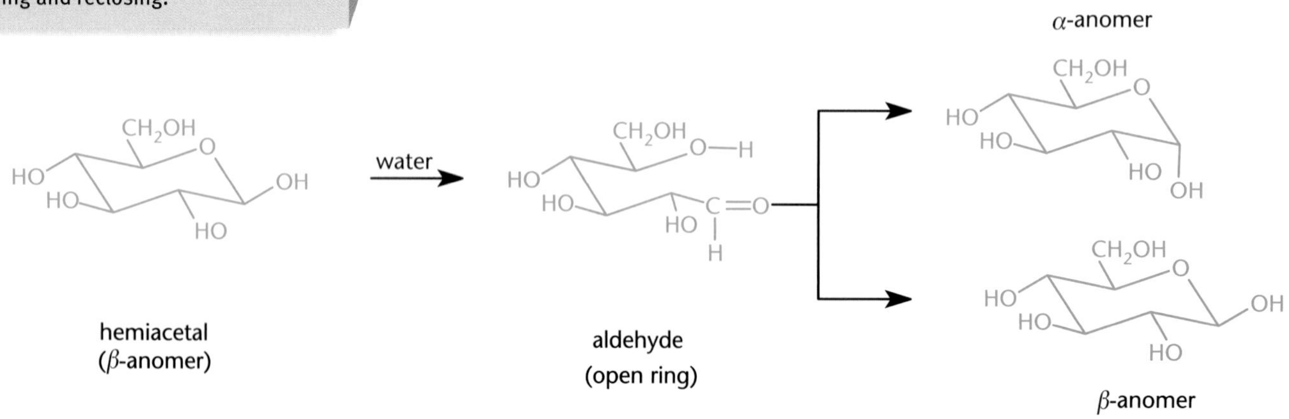

hemiacetal (β-anomer)

water

aldehyde (open ring)

α-anomer

β-anomer

Figure 14.7

C. MONOSACCHARIDE REACTIONS

1. Ester Formation

Monosaccharides contain hydroxyl groups and can undergo many of the same reactions as simple alcohols. Therefore, they may be converted to either esters or ethers. In the presence of acid anhydride and base, all of the hydroxyl groups will be esterified. The following reaction is an example of glucose esterification.

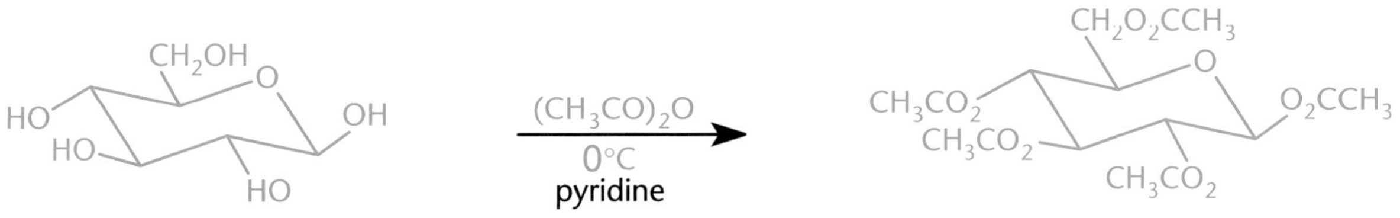

β-D-Glucose $\xrightarrow[\text{pyridine}]{(CH_3CO)_2O,\ 0°C}$ Penta-O-acetyl- β-D-glucose

Figure 14.8

2. Oxidation of Monosaccharides

As they switch between anomeric configurations, the hemiacetal rings spend a short period of time in the open-chain aldehyde form. Like all aldehydes, these can be oxidized to carboxylic acids called **aldonic acids.** Thus, the aldoses are reducing agents. Any monosaccharide with a hemiacetal ring (–OH on C–1) is considered a **reducing sugar** and can be oxidized. Both Tollen's reagent and Benedict reagent can be used to detect the presence of reducing sugars. A positive Tollen's test involves the reduction of Ag^+ to form metallic silver. When Benedict reagent is used, a red precipitate of Cu_2O indicates the presence of a reducing sugar. Ketose sugars are also reducing sugars and give positive Tollen's and Benedict tests, because they can isomerize to aldoses via keto-enol shifts.

MCAT SYNOPSIS

Key reactions of monosaccharides include:

- ester formation
- oxidation
- glycosidic reactions

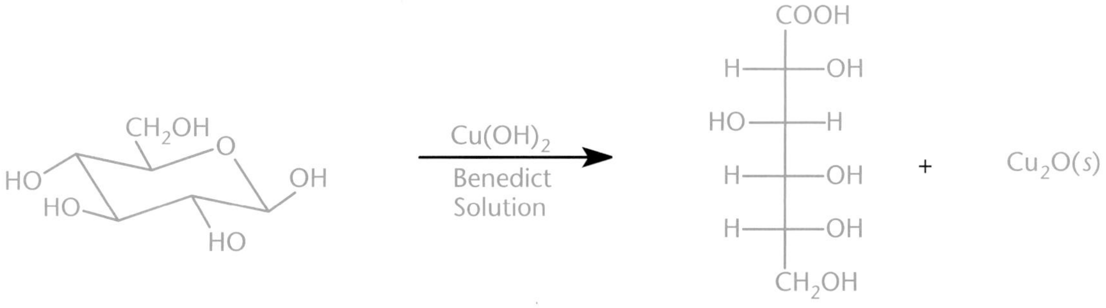

β-D-Glucose $\xrightarrow[\text{Benedict Solution}]{Cu(OH)_2}$ D-Gluconic Acid (an aldonic acid) + $Cu_2O(s)$ (red solid)

Figure 14.9

Teacher Tip

This reaction is really just a dressed-up S_N2 reaction with the sugar acting as the nucleophile.

3. Glycosidic Reactions

Hemiacetal monosaccharides will react with alcohols under acidic conditions. The anomeric hydroxyl group is transformed into an alkoxy group, yielding a mixture of the alpha and beta acetals. The resulting bond is called a **glycosidic linkage,** and the acetal is known as a **glycoside.** An example is the reaction of glucose with ethanol.

Glycosides do not mutarotate and are stable in water.

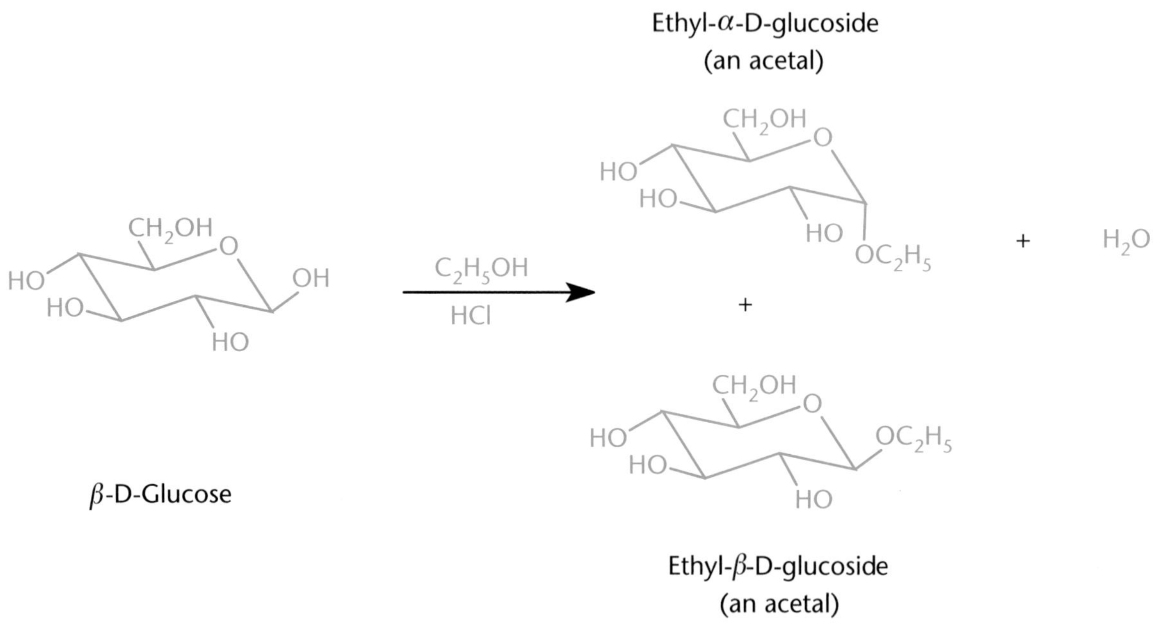

Figure 14.10

DISACCHARIDES

Teacher Tip

In lactose intolerance, a person is missing the lactase enzyme, which breaks the disaccharide lactose into two glucose molecules.

As discussed above, a monosaccharide may react with alcohols to give acetals. When that alcohol is another monosaccharide, the product is called a **disaccharide.** The formation of a disaccharide is shown below.

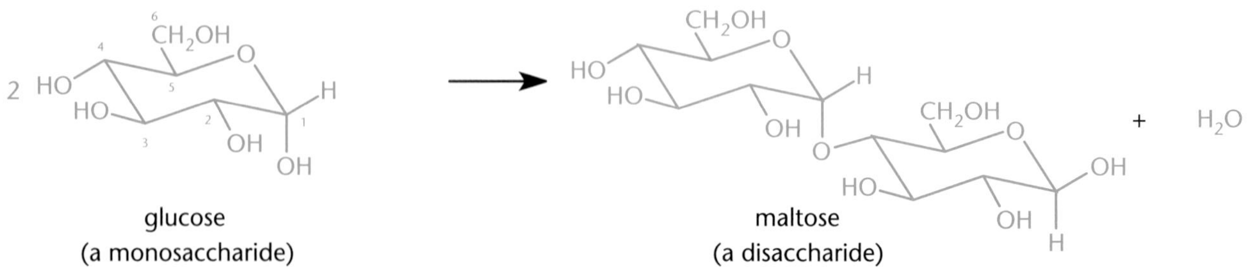

Figure 14.11

The most common glycosidic linkage occurs between C–1 of the first sugar and C–4 of the second, and is designated as a 1,4′ link. 1,6′ and 1,2′ bonds are also observed. The glycosidic bonds may be either alpha or beta, depending on the orientation of the hydroxyl group on the anomeric carbon.

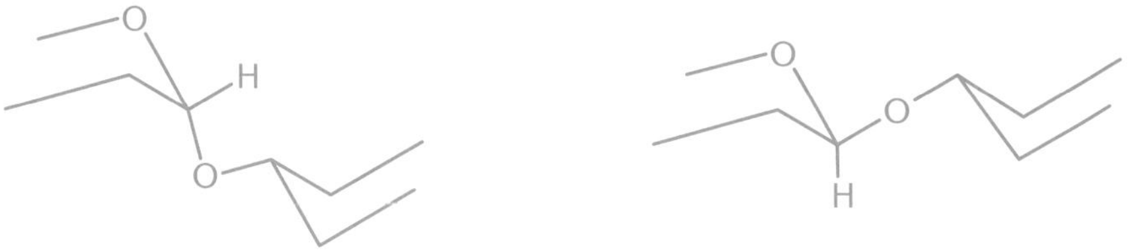

α-glycosidic linkage

β-glycosidic linkage

Figure 14.12

These glycosidic linkages can often be cleaved in the presence of aqueous acid. For example, the glycosidic linkage of maltose, a disaccharide, can be cleaved to yield two molecules of glucose.

POLYSACCHARIDES

Polysaccharides are formed via linkage of monosaccharide units with glycosidic bonds. The three most important biological polysaccharides are **cellulose, starch,** and **glycogen.** Cellulose is comprised of D-glucose linked by 1,4′-beta-glycosidic bonds. Cellulose is the structural component of plants. Starch stores energy in plants and glycogen stores energy in animals; both are formed by linking glucose units in 1,4′-alpha-glycosidic bonds, with occasional 1,6′-alpha-glycosidic bonds creating branches. While all three are composed of glucose subunits, the orientation about the anomeric carbon gives them biological differences. Cellulose cannot be digested by humans, while starch and glycogen can, and are important energy sources for living organisms.

MCAT SYNOPSIS

Key biological polysaccharides:
cellulose (1,4′ beta);
starch and glycogen (mostly 1,4′ alpha; some 1,6′ alpha).

CH$_2$OH OH CH$_2$OH
O HO O O
HO O HO
OH CH$_2$OH OH

Cellulose, a 1,4′, -β-D-Glucose polymer

CH$_2$OH
O
O
HO
OH CH$_2$OH
O O
HO
OH CH$_2$OH
O O
HO
OH
O

Starch, a 1,4′, -α-D-Glucose polymer

PRACTICE QUESTIONS

1. What description best fits the pair of sugars shown below?

CH_2OH
H — OH
H — OH
HO — H
CHO

CH_2OH
H — OH
H — OH
OHC — OH
H

A. They are enantiomers.
B. They are diastereomers.
C. They are meso compounds.
D. They are identical.

2. Which of the following sugars will yield a positive Tollen's test?

A. HOH_2C, O, OCH_3, OH, OH

B. OH, OH, O, HO, OAc, HO

C. HO, O, OH, OH, OH

D. HO_2C, OH, CO_2H, OH

3. Galactose is the C–4 epimer of glucose; which structure below is galactose?

A.
CHO
H — OH
HO — H
HO — H
H — OH
CH_2OH

B.
CHO
H — OH
H — OH
H — OH
H — OH
CH_2OH

C.
CHO
HO — H
HO — H
H — OH
H — OH
CH_2OH

D.
CHO
H — OH
HO — H
H — OH
HO — H
CH_2OH

4. Under strongly acidic conditions, aldoses become oxidized to dicarboxylic acids called *aldaric acids*. An unknown pentose X, which is optically active, produces an optically inactive aldaric acid upon treatment with HNO_3. What is the structure of pentose X?

A.
CHO
H — OH
HO — H
HO — H
CH_2OH

B.
CHO
HO — H
HO — H
H — OH
CH_2OH

C.
CH_2OH
HO — H
HO — H
H — OH
CHO

D.
CHO
H — OH
H — OH
H — OH
CH_2OH

CHAPTER 15

AMINO ACIDS, PEPTIDES, AND PROTEINS

Proteins are large polymers composed of many amino acid subunits. Proteins have diverse biological roles; for example, they provide structure (keratin, collagen), regulate body metabolism via hormonal control (insulin), and serve as catalysts (enzymes).

TEACHER TIP

Many Organic Chemistry topics can be tested with amino acids and proteins: carboxylic acid derivatives (peptide bond = amide linkage), hydrogen bonding, electrophoresis, stereochemistry, and acid-base properties. Expect to be tested on the basics, even with complicated molecules.

AMINO ACIDS

Amino acids contain an amine group and a carboxyl group attached to a single carbon atom (the alpha carbon atom). The other two substituents of the alpha carbon are usually a hydrogen atom and a variable side-chain referred to as the **R-group.**

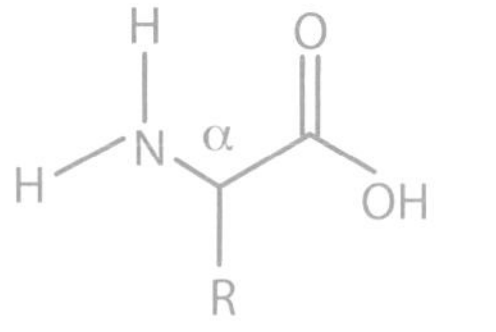

H, H, N, α, O, OH, R

Figure 15.1

The alpha carbon is a chiral center (except in glycine, the simplest amino acid, where R=H), and thus all amino acids (except for glycine) are optically active. Naturally-occurring amino acids (of which there are 20) are L-enantiomers (see chapters 2 and 14).

MCAT SYNOPSIS

Except for glycine, all amino acids are chiral.

By convention, the Fischer projection for an amino acid is drawn with the amino group on the left.

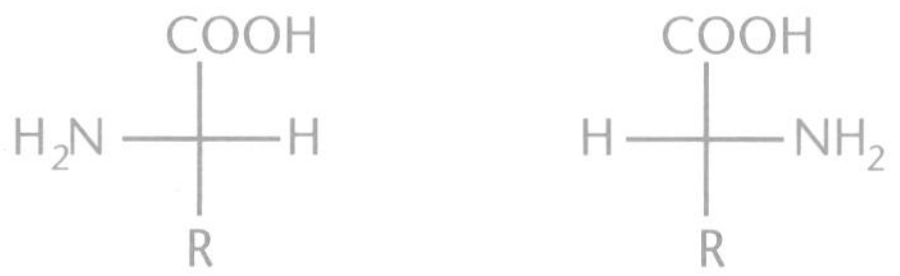

COOH, H_2N, H, R — L-amino acid

COOH, H, NH_2, R — D-amino acid

Figure 15.2

A. ACID-BASE CHARACTERISTICS

Amino acids have an acidic carboxyl group and a basic amino group on the same molecule (see General Chemistry, chapter 10 for a discussion of acids and bases). As a result, when they are in solution, amino acids sometimes take the form of dipolar ions, or **zwitterions** (from the German *zwitter*, "hybrid"). The two halves of the molecules neutralize each other, so that at neutral pH they exist in the form of internal salts.

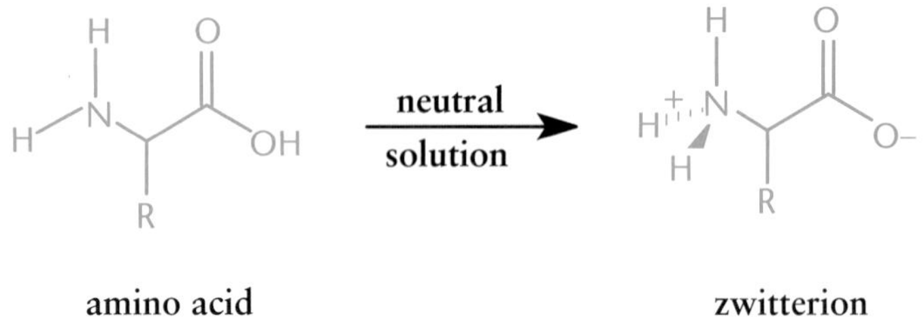

neutral solution

amino acid

zwitterion

Figure 15.3

Amino acids are **amphoteric**; *i.e.,* they may act as either acids or bases, depending on their environment. Amino acids in acidic solution are fully protonated. Because they have two protons that can dissociate—one from the carboxyl group and one from the amino group—amino acids have at least two dissociation constants, K_{a1} and K_{a2}.

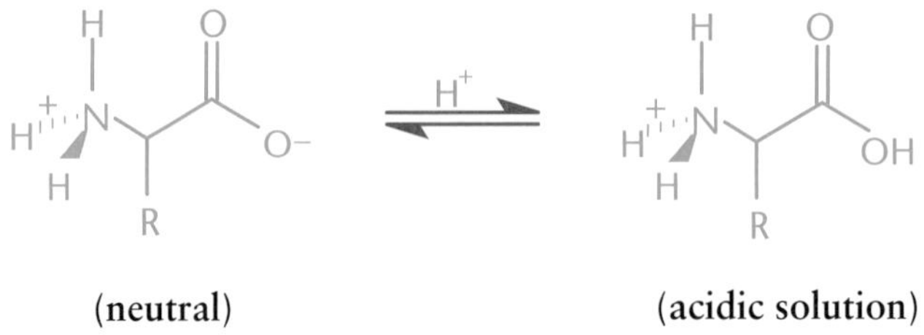

H^+

(neutral)

(acidic solution)

Figure 15.4

Amino acids in basic solution are deprotonated. They have two proton-accepting groups and, therefore, at least two dissociation constants, K_{b1} and K_{b2}.

OH^-

$+ \; H_2O$

(neutral)

(basic solution)

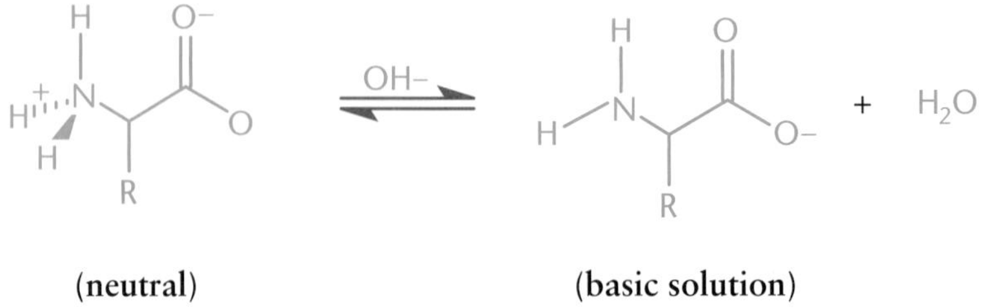

Figure 15.5

MCAT SYNOPSIS

At the isoelectric point, an amino acid is uncharged.

At low pH, the amino acid carries an excess positive charge, and at high pH, the amino acid carries an excess negative charge. The intermediate pH, at which the amino acid is electrically neutral and exists as a zwitterion, is the **isoelectric point (pI)**, or **isoelectric pH,** of the amino acid.

The isoelectric pH lies between pK_{a1} and pK_{a2}.

B. TITRATION OF AMINO ACIDS

Because of their acidic and basic properties, amino acids can be titrated. The titration of each proton occurs as a distinct step resembling that of a simple monoprotic acid. The titration curve of glycine is shown in Figure 15.7.

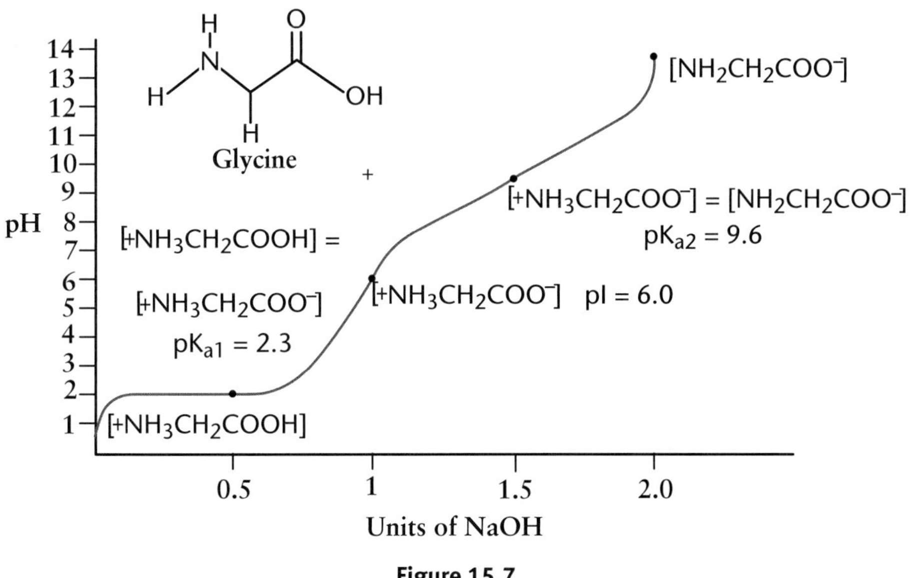

Figure 15.7

A 1M glycine solution is acidic; the glycine exists predominantly as $^+NH_3CH_2COOH$. The amino acid is fully protonated and carries a positive charge. As the solution is titrated with NaOH, carboxyl groups lose a proton. During this stage, the amino acid acts as a buffer and the pH changes very slowly. When 0.5 mol of base has been added to the amino acid solution, the concentrations of $^+NH_3CH_2COOH$ and $^+NH_3CH_2COO^-$ (its zwitterion) are equimolar. At this point the pH is equal to the pK_{a1}, and the solution is buffered against pH changes.

As more base is added, all of the carboxyl groups are deprotonated. The amino acid loses buffering capacity, and thus the pH rises more rapidly. When 1 mol of base has been added, glycine exists predominantly as $^+NH_3CH_2COO^-$. The amino acid is now electrically neutral; the pH is equal to glycine's pI.

MCAT Synopsis

Titration with base: first the carboxyl group is deprotonated, then the amino group.

Glycine passes through a second buffering stage during which pH change is slow because continued titration deprotonates amino groups. When 1.5 mol of base have been added, the concentrations of $^{+}NH_3CH_2COO^-$ and $NH_2CH_2COO^-$ are equimolar, and the pH is equal to pK_{a2}.

MCAT SYNOPSIS

Amino acids pass through at least two buffering stages, one at each pK_a.

As another 0.5 mol of base is added, all of the amino groups are deprotonated to $NH_2CH_2COO^-$; glycine is now completely deprotonated.

Certain things should be noted about the titration of amino acids:

1. When adding base, the carboxyl group loses its proton first; after all of the carboxyl groups are fully deprotonated, the amino group loses its acidic proton.
2. Two moles of base must be added in order to deprotonate one mole of most amino acids. The first mole deprotonates the carboxyl group, while the second mole deprotonates the amino group.
3. The buffering capacity of the amino acid is greatest at or near the two dissociation constants, K_{a1} and K_{a2}. At the isoelectric point, its buffering capacity is minimal.
4. It is possible to perform the titration in reverse, from alkaline pH to acidic pH, with the addition of acid; the sequence of events is reversed.

TEACHER TIP

Review acids, bases, and the Henderson-Hasselbalch equation more closely.

C. HENDERSON-HASSELBALCH EQUATION

The ratio of an amino acid's ions are dependent on pH. The **Henderson-Hasselbalch equation** defines the relationship between pH and the ratio of conjugate acid to conjugate base, and provides a mathematical expression for the dissociation constants of amino acids.

$$pH = pK_a + \log \frac{[\text{conjugate base}]}{[\text{conjugate acid}]}$$

When the pK_{a1} of glycine is known, the ratio of conjugate acid to conjugate base for a particular pH can be determined. For example, at pH 3.3, glycine which has a pK_a of 2.3, will have the ratios:

$$3.3 = 2.3 + \log \frac{[^{+}H_3NCH_2COO^-]}{[H_3N^+CH_2COH]}$$

MCAT SYNOPSIS

The best buffering occurs within one pH unit of the pK_a.

$$\text{By subtraction: } \log \frac{[H_3N^+CH_2COO^-]}{[H_3N^+CH_2COOH]} = 1$$

$$\text{The antilog of } 1 = 10, \text{ thus: } \frac{[H_3N^+CH_2COO^-]}{[H_3N^+CH_2COOH]} = \frac{10}{1}$$

So, in this example, there are 10 times as many zwitterions as there are of the fully protonated form.

The Henderson-Hasselbach equation can be used experimentally to prepare buffer solutions of amino acids. The best buffering regions of amino acids occur within one pH unit of the pK_a or pK_b. For example, the carboxyl group of glycine, which has a pK_a of 2.6, shows high buffering capacity between pH 1.6 and 3.6.

D. AMINO ACID SIDE-CHAINS

Amino acid side-chains (R-groups) give chemical diversity to the backbone of the amino acid molecule. They also give proteins some distinguishing features. The twenty amino acids are classified according to whether their side chains are **nonpolar, polar** (but uncharged), **acidic,** or **basic.**

TEACHER TIP

Do not memorize all the amino acids. You are not expected to know them for the exam. Just understand the concepts involved in these different types of side-chains and how they interact.

1. Nonpolar Amino Acids

Nonpolar amino acids have R-groups that are saturated hydrocarbons. The R-groups are hydrophobic and decrease the solubility of the amino acid in water. Amino acids with nonpolar side-chains are usually found buried within protein molecules, away from the aqueous cellular environment.

MCAT SYNOPSIS

Nonpolar amino acids are often found at the core of globular proteins or in transmembrane regions of proteins that are in contact with the hydrophobic portion of the phospholipid membrane.

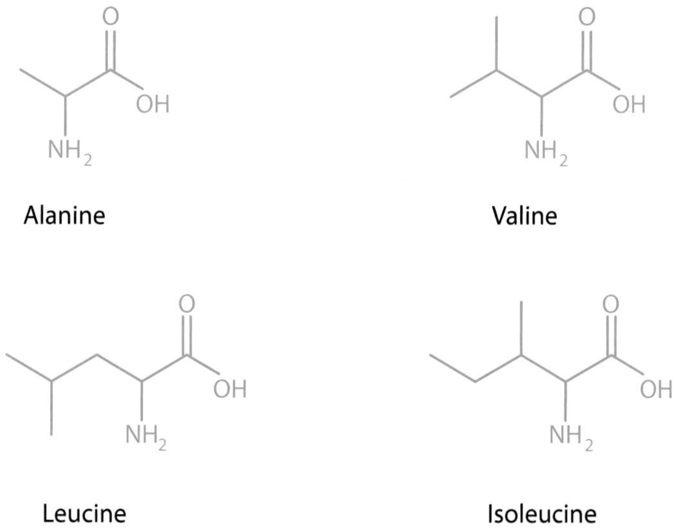

O OH NH_2

Alanine

O OH NH_2

Valine

O OH NH_2

Leucine

O OH NH_2

Isoleucine

Figure 15.8a

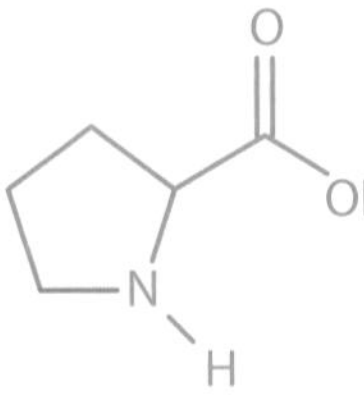

Proline

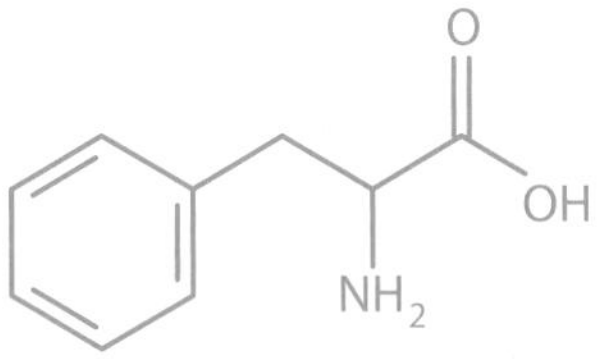

Phenylalanine

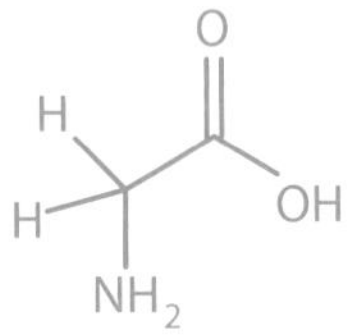

Glycine

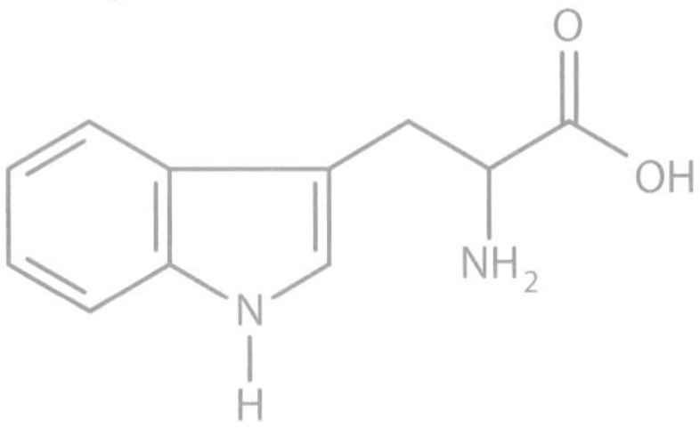

Tryptophan

Figure 15.8b

MCAT Synopsis

The other types of amino acids (polar, acidic, and basic) are found in regions of proteins that are exposed to the aqueous, polar environment.

2. Polar Amino Acids

Polar amino acids have polar, uncharged R-groups that are hydrophilic, increasing the solubility of the amino acid in water. They are usually found on protein surfaces.

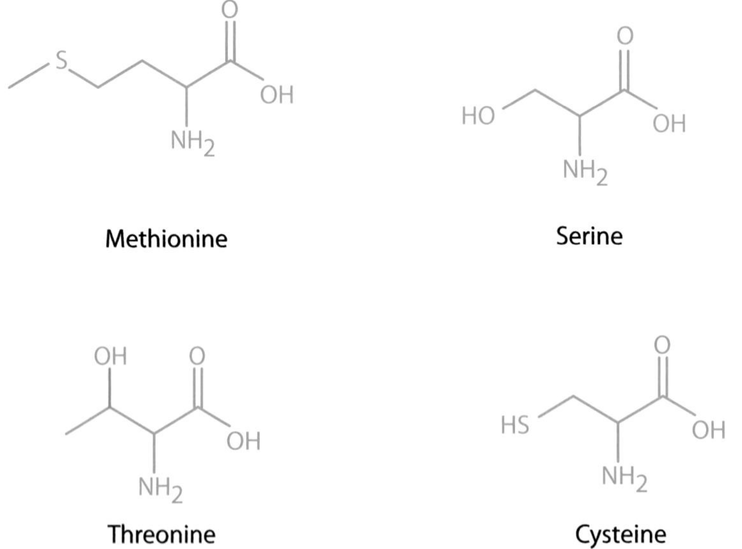

Figure 15.9a

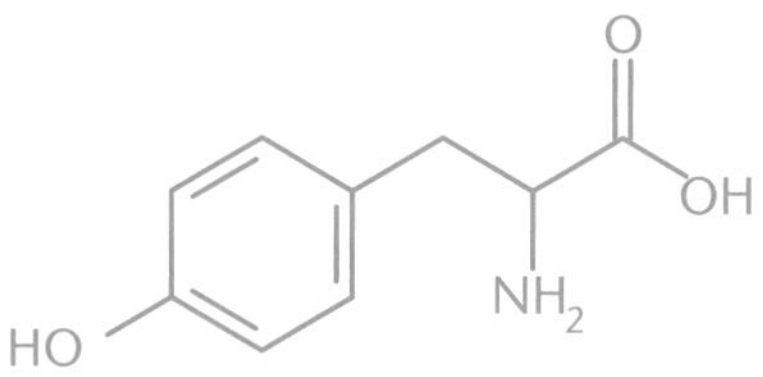

Tyrosine

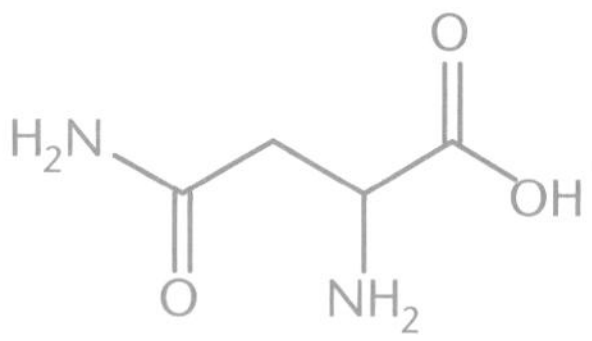

Asparagine

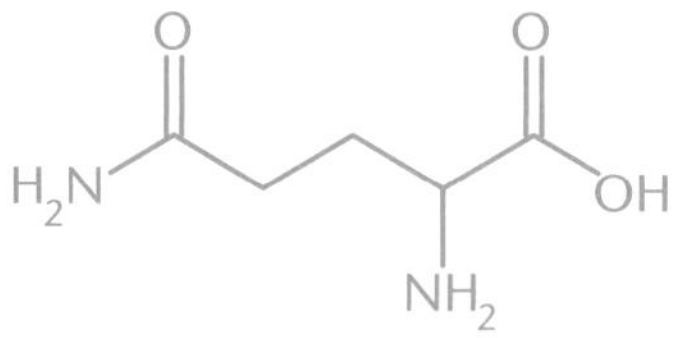

Glutamine

Figure 15.9b

3. Acidic Amino Acids

Amino acids whose R-group contains a carboxyl group are called acidic amino acids. They have a net negative charge at physiological pH (pH 7.4),

Aspartic Acid

Glutamic Acid

(Salt is Aspartate)

(Salt is Glutamate)

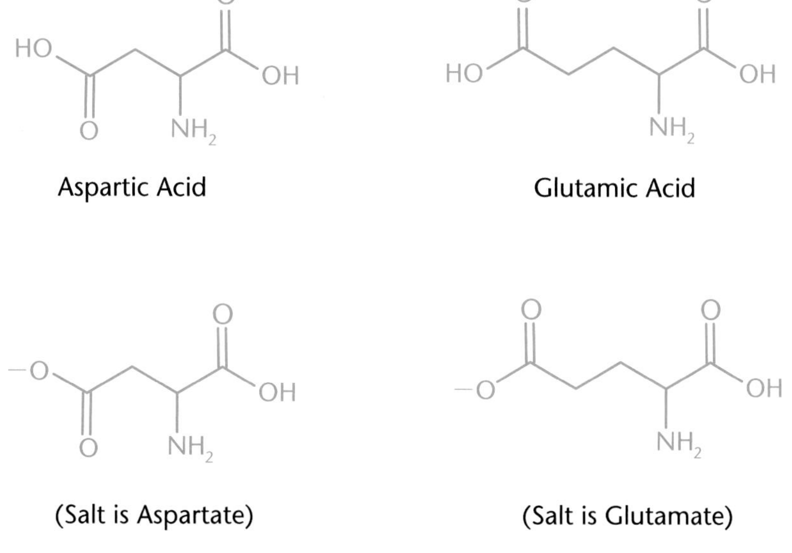

Figure 15.10

Aspartic acid and glutamic acid each have three groups that must be neutralized during titration (two –COOH and one $-NH_3^+$). Therefore, their titration curve is different from the standard curve for amino acids (exemplified by glycine). The molecule has three distinct dissociation

> **MCAT SYNOPSIS**
>
> Acidic amino acids have a negative charge at physiologic pH (pH 7.4). They have three distinct pK_a's.

constants (pK_{a1}, pK_{a2}, and pK_{a3}) although the neutralization curves of the two carboxyl groups overlap to a certain extent.

Because of the additional carboxyl group, the isoelectric point is shifted toward an acidic pH. Three moles of base are needed to deprotonate one mole of an acidic amino acid.

MCAT SYNOPSIS

At physiological pH, basic amino acids have a net positive charge. They also have three dissociation constants.

4. Basic Amino Acids

Amino acids whose R-group contains an amino group are called basic amino acids and carry a net positive charge at physiological pH.

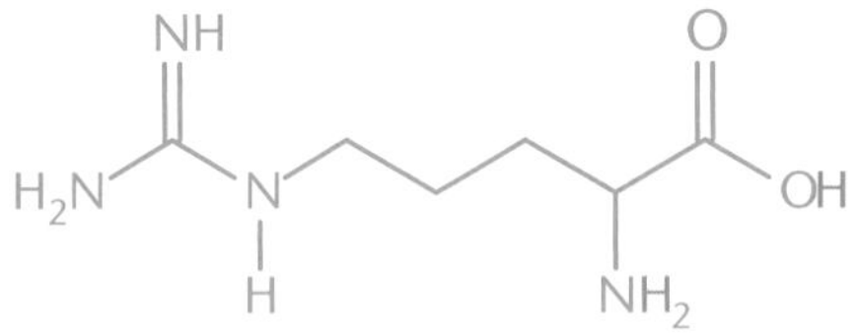

Arginine

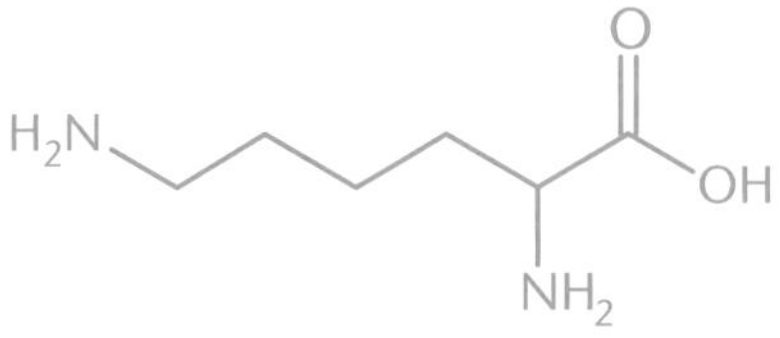

Lysine

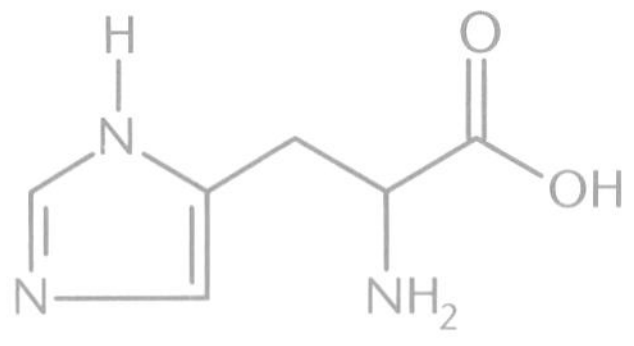

Histidine

Figure 15.11

The titration curve of amino acids with basic R-groups is modified by the additional amino group that must be neutralized. Although basic amino acids have three dissociation constants, the neutralization curves for the two amino groups overlap. The isoelectric point is shifted toward an alkaline pH. Three moles of acid are needed to neutralize one mole of a basic amino acid.

Understanding titration curves and isoelectric points helps predict the charge of particular amino acids at a given pH. For example, in a mixture of glycine, glutamic acid, and lysine at pH 6.0, glycine will be neutral, glutamic acid will be negatively charged, and lysine will be positively charged.

PEPTIDES

Peptides are composed of amino acid subunits, sometimes called **residues,** linked by **peptide bonds.** Peptides are small proteins (the distinction between a peptide and protein is vague). Two amino acids joined together form a **dipeptide,** three form a **tripeptide,** and many amino acids linked together form a **polypeptide**.

A. REACTIONS

Amino acids are joined by **peptide bonds** (amide bonds) between the carboxyl group of one amino acid and the amino group of another. This bond is formed via a condensation reaction (a reaction in which water is lost). The reverse reaction, hydrolysis (cleavage with the addition of water) of the peptide bond, is catalyzed by an acid or base.

Certain enzymes digest the chain at specific peptide linkages. For example, **trypsin** cleaves at the carboxyl end of arginine and lysine; chymotrypsin cleaves at the carboxyl end of phenylalanine, tyrosine, and tryptophan.

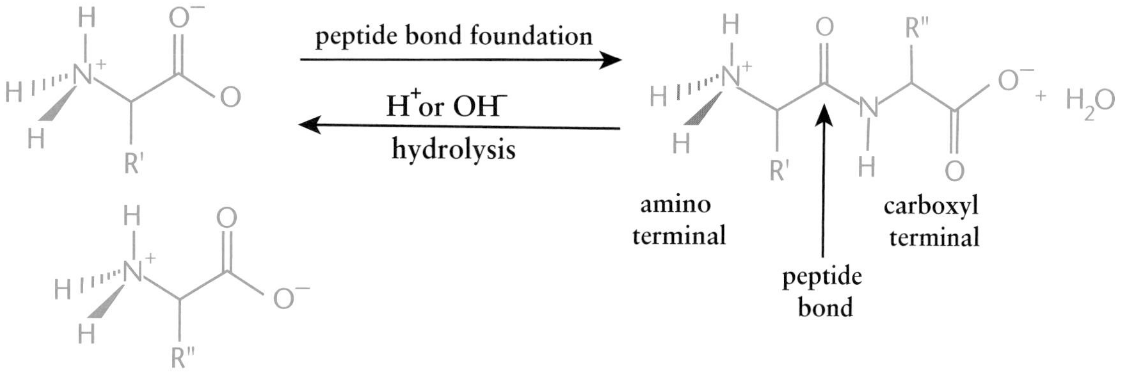

Figure 15.12

B. PROPERTIES

The terminal amino acid with a free alpha-amino group is known as the **amino-terminal** or **N-terminal** residue, while the terminal residue with a free carboxyl group is called the **carboxy-terminal** or **C-terminal** residue. By convention, peptides are drawn with the N-terminal end on the left and the C-terminal end on the right.

Amides have two resonance structures, and the true structure is a hybrid with partial double-bond character. As a result, rotation about the C–N bond is restricted. The bonds on either side of the peptide unit, however, have a great deal of rotational freedom.

MCAT Synopsis

Rotation is limited around the peptide bond because resonance gives the C–N bond partial double-bond character.

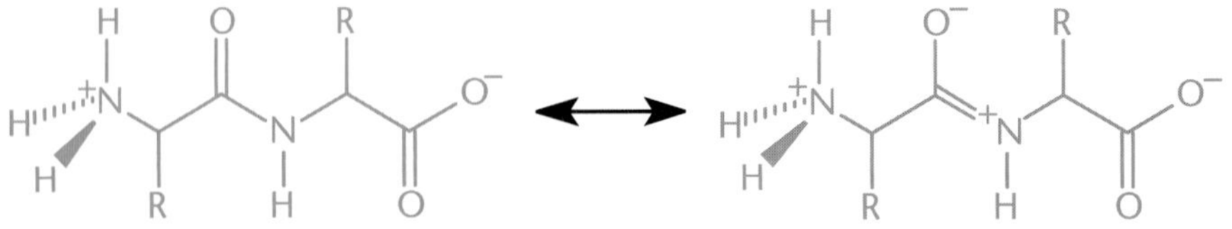

Figure 15.13

TEACHER TIP

Be familiar with the primary, secondary, tertiary, and quaternary structure elements of protein and the factors that affect them.

PROTEINS

Proteins are polypeptides that can range from only a few to more than a thousand amino acids in length. Proteins serve many diverse functions in biological systems, acting as enzymes, hormones, membrane pores, receptors, and elements of cell structure. Four structural levels of protein structure—**primary, secondary, tertiary,** and **quaternary**—are described below.

A. PRIMARY STRUCTURE

The primary structure of the protein refers to the sequence of amino acids, listed from the N-terminal to the C-terminal, and covalent bonds between residues in the chain. The most common of these bonds is a disulfide bond; two **cysteine** molecules become oxidized to form **cystine,** which has a disulfide bond. Disulfide bonds create loops in the protein chain.

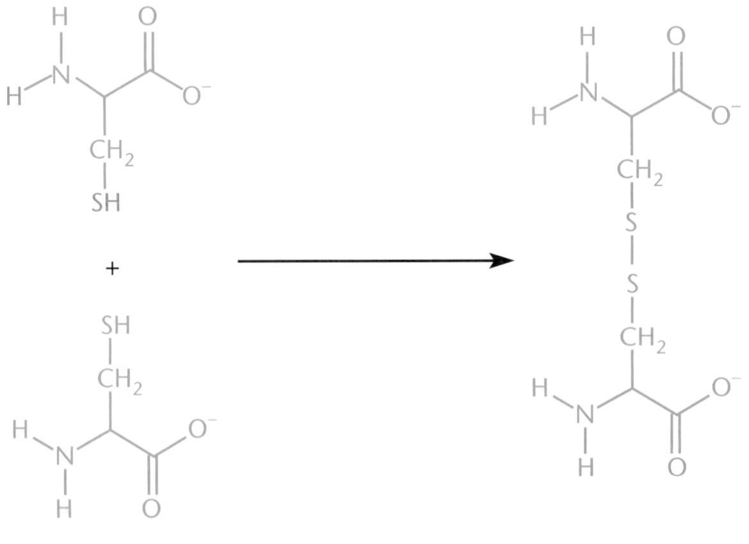

cysteine

cystine

Figure 15.14

The higher-level structures of a protein are dependent on the primary sequence; in other words, a protein will assume whatever secondary, tertiary, and quaternary structures are most energetically favorable given its primary structure and environment. The primary structure of a protein can be determined using a laboratory procedure called **sequencing.**

B. SECONDARY STRUCTURE

The secondary structure of a protein refers to the local structure of neighboring amino acids, governed mostly by hydrogen bond interactions within and between peptide chains. The two most common types of secondary structures are the **α-helix** and the **β-pleated sheet.**

1. α-Helix

α-helix is a rodlike structure in which the peptide chain coils clockwise about a central axis. The helix is stabilized by intramolecular hydrogen bonds between carbonyl oxygen atoms and amine hydrogen atoms four residues away. The side-chains point away from the structure's core and interact with the cellular environment. A typical protein with this structure is **keratin,** which is found in feathers and hair.

2. β-Pleated Sheet

In β-pleated sheets, the peptide chains lie alongside each other in rows. The chains are held together by intramolecular hydrogen bonds between carbonyl oxygen atoms on one peptide chain and amine hydrogen atoms on another. In order to accommodate the maximum number of hydrogen bonds, the β-pleated sheet assumes a rippled, or pleated, shape. The R-groups of the amino residues point above and below the plane of the β-pleated sheet. Silk fibers are composed of β-pleated sheets.

TEACHER TIP

Hydrogen bonds show up in all kinds of interesting places! Be on the lookout for these strong interactions and how they might play a role.

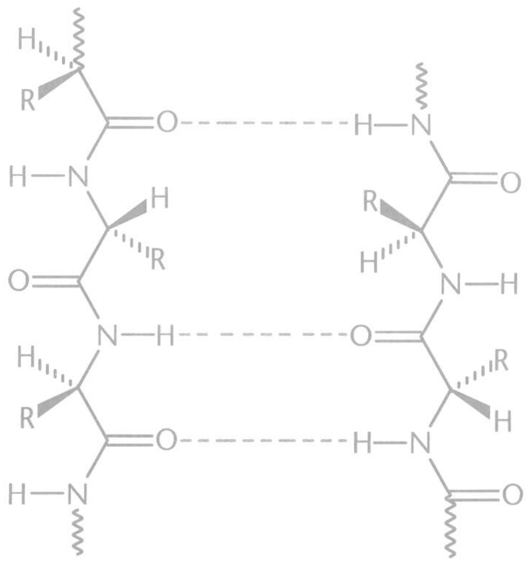

Figure 15.15: β-Pleated Sheet

MCAT Synopsis

- Primary structure consists of the amino acid sequence and covalent bonds.
- Secondary structure describes hydrogen bonding (α-helix and β-pleated sheets).
- Tertiary structure is the three-dimensional shape of the protein.
- Quaternary structure is the arrangement of polypeptide subunits.
- Conjugated proteins have prosthetic groups.

C. TERTIARY STRUCTURE

Tertiary structure refers to the three-dimensional shape of the protein, as determined by hydrophilic and hydrophobic interactions between the R-groups of amino acids that are far apart on the chain.

Certain individual amino acids have significant effects on tertiary structure. For instance, disulfide bonds will cause loops and twists. Proline, because of its shape, cannot fit into an α-helix, and its presence causes a kink in the chain.

Amino acids with hydrophilic (polar and charged) R-groups tend to arrange themselves toward the outside of the protein, where they interact with the aqueous cellular environment. Amino acids with hydrophobic R-groups tend to be found close together, protected from the aqueous environment by polar amino and carboxyl groups.

Proteins are divided into two major classifications on the basis of tertiary structure. **Fibrous proteins,** such as **collagen,** are found as sheets or long strands, while **globular proteins,** such as **myoglobin,** are spherical in shape.

D. QUATERNARY STRUCTURE

Some proteins contain more than one polypeptide subunit. The quaternary structure refers to the way in which these subunits arrange themselves to yield a functional protein molecule. **Hemoglobin,** which is composed of four polypeptide chains, possesses quaternary structure.

E. CONJUGATED PROTEINS

Some proteins, known as **conjugated proteins,** derive part of their function from covalently attached molecules called **prosthetic groups.** Prosthetic groups may be organic molecules or metal ions. Many vitamins are prosthetic groups. Proteins with lipid, carbohydrate, and nucleic acid prosthetic groups are called **lipoproteins, glycoproteins,** and **nucleoproteins,** respectively. Prosthetic groups play major roles in determining the function of the proteins with which they are associated. For example, the **heme group** carries oxygen in both myoglobin and hemoglobin. The heme is composed of an organic porphyrin ring with an iron atom bound in the center. Hemoglobin is inactive without the heme group.

F. DENATURATION OF PROTEINS

Denaturation, or **melting,** is a process in which proteins lose their three-dimensional structure and revert to a **random-coil** state. Denaturation can be caused by detergent, or by changes in pH, temperature, or solute concentration. The weak intermolecular forces keeping the protein stable and functional are disrupted. When a protein denatures, the damage is usually permanent. However, certain gentle denaturing agents do not permanently disrupt the protein. Removing the reagent might allow the protein to **renature** (regain its structure and function).

MCAT Synopsis

Denaturation is the loss of three-dimensional structure.

PRACTICE QUESTIONS

1. Which of the following statements is NOT correct about protein structure?

A. Primary structure is formed by ionic bonds.
B. Secondary structure is formed by disulfide bonds.
C. Tertiary structure is formed by hydrophobic interactions.
D. Quaternary structure is formed by two or more peptides/protein subunits.

2. Which reaction sequence below correctly describes a Strecker synthesis of amino acids?

A. RCHO $\xrightarrow[NH_3]{CN^-}$ $\xrightarrow{H_3O^+}$

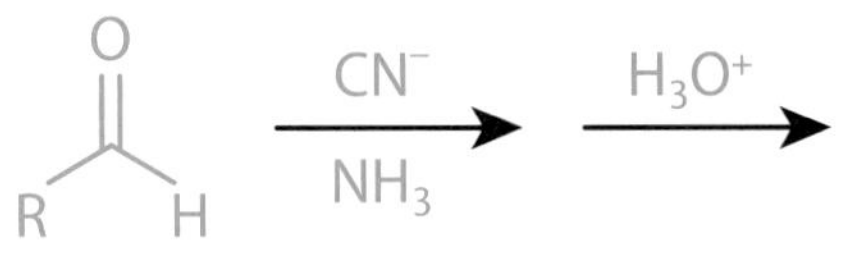

B. RCHO $\xrightarrow{H_3O^+}$ $\xrightarrow[NH_3]{CN^-}$

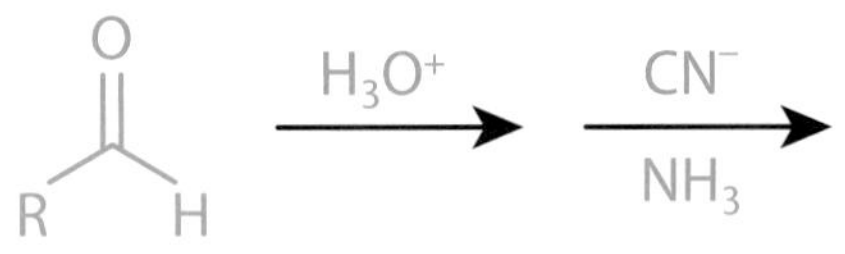

C. RCOOH $\xrightarrow[NH_3]{CN^-}$ $\xrightarrow{H_3O^+}$

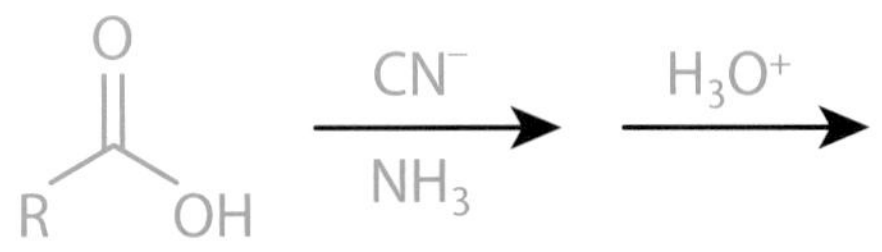

D. RCOOH $\xrightarrow{H_3O^+}$ $\xrightarrow[NH_3]{CN^-}$

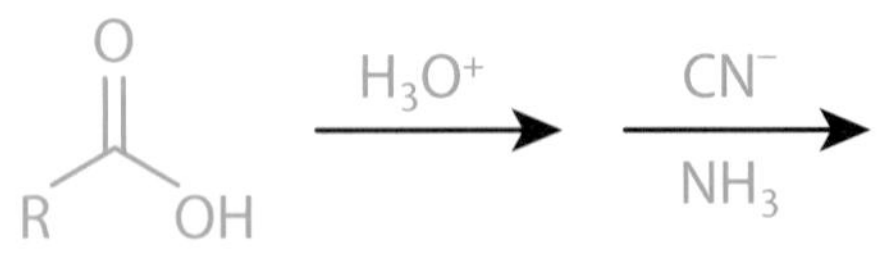

3. Which of the following is true about Edman degradation?

A. It is useful for sequencing proteins like myoglobin, which contains 153 amino acids.
B. Individual amino acids are cleaved from the carboxy terminus of the peptide.
C. A benzyl alcohol is used in the reaction.
D. Phenylisothiocyanate is used in the reaction.

4. The molecule shown below is treated with NaN_3 in base, followed by H_2 over palladium, and finally aqueous acid. One of the intermediates forms a ring. What is the product formed?

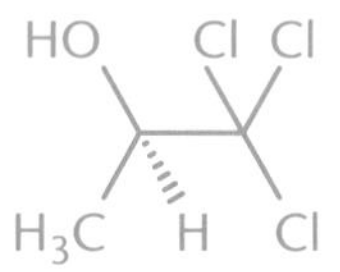

HO, Cl Cl, H_3C, H, Cl

A. Racemic alanine
B. R-alanine
C. S-alanine
D. Glycine

5. Which of the statements below is NOT true about protein denaturation?

A. Sonication affects hydrogen bonds.
B. Changing pH affects ionic attractive forces.
C. CNBr affects methionine residues.
D. Urea affects noncovalent bonds.

Part II
Practice Sections

INSTRUCTIONS FOR TAKING THE PRACTICE SECTIONS

Before taking each Practice Section, find a quiet place where you can work uninterrupted. Take a maximum of 70 minutes per section (52 questions) to get accustomed to the length and scope.

Keep in mind that the actual MCAT will not feature a section made up of Organic Chemistry questions alone, but rather a Biological Sciences section made up of both Organic Chemistry and Biology questions. Use the following three sections to hone your Organic Chemistry skills.

Good luck!

PRACTICE SECTION 1

Time—70 minutes

QUESTIONS 1–52

Directions: Most of the questions in the following Organic Chemistry Practice Section are organized into groups, with a descriptive passage preceding each group of questions. Study the passage, then select the single-best answer to the question in each group. Some of the questions are not based on a descriptive passage; you must also select the best answer to these questions. If you are unsure of the best answer, eliminate the choices that you know are incorrect, then select an answer from the choices that remain.

Period	1 IA 1A	2 IIA 2A	3 IIIB 3B	4 IVB 4B	5 VB 5B	6 VIB 6B	7 VIIB 7B	8	9 VIII 8	10	11 IB 1B	12 IIB 2B	13 IIIA 3A	14 IVA 4A	15 VA 5A	16 VIA 6A	17 VIIA 7A	18 vIIIA 8A
1	1 H 1.008																	2 He 4.003
2	3 Li 6.941	4 Be 9.012											5 B 10.81	6 C 12.01	7 N 14.01	8 O 16.00	9 F 19.00	10 Ne 20.18
3	11 Na 22.99	12 Mg 24.31											13 Al 26.98	14 Si 28.09	15 P 30.97	16 S 32.07	17 Cl 35.45	18 Ar 39.95
4	19 K 39.10	20 Ca 40.08	21 Sc 44.96	22 Ti 47.88	23 V 50.94	24 Cr 52.00	25 Mn 54.94	26 Fe 55.85	27 Co 58.47	28 Ni 58.69	29 Cu 63.55	30 Zn 65.39	31 Ga 69.72	32 Ge 72.59	33 As 74.92	34 Se 78.96	35 Br 79.90	36 Kr 83.80
5	37 Rb 85.47	38 Sr 87.62	39 Y 88.91	40 Zr 91.22	41 Nb 92.91	42 Mo 95.94	43 Tc (98)	44 Ru 101.1	45 Rh 102.9	46 Pd 106.4	47 Ag 107.9	48 Cd 112.4	49 In 114.8	50 Sn 118.7	51 Sb 121.8	52 Te 127.6	53 I 126.9	54 Xe 131.3
6	55 Cs 132.9	56 Ba 137.3	57 La* 138.9	72 Hf 178.5	73 Ta 180.9	74 W 183.9	75 Re 186.2	76 Os 190.2	77 Ir 190.2	78 Pt 195.1	79 Au 197.0	80 Hg 200.5	81 Tl 204.4	82 Pb 207.2	83 Bi 209.0	84 Po (210)	85 At (210)	86 Rn (222)
7	87 Fr (223)	88 Ra (226)	89 Ac~ (227)	104 Rf (257)	105 Db (260)	106 Sg (263)	107 Bh (262)	108 Hs (265)	109 Mt (266)	110 --- 0	111 --- 0	112 --- 0		114 --- 0		116 --- 0		118 --- 0

Series														
Lanthanide Series*	58 Ce 140.1	59 Pr 140.9	60 Nd 144.2	61 Pm (147)	62 Sm 150.4	63 Eu 152.0	64 Gd 157.3	65 Tb 158.9	66 Dy 162.5	67 Ho 164.9	68 Er 167.3	69 Tm 168.9	70 Yb 173.0	71 Lu 175.0
Actinide Series~	90 Th 232.0	91 Pa (231)	92 U (238)	93 Np (237)	94 Pu (242)	95 Am (243)	96 Cm (247)	97 Bk (247)	98 Cf (249)	99 Es (254)	100 Fm (253)	101 Md (256)	102 No (254)	103 Lr (257)

PASSAGE I (QUESTIONS 1–7)

Alcohols and ethers are functional groups that can also be thought of as substituted water molecules. When one hydrogen of water is replaced with a hydrocarbon, it becomes an alcohol and when both are substituted, the molecule becomes an ether. When substitution of water yields an alcohol, the result is a polar molecule capable of hydrogen bonding in solutions, but its polarity and ability to form hydrogen bonds decrease as the length of hydrocarbon increases. Ethers, in contrast, are relatively nonpolar and the hydrogen bonds that they form are too weak to appreciably affect their boiling points. The reactivity of alcohols is influenced by the electron-releasing property of carbons and electron withdrawing power of halides attached to the hydrocarbon.

1. Which of the following is the best example of a dehydration reaction through a carbonium ion?

A. $H_3C\text{–}CH_2CH_2CH_2\text{–}OH \xrightarrow{HCl} H_3C\text{–}CH=CH\text{–}CH_3$

B. $H_3C\text{–}CH_2CH_2CH_2\text{–}OH \xrightarrow[H_2SO_4]{NaBr} H_3C\text{–}CH_2CH_2CH_2\text{–}Br$

C. $H_3C\text{–}CH_2\text{–}OH \xrightarrow[\Delta]{Cu} H_3C\text{–}CH=O$ (H)

D. $H_3C\text{–}CH_2CH_2CH_2\text{–}Cl \xrightarrow{KOH} H_3C\text{–}CH_2\text{–}CH=CH_2$ (H, H)

2. Which of the following structures is most amenable to O–H bond cleavage by active metals?

A. $CH_3-CH_2-C(CH_3)(H)-OH$

B. $CH_3-CH_2-C(CH_3)(CH_3)-OH$

C. CH_3OH

D. $CH_3CH_2CH_2-OH$

3. Which of the following compounds would react to form a tertiary alcohol by the Grignard reaction?

A. $H-C(H)=O$

B. $CH_3-CH_2-C(H)=O$

C. $CH_3-C(CH_3)=O$

D. $CH_3-C(H)=O$

4. Which of the following compounds would be expected to have the highest boiling point?

A. $CH_3CH_2CH_2CH_2CH_3$
B. $CH_3CH_2\text{-O-}CH_2CH_3$
C. $CH_3CH_2CH_2Cl$
D. $CH_3CH_2CH_2OH$

5. In the presence of a hydrogen halide and acid, which substrate will undergo an S_N1 substitution reaction most rapidly?

A. CH_3-OH

B. CH_3CH_2OH

C. $CH_3-C(H)(OH)-CH_3$

D. $CH_3-C(CH_3)(OH)-CH_3$

6. Which of the following compounds is LEAST likely to be an intermediate in the synthesis of sec-butyl alcohol from ethanol and a Grignard reagent?

A. CH_3CH_2Br
B. CH_3CH_2MgBr
C. CH_3–$CH_2C(CH_3)$=O
D. CH_3CH_2–CH(OMgBr)CH_3

7. What halide compound will NOT form an ether with a Williamson synthesis?

A. CH_3Br

B. Br (bromobenzene)

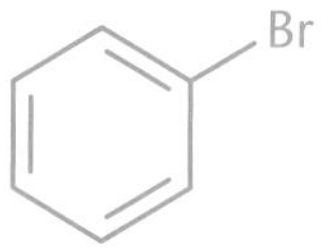

C. CH_2Br (benzyl bromide)

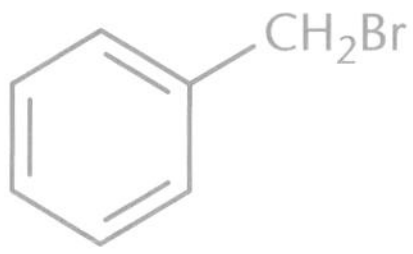

D. H_3C, CH_3, Br (2-bromopropane)

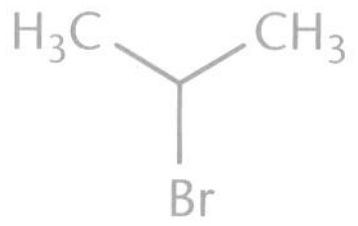

PASSAGE II (QUESTIONS 8–15)

A student investigates the substitution kinetics of two alkyl halides, shown in the figure below (reactions 1 and 2). He uses acetone as a solvent, and finds that the rate equation for both reactions is consistent with S_N2 kinetics. To his surprise, however, the stereochemistry in reaction 1 remains the same throughout the substitution, with no inversion occurring overall.

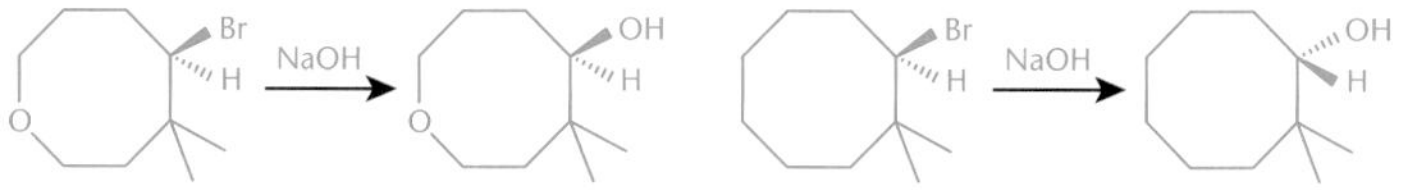

Br, H, O —NaOH→ OH, H, O

Reaction 1

Br, H —NaOH→ OH, H

Reaction 2

In a separate experiment, the student switches the solvent to isopropanol, and measures the kinetics of each reaction. He finds that the rate equation for both reactions is consistent with S_N1 kinetics. In addition to the usual S_N1 products, there are several additional products that result from alkyl group shifts. The rates of each substitution reaction are listed in the table below.

Reaction	Rate in Acetone (Ms^{-1})	Rate in Isopropanol (Ms^{-1})
1	2000	175
2	180	175

8. Which of the following is a suitable substitution for acetone?

A. O, N (N,N-dimethylacetamide)

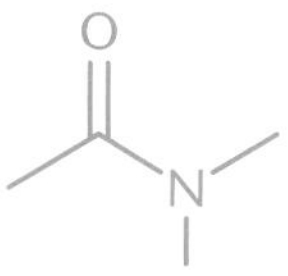

B. OH, O (propanoic acid)

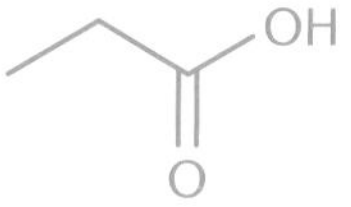

C. OH (cyclohexanol)

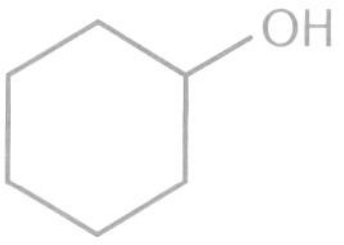

D. (benzene)

9. The student deduces that in the presence of acetone (reaction 1), the oxygen atom takes part in substitution as a separate nucleophile, before the addition of hydroxide. What is the correct sequence for the change in stereochemistry?

A. S to R to S
B. R to S to R
C. R to R to S
D. S to S to R

10. Which of the following correctly illustrates the intermediate formed from oxygen attack?

A.
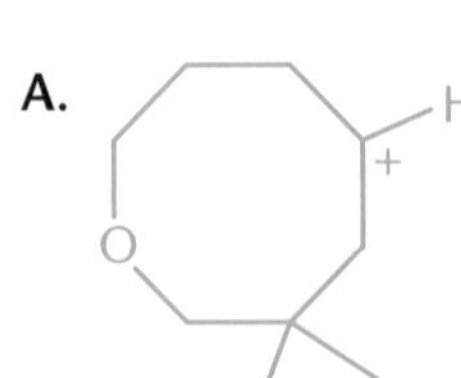

B.
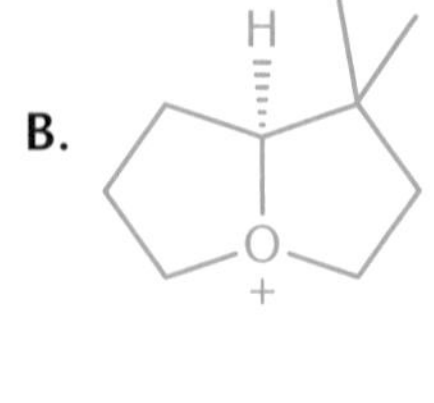

C.
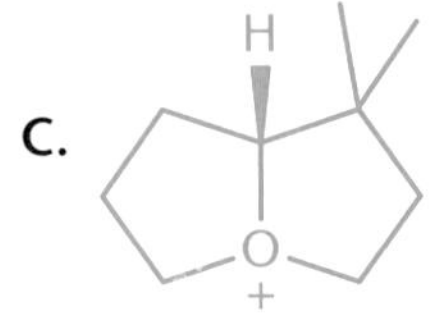

D.
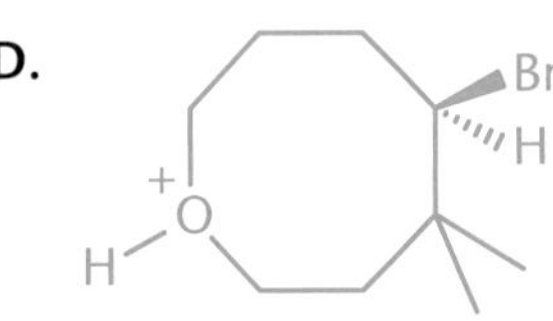

11. For reaction 2, why is the rate in acetone slightly faster than in isopropanol?

A. S_N2 reactions occur over two steps, while S_N1 reactions occur in one step.
B. S_N2 reactions occur in one step, while S_N1 reactions occur over two steps.
C. The presence of the oxygen atom speeds up reaction 2 in acetone.
D. The absence of the oxygen atom slows down reaction 2 in isopropanol.

12. Why are polar protic solvents preferred in S_N1 reactions?

A. The carbocation formed is stabilized by salvation.
B. The incoming nucleophile is stabilized by salvation.
C. The carbocation formed is stabilized by protons donated by the solvent.
D. The leaving group is destabilized by solvation.

13. Why does racemization occur during S_N1 reactions?

A. The incoming nucleophile racemizes the alkyl halide, before any substitution occurs.
B. The incoming nucleophile can attack from either side of the carbocation, which is sp^2-hybridized.
C. The incoming nucleophile can attack from either side of the carbocation, which is sp-hybridized.
D. The alkyl halide racemizes spontaneously before any reaction occurs.

14. What is the driving force for alkyl group shifts during S_N1 reactions?

A. Formation of secondary carbocations
B. Formation of primary carbocations
C. Formation of a stable tertiary radical
D. Formation of tertiary carbocations

15. Which of the following are possible S_N1 products from reactions 1 and 2?

I
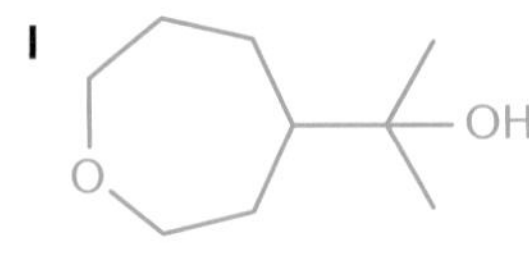

compound I

II

compound II

III

compound III

A. I only
B. II only
C. II and III
D. I and III

QUESTIONS 16–19 ARE NOT BASED ON A DESCRIPTIVE PASSAGE.

16. The cytosolic aspect of the eukaryotic cell membrane has which of the following chemical properties?

A. Hydrophilic
B. Hydrophobic
C. Nonpolar
D. Insoluble

17. Optically active compounds that rotate plane-polarized light counterclockwise are prefixed with

A. R.
B. S.
C. D.
D. L.

18. Which of the following compounds is a mirror image of itself?

A. Anomer
B. Epimer
C. Meso compound
D. Geometric isomer

19. What is the degree of unsaturation for a molecule with the molecular formula C20H40?

A. 24
B. 22
C. 28
D. 20

PASSAGE III (QUESTIONS 20–29)

Carbohydrates are one of the primary chemical classes that sustain life. Glucose provides energy for cellular respiration and metabolism. "Carbohydrates" is a term that includes both the simple sugars (monosaccharides) and linked monosaccharides (disaccharides and polysaccharides). Monosaccharides are polyhydroxy aldehydes, or polyhydroxy ketones, and are classified as trioses, tetroses, pentoses, and hexoses, according to the number of carbons in their structure. Monosaccharides can reduce Benedict's or Tollen's reagent and are therefore known as reducing sugars. However, reduction requires that the hemi-acetal or carbonyl group, for aldehydes or ketones, respectively, be in the free form.

20. Which set of descriptors is accurate for the monosaccharide structure shown below in its open and ring forms?

A. D aldose, pentose, pyranose ring, α anomer
B. D aldose, pentose, furanose ring, β anomer
C. L ketose, pentose, furanose ring, α anomer
D. L aldose, hexose, furanose ring, α anomer

21. In the open and ring structures in the previous question, which carbons are chiral centers in the open and ring forms, respectively?

A. C3 and C4; C3 and C4
B. C1, C3, and C4; C1, C3, C4 and C5
C. C3 and C4; C1, C3, and C4
D. C1, C2, and C5; C2, and C5

22. Which of the following structure(s) in Figure 2 are nonreducing sugars?

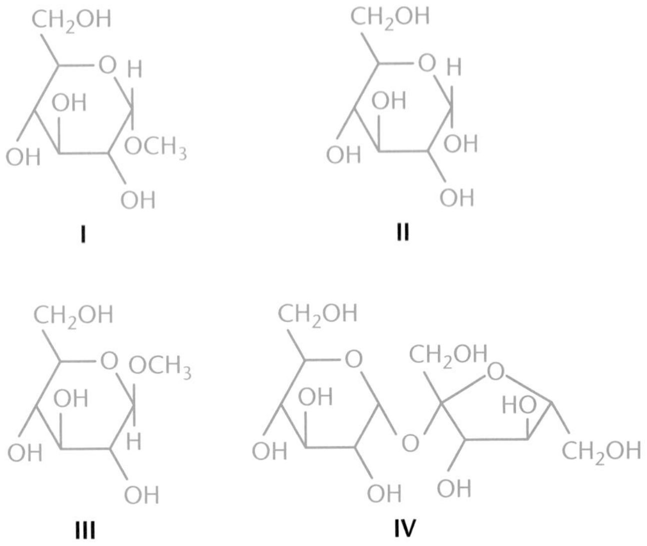

A. I
B. II, III
C. IV
D. I, III, and IV

23. Fehling's solution, Tollen's reagent, and bromine water will all oxidize glucose.

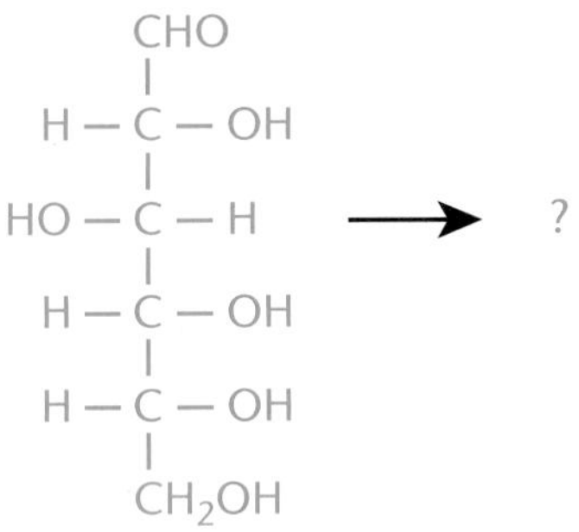

Figure 3

Which of the following structures shown in Figure 4 represents the only product produced by oxidizing glucose with bromine water?

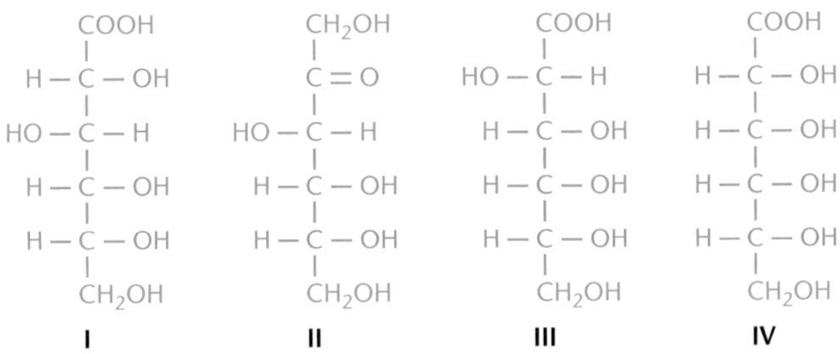

Figure 4

A. I
B. II
C. III
D. IV

24. Which sequence of treatments would yield the structure shown below from fructose?

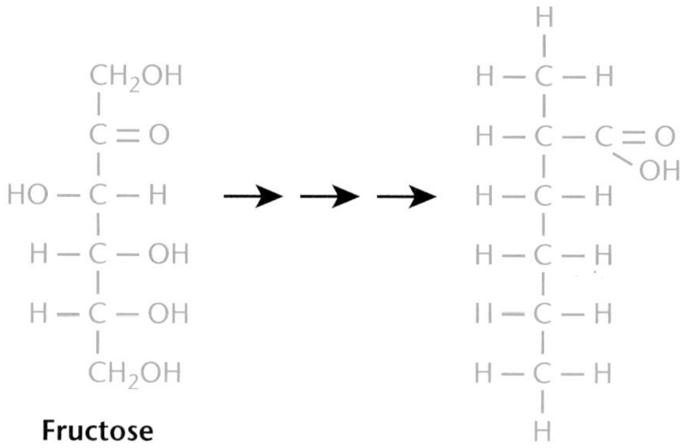

Fructose

A. Acetic anhydride → hydrolysis → HI, heat →
B. HCN → HI, heat → hydrolysis →
C. HCN → hydrolysis → HI, heat →
D. H_2, Ni → HI, heat →

25. What is observed, respectively, by 1) treating glucose with acetic anhydride, or 2) treating glucose with hydrogen and nickel, then with acetic anhydride?

A. 4 hydroxyl groups; 5 hydroxyl groups
B. 5 hydroxyl groups; 4 hydroxyl groups
C. 5 carbonyl groups; 6 hydroxyl groups
D. 1 carbonyl group; 4 hydroxyl groups

26. Which of the compounds shown below will NOT form the same structure as the other three upon treatment with phenylhydrazine followed by warm acid?

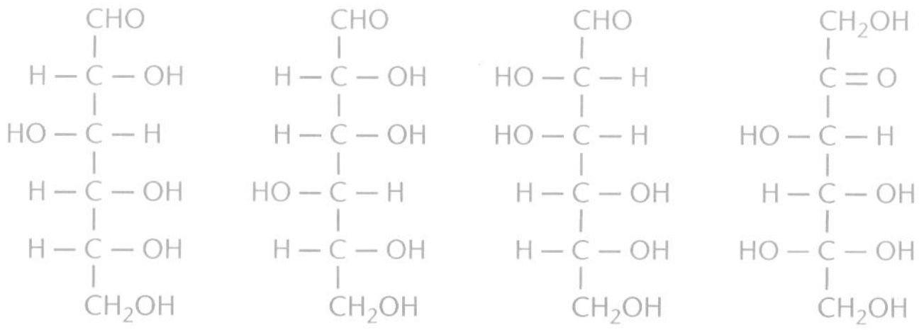

I Glucose, II Gulose, III Mannose, IV Fructose

A. I
B. II
C. III
D. IV

27. Which of the following statements is true of the ATP molecule shown below?

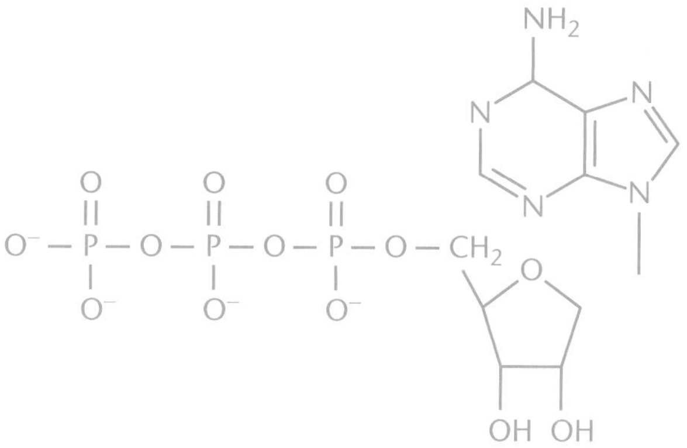

Adenosine Triphosphate (ATP)

A. ATP is a glycoside.
B. ATP is a sugar ester.
C. It has a phosphodiester linkage.
D. A and B only

28. The phosphodiester linkage between sugars in DNA is relatively resistant to alkaline hydrolysis compared to the similar linkage in RNA. Which of the factors below contributes to this fact?

A. The triphosphate is a triprotic acid.
B. The –OH group on C2 of ribose can be attacked by an unbound –OH group on the triphosphate.
C. The lack of an –OH group on C2 of deoxyribose removes a target for rearrangement of the triphosphate ester linkage.
D. All of the above

29. What product is expected after treatment of β-D-(+)-glucose with methanol and HCl?

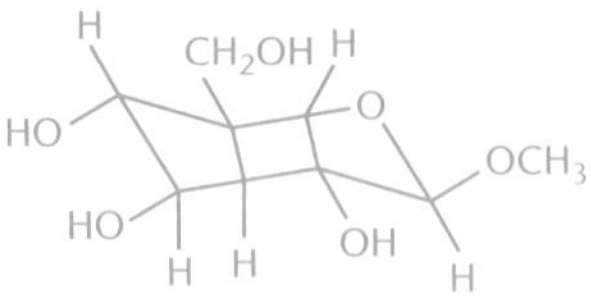

I 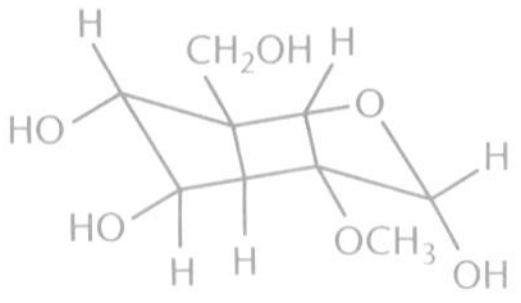 II 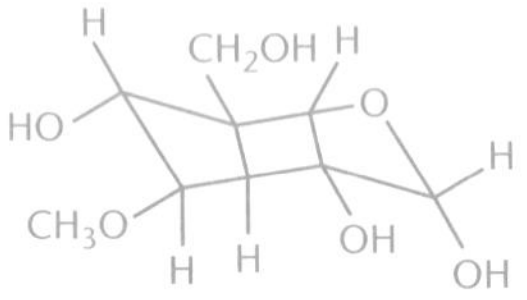 III 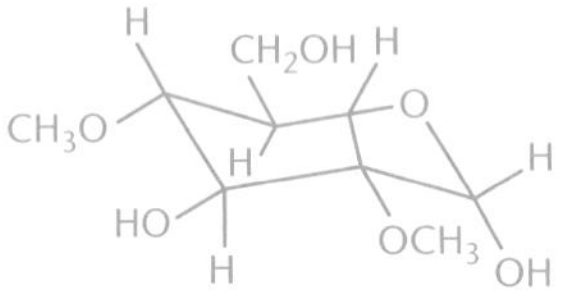 IV

A. I
B. II
C. III
D. IV

QUESTIONS 30–32 ARE NOT BASED ON A DESCRIPTIVE PASSAGE.

30. Which of the following halogens, if reacted with isobutane in the presence of light, will produce a compound with a tertiary carbon?

A. Fluorine
B. Bromine
C. Chlorine
D. Iodine

31. Alcohols most commonly react via bimolecular nucleophilic substitution.

Which of the following does NOT describe this type of reaction?

I. The rate-limiting step has a molecularity of two.
II. The reaction produces a racemic mixture of products.
III. An inversion of absolute configuration occurs

A. I and II only
B. II and III only
C. II only
D. I, II, and III

32. Which of the following will most readily react with an amine to form an amide?

A. Acyl chloride
B. Ester
C. Carboxylic acid
D. Acid anhydride

PASSAGE IV (QUESTIONS 33–39)

The citric acid cycle, or Kreb's cycle, is an enzymatic pathway that is important for cellular respiration. An integral part of the electron transport chain, the enzymes in this pathway combine pyruvate, the product from glycolysis, with oxaloacetate to form citrate, which is degraded back to oxaloacetate through a series of reactions. The energy from these reactions is used to generate high-energy molecules such as ATP and NADH or NADPH. The products of the citric acid cycle include several mono-, di- and tricarboxylic acids, including citric acid, succinic acid, and oxaloacetic acid.

The citric acid cycle is found in various organisms from humans to bacteria, though there are differences in the structure of the intermediates. Herbicides and pesticides have been designed to take advantage of these differences to inhibit the citric acid cycle. Some of these inhibitors are shown below.

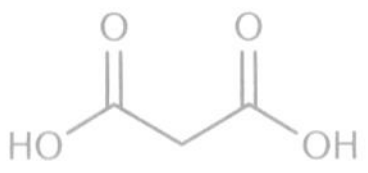

Malonic acid 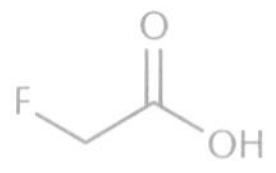 Fluoroacetic acid 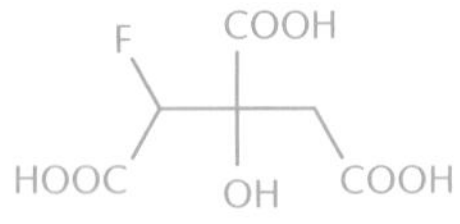 Fluorocitric acid

Various physical and chemical properties have been determined for intermediates of the citric acid cycle as well as for putative inhibitors. Elucidation of these properties is important for chemical and biological applications.

33. Which of the following can most effectively synthesize malonic acid from acetic acid?

A. Br_2/PBr_3, then NaCN, and finally aqueous acid
B. Excess methanol in aqueous acid
C. Base, followed by formic acid, then acid neutralization
D. $KMnO_4$

34. Although there are known inhibitors of the citric acid cycle, the pH of mitochondrial matrix can alter the charges on various carboxylic acids, based on the pH, which may have an affect on the rate of the reactions taking place within the cycle. Which of the following pairs incorrectly describes their relative acidities?

A. O OH < O OH O_2N

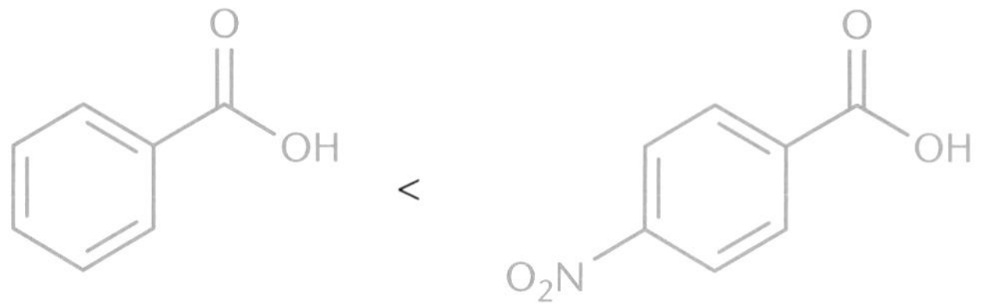

B. O OH < O OH H_3CO

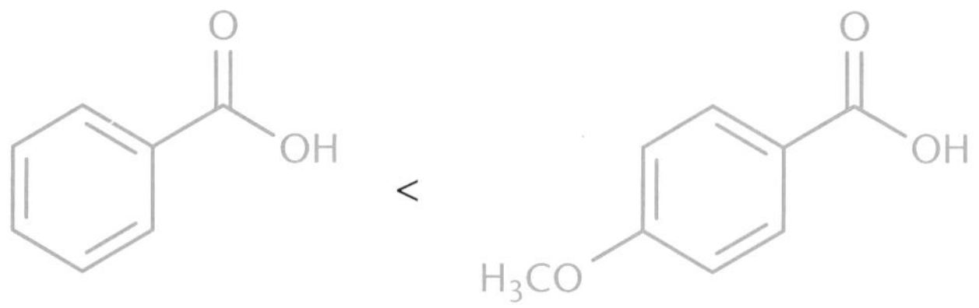

C. O OH > O OH H_3C

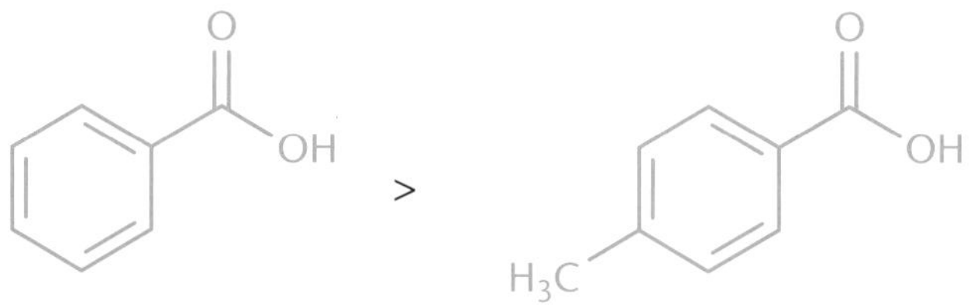

D. O OH Cl > O OH Cl

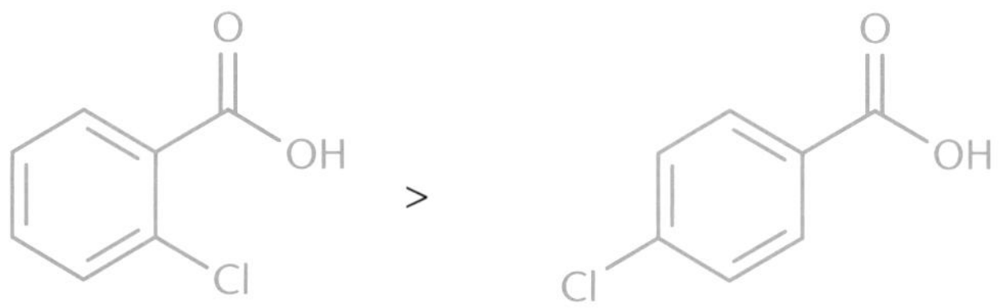

35. Isocitric acid (below) is one of the intermediates of the citric acid cycle. Which of the following names is the correct IUPAC name for isocitric acid?

A. O CH_3 O H_3C CH_3 CH_3

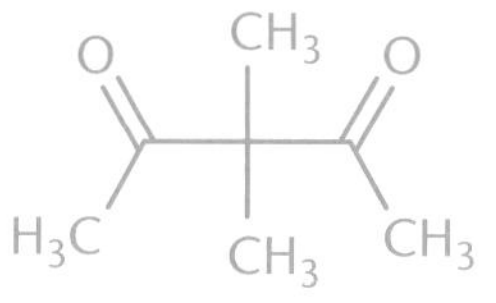

B. O H_3C CH_3

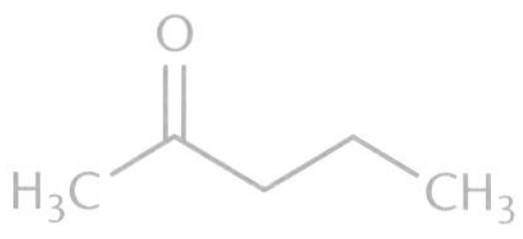

C. O O H_3C CH_3

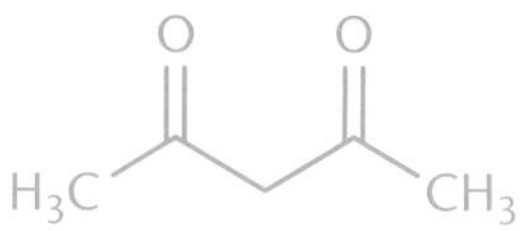

D. O O H_3C CH_3

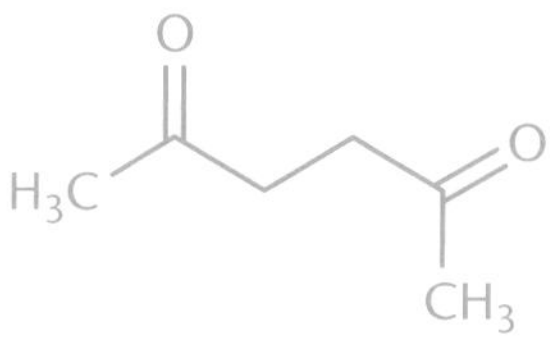

A. Tricarboxyl-2-pentanol
B. 2-hydroxy-3-carboxypentadicarboxylic acid
C. 1-hydroxypropane-1,2,3-tricarboxylic acid
D. 2-hydroxy-3-oxo-pentadicarboxylic acid

36. Which of the following statements is NOT correct?

A. Fluoroacetic acid is more acidic than chloroacetic acid is.
B. Trifluoroacetic acid is more acidic than fluoroacetic acid is.
C. Succinic acid ($HOOCCH_2CH_2COOH$) is more acidic than malonic acid is.
D. 2-fluorobutanoic acid is more acidic than 4-fluorobutanoic acid is.

37. Which of the following reactions described below is unlikely to occur in the presence of heat?

A. 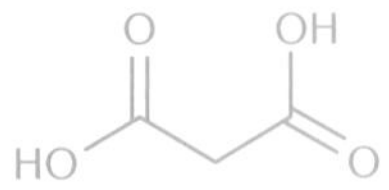 forms a monocarboxylic acid

B. 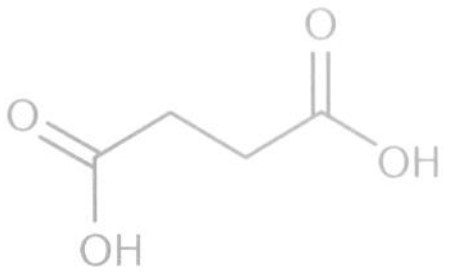 forms a cyclic compound

C. 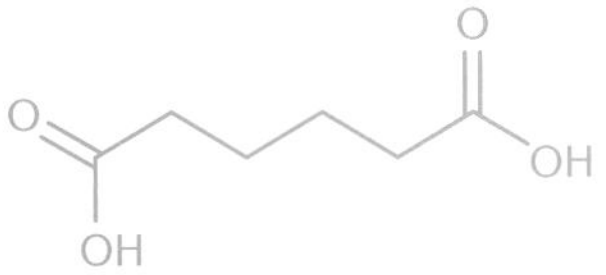 forms a cyclic compound

D. 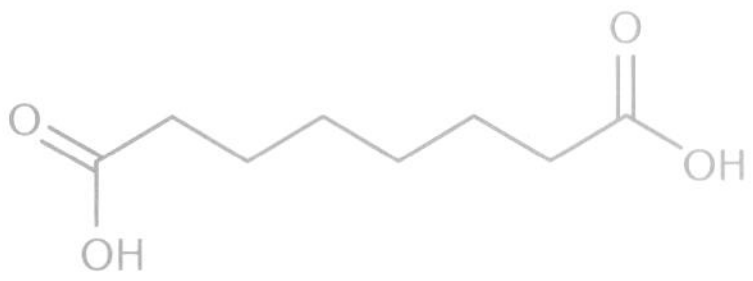 forms a cyclic compound

38. Adipic acid and succinic acid can be synthesized from tetrahydrofuran (below). Which of the following statements is NOT true of these syntheses?

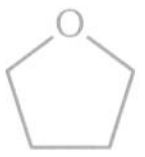

THF 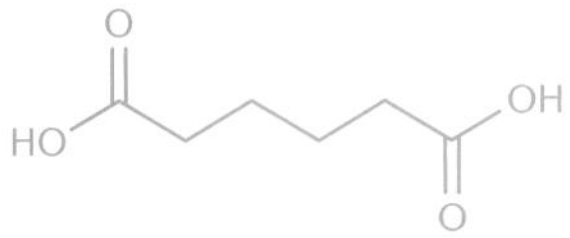   Adipic acid 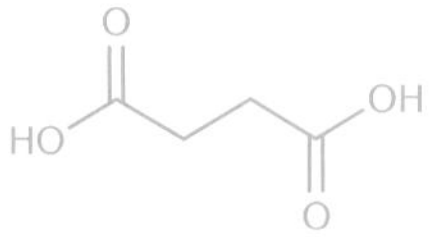   Succinic acid

A. THF is treated with concentrated HI.
B. There is an oxidation step in the synthesis of adipic acid.
C. There is dicarbonation in the synthesis of adipic acid.
D. A diol intermediate forms in the synthesis of succinic acid.

39. A bacterium is found to have an enzyme that cleaves fluorocitric acid into fluoroacetic acid and oxaloacetate. Which of the following is the simplest mechanism leading to cleavage?

A. Removing hydrogen from the alcohol group
B. Nucleophilic attack by threonine side chain on carbonyl carbon
C. Nucleophilic attack by cysteine side chain on carbonyl carbon
D. Fluoride ion acting as nucleophile

PASSAGE V (QUESTIONS 40–46)

Without the aid of spectroscopy or polarimetry, Emil Fischer was able to determine the absolute structure of glucose using several simple reactions. One of these reactions, the *Ruff degradation*, shortens aldoses by removing the aldehyde group as carbon dioxide via oxidation to carboxylic acids (Figure 1). Sugars can also be oxidized to aldaric acids in the presence of nitric acid (Figure 2). Fischer also developed a method of interchanging the end groups of any sugar without affecting the stereochemistry of the other chiral centers (Figure 3). Finally, the *Kiliani-Fischer synthesis* lengthens a sugar molecule by one carbon atom (Figure 4).

$$\text{CHO}-(\text{CHOH})_n-\text{CH}_2\text{OH} \xrightarrow[\text{2. } H_2O_2,\ Fe_2(SO_4)_3]{\text{1. } Br_2,\ H_2O} \text{CHO}-(\text{CHOH})_{n-1}-\text{CH}_2\text{OH} + CO_2$$

Figure 1

$$\text{CHO}-(\text{CHOH})_n-\text{CH}_2\text{OH} \xrightarrow{HNO_3} CO_2H-(\text{CHOH})_n-CO_2H$$

Figure 2

$$\text{CHO}-(\text{CHOH})_n-\text{CH}_2\text{OH} \xrightarrow{\text{Several steps}} \text{CH}_2\text{OH}-(\text{CHOH})_n-\text{CHO}$$

Figure 3

$$\text{CHO}-(\text{CHOH})_n-\text{CH}_2\text{OH} \xrightarrow[\text{2. } H_3O^+]{\text{1. HCN}} \text{CHO}-(\text{CHOH})_{n+1}-\text{CH}_2\text{OH}$$

Figure 4

Before determining the structure of glucose, Fischer knew that glucose is an optically active aldohexose that can be degraded to D-(+)-glyceraldehyde. Fischer also devised a two-dimensional representation of three-dimensional molecules, now known as the Fischer projection, which is particularly useful for describing sugars and their derivatives, by readily providing stereochemical information.

40. What is the IUPAC name for D-(+)-glyceraldehyde, shown below?

CHO
H —+— OH
CH₂OH

A. (2R)-2,3-Dihydroxypropanal
B. (2R)-1,2-Dihydroxypropan-3-al
C. (2S)-1,2-Dihydroxypropan-3-al
D. (2S)-2,3-Dihydroxypropanal

41. Ruff degradation of D-(+)-glucose and D-(+)-mannose gives the same aldopentose (D-(-)-arabinose). Which of the following does this suggest?

A. Glucose and mannose are enantiomers.
B. Glucose and mannose are C3 epimers.
C. Glucose and mannose are C2 epimers.
D. Glucose and mannose are identical.

42. To differentiate between glucose and mannose, Fischer interchanges the end groups of those sugars (Figure 3). When this reaction is performed on D-(+)-mannose, the product is again D-(+)-mannose; which of the following sugars is D-(+)-mannose?

A.
CHO
H —+— OH
H —+— OH
HO —+— H
HO —+— H
CH_2OH

B.
CHO
H —+— OH
HO —+— H
H —+— OH
HO —+— H
CH_2OH

C.
CHO
H —+— OH
HO —+— H
H —+— OH
H —+— OH
CH_2OH

D.
CHO
HO —+— H
HO —+— H
H —+— OH
H —+— OH
CH_2OH

43. Suppose that when performing the reaction shown in Figure 1, the reagents in step 1 are replaced by HNO_3. What is the most likely change observed in the product?

A. The functional groups on either end will be switched.
B. The products are two smaller carboxylic acids.
C. The product contains two fewer carbon atoms than the reactant.
D. The product is optically inactive, since all the –OH group is oxidized.

44. A Kiliani-Fischer synthesis is performed on D-(+)-glyceraldehyde. Which of the molecules below correctly illustrates the intermediate after step 1?

A. CN / HO—H / H—OH / CH_2OH

B. CH_2NH_2 / HO—H / H—OH / CH_2OH

C. H, NH / HO—H / H—OH / CH_2OH

D. CH_2CN / H—OH / CH_2OH

45. When a Kiliani-Fischer synthesis is performed on D-(+)-glyceraldehyde, there are two tetroses possible. What is the relationship between them?

A. They are enantiomers.
B. They are structural isomers.
C. They are geometric isomers.
D. They are diastereomers.

46. Suppose that instead of D-sugars, L-sugars are the most common naturally occurring sugars. How does this affect the optical rotation of the corresponding aldohexoses?

A. The optical rotation of the L-sugars has the same magnitude as D-sugars, but they have opposite signs.
B. The optical rotation of the L-sugars is twice the magnitude of D-sugars, but they have the same sign.
C. The optical rotation of the L-sugars has the same magnitude and sign as the D-sugars.
D. There is no correlation between optical rotation and L/D designations.

PASSAGE VI (QUESTIONS 47–52)

Carbon is one of the most abundant elements on Earth and is a major component of all organisms. Carbon has four valence electrons available for bonding, making it possible for carbon to join with an array of other elements to potentially form an infinite number of compounds. For these reasons, the analysis and synthesis of carbon-based compounds plays a key role in the pharmaceutical industry.

Morgan and colleagues are attempting to develop a new drug with analgesic and antipyretic properties, which will out-compete those currently on the market. To do this, they have developed several structures in an attempt to increase the absorption rate of the ingested drug. The drug designers hope that the added hydroxyl and carbonyl groups will allow for increased hydrogen bonding with polar water molecules inside the human body. If this is the case, then perhaps it will be easier for the drug to cross biological barriers, such as the lumen of the stomach, and be carried in the blood to its targets.

Drug A

Drug B

47. Despite having different structures, drugs A and B shown below have a common feature on their IR spectra. Which of the following is a correct description of that feature?

A. Both drugs have an absorption band at 2,200 cm^{-1}.
B. Both drugs have a broad absorption centered at 3,500 cm^{-1}.
C. Both drugs have a characteristic double absorption band at 2,850 and 2,750 cm^{-1}.
D. Both drugs have a large overtone that spans 3,500 to 2,500 cm^{-1}.

48. What is the correct electron configuration for carbon?

A. $1s^2\ 2s^2\ 2p^2$
B. $1s^2\ 2s^2$
C. $1s^2\ 2s^2\ 2p^6\ 3s^2\ 3p^2$
D. $1s^2\ 2s^2\ 2p^6$

49. How would one best describe the overlap of orbitals that is required to form pi bonds seen in the structure of both drugs?

A. Parallel overlap of two s orbitals
B. Overlap of one s and one p orbital
C. Perpendicular overlap of two p orbitals
D. Parallel overlap of two p orbitals

50. For each hydrogenation reaction below, energy is released per double bond reduced. In which reaction will the energy per double bond be most negative?

A.

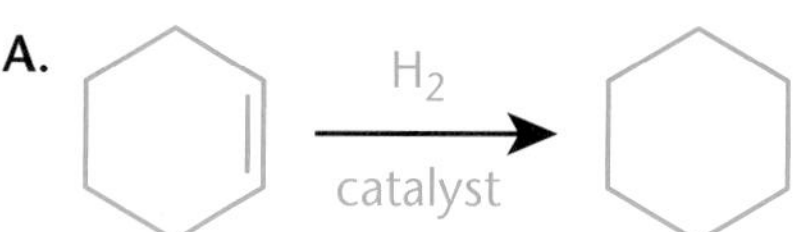

B.

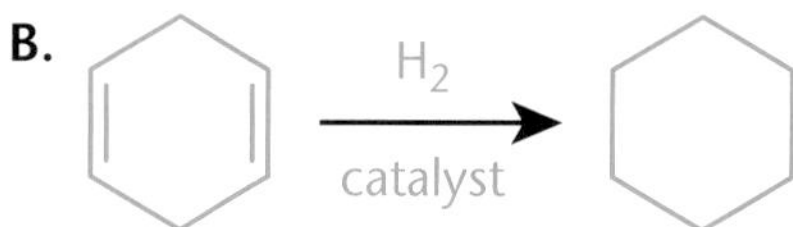

C.

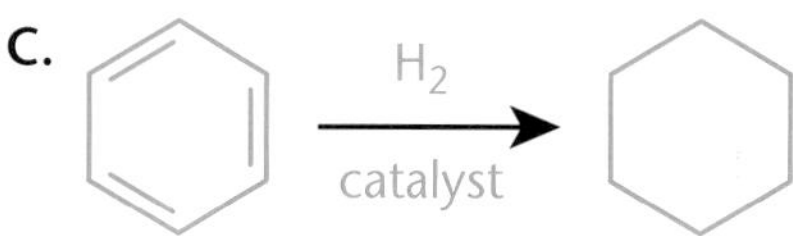

D. The energy is always equal for each individual double bond.

51. While attempting to manufacture drug A, a chemist isolates an impurity. He analyzes the molecule in order to determine the structure of several bonds in question. An image of the molecule can be seen below.

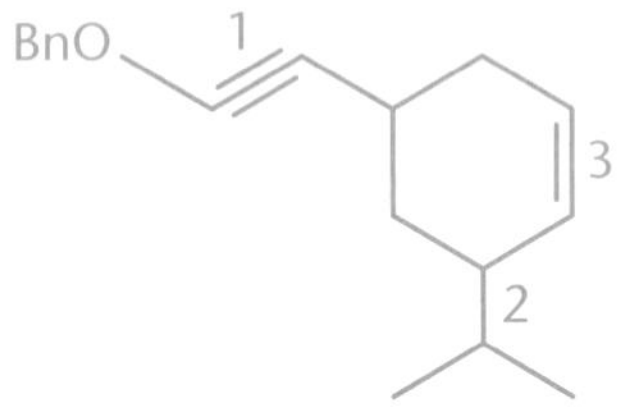

Which of the following is most likely true?

A. The bond lengths increase in the order of 2<3<1, while the bond strengths increase in the order of 1<3<2.

B. The bond lengths decrease in the order of 2>3>1, while the bond strengths decrease in the order of 1>3>2.

C. The bond lengths increase in the order of 1<3<2, while the bond strengths increase in the order of 1<3<2.

D. The bond lengths decrease in the order of 2>3>1, while the bond strengths increase in the order of 1<3<2.

52. A chemist hopes to create a method of deactivating the drugs in order to prevent their quick absorption through the lumen of the stomach. Which of the following treatments should he investigate as a basis for this task?

A. Hydrogenation (H_2 over Pd)

B. Forming methyl esters from all the carboxylic acid groups present

C. Reduction with $LiAlH_4$

D. Substitution with $SOCl_2$

PRACTICE SECTION 2

Time—70 minutes

QUESTIONS 1–52

Directions: Most of the questions in the following Organic Chemistry Practice Section are organized into groups, with a descriptive passage preceding each group of questions. Study the passage, then select the single-best answer to the question in each group. Some of the questions are not based on a descriptive passage; you must also select the best answer to these questions. If you are unsure of the best answer, eliminate the choices that you know are incorrect, then select an answer from the choices that remain.

Period	1 IA 1A	2 IIA 2A	3 IIIB 3B	4 IVB 4B	5 VB 5B	6 VIB 6B	7 VIIB 7B	8	9 VIII 8	10	11 IB 1B	12 IIB 2B	13 IIIA 3A	14 IVA 4A	15 VA 5A	16 VIA 6A	17 VIIA 7A	18 vIIIA 8A
1	1 H 1.008																	2 He 4.003
2	3 Li 6.941	4 Be 9.012											5 B 10.81	6 C 12.01	7 N 14.01	8 O 16.00	9 F 19.00	10 Ne 20.18
3	11 Na 22.99	12 Mg 24.31											13 Al 26.98	14 Si 28.09	15 P 30.97	16 S 32.07	17 Cl 35.45	18 Ar 39.95
4	19 K 39.10	20 Ca 40.08	21 Sc 44.96	22 Ti 47.88	23 V 50.94	24 Cr 52.00	25 Mn 54.94	26 Fe 55.85	27 Co 58.47	28 Ni 58.69	29 Cu 63.55	30 Zn 65.39	31 Ga 69.72	32 Ge 72.59	33 As 74.92	34 Se 78.96	35 Br 79.90	36 Kr 83.80
5	37 Rb 85.47	38 Sr 87.62	39 Y 88.91	40 Zr 91.22	41 Nb 92.91	42 Mo 95.94	43 Tc (98)	44 Ru 101.1	45 Rh 102.9	46 Pd 106.4	47 Ag 107.9	48 Cd 112.4	49 In 114.8	50 Sn 118.7	51 Sb 121.8	52 Te 127.6	53 I 126.9	54 Xe 131.3
6	55 Cs 132.9	56 Ba 137.3	57 La* 138.9	72 Hf 178.5	73 Ta 180.9	74 W 183.9	75 Re 186.2	76 Os 190.2	77 Ir 190.2	78 Pt 195.1	79 Au 197.0	80 Hg 200.5	81 Tl 204.4	82 Pb 207.2	83 Bi 209.0	84 Po (210)	85 At (210)	86 Rn (222)
7	87 Fr (223)	88 Ra (226)	89 Ac~ (227)	104 Rf (257)	105 Db (260)	106 Sg (263)	107 Bh (262)	108 Hs (265)	109 Mt (266)	110 --- ()	111 --- ()	112 --- ()		114 --- ()		116 --- ()		118 --- ()

Lanthanide Series*	58 Ce 140.1	59 Pr 140.9	60 Nd 144.2	61 Pm (147)	62 Sm 150.4	63 Eu 152.0	64 Gd 157.3	65 Tb 158.9	66 Dy 162.5	67 Ho 164.9	68 Er 167.3	69 Tm 168.9	70 Yb 173.0	71 Lu 175.0
Actinide Series~	90 Th 232.0	91 Pa (231)	92 U (238)	93 Np (237)	94 Pu (242)	95 Am (243)	96 Cm (247)	97 Bk (247)	98 Cf (249)	99 Es (254)	100 Fm (253)	101 Md (256)	102 No (254)	103 Lr (257)

PASSAGE I (QUESTIONS 1–8)

The Wieland-Miescher ketone (Figure 1) is one of the most versatile building blocks in synthetic chemistry, found in the synthesis of many natural products, a majority of which are medically relevant. These products have diverse applications and include compounds ranging from antimicrobial to anticancer agents. The Wieland-Miescher ketone is prepared from two other commonly used building blocks, shown below, via a Robinson annulation.

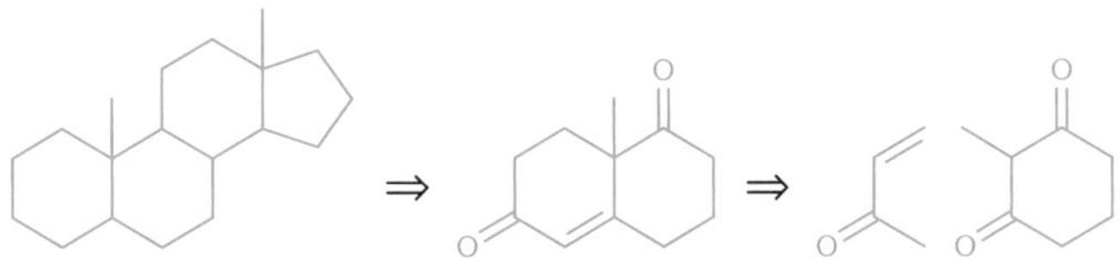

Androstane ⇒ Wieland-Miescher ketone ⇒ I II

Figure 1

One of the earliest uses of the Wieland-Miescher ketone was in the synthesis of steroids, because it contains two of the four rings in the steroid skeleton. An example is the synthesis of androstane, the steroid hydrocarbon backbone, accessible from two other precursor molecules (compounds III and V; Figures 2 and 3).

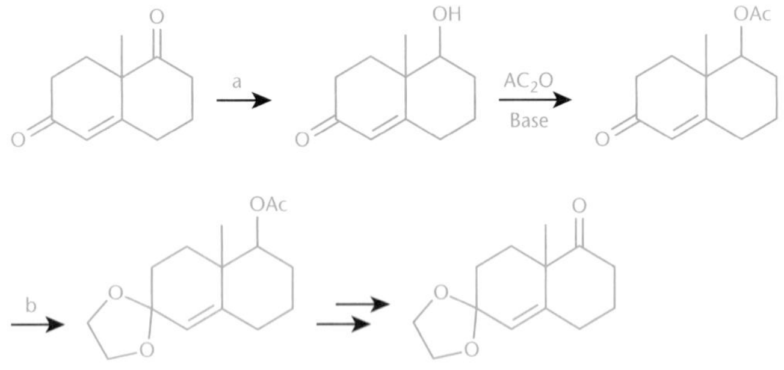

O → a → OH → AC_2O, Base → OAc → b → OAc → O

Figure 2

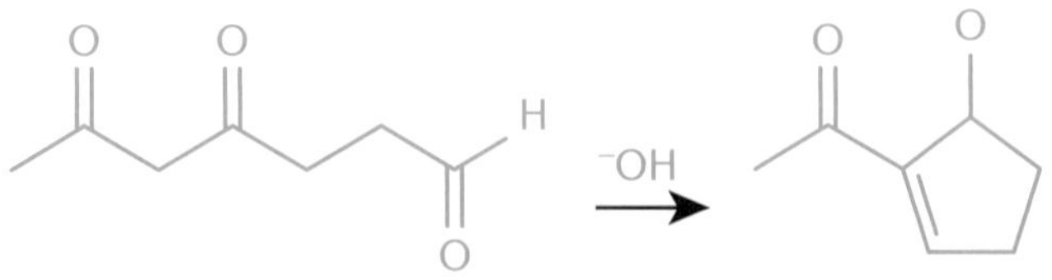

IV → ^{-}OH → V

Figure 3

1. What is the IUPAC name of compound I?

   A. 3-buten-2-one
   B. 1-buten-3-one
   C. Vinyl methyl ketone
   D. 2-buten-2-one

2. Which of the following can selectively reduce the ketone shown in reaction a in Figure 2?

   A. $LiAlH_4$
   B. Ag_2O
   C. $NaBH_4$
   D. H_2NNH_2

3. After formation of the ester, the remaining ketone needs to be protected (reaction b). Which of the following converts the ketone to the acetal shown in Figure 2?

   A. 2 CH_3OH, H_3O^+
   B. $HOCH_2CH_2OH$, H_2O
   C. 2 C_2H_5OH, H_3O^+
   D. $HOCH_2CH_2OH$, H_3O^+

4. What is the IUPAC name of compound IV?

   A. 3,5-dioxohexanal
   B. 4,7-oxoheptan-2-one
   C. 4,6-dioxoheptanal
   D. 1,4, 6-trioxoheptane

5. Which enol of compound IV contributes to the formation of compound V?

   A. 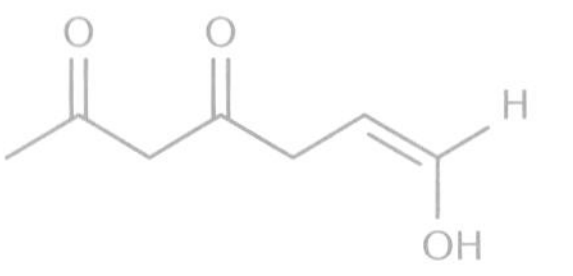 B. 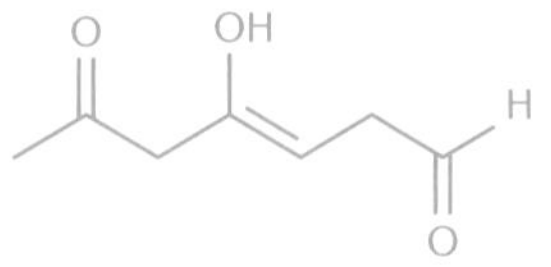 C. 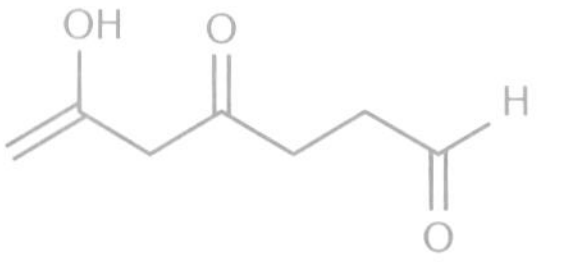 D.

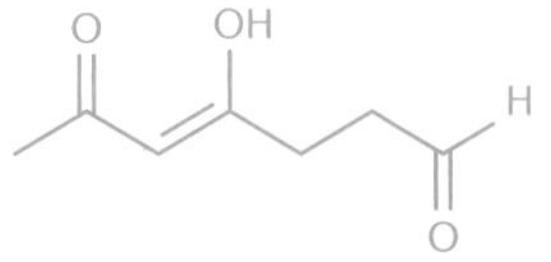

6. In the figure below, what reaction is occurring in the coupling between compounds III and V to form the steroid backbone?

A. Ketal formation
B. Robinson annulation
C. Wolff-Kishner reduction
D. Michael addition

7. What reagent is used to deprotect the ketone (reaction d) shown in Figure 4?

A. H_2O_2
B. NaOH
C. H_3O^+
D. CrO_3

8. The final step to forming androstane involves the complete reduction of all the ketone groups present (reaction e). Which of the following reagents can be used?

A. Hg(Zn), HCl
B. $(C_6H_5)_3P{=}CH_2$
C. Ag_2O
D. HCN

PASSAGE II (QUESTIONS 9–15)

Salicylic acid (Figure 1a) is an important precursor in the synthesis of various pharmaceuticals, artificial flavors, and preservatives. It is formed when sodium phenolate is combined with carbon dioxide under heat and pressure, in the presence of a base. Both its carboxyl and hydroxyl groups have proven useful targets for synthetic modification. For example, the hydroxyl group of salicylic acid reacts with acetic acid to form acetylsalicylic acid, better known as aspirin. The versatility of salicylic acid is further demonstrated by the ease with which the carboxyl group forms esters with various alcohols. Some esters of salicylic acid produce molecules that absorb UV light for use in suntan lotions, while other esters are used as antiseptic and antipyretic agents. In addition to esters, amides that are formed from salicylic acid have been shown to have practical applications. A family of compounds related to salicylanilide (Figure 1b) consists of salicylic acid-related amides in which one or more hydrogen atoms are replaced by a benzene ring. Brominated salicylanilides are used as disinfectants with antibacterial and antifungal activities. Some salicylanilide derivatives are used as pesticides while others, like oxyclozanide and rafoxanide, have antihelminthic properties.

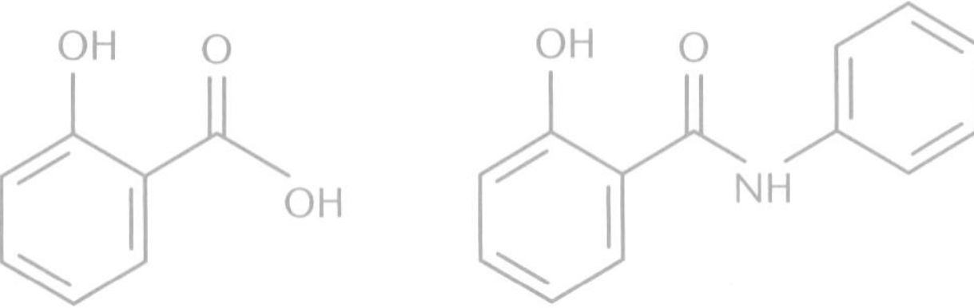

Figure 1a **Figure 1b**

A compound that is structurally related to salicylanilide and salicylic acid is acetanilide (Figure 2a). Acetanilide has antipyretic and analgesic properties and was previously marketed under the brand name Antifebrin. The well-known analgesic acetaminophen (Figure 2b) differs from acetanilide by only one hydroxyl group.

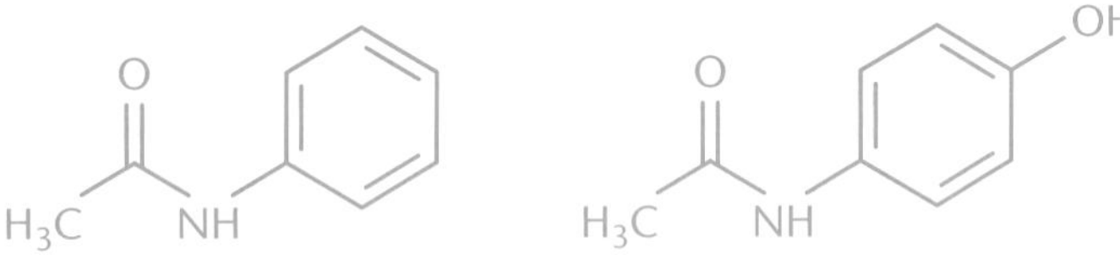

Figure 2a **Figure 2b**

9. Using a purified enzyme preparation, a scientist discovers that salicylanilide acts as a suicide substrate, and is metabolized to aniline. To confirm her observations, she measures the concentration of aniline in the test medium following the assay. Which amino acid residue is least likely to be responsible for the mechanism of enzyme inhibition?

A. Leucine
B. Serine
C. Cysteine
D. Lysine

10. What is the major product of salicylanilide and $LiAlH_4$?

Isocitric Acid

11. A chemist is attempting a novel synthesis of salicylanilide in which benzoic acid is formed from phenol. Which of the following is true?

A. KCr_2O_7, H_2SO_4, water → excellent yield
B. Bleach, acetic acid → good yield
C. CrO_3-pyridine, CH_2Cl_2 → good yield
D. None of the above

12. In an analogue of salicylanilide, the amide bond has been replaced with an ester bond (the nitrogen atom is now oxygen). This analogue is heated with NaOH and then acidified. Which of the following are among the major products?

A.

B.

C.

D.

13. If the molecule in Figure 3 below undergoes a Hofmann rearrangement, what is the product?

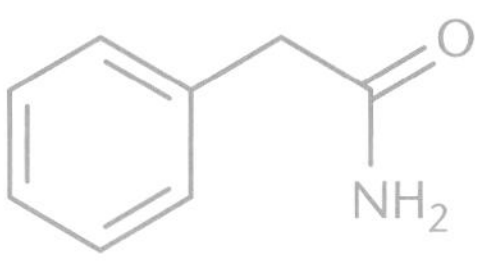

Figure 3

A.

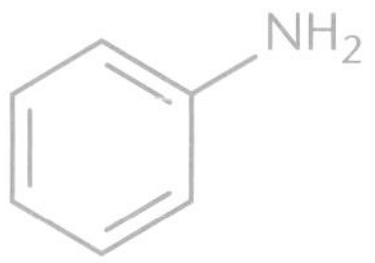

B.

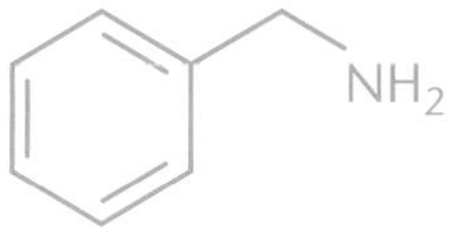

C.

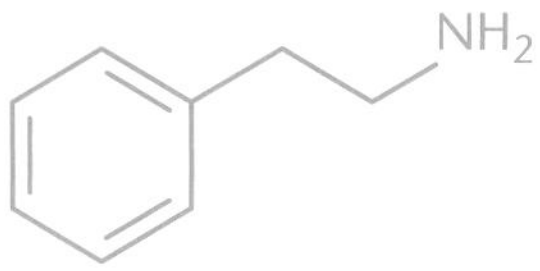

D.

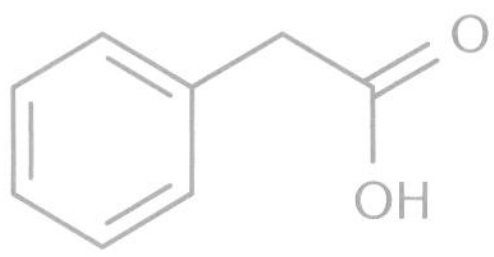

14. What is the IUPAC name for salicylanilide?

A. 2-hydroxy-N-phenyl-benzamide
B. 3-hydroxybenzanilide
C. 3-oxo-3-anilido-phenol
D. 3-hydroxy-1-cyano-N-phenylbenzoic acid

15. Which of the following syntheses gives the highest yield of acetanilide?

A.

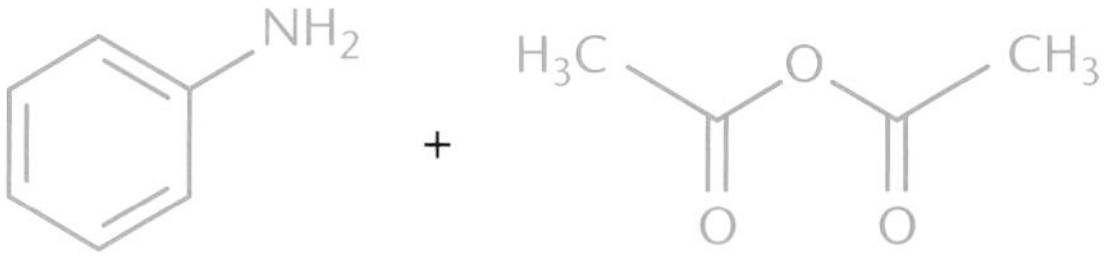

B.

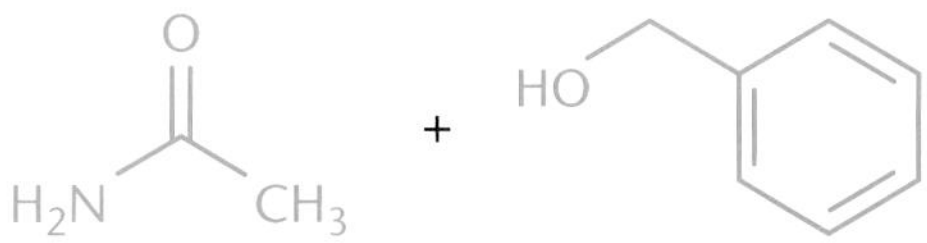

C.

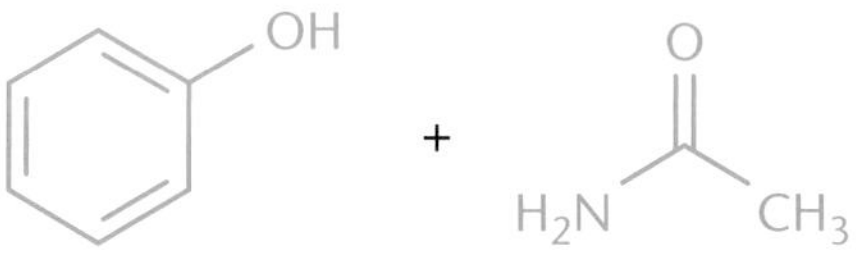

D.

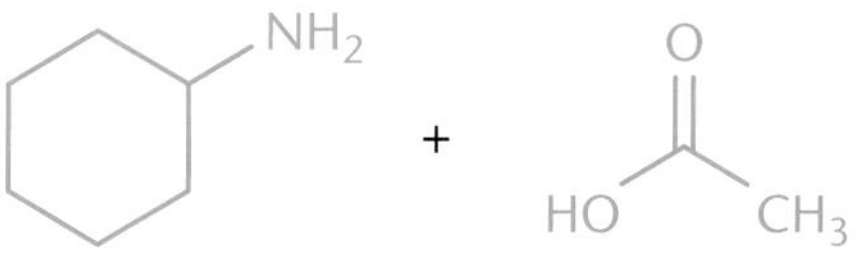

QUESTIONS 16–19 ARE NOT BASED ON A DESCRIPTIVE PASSAGE.

16. Which of the following reactions is not characteristic of a carboxylic acid?

A. Nucleophilic substitution
B. Decarboxylation
C. Esterification
D. Nucleophilic addition

17. Nitriles are hydrolyzed to amines under mild polar conditions and mild heat.

What is the product of the same reaction under more extreme polarity (very acidic or basic) and higher temperatures?

A. Aldehyde
B. Ester
C. Carboxylic acid
D. Ketone

18. The partial double-bond character of the peptide bonds formed between amino acids in a polypeptide has its most significant impact on which enzyme structure?

A. Primary
B. Secondary
C. Tertiary
D. Quaternary

19. What is the maximum number of isomeric pairs that can be formed from mononitration of chlorobenzene?

A. 1
B. 2
C. 3
D. 4

PASSAGE III (QUESTIONS 20–28)

Mass spectrometry (MS) involves the bombardment of the original molecule (M) with electrons, to form radical cations:

$$M + e^- \rightarrow M^{+\bullet} + 2e^-$$

Radical cations fragment to smaller pieces, and only stable cation fragments are detected for the mass spectrum, at their mass/charge (m/z) ratio (for simplicity, only fragments with charge = +1 will be considered). Several common fragmentation patterns are listed in Table 1.

Table 1

McLafferty Rearrangement	
α-cleavage	
Alkanes	Cleavage to give most stable carbocation
Alkenes	Cleavage to give allylic cations
Alcohols	Cleavage of —OH via loss of H_2O; α-cleavage
Amines	α-cleavage

A student obtains a mass spectrum of compound Y, with molecular formula $C_6H_{10}O$, and key fragments occur at m/z values of 41 and 29, as well as two smaller peaks occurring at m/z 57, and 43. Through more tests on compound Y, the student deduces that compound Y contains a cyclobutane ring, an aldehyde group, and a methyl group. The student also finds from the mass spectrum that:

(1) a McLafferty Rearrangement takes place, *before any fragmentation occurs*;

(2) the parent peak is the base peak.

20. On a mass spectrum, abundances are measured relative to the

A. parent peak.
B. smallest peak.
C. number of possible fragments.
D. base peak.

21. At what m/z value does the base peak for compound Y occur?

A. 94
B. 96
C. 98
D. 100

22. The enol fragment resulting from McLafferty rearrangements typically isomerizes to what type of compound?

A. Carbonyls
B. Alcohols
C. Epoxides
D. Carboxylic acids

23. Given that a McLafferty rearrangement takes place before other fragmentation occurs, what is the most likely structure of compound Y?

A.

B.

C.

D.

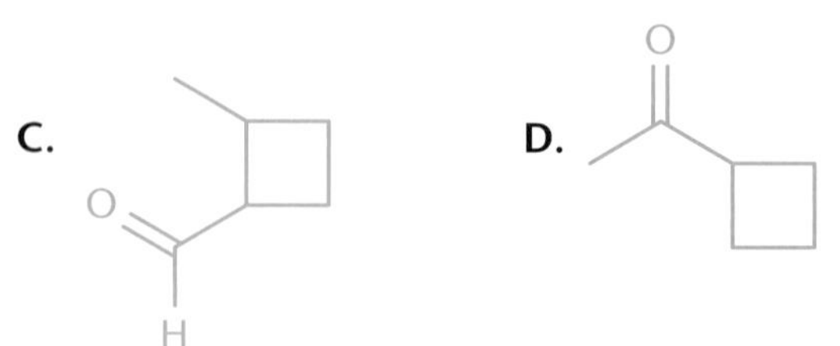

24. The key fragment at m/z 41 corresponds most likely to which structure?

A. 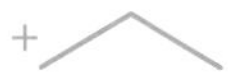 B. 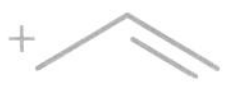 C. 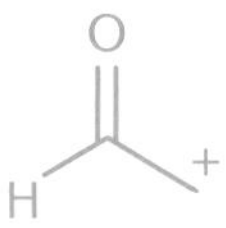 D.

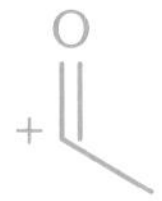

25. The key fragment at m/z 29 corresponds most likely to which structure?

A. $H{-}C{\equiv}O^+$ B. $H_2C{=}CH_2$

C. $H_3C{-}^+$ D. $C{\equiv}O^+$

26. In a separate experiment, the student obtains the mass spectrum of compound Z, also with the molecular formula $C_6H_{10}O$. To her surprise, there is no parent peak, though there is a base peak at m/z 80 and a peak at m/z 31.

What functional group does compound Z most likely contain?

A. Alcohol
B. Ketone
C. Ether
D. Aldehyde

27. The key fragment at m/z 31 corresponds to which of the following structures?

A. $[C_2H_6]^{+\bullet}$ B. $[H_2C{-}NH_2]^{+\bullet}$

C. $[H_2C{=}O]^{+\bullet}$ D. $[HN{=}NH]^{+\bullet}$

28. The base peak at m/z 80 comes from the most stable carbocation fragment. Which of the following structures corresponds to the base peak?

A. 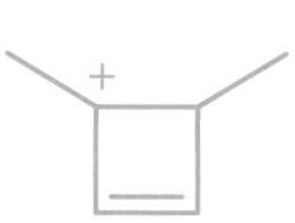 B. 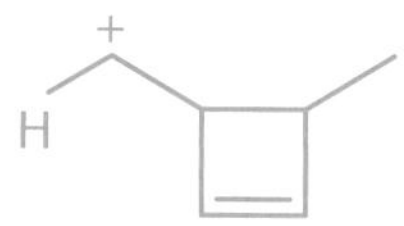 C. D.

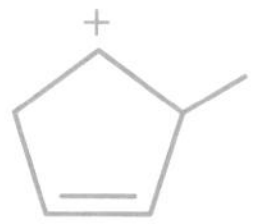

PASSAGE IV (QUESTIONS 29–36)

Compound I, with molecular formula C_7H_{12}, is an optically active molecule with one stereocenter. It is found to react with two molecules of hydrogen to give compound II, also optically active with one stereocenter.

When compound I is reacted with acidic potassium permanganate over heat, carbon dioxide is emitted, and compound III, with formula $C_6H_{12}O_2$, is also formed. Compound III is also optically active and is found to react with acidic methanol to form an optically active compound IV, with formula $C_7H_{14}O_2$.

The IR spectrum for compound III contains a broad absorbance band that spans approximately 1000 wavenumbers, as well as a sharp absorbance at 1,720 cm^{-1}. The ^{1}H-NMR spectrum for compound III contains a characteristic singlet at 12 ppm. Several IR bond-stretching frequencies and ^{1}H-NMR chemical shifts are listed.

IR		¹H NMR	
Bond	Stretching frequency (cm^{-1})	Type of proton	Chemical shift (ppm)
C—O	1000–1250	—CH_3 (aliphatic)	0–1.5
C=O	1650–1740	—CH_2— (aliphatic)	1.5–3
O—H (alcohol)	3400	=CH_2 (alkene)	5–7
O—H (acid)	2500–3500	CHO (aldehyde)	9–10
C=C	1400–1600	—OH (acid)	10–13

29. What are the degrees of unsaturation of compound I?

A. 0
B. 1
C. 2
D. More information is needed.

30. Which of the following is a possible structure for compound I?

A. 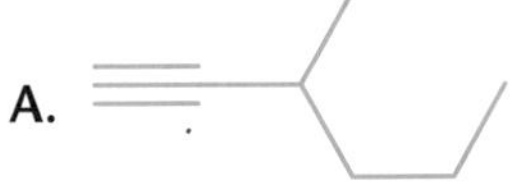

B. 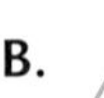

C. 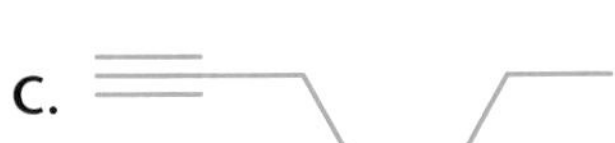

D. 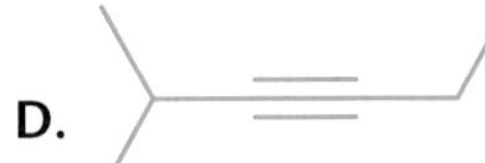

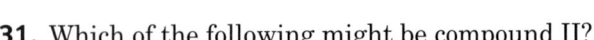

31. Which of the following might be compound II?

A. Heptane
B. 3-methylhexane
C. 2,2-dimethylpentane
D. 2-methylhexane

32. Given compound III's spectral information, what functional group does it most likely contain?

A. Carboxylic acid
B. Aldehyde
C. Ketone
D. Alcohol

33. Which of the following is a suitable catalyst for the conversion of compound I to compound II?

A. Aluminum
B. Magnesium
C. Platinum
D. Lithium

34. Using IR spectroscopy only, what will be an indication that conversion from compound I to compound II was successful?

A. Appearance of a sharp absorbance band at 1,720 cm^{-1}
B. Disappearance of a broad absorbance band at 3,400 cm^{-1}
C. Appearance of a sharp absorbance band at 960 cm^{-1}
D. Disappearance of a sharp absorbance band at 2,200 cm^{-1}

35. Suppose that instead of acidic potassium permanganate with heat, ozone, followed by aqueous workup, is used on compound I. Which of the following are possible products?

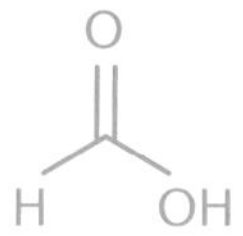

compound V

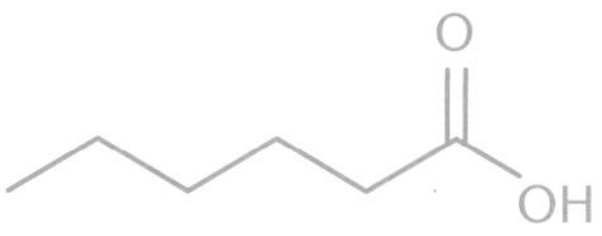

compound VI

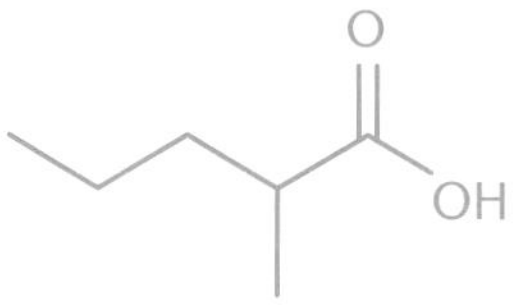

compound VII

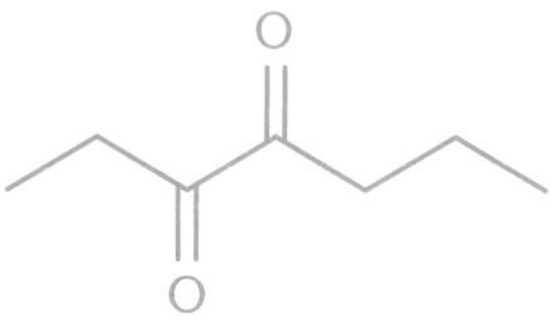

compound VIII

A. V only
B. VIII only
C. V, VI, and VIII
D. V and VII

36. Using ^{1}H-NMR spectroscopy only, what will be an indication that conversion from compound III to compound IV is successful?

A. Appearance of a singlet at 4 ppm, with the singlet at 12 ppm remaining
B. Disappearance of the singlet at 12 ppm only
C. Appearance of a singlet at 4 ppm, with the disappearance of the singlet at 12 ppm
D. Appearance of a doublet at 12 ppm

QUESTIONS 37–39 ARE NOT BASED ON A DESCRIPTIVE PASSAGE.

37. How many peaks are there in an H-NMR spectrum of 2-methyl-2-butene?

A. 2
B. 4
C. 5
D. 10

38. Which of the following is a product of the reaction between propylmagnesium bromide and ethyne?

A. 1-pentyne
B. Propane
C. 1-pentene
D. Propene

39. What is the major product of the following reaction?

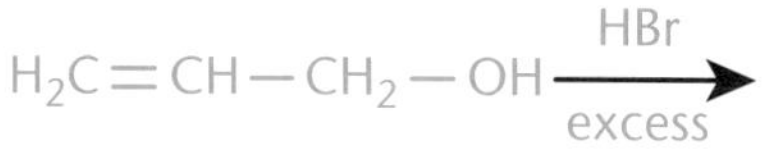

$$H_2C{=}CH{-}CH_2{-}OH \xrightarrow[\text{excess}]{\text{HBr}}$$

A. 2,4-dibromopropane
B. 1-bromoprop-3-ene
C. 2-bromopropan-3-ol
D. 2-hydroxypropan-3-ol

PASSAGE V (QUESTIONS 40–47)

Qualitative organic analysis is a process often employed by chemists in order to identify unknown compounds of interest. Though its origins are in the lab, chemical analysis plays an important and practical role in areas such as medicine, environmental monitoring, and forensic science. Identification of substances revolves around a set of known properties associated with specific functional groups. The difficulty of verifying a substance's identity lies in the fact that there are millions of chemically and structurally unique compounds in the world, which, to the naked eye, have very few distinguishable features. In order to simplify the daunting task of sifting through each possibility, it is the chemist's duty to develop a logical and well-planned method for analysis.

As a final assignment for his chemistry lab, a student is given a set of unknown compounds and must identify each one using the techniques he learned throughout the course. The student performs solubility tests to divide the unknowns into broad categories, before testing with several reagents in order to identify functional groups. Brady's reagent (2,4-Dinitrophenylhydrazine) is a commonly used compound, which produces a yellow or red precipitate when in the presence of a carbonyl group of ketones or aldehydes. Once a carbonyl is identified, the Tollen's test can be used to make a distinction between aldehydes and ketones. Silver nitrate (Tollen's reagent) is used to oxidize the carbonyl of an aldehyde forming a carboxylic acid and an easily idenitifiable silver mirror. Once the presence of such functional groups is verified, infrared spectroscopy can then be utilized to further predict the structure. After running a series of tests on each of his unknowns, the student proposes the structures shown in Figures 1a, 1b, and 1c.

Substance A

Figure 1a

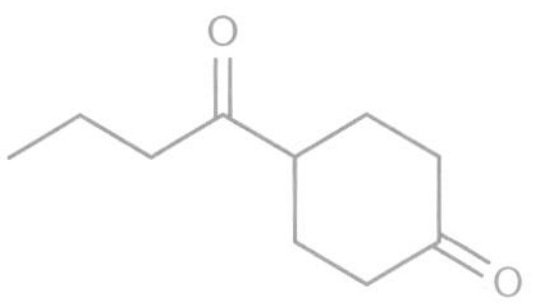

Substance B

Figure 1b

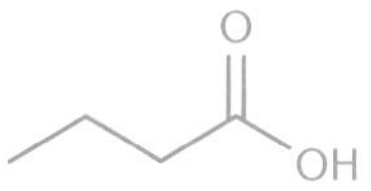

Substance C

Figure 1c

40. What is the appropriate IUPAC name for the predicted structure of substance A?

A. 4,4-dimethyl-5-pentaldehyde
B. 5-(4,4 dimethyl)-pentaldehyde
C. 2, 2-dimethylpentanal
D. 4,4-dimethylpentanal

41. A Grignard reagent is used in the reaction below. What is the IUPAC name for the product that would be produced by this reaction?

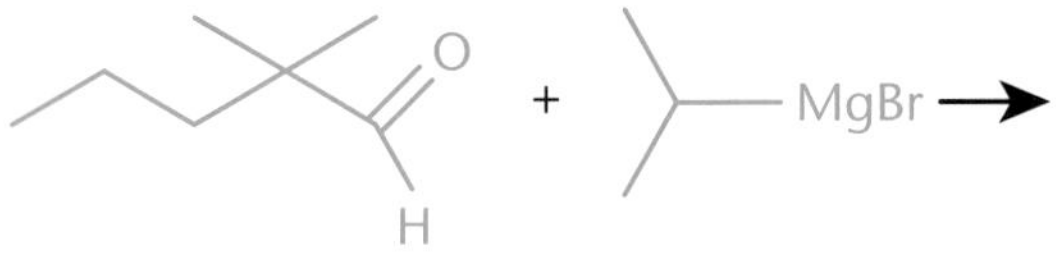

Substance A

A. 2,4,4-trimethylheptan-3-ol
B. 3-(2-ethyl-4-dimethyl)-hexanol
C. 2,4,4 trimethyl-heptane alcohol
D. 5-(4,4,6-trimethyl)-heptanol

42. The student is told that he can synthesize substance C by treating butanenitrile with aqueous acid. Which of the structures below correctly depicts butanenitrile?

A.

B.

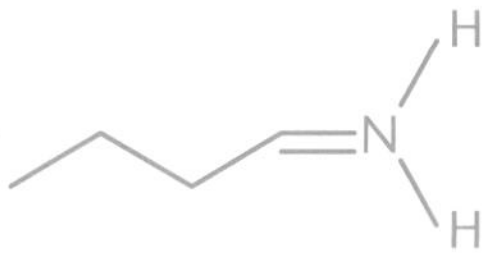

C.

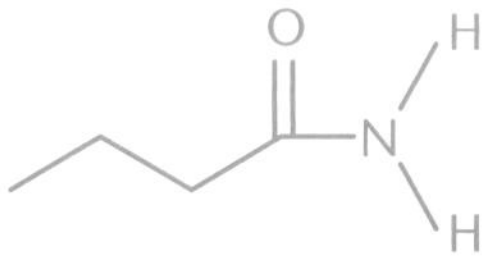

D.

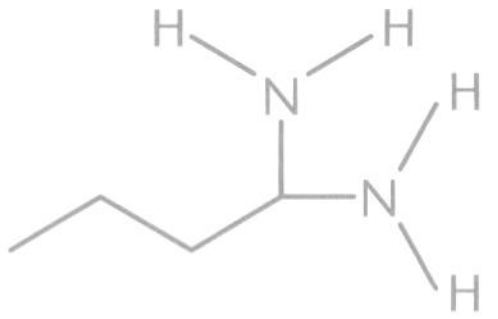

43. Substance B is subjected to a reaction and the product is given below. What is the correct IUPAC name for this product?

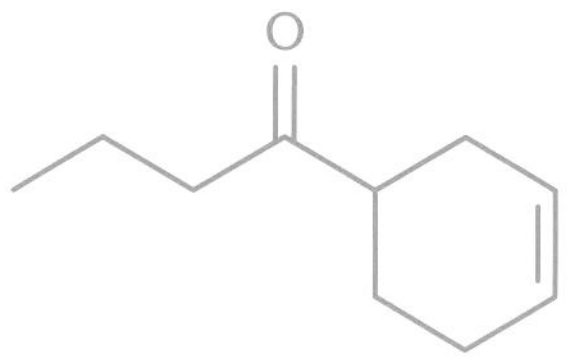

A. 1-hexane-2-butanone
B. 5-hexane-4-butanone
C. 1-(1-butanone)-cyclohex-3-ene
D. Butanone-cyclohexen

44. The product from the previous question is subjected to a reaction that opens the ring structure by breaking the double bond. This produces a final product that maintains the carbonyl but now has a saturated carbon chain in place of the ring. What is the name of this new product?

A. 4-decanone
B. 4-(3-propyl)-heptanone
C. 5-(4-ethyl)-octanone
D. 4-(5-ethyl)-octanone

45. During the course of analysis, the student uses Brady's reagent on all three unknowns. Mixing Brady's reagent with which of the following would cause a yellow or red precipitate?

A. Substance A only
B. Substance A and C only
C. Substance B and C only
D. Substance A and B only

46. A fourth unknown is given to you and you are told that there is only one functional group on this molecule. When it is mixed with 2,4-DNPH, a yellow crystal falls out of solution. This same unknown is then combined with Tollen's reagent, which fails to produce a silver mirror. If this unknown is mixed with a Wittig reagent, the most likely product to form would be a(n)

A. aldehyde.
B. ketone.
C. alkene.
D. alkyne.

47. One of the unknowns displayed the following stretches on the IR spectrum:

1,200 cm^{-1} strong
1,760 cm^{-1} strong
Broad stretch in the region between 3,500–2,500 cm^{-1}

With this information in hand, what can be said about this compound?

A. Mixing this unknown with Tollen's reagent will produce a silver coat on the test tube glass.
B. Addition of excess alcohol to this unknown in the presence of acid and heat will result in ester formation.
C. When reacted with 2,4-DNPH a red precipitate falls out of solution.
D. Reaction with $LiAlH_4$ in a THF solution will result in the formation of an alcohol.

PASSAGE VI (QUESTIONS 48–52)

Some of the most abundant neurotransmitters in the central nervous system (CNS) are amino acids. For example, glutamate and aspartate are responsible for most of the excitatory neurotransmission in brain and spinal cord, respectively, while glycine, the simplest of the essential amino acids, is a major inhibitory neurotransmitter of spinal cord. In addition, GABA or gamma-aminobutyrate, while not one of the 20 essential amino acids, is the most abundant inhibitory neurotransmitter in the CNS. Disruptions in the regulation of these amino acids can lead to various diseases of the CNS. For instance, excessive stimulation of ionic glutamate receptors can lead to excitotoxic neuron death.

Glutamate is converted to GABA in the brain by the enzyme L-glutamate decarboxylase (GAD). This enzyme removes the carboxylic acid group in the amino acid backbone, as CO_2 (Figure 1). There are two main isoforms of the GAD in the brain: GAD1 and GAD2 or GAD67 and GAD65, where the numbers signify the enzyme's weight in kD. Abnormalities of these enzymes have been discovered in various conditions including epilepsy and schizophrenia.

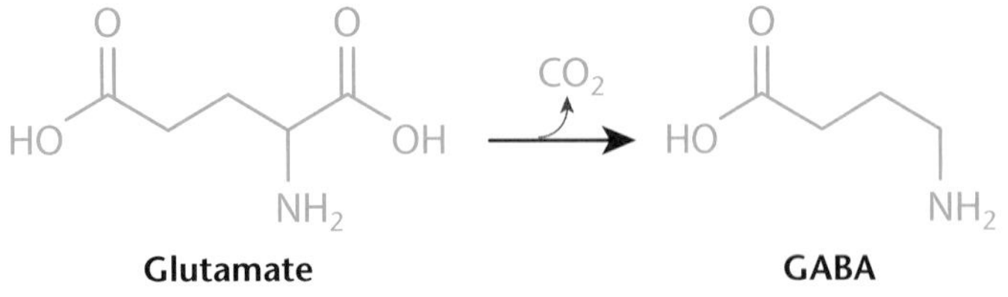

HO OH NH2 — CO_2 → HO NH2

Glutamate GABA

Figure 1

Without an enzyme, simple carboxylic acids rarely undergo decarboxylation. GAD requires pyridoxal 5′-phosphate (PLP) (Figure 2) as a cofactor to effect decarboxylation. A lysine residue in GAD forms a Schiff base with the aldehyde group of PLP. As with many enzymes, after GAD catalyzes decarboxylation, the cofactor remains unchanged.

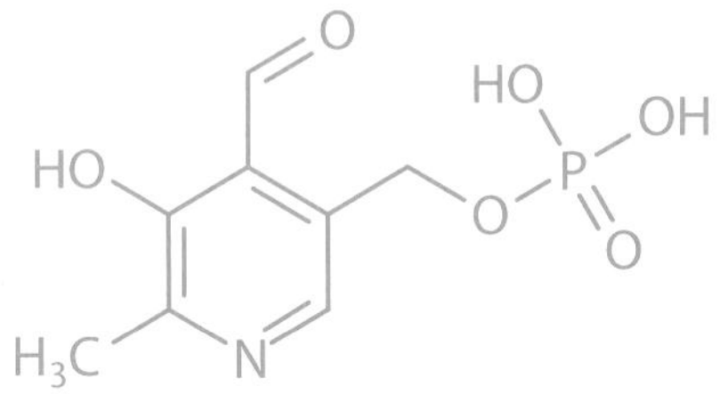

O HO OH HO O P O H_3C N

Figure 2

Table 1

Amino acid	pK_{a1}	pK_{a2}	pK_{a3}
Glycine	2.34	9.60	
Aspartic acid	1.88	3.65	9.60
Glutamic acid	2.19	4.25	9.67

48. A mixture of glycine, aspartate, glutamate, and other amino acids is placed in a well in the center of an electrophoresis gel. When current is applied to the bath at pH 4, which of the following accurately describes the action of glycine?

A. Glycine will migrate toward the cathode.
B. Glycine will migrate toward the anode.
C. Glycine will not migrate, because its net charge is zero.
D. Unlike peptides and proteins, single amino acids cannot migrate in an electric field.

49. You plan to separate a solution of glycine and aspartic acid (below) into individual amino acids. What pH would you choose for the electrophoresis buffer?

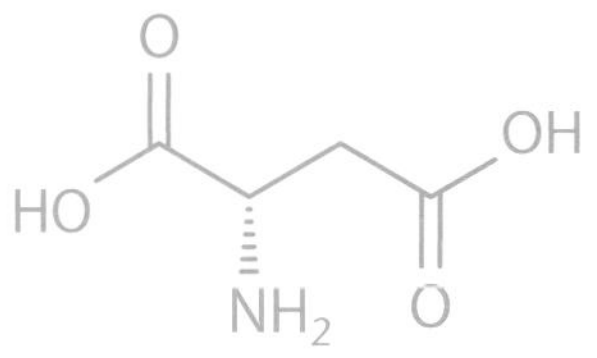

A. 1.88
B. 2.19
C. 2.34
D. 2.77

50. The decarboxylation mechanism requires the formation of a Schiff base. Which of the following most closely resembles a Schiff base?

A. $R_1R_2C{=}N{-}H$
B. $R_1R_2C{=}N{-}NH_2$
C. $R_1R_2C{-}NH{-}R_3$
D. $R_1N{=}NR_2$

51. Mechanistically, how would a lysine residue in GAD most likely begin to form an imine with the aldehyde group in PLP?

A. The amine of the lysine side chain would bond to the carbonyl carbon of PLP by nucleophilic attack.
B. Oxygen in water would nucleophillically attack the aldehyde group of PLP.
C. The carbonyl carbon loses its proton to the amine on the lysine backbone.
D. The carboxylic acid of the lysine residue donates a proton to the carbonyl oxygen to facilitate nucleophilic attack on the carbonyl carbon.

52. In the absence of GAD and PLP, which of the following molecules can undergo decarboxylation, with heating only?

A. Glutamic acid
B. 3-oxo-2-aminobutyric acid
C. 2-aminoethanoic acid
D. Aspartic acid

PRACTICE SECTION 3

Time—70 minutes

QUESTIONS 1–52

Directions: Most of the questions in the following Organic Chemistry Practice Section are organized into groups, with a descriptive passage preceding each group of questions. Study the passage, then select the single-best answer to the question in each group. Some of the questions are not based on a descriptive passage; you must also select the best answer to these questions. If you are unsure of the best answer, eliminate the choices that you know are incorrect, then select an answer from the choices that remain.

Period	1 IA 1A	2 IIA 2A	3 IIIB 3B	4 IVB 4B	5 VB 5B	6 VIB 6B	7 VIIB 7B	8 VIII 8	9 VIII 8	10 VIII 8	11 IB 1B	12 IIB 2B	13 IIIA 3A	14 IVA 4A	15 VA 5A	16 VIA 6A	17 VIIA 7A	18 vIIIA 8A
1	1 H 1.008																	2 He 4.003
2	3 Li 6.941	4 Be 9.012											5 B 10.81	6 C 12.01	7 N 14.01	8 O 16.00	9 F 19.00	10 Ne 20.18
3	11 Na 22.99	12 Mg 24.31											13 Al 26.98	14 Si 28.09	15 P 30.97	16 S 32.07	17 Cl 35.45	18 Ar 39.95
4	19 K 39.10	20 Ca 40.08	21 Sc 44.96	22 Ti 47.88	23 V 50.94	24 Cr 52.00	25 Mn 54.94	26 Fe 55.85	27 Co 58.47	28 Ni 58.69	29 Cu 63.55	30 Zn 65.39	31 Ga 69.72	32 Ge 72.59	33 As 74.92	34 Se 78.96	35 Br 79.90	36 Kr 83.80
5	37 Rb 85.47	38 Sr 87.62	39 Y 88.91	40 Zr 91.22	41 Nb 92.91	42 Mo 95.94	43 Tc (98)	44 Ru 101.1	45 Rh 102.9	46 Pd 106.4	47 Ag 107.9	48 Cd 112.4	49 In 114.8	50 Sn 118.7	51 Sb 121.8	52 Te 127.6	53 I 126.9	54 Xe 131.3
6	55 Cs 132.9	56 Ba 137.3	57 La* 138.9	72 Hf 178.5	73 Ta 180.9	74 W 183.9	75 Re 186.2	76 Os 190.2	77 Ir 190.2	78 Pt 195.1	79 Au 197.0	80 Hg 200.5	81 Tl 204.4	82 Pb 207.2	83 Bi 209.0	84 Po (210)	85 At (210)	86 Rn (222)
7	87 Fr (223)	88 Ra (226)	89 Ac~ (227)	104 Rf (257)	105 Db (260)	106 Sg (263)	107 Bh (262)	108 Hs (265)	109 Mt (266)	110 --- ()	111 --- ()	112 --- ()		114 --- ()		116 --- ()		118 --- ()

Lanthanide Series*	58 Ce 140.1	59 Pr 140.9	60 Nd 144.2	61 Pm (147)	62 Sm 150.4	63 Eu 152.0	64 Gd 157.3	65 Tb 158.9	66 Dy 162.5	67 Ho 164.9	68 Er 167.3	69 Tm 168.9	70 Yb 173.0	71 Lu 175.0
Actinide Series~	90 Th 232.0	91 Pa (231)	92 U (238)	93 Np (237)	94 Pu (242)	95 Am (243)	96 Cm (247)	97 Bk (247)	98 Cf (249)	99 Es (254)	100 Fm (253)	101 Md (256)	102 No (254)	103 Lr (257)

PASSAGE I (QUESTIONS 1–8)

The carbonyl group, C=O, is central to the chemistry of aldehydes and ketones. Even though aldehydes are distinguished from ketones by only a hydrogen atom, their reactivities are dissimilar enough that they can be differentiated by chemical means. For example, aldehydes can be more easily oxidized compared to ketones, and aldehydes are more reactive toward nucleophilic addition. The structure of aldehydes and ketones include the central carbonyl carbon being bonded to three other groups: oxygen, by a double (s + p) bond, and two others by s bonds. The three bonds are coplanar, with bond angles of 120°. In addition, the electronegative oxygen atom in aldehydes and ketones unequally shares electrons, creating polar compounds.

Nucleophilic addition is a prominent reaction with aldehydes and ketones. The mechanism includes a transition state where the reactant molecule changes from a trigonal planar to a tetrahedral geometry, after nucleophilic attack at the carbonyl carbon atom, which has a partial positive charge. The Cannizzaro reaction is an example of nucleophilic addition that occurs when an aldehyde containing no α-hydrogen is allowed to react with aqueous or alcoholic hydroxides at room temperature; the aldehyde self-oxidizes, yielding an alcohol and a salt of a carboxylic acid.

1. A mixture of two alcohols, $CH_3CH_2CH_2CH_2OH$ and $CH_3CH_2CH(OH)CH_3$, is treated with pyridinium dichromate (PDC) in the presence of sulfuric acid to give a mixture of compounds. Reaction of this mixture with Tollen's reagent would give which of the following products?

A. O

B. H, O

C. O, OH

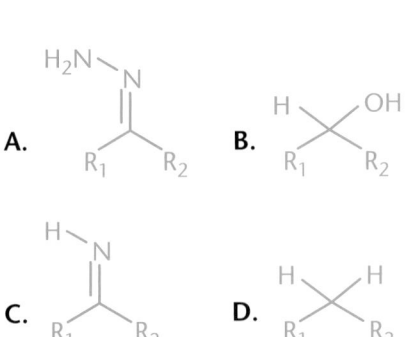

D. OH

2. Aldehydes and ketones can be reduced to their corresponding alcohols and/or hydrocarbons with suitable reducing agents. What is the final product of the reaction sequence shown below?

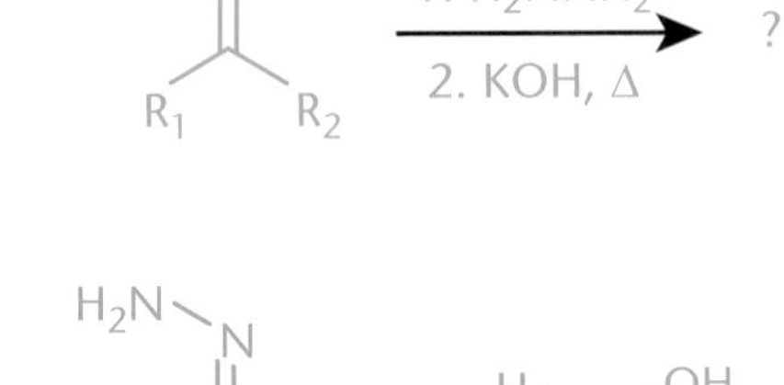

A. H_2N, N, R_1, R_2

B. H, OH, R_1, R_2

C. H, N, R_1, R_2

D. H, H, R_1, R_2

3. What compound results when ethyl methyl ketone reacts with HCN followed by treatment with sulfuric acid and heat?

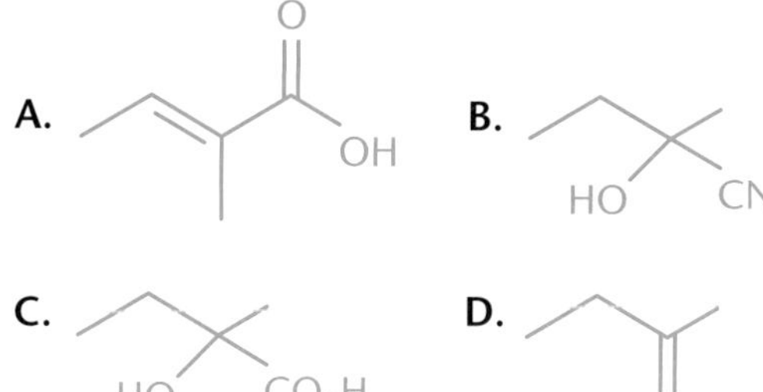

4. Which would be a product of a reaction with aqueous or alcoholic hydroxides and acetaldehyde?

A. O, O^-Na^+

B. OH

C. O, O^-Na^+

D. OH, O, H

5. In the reaction above, what is the nucleophile involved in the mechanism?

A. ^-OH

B. $[CH_2CHO]^-$

C. O^-, O, H

D. OH, O, H

6. If β-hydroxybutyraldehyde produced from an aldol condensation is reacted with dilute acid, which of the following would be a resulting product?

A. CHO

B. CO_2H

C. C=O

D. C=O

7. Aldol condensation is useful in the synthesis of larger molecules from smaller precursors. What sequence of reactions would result in using acetaldehyde to make n-butyraldehyde?

A. Aldol condensation to β-hydroxybutyraldehyde, hydrogenation to n-butyl alcohol, oxidation to n-butyraldehyde

B. Aldol condensation to β-hydroxybutyraldehyde, dehydration to 2-butenal, oxidation to n-butyraldehyde

C. Aldol condensation to β-hydroxybutyraldehyde, dehydration to 2-butenal, hydrogenation of the alkene to n-butyraldehyde (Hydrogenation only reduces *aromatic* carbonyl compounds *e.g.*, benzaldehyde, acetophenone, etc.)

D. Hydrogenation to ethyl alcohol, oxidation to acetone, aldol condensation to n-butyraldehyde

8. A Perkin condensation adds anhydrides to aromatic aldehydes in the presence of a base to give α, β-unsaturated acids. The corresponding saturated acid can then be made by hydrogenation of the carbon-carbon double bond. Which compound, in addition to acetic anhydride, represents the starting compound if the end product of a Perkin condensation produces the compound shown below?

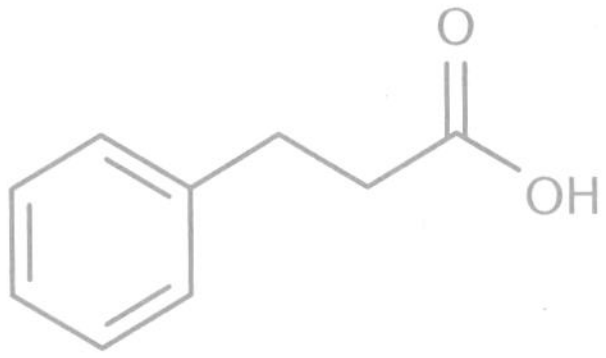

A.

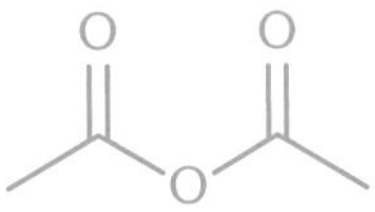

B.

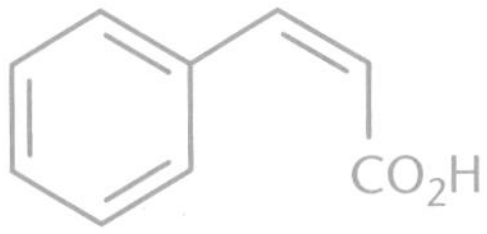

C.

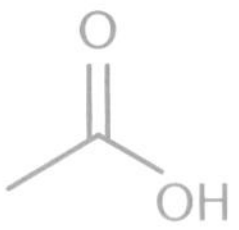

D.

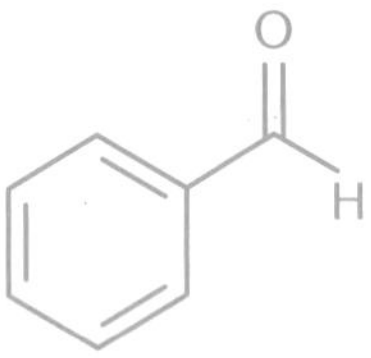

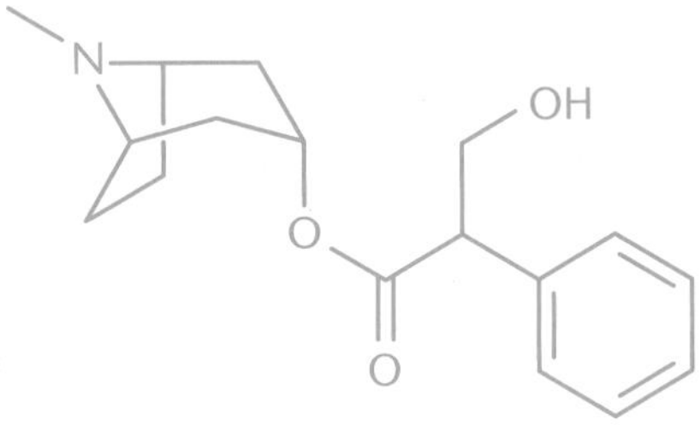

Atropine

Figure 1a

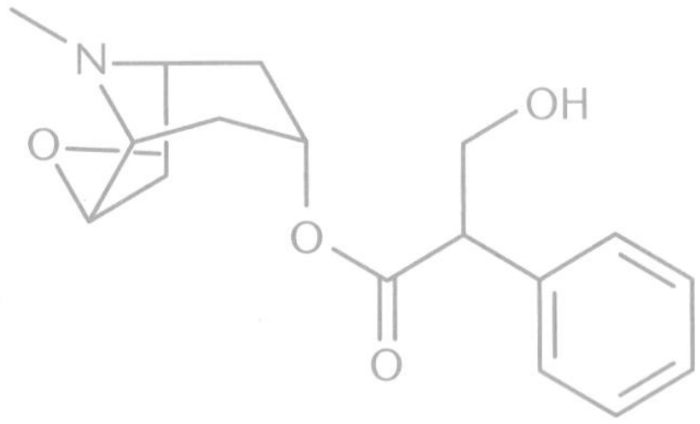

Scopolamine

Figure 1b

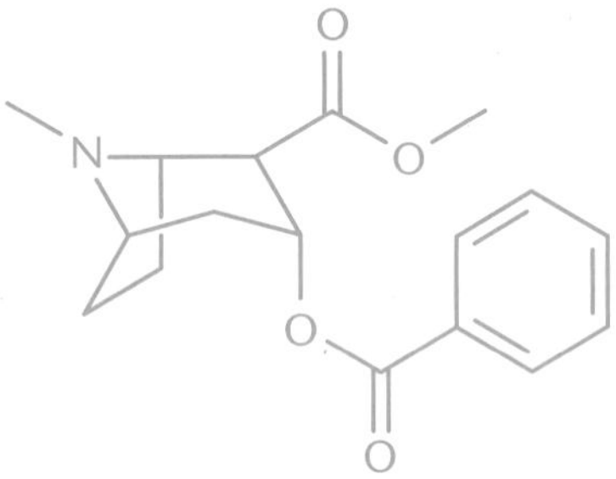

Cocaine

Figure 1c

PASSAGE II (QUESTIONS 9–15)

Atropine (Figure 1a) is a widely administered alkaloid drug used as a depressant of the parasympathetic nervous system, effective in the treatment of cardiac arrest, as well as being a popular drug in ophthalmology for pupil dilation. Atropine is categorized as a tropane alkaloid, in the same group as other drugs such as scopolamine and cocaine.

Atropine and other tropane alkaloids can be conveniently derived from tropinone (figure 2), a symmetric bicyclic nitrogenous ketone. In 1917, Sir Robert Robinson reported a facile synthesis of tropinone from succinaldehyde, methylamine, and acetone dicarboxylic acid.

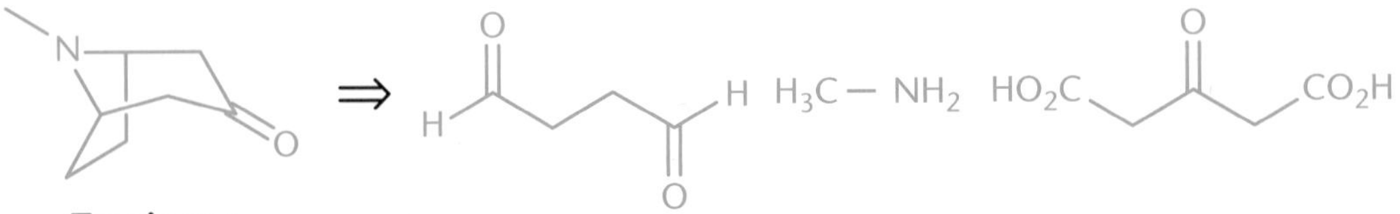

Figure 2

A proposed mechanism begins with the formation of a Schiff base between succinaldehyde and methylamine, followed by nucleophilic addition of the Schiff base to the second aldehyde group to form the five-membered ring (Figure 3). The remaining mechanism is illustrated below.

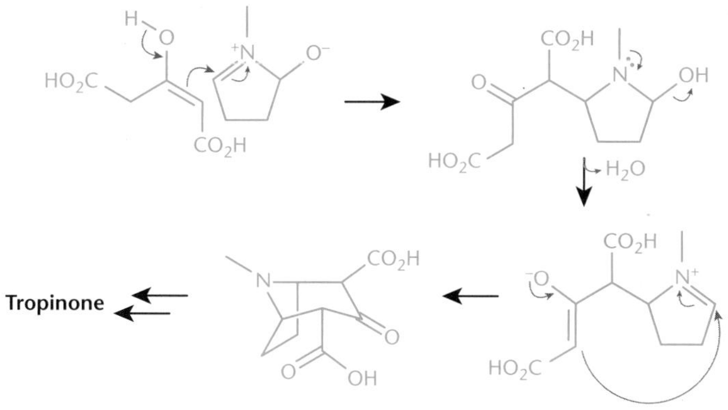

Figure 3

9. Which of the following structures illustrates the Schiff base initially formed between succinaldehyde and methylamine?

A.

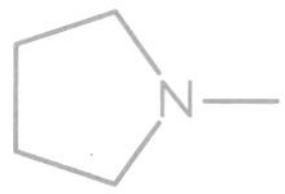

B.

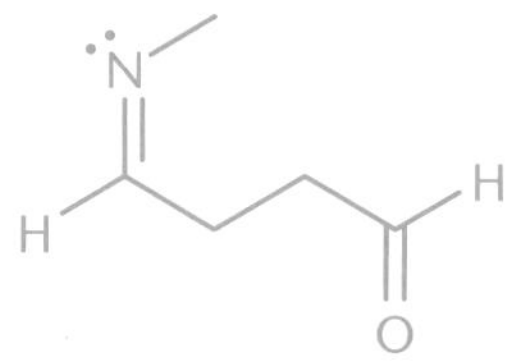

C.

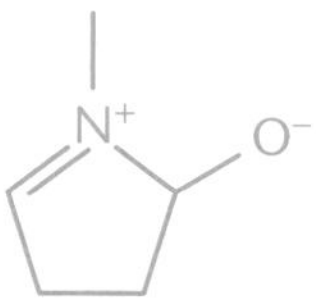

D.

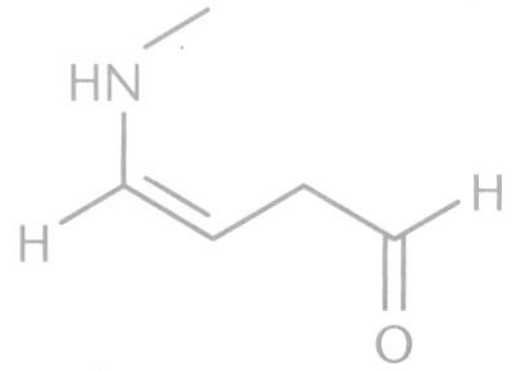

For questions 10 and 11, please refer to the reaction shown below.

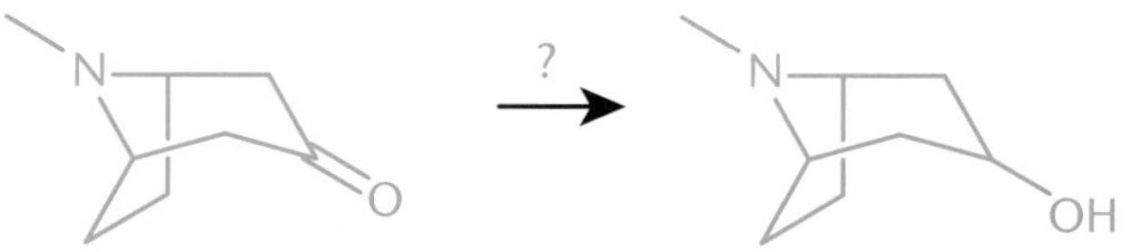

10. Which of the following reagents would be most suitable for the transformation above?

A. $Na_2Cr_2O_7$
B. $NaBH_4$
C. BH_3/THF, followed by H_2O_2/NaOH
D. HBr

11. What is a suitable name for the product shown?

A. Tropinol
B. Tropane
C. Tropene
D. Tropinamine

12. The active form of atropine is synthesized by the addition of the molecule shown below. What is the IUPAC name?

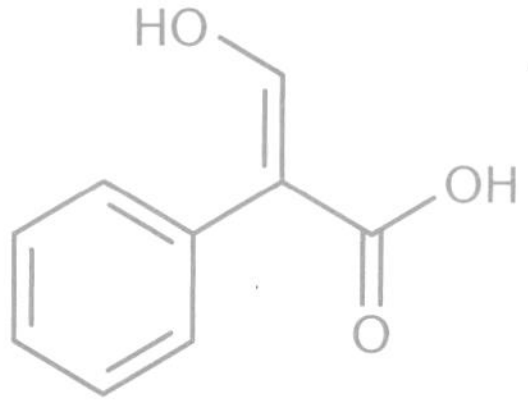

A. (S)-3-Hydroxy-2-phenylethanoic acid
B. (S)-3-Hydroxy-2-phenylpropanoic acid
C. (R)-2-Hydroxy-3-phenylbutanoic acid
D. (R)-3-Hydroxy-2-phenylpropanoic acid

13. How many distinct ^{1}H-NMR signals are observed in the spectrum of tropinone?

A. 7
B. 8
C. 4
D. 5

14. How many distinct ^{13}C NMR signals are observed in the spectrum of tropinone?

A. 5
B. 7
C. 10
D. 8

15. It would seem more logical to use acetone as a starting material, as the final steps to tropinone (not shown) can be avoided. Which of the following explains why acetone dicarboxylic acid is used instead of acetone?

I. It is a better electrophile than acetone is.
II. Its enol is more stable than that of acetone is.
III. The a-protons are more acidic than acetone is.
IV. The b-protons are more acidic than acetone is.

A. I only
B. III only
C. II and III
D. II and IV

QUESTIONS 16–18 ARE NOT BASED ON A DESCRIPTIVE PASSAGE.

16. How many absorption peaks will the following compound have?

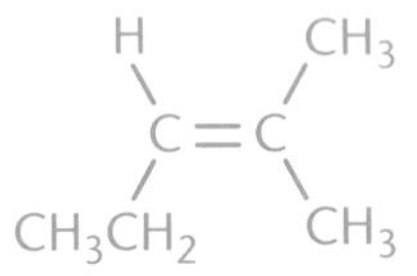

A. 5
B. 6
C. 7
D. 8

17. Which of the following steps would never form a radical in a radical halogenation reaction?

A. Initiation
B. Elongation
C. Propagation
D. Termination

18. Triglycerides include which of the following?

A. Glycerol and fatty esters
B. Esters, alcohols, and phospholipids
C. Fatty acids, ester, and alcohols
D. Glycerol and fatty acids

PASSAGE III (QUESTIONS 19–26)

A student is developing a new “orange azo dye” for a science fair project. He plans to synthesize a part of the dye molecule, which is colorless, and unveil the color at the science fair. He decides to start his synthesis with benzoic acid, but unfortunately, he only has benzene and phenol as aromatic starting materials. The synthesis of the colorless precursor is illustrated below.

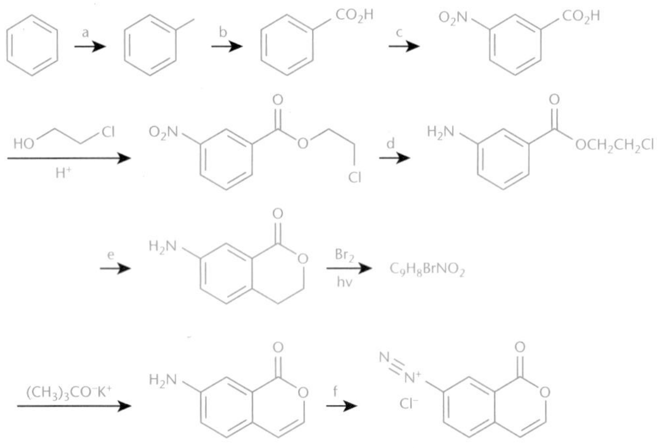

19. As shown in the figure above, benzoic acid can be synthesized from benzene in two steps. What two reactions (a and b) are needed?

A. Step 1: CH_3Cl, $AlCl_3$; Step 2: $KMnO_4$, heat
B. Step 1: CH_3OH, Al_2O_3; Step 2: $KMnO_4$, heat
C. Step 1: CH_3Cl, $AlCl_3$; Step 2: PCC
D. Step 1: CH_3COCl, $AlCl_3$; Step 2: CrO_3

20. What reagents are required for reaction c?

A. HNO_2
B. Concentrated HNO_3 and H_2SO_4
C. $NaNO_2$
D. Concentrated HNO_3

21. Which of the following reagents can be used in reaction d?

I. H_2, Pt
II. Sn, H_2SO_4
III. Zn, HCl

A. I only
B. II only
C. II and III
D. I, II, and III

22. How do amine groups direct subsequent reactions in the benzene ring?

A. Deactivate the ring, *ortho*- or *para*-directing
B. Activate the ring, *meta*-directing
C. Activate the ring, *ortho*- or *para*-directing
D. Deactivate the ring, *meta*-directing

23. Which of the following Lewis acids below can best catalyze reaction e?

I. BCl_3
II. $AlCl_3$
III. $PbCl_4$
IV. $[NiCl_4]^{2-}$

A. II only
B. IV only
C. I and II
D. III and IV

24. Which compound below, with molecular formula $C_9H_8BrNO_2$, is the correct structure of the product of reaction e after radical monobromination?

A. 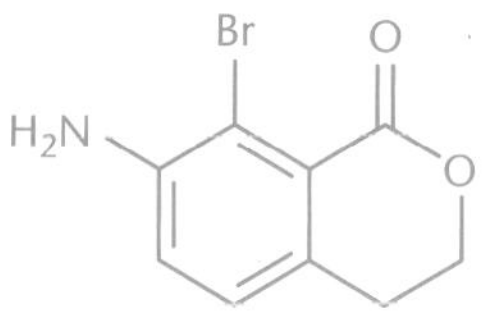
H2N
Br
O
O

B. 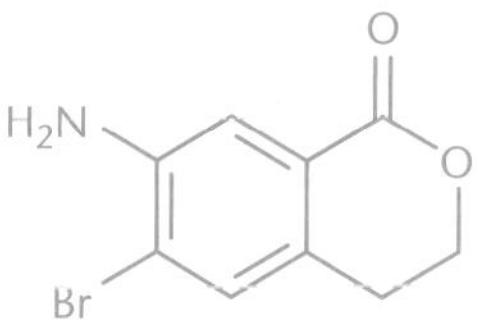
H2N
O
O
Br

C. 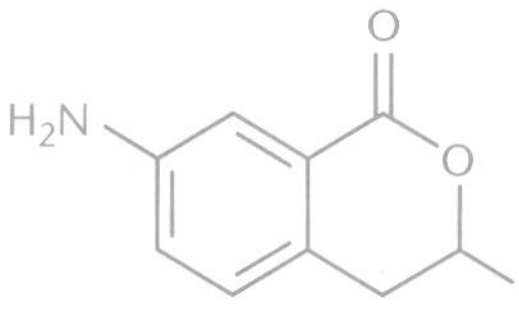
H2N
O
O
Br

D. 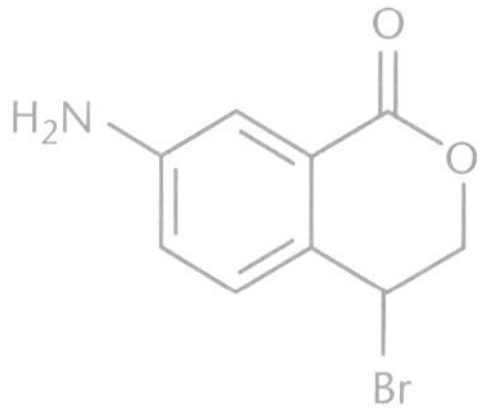
H2N
O
O
Br

25. At the science fair demonstration, the student treats the diazonium salt with phenol to form the orange azo dye. He knows, however, that he needs to somehow activate the phenol first before nucleophilic aromatic substitution can occur. What reagent can activate phenol?

A. HCl
B. H_2O
C. NaH
D. H_3O^+

26. After working up with mild aqueous acid, what is the structure of the orange azo dye?

A. 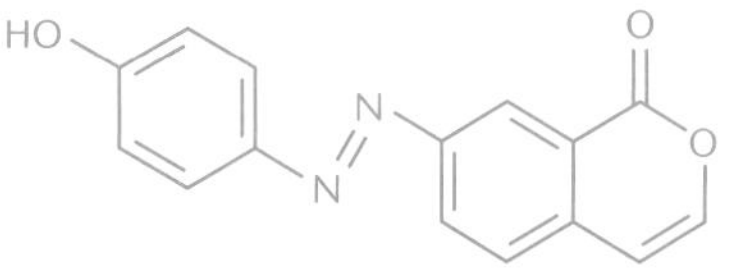
HO
N
N
O
O

B. 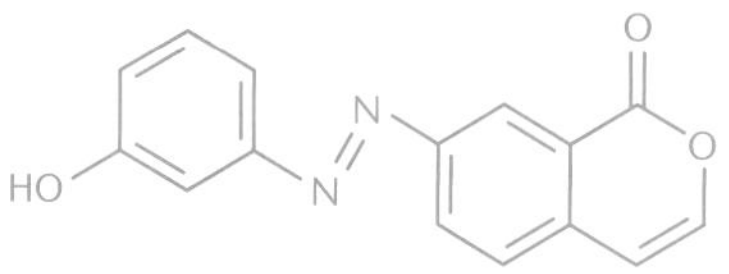
HO
N
N
O
O

C. 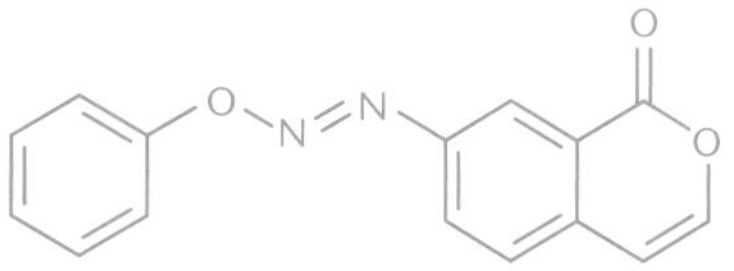
O
N
N
O
O

D. 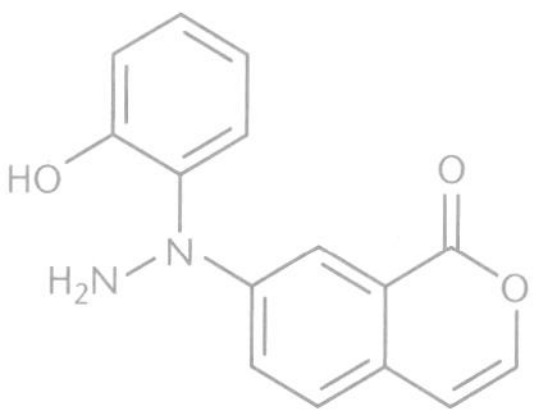
HO
H2N
N
O
O

PASSAGE IV (QUESTIONS 27–36)

A student attempts to separate a mixture of acetaminophen, amantadine, aspirin, caffeine, and ethenzamide (Figures 1a, 1b, 1c, 1d, and 1e).

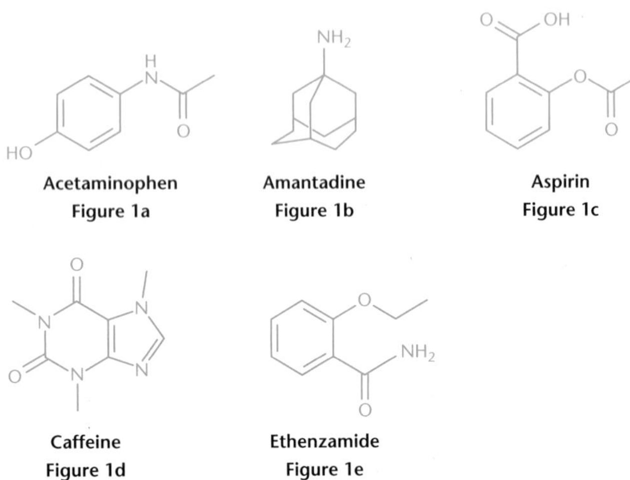

Acetaminophen Figure 1a

Amantadine Figure 1b

Aspirin Figure 1c

Caffeine Figure 1d

Ethenzamide Figure 1e

At her disposal are several solvents; their densities and boiling points are listed in Table 1.

Table 1

Solvent	Density (g/mL)	Boiling point (°C)
Water	1.0	100
Ethanol	0.8	78.0
Chloroform	1.5	61.0
Diethyl ether	0.7	35.0

As a reference, the student constructs a flow chart illustrating her separation process (Figure 2.)

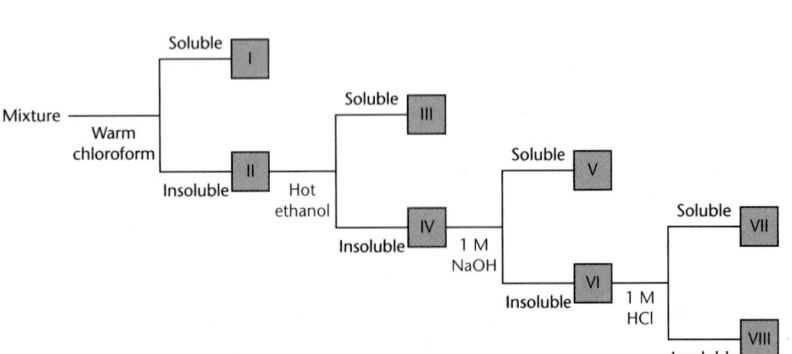

Mixture
Warm chloroform
Soluble I
Insoluble II
Hot ethanol
Soluble III
Insoluble IV
1 M NaOH
Soluble V
Insoluble VI
1 M HCl
Soluble VII
Insoluble VIII

Figure 2

27. What compound belongs in box I of Figure 2?
    A. Amantadine
    B. Aspirin
    C. Ethenzamide
    D. Caffeine

28. What compound belongs in box III of Figure 2?
    A. Acetaminophen
    B. Caffeine
    C. Ethenzamide
    D. Amantadine

29. Which of the following sets of ^{1}H NMR data corresponds to aspirin?
    A. d 2.0 (singlet, 3H), d 6.7 (doublet, 2H), d 7.4 (doublet, 2H), d 9.2 (singlet, 1H), d 9.6 (singlet, 1H)
    B. d 3.2 (singlet, 3H), d 3.4 (singlet, 3H), d 3.9 (singlet, 3H), d 7.9 (singlet, 1H)
    C. d 2.3 (singlet, 3H), d 7.1 (doublet, 1H), d 7.3 (triplet, 1H), d 7.6 (triplet, 1H), d 7.9 (doublet, 1H)
    D. d 1.1 (triplet, 3H), d 4.1 (quartet, 2H), d 7.3–7.5 (multiplet, 4H), d 7.9 (doublet, 2H)

30. Given that aspirin is soluble in 1 M NaOH, which of the structures below corresponds to the dissolved species?

A.

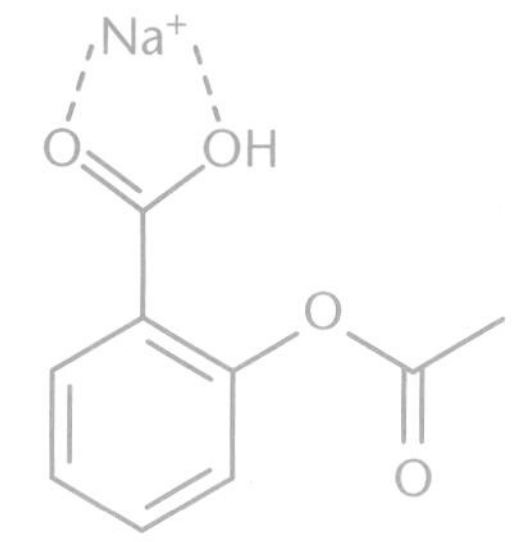

B.

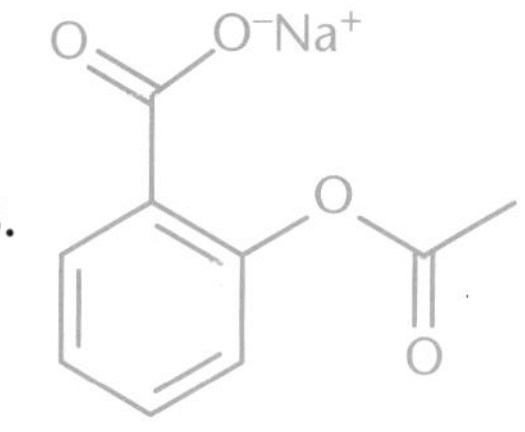

C.

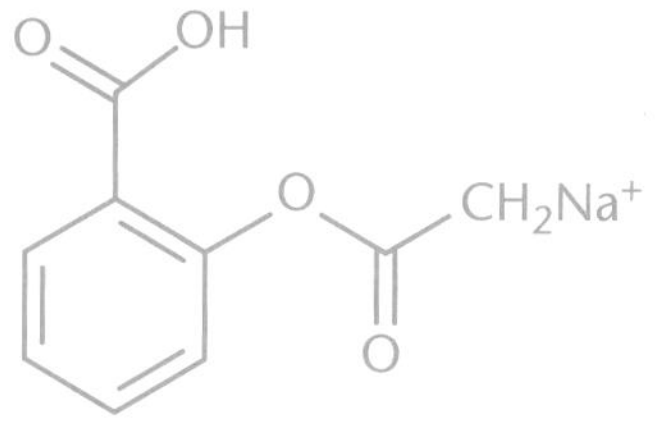

D.

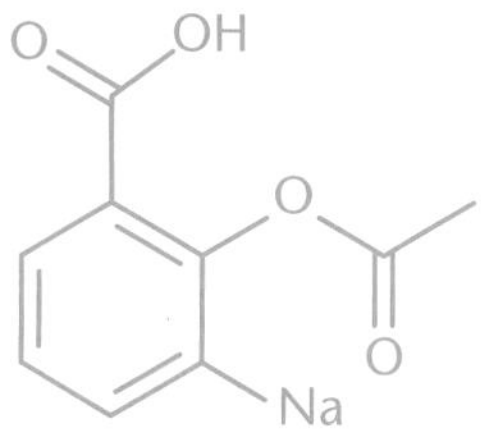

31. What pair of compounds is being separated in the final step (addition of 1 M HCl)?

A. Amantadine and caffeine
B. Amantadine and ethenzamide
C. Acetaminophen and ethenzamide
D. Acetaminophen and aspirin

32. How many different signals are observed in the ^{13}C NMR spectrum for acetaminophen?

A. 8
B. 5
C. 7
D. 6

33. Suppose that the student accidentally adds $LiAlH_4$ to the initial mixture. Which of the following compounds will undergo reduction?

I. Amantadine
II. Acetaminophen
III. Aspirin
IV. Ethenzamide

A. I only
B. III only
C. II and IV
D. II, III, and IV

34. The structure of ibuprofen is given in the figure below. If ibuprofen is added to the initial mixture, at which box in Figure 2 above does it appear?

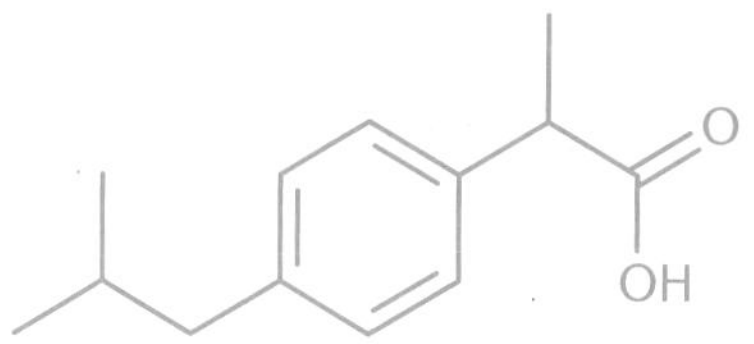

A. I
B. III
C. V
D. VII

35. Suppose the initial mixture is treated with sodium hydride (NaH), followed by methyl iodide. Which of the steps in Figure 2 will not separate any compounds?

I. 1 M HCl
II. 1M NaOH
III. Warm chloroform
IV. Hot ethanol

A. III only
B. IV only
C. I and II
D. I and IV

36. Another student decides to separate the same mixture of compounds using the same solvents, but in a different order. Which of the variations below can still give complete separation of the mixture into individual compounds?

A. 1 M HCl, followed by hot ethanol, 1 M NaOH, and warm chloroform last
B. 1 M NaOH first, followed by hot ethanol, warm chloroform, and 1 M HCl last
C. 1 M HCl first, followed by warm chloroform, 1 M NaOH, and hot ethanol last
D. 1 M NaOH, followed by 1 M HCl, hot ethanol, and warm chloroform last

QUESTIONS 37–39 ARE NOT BASED ON A DESCRIPTIVE PASSAGE.

37. In a room temperature sample of *cis*-1,2-dibromocyclohexane in a chair conformation, the configuration of the chlorines will

A. be axial.
B. be equatorial.
C. alternate between axial and equatorial switching conformations at the same time.
D. alternate between axial and equatorial switching conformations at different times.

38. Which of the following compounds produces the most heat per mole of compound when reacted with oxygen?

A. CH_4
B. C_2H_6
C. Cyclohexane
D. Cycloheptane

39. Using gel electrophoresis, a scientist can separate a mixture of amino acids by subjecting them to an electric field. The strength and direction of the electric field is determined by the net charge of the amino acid. If a solution of four different amino acids at a pH of 8. underwent gel electophoresis, which of the following would move furthest in the direction of the anode?

A. Glutamate
B. Glutamine
C. Lysine
D. Histidine

PASSAGE V (QUESTIONS 40–47)

Methylphenidate is a drug used primarily to treat children with attention deficit hyperactivity disorder. While the precise mechanism of action is unclear, it is known to inhibit monoamine neurotransmitter reuptake in a noncompetitive manner. Paradoxically, when the compound is administered to laboratory animals or healthy human volunteers it acts as a stimulant and increases locomotor activity. The molecule has two stereocenters and the configuration of these greatly impacts the efficacy and side effects of the molecule. Studies have demonstrated that d-*threo*-methylphenidate is the most potent isomer. In order to study the effects of the various enantiomers and diastereomers, asymmetric syntheses have been employed. Utilizing a starting compound that is chiral can reduce the need to resolve enantiomers and produce an enantiomerically pure product. The various isomers of methylphenidate or methyl-2-phenyl-2-(2′-piperidyl)-acetate are shown.

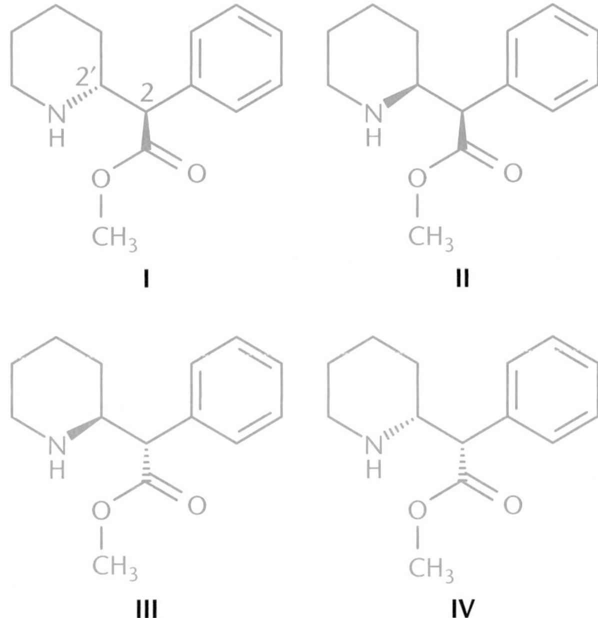

40. For her thesis, a graduate student uses a seven-step chiral synthesis to produce methylphenidate, which will be used in various experiments. After the fourth step, the product has an observed optical rotation. After the fifth step, however, the optical rotation of the product was one-half of the previously observed value. What accounts for this discrepancy?

A. The current solution is half the concentration of previous syntheses.
B. Her starting compound was the opposite chirality.
C. The sample tube of the polarimeter is twice the length.
D. Both B and C

41. Which compound in the figure above is (2R, 2′R)-(+)-*threo*-methyl-α-phenyl-α-(2-piperidyl) acetate, also known as d-threo-methylphenidate?

A. I
B. II
C. III
D. IV

42. Which of the compounds in the figure are structural (constitutional) isomers?

A. I and II
B. II and III
C. I and III
D. None of the above

43. Which of the compounds in the figure are stereoisomers?

A. I and II
B. II and III
C. I and III
D. All of the above

44. Which of the molecules shown are diastereomers?

A. I and II
B. II and IV
C. I and III
D. None of the above

45. While devising an asymmetric, multistep synthesis, a student proposes an S_N2 reaction at a chiral atom. Both the beginning reactant and final product have an R orientation. What will his mentor most likely tell him?

A. Proceed; the dehydration of a tertiary alcohol with strong base is an S_N2 reaction.
B. Halt; the S_N2 will invert the stereocenter.
C. Proceed; the S_N2 will not invert the stereocenter.
D. Both A and C.

46. Which of the following can exist as geometric isomers?

A. 1-bromo-1-pentyne
B. 1, 2-dibromopentane
C. 1-bromo-1-pentene
D. None of the above

47. Which of the following most likely explains why d-*threo*-methylphenidate is the most potent stereoisomer for inhibiting dopamine reuptake *in vitro*?

A. This isomer most readily crosses the blood-brain barrier.
B. This isomer binds most effectively to the dopamine reuptake transporter.
C. This isomer most closely mimics dopamine.
D. None of the above

PASSAGE VI (QUESTIONS 48–52)

Bonds in organic chemistry are mostly covalent bonds, sharing electrons. Electrons occupy orbitals consisting of electron pairs with opposite spins. Orbitals occupy shells, or energy levels. Electrons in the outer shell of an atom, the valence electrons, largely determine the bonding characteristics of the atom, and usually adhere to the octet rule. The octet rule states that, for an atom to be stable, its outer electron shell must be occupied by eight electrons. Covalent bonds also usually obey the octet rule. Thus, eight electrons in the outer shell of each of the bonded atoms form a stable, nonreactive molecule. Lewis structures are commonly used to show the valence electrons with dots representing electrons of the outer shell. For example, the Lewis structure for carbon, as the neutral atom presented in the periodic table, would be represented as shown in Figure 1.

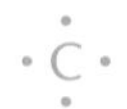

Figure 1

From Lewis structures, the electron domains of a molecule can be counted. According to the valence shell electron-pair repulsion (VSEPR) model, the shape of a molecule can be determined by first drawing its Lewis structure and counting the number of electron domains, then arranging those domains around the central atom such that their repulsions of one another are minimized. Electron domains consist of 1) each single bond; 2) each double bond; 3) each triple bond; and 4) each nonbonding electron pair on the central atom. Finally, the electron domains are positioned such that the atoms form a molecular geometry. Much like balloons (representing electron domains) would position themselves when tied together, electron domains position themselves according to their repulsion to each other. Domain numbers around a central atom determine geometries (see Table 1). (Note: One or two nonbonding domains on the central atom will alter the bond angles due to repulsion of the bonding domains.)

Domain number	Geometry	Depiction
2	Linear	
3	Trigonal planar	
4	Tetrahedral	
5	Trigonal bypyramidal	
6	Octahedral	

Once the geometry of the molecule has been determined, the hybrid orbitals necessary to accommodate their electron's geometric arrangement can be specified.

48. Table 2 shows the categories of electron assignments corresponding to values for the three quantum numbers *n* (which defines the energy level), *l* (which defines the shape of the electrons orbitals), and m_l (which defines the orientation of the orbitals is space). Organic molecules are composed mainly of the atoms carbon (atomic number 6), hydrogen (atomic number 1), nitrogen (atomic number 7), and oxygen (atomic number 8). Which of the following atoms has a valence electron possessing a spherical-shaped orbital?

n (shell)	*l* values	subshell	m_l values	No. orbitals (subshell)	No. orbitals (shell)
1	0	1s	0	1	1
2	0	2s	0	1	
2	1	2p	1, 0, –1	3	4
3	0	3s	0	1	
3	1	3p	1, 0, –1	3	
3	2	3d	2, 1, 0, –1, –2	5	9

A. Hydrogen
B. Carbon
C. Nitrogen
D. Oxygen

49. Carbon, with an atomic number of 6, and oxygen, atomic number 8, can form carbon dioxide, a molecule critical for life on earth. When more than one Lewis structure is possible for a molecule, assigning formal charges may help decide which structure is correct. The preferred Lewis structure is the one with atoms bearing the charge closest to zero, and in which any negative charges are assigned to the more electronegative atom(s). What is the preferred Lewis structure for carbon dioxide (CO_2)?

A. O::C::O
B. O:C:O
C. :O::C::O:
D. :O:C:::O:

50. Bonds between any two atoms in a molecule vary little in their energy from molecule to molecule. For example the bond between carbon and hydrogen in propane varies little in energy from the same bond within methane. Thus, tables of average bond enthalpies between specific atoms can be accurate enough to provide valid comparisons of relative bond energies among fuel molecules, expressing the energy as kJ/mole. Remember that the reaction in gas plus oxygen yields carbon dioxide and water. Given the enthalpy values below, which of the following gases is the most efficient fuel on a per mole basis?

Bond	Enthalpy (kJ/mole)
C—H	413
C—C	348
O—O	146
C=O	799
O—H	463

A. Methane
B. Ethane
C. Propane
D. Butane

51. Using the VSEPR model rules, what shape would you predict for the carbon dioxide (CO_2) molecule?

A. Linear
B. Trigonal planar
C. Tetrahedral
D. Trigonal bipyramidal

52. According to the VSEPR model described above, what shape would you ascribe to the methane (CH_4) molecule?

A. Linear
B. Trigonal planar
C. Tetrahedral
D. Trigonal bipyramidal

Answers and Explanations

CHAPTER PRACTICE QUESTIONS

CHAPTER 1: NOMENCLATURE

1. A

The longest chain contains six carbon atoms and the carboxylic acid has the highest priority, so the basic structure is a hexanoic acid. A methyl group and a phenyl group are bonded to the fourth carbon of the backbone making the correct answer 4-methyl-4-phenyl-hexanoic acid. (D) is incorrect, as benzene is not of higher priority than the acid. Further, the carboxylic acid group is misnamed in this choice. (C) is incorrect because no aldehydes are present. Finally, (B) is incorrect because the longest chain con tains six, not five carbon atoms.

2. C

The parent compound, with the ketone group bonded to a cyclohexane ring having the highest priority, is a cyclohexanone. Starting at the carbonyl group and counting clockwise, the chloride is given a 2- position, and the phenyl group a 5- position. The ketone, not the alkane (A), has highest priority. (B) is incorrect: the prefixes *ortho-*, *meta-*, and *para-* are used only for disubstituted benzenes. IUPAC naming dictates that substituents should be numbered such that the sum is as low as possible (D).

3. B

Starting from the anomeric carbon (the hemiacetal), the sugar is an a-sugar because the anomeric –OH group is pointing downward and trans- to the $-CH_2OH$ group, so (C) and (D) are incorrect. The Haworth projection does not readily provide whether the sugar is originally D or L (A).

4. D

The parent compound is an ethyl ester, and the longest chain not counting the ethyl group contains three carbons, so the parent compound is an ethyl propanoate. The third carbon also has two substituents (ketone and benzene ring), and ethyl 3-oxo-3-phenylpropanate accurately addresses those substituents. (C) contains no carboxylic acid in the molecule. Ether (A) and alkane (B) do not have the correct suffix for an ester.

5. C

Among the numerous functional groups, the carboxylic acid has the highest priority, so the parent compound ends with an –oic acid suffix. (A) denotes an alcohol, (B) a halide, and (D) an alkyne, all of which are of lower priority than a carboxylic acid and would not be an appropriate suffix for the molecule.

HIGH-YIELD SIMILAR QUESTIONS

Nomenclature

1. The word “ethyl” would be replaced with whatever was attached to the ester oxygen.
2. The two products would be (1*R*, 2*S*)-2, 5, 5-trimethylcyclohexanol and (1*S*, 2*S*)-2, 5, 5-trimethylcyclohexanol.

OH
Me
(R)
(S)
Me
Me

OH
Me
(S)
(S)
Me
Me

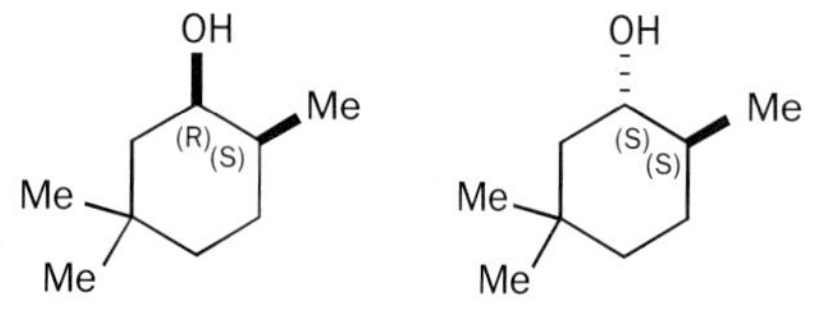

3. The two products are (R,Z)-6-chloro-6-cyclopentyl-N-methylhex-5-en-2-amine and (S, Z)-6-chloro-6-cyclopentyl-N-methylhex-5-en-2-amine. (Try saying those ten times fast!)

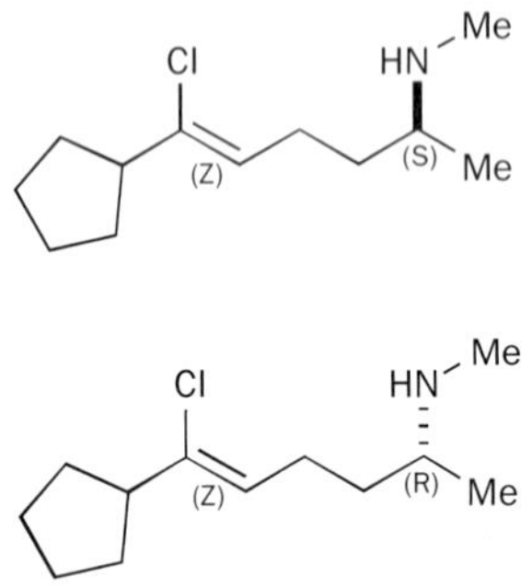

Cl HN Me (Z) (S) Me

Cl HN Me (Z) (R) Me

CHAPTER 2: ISOMERS

1. C

To answer this question correctly—and avoid picking (B)—you must remember that atoms other than carbon can be chiral. By definition, a chiral center is an atom that is bonded to four different atoms or groups of atoms; in addition to carbon, nitrogen, phosphorus, sulfur, and other atoms can also be chiral centers. There are two chiral centers in this molecule—a carbon and a nitrogen—adjacent to each other in the pyrrolidine ring.

2. B

The 4,4-dimethyl-3-phenylpentane-2-ol molecule is presented in the Newman projection. Drawing the alcohol in straight chain form, keeping in mind that the hydrogen atoms are *trans-* to each other, and the hydroxyl group is *trans-* to the *t*-butyl group, gives:

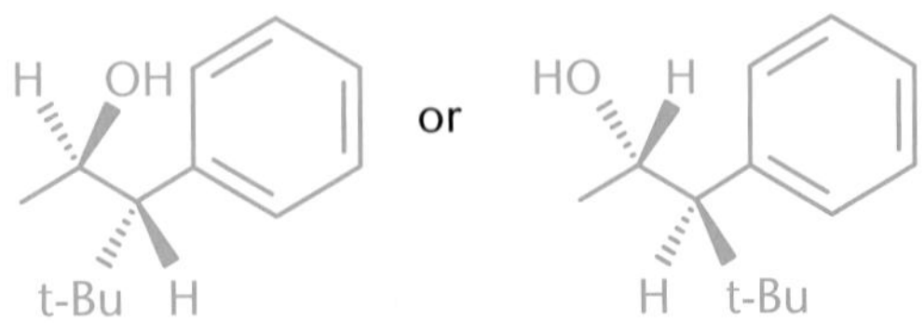

H OH t-Bu H or HO H H t-Bu

Because the stereocenters are at C2 and C3, (A) and (C) are incorrect. Starting with C2, assigning priority gives –OH as 1, C bonded to rest of compound as 2, the methyl group as 3, and H as 4, for a 2R configuration for the left alcohol, or 2S for the right alcohol. Assigning priorities to C3 gives: C bonded to the adjacent –OH is 1, C of the benzene is 2, C of tert-butyl group is 3 and H is 4, to give 3S for the left alcohol, or 3R for the right alcohol. Because (B) refers to the left alcohol, it is the correct answer.

3. D

While this is a bulky, complex molecule, the incorrect (true) statements can be eliminated quickly. (A) is true, because the molecule contains both an amine and a carboxylic acid. (B) is also true, in that nitrogen bound to two hydrogens defines a primary amine. Moreover, a benzene ring with an –OH group is referred to as a phenol. (C) is also correct because the carboxylic acid is the highest priority functional group in the molecule leading to the molecule being named with either the suffix "–oic acid." This leaves (D) as the false statement: The maximum number of stereoisomers that a molecule may have is 2^n, where n is the number of stereogenic atoms. There are four stereocenters in the compound, shown by asterisks below, giving $2^4 = 16$ possible stereoisomers. For 32 stereoisomers, there needs to be five stereocenters present.

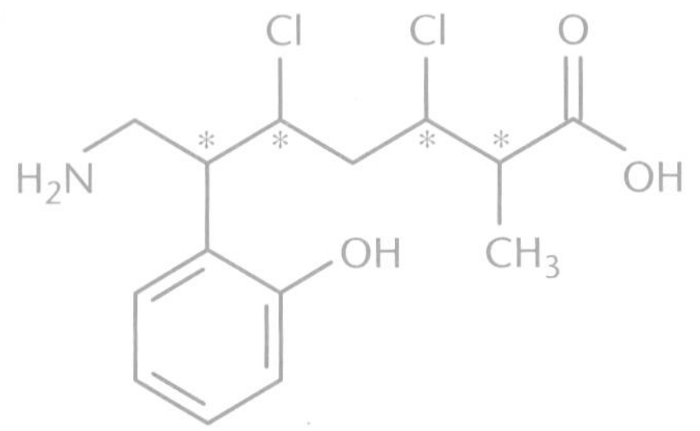

Cl Cl O H_2N OH OH CH_3

4. B

The addition of bromine across a double bond gives a *trans*-dibromo product, because each bromide is added sequentially, with the initial formation of a bromonium (Br^+) intermediate, where the first bromide forms bonds to both carbon atoms. Nucleophilic attack of the second bromide occurs in a S_N2 fashion, such that the bromine atoms are on opposite sides; *cis*-dibromo products cannot form, so (A) and (C) are incorrect. Because both bromines are added, (D) is incorrect.

HIGH-YIELD SIMILAR QUESTIONS

Isomers

1. The two alkenes are geometric isomers (and therefore diastereomers as well).
2. Yes, hydrogenation would destroy the distinction between E and Z alkenes to give the same molecule.
3. Because the two geometric isomers are diastereomers, they would have different physical properties (different melting points, boiling points, solubilities, etc.). After hydrogenation, they would have the same properties because they would be the same molecule.

Meso Compounds

1. Only the middle compound would give rise to an achiral polyol upon reduction.

Fischer Projections

Questions 1 and 2:

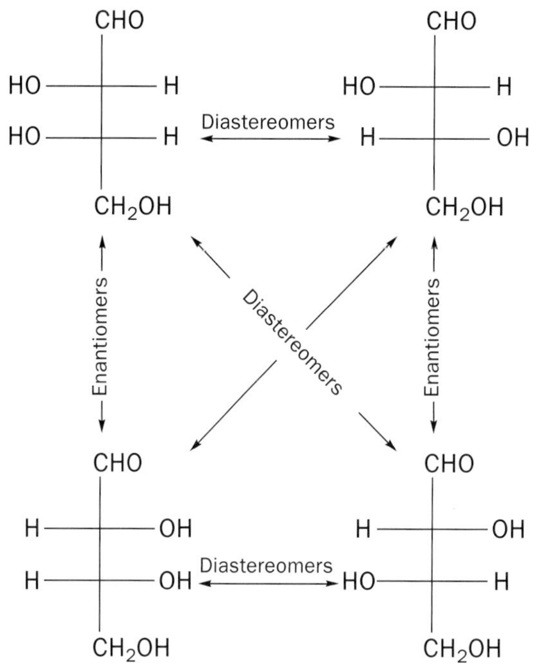

CHO; HO—H; HO—H; CH_2OH ←Diastereomers→ CHO; HO—H; H—OH; CH_2OH

Enantiomers / Diastereomers / Diastereomers / Enantiomers

CHO; H—OH; H—OH; CH_2OH ←Diastereomers→ CHO; H—OH; HO—H; CH_2OH

3. The two products are enantiomers.

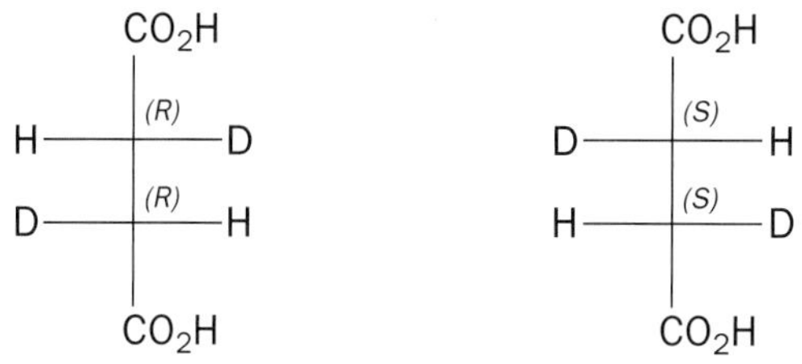

CO_2H; H—(R)—D; D—(R)—H; CO_2H

CO_2H; D—(S)—H; H—(S)—D; CO_2H

CHAPTER 3: BONDING

1. C

Single bonds consist of sigma bonds only, which are sp^3 hybridized and in a tetrahedral geometry, and have bond angles of 109.5°. Double bonds have one sigma and one pi bond, and are sp^2 hybridized with a bond angle of 120° (trigonal planar geometry.) Triple bonds have one sigma bond and two pi bonds, and are sp hybridized with a bond angle of 180°. (A) and (B) refer to double bonds. (C) correctly lists the bond angle for a single bond.

2. A

Carbon dioxide is linear and therefore the dipole forces oppose and negate each other. The same is true for $BeCl_2$: even though the Be–Cl bond is polar, the linearity of the molecule leaves no net dipole moment. (C) is incorrect because the lone pair of electrons in NH_3 adds to the net dipole moment, while the lone pair in NF_3 opposes the dipole effect of the N–F bonds. SO_2 has two lone pairs, and is not linear (SO_2 has the same geometry as H_2O, which has a substantial dipole moment).

3. C

While both H_2O and HF participate in hydrogen bonding, the structure of water allows it to form a greater number of H–bonds than HF. This increased H–bonding leads to an increase in boiling point, so (A) is incorrect. Similarly, the -OH in 1-butanol forms H–bonds while the central oxygen atom of its isomer, diethyl ether, does not, so (D) is incorrect. (B) is also incorrect because ammonia can form various hydrogen bonds with water while methane cannot (see below). DMSO, or dimethylsulfoxide, is a polar molecule but it does not participate in hydrogen bonding; rather, it dissolves ions by ion-dipole attraction (see below).

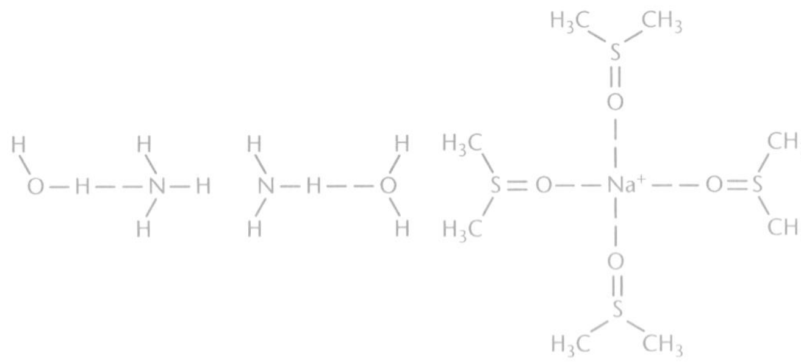

4. D

Benzene has a delocalized pi system, and all of the carbon atoms are sp^2 hybridized, thus (A) is incorrect. 1-butyne has single and triple bonds, which means it exhibits both sp and sp^3 hybridization, making (B) incorrect. Propene has single and double bonds, corresponding to sp^3 and sp^2 hybridized orbitals, so (C) is incorrect. 2,3-hexadiene is a cumulene, where the two alkenes are directly adjacent to each other, the carbon between the two alkenes is sp hybridized, with a bond angle of 180°. Because the remainder of the molecule contains sp^2 and sp^3 hybridized orbitals, (D) is correct.

CHAPTER 4: ALKANES

1. A

A general rule of thumb is that branching decreases the boiling point of any particular alkane, due to sterics, leading to weaker van der Waals interactions, so (D) is incorrect. In (C), the wrong isomer is paired with the reason. n–Octane (left molecule), being linear and having more places to interact with other molecules through van der Waals forces, means its boiling point is higher than 2,3,4-trimethylpentane (right molecule). (B) is incorrect because the electronegativity difference between C–H bonds in different alkane isomers is the same, or negligible.

2. D

For Grignard reagents to be destroyed, the reaction media must be sufficiently acidic. However, hydrogen atoms in alkanes are among the least acidic protons, regardless of location. Therefore, (D) is correct.

3. D

The Wurtz reaction is the sodium-promoted coupling of two alkyl halides to form an alkane: 2 R–X + 2 Na → 2 R–R + 2 Na–X where X=Br or Cl. Starting with 1,3-dichlorocyclobutane, both chlorides leave the reactant and a single C–C bond is formed, resulting in the strained ring shown in (D). (A) could apply if the reaction mixture contained $ClCH_3$; however, in that case it would not be the major product. No new bonds (B) are being formed (only reduction of chloride groups have occurred). (C) is not a possible product from 1,3-dichlorocyclobutane.

4. C

A Wurtz reaction is useful in the preparation of symmetric alkanes, with an even number of carbons. Note that the resulting alkane will have an even number of carbon atoms, regardless of the starting alkyl halide.) The alkanes in (A) and (B) contain an odd number of carbon atoms. The alkane in (C) could be formed by: 2 $(CH_3)_2CHCH_2X$ + 2 Na → C_8H_{18} + 2 NaCl. (D) is incorrect because the alkane is asymmetric and it is difficult to form only that product from two alkyl halides with different structures.

5. D

All of these methods could be used to reduce an alkyl halide to its corresponding alkane. In (A) and (B), a hydrogen atom replaces the chlorine atom reducing it to the alkane. (C) describes a Grignard reaction with the Mg forming an organometallic with the reactant followed by a reaction with water to form the alkane.

HIGH-YIELD SIMILAR QUESTIONS

Nucleophilicity Trends

1. The molecules in order of increasing nucleophilicity are: acetonitrile < pyridine < DMAP < triethylamine.
2. In methanol, the nucleophilicity order is I > Br > Cl > F. In DMSO, it would be F > Cl > Br > I.
3. The ordering of increasing nucleophilicity in methanol is: $Ph_3N < Et_3N < Ph_3P < Et_3P < Et_3As$. Triphenylamine and triphenylphosphine are less nucleophilic than triethylamine and triethylphosphine, respectively, because with the phenyl analogs the lone pair can be delocalized into the three phenyl rings, making the lone pair more stable and therefore less reactive (and less nucleophilic). As for the triethyl compounds, the amine is less nucleophilic than the phosphine, which is less nucleophilic than the arsine, because nitrogen is surrounded by more solvent molecules *via* hydrogen bonds, and therefore it is harder for the lone pair to react because it is stabilized by hydrogen bonding. Triphenylarsine is the most nucleophilic because it is least surrounded by solvent.

Substrate Reactivity: S_N1 Reactions

1. The resulting tropenyl (cycloheptatrienyl) cation is aromatic.
2. The products isolated would be a mixture of 1-methoxybutane (methyl butyl ether), 2-methoxybutane (methyl *sec*-butyl ether), and 2-methoxy-2-methylpropane (*tert*-butyl methyl ether; this one is a bit tricky to figure out).
3. 1-Iodocyclopropene is much more reactive because the carbocation generated when the iodide leaves is aromatic.

CHAPTER 5: ALKENES AND ALKYNES

1. D

The longest straight chain contains six carbons, so (B) and (C) are incorrect. Between (A) and (D), proper IUPAC naming requires that the sum be as low as possible. The sum of numbers in (A) is 10 while in (D) it is eight, so (A) is incorrect. The substitution at the alkene is Z, because the two groups with the higher priority are on the same side of the alkene.

2. A

Hydrogenation with Lindlar's catalyst will partially reduce triple bonds, giving alkenes (B) and (D).

The addition of hydrogen occurs in a *syn* fashion *i.e.,* both hydrogen atoms are added on the same side, and so the alkene formed will have a Z geometry (see below), so (C) is incorrect.

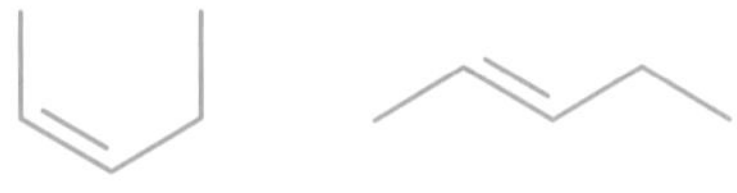

Z-2-pentene E-2-pentene

3. C

At –78°C, the addition of bromine across a diene gives the *kinetic* product *i.e.,* a 1,4-addition. (B) is the *thermodynamic* product (1,2-addition). At lower temperatures, intermediates become more long-lived, allowing rearrangements to occur (see below). Bromine cannot be added to the same carbon (A). The double bond is broken with the addition of bromine (D).

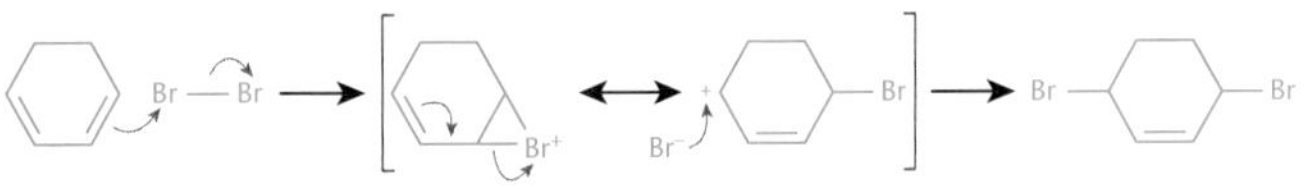

4. D

(A) and (B) add across the triple bond to yield aldehydes with terminal alkynes, and ketones with internal alkynes, so they are incorrect. Acidic $KMnO_4$ will cleave triple bonds with concurrent oxidation, giving carboxylic acids and carbon dioxide (with terminal alkynes) (C).

5. B

The addition of HBr across 1-pentene gives 1-bromopentane, making (A) incorrect. To yield 2-bromopentane, the reaction mechanism needs to proceed by radical addition, and peroxides are known to easily generate radicals, so (B) is correct. Heating the mixture (C) has no effect on dictating anti-Markovnikov addition, and (D) will cause formation of *trans*-1,2-dibromopentane.

CHAPTER 6: AROMATIC COMPOUNDS

1. C

The order of reactions is Friedel-Crafts acylation, Friedel-Crafts alkylation, Williamson ether synthesis, and Clemmenson reduction (see below.)

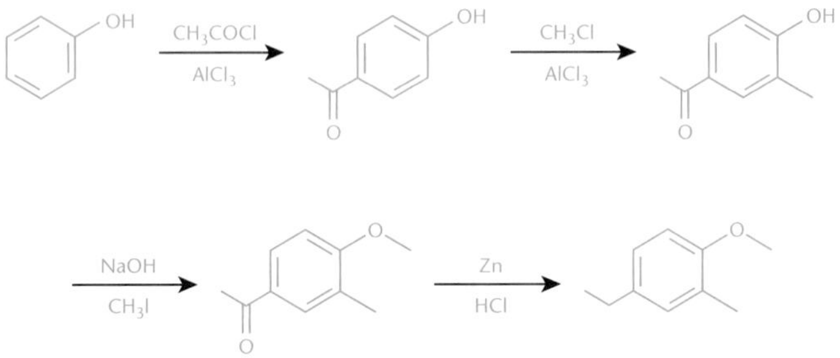

(A) refers to the penultimate product above, while (B) implies that the Williamson ether synthesis furnishes the benzene with an additional methyl group. (D) implies that a chloride from HCl is added to benzene.

2. A

The ammonium group, with a positive charge on nitrogen, deactivates the benzene by pulling electron density away from the ring, directing subsequent groups to the *meta* positions. (B) refers to groups that donate electron density into the benzene ring *e.g.,* alcohols, amines, and so on., while (C) refers to halogens. *Meta*-directing groups cannot activate the ring (D).

3. B

The formula for aromaticity follows Hückel's Rule, which states that the number of π electrons equals $4n + 2$, where n is an integer. Counting two electrons per double bond or sp^2 atom: item I has eight electrons, item II has 10 (including the lone pair on nitrogen), and item III has eight. Only item II gives an integer for n (4), while I and III give $n = 1.5$.

4. A

NBS, or N-bromosuccinimide is a reagent used in radical bromination. Benzene rings themselves rarely undergo radical reactions because radical formation would result in a loss of aromatic stabilization (C) and (D). The most stable radical for ethyl benzene is the benzyl radical (see below), so bromine will most likely be added to that position, making (A) the correct answer. The product in (B) implies that an unstable primary radical is formed as an intermediate.

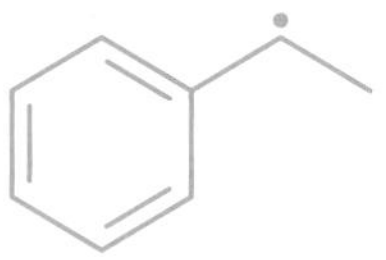

5. D

The key to answering this question is to decide where the carbonyl group is situated given the chemical shifts. The multiplet at d 7.20 corresponds to the five protons in the benzene ring. (C) can be quickly disregarded because there is no signal that corresponds to the aldehyde proton. (B)'s structure cannot produce a singlet on the ^{1}H NMR spectrum. The spectrum for (A)'s structure will not have a quartet.

HIGH-YIELD SIMILAR QUESTIONS

Electrophilic Aromatic Substitution

1.

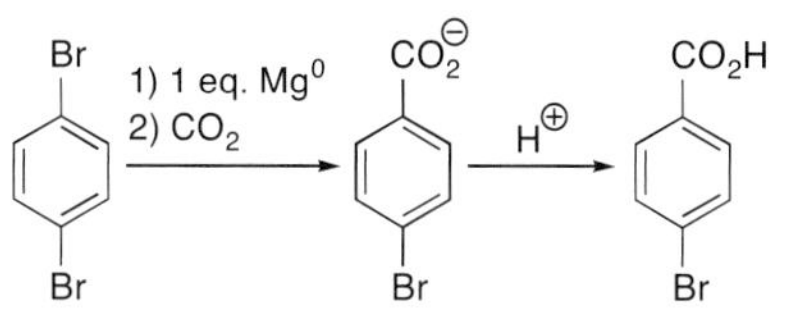

Br, Br; 1) 1 eq. Mg^0 2) CO_2 → $CO_2^{\ominus}$, Br; $H^{\oplus}$ → CO_2H, Br

2. Either *ortho* or *para* to the methoxy group.

3.

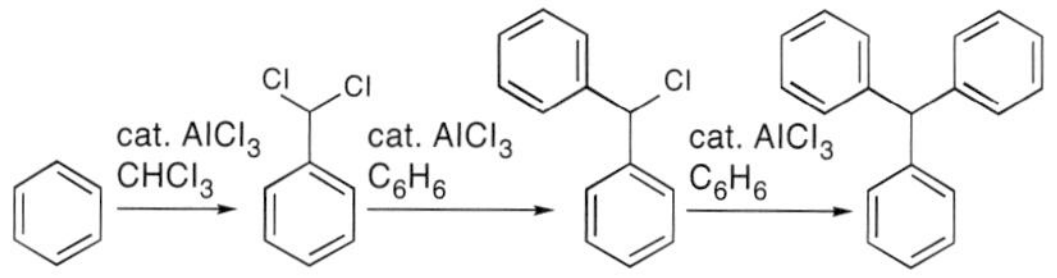

cat. $AlCl_3$, $CHCl_3$ → Cl, Cl; cat. $AlCl_3$, C_6H_6 → Cl; cat. $AlCl_3$, C_6H_6 →

Identifying Structure of Unknown Aromatic

1. Either strong aqueous acid or strong aqueous base would hydrolyze the aromatic amide back to the aromatic amine.
2. The ketone is conjugated with the aromatic ring, and therefore more stable and lower in energy. Because $E = hf = hc/\lambda$, lower energy means a lower wavenumber stretch in the IR.
3. The unstable primary carbocation is converted into a more substituted and therefore more stable secondary carbocation.

CHAPTER 7: ALCOHOLS AND ETHERS

1. C

mCPBA is used to form epoxides, which occurs in a *syn* fashion. Starting with E-2-pentene, two products, a pair of enantiomers, are possible:

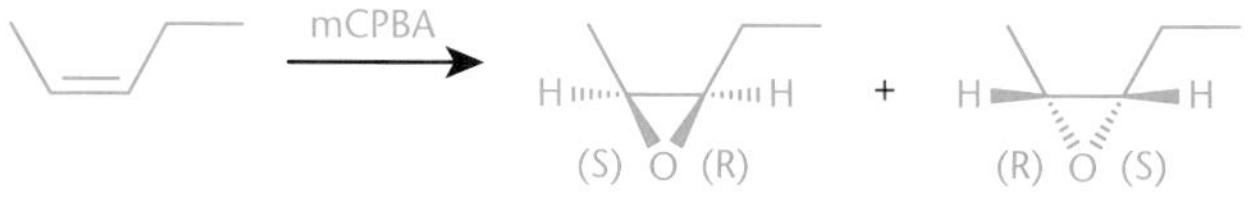

mCPBA → H, H, (S) O (R) + H, H, (R) O (S)

Item I is incorrect, as formation of a 2(R), 3(R) product implies that epoxidation occurs in an *anti*-fashion. Item IV is also incorrect, as a 2(S), 3(S) product is the enantiomers of 2(R), 3(R), which does not form. Because those items are incorrect, the answer here must be (C).

2. A

In the presence of strong acids, ethers are cleaved, via protonation of the oxygen atom, followed by a

S_N2 reaction by the bromide ion, forming an alkyl halide and an alcohol. However, because benzene cannot undergo S_N2 reactions, the bromide ion can only attack on the propyl side of the ether, forming phenol and bromopropane:

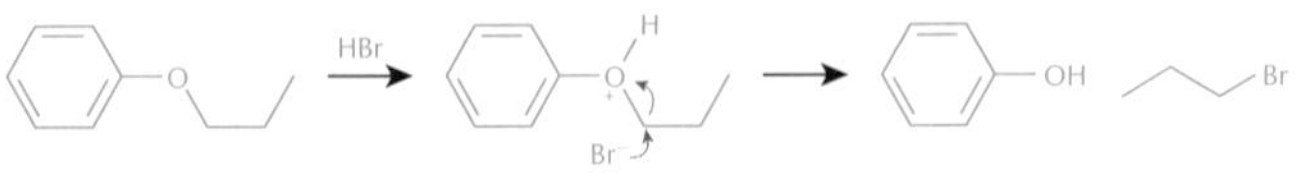

(B) and (C) require bromide to attack the benzene carbon in an S_N2 fashion. Hydrocarbons do not form during ether cleavage (D).

3. D

Primary and secondary alcohols can undergo oxidation, while tertiary alcohols (A) cannot. Ketones and carboxylic acids (B) and (C) cannot be further oxidized.

4. C

Acid-catalyzed dehydration of tertiary alcohols proceeds by E1, via the formation of a stable tertiary carbocation. There are three products possible:

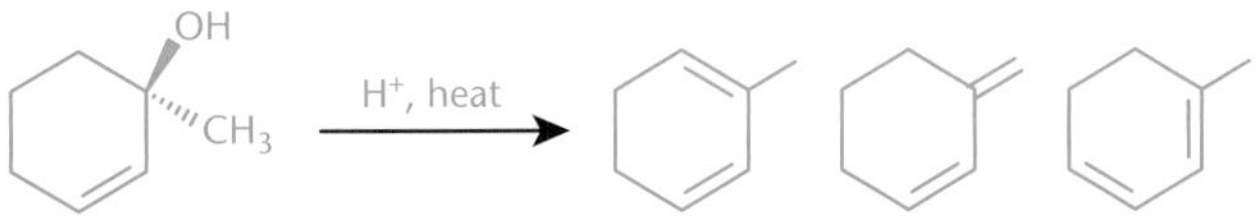

The third product comes from a separate resonance form.

5. D

The product comes from a base catalyzed opening of the epoxide. (A) and (C) are acidic conditions, while bromomethane alone (B) is unlikely to elicit any ring opening (a catalyst is required). Base catalysis (D), with sodium methoxide as the base, can effectively open the epoxide ring and furnish the methyl ether in the correct position.

CHAPTER 8: ALDEHYDES AND KETONES

1. D

Hydrazine is nucleophilic, and attacks the carbonyl carbon of both molecules, forming a negatively charged oxide intermediate. However, for benzoyl chloride, the C=O double bond is reformed, and chloride is displaced as it is a good leaving group. (D) is an example of a substitution reaction. Benzaldehyde, on the other hand, forms a hydrazone with hydrazine, via nucleophilic addition, and condensation (the carbonyl oxygen atom leaves as water). Benzaldehyde and benzoyl chloride undergo different reactions (A), the final products are clearly different (B), and the reaction types have been transposed (C).

2. A

Oxygen 2 is initially protonated (activated to leave as water), followed by nucleophilic attack by the alcohol group (oxygen 3) on the carbonyl carbon atom. The cyclic product, a lactone, contains oxygens 1 and 3, so (A) is correct. While oxygen 2 could act as a nucleophile, it cannot attack the carbonyl group it is bonded to (B). (C) requires water to be a nucleophile, and thus a cyclic product will not form. Finally, radioisotope labeling of the oxygen atoms could be used to effectively determine which atom is incorporated into each molecule, so (D) is incorrect.

3. B

In the reaction, perchloric acid only serves to provide protons—not oxygen atoms—to the reactant, the methyl enol ether of acetone, so (D) is true. Mechanistically, in the acidic environment, the alkene becomes protonated, and oxygen forms a C=O double bond with the newly formed carbocation. The oxygen atom is temporarily positively charged, opening up the central carbon atom to nucleophilic attack by water. This means that (C) is true. The newly added water transfers a proton to the methoxy group to form methanol, which is a good leaving group and yields the two products listed. Therefore the oxygen atom of the enol ether will actually be found in methanol, not acetone, so (A) is true and (B) is false, making it the correct choice.

4. D

The structure of 3-ethylhept-6-en-3-ol is shown below:

An anhydrous environment implies that Grignard reagents are being used. Because various Grignard reagents are present among the choices, all of them are feasible. (A) and (B) both produce the product required, the only difference being the initial Grignard reagent. (C) also produces the same product, because Grignard reagents will alkylate esters to completion, forming tertiary alcohols. Because (A), (B), and (C) give 3-ethylhept-6-en-3-ol, (D) is correct.

5. C

A Robinson Annulation forms a new six-membered ring via a Michael addition (*e.g.,* nucleophilic addition to a, β-unsaturated ketones), followed by an aldol condensation; therefore, the progression of steps in (C) is correct. A substitution is not involved in ring formation.

CHAPTER 9: CARBOXYLIC ACIDS

1. C

1-Bromopentane can be used to synthesize hexanoic acid in either of the "step-up" reactions listed in (A) and (B). The additional carbon comes from CO_2 (A) or –CN (B). When 1-heptyne is oxidized in aqueous acidic permanganate, the terminal carbon is lost as CO_2, and the remaining molecule is hexanoic acid. Cyclohexene can also be oxidized by $KMnO_4$, but the product is a dicarboxylic acid formed from oxidative cleavage of the double bond, to give adipic acid (1,6-hexanedioic acid) (C) is the correct choice.

2. C

PCl_3, PCl_5, and $SOCl_2$ are all sufficiently reactive to donate a chloride atom to a carboxylic acid to form the acyl chloride. The C–Cl bond of carbon tetrachloride, a common solvent rather than a reagent, is quite stable and is not a good source of Cl^- nucleophiles.

3. A

Lithium aluminum hydride ($LiAlH_4$) is an effective reducing agent for carboxylic acids. It is also very reactive with water, so performing the reaction as listed in (B) does not work. While sodium tetrahydroborate is a reducing agent, it is not strong enough to reduce carboxylic acids.

4. D

The reaction described is a Fischer esterification where the –OH group of ethanoic acid is first protonated to form water, which is a good leaving group. The oxygen atom of ethanol then attacks the carbonyl carbon of ethanoic acid nucleophilically, ultimately displacing water to form ethyl acetate.

The acid catalyst is regenerated from the proton of ethanol. While acetic anhydride can form via the coupling of two acetic acid molecules, it would not be a major product given the conditions listed in the question (A). Ethers and alkenes do not form under these conditions either, (B) and (C).

5. B

The reaction takes place according to the figure below. The labeled carbon ends up in the second position. The molecule in (A) could be produced by treating methyliodide with Mg and then reacting the product with an oxirane followed by reduction with permanganate. (C) could be obtained by treating chloroethane with Mg and proceeding with carbonation. Multiple labeled carbon molecules are required in order to obtain the molecule in (D).

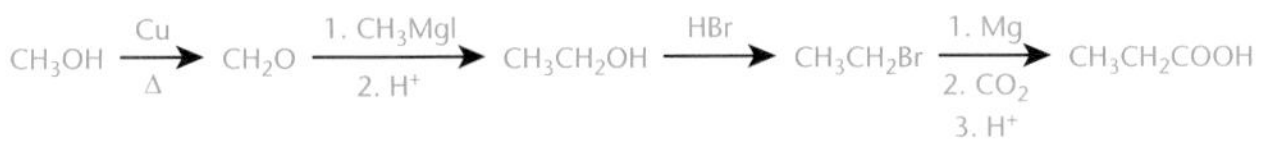

$$CH_3OH \xrightarrow[\Delta]{Cu} CH_2O \xrightarrow[2.\ H^+]{1.\ CH_3MgI} CH_3CH_2OH \xrightarrow{HBr} CH_3CH_2Br \xrightarrow[2.\ CO_2\ \ 3.\ H^+]{1.\ Mg} CH_3CH_2COOH$$

CHAPTER 10: CARBOXYLIC ACID DERIVATIVES

1. A

Rotation about the C–N bond in (A) is significantly hindered, so much so that it produces two peaks by PMR (see below). The C–C and C–O bonds rotate freely and would not exist as optical diastereomers.

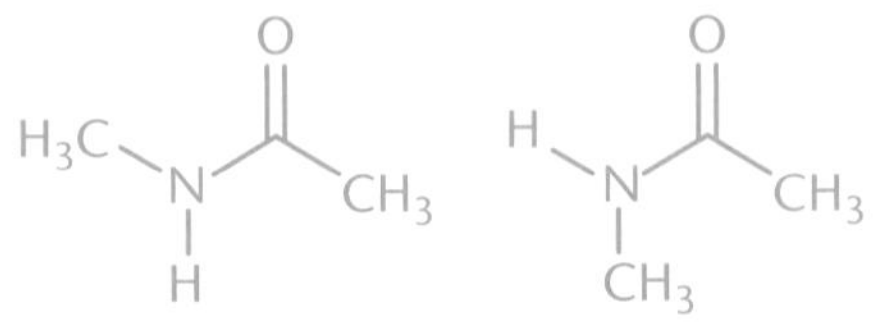

E-isomer: $H_3C-NH-C(=O)-CH_3$

Z-isomer: $H-N(CH_3)-C(=O)-CH_3$

E-isomer **Z-isomer**

2. D

There is a hierarchy to the reactivity of carboxylic acid derivatives, which dictates how reactive they are toward nucleophilic attack. This order, from highest to lowest, is the following:

Acid chlorides > anhydrides > esters > amides

In practical terms this means that derivatives of higher reactivity can form derivatives of lower activity, but not the opposite. Acid chlorides are more reactive with than anhydrides and esters (A) and (B). Anhydrides are more reactive than amides (C). Nucleophilic attack of an ester cannot result in the corresponding anhydride.

3. C

Halide ions are excellent leaving groups and acyl halides are very reactive compounds. Halide groups in acyl halides are open neither to nucleophilic (A) nor electrophilic attack (B). It is the carbonyl carbon that favors nucleophilic attack. Rotation about the C=O (D) is irrelevant, as it is not specific to acyl halides.

4. A

A Fischer esterification involves refluxing a carboxylic acid and a primary or secondary alcohol with an acid catalyst. Under these conditions, the carbonyl carbon is open to attack by the oxygen atom in the alcohol acting as a nucleophile. The rate of this reaction is dependant of the amount of sterics at and around the carbonyl carbon. The molecule in (A) is the least sterically hindered, thus the reaction will take place most rapidly. (B), (C), and (D) have increasing amounts of steric crowding, which correlate with decreasing rates of esterification.

5. D

The presence of the oxygen atom in the carbonyl group makes the adjacent carbon more electrophilic (and thus more reactive) toward nucleophilic attack than an alkyl halide. The transition state formed when an acyl chloride undergoes a nucleophilic reaction is less sterically hindered than the transition state produced by the primary alkyl halide reaction (B). The pi bond of the carbonyl group requires less energy to break than the sigma bond of the alkyl chloride (C). The more electronegative an atom or group, the better leaving group it is. The rate of reaction is increased by the relative positive charge of the carbon (electrophile) that is being attacked by the nucleophile. If the chloride in the alkyl halide is more electronegative than the Cl in the acyl halide, then the reaction of the alkyl halide should progress more rapidly. Therefore (D) is the correct answer.

HIGH-YIELD SIMILAR QUESTIONS

Intramolecular Ring Closures

1.

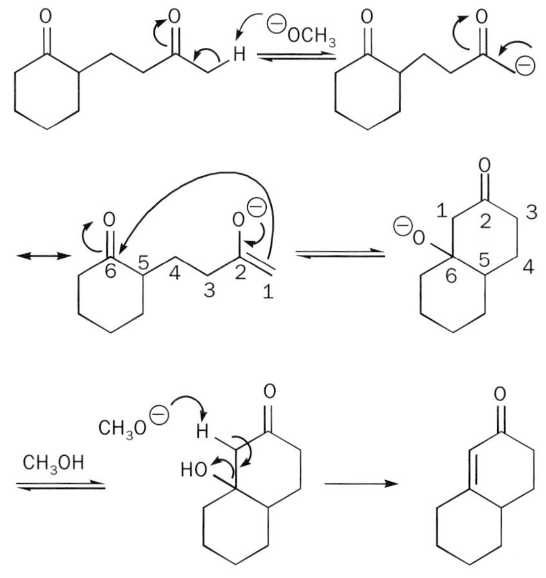

O O $^{\ominus}OCH_3$ H O O

O 6 5 4 3 2 1 O 1 2 3 O 6 5 4

CH_3OH $CH_3O^{\ominus}$ H HO O O

2.

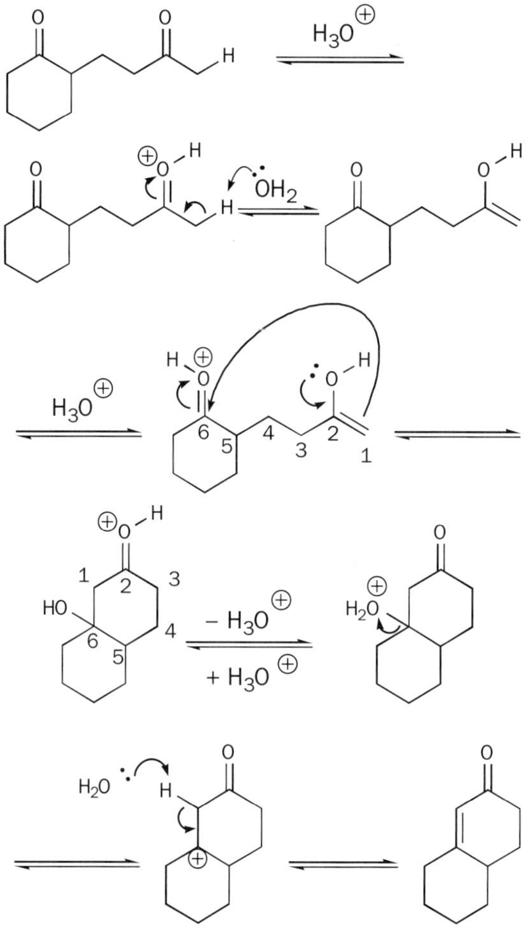

O O H $H_3O^{\oplus}$

O $^{\oplus}O$–H $\ddot{O}H_2$ H O O–H

$H_3O^{\oplus}$ H $\oplus$ O 6 5 4 3 2 1 O–H

$^{\oplus}O$–H 1 2 3 HO 4 6 5 $-\ H_3O^{\oplus}$ $+\ H_3O^{\oplus}$ $H_2O^{\oplus}$ O

H_2O H O O

3.

HO H $EtO^{\ominus}$ O H O O

H O H O

H $O^{\ominus}$ EtOH H OH O O

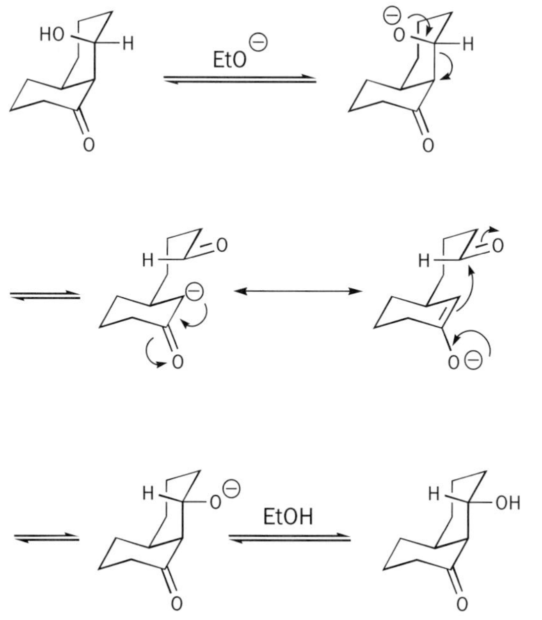

CHAPTER 11: AMINES AND NITROGEN-CONTAINING COMPOUNDS

1. C

All groups (except hydrogen atoms) bonded to nitrogen need to be specified by the N- prefix, followed by the group. This prefix is repeated for each group. (A) fails to provide a N- prefix per methyl substituent, while (B) uses no prefixes. (D) does not specify the position of the amino substituent.

2. A

The nitrogen atoms in pyrrolidine and pyrrole have one lone pair (with three bond pairs) to remain neutral, so (C) and (D) are incorrect. An anti-aromatic system has 4n electrons, where *n* is an integer. Because pyrrolidine lacks such a system, (B) is incorrect. Pyrrole is indeed aromatic, because there are 6p electrons, counting the lone pair on the nitrogen. The lone pair is part of a stable benzene-like electron system, which explains the extremely low basicity.

3. D

This is an exhaustive methylation reaction, with the amine tethered to the alkene, instead of being an individual product. (B) is incorrect, because the reaction is incomplete. (A) is also incorrect, because the methyl groups are not removed. (C) is incorrect given the starting amine.

4. C

The intermediate for a reductive amination is an imine, formed between a carbonyl group and a primary amine. (A) is incorrect, because nowhere during imine formation does an ammonium ion form, while (B) is incorrect because it is piperidine itself. Finally, (D) is an enamine, formed between a carbonyl group and a *secondary* amine. The starting material does not have any secondary amines present.

5. B

A nitrene is the nitrogen equivalent of a carbene, a highly reactive *neutral* species.

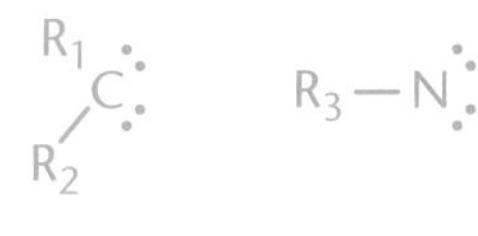

Carbene **Nitrene**

CHAPTER 12: PURIFICATION AND SEPARATION

1. B

Isoelectric focusing exploits the isoelectric point of proteins, which are separated based on pH only. Separation by mass (A) is an important principle for SDS-PAGE. (C) is incorrect because separation by charge is the basis for any electrophoresis. (D) is incorrect because molecules tend to "tumble," or move freely, during electrophoresis, making molecule shape an inaccurate tool for resolution.

2. C

R_f, or retention value, is a quotient between the distance moved by the spot (sample) over the distance moved by the solvent front. In other words, the closer the spot is to the solvent front, the larger the R_f. The polarity of each compound is given, as well as the solvent system used, both of which point to compound III as being the top spot. (B) is incorrect, as the second largest R_f can belong to either compound I or IV, both less polar than III. The spot with the smallest R_f (A) belongs to compound II, the most nonpolar compound amongst the four.

3. B

SDS is a detergent, and will digest proteins, forming micelles with uniform negative charges. Because the protein is sequestered within the micelle, other factors such as charge of the protein, and shape play minimal roles during separation; in essence, the protein micelles can be modeled as being spheres of different sizes. SDS has no effect on the gel matrix (polyacrylamide), so (A) and (C) are incorrect (reducing agents, like mercaptoethanol, are used to break up multiunit proteins.) (D) incorrectly describes the micelles as being positively charged.

4. A

Because methylene chloride is denser than brine (saltwater), the organic layer will settle at the bottom of the funnel, making (C) incorrect. (B) is also incorrect; methylene chloride is nonpolar, so it cannot mix with brine.

HIGH-YIELD SIMILAR QUESTIONS

Isoelectric Focusing

1. It will migrate toward the cathode.
2. pI = (pKa of COOH1 + pKa of COOH2)/2
3. Zwitterion form

Extraction

1. Benzoic acid is a stronger acid than phenol, thus a weak base can be used to deprotonate benzoic acid and move it into the aqueous phase.
2. p-Nitrophenol and phenol will be deprotonated by the strong base and will move into the aqueous phase.

Chromatography

1. 3 cm
2. In a more basic environment, more proteins will have a greater negative charge increasing their affinity to the anion exchanger.
3. Electrophoresis is a technique that can separate proteins based on size.

CHAPTER 13: SPECTROSCOPY

1. C

Alkyl benzenes commonly break apart to form a benzyl fragment (m/z 91), which rearranges to a *tropylium* fragment, which is aromatic (the empty p-orbital is part of the continuous p-system). It can also be found by calculating the weights of the fragments for each choice: 105 for (A), 104 for B (note the structure is cyclooctatetraene, which is antiaromatic), and 103 for (D).

2. B

The region in question often gives information about the types of alkyl groups present. Specifically, an ethyl group will give a characteristic triplet (for the methyl group, which is coupled to $-CH_2$), and a quartet (for $-CH_2$, which is coupled to the methyl group), while a septet (for the –CH group, which is coupled to two methyl groups) and a doublet (for the two methyl groups coupled to –CH) are characteristic of an isopropyl group. (C) is incorrect since the alkyl group to peak relationship is reversed, while the alcohol hydrogen (D) is an unreliable check because that peak can occur anywhere between 0–10 ppm, depending on the alcohol.

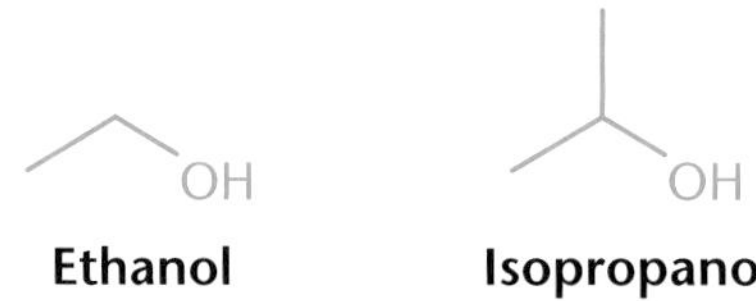

Ethanol   Isopropanol

3. C

The molecule is symmetric, with a mirror plane present that bisects the nitrogen and carbon atoms in the center ring, so many carbon atoms will have identical chemical shifts in the ^{13}C NMR spectrum. There is one signal for the outermost four carbon atoms, one signal for the four carbon atoms in the middle of the outer rings, one signal for the bridgehead carbon atoms, and finally 1 signal for the carbon in the center ring, for a total of 4 ^{13}C signals. (A), (B) and (D) fail to account fully for the mirror plane giving rise to identical signals.

4. A

In conjugation with double bonds, carbonyl groups (C=O) tend to absorb at lower wave numbers because the delocalization of p-electrons causes the C=O bond to lose double bond character; that shifts the stretching frequency closer to C–O stretches, which occur between 1,000–1,250 cm^{-1}. For that reason, (B) and (C) are incorrect. For the C=O stretch to disappear (D), the bond would need to be fully broken, which is not something that happens during conjugation.

HIGH-YIELD SIMILAR QUESTIONS

NMR Spectroscopy

1.

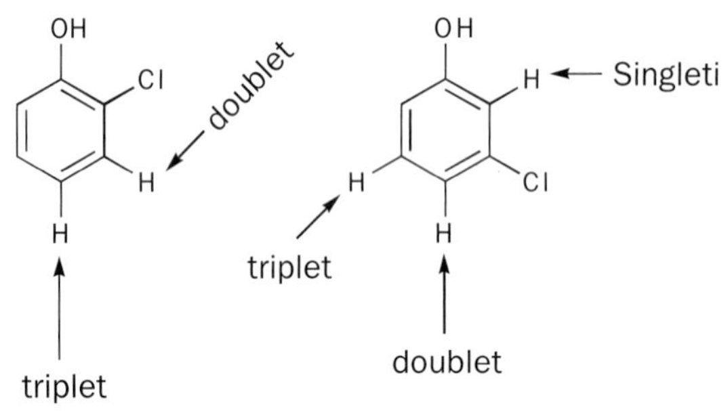

2. Alcohols (and amine) protons tend to have very broad shapes, rather than sharp, well defined peaks. This is due to the fact that they exchange protons with residual water in the solvent.
3. In general, the aromatic protons wouldn't be shifted as far downfield, because iodine is less electronegative than chlorine.

Combined Spectroscopy: IR and NMR

1. You only have six carbons to work with, so any rings present would have to be small, meaning that they would have a great deal of angle strain. This would make having multiple rings in the unknown very unlikely.
2. The carbonyl IR stretch would be closer to 1700 (*i.e.,* weaker). The resonance donation of the ester alkoxide makes the C=O bond more unstable and therefore higher in energy.
3. The methyl ketone protons would be further upfield in the NMR (closer to 2 ppm than 4 ppm). This is because the partial positive charge on the carbonyl carbon is less electron withdrawing than a highly electronegative oxygen.

CHAPTER 14: CARBOHYDRATES

1. D

The easiest way to answer this question is to determine the stereochemistry of C2 (counting from the aldehyde), which for both sugars is R. Because the other chiral carbons for both sugars are the same, they are identical; (A) and (B) are incorrect. (C) is incorrect because there is no internal plane of symmetry.

2. C

(A) and (B) are incorrect because there are no hemiacetals present. For sugars in straight chain form, a reducing sugar contains groups at either end of the chain which can be oxidized; (D) is incorrect with two carboxylic acids, which cannot be oxidized further. (C) is a reducing sugar, via ketone-enol tautomerism.

3. A

Galactose is a diastereomer of glucose, with the stereochemistry at C4 (counting from the aldehyde) reversed. Being able to identify C4 is enough to answer this question, even if you do not remember what glucose looks like. Because (B), (C) and (D) have identical stereochemistry at C4, they are incorrect.

4. D

To answer this question, replace the ends of each sugar with carboxylic acids, and then find the meso sugar. (B) is incorrect because the aldaric acid remains optically active (no internal mirror plane), while (A) and (C) are identical (one is the 180° flip of the other).

CHAPTER 15: AMINO ACIDS, PEPTIDES, AND PROTEINS

1. B

The primary structure of proteins is simply the chain of amino acids linked by covalent (peptide) bonds (A). Tertiary structure (C) is indeed formed by hydrophobic interactions, in addition to hydrogen bonding, salt bridges, and disulfide bonds. Secondary structure (B), such as a-helices and b-sheets, does not depend on formation of disulfide bonds, so it is the correct answer.

2. A

(C) and (D) are incorrect because Strecker synthesis converts aldehydes, not carboxylic acids, into amino acids. The aldehyde is first converted to an imine with ammonia, followed by nucleophilic attack with cyanide to form an a-aminonitrile. The nitrile is subsequently hydrolyzed to a carboxylic acid. (B) reverses the reaction steps.

3. D

The Edman degradation is useful only in sequencing proteins up to a maximum of 50 amino acids in length. Myoglobin (A) is too big to be sequenced effectively by Edman degradation. Edman degradation also cleaves amino acids from the amino terminus of the peptide (B). A benzyl alcohol (C) is used in a Bergmann degradation.

4. C

The oxygen atom of the alcohol is deprotonated in the presence of base, and is able to create an epoxide ring and displace one of the chloride atoms. The azide group ($-N_3$) opens the ring near the methyl group, and a second chloride is displaced to form an acid chloride. After reduction of the azide, and hydrolysis of the acid chloride, alanine is formed. (D) is incorrect. Because the reaction proceeds through an oxirane ring, the chirality is preserved but the stereochemistry changes from R to S (azide attack proceeds by S_N2), thus (C) is the correct answer.

5. C

(A), (B), and (D) are true of protein denaturation: sonication creates heat and excess molecular motion, which disrupts H-bonds and van der Waals forces; changes in pH can protonate or deprotonate specific protein residues, thereby changing their interactions with other ionic species; and urea is a powerful denaturant, and one of the ways in which it acts is by interfering with noncovalent bonds. (C) does not directly refer to denaturation, but rather to cleavage of the protein at methionine residues with cyanogen bromide (CNBr).

PRACTICE SECTIONS

PRACTICE SECTION 1

1. A	19. B	37. D
2. C	20. B	38. B
3. C	21. C	39. A
4. D	22. D	40. A
5. D	23. A	41. C
6. C	24. C	42. D
7. B	25. C	43. C
8. A	26. B	44. A
9. B	27. D	45. D
10. B	28. D	46. D
11. B	29. A	47. D
12. A	30. B	48. A
13. B	31. C	49. D
14. D	32. A	50. B
15. D	33. A	51. B
16. A	34. B	52. B
17. D	35. C	
18. C	36. C	

ANSWER KEY

PASSAGE I

1. A

Dehydration reactions can occur in the presence of acid and heat. An alkene is formed following the dissociation of a protonated alcohol, ROH_2^+, through a carbonium ion. The loss of a hydrogen ion from the carbonium ion completes the reaction. However, the carbonium ion may rearrange itself to form on another carbon to increase stability. The formation of 2-butene from n-butyl alcohol (the product and reactant, respectively, in (A)) is a good example of this phenomenon. (B) is incorrect, although it could be regarded as dehydration. The bromine from sodium replaces the protonated alcohol to yield the n-butyl bromide by the S_N2 mechanism. Answers (C) and (D) are incorrect because they are oxidations, not dehydrations.

2. C

Under certain circumstances, the –OH group of alcohols can become deprotonated thereby causing them to behave as acids. Active metals such as sodium, aluminum, and potassium form alkoxides (RO^-) which bond to the metal atom and release hydrogen gas. More carbons on an alcohol increases the electron releasing (inductive) effect and tends to increase the negative charge on the oxygen atom of the –OH group. This results in a tighter bond between the hydrogen and oxygen, and a weaker acid. C is correct because, as a primary alcohol with only one carbon, the hydrogen ion is more likely to be replaced by the metal than (A), which is a secondary alcohol or (B), which is a tertiary alcohol. (D), while it is a primary alcohol, has more carbons and thus a greater inductive effect than methanol.

3. C

Grignard reagents form alcohols by attacking carbonyl carbons as a nucleophile. The oxygen atom of the carbonyl group becomes the –OH group of the alcohol. (C) is the only ketone among the choices and will form a tertiary alcohol after nucleophilic attack. (A) would form a primary alcohol, and (B) and (D) would form secondary alcohols upon addition of the Grignard reagent.

4. D

Hydrogen bonding between molecules tends to increase the boiling point because greater energy (higher temperature) is required to break the hydrogen bonds. Because all of the choices have similar molecular weights this property cannot account for a difference in boiling point. Other intermolecular forces that affect boiling point are much less important when comparing these four molecules.

5. D

The S_N1 mechanism proceeds through a carbonium ion, and the stability of that carbonium ion intermediate determines the reactivity. The order of carbonium ion stability is allyl > benzyl > 3° > 2° > 1°< methyl. (D) is correct because, as a tertiary alcohol, it is most likely to react via an S_N1 mechanism. (A) and (B) are primary alcohols and (C) is a secondary alcohol and would more likely undergo an S_N2 reaction.

6. C

Because ethanol is the starting material and the product is sec-butyl alcohol, it would be reasonable to make both the Grignard reagent and an aldehyde from ethanol since Grignard reagents add to aldehydes to form secondary alcohols. (C) is the best choice because the molecule already contains four carbons and the Grignard reagent will add at least one additional carbon. (A) is formed when making the Grignard reagent from ethanol. (B) is the Grignard reagent. (D) is the final intermediate and occurs immediately prior to loss of MgBr to form sec-butyl alcohol.

7. B

The bond between bromine and the aryl ring of bromobenzene is unreactive to nucleophilic substitution, and therefore, an ether cannot be formed by the Williamson synthesis. An alkoxide or phenoxide ions will react with methyl bromine (A) to form an ether as will benzyl chloride and 2-bromopropane, (C) and (D) respectively.

PASSAGE II

8. A

Acetone is a polar aprotic solvent, while (B) and (C) are polar protic solvents, so they are not suitable for S_N2 reactions. (D) is nonpolar, so it is unlikely to dissolve the reactants and products.

9. B

For reaction 1 in acetone, the stereochemistry of the initial reactant and product is (R). Because S_N2 kinetics are observed, an inversion must occur between each substitution, or a switch from R to S to R. (A) has the stereochemistry reversed, while (C) and (D) do not account for two rounds of inversion.

10. B

Information provided in the question immediately discounts answers A (S_N1 intermediate) and D. The stereochemistry of the intermediate in (C) is (R), which is incorrect since an inversion must occur.

11. B

The presence of the oxygen atom has a minimal effect on the rate values for reaction 2 compared to reaction 1, so answers (C) and (D) are incorrect. (A) is incorrect because the number of steps for each substitution reaction is reversed.

12. A

The function of the solvent in S_N1 reactions is to stabilize the intermediate by solvation; in this case a carbocation. The incoming nucleophile (B) plays no role in affecting the rate, while protons (C) cannot stabilize another positively charged species. Destabilizing the leaving group (D) will likely slow down S_N1 reactions.

13. B

The carbocation intermediate is flat, with the empty p-orbital perpendicular to the three bond pairs. As such, the incoming nucleophile has access to the carbocation from either side of the plane, leading to racemization. The nucleophile itself has no effect on the initial alkyl halide (A) in S_N1 reactions, while (D) is incorrect since a chiral compound cannot racemize spontaneously. (C) refers to the carbocation as being sp-hybridized, which is incorrect.

14. D

A tertiary carbocation is more stable than primary and secondary carbocations due to inductive effects, so answers (A) and (B) are incorrect. (C) is incorrect because radicals do not form during S_N1 reactions.

15. D

Possible alkyl shifts leading to more stable carbocations are shown below. Compound II is incorrect, since the –OH group is in the wrong position, so answers (B) and (C) are incorrect. (A) is incorrect because it is not the only product possible.

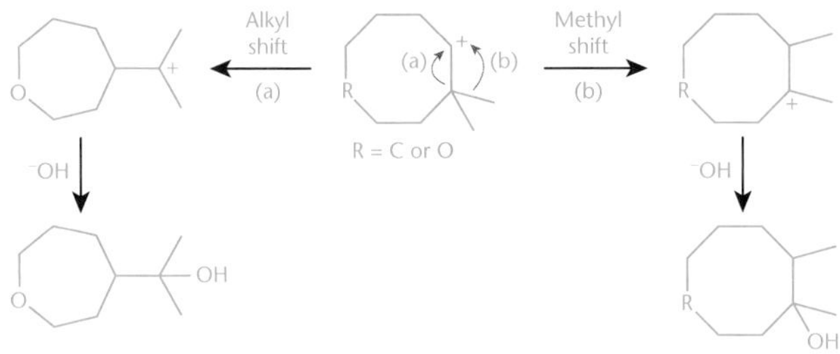

QUESTIONS 16–19

16. A

Choices (B) and (C) are wrong for the same reason and thus the savvy test taker could have eliminated both of them at the same time. The phosholipid bilayer's interior is nonpolar, but the sides that face either the external environment or the internal environment of the cell are polar. Choice (D) is wrong because insoluble is a relative term and no solvent was mentioned the question stem.

17. D

Laevorotatory compounds are defined as optically active compounds that rotate plane-polarize light in a counterclockwise fashion. Dextrorotatory compounds rotate it in a clockwise direction. Neither the R nor the S designation indicated the direction of rotation of plane-polarized light; rather, they indicate the orientation of groups around a chiral carbon.

18. C

Meso compounds by definition have an internal plane of symetry and thus can be mirror images of each other. (A) and (B) can be eliminated because an anomer is a special class of epimer and thus both terms refer to similar stereoisomeric relationships. (D) is wrong because geometric isomers need not be symmetric.

19. B

A perfectly saturated hydrocarbon has 2n + 2 hydrogens for n carbons. In the above example, this computes to 42 hydrogens implying that 22 degrees of unsaturation exist. Choices (A) and (D) arise from forgetting that the formula is $2n + 2$ and not just $2n$ (which would make an alkene).

PASSAGE III

20. B

The monosaccharide is (D) because the chiral carbon furthest from the carboxyl group is to the right in the open structure; it is an aldose rather than ketose because the open chain form shows that the carbon atom number one is an aldehyde; it is a pentose because it has five carbons; it is a furanose ring because it is a five-membered ring (including the oxygen) named after furan; it is β because the number 1 carbon atom hydroxyl is on the same side of the ring as the CH_2OH group. (A) is incorrect because it contains pyranose ring and the α anomer as descriptors. (C) is incorrect because it contains L, ketose, and α anomer as descriptors. (D) is incorrect because it contains L, hexose, and α anomer as descriptors (all descriptors are explained with the correct above).

21. C

Carbons are numbered with carbon number 1 (C1) as the carbonyl carbon, then carbons are numbered sequentially going away from the carbonyl carbon. Chiral centers are asymmetric carbons, meaning that all four bonds are to different atoms or groups. The open ring has two asymmetric carbons, C3 and C4, and the ring structure has three (C1, C3, and C4), having gained one when carbons 5 and 1 joined to form the ring structure. (A) is incorrect, as the ring structure has three (C1, C3, & C4) asymmetric carbons. (B) is incorrect, as C1 is not asymmetric on the open structure, and C5 is not asymmetric. (D) is incorrect, as the answers are the reverse of the correct answers, giving the symmetric carbons rather than the asymmetric carbons.

22. D

Monosaccharides are reducing sugars because they are either aldehydes or ketones with an α-hydroxyl group, either of which are able to reduce Benedict's or Tollen's reagents. Structures I and III, however, have a methyl group added to the oxygen at the C1 carbon, so the sugar is no longer an aldehyde and the methyl group destroys the reducing power of the aldehyde group. Therefore, structures I and III are non-reducing. Disaccharides are often reducing sugars because they are in equilibrium with their open structures which allows the OH groups of the C1 and C2 carbons to participate in reduction. However, the Oxygen atoms attached to the C1 and C2 carbons in structure IV (which is sucrose) are tied up in the glycosidic linkage and therefore are unable to form the open structure and provide reducing power. Therefore, structures I, III, and IV are all nonreducing sugars. (A) is incorrect because it is incomplete because structures III and IV are not included. (B) is incorrect because it (glucose) is a reducing sugar. (C) is incorrect because it is incomplete because it does not include structures I and III.

23. A

Bromine water is acidic and thus does not allow isomerization to take place as do the alkaline solutions provided by Fehling's (Benedict's) solution and Tollen's reagent. (B) is incorrect because it does not show the C1 carbon to have been oxidized and a double bond to oxygen has formed at C2. (C) is incorrect because it shows isomerization that changes the hydroxyl at C2 to the β orientation, and the orientation of the hydroxyl at C3 has changed to α. (D) is incorrect because isomerization has resulted in the switch to α-hydroxyl to β-hydroxyl at the C3 carbon.

24. C

The first reaction is with HCN to form the cyanohydrin at the C2 carboxyl, which is then hydrolyzed to the hydroxy acid. Upon treatment with hydrogen iodide and heat, the hydroxyls are reduced to hydrogens, yielding the final product, α-methylcaproic acid. (A) is incorrect because acylation would have added an acyl group to each hydroxyl group. (B) is incorrect because after the cyanohydrin is formed by reaction with HCN, reaction with HI next would reduce hydroxyls to hydrogens, but leave the cyanohydrin intact. Hydrolysis treatment would then produce the unsaturated hydroxy acid. (D) is incorrect because if fructose is first reduced with H_2 and nickel, it would change carbonyl to a hydroxyl, then HI and heat treatment would change reduce the alcohols to hydrogens, but add iodine to the C2 carbon.

25. C

Acylation of glucose with acetic anhydride results in the formation of an acyl linkage to each hydoxyl group in the glucose molecule, which is 5 hydroxyls in glucose. Reduction of glucose with hydrogen and nickel reduces the carbonyl, changing to another hydroxyl, and allowing a subsequent acylation reaction to yield 6 hydroxyls per glucose molecule. (A) is incorrect, as both answers are one short of the correct number of hydroxyls observed for the corresponding treatments. (B) is incorrect because the second treatment shows there to be 6 hydroxyls, not four. (D) is incorrect because neither treatment is specific for the carbonyl group, and the second part of the answer is wrong for the corresponding treatment.

26. B

An excess of phenylhydrazine reacts with aldose and ketose sugars to produce an osazone that can then have the phenylhydrazine group removed by warm acid to give an osone. This activity destroys differences based on the C2 carbon. Because glucose, mannose, and fructose differ only at C2, they will all yield the same osazone after reacting with phenylhydrazine, and after subsequent treatment with warm acid, the same osone structure will result for the three compounds. Gulose, however, differs at the C4 carbon, and thus its structure will differ from the other three structures. (A) is incorrect because it will have the same osazone and osone structure as mannose and fructose. (C) is incorrect because it will have the same osazone and osone structure as as glucose and and fructose. (D) is incorrect because it will have the same osazone and ozone structure as glucose and mannose.

27. D

A sugar can be reacted with other compounds to form glycosides through a glycosidic bond, which is basically an ether linkage (R–O–R). The other compound can be an alcohol, a thio, or an amine. The triphosphate is an ester linkage but not a diester linkage, as would be true if one of the O^- groups were to form another ester linkage with a second molecule, such as another ribose. The latter occurs in RNA and DNA. (A) and (B) are incomplete. (C) is incorrect as the triphosphate is linked in an ester linkage, not a diester linkage.

28. D

Phosphoric acid is a triprotic acid, because it has three–OH groups. It can form the anhydrides di- or triphosphoric acid, which also have multiple –OH groups that form ester linkages with the –OH groups of sugars. Ribose molecules in RNA and DNA are held together by the phosphodiester bonds from the 5′ carbon of one ribose to the 3′ OH of an adjacent ribose. The –OH groups of the phosphoric acid can form an unstable cyclic bond with the 3′ and 2′ OH groups of ribose under alkaline conditions, resulting in strand breakage in RNA. Because deoxyribose does not have an OH group at the 2′ sugar, it is not susceptible to the cyclic ester formation by phosphoric acid. The other answer choices are correct but incomplete.

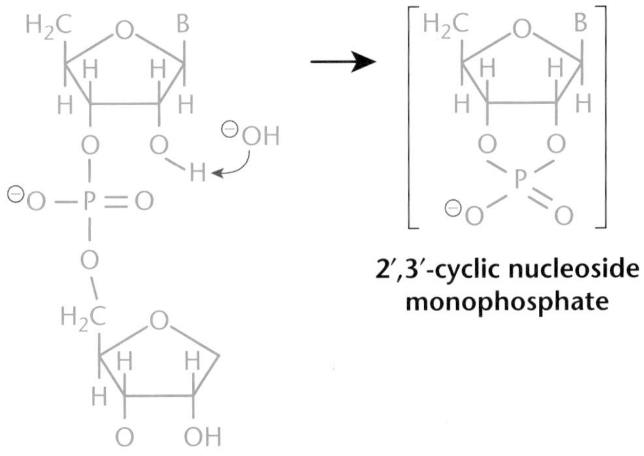

2′,3′-cyclic nucleoside monophosphate

29. A

Methylation occurs at the C1 carbon, which is, of course, the aldehyde (strictly speaking, the hemiacetal) group. Methylation of the other carbons occurs under alkaline conditions with methyl sulfate. (B) is wrong because methylation occurs only at the C1 carbon. (C) is incorrect because methylation occurs only at the C1 carbon under these conditions. (D) is also wrong for the same reason.

QUESTIONS 30–32

30. B

Bromine is selective for secondary and tertiary carbons whereas fluorine (A) and chlorine (C) prefer primary carbons. Iodine (D) rarely reacts via free radical halogenation because its large atomic radius makes it the most stable halogen in ionic form.

31. C

What are the characteristics of a bimolecular nucleophilic substitution reaction? Because item II appears in all of the choices, it makes sense to evaluate I or III. Both of those are characteristic of S_N2 reactions, so neither can be correct. That leaves (C) as the only valid option.

32. A

Which class of carbonyls is the most reactive? The electronegativity of the halogen group accentuates the nucleophilic character of the already polar carbonyl carbon increasing its susceptibility to electrophilic attack. Furthermore, halogens are among the best leaving groups.

PASSAGE IV

33. A

The methyl group of acetic acid is brominated during the first step, after which the bromide is substituted with a cyanide group. Hydrolysis with aqueous acid converts the –CN to –COOH. Excess methanol in aqueous acid (B) is incorrect, as this reaction forms an ester. While base, followed by formic acid, then acid neutralization (C) is a possible procedure, it is unlikely to synthesize malonic acid in high yields because the carboxylic acids present would affect the reactivities of the base. $KMnO_4$ (potassium permanganate) (D) is a strong oxidizer and can form carboxylic acids; however, it cannot add carbon atoms to acetic acid to form malonic acid.

34. B

The acidity of carboxylic acids increases with increased stability of the conjugate base. Because nitro groups are electron withdrawing, they stabilize the conjugate base by inductive effects, so (A) is a correct inequality, and an incorrect choice. A methyl group in the para position is actually destabilizing, as it donates electrons into the benzene ring, resulting in a weaker acid, so (C) is incorrect. A chloride in the ortho position stabilizes the base more than when it is in the *meta* or *para* positions, so (D) is incorrect. The oxygen atom in the para-substituted methoxy group in (B) actually donates electron density to the overall molecule, makes the proton less likely to leave, and makes it less acidic than benzoic acid.

35. C

In molecules that have three or more carboxylic acid groups, the carboxylic acids are no longer counted in the main alkane backbone but are named using a carboxylic acid suffix. In isocitric acid, the alkane chain is propane (three carbons) and the number one carbon has an –OH group. The carboxylic acids are considered substituents at carbons 1, 2, and 3 on the propane chain. Tricarboxyl-2-pentanol (A) incorrectly indicates that an alcohol has higher priority than a carboxylic acid. The *oxo-* in (D) denotes a carbonyl group, not a carboxylic acid. (B) erroneously includes carbons from the carboxylic acids in the main alkane chain.

36. C

Fluorine is more electronegative than chlorine, and its presence near the carboxylic acid is more electron-withdrawing making fluoroacetic acid more acidic. Three electronegative atoms enhance the effect making (B) a true statement. The effect of this electron withdrawing ability decreases as distance from the acidic proton increases; therefore, 2-fluorobutanoic acid is more acidic than 4-fluorobutanoic acid. The additional alkyl group in succinic acid works to slightly destabilize the conjugate base when compared to malonic acid. Malonic acid is the more acidic compound thus (C) is the correct choice.

37. D

When heated, the dicarboxylic acid in (A) forms acetic acid and carbon dioxide. In (B), the structure lends itself to the formation of a cyclic anhydride, namely succinic anhydride. In (C), a seven-membered lactone forms. (D)'s dicarboxylic acid, suberic acid, would not form a nine-membered lactone ring, because a nine-membered ring is not as energetically favorable as it is in the cases with five- or seven-membered rings. Suberic acid is more likely to form straight-chain polymeric anhydrides when heated.

38. B

THF and succinic acid have four carbon molecules while adipic acid contains six carbons. While there is more than one way to perform these syntheses, (B) is incorrect. The oxidation step is not needed in the synthesis of adipic acid. Both reactions start with HI (A), which opens the THF ring and leaves iodide atoms on each end of the chain. The addition of two CO_2 molecules (carbonation) converts the iodinated intermediate into a dicarboxylic acid, namely adipic acid. Because succinic acid does not require additional carbons, base is applied to make a diol (D), which is then oxidized.

39. A

By binding molecules in specific configurations and lowering reaction energies, enzymes are able to catalyze organic reactions. In this case, the simplest organic reaction is to deprotonate the alcohol in fluorocitrate. The oxygen anion that remains forms a carbonyl with the carbon atom it is bonded to, and fluoroacetic acid is the leaving group; oxaloacetic acid is the other product. Because enzymes can sometimes catalyze reactions that are not feasible using other catalysts, complicated mechanisms could exist for (B), (C), and (D). However, if the oxygen in threonine—the sulfur in cysteine—or the fluoride ion were to act as nucleophiles, the products would not be formed in a single step.

PASSAGE V

40. A

At C2, the order of substituent priority, in decreasing order, is the following: –OH, –CHO, $-CH_2OH$, and –H. The substituents form a counterclockwise turn, which would imply 2S; however, the hydrogen atom is on a horizontal bond in a Fischer projection, which can be represented as a wedge, so the actual configuration is 2R. In addition, the longest chain contains three carbon atoms, with the aldehyde having higher priority than the alcohol groups, so the compound name is as given in (A).

41. C

Ruff degradation removes aldehyde groups as CO_2, shortening sugars by one carbon atom (see Figure 1); the carbon directly adjacent to the starting aldehyde group now becomes the new aldehyde. If, D-(-)-arabinose can be formed from either D-(+)-glucose or D-(+)-mannose, then this implies that only the stereochemistry at C2 is different ((D) is incorrect), which becomes the aldehyde group in arabinose. Therefore, D-(+)-glucose and D-(+)-mannose must be C2 epimers. If glucose and mannose were C3 epimers (B), then one round of Ruff degradation would produce different aldopentoses. If glucose and mannose were enantiomers (A), then all their stereocenters would have opposite configurations to one another, and removing the aldehyde group would still give a distinct pair of enantiomeric aldopentoses.

42. D

Because the passage concentrates on D-sugars only, (A) and (B) can be discounted. (C) is incorrect, as the reactant and products are different.

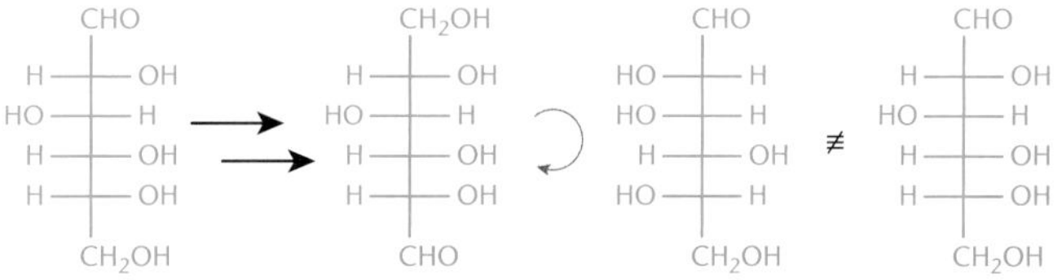

Interchanging the end groups of (D), followed by 180° rotation, gives the same sugar.

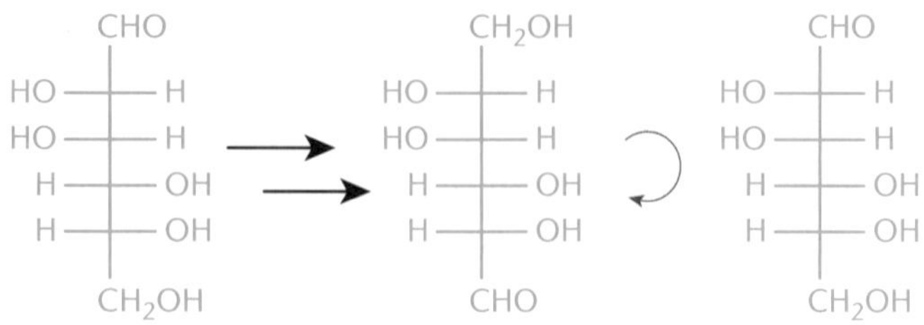

43. C

HNO_3 oxidizes both end groups to carboxylic acids, as seen in Figure 2. Because HNO_3 does not oxidize all –OH groups present, (D) is incorrect. Treatment of the dicarboxylic acid with reaction steps shown Figure 1 will therefore remove a CO_2 molecule from both ends, giving a product with two fewer carbon atoms than the reactant (C). Because the functional groups on both ends of the molecule are fully oxidized to carboxylic acids, switching functional groups (A) would not occur. Ruff degradation does not break up the reactant sugar (step 2 is responsible for oxidizing the carboxylic acid to carbon dioxide), so (B) is incorrect.

44. A

Addition of HCN to aldehydes forms cyanohydrins, via nucleophilic attack of the cyanide ion on the carbonyl carbon atom. The proton is transferred to oxygen to form an alcohol. (B) results from treatment of a cyanohydrin with lithium aluminum hydride (reduction of the cyanide group), while (C) is the intermediate that leads to (B), so they are both incorrect. Finally, because HCN is not a reducing agent, it cannot readily replace alcohol groups with hydrogen, so (D) is incorrect.

45. D

Because the addition of HCN is not stereoselective, the stereochemistry of the cyanohydrin carbon can be R or S. In addition, the other chiral carbon atom in glyceraldehyde has a fixed stereochemistry (R), so the pair of tetroses are diastereomers, where only one stereocenter has a different configuration. Because the definition of diastereomers excludes enantiomers (A). Structural isomers (B) have the same general formula, but the atoms/molecules are arranged differently, which is not the case with pairs of sugars. Geometric isomers (C) refer to *cis-/trans*-isomerism such as those seen in vicinal substituted alkenes, not sugars.

46. D

A common mistake is to assume that once D or L is known for a particular sugar, its optical rotation can be easily predicted. However, the optical rotation for any molecule can only be determined experimentally, and does not depend on D/L, or R/S configurations. For example, it is only by chance that in nature, glucose exists in a D-(+)- configuration.

PASSAGE VI

47. D

Because both drugs contain carboxylic acid groups, which can take part in extensive hydrogen bonding with each other, their IR spectra contains a very broad absorption band that spans 3,500 to 2,500 cm^{-1},which corresponds to the acid O–H bond stretch. (A) describes carbon-carbon triple bond stretches, while (B) corresponds to alcohol O–H stretches. Finally, (C) describes aldehyde C–H stretches, which is present only in drug A.

48. A

Carbon is a p-block element, so the highest occupied orbital is a p orbital. Elemental carbon contains six electrons (*i.e.*, its atomic number), and filling up the orbitals via the Aufbau principle, there are two electrons in the 1s orbital, two in the 2s orbital, and two in the 2p orbital, i.e., $1s^2\ 2s^2\ 2p^6$. (A) is correct.

49. D

A pi bond forms by the parallel (side-to-side) overlap of two p orbitals. No s orbitals are involved in pi bond formation (A) and (B). Perpendicular overlap of p orbitals (C) cannot result in bonds.

50. B

Negative (exothermic) energy is a measure of stability: the more negative a reaction is, the less stable the initial reactant is. Thus, a molecule that is initially very stable will release less energy during an exothermic reaction. (C) is incorrect, because benzene rings are more stable than rings with unconjugated pi bonds, so energy released is less than choices (A) and (B). 1,3-cyclohexadiene (B) is less stable than cyclohexene (A) due to increased ring strain and sterics (double bonds are shorter than single bonds), so (B) releases more energy upon hydrogenation.

51. B

The strength of carbon-carbon bonds is directly correlated to the number of times they are bonded to each other. Triple bonds are strongest, followed by double bonds, and then single bonds. Triple bonds are also the shortest, followed by double bonds, and then single bonds (the longest). (B) correctly describes, in decreasing order, both bond strength and bond length.

52. B

The most convenient way to deactivate the drugs is to reduce their polarity; forming esters can effectively reduce absorption through the lumen. Hydrogenation (A) is unlikely to have any effect on polarity, since the double bonds present are not affected. Reduction to primary alcohols (C) will greatly increase the polarity of the drugs. Substitution with $SOCl_2$ (D) converts the drugs to acid chlorides, which are unreliable as drugs since they are highly reactive.

PRACTICE SECTION 2

ANSWER KEY

1. A	19. C	37. B
2. C	20. D	38. C
3. D	21. C	39. A
4. C	22. A	40. C
5. D	23. C	41. A
6. B	24. B	42. A
7. C	25. A	43. C
8. A	26. A	44. D
9. A	27. C	45. D
10. D	28. C	46. C
11. D	29. C	47. B
12. C	30. A	48. A
13. B	31. B	49. D
14. A	32. A	50. A
15. A	33. C	51. A
16. D	34. D	52. B
17. C	35. D	
18. B	36. C	

PASSAGE I

1. A

(C) is incorrect because the substituents are not in alphabetical order. (B) is incorrect because the alkene—part of the longest carbon chain—is not given priority. (D) is incorrect because the numbering is not correct (in fact, the compound would contain a carbon with five bonds.)

2. C

(B) is an oxidizing agent. (D) is incorrect because a hydrazone is formed, with no reduction occurring. $LiAlH_4$ is a much stronger reducing agent than $NaBH_4$, and can reduce both ketones present to alcohols.

3. D

The ketone group is protected as an acetal, and an alcohol in the presence of aqueous acid is used. (B) is incorrect, because acid is a required catalyst.

4. C

The longest chain contains seven carbon atoms, with the aldehyde having a higher priority than the ketone groups. The oxo prefix in (B) cannot refer to the aldehyde and only one of the ketones.

5. D

The simplest way to answer this question is to recognize which protons are the most acidic (the ones between the two ketone groups) for enol formation. (B) and (C) are incorrect because those enols will not produce five-membered rings. (A) is incorrect because the aldehyde is not present in compound V.

6. B

The coupling between compounds III and V occurs in the same way as the coupling between compounds I and II. There is no ketone group protection, so (A) is incorrect, and because no reduction of ketone groups is occurring, (B) is incorrect. (D) is incorrect since it is part of (A).

7. C

Aqueous acids are sufficient enough to remove acetals, which are stable in bases (B), as well as oxidizing agents (A) and (D).

8. A

(B) is used for Wittig reactions, which add carbon atoms to carbonyl groups, while (C) is an oxidant. (D) is used for cyanohydrin formation. (A) contains the reagents needed for a Clemmensen reduction.

PASSAGE II

9. A

Given the favorable energies achieved through catalysis by enzymes, salicylanilide is undergoing nucleophilic attack at the carbonyl carbon, because aniline is being formed. Of the residues listed, leucine (A) is least likely to be participating in this reaction because its alkyl side chain does not contain an acceptable nucleophile. In contrast, the other amino acids have potential nucleophiles in their side chains: serine has an oxygen atom, cysteine has a sulfur atom, and lysine has a nitrogen atom, all of which could act as nucleophiles.

10. D

When lithium aluminum hydride is introduced to an amide bond, it reduces the carbonyl carbon completely (the oxygen atom is removed) while leaving the nitrogen atom; RCONHR' + $LiAlH_4$ → RCH_2 NH_2R'. (A) is the result of an –OH group acting as a nucleophile. (B) does not account for the carbonyl carbon that remains after reduction. (C) shows the formation of an ester linkage.

11. D

The groups of reactants and reagents shown are able to oxidize aliphatic alcohols, not phenol. When combined with the reagents in (A) and (B), primary alcohols are oxidized to carboxylic acids. CrO_3^- pyridine, CH_2Cl_2 (choice C) would oxidize a primary alcohol to an aldehyde.

12. C

When an ester bond is heated with a strong base such as NaOH, the hydroxide group acts as a nucleophile and attacks the carbonyl carbon. The leaving group is the alcohol formed from the noncarbonyl oxygen (after acidification). In the case of salicylanilide, the major products of this synthesis are phenol (C) and salicylic acid. (A) is close to salicylic acid but incorrect, because it cannot be formed from saponification of phenyl 2-hydroxybenzoate. (D) is too far reduced to be a possible product. It is conceivable that the product salicylic acid goes on to form a ring under these conditions. However, if the OH group were to act as a nucleophile on the carboxylic acid, the ring formed would be a four-membered ring, not five-membered as shown.

13. B

A Hofmann rearrangement converts a primary amide to a primary amine with the loss of one carbon, as in (B). (A) reflects a loss of two carbons. While the amide is converted to an amine, (C) does not account for the loss of a carbon. (D) is incorrect because a Hofmann rearrangement does not convert amides to carboxylic acids.

14. A

The amide group has fairly high priority among functional groups in that it is higher than alcohol, phenyl, and alkyl groups. However, among carboxylic acid derivatives it is the lowest. Because there is an amide group, (A) is correct. An alternate name is 2-hydroxybenzanilide, which is similar to (B) 3-hydroxybenzanilide. (C) does not account for the priority of the amide group over the alcohol group, and (D) erroneously describes a carboxylic acid, which is distinct from an amide.

15. A

Aniline and acetic anhydride (A) combine to form acetanilide. The amino group of aniline attacks one of the carbonyl groups of acetic anhydride with acetate as the leaving group. Amides are relatively unreactive species and (B) and (C) would not result in acetanilide. The reaction in (D) creates an amide group very similar to acetanilide. However, instead of aniline, the reaction uses cyclohexane amine.

QUESTIONS 16–19

16. D

While nucleophilic addition could theoretically occur in a carboxylic acid, many other compounds—even alkanes—undergo this type of reaction, so (D) is not specific to carboxylic acids.

17. C

High temperature and extreme basicity or acidity create highly oxidative conditions. These favor the formation of the most oxidized compound: a carboxylic acid.

18. B

A peptide bond is said to have partial double bond character. To answer this question, you must understand that pi bonds prevent rotation about the axis of the bond. The α-helices and β-pleats that compose a protein's secondary structure are explained by this rigidity of peptide bonds.

19. C

The addition of one nitrate group breaks the symmetry of chlorobenzene. Because the nitrate group can add on to the 1,2,3,4 carbons (5,6 are indistinguishable from 2,3). One might initially think (D) to be correct. However, the chlorine at position one forces the incoming nitrate, were it to add there, into one conformation. If the nitrate added at position one, then it would be on the opposite side of the carbon skeleton (remember that benzene is planar) and so both 'isomers' would appear exactly the same. However, for addition at positions 2, 3, 4 the nitrate group could add on either *cis* or *trans* to the chlorine thus creating an isomeric pair.

PASSAGE III

20. D

The base peak is by definition designated 100 percent abundant and all other peaks are measured relative to it. (C) is incorrect, because the number of possible fragments are different for different compounds, while (A) is incorrect, because the parent peak is not always evident on a mass spectrum. Finally, (B) is incorrect, because the smallest peak will give relative abundances of larger peak at more than 100 percent, which is impossible.

21. C

According to the passage, the base peak is the parent peak of compound Y, so this is a simple calculation based on the molecular formula $C_6H_{10}O$:

$$m/z = (6 \times 12) + (10 \times 1) + (16 \times 1) = 72 + 10 + 16 = 98$$

22. A

An enol isomerizes to carbonyl compounds due to keto-enol tautomerization. (D) is incorrect, because a carboxylic acid cannot be formed with a single oxygen atom, while (B) is incorrect, because the alkene will have to be reduced to form an alcohol, and reduction does not happen spontaneously. (C) is incorrect, because an epoxide is strained, and isomerization to it represents an uphill (unfavorable) climb in energy.

23. C

A very particular arrangement of atoms (see Question 6) is needed for a McLafferty arrangement. Answers (A), (B), and (D) are incorrect, since the arrangement of atoms does not allow a McLafferty rearrangement to take place.

24. B

An allylic cation, from an α-cleavage (see below) is stable due to resonance, and corresponds to m/z 41. (A) is incorrect, because its m/z is 43, not 41. Answers (C) and (D) are incorrect for the same reason.

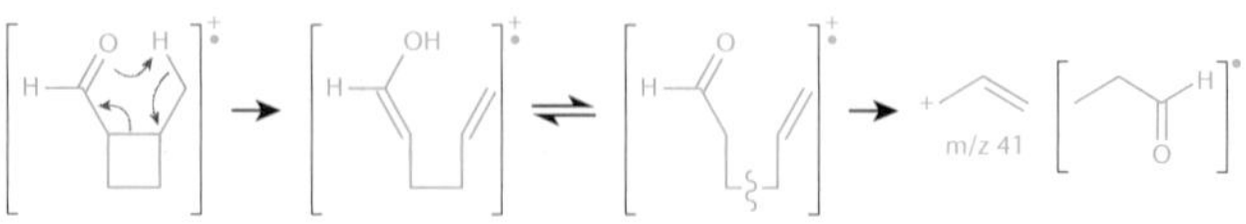

m/z 41

25. A

The fragment at m/z 29 comes from an α-cleavage of the aldehyde group, forming a carbocation which can be resonance stabilized by the lone pairs on oxygen. Answers (B) and (D) are incorrect, because their m/z values are 28, not 29, while a primary ethyl carbocation (C) cannot stabilize by resonance, and thus is unlikely to appear on a mass spectrum.

26. A

According to the passage, alcohols readily lose the –OH group (as water) in the mass spectrum, and so the parent peak will either be small or not present. Another hint comes from m/z 80, which happens to correspond to m/z 98 – 18, or the molecular ion losing water. No ether group (C) would have a mass of 18. A methoxy group, the smallest possible ether, would result in 31 being subtracted from the molecular ion peak. Similarly, ketone (B) and aldehyde (D) do not readily lose their oxygen atom as water.

27. C

The m/z 29 fragment comes from the α-cleavage of the alcohol. (A) and (D) are incorrect because their m/z values are 30. (B) is incorrect because compound Z does not contain a nitrogen atom.

28. C

(B) and (D) are incorrect because primary and secondary carbocations are less stable than allylic cations (A) and (C.) However, (A) is incorrect; a cyclobutene ring will have a much higher ring strain than a cyclopentene ring, and so it is less stable than (C).

PASSAGE IV

29. C

Because compound I reacts with *two* molecules of hydrogen, compound I has two degrees of unsaturation. A more definitive way to deduce the answer is to follow the equation below:

$$\text{Degrees of unsaturation} = \frac{2C + 2 - H - X + N}{2}$$

Where C is the number of carbon atoms, H is the number of hydrogen atoms, X is the number of halides, and N the number of nitrogen atoms.

30. A

Compound I is optically active; because straight chain compounds cannot be optically active, (B) and (C) are incorrect. (D) is also incorrect, because there are no chiral carbon atoms.

31. B

(B) is the only molecule with a chiral carbon atom. The other answer choices are not optically active.

32. A

The structure can be verified by information provided in the table: a sharp absorbance at 1,720 cm^{-1}, combined with the broad overtone between 2,500–3,500 cm^{-1} is indicative of a carboxylic acid. The single piece of ^1H-NMR information also points to (A). (D) is incorrect: alcohols indeed have an IR absorbance at 3,400 cm^{-1}, but there is no large overtone. (B) and (C) are incorrect because the IR spectra for those also lack the broad absorbance.

33. C

Hydrogenation is occurring, so a suitable metal is needed for an adsorbent surface. Platinum is a relatively inactive metal, making it an excellent catalyst. All the other metals are too reactive themselves to be catalysts.

34. D

The IR spectrum for compound II should not have an absorbance band corresponding to the carbon-carbon triple bond stretch, which occurs at approximately 2,200 cm^{-1}. (A) implies that a carbonyl group has formed. (B) refers to an alcohol group. (C) is incorrect because carbon-carbon triple bonds stretches do not occur at such a low wave number.

35. D

Ozone cleaves triple bonds, and with aqueous workup yields two carboxylic acids. Because compound III is chiral, at least one of the products from ozonolysis should also be chiral, which in this case is compound VII. (B) and (C) are incorrect because VIII comes from an internal alkyne, while VI comes from an achiral terminal alkyne. Compound V (A) is not the sole product formed from the cleavage of a terminal alkyne.

36. C

An esterification is occurring, so disappearance of the hydrogen singlet of the carboxylic acid proton (at 12 ppm) indicates that the reaction is successful. (A) is incorrect, while (B) is only partially correct, because the ^1H-NMR spectrum for compound IV will also include a singlet for the methyl group protons; (C) sufficiently includes both the disappearance and appearance of the corresponding singlets. (D) is also incorrect: the carboxylic acid proton singlet does not couple to other protons, and the presence of that signal implies that no reaction takes place.

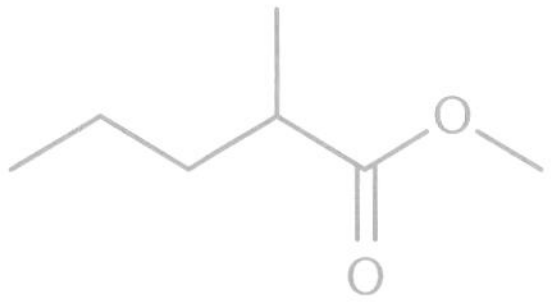

O O

Compound IV
($C_7H_{14}O_2$)

QUESTIONS 37–39

37. B

The unique hydrogen environments are as follows: one hydrogen bonded immediately to the alkene and each of the three methyl groups occupies a unique environment because there is no free rotation around a double bond thus preventing symmetry in the local electronic environment. (A) assumes that all methyls are electronically equivalent.

38. C

This is an example of a Grignard reaction. Because the products of such reactions have a carbon chain equal to the sum of the carbon chains of the reactants, (B) and (D) can be eliminated. Because the Grignard reaction is a reduction reaction, ethyne should be converted into ethene, making (C) more likely than (A).

39. A

Both the alcohol and alkene moieties react with HBr. The alkene reacts to form the more stable carbocation and the alcohol reacts by the S_N2 mecha-nism to substitute the halogen for the hydroxyl group.

PASSAGE V

40. C

The longest chain contains five carbon atoms, and because the aldehyde group has the highest priority, the parent compound is a pentanal. In addition, because the aldehyde has the highest priority, it is assigned as carbon 1, which implies that the adjacent carbon with two methyl groups bonded to it is carbon 2. IUPAC naming requires that numbering redundancies be included for all substituents, giving 2,2-dimethylpentanal, or (C). The other choices don't give the aldehydes group the highest priority.

41. A

This question gives you the mechanism with which Grignard reagents work. The nucleophile in this case is the isopropyl group, which attacks the carbonyl carbon atom, which ultimately forms a secondary alcohol upon acidic workup.

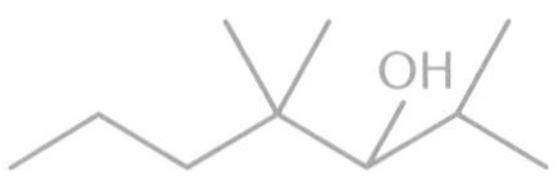

To name this alcohol, the longest chain contains seven carbon atoms, and labeling the rightmost carbon atom as number 1 gives three methyl groups (on carbons 2, 4, and 4), while the hydroxyl group is on carbon 3, to give 2, 4, 4-trimethylheptan-3-ol (remember that substituents are named alphabetically, and that the numbers give the lowest possible sum). (D) is incorrect because the numbers are counted from the leftmost carbon atom, while (B) fails to account for the longest chain present. (C) fails to provide the position of the alcohol group.

42. A

The question provides a reaction that nitriles can undergo, namely, hydrolysis of the C–N triple bond by aqueous acid to form carboxylic acids. A nitrile contains cyanide (–C≡N) as the main functional group. (C) is an amide, while (B) is an imine. (D) is a diamine.

43. C

We have a six-member ring that has one double bond. This is classified as a cyclohexene (*cyclo-* for the ring structure; *hex-* meaning six carbons; *-ene* indicating the double bond). The ring is our main structure and thus the carbon chain will be treated as a substituent. (A) and (B) are incorrect; butanone is identified as the main structure and the cyclohexen is misidentified. We see that it is composed of four carbons and has a carbonyl attached with and adjacent alkyl group. Thus, the name of the substituent will be 1-butanone (*but-* meaning four; *-one* indicating a ketone; and one indicating that the ketone is positioned on the first carbon). Now that we know the substituent's name we can complete it by referencing location. Because the butonone is the only substituent, the carbon it attaches to will be carbon 1 by default. If the 1-butanone is on the first carbon, then that means our double bond is on the third carbon. This should be indicated before the *–en* ending when identifying the cyclohexen molecule. Thus, the complete name of the structure is 1-(1-butanone)-cyclohex-3-en. (D) is incorrect as there is no reference to substituent location.

44. D

This question requires you to draw out a new structure for the proposed product. The question tells you that the double bond has been broken, opening the hexe-3-en ring. This leaves the previous butanone structure with a saturated carbon chain (no double bonds) in place of the ring. So you need to draw out the new structure and name the molecule. Because the double bond was between the third and fourth carbon of the hexane ring, there will be two new carbon chains of differing lengths.

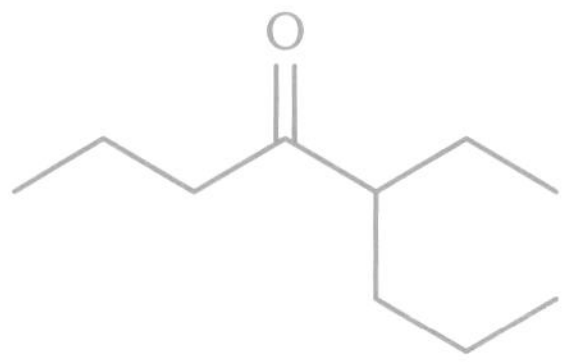

Remember to choose the carbon chain that is longest when naming your structure. Here you see that the longest chain consists of eight carbons. (A) is incorrect because all 10 carbons are not part of one continuous chain; in (B), the seven-member chain is not the longest continuous chain. If we number the carbons so that the high priority substituent has the lowest number, we are left with 4-(5-ethyl)-octanone. (C) is incorrect as the carbonyl is given the higher number.

45. D

Brady's reagent will produce a yellow or red precipitate when in the presence of aldehydes and ketones. (D) is the only choice that includes both of these functional groups.

46. C

According to the question, the fourth unknown forms a precipitate with Brady's reagent, but no silver mirror is observed with Tollen's reagent, so the unknown most likely contains a ketone group. One of many reactions that ketones can undergo is the Wittig reaction, which forms alkenes (C). (A) and (B) are meant to confuse you; several of the tests would first lead you to the conclusion that the molecule may be an aldehyde or ketone and you may forget to consider the Wittig reaction. (D) tests your knowledge of the difference between an alkene (double bond) and an alkyne (triple bond).

47. B

A strong absorbance at 1,200 cm^{-1} indicates the presence of a C–O single bond. The strong absorbance at 1,760 cm^{-1} indicates a carbonyl group (C=O stretching.) The broad stretch that spans 3,500–2,500 cm^{-1} indicates the O–H bond of a carboxylic acid (do not confuse this with a strong absorbance at 3,400 cm^{-1}, which indicates an alcohol or phenol O–H stretch.) Information from the IR spectrum points to substance C, the carboxylic acid. Were this mixed with Tollen's reagent, no silver mirror (A) would be produced (because it's not an aldehyde). Adding alcohol to a carboxylic acid and applying heat does indeed form an ester (B). Carboxylic acids do not react with Tollen's reagent (2,4-DNPH) and thus there should be no precipitate (C). $LiAlH_4$ would cause an alcohol formation when mixed with a ketone or an aldehyde, not a carboxylic acid (D).

PASSAGE VI

48. A

Charged molecules, such as amino acids, will migrate to either electrode when placed in an electric field, so (D) is not correct. The motility of molecules in an electric field also depends on their net charge:

glycine exists in one of three states that change with increasing pH (low pH: $NH_3^+CH_2COOH$, pI: $NH_3^+CH_2COO^-$, high pH: $NH_2CH_2COO^-$). For glycine, the isoelectric point is the mean of pKa_1 and pKa_2 or (9.60 + 2.34)/2 = 5.97. Because the electrophoresis is taking place at pH 4, glycine is in its fully protonated form ($NH_3^+CH_2COOH$), and will migrate toward the cathode (A), or the negative terminal. (B) would be correct at a pH above 5.97, while (C) would be correct at a pH of 5.97.

49. D

The pH of the electrophoresis buffer should be configured so as to draw one amino acid toward the cathode, one to the anode (or one to remain stationary. The isoelectric point for glycine is (9.60 + 2.34)/2 = 5.97, and the pI of aspartic acid, using pKa_1 and pKa_2, is (1.88 + 3.65)/2 = 2.77. Performing the electrophoresis at pH 2.77 would draw glycine toward the cathode, and glutmate would remain stationary. Any other pH would draw both amino acids toward the cathode.

50. A

A Schiff base, also known as an imine, has a general formula like that of (A), and can be formed from a primary amine and a carbonyl compound. (C) is a secondary amine, and (D) is a diazene group. (B) is incorrect, because the structure corresponds to a hydroazone.

51. A

The aldehyde group in PLP must be converted into a Schiff base in order to decarboxylate glutamic acid. Without knowing the reaction mechanism, it can be surmised that the active site lysine in GAD participates in the decarboxylation of glutamate via Schiff base formation, using its side chain amine group. The mechanism begins with the N atom of lysine's ε-amino group (side chain amino) making the nucleophilic attack on the aldehyde as described in (A). (C) and (D) can be ruled out since the α-amino group and the carboxylic acid are in the peptide backbone, and are unlikely to participate in catalysis. (B) does not make sense mechanistically as a geminal diol is being formed, which does not contribute to the progress of the reaction.

52. B

In the absence of the appropriate enzyme and cofactor, aspartic and glutamic acid does not decarboxylate spontaneously, or even with heating, so (A) and (D) are incorrect. For this question, a beta-oxo acid (B) can effectively be decarboxylated upon heating. 2-aminoethanoic acid (C) is the IUPAC name for glycine, which like aspartic and glutamic acid, does not lose CO_2 readily.

PRACTICE SECTION 3

ANSWER KEY

1. C
2. D
3. A
4. D
5. B
6. A
7. C
8. D
9. B
10. B
11. A
12. B
13. C
14. A
15. C
16. B
17. D
18. D
19. A
20. B
21. D
22. C
23. C
24. D
25. C
26. A
27. D
28. A
29. C
30. B
31. B
32. D
33. D
34. C
35. B
36. A
37. C
38. D
39. A
40. A
41. A
42. D
43. D
44. A
45. B
46. C
47. B
48. A
49. C
50. A
51. A
52. C

PASSAGE I

1. C

Tollen's reagent oxidizes aldehydes but not ketones to give the corresponding carboxylic acid. Because $CH_3CH_2CH_2CH_2OH$ is a primary alcohol, it is oxidized to a mixture of an aldehyde and a carboxylic acid, in contrast to $CH_3CH_2CH(OH)CH_3$ which, as a secondary alcohol, is oxidized to a ketone. (A) is the unreacted ketone formed from oxidation of the secondary alcohol. (B) is the reactant upon which Tollen's reagent reacts, not the product of the reaction. (D) is unreacted secondary alcohol.

2. D

In the presence of base and heat, the addition product, a hydrazone, is unstable, and progresses to the alkane. (A) is incorrect, though it would be correct if the reaction environment were acidic. In basic environment, however, it is an unstable intermediate. (B) is the alcohol and would not be made under the conditions shown. (C) is incorrect, as the complete molecule of hydrazine adds to the reactant in the intermediate step, as in (A).

3. A

Acid hydrolysis of the 2-butanone cyanohydrin (B) produces 2-methyl-2-butenoic acid, which in turn resulted from the nucleophilic addition of –CN to the carbonyl carbon of methyl ethyl ketone (D). (C) is the unstable intermediate formed from hydrolysis of the cyanohydrin leading to the final product.

4. D

When a α-hydrogen exists on the aldehyde or ketone, the presence of a dilute base or dilute acid results in an aldol condensation, and two molecules of acetaldehyde combine to form β-hydroxybutyraldehyde. (A) is a salt of the carboxylic acid of butyraldehyde that would result had the reactant been butyraldehyde and had there been no α-hydrogen. (B) is the alcohol that would result had there been no α-hydrogen. (C) is a salt of the carboxylic acid that would result had there been no α-hydrogen.

5. B

The reaction is done in a basic environment, and the hydroxide ion removes a hydrogen ion from the α-hydrogen of acetaldehyde to create a carbanion, the nucleophilic reagent which attacks a second acetaldehyde's carbonyl carbon. (A) is the hydroxide ion that abstracts the hydrogen ion from the α-hydrogen of acetaldehyde to form the nucleophilic reagent. (C) is the resulting ion formed by the nucleophilic attack but before hydrolysis to the final product. (D) is the final product.

6. A

The aldol is dehydrated to form 2-butenal (crotonaldehyde). The reaction places the double bond between the α and β carbons. (B) is a carboxylic acid, which is not the type of product expected from dehydration from an aldol. (C) and (D) place the double bond incorrectly.

7. C

Aldol condensation of two molecules of acetaldehyde is the first step to yield the 4-carbon compound under basic conditions, and hydrolysis yields 2-butenal followed by hydrogenation of the alkene to give butyraldehyde. (A) skips the dehydration to 2-butenal step. (B) skips the hydrogenation to n-butyl alcohol step. (D) is incorrect because, for one thing, acetone cannot be accessed from ethyl alcohol via aldol condensation.

8. D

Benzaldehyde reacts with acetic anhydride to give cinnamic acid, which can then be hydrogenated with molecular hydrogen and nickel catalyst to give hydrocinnamic acid. (A) is incorrect because, although a starting material (acetic anhydride), the question asks for the other starting compound. (B) is the result of the condensation reaction but not of the hydrogenation reaction. (C) accepts the hydrogen released in the condensation, but is not the product of the condensation or the hydrogenation.

PASSAGE II

9. B

A Schiff base (aka imine) is formed between a primary amine and carbonyl group, with the loss of a water molecule. (A) is not an imine (it is just a regular amine). (C) is incorrect because the five-membered ring is formed after initial Schiff base formation. (D) is incorrect: the molecule is an enamine, formed between a secondary amine and carbonyl group.

10. B

A reduction is occurring, and (B) is the only reducing group among the choices. (A) is an oxidizing agent, (C) is used for hydroboration and hydroxylation of alkenes, and (D) is typically used for, among other reactions, bromination of alkenes.

11. A

The product contains an alcohol functional group, so the name should contain the suffix *–ol*, in keeping with naming tropinone with the suffix *–one* implying the ketone group. Tropane (B) is correct only if the ketone group is removed, while tropene (C) is incorrect because no alkenes are present. Tropinamine (D) implies that an additional amine group is present.

12. B

The longest chain contains three carbon atoms, with the carboxylic acid having the highest priority, so the parent compound is propanoic acid; (A) is incorrect. The stereochemistry of C2 (see illustration) is S, so (C) and (D) are incorrect.

13. C

Because tropinone is a symmetric molecule, with a plane of symmetry that bisects the carbonyl group and nitrogen, there are several signals that occur at identical chemical shifts. Starting at the carbons alpha to the carbonyl group (see below), there is one signal for the alpha protons, one for the beta protons, one for the gamma protons, and one for the methyl group on the nitrogen atom, for a total of 4 ^{1}H-NMR signals.

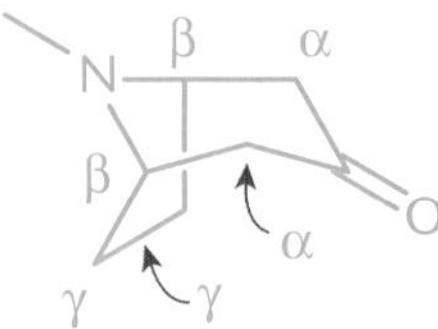

14. A

Using the same plane of symmetry that bisects the carbonyl group and the nitrogen as above, and starting from the carbonyl carbon, there is one signal for the carbonyl, one for carbons in the alpha position, one for the beta-carbons, one for the gamma carbons, and one for the methyl group on nitrogen, for a total of five distinct ^{13}C NMR signals.

15. C

Because the enol is attacking, it cannot be an electrophile, so item I is incorrect. The formation of an enol depends on the acidity of the protons alpha to the carbonyl group, and more carbonyl groups that flank such protons increases their acidity. Therefore, item III is correct. Finally, if the α-protons are more acidic, then the enol will be formed more easily, implying an increase in stability, making item II correct. β-protons (item IV) are too distant from the carbonyl group to affect acidity. With items II and III correct, that means (C) is the answer.

QUESTIONS 16–18

16. B

The unique environments are as follows: the hydrogen common immediately off the alkene, each methyl group immediately attached to the alkene has its own peak as there is no free rotation around a double bond and because the other groups attached to the alkene group obviate symmetry, there are two distinct chemical environments, the ethyl group gives three peaks, one for the methyl hydrogens and one for each hydrogen of the intermediate carbon.

17. D

The question requires you to know that in a radical halogenation reaction, the initiation and propagation steps (A) and (C) give rise to molecules with unpaired electrons. Only termination (D) will end the process, yielding molecules with no free radicals. Elongation (B) is not a step in radical halogenation.

18. D

The question requires you to know the chemical structure of a triglyceride. Triglycerides are composed of fatty acids and the three-carbon backbone of glycerol.

PASSAGE III

19. A

The two reactions used to convert benzene to benzoic acid in this case is a Friedel-Crafts alkylation, followed by side-chain oxidation. Only (A) contains the required reagents for those reactions. PCC (C) is not strong enough an oxidant, (D) lists a Friedel-Crafts *acylation* as the first step, and the first step of (B) does not lead to alkylation.

20. B

Two concentrated acids (nitric and sulfuric) are needed for nitration to occur; the actual active species is a nitroso ($^{+}NO_2$) cation. (A) and (C) are incorrect because, in those cases, NO_2 exists as an anion. (D) is incorrect because a nitroso ion cannot form spontaneously from nitric acid (sulfuric acid is required for activation of nitric acid).

21. D

The reduction of aromatic nitro compounds to amines can be performed by either hydrogenation (item I) or treatment with an active metal in an acidic media (items II and III). Because all items are correct, (D) is correct.

22. C

Meta-directing groups deactivate benzene rings by withdrawing electron density, so (B) is incorrect. Conversely, *ortho*- and *para*-directing groups activate benzene rings by donating electron density by resonance and/or inductive effects, so (A) is incorrect. Because an amine group contains a lone pair on nitrogen, it can donate electrons into the benzene ring by resonance, so (D) is incorrect.

23. C

A good Lewis acid, for example, is one where the molecule is electron deficient, such as salts formed by Group III elements, including boron (item I) and aluminum (item II). Items III and IV are weaker Lewis acids than items I and II, because the metals are less electron deficient. Because items I and II are correct, the answer is (C).

24. D

Benzene rings rarely undergo radical reactions, since aromaticity is destroyed to give a very high energy radical, so (A) and (B) are incorrect. Radicals that can delocalize into the benzene ring, such as a benzyl radical, however, are highly stable, and (D) comes from the radical bromination of its corresponding benzyl radical. (C) is incorrect because bromine is in the wrong position.

25. C

Among the choices, only NaH (sodium hydride) can activate phenol via deprotonation of the alcohol group, to form sodium phenoxide and gaseous hydrogen. A negatively charged phenoxide is more likely to undergo electrophilic aromatic substitution (*para*-directed) than phenol itself, which has no charge. HCl and H_3O^+ (A) and (D) protonate phenol, giving it a positive charge, which will deactivate the benzene ring. Phenol is not activated in water (B), and is only sparingly soluble.

26. A

Phenol (or phenoxide) is an *ortho-/para*-directing group by resonance, so (B), a *meta*-substituted product, is incorrect. The oxygen atom is unlikely to attack the nitrogen atom, both electronegative elements, directly, so (C) is incorrect. In (D), phenol has been added to the wrong nitrogen atom (besides, the product is not an azo dye).

PASSAGE IV

27. D

Of the compounds in the starting mixture, caffeine is the most nonpolar, so it will dissolve in warm chloroform. The other choices contain some sort of polar functional group or arrange the slightly polar groups such that the molecule overall has a degree of polarity (amine group in amantadine, carboxylic acid in aspirin, and amide and ether groups in ethenzamide).

28. A

With caffeine already separated, (B) is incorrect. For this question, it is sufficient to realize that hot ethanol will most likely dissolve acetaminophen over the other two choices, due to the presence of the phenol group.

29. C

Because none of the choices lists a signal which corresponds to a carboxylic acid proton—which occurs between δ10–13—it may be easier to discern which choices are incorrect as a result of specific signals. (D) is incorrect, as the first two signals (triplet and quartet) are indicative of an ethyl group, which is present only in ethenzamide. (B) is also incorrect, since the singlets that integrate to three protons correspond to the N-bonded methyl groups in caffeine. (A) is incorrect because the two doublets that occur in the phenyl proton region strongly suggest a *para*-substituted benzene, which is observed in the structure for acetaminophen.

30. B

The solubility of aspirin in NaOH is a result of deprotonation leading to formation of a charged species in an aqueous solution. The most acidic proton is in the carboxylic acid group, rather than the α-protons (C) or the phenyl protons (D). While the association of sodium ions to oxygen atoms does occur (A), no actual deprotonation is occurring, so it is incorrect.

31. B

The answer should be apparent from your work in answering the previous four questions. Aspirin (D) cannot appear in the final separation. Caffeine (A) is separated after the addition of warm chloroform. Acetaminophen (C) dissolves in hot ethanol.

32. D

Because acetaminophen is a *para*-substituted benzene, some of the phenyl carbon atoms will have identical ^{13}C NMR signals. There are a total of six distinct signals (see below.) The other answers fail to account for symmetry.

33. D

$LiAlH_4$ is a strong reducing agent, able to reduce amides, esters, and carboxylic acids into their corresponding amines and alcohols. Because acetaminophen and ethenzamide contain amides, and aspirin contains a carboxylic acid and an ester, they can be reduced by $LiAlH_4$. Amines groups are unaffected by $LiAlH_4$, so item I is incorrect. (D) is correct.

34. C

Ibuprofen contains a carboxylic acid group, so it is expected that, like aspirin, it will dissolve in NaOH. In addition, it is insoluble in chloroform, ethanol, and HCl.

35. B

The reaction sequence of sodium hydride, followed by methyl iodide is able to form ethers (with the hydroxyl group in acetaminophen) or esters (with the carboxylic acid group in aspirin.) As such, hot ethanol will unlikely be able to dissolve the methyl ether of acetaminophen. The methyl ester of aspirin, however, can be converted back to the carboxylate via saponification, so (C) is incorrect. As for (A) and (D), the reaction conditions in the question will not affect caffeine, amantadine, and ethenzamide.

36. A

NaOH will dissolve in both aspirin and acetaminophen (NaOH will deprotonate the hydroxyl group in acetaminophen), so any answer choice which uses NaOH before hot ethanol is incorrect (B), (C), and (D).

QUESTIONS 37–39

37. C

Because the substituents are bulky, both will want to be equatorial; however because the compound is *cis* on two adjacent carbons only one substituent can exist in either configuration. They will switch at the same time because the change in one's configuration provides the energy to simultaneously change the other's configuration.

38. D

In the combustion reaction, the hydrocarbon is usually the limiting reagent. Because carbon is present in at least an equimolar amount with hydrogen in all hydrocarbons, the compound that has the greatest moles of carbon will produce the greatest heat (the combustion of a hydrocarbon is an exothermic reaction). The fact that both (C) and (D) have ring structures is not relevant, as cycloheptane clearly has more carbons than any of the other choices.

39. A

What type of amino acid moves toward the anode? Any acidic amino acid. The only acidic amino acid listed is glutamate, the ionized form of glutamic acid. Lysine (C) and histidine (D) are basis (*i.e.*, cations) at or near physiologic pH. Glutamine (B) is uncharged.

PASSAGE V (QUESTIONS 40–47)

40. A

The observed optical rotation is dependent on the concentration of the solution and the length of the polarimeter tube. As the concentration of the solution increases, the number of molecules that can alter the path of light increases. By the same principle, the longer the polarimeter tube, the more molecules there will be in the light's path. Therefore, observed rotation is proportional to solution concentration and tube length. If the solution is half the concentration as before, the student's reading is reduced by a factor of two. Doubling the length of the polarimeter tube (C) doubles the optical rotation. If she starts with a molecule of the opposite chirality, her polarimeter reading will have the same magnitude but in the opposite direction.

41. A

It would be convenient to draw the hydrogen atoms of C2 (with a dash) and C2′ (with a wedge) before designating their stereochemistry. Ignoring the (+) and the *threo-* prefixes, the stereochemistry of C2 in compound I is R (priority of groups at C2 in decreasing order being the ester oxygen, the piperidine nitrogen, the benzene ring, and the hydrogen atom), while the stereochemistry of C2′ is also R (priority being the nitrogen atom, the carbon bounded to the ester and the benzene, $-CH_2^-$, and the hydrogen atom).

42. D

A structural or constitutional isomer is one in which the chemical formula is the same, though the atoms/molecules are arranged differently in space (for example, C_4H_{10} could describe n-butane or 2-methylpropane). The listed compounds are stereoisomers of each other, not constitutional isomers.

43. D

Stereoisomers have the same structure overall, but different stereochemistry at chiral carbon atoms. The theoretical number of stereoisomers for any molecule is 2^n, where n is the number of stereocenters. Because methylphenidate has two stereocenters, there are 2^2, or four stereoisomers, or compounds I–IV in Figure 1.

44. A

To identify diastereomers, the most straightforward way is to decide which pairs of compounds only have *one* of their chiral configurations switched, as opposed to both *i.e.,* pairs of compounds that are not enantiomers are diastereomers. Of the molecules listed, I and II are diastereomers, as are I and IV, III and IV, and II and III.

45. B

(C) is incorrect because S_N2 reactions always result in inversion of stereocenters. (A) incorrectly refers to dehydration reactions as proceeding via a S_N2 mechanism (dehydration with strong bases proceed by E2).

46. C

By definition, geometric isomers refer to *cis-/trans-* or E-/Z-isomers of substituted alkenes, which applies only to (C). Furthermore, alkenes prevent the rotation of the atoms bonded to the first and third carbons. In this case H and Br are the atoms bonded to the one carbon of the double bond, and H and C_3H_7 are bound to the other carbon. Depending on how those four molecules are arranged, 1-bromo-1-pentene can exist as enantiomers. (A) and (B) are incorrect, as there are no chiral atoms and no nonsuperimposible mirror images.

47. B

According to the passage, methylphenidate acts at monoamine transporters in a noncompetitive manner. This means that its mechanism of action does not involve competition with dopamine. Because the molecular similarities of methylphenidate to dopamine are irrelevant (and nonexistent, really), (C) is incorrect. Because the activity is being assessed *in vitro*, the ability of methylphenidate to cross the blood-brain barrier (BBB) is not relevant to the question, so (A) is incorrect.

PASSAGE VI

48. A

Hydrogen is the correct answer. The valence electrons are those in the outer electron shell of the atom. The atomic number provides the value for the number of electrons in the atom. Pauli's exclusion principle restricts the number of electrons in an orbital to two. Therefore, hydrogen's one electron is in the 1s orbital which also composes the outer shell. The s orbitals are spherically shaped by definition.

49. C

Each dot in a Lewis structure represents one electron, and each atom can be shown to have eight valence electrons, satisfying the octet rule that an outer electron shell of eight electrons is needed for chemical stability. (A) does not account for eight valence electrons for both carbon and oxygen. With (B) and (D), there should be no hydrogens, plus carbon and oxygen should each have eight electrons.

50. A

Methane has the maximum ratio of hydrogens to carbons of any molecule since all four valence electrons of carbon are bonded to a hydrogen. C–H bonds are higher in energy than C–C bonds. Thus, any substitution of hydrogens for carbons reduces the bond energies contained in the molecule; the longer the molecule, the lower its potential energy compared to methane. Ethane has two carbons per molecule, propane has three, and butane has four.

51. A

The Lewis structure for the CO_2 molecule is:

:O: :C: :O:

The number of electron domains around the central atom is two, and they are bonding domains. There are no nonbonding domains on the central atom. The electrons on the two oxygen atoms are not on the central atom and thus do not define the geometry of this molecule. (A) is correct.

52. C

The CH_4 molecule has four electron domains, one each for the four carbon-hydrogen bonds around the central atom carbon. There are no nonbonding electron pairs. Thus, the four electron domains dictate a tetrahedral shape. A linear shape is dictated by two electron domains, a trigonal planar by three, and a trigonal bipyramidal shape by five. The Lewis structure for the CO_2 molecule is:

H
H:C:H
H

The number of electron domains around the central atom is two, and they are bonding domains. There are no nonbonding domains on the central atom. The electrons on the two oxygen atoms are not on the central atom and thus do not define the geometry of this molecule.

INDEX

D

E

F

G

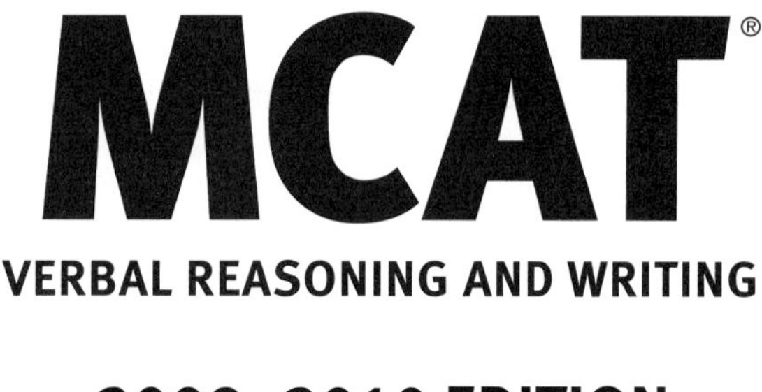

2009–2010 EDITION

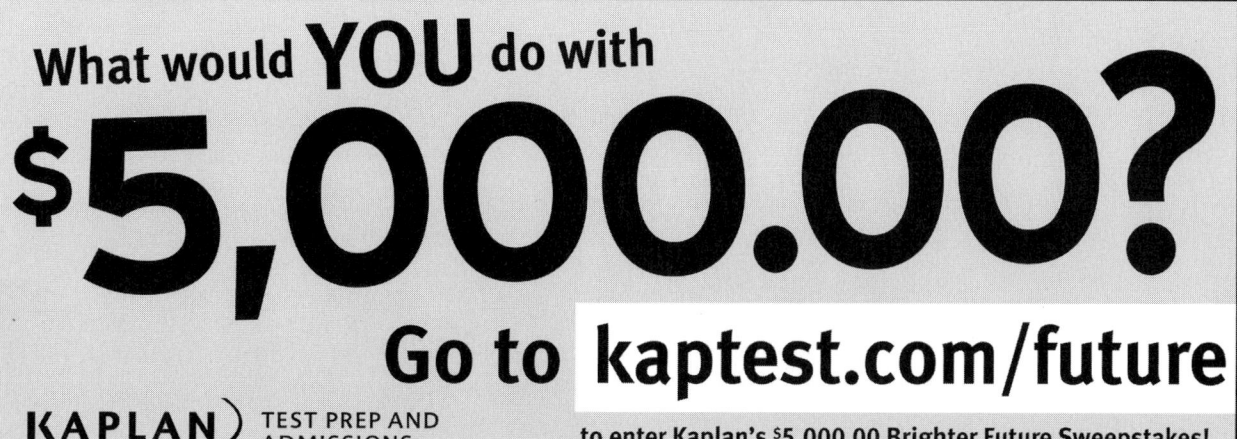

Related Titles

Kaplan MCAT Biology 2009–2010
Kaplan MCAT General Chemistry 2009–2010
Kaplan MCAT Organic Chemistry 2009–2010
Kaplan MCAT Physics 2009–2010

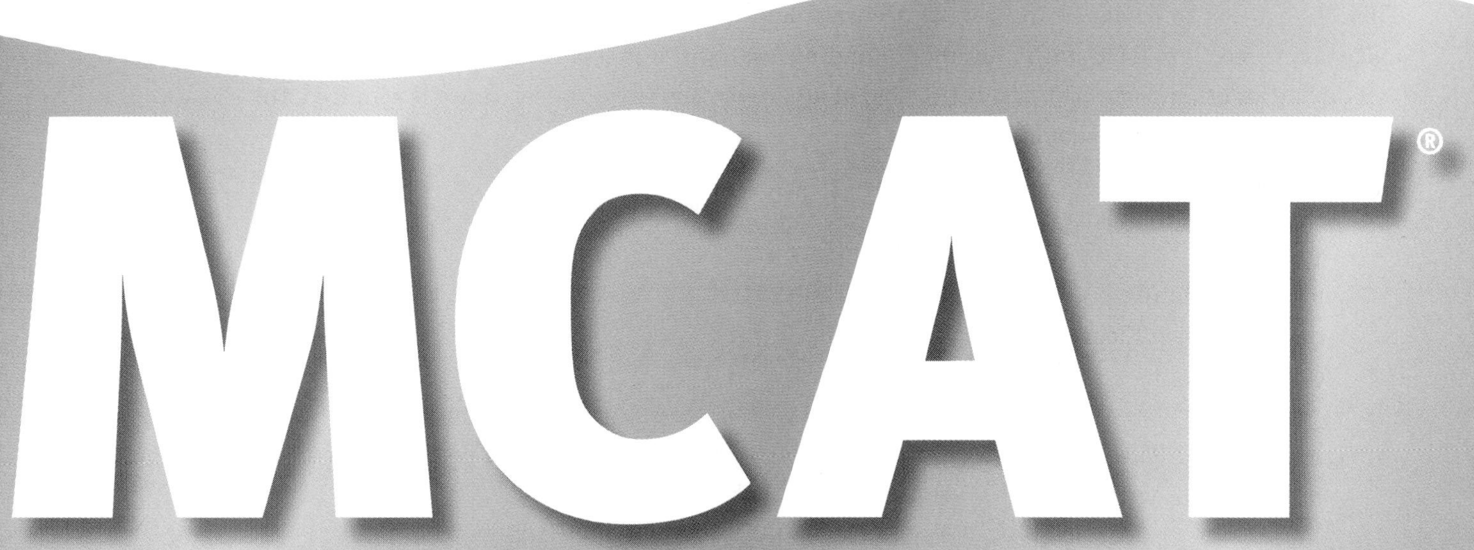

MCAT®
VERBAL REASONING & WRITING

2009–2010 EDITION

The Staff of Kaplan

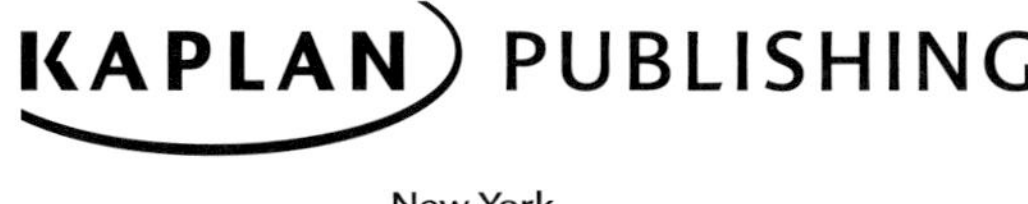

New York

Published by Kaplan Publishing, a division of Kaplan, Inc.
1 Liberty Plaza, 24th Floor
New York, NY 10006

Printed in the United States of America

10 9 8 7 6 5 4 3 2 1

ISBN: 978-1-4277-9876-3

Kaplan Publishing books are available at special quantity discounts to use for sales promotions, employee premiums, or educational purposes. Please email our Special Sales Department to order or for more information at kaplanpublishing@kaplan.com, or write to Kaplan Publishing, 1 Liberty Plaza, 24th Floor, New York, NY 10006.

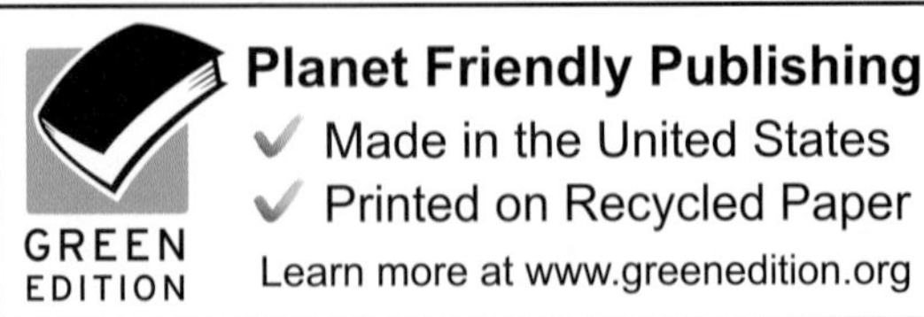

- Manufacturing books in the United States ensures compliance with strict environmental laws and eliminates the need for international freight shipping, a major contributor to global air pollution. Printing on recycled paper helps minimize our consumption of trees, water and fossil fuels.
- Trees Saved: 43 • Air Emissions Eliminated: 3,782 pounds
- Water Saved: 16,677 gallons • Solid Waste Eliminated: 1,640 pounds

Contents

How to Use this Book

Kaplan Verbal Reasoning and Writing, along with the other four books in our MCAT subject review series, brings the Kaplan classroom experience right into your home!

Kaplan has been preparing premeds for the MCAT for more than 40 years in our comprehensive courses. In the past 15 years alone, we've helped over 400,000 students prepare for this important exam and improve their chances of medical school admission.

Think of Kaplan's five MCAT subject books as having a private Kaplan teacher right by your side! We've created a team of the **top MCAT teachers in the country**, who have read through these comprehensive guides. In the sidebars of every page, they offer the same tips, advice, and test day insight that they offer in their Kaplan classroom.

Pay close attention to **Teacher Tip** sidebars like this:

TEACHER TIP

Did you know that many medical schools consider your MCAT Verbal score the most important of the section scores? That's because the Verbal section reflects what you will do as a doctor—think critically!

When you see them, you know what you're getting the same insight and knowledge that students in Kaplan MCAT classrooms across the country receive.

After these teachers walk you through the book, practice with questions at the end of each chapter and three practice sections at the end of the book.

We're confident that this guide, and our award-wining Kaplan teachers, can help you achieve your goals of MCAT success and admission into medical school!

Good luck!

EXPERT KAPLAN MCAT TEAM

Marilyn Engle

MCAT Master Teacher; Teacher Trainer; Kaplan National Teacher of the Year, 2006; Westwood Teacher of the Year, 2007; Westwood Trainer of the Year, 2007; Encino Trainer of the Tear, 2005

John Michael Linick

MCAT Teacher; Boulder Teacher of the Year, 2007; Summer Intensive Program Faculty Member

Dr. Glen Pearlstein

MCAT Master Teacher; Teacher Trainer; Westwood Teacher of the Year, 2006

Matthew B. Wilkinson

MCAT Teacher; Teacher Trainer; Lone Star Trainer of the Year, 2007

INTRODUCTION TO THE MCAT

THE MCAT

The Medical College Admission Test, affectionately known as the MCAT, is different from any other test you've encountered in your academic career. It's not like the knowledge-based exams from high school and college, whose emphasis was on memorizing and regurgitating information. Medical schools can assess your academic prowess by looking at your transcript. The MCAT isn't even like other standardized tests you may have taken, where the focus was on proving your general skills.

Test Tip

The MCAT places more weight on your thought process. However you must have a strong hold of the required core knowledge. The MCAT may not be a perfect gauge of your abilities, but it is a relatively objective way to compare you with students from different backgrounds and undergraduate institutions.

Medical schools use MCAT scores to assess whether you possess the foundation upon which to build a successful medical career. Though you certainly need to know the content to do well, the stress is on thought process, because the MCAT is above all else a thinking test. That's why it emphasizes reasoning, critical and analytical thinking, reading comprehension, data analysis, writing, and problem-solving skills.

The MCAT's power comes from its use as an indicator of your abilities. Good scores can open doors. Your power comes from preparation and mindset, because the key to MCAT success is knowing what you're up against. And that's where this section of this book comes in. We'll explain the philosophy behind the test, review the sections one by one, show you sample questions, share some of Kaplan's proven methods, and clue you in to what the test makers are really after. You'll get a handle on the process, find a confident new perspective, and achieve your highest possible scores.

ABOUT THE MCAT

Information about the MCAT CBT is included below. For the latest information about the MCAT, visit www.kaptest.com/mcat.

MCAT CBT

Format	U.S. — All administrations on computer International — Most on computer with limited paper and pencil in a few isolated areas
Essay Grading	One human and one computer grader
Breaks	Optional break after each section
Length of MCAT Day	Approximately 5.5 hours
Test Dates	Multiple dates in January, April, May, June, July, August, and September Total of 24 administrations each year.
Delivery of Results	Within 30 days. If scores are delayed notification will be posted online at www.aamc.org/mcat Electronic and paper
Security	Government-issued ID Electronic thumbprint Electronic signature verification
Testing Centers	Small computer testing sites

PLANNING FOR THE TEST

As you look toward your preparation for the MCAT consider the following advice:

Complete your core course requirements as soon as possible. Take a strategic eye to your schedule and get core requirements out of the way now.

Take the MCAT once. The MCAT is a notoriously grueling standardized exam that requires extensive preparation. It is longer than the graduate admissions exams for business school (GMAT, $3^1/_2$ hours), law school (LSAT, $3^1/_4$ hours) and graduate school (GRE, $2^1/_2$ hours). You do not want to take it twice. Plan and prepare accordingly.

TEST TIP

Go online and sign up for a local Kaplan Pre-Med Edge event to get the latest information on the test.

THE ROLE OF THE MCAT IN ADMISSIONS

More and more people are applying to medical school and more and more people are taking the MCAT. It's important for you to recognize that while a high MCAT score is a critical component in getting admitted to top med schools, it's not the only factor. Medical school admissions officers weigh grades, interviews, MCAT scores, level of involvement in extracurricular activities, as well as personal essays.

In a Kaplan survey of 130 pre-med advisors, 84% called the interview a "very important" part of the admissions process, followed closely by college grades (83%) and MCAT scores (76%). Kaplan's college admissions consulting practice works with students on all these issues so they can position themselves as strongly as possible. In addition, the Association of American Medical Colleges (AAMC) has made it clear that scores will continue to be valid for 3 years, and that the scoring of the computer-based MCAT will not differ from that of the paper and pencil version.

REGISTRATION

The only way to register for the MCAT is online. The registration site is: www.aamc.org/mcat.

You will be able to access the site approximately 6 months before your test date. Payment must be made by MasterCard or Visa.

Go to www.aamc.org/mcat/registration.htm and download *MCAT Essentials* for information about registration, fees, test administration, and preparation. For other questions, contact:

MCAT Care Team
Association of American Medical Colleges
Section for Applicant Assessment Services
2450 N. St., NW
Washington, DC 20037
www.aamc.org/mcat
Email: mcat@aamc.org

You will want to take the MCAT in the year prior to your planned start date. Don't drag your feet gathering information. You'll need time not only to prepare and practice for the test, but also to get all your registration work done.

ANATOMY OF THE MCAT

TEST TIP

The MCAT should be viewed just like any other part of your application: as an opportunity to show the medical schools who you are and what you can do. Take control of your MCAT experience.

Before mastering strategies, you need to know exactly what you're dealing with on the MCAT. Let's start with the basics: The MCAT is, among other things, an endurance test.

If you can't approach it with confidence and stamina, you'll quickly lose your composure. That's why it's so important that you take control of the test.

The MCAT consists of four timed sections: Physical Sciences, Verbal Reasoning, Writing Sample, and Biological Sciences. Later in this section we'll take an in-depth look at each MCAT section, including sample question types and specific test-smart hints, but here's a general overview, reflecting the order of the test sections and number of questions in each.

Physical Sciences

Time	70 minutes
Format	• 52 multiple-choice questions: approximately 7–9 passages with 4–8 questions each • approximately 10 stand-alone questions (not passage-based)
What it tests	basic general chemistry concepts, basic physics concepts, analytical reasoning, data interpretation

Verbal Reasoning

Time	60 minutes
Format	• 40 multiple-choice questions: approximately 7 passages with 5–7 questions each
What it tests	critical reading

Writing Sample

Time	60 minutes
Format	• 2 essay questions (30 minutes per essay)
What it tests	critical thinking, intellectual organization, written communication skills

Biological Sciences

Time	70 minutes
Format	• 52 multiple-choice questions: approximately 7–9 passages with 4–8 questions each • approximately 10 stand-alone questions (not passage-based)
What it tests	basic biology concepts, basic organic chemistry concepts, analytical reasoning, data interpretation

TEST TIP

There's no penalty for a wrong answer on the MCAT, so NEVER LEAVE ANY QUESTION BLANK, even if you have time only for a wild guess.

The sections of the test always appear in the same order:

Physical Sciences
[optional 10-minute break]
Verbal Reasoning
[optional 10-minute break]
Writing Sample
[optional 10-minute break]
Biological Sciences

SCORING

Each MCAT section receives its own score. Physical Sciences, Verbal Reasoning, and Biological Sciences are each scored on a scale ranging from 1–15, with 15 as the highest. The Writing Sample essays are scored alphabetically on a scale ranging from J to T, with T as the highest. The two essays are each evaluated by two official readers, so four critiques combine to make the alphabetical score.

TEST TIP

The percentile figure tells you how many other test-takers scored at or below your level. In other words, a percentile figure of 80 means that 80 percent did as well or worse than you did, and that only 20 percent did better.

The number of multiple-choice questions that you answer correctly per section is your "raw score." Your raw score will then be converted to yield the "scaled score"—the one that will fall somewhere in that 1–15 range. These scaled scores are what are reported to medical schools as your MCAT scores. All multiple-choice questions are worth the same amount—one raw point—and *there's no penalty for guessing*. That means that *you should always select an answer for every question, whether you get to that question or know the answer not!* This is an important piece of advice, so pay it heed. Never let time run out on any section without selecting an answer for every question.

Your score report will tell you—and your potential medical schools—not only your scaled scores, but also the national mean score for each section, standard deviation, national scoring profile for each section, and your percentile ranking.

WHAT'S A GOOD SCORE?

There's no such thing as a cut-and-dry "good score." Much depends on the strength of the rest of your application (if your transcript is first-rate, the pressure to strut your stuff on the MCAT isn't as intense) and on where you want to go to school (different schools have different score expectations). Here are a few interesting statistics:

For each MCAT administration, the average scaled scores are approximately 8 for Physical Sciences, Verbal Reasoning, and Biological Sciences, and N for the Writing Sample. You need scores of at least 10–11 to be considered competitive by most medical schools, and if you're aiming for the top you've got to do even better, and score 12 and above.

You don't have to be perfect to do well. For instance, on the AAMC's Practice Test 5R, you could get as many as 10 questions wrong in Verbal Reasoning, 17 in Physical Sciences, and 16 in Biological Sciences and still score in the 80th percentile. To score in the 90th percentile, you could get as many as 7 wrong in Verbal Reasoning, 12 in Physical Sciences, and 12 in Biological Sciences. Even students who receive perfect scaled scores usually get a handful of questions wrong.

It's important to maximize your performance on every question. Just a few questions one way or the other can make a big difference in your scaled score. Here's a look at recent score profiles so you can get an idea of the shape of a typical score distribution.

Physical Sciences		
Scaled Score	Percent Achieving Score	Percentile Rank Range
15	0.1	99.9–99.9
14	1.2	98.7–99.8
13	2.5	96.2–98.6
12	5.1	91.1–96.1
11	7.2	83.9–91.0
10	12.1	71.8–83.8
9	12.9	58.9–71.1
8	16.5	42.4–58.5
7	16.7	25.7–42.3
6	13.0	12.7–25.6
5	7.9	04.8–12.6
4	3.3	01.5–04.7
3	1.3	00.2–01.4
2	0.1	00.1–00.1
1	0.0	00.0–00.0
Scaled Score Mean = 8.1 Standard Deviation = 2.32		

Verbal Reasoning		
Scaled Score	Percent Achieving Score	Percentile Rank Range
15	0.1	99.9–99.9
14	0.2	99.7–99.8
13	1.8	97.9–99.6
12	3.6	94.3–97.8
11	10.5	83.8–94.2
10	15.6	68.2–83.7
9	17.2	51.0–68.1
8	15.4	35.6–50.9
7	10.3	25.3–35.5
6	10.9	14.4–25.2
5	6.9	07.5–14.3
4	3.9	03.6–07.4
3	2.0	01.6–03.5
2	0.5	00.1–01.5
1	0.0	00.0–00.0
Scaled Score Mean = 8.0 Standard Deviation = 2.43		

TEST TIP

The raw score of each administration is converted to a scaled score. The conversion varies with administrations. Hence, the same raw score will not always give you the same scaled score.

Writing Sample		
Scaled Score	Percent Achieving Score	Percentile Rank Range
T	0.5	99.9–99.9
S	2.8	94.7–99.8
R	7.2	96.0–99.3
Q	14.2	91.0–95.9
P	9.7	81.2–90.9
O	17.9	64.0–81.1
N	14.7	47.1–63.9
M	18.8	30.4–47.0
L	9.5	21.2–30.3
K	3.6	13.5–21.1
J	1.2	06.8–13.4
		02.9–06.7
		00.9–02.8
		00.2–00.8
		00.0–00.1
75th Percentile = Q 50th Percentile = O 25th Percentile = M		

Biological Sciences		
Scaled Score	Percent Achieving Score	Percentile Rank Range
15	0.1	99.9–99.9
14	1.2	98.7–99.8
13	2.5	96.2–98.6
12	5.1	91.1–96.1
11	7.2	83.9–91.0
10	12.1	71.8–83.8
9	12.9	58.9–71.1
8	16.5	42.4–58.5
7	16.7	25.7–42.3
6	13.0	12.7–25.6
5	7.9	04.8–12.6
4	3.3	01.5–04.7
3	1.3	00.2–01.4
2	0.1	00.1–00.1
1	0.0	00.0–00.0
Scaled Score Mean = 8.2 Standard Deviation = 2.39		

WHAT THE MCAT REALLY TESTS

It's important to grasp not only the nuts and bolts of the MCAT, so you'll know *what* to do on test day; but also the underlying principles of the test, so you'll know *why* you're doing what you're doing on test day. We'll cover the straightforward MCAT facts later. Now it's time to examine the heart and soul of the MCAT, to see what it's really about.

THE MYTH

Most people preparing for the MCAT fall prey to the myth that the MCAT is a straightforward science test. They think something like this:

> *"It covers the four years of science I had to take in school: biology, chemistry, physics, and organic chemistry. It even has equations. OK, so it has Verbal Reasoning and Writing, but those sections are just to see if we're literate, right? The important stuff is the science. After all, we're going to be doctors."*

Well, here's the little secret no one seems to want you to know: The MCAT is not just a science test; it's also a thinking test. This means that the test is designed to let you demonstrate your thought process, not just your thought content.

The implications are vast. Once you shift your test-taking paradigm to match the MCAT modus operandi, you'll find a new level of confidence and control over the test. You'll begin to work with the nature of the MCAT rather than against it. You'll be more efficient and insightful as you prepare for the test, and you'll be more relaxed on test day. In fact, you'll be able to see the MCAT for what it is rather than for what it's dressed up to be. We want your test day to feel like a visit with a familiar friend instead of an awkward blind date.

THE ZEN OF MCAT

Medical schools do not need to rely on the MCAT to see what you already know. Admission committees can measure your subject-area proficiency using your undergraduate coursework and grades. Schools are most interested in the potential of your mind.

In recent years, many medical schools have shifted pedagogic focus away from an information-heavy curriculum to a concept-based curriculum. There is currently more emphasis placed on problem solving, holistic thinking, and cross-disciplinary study. Be careful not to dismiss this important point, figuring you'll wait to worry about academic trends until you're actually in medical school. This trend affects you right now, because it's reflected in the MCAT. Every good tool matches its task. In this case the tool is the test, used to measure you and other candidates, and the task is to quantify how likely it is that you'll succeed in medical school.

Your intellectual potential—how skillfully you annex new territory into your mental boundaries, how quickly you build "thought highways" between ideas, how confidently and creatively you solve problems—is far more important to admission committees than your ability to recite Young's modulus for every material known to man. The schools assume they can expand your knowledge base. They choose applicants carefully because expansive knowledge is not enough to succeed in medical school or in the profession. There's something more. And it's this "something more" that the MCAT is trying to measure.

Every section on the MCAT tests essentially the same higher-order thinking skills: analytical reasoning, abstract thinking, and problem solving.

Most test-takers get trapped into thinking they are being tested strictly about biology, chemistry, etc. Thus, they approach each section with a new outlook on what's expected. This constant mental gear-shifting can be exhausting, not to mention counterproductive. Instead of perceiving the test as parsed into radically different sections, you need to maintain your focus on the underlying nature of the test: It's designed to test your thinking skills, not your information-recall skills. Each test section thus presents a variation on the same theme.

WHAT ABOUT THE SCIENCE?

With this perspective, you may be left asking these questions: "What about the science? What about the content? Don't I need to know the basics?" The answer is a resounding "Yes!" You must be fluent in the different languages of the test. You cannot do well on the MCAT if you don't know the basics of physics, general chemistry, biology, and organic chemistry. We recommend that you take one year each of biology, general chemistry, organic chemistry, and physics before taking the MCAT, and that you review the content in this book thoroughly. Knowing these basics is just the beginning of doing well on the MCAT. That's a shock to most test-takers. They presume that once they recall or relearn their undergraduate science, they are ready to do battle against the MCAT. Wrong! They merely have directions to the battlefield. They lack what they need to beat the test: a copy of the test-maker's battle plan!

TEST TIP

Don't think of the sections of the MCAT as unrelated timed pieces. Each is a variation on the same theme, since the underlying purpose of each section and of the test as a whole is to evaluate your thinking skills. Memorizing formulas won't boost your score. Understanding fundamental scientific principles will.

You won't be drilled on facts and formulas on the MCAT. You'll need to demonstrate ability to reason based on ideas and concepts. The science questions are painted with a broad brush, testing your general understanding.

TAKE CONTROL: THE MCAT MINDSET

In addition to being a thinking test, as we've stressed, the MCAT is a standardized test. As such, it has its own consistent patterns and idiosyncrasies that can actually work in your favor. This is the key to why test preparation works. You have the opportunity to familiarize yourself with those consistent peculiarities, to adopt the proper test-taking mindset.

TEST TIP

Those perfectionist tendencies that make you a good student and a good medical school candidate may work against you in MCAT Land. If you get stuck on a question or passage, move on. Perfectionism is for medical school—not the MCAT. And you don't need to understand every word of a passage before you go on to the questions—what's tripping you up may not even be relevant to what you'll be asked.

The following are some overriding principles of the MCAT Mindset that will be covered in depth in the chapters to come:

- Read actively and critically.
- Translate prose into your own words.

- Save the toughest questions for last.
- Know the test and its components inside and out.
- Do MCAT-style problems in each topic area after you've reviewed it.
- Allow your confidence to build on itself.
- Take full-length practice tests a week or two before the test to break down the mystique of the real experience.
- Learn from your mistakes—get the most out of your practice tests.
- Look at the MCAT as a challenge, the first step in your medical career, rather than as an arbitrary obstacle.

And that's what the MCAT Mindset boils down to: Taking control. Being proactive. Being on top of the testing experience so that you can get as many points as you can as quickly and as easily as possible. Keep this in mind as you read and work through the material in this book and, of course, as you face the challenge on test day.

Now that you have a better idea of what the MCAT is all about, let's take a tour of the individual test sections. Although the underlying skills being tested are similar, each MCAT section requires that you call into play a different domain of knowledge. So, though we encourage you to think of the MCAT as a holistic and unified test, we also recognize that the test is segmented by discipline and that there are characteristics unique to each section. In the overviews, we'll review sample questions and answers and discuss section-specific strategies. For each of the sections—Verbal Reasoning, Physical/Biological Sciences, and the Writing Sample—we'll present you with the following:

- **The Big Picture**
  You'll get a clear view of the section and familiarize yourself with what it's really evaluating.
- **A Closer Look**
  You'll explore the types of questions that will appear and master the strategies you'll need to deal with them successfully.
- **Highlights**
  The key approaches to each section are outlined, for reinforcement and quick review.

Part I
Verbal Reasoning

CHAPTER 1

INTRODUCTION TO VERBAL REASONING

Many test-takers find the Verbal section of the MCAT to be the most challenging and, yes, frightening. So here's the first strategy you need to know: don't panic! The Verbal section tests your reading, thinking, and writing abilities. You've already mastered these skills. If you hadn't, you wouldn't be studying for the MCAT right now. So you're not being asked to learn something new and mysterious, then quickly turn it into MCAT points. You're asked to use the skills you have, but tweaked for the MCAT. That's why you're reading this book. So don't worry. We'll demystify MCAT Verbal by identifying exactly what makes it such a challenging section. Then we'll introduce you to Verbal Reasoning **THE KAPLAN WAY**—reading for structure, not detail. On Test Day, you'll be prepared with a powerful arsenal of analytical tactics from our Verbal Reasoning chapters, lessons, and Training Library. You *can* improve your critical reading between now and Test Day; we'll show you how!

TEACHER TIP

Have confidence; you can do this!

The passages you'll confront on Test Day probably won't be fun to read. Odds are, they'll be boring. If they're too engaging, check the cover. You may be taking the wrong test. As part of the challenge, you must be able to concentrate and glean meaning from the text, regardless of its nature. This means working through your resistance to dry passages and overcoming any anxiety or frustration. The more control you can muster, the quicker you can move through each passage, through the questions, and to a higher score.

Don't make the mistake that so many MCAT participants make in underestimating the challenge of the Verbal Reasoning section. Sometimes it falls under the shadow cast by the looming science sections. Also, students figure that there isn't anything to "study" for this section. It's true that studying for content isn't going to get you points on MCAT, but studying for strategy will. Verbal Reasoning is conquered with strategy, and you need to know what that strategy is and how to apply it effectively. Be aware that the scoring gradient for Verbal Reasoning is very steep. It's hard to get a good score so you can't afford to be cavalier. Some medical

TEACHER TIP

Did you know that many medical schools consider your MCAT Verbal score the most important of the section scores? That's because the Verbal section reflects what you will do as a doctor—think critically!

schools add all your MCAT scores together for a composite score; if you blow off Verbal Reasoning, you could kill your composite. Practice Verbal Reasoning as you would the other test sections, and challenge yourself to acquire the specialized reading skills required on the MCAT.

THE ANATOMY OF THE PASSAGE

MCAT Verbal Reasoning passages cover a great variety of subjects. Past MCATs have had passages on everything from Native American life in Alaska to Sartre's philosophy. Should you be worried about your possible unfamiliarity with such topics? No way! For one thing, any information you need to answer the questions is in the passage itself. All you have to do is concentrate on reading and thinking critically. Even better, regardless of whether you're dealing with a humanities, social science, or science text, every passage can be handled easily if you follow some general principles... the ones we will cover in the next chapter, Reading the Kaplan Way. But first, we'll look at how our everyday reading differs from the active reading you'll do on MCAT Verbal.

READING ON THE MCAT VERSUS EVERYDAY READING

Ordinarily, we read for one or both of two simple reasons: to learn something or to pass the time pleasantly. Needless to say, neither of these reasons has anything to do with the MCAT. Furthermore, on a daily basis we tend to read for content. "What's the deeper meaning here?" we ask ourselves, or "What's this book about?" But anyone who tries to read for content during the MCAT is missing the point. There's just no time under strict test conditions to understand everything that's written—and, as we'll see, there's no payoff in it, either.

So what does MCAT reading, as distinct from everyday reading, involve? Broadly stated, it involves two things:

Reading for author **PURPOSE**—the "why" of the text
Reading for passage **STRUCTURE**—the "how" of the text

Almost every single MCAT Verbal Reasoning question fundamentally hinges on your ability to step back from the text and analyze why the author is writing in the first place, and how she puts her text together.

Why so? Why does the MCAT test these particular skills?

Here's the deal: Demanding that we figure out the author's purpose and the passage's structure is the best way to test how each of us thinks about the prose we read. And thinking is always being tested, one way or another, on every MCAT question.

Look at it this way. You have probably written a term paper that begins something like this:

> *The purpose of this paper is to examine the Christian imagery employed by John Milton in Paradise Lost, and then to compare it to the pagan imagery in Paradise Regained. I will show that Milton's views of divinity and predestination, in particular, underwent a metamorphosis, as he....*

Most of us would say, "Sure, I was taught to begin papers with that kind of statement of intent. And yes, I was also told to describe how I planned to achieve that purpose." In other words, most of us were trained to announce our *why* and *how* right at the beginning of the paper.

Now there are good reasons, of course, to urge students to write in this fashion. If you (the student writer) lay out the why and how of your paper up front, you're more likely to write with unity and clarity as you go along. Moreover, announcing what you've set out to do helps the grader evaluate whether you've done it. (Remember this when you start to learn the writing sample.)

However, more sophisticated writing—like the prose you'll see on the MCAT—doesn't always reveal its secrets quite so explicitly. Authors always have a purpose, of course, and always have a structural plan for carrying out that purpose. But sophisticated writers may not announce their purpose, which puts an extra burden on the reader to analyze what's stated, read between the lines, and draw inferences.

So, in order to set up the questions—to test how we think about the prose we read—the MCAT editors omit or disguise the statement of purpose, and challenge us to unpack it. Consider this first sentence of a typical passage:

> The great migration of European intellectuals to the United States in the second quarter of the twentieth century prompted a transmutation in the character of Western social thought.

Teacher Tip

Reading the Kaplan Way is reading with a strategic approach. It's this approach to the passage, rather than how much you really understand, that gets you points on the MCAT.

See? We can figure out why the author is writing: His purpose, we might say, is *"to explore how the arrival of European eggheads during the period 1926–1950 changed Western social thought"* (your phrasing might be a bit different, but the gist is probably the same). So there is a definite purpose and structure here; we just have to work a little harder at figuring them out than we're used to. In the next chapter, Reading the Kaplan Way, we'll learn to execute a scientific protocol of sorts that will allow us to find the purpose and structure of any passage the MCAT gives us on Test Day.

CHAPTER 2

READING THE KAPLAN WAY

PRINCIPLES THAT WILL REWARD YOU

MCAT Verbal Reasoning tests your understanding of what an author is thinking and doing. Therefore, your focus as you read must always be on the author. The test writers want you to look beyond content—they want you to draw conclusions about the *why* and *how* of the text, not the *what*. In other words, why has it been written and how has it been put together? **Detail questions**—those that ask about the what—are very rare indeed on the MCAT. By contrast, questions that ask about the why and the how—global, deduction, evaluation, application, and incorporation questions—are the mainstay of the Verbal Reasoning section. That's where critical thinking skills come into play.

The passage exists only because the author has a specific purpose in mind. Therefore, as you read, you need to keep asking yourself, "Why?" "Why are you telling me this, author? Why are you discussing this theory? Why are you citing this opinion? Why are you including this particular detail at this place in the text?" Keep in mind that the author's purpose is usually to convince his reader to accept his specific ideas. Even when the text is more objective—a descriptive "storytelling" text—you have to keep asking why and how, not what.

Teacher Tip

Know what's important in the passage and what isn't. For humanities and many social sciences, it's ALL about the author.

Details are in the passage only to illustrate what the author is thinking or doing. Therefore, read over details quickly; read them more closely only when questions demand it. There's no payoff in just "getting through the passage" without comprehension; on the other hand, trying to assimilate all of the content is a waste of time. Instead, boil the passage down to its basics.

Teacher Tip

When you read for the MCAT, you're not reading to learn or remember anything. You don't even need to understand everything. You just want to paraphrase the gist of each paragraph so you can use the passage efficiently to research answers.

Paragraphs are the fundamental building blocks of the passage. Therefore, as you read, take note of paragraph topics rather than specifics. Ask yourself, "What's the purpose of this paragraph? How does it fit into the overall structure of the passage?" For example, does this paragraph capture the author's main idea or rather a small supporting example? Is the author using an analogy to strengthen her point or to refute someone else's contrary idea?

THE SKILLS BEHIND THE PRINCIPLES

In order to apply these critical reading principles, you have to develop MCAT-specific critical reading skills. The next section of this chapter is designed to help you with this process. We'll explain the concepts and give you drills to help you sharpen the necessary skills.

TEACHER TIP

When you summarize a paragraph, you put the gist, or purpose, into your own words. Make a map by writing down this paraphrase on your scratch paper. Don't try to remember what you read; MCAT passages are much too dense to do that well. Write what you need to know in the map.

Pause frequently to summarize. Don't glaze!

A good summary captures the contents of a block of text in a few words or a sentence without losing any of the text's basic ideas. Consider the following block of text:

> Most of the developed countries are now agreed on the need to take international measures to reduce carbon emissions into the atmosphere. Despite this consensus, a wide disagreement among economists as to how much emission reduction will actually cost continues to impede policy making. Economists who believe that the energy market is efficient predict that countries that reduce carbon emission by as little as 20 percent will experience significant losses to their gross national product. Those who hold that the market is inefficient, however, estimate that costs will be much lower....

TEACHER TIP

When you map, don't worry about spelling, grammar, word choice, or punctuation. It doesn't even need to be in English. Nobody is going to read this map but you. Just use your words, symbols—or whatever—to write the purpose of the paragraph.

A good summary of this text would be something like: *An international policy to reduce carbon emissions has been held up by arguments about how much it would cost.* That's the basic idea here; the rest is just detail.

MCAT answer choices are frequently just paraphrases of what was stated in the passage. Learn to paraphrase and you'll learn to be attuned to correct answer choices.

TEACHER TIP

Paraphrase and map after each paragraph. Don't map before reading the entire paragraph, and don't wait until the end of the passage. Mapping takes practice. Initially you'll go slowly, but don't give up; this is an important strategy that must be mastered and applied.

The key to reading MCAT passages successfully will be to leave behind the habit of reading passively, letting the words glide by, even as your mind wanders to other subjects (like your anxieties about getting into med school, for instance). With these tools, you will learn to read more actively, pausing frequently to quickly summarize and paraphrase what you've just read. **A good reader checks her understanding frequently without getting bogged down on any one section.**

FIND THE TOPIC, SCOPE, AND PURPOSE

Finding the topic, scope, and purpose will force you to check your understanding of each paragraph. Let's define our terms:

The **topic** is the author's basic subject matter: World War I, volcanoes, or Charles Dickens's *Bleak House*.

The **scope** is the specific aspect of the topic on which the author focuses: the causes of World War I, competing theories about predicting volcanic eruptions, or Dickens's critique of the English legal system.

The **purpose** is the reason why the author wrote the passage: to dispute a common belief about the causes of World War I, to describe competing theories about predicting volcanic eruptions, or to support Dickens's critique of the English legal system.

Identifying these parameters of a passage makes it easier to attack. While reading Verbal Reasoning passages, most MCAT test-takers have two maladaptive tendencies: (1) the tendency to glaze over, so that they realize when their eyes reach the end of a paragraph that they weren't really paying attention, and (2) the tendency to read for detail instead of structure, so that they get bogged down when faced with a patch of dense text or a cluster of thorny details. Because MCAT Verbal passages are challenging, both of these tendencies will be an issue for most test-takers; you can learn to manage both by doing active tasks (finding topic, scope, and purpose for instance) which will keep you attentive and attuned to structure. And, with practice, you'll find yourself getting "glazed and bogged" less and less.

You already learned to map the gist of each paragraph. When you're finished reading the entire passage, map the overall topic, scope, and purpose. If you were to map the previous paragraph, you'd come up with the following:

Topic: verbal reasoning

Scope: topic, scope, purpose

Purpose: to explain topic, scope, and purpose for verbal reasoning

TEACHER TIP

To find scope, ask yourself the question, "What about the topic?" If the topic is MCAT Verbal Reasoning, what about it? You're reading about the definitions of topic, scope, and purpose. That's the scope. It's important to note this because many wrong answers go out of scope.

TEACHER TIP

To find purpose, ask yourself if the author is neutral or has a point of view. If he's neutral, he'll start with a neutral verb such as "explain" "describe," "show," or " compare." If he has a point of view, he'll use language such as "advocate," "criticize," or "support." Always write purpose starting with a verb. For one thing, a verb shows action, and the purpose is the reason why the author acted to write the passage. Not only that, but on the rare occasion when the test-maker gives you a purpose question, he may start each answer with a verb. If you know the author is neutral and your purpose verb reflects that, all you have to do is get rid of any answer that doesn't start with a neutral verb.

When you map, you can't glaze; you're forced to stop, think, and write after each paragraph.

TEACHER TIP

The purpose of each paragraph is the "why," not the "what." Ask why the author wrote this. What's the gist of what he's trying to tell you? Then write it in as your paraphrase of the paragraph.

For most passages, the topic and scope remain the same in the passage. However, within the overall purpose of the passage, each paragraph has its own unique purpose, and we will discuss this in greater detail in the next section. In the next section, we'll focus on an irreducible property of every paragraph: its purpose.

DRILL #1: FINDING TOPIC, SCOPE, AND PURPOSE

Directions: Read each of these paragraphs actively, assigning a topic, scope, and purpose to each in your own words. Then, using your own interpretation of each paragraph, match each of the numbered statements on page 26 with a paragraph that it best describes. There may be more than one correct statement for each text. Not every statement necessarily matches up with one of the texts.

TEACHER TIP

You already know that purpose is key to the author's reason for writing the passage. Remember to first ask yourself if the author is neutral or has a point of view, and watch for contrast keywords and phrases to clue you in.

A. At the Battle of Gettysburg in July 1863, 75,000 Confederate troops faced 90,000 Union soldiers in one of the largest battles of the American Civil War. For two days, both armies suffered heavy casualties in constant fighting, without either gaining a clear advantage. On the third and final day of the battle, Confederate forces mounted one last effort to penetrate Union lines. But the attempt ended in complete failure, forcing Confederate troops to withdraw far to the south....

B. In January 1863, seven months before the decisive Battle of Gettysburg, President Lincoln issued the Emancipation Proclamation, in which he declared an end to slavery in the United States. Some historians cite Lincoln's edict as proof that he wanted to do away with slavery because he considered it morally repugnant. While Lincoln certainly opposed the institution on ethical grounds, the timing of the proclamation suggests that he was out to weaken the Confederacy rather than to undertake a moral crusade....

TEACHER TIP

"While" is a nice contrast keyword, isn't it? So Lincoln wasn't out to lead a moral crusade but rather to weaken the opposition. That's what the author is *really* writing about.

C. Gettysburg was a turning point in the Civil War. Before the battle, Confederate forces under General Robert E. Lee had defeated their Union counterparts in a string of major engagements. After the battle, however, Union forces took the initiative, finally defeating the Confederacy less than two years later. By invading Union territory, the Confederate leadership had sought to shatter the Union's will to continue the war and to convince European nations to recognize the Confederacy as an independent nation. Instead, the Union's willingness to fight was strengthened and the Confederacy squandered its last chance for foreign support....

D. The Confederacy had hoped that France and Great Britain would intervene militarily on its side in order to restore the European-American cotton trade. But once President Lincoln issued the Emancipation Proclamation—which changed the focus of the Civil War from a conflict over states' rights to one over slavery—both the French and British concluded that their status in the international community would be jeopardized were they, in effect, to support slavery...

1. argue that the outcome of the Battle of Gettysburg undermined the Confederacy's military and political goals in the Civil War
2. discuss the course of one of the most important battles of the Civil War
3. point out that Lincoln's primary motive for delivering the Emancipation Proclamation was to strengthen the Union in its struggle with the Confederacy
4. describe the effect of the Emancipation Proclamation on the Confederacy's foreign relations
5. convey a sense of the close relations that existed between the Confederacy and European nations before the Battle of Gettysburg
6. settle an ongoing debate among historians about the importance of the Emancipation Proclamation to the Confederacy's defeat at the Battle of Gettysburg
7. propose that the Battle of Gettysburg played a crucial part in changing the course of the Civil War
8. refute the view that the Emancipation Proclamation stemmed from Lincoln's desire to destroy slavery
9. explain the cotton trade's role in turning the international community against the Confederacy
10. show that the Union won the Battle of Gettysburg because it had more troops than the Confederacy

TEACHER TIP

Note that each purpose statement starts with a verb. That's why your purpose statement should also start with a verb. If you described the purpose with a neutral verb, you can quickly eliminate any statement which starts with a point of view verb, and vice-versa. How fast is that?!

ANSWERS TO DRILL #1

Statements 1 and 7 match up with text C: topic is the Battle of Gettysburg; scope is the battle's role in determining the outcome of the Civil War; and purpose is to assert that Gettysburg was a turning point in the eventual defeat of the South and victory of the North.

Statement 2 matches up with text A: topic is the Battle of Gettysburg; scope is the battle itself, and purpose is to describe what happened during the battle.

Statements 3 and 8 match up with text B: topic is the Emancipation Proclamation; scope is Lincoln's motive for issuing the proclamation; and purpose is to argue that Lincoln did so in order to weaken the Confederacy.

Statement 4 matches up with text D: topic is Confederate foreign relations; scope is the connection between the Emancipation Proclamation and Confederate foreign relations; and purpose is to describe the effect of the proclamation on Confederate foreign relations.

Statement 5 doesn't match up with any text: texts C and D mention Confederate–European relations, but neither of them speaks of close relations before Gettysburg.

Statement 6 doesn't match up with any text: none of the texts refers to a debate among historians.

Statement 9 doesn't match up with any text: only text D refers to the cotton trade, but it doesn't draw any connection between the cotton trade and the international community's rejection of the Confederacy.

Statement 10 doesn't match up with any text: text A mentions the number of troops each side deployed at Gettysburg, but its purpose isn't to argue that the Union won at Gettysburg because it had more troops.

THE IMPORTANCE OF PURPOSE

When a group of sentences is set together by indentation (such as a paragraph), this is a significant event. It means that these sentences all have something in common, a distinct unifying idea that justifies setting them together. Each paragraph, then, must always serve a purpose in the larger context of the passage: an author never writes just to pass the time, but rather to make a point. In other words, the **purpose** of a paragraph is the major point the author wants you to take away—e.g., *"World War I was caused by European competition for overseas colonies, not by alliance arrangements in Europe"*; or *"so-and-so's theory of volcanic eruptions is the most credible because of such-and-such"*; or *"Dickens's critique of the English legal system was flawed by his inability to understand legal arguments."* **As an MCAT test-taker, it is most important that you grasp this purpose in order to ace the questions.** Of course, the author must achieve his purpose with supporting evidence, and this evidence will come in the form of details. What is not important for you as an MCAT test-taker is to memorize these details while you read the passage, because you are free to relocate them if a question requires you to do so. Because you will read for structure, not detail, you will be able to relocate relevant details quickly.

TEACHER TIP

Determining and mapping purpose are absolutely vital to understanding the author.

DRILL #2: DISTINGUISHING THE PURPOSE OF A PARAGRAPH FROM SUPPORTING DETAILS

Instructions: In your own words, jot down the purpose and the supporting details of each paragraph.

TEACHER TIP

Step back from this paragraph and determine the gist of what the author wants you to know.

1. In the early 20th century, impoverished southern black farmers migrated in large numbers to northern cities in search of steady employment. With a rapidly expanding industrial base, Chicago was the destination for much of this wave of emigration. Many of these farmers were eventually able to find jobs in Chicago's factories, but life was not easy for them. They received very low wages for long hours of physically demanding work. Moreover, they were often torn from their families, with wives and children left behind out of economic necessity. And though discrimination was less intense in the North than in the South, black migrants were still subject to unfair treatment in matters of pay, promotion, and job security.

TEACHER TIP

You did, of course, ask yourself whether the author is neutral or has a point of view, and started purpose with a verb, didn't you? Way to go!

Purpose: ____

Supporting Details: ____

TEACHER TIP

Did you note the contrast word "but"? That will introduce you to the author's purpose in writing this paragraph.

2. Theropods, or three-toed dinosaurs, were traditionally thought of as unsociable, land-bound creatures who preferred to scavenge than to hunt. But recently uncovered fossil evidence has led to a thorough reassessment of this view. The discovery of numerous sets of three-toed tracks at many fossil sites, for instance, has convinced paleontologists that theropods moved in packs, at least when feeding. Furthermore, some fossil sites were under water when dinosaurs roamed the earth, indicating that theropods could swim. In fact, paleontologists now think that they were excellent swimmers who experienced little trouble capturing prey in the water. Their ability to swim has also undermined the belief that they were scavengers rather than hunters, because scavengers look for carrion on land, not in the water.

TEACHER TIP

Don't get bogged down in details; they don't show up in many questions. Focus on the author's purpose instead.

Purpose: ____

Supporting Details: ____

3. The poetry of the earliest Greeks was completely impersonal. It was folk poetry, whose purpose was to express the thoughts and feelings of the entire community. During the later age of heroes, however, the focus of Greek poetry switched from the community to the individual. This poetry celebrates the lives of important personages

such as kings and warriors. In so doing, it reflects the changing nature of ancient Greek life: a society that had initially been free of stark class differences eventually developed a hierarchical structure, with a small ruling elite in control of the masses.

Purpose: ______________________________

Supporting Details: ______________________________

TEACHER TIP

Did you catch the contrast keyword this time? Good for you!

ANSWERS TO DRILL #2

TEACHER TIP

Finding purpose and writing it down with an initial verb will score you points on the MCAT. It's going to make all the difference in getting the right answer for global questions (main idea) and inference questions.

1. **Purpose:** to argue that poor black farmers who migrated to Chicago in search of jobs often found employment, but life remained difficult for them

   Supporting details: low wages for hard work, family separation, job discrimination

2. **Purpose:** to describe new finding about therapods

   Supporting details: they were sociable (numerous sets of fossil tracks) and could swim (underwater tracks)

3. **Purpose:** to argue that change in Greek poetry showed societal change from community emphasis → individual.

   Supporting details: folk poetry was the norm in early Greek society when no classes existed; heroic poetry became the norm later when society was ruled by a small elite of warriors and kings

CHAPTER 3

KEYWORDS

Keywords and phrases are just that: keys to open the locks which tell you the passage structure and author's intent. These are the important points to know when reading an MCAT passage. The rest is detail, which may or may not be important depending on whether there are related questions.

Teacher Tip

It's not a question of saying: "Aha—here's a keyword!" It's more an issue of what that keyword tells you about the paragraph.

Let's take a little quiz on keywords. Read the paragraph below as you normally would, then answer the question that follows.

> *Although keywords pop up all the time, we seldom pay attention to them. In fact, sometimes we skip right over them. Consequently, they don't seem important. But they are very important. Why? Because they help you to be an active, critical reader who scores well on the verbal section of the MCAT.*

Here's the quiz question: how many keywords did you see in this passage, and more important, were you able to use them to quickly get structure and author intent? Let's look at the paragraph again, sentence by sentence, and read critically.

Although keywords pop up all the time, we seldom pay attention to them.

The sentence starts with a contrast keyword, "although." This tells you that there's opposition here: we see the keywords but we don't read them critically. The author's topic is *keywords*.

Teacher Tip

Contrast keywords are the most important in any MCAT passage. They indicate the author's purpose, point of view, and voice. Remember, it's ALL about the author!

In fact, sometimes we skip right over them.

"In fact" is a continuation keyword; we're getting more of the same. But once you know what the issue is—in this case, keywords—you don't need much more of the same. This is not a particularly important sentence and you don't need to spend a lot of time on it.

Teacher Tip

When you see a continuation keyword, you can speed up your reading. You don't need to carefully read more of the same.

Consequently, they don't seem important.
"Consequently" indicates someone's conclusion, though not necessarily the author's. Here the conclusion seems to be from those who don't read keywords carefully.

TEACHER TIP

See how contrast keywords signal author purpose? Write that purpose in your map.

But they are very important.
Ah, another contrast word. This one indicates scope—the author's intent in writing about the topic. Now we know the author's voice—his point of view: *keywords are important.*

Why?
Rhetorical questions are lovely. Since they exist only as a literary device to allow the author to continue with his real purpose, they act as another clue to author's point of view.

TEACHER TIP

Always read the entire paragraph and passage. Just know what parts are important so you can read quickly over the less important ones. That will save you time.

Because they help you to be an active, critical reader who scores well on the verbal section of the MCAT.
"Because" is an evidence keyword and introduces the author answering his own rhetorical question. But you knew that would come next, didn't you? When you read actively, you're marching right up there with the author, not trying to play catch-up. That allows you to read faster and with more understanding.

So what does the critical reader take from this paragraph? **Keywords are important to gain points on MCAT verbal.** That's it. The rest is background and detail.

TYPES OF KEYWORDS

TEACHER TIP

Pay attention to conclusion keywords when you see them, but don't expect they'll always sum up the passage. Why not? Because passages are lifted from longer works, so the end of a passage is not necessarily the end of the book, chapter, or wherever it comes from. Rest assured, though, that everything you need to answer the questions correctly is in the passage.

The most important types of keywords are **Conclusion, Evidence, Contrast**, and **Emphasis**, because these are the ideas that will lead you to relevant text to answer the questions. There are other important types as well: **Continuation, Illustration, and Sequence**.

CONCLUSION KEYWORDS signal that the author is about to sum up or announce her thesis. The most common one is *therefore,* to which we can add:

- thus
- believes
- consequently
- we can conclude that

- in conclusion
- so
- it can be seen that
- Toynbee claims that

Since these keywords have to do with the author's logic, it's no wonder they're especially crucial for Verbal Reasoning

EVIDENCE KEYWORDS signal that the author is about to provide support for a point. Here are the four most common evidence keywords:

- because
- for
- since
- the reason is that

CONTRAST KEYWORDS, of course, signal an opposition or shift. There are lots of these words:

- but
- however
- although
- not
- nevertheless
- despite
- alternatively
- unless
- though
- by contrast
- yet
- still
- otherwise
- while
- notwithstanding

Contrast Keywords are among the most significant in Verbal Reasoning because so many passages are based on contrast or opposition. Almost certainly, something important is happening when a contrast keyword shows up.

TEACHER TIP

"These keywords indicate the idea of 'more of the same"; evidence for what the author has already said. Thus, they tend to indicate details. And what do you do with details? Not much, other than to note where they are so you can refer to them if needed.

TEACHER TIP

Some more subtle contrast words are traditionally, initially, and originally. They always indicate something's going to change. That change is what the author is going to focus on.

EMPHASIS KEYWORDS may be the most welcome. If we're supposed to read for the author's point of view—and we are—what better way than to stumble across words and phrases whose sole purpose is to announce *"I, the author, find this important"?* Note these:

- above all
- most of all
- primarily
- in large measure
- essentially
- especially
- particularly
- indeed

TEACHER TIP

These words serve essentially the same purpose as evidence words. Don't spent lots of time worrying about what's being continued.

CONTINUATION KEYWORDS announce that more of the same is about to come. "And" is probably the most common one in the English language. Others include:

- also
- furthermore
- in addition
- as well as
- moreover
- plus
- at the same time
- equally

Also (there's a signal for you!), the appearance of a colon serves a similar purpose: It indicates that what is to follow will expand upon—or continue—what came before.

ILLUSTRATION KEYWORDS signal that an example is about to arrive. "One example" and "for instance" are the most obvious. But think about these:

- As Maya Angelou says,
- For historians,
- In the words of Hannah Arendt,
- According to these experts,
- To Proust,

In each case, what's about to follow is an example of that person's thinking.

SEQUENCE KEYWORDS are the author telling you *"Hey, there's some sort of order at work here."* Some examples are:

- Secondly (thirdly, fourthly, etc.)
- Next,
- Finally,
- On the one hand,
- Recently,

TEACHER TIP

These are helpful words, when used (which is seldom). They allow you to map a passage as, for example, "¶1 Step 1, ¶2 Step 2 ¶3 Step 3". Nice and easy.

KEYWORDS EXERCISE

The best MCAT test-takers are attentive to purpose and structure at every moment, and when keywords come along, they tend automatically to anticipate where the author will take the passage next. As a result, the reader stays ahead of the author, rather than behind, and is less likely to get confused by dense detail or to lose sight of the structure as a whole.

TEACHER TIP

Learn to pay attention to keywords and what they tell you about the author and the structure of the passage. Your MCAT Verbal score will thank you for it.

DIRECTIONS: Each of the following pieces of text—any of which might be found in a Verbal Reasoning passage—ends with a familiar keyword. After you read it, try to formulate an idea of what ought to follow the keyword; then look at the three possibilities listed. Choose the one of the three that would most logically complete the sentence:

1. The latest research seems to suggest that people who consume alcohol in moderation may be healthier, on average, than either those who never drink or heavy drinkers. Hence,
   A. people who enjoy a single glass of wine with dinner need not fear that they are endangering their health.
   B. at least one clinical study rates both non-drinkers and heavy drinkers as less psychologically stable compared with moderate drinkers.
   C. without more data, it would be premature to change one's lifestyle on the basis of these findings.

2. The photograph being copied must be in good condition; otherwise,
   A. it should be examined with a magnifying glass under strong white light.
   B. its dimensions must be identical to those of the desired duplicate.
   C. the duplicate will exhibit the same scratches or smears as the original.
3. The fresco was completed after Giotto's death by an apprentice whose skills were not quite up to the task, and
   A. he clearly attempted to imitate the master's strokes.
   B. neither the perspective nor the colors are convincing.
   C. he had studied with the master for only a short time.
4. The evidence suggesting that the two species of felines may have existed simultaneously on the African veldt is purely circumstantial. For example,
   A. with no direct proof to the contrary, many experts still believe that the giant cats died out long before their smaller relatives appeared.
   B. fossil traces of both species have been found in separate areas in sediments that are thought to have been laid down by the same floodwaters.
   C. since all of the giant fossils found so far have been male, some scientists suspect that the smaller ones represent the females and young of the same sexually dimorphic species.
5. Only one day-care facility in this city bases its fees on a sliding scale according to family income, and there are over 300 children on its waiting list. Consequently,
   A. it is nearly impossible for most poor mothers to work outside the home while providing care for their children.
   B. the blame for the lack of affordable child care alternatives must be placed on state legislators, who have stymied every attempt to redress the situation.
   C. the number of high- and middle-income families who place their pre-school children in day care primarily to give them an educational advantage continues to rise.

6. The purpose of the proposed advertising campaign is, first, to increase public awareness of the company's new logo. For instance,
   A. it is hoped that the new commercials will reinforce brand loyalty among consumers.
   B. a major portion of the budget has been allocated to create a striking and memorable design.
   C. television viewers should be able to identify the design correctly after seeing the commercial only once.
7. Tobacco companies often advertise cigarettes with filter tips or with lower levels of tar and nicotine as "lighter," implying that they are less damaging to health than regular cigarettes. But
   A. several studies have shown that people who smoke such cigarettes tend to inhale more deeply, thereby delivering at least as much tar and nicotine to their lungs as if they were smoking regular cigarettes.
   B. in manufacturing and marketing these products, the tobacco companies are responding to the widespread awareness and fear, even among habitual smokers, of the harmful effects of smoking.
   C. the impression created by these advertisements is that people—particularly young women—who care about their health may smoke these cigarettes without having to worry about developing cancer or emphysema.
8. Many methods of contraception work by preventing sperm from fertilizing the ovum. Alternatively,
   A. latex condoms and diaphragms present physical barriers to sperm; the contraceptive efficacy of these methods can be increased chemically via spermicides.
   B. these methods, however varied their mechanisms, are all prophylactic in nature, in that no embryo is ever created.
   C. pregnancy can be averted after fertilization by causing the fertilized egg to be expelled from the body, rather than implanting in the uterine wall.
9. That Nabokov's novels found a mass audience in the United States, a country in which relatively few people study foreign languages, is mystifying, especially given
   A. his appeal to academics and literary critics.
   B. his penchant for multilingual puns.
   C. the ribald adult content of his books.

TEACHER TIP

Every time you see practice drills or questions for passages, you'll also see explanations of right and wrong answers. Study these, even if you got the answer right. You want to make sure you know why the answer is right and why others are wrong.

ANSWER EXPLANATIONS

1. **A**

Hence is a conclusion keyword, and (A) is the only one of the choices that can reasonably be deduced from the previous sentence. (B) provides additional evidence along the same lines, and would more logically follow a continuation keyword like "moreover." (C), which takes a different view, would probably start off with a contrast keyword like "however."

2. **C**

The contrast keyword "otherwise" warns of some undesired consequence to follow if the photo is in bad shape; (C) fits the bill. (A) is a precondition to ensure that the original photo is okay; it should take a conclusion keyword like "therefore." (B) describes a second requirement that's distinct from the photo's condition; it needs a continuation keyword like "also" to set it up.

3. **B**

"And" expresses continuation, another piece of evidence that points in the same direction. Replacing "and" with a wordier evidence keyword, such as "as evidenced by the fact that," would make (B) even more clearly correct. contrast keyword "although" would more appropriately introduce (A), which expresses a subtle contrast (the apprentice didn't succeed, though he tried). (C) attempts to explain why the apprentice wasn't up to snuff; an evidence keyword like "since" should set up this choice.

4. **B**

"For example," one of the most common illustration keywords, sets the stage for (B), a specific piece of the circumstantial evidence mentioned in the first part of the sentence. (A) suggests an opposing conclusion— that the two species did not coexist—and would probably be introduced by a conclusion keyword like "thus." (C) reinforces the main clause's statement that only circumstantial evidence supports the conclusion that the two species coexisted; this choice raises additional evidence pointing to an alternative conclusion, and would be more effectively set up by the continuation keyword "in addition."

5. **A**

The conclusion keyword "consequently" leads nicely to (A), a natural result of the first sentence. Placing blame, (B), is not a result but a conclusion, but it can't be introduced by a conclusion keyword because it's buttressed by new evidence (the legislators have stymied every attempt to redress the situation). Emphasis keywords like "in large measure" would serve better. (C) discusses a simultaneous but different trend. At the same time, a continuation keyword with subtle overtones of contrast would set it up better.

6. **C**

Illustration keywords "for instance" should lead to an example of how the campaign would increase public awareness; (C) would be a reasonable result to hope for. A sequence keyword like "secondly" would more effectively indicate that (A) raises a new issue, brand loyalty, that is an additional purpose of the campaign, unrelated to public awareness. (B) requires a conclusion keyword like "hence" to show that the previously stated objective mandates a hefty design budget for the new logo.

7. **A**

"But," one of the bluntest contrast keywords in the English language, leads to (A), an outcome diametrically opposed to the claims in the cigarette ads. (B) is an attempt to infer why the tobacco companies would make such claims; conclusion keywords like "it can be concluded that" would clarify the logical connection. (C) continues the train of thought begun in the previous sentence, summarizing the subtext of the advertisements; emphasis keywords like "above all" would work well here.

8. **C**

The contrast keyword "alternatively" has to introduce contraceptive methods that don't rely on preventing fertilization; (C), preventing implantation after the fact, is a good alternative. (A), which describes specific contraceptive methods that prevent fertilization, would be better introduced by an illustration keyword like "for example." An emphasis keyword like "essentially" would help (B) point out what all these methods have in common.

9. **B**

"Especially" is another emphasis keyword. (B) is the only choice that would make Nabokov's mass appeal in a linguistically provincial country even more mystifying. His appeal to academic and literary critics might explain his mass readership, or at least render it less mystifying; (A) should thus be introduced by a contrast keyword like "despite." (C) would tend to work in favor of Nabokov's mass appeal, rather than against it; a combination of contrast and evidence keywords—something like "though perhaps understandable, given"—would make for a better transition

Teacher Tip

Rule of thumb: it should take you twice as long to review explanations as it takes to answer the questions.

CHAPTER 4

THE VERBAL REASONING QUESTION TYPES

Now that you know the Kaplan strategy for managing the passage, it's time to turn your attention to the questions. There are several classic question types that show up over and over on the MCAT, so it's helpful to be able to identify what type you're dealing with. Each question type is tackled with a slightly different approach. These targeted and efficient approaches save you time, stress, and uncertainty. Before we start, here are a few tips to remember:

1. There are no points in the passages. The longer you take to read or reread (please don't), the less time you have for the questions. Fewer questions answered correctly = lower MCAT score. Read quickly, in about 4 to 4.5 minutes. All you want from the read is a structural map. Your real goal is to get to the questions and answer them correctly.
2. Slow down when you get to the questions and answers. Misreading here can mean wrong answers.
3. Predict! After you research the information you need to answer a question, try to predict the general direction of the right answer. You won't come up with the test-maker's words, of course, but you'll know what you're looking for. Do, however, stay flexible.
4. Attack the question! Don't creep up on it with fear and loathing. Barge right in with confidence (after all, you're using the time-tested Kaplan strategy). You can do this!
5. Don't let a difficult passage or question drag you down. Almost everyone's going to get something wrong; just shrug it off and move on. Every question is another opportunity to get another point.

TEACHER TIP

There is always one right and three wrong answers to an MCAT question. If you don't predict and have a sense of what the answer should look like, you'll read all four answers, hoping that one jumps out at you. In reality then, you're reading three wrong answers carefully. Definite waste of time! Avoid this by predicting first.

Take a look at the Verbal Reasoning question types and strategies identified and defined below. Practice recognizing them and keep using the strategies. You'll love the bump in your MCAT score.

VERBAL REASONING QUESTION TYPES

Every question type requires that you identify one or both of the following:

1. **Main Idea**
   - Questions that ask for the "central thesis," "primary purpose," or "main idea."
   - The correct answer will reflect the overall scope and purpose.

Teacher Tip

To answer main-idea questions, just refer to your topic, scope and purpose—backward. Start with purpose. After all, the author's purpose is to tell you his main idea. With practice, answering these questions will be fast and easy.

2. **Detail**
   - Questions that ask what was stated in the passage.
   - The correct answer will be very close to the text in the passage.
   - These questions are relatively rare today.
   - When they do appear, they often come in the form of scattered detail: "All of the following arguments are made in the passage EXCEPT. . . ."

Teacher Tip

Look for words such as "according to" or "as stated in the passage" to ID detail questions. Refer to your map to home in on the paragraph that contains the answer, re-read the relevant information in the paragraph, predict, then match your prediction with an answer choice.

The most common Verbal Reasoning questions ask more:

3. **Deduction**
   - Questions that require you to identify assumptions or logical conclusions from your broader understanding of the passage.
   - Creative interpretation isn't rewarded here. The correct answer will definitely be based on the passage.

Teacher Tip

These are the inference and assumption questions. Don't panic—these questions may look hard but the right answer is still supported in the passage. Rely on your map, your re-read of the relevant information, and your prediction.

4. **Evaluation**
   - Questions that ask how the author put together the argument.
   - Correct answers stick to the scope of the argument and identify how the author moves between evidence and conclusion.

5. **Application**
   - Questions that ask you to apply the ideas in the passage to a different situation or context.
   - These may seem to encourage creative interpretations, but don't be fooled! Correct answers stick closely to the ideas in the passage.

6. **Incorporation**
   - Questions that ask you to incorporate new information into reasoning found in the passage.

Teacher Tip

Incorporation questions usually end up as "strengthen" or "weaken." The first thing you need to do is ask yourself what the author's ideas are, then look for evidence that will either support or weaken those ideas.

THE QUESTION TYPES IN VITRO

There are lots of ways the test-makers can ask a question and you can be pretty sure that they'll stay away from the most direct, comprehensible language. No, they're not trying to trick you but hey, this is a test, right? It's designed to use your critical thinking skills—which would not really be tested if the questions were obvious and easy. Take a look at some common ways the test-maker phrases different question types.

DEDUCTION

1. The author of the passage would most likely agree that:
   A. The post-1991 MCAT is superior to the pre-1991 MCAT.
   B. Wilson's theory is over-reaching but represents a desirable ideal.
   C. Because causality is so diffuse, a consilient understanding of science is probably unattainable.
   D. The MCAT is the best predictor of performance in medical school.

TEACHER TIP

The more vague terms—"most likely agree" or "it can be inferred"—signal deduction questions.

EVALUATION

2. The author mentions "third-order discontinuities" primarily in order to:
   A. provide support for the theory of plate tectonics.
   B. account for breaks in magma chambers.
   C. present evidence in support of the magma-supply model.
   D. discredit the notion that ridge morphology depends on magma supply.

TEACHER TIP

Keep your eyes on the word "in order to" at the end of the question. They signal a question asking "why?" Research the quoted phrase and ask yourself what function it has in the passage. In other words, why is it there?

APPLICATION

3. Which of the following would be an example of consilience according to Wilson?
   A. A scholar composes a poem about the passing of a vesicle from ER to cis-Golgi.
   B. A neurologist studies neural patterns in the brain of a talented composer.
   C. A historian tests her hypothesis about the causes of revolution by comparing economic data from several nations, some of which later revolted.
   D. An economist studies the writing of William Carlos Williams.

TEACHER TIP

Remember learning, when you were a kid, not to touch the hot stove because hot things burn? At any age thereafter, you knew not to touch hot things because they burn. You applied information from one situation to another. That's what an application question requires you to do.

TEACHER TIP

This is a strengthen question, and note what a lovely question it is. The test-maker actually gives you the author's claim (Winston was a traitor). Now go research his support in the passage, and choose an answer that similarly supports the claim.

INCORPORATION

4. Based on information in the passage, which of the following new discoveries would best support the author's claim that Winston was a traitor?
   A. A black sword under the sea chest
   B. A red waistband and flannel waistcoat
   C. The absence of gunpowder in the tunnel
   D. Mutinous sailors stranded in the Pacific

TEACHER TIP

See how Roman numeral I shows up three times in the answer? Why not start there? Research the answer (first read the question, of course) and determine if Roman numeral I is in the passage. If not, the answer has to be B. Roman numeral questions hold the seeds of their own demise!

DETAIL

5. According to the passage, American migrants in the mid-1840s often:
   I. doubted the economic potential of the Great Plains.
   II. had an overly optimistic image of the Great Plains.
   III. were misinformed by newspaper stories.
   A. I only
   B. II only
   C. I and III only
   D. I, II, and III

TEACHER TIP

The words "central thesis" are just another way to ask a global (main idea) question. Read your mapped-out purpose, scope, and topic in that order. That's the prediction you're going to match with the correct answer.

GLOBAL

6. The author's central thesis is that:
   A. Consilience is a jumping together of multiple distinct thought processes to arrive at a similar conclusion.
   B. MCAT consilience should supplant the dominant modes of inquiry of those disciplines which it has not yet conquered.
   C. Wilsonian consilience may be impractical, but MCAT consilience is a worthy goal.
   D. Whewell would have contested Wilson's interpretation of consilience.

CLASSIC WRONG ANSWERS

The MCAT test-makers are very nice people. No, really—they are! They don't play tricks on you. They don't, for example, give you a question with no correct answer, or more than one correct answer. The test-makers give you one, and only one, right answer. One right, four rotten—every time. They're also very consistent in the kinds of wrong answers they provide. It's like a pattern. We can predict a pattern because it's consistent and the same thing applies to wrong-answer patterns. Since we can learn the wrong-answer patterns, we can avoid them. Here's what you need to know about wrong-answer patterns.

FAULTY USE OF DETAIL (FUD)

This will be a detail that's in the passage but is not the right detail for the question asked. If the test-maker, or your map, points you to a particular paragraph, stay there. If you research all over the passage, you may find a nice detail but it won't be the one you need. You won't be surprised to learn that FUDs show up a lot in science passages, where you can anticipate lots of detail questions.

> **TEACHER TIP**
>
> FUDs are classic wrong answers for main-idea questions. You're looking for an answer that encompasses the entire passage, which a detail can't do. Never choose a detail as the answer to a main-idea question.

OUT-OF-SCOPE (OS)

An out-of-scope answer is outside the parameters of the passage. It may sound good—it may reflect something you know or believe—but if it isn't in or reflected in the passage, it isn't right. You can be absolutely sure that the correct answer is supported in the passage, so always check your answer with the passage.

> **TEACHER TIP**
>
> OS answers are particularly common for inference and deduction questions, and they also show up in main-idea answer choices. Avoid them by remembering that the right answer must be true, at least according to the author, based on what he says in the passage. Unfortunately, what YOU think should be true doesn't count.

EXTREME

The MCAT test-maker doesn't often give you passages in which an author expresses very extreme ideas, such as "All students always do well on the MCAT verbal section." Consequently, answers using extreme words ("all," "always") are usually wrong. The only time they're right is when the author is extreme, but we already know that's pretty rare. Train yourself to recognize extreme words and you'll save yourself a lot of wasted time.

> **TEACHER TIP**
>
> Want some more extreme words? How about "no," "never," "impossible," or ANY word which leaves you nothing in between the extremes. But be careful; don't just look at the word. Look at context, too. Note, for instance, the difference between the extreme "no" and the possible "almost no . . ."

OPPOSITE

This is just what you think it is—an answer that's wrong because it's the opposite of what the passage says. It's a common trap for questions that ask what the author doesn't do ("the author uses all literary devices EXCEPT…), and it's an easy trap to fall into if you've just skimmed over the question.

The test-maker always lays a trap for the student who thinks he remembers what he read. There will be at least one answer that is memorable from the passage because it uses a stand-out word or phrase or idea. The sloppy student says, "Yeah, I remember that so it must be the right answer." Nope. Memory is notoriously faulty. Always go back to your map and the passage to check out the possible answers. But practice will show you that it's usually easy to get rid of one or two answer choices, often because they incorporate classic wrong-answer patterns. Eliminate those right away and research the two or three possibilities that remain.

> **TEACHER TIP**
>
> If you get stuck between two answers, don't compare them because there's no such thing as good, better, best. There's only right and wrong. Instead, challenge yourself to "show me." Go back and see which answer is supported in the passage. The right one is supported, the wrong one isn't. It's that simple.

Part II
The Essay

CHAPTER 5

INTRODUCTION TO THE ESSAY

ABOUT THIS SECTION

This section introduces you to the five-step approach to writing an essay and gives you a chance to practice your new skills. Note that the skills involved in producing a good essay in 30 minutes cannot be learned instantly; it takes time and practice to assimilate our method.

Teacher Tip

Following the Kaplan method takes the worry and tension out of writing the MCAT essay.

Chapter 5 provides you with important information about the MCAT essay assignment as well as a summary of Kaplan's to essay-writing approach.

Chapter 6 takes you through Kaplan's Five-Step Method, one step at a time.

Chapter 7 provides you with practice essay assignments to give you the opportunity to become expert at the whole five-step process. You can develop your critical skills by comparing your own essays with others written by students on the same topics.

ABOUT THE MCAT WRITING SAMPLE

The essay section of the MCAT contains two 30-minute timed essays which you will type on the computer. After you work on the first essay question for 30 minutes, the clock will stop and you will be unable to continue writing. You'll be told to go on to the second essay question, for which you will be allowed another 30 minutes. It will be up to you to pace yourself during each 30-minute period and not get bogged down.

You must write on the assigned topic. You must write in English, not a foreign language, and you must try to accomplish everything the instructions require.

Teacher Tip

The MCAT essay requirements are not the same as most other essays you've written. You need a method and strategy to write a successful essay.

THE WRITING SAMPLE'S PURPOSE AND FORMAT

The writing sample tests your ability to:

1. develop a central idea,
2. synthesize ideas,
3. express ideas logically and cohesively, and
4. write clearly, using standard written English and proper punctuation.

In other words, it tests your ability to write a good brief essay. Of course, you are not expected to produce final-draft quality—the MCAT readers know you have only 30 minutes to write. But don't assume this means they have low standards. When you read the sample essays in the MCAT student manual, you'll see that the test-makers' expectation of a good essay really *is* a good essay.

Teacher Tip

MCAT essays never ask you for academic information in any of these categories. The prompts are broad and can be interpreted in many ways.

THE 10 WRITING SAMPLE CATEGORIES

Past writing sample statements have all fallen into one of the following broad categories:

- Advertising/Media Business
- Education/the Mind/Government
- History
- International Politics
- Law
- National Politics
- Science/Technology
- Sociology

Each essay question will have the same format: a statement followed by a set of instructions containing three distinct tasks. Each question will look something like this:

Consider this statement:

True leadership leads by example rather than by command.

Write a unified essay in which you perform the following tasks. Explain what you think the above statement means. Describe a specific situation in which true leaders lead by command rather than by example. Discuss what you think determines when a leader should lead by example or by command.

THE STATEMENT

The statement you are given may be an opinion, widely shared belief, philosophical dictum, or assertion about general policy concerns in such areas as history, political science, business, or law.

You can be sure that the statement will *not* concern scientific or technical topics (e.g., biology, physics, or chemistry), your reasons for entering the medical profession, emotionally charged religious or social issues (e.g., abortion), or obscure social or political issues that might require specialized knowledge. In fact, you will not need any specialized knowledge to do well on this part of the MCAT.

TEACHER TIP

The essays are, first and foremost, writing samples for medical schools to assess how well you think, organize, communicate, and support ideas.

THE INSTRUCTIONS

Though worded slightly differently each time, the instructions which follow the statement will ask you to perform these tasks in a unified essay:

> **Task 1: Provide your interpretation or explanation of the statement.**
>
> **Task 2: Offer a concrete example (hypothetical or actual) that illustrates a point of view directly opposite to the one expressed in the statement.**
>
> **Task 3: Explain how the conflict between the viewpoint expressed in the statement and the viewpoint you described for task 2 might be resolved.**

These tasks give you quite a lot to complete in a scant 30 minutes. It's a good idea, therefore, to approach this section prepared for what you'll find. That's where this booklet and the writing lessons will help: they'll familiarize you with the section and give you a firm sense of how to accomplish all necessary tasks. Actually, once you know what you're doing, the three tasks make your job somewhat easier since they "design" your essay for you (a good part of the battle!).

TEACHER TIP

Save time by learning the essay instructions before test day. They are always the same except for reference to the given statement.

FREQUENTLY ASKED QUESTIONS ABOUT THE WRITING SAMPLE

Question:
Is there a right or wrong answer to these essay questions?

Answer:
No. Essays won't be judged on whether or not the readers agree with your position or think your points true. Furthermore, the instructions won't ask you to take a position regarding the statements you discuss. If you feel that offering your position on the statement or a related issue will make a better essay, that's fine. But don't feel pressured to agree or disagree with the statement.

TEACHER TIP

At some future time, a computer—a so-called e-rater—will take the place of one human reader. But not yet.

Question:
Who grades my essays?

Answer:
Two readers read each essay and score them independently—that means neither scorer knows how the other graded your essay. If the two scorers differ by more than a point (on a six-point scale), a third scorer is called in as a final judge.

Question:
What kind of score will be reported?

Answer:
Once the readers have graded your essays, the total scores for both essays are added together. This combined score will then be converted into an alphabetic rating (ranging from J to T) and sent to you and the medical schools that receive your other MCAT information. The medical schools will also get percentile information on how well you did compared to your peers. For more information on what constitutes a particular point score (say a score of 4 rather than 6 on any particular essay), consult your MCAT Student Manual, which contains detailed descriptions of what level of accomplishment each score represents.

TEACHER TIP

Overall, the average essay score is 4. To score in at least the average range, all three tasks must be addressed.

Question:
What's a good score?

Answer:

Statistically speaking, there will be very few 6-point essays. An essay of 4 or 5 would place you at the upper range of those taking this exam. But a good score is a personal estimation. After all, if you have very weak writing skills and pump up your skills using the Kaplan materials, you may feel very good about getting a score of 3—and you'd be right to feel that way. However, be aware that the average MCAT essay score is 4, so you'll want to improve your writing skills to reach at least the average score.

Question:

How are my essays graded?

Answer:

Your readers will use a holistic grading technique. This means that each reader supplies a single numeric score for the essay as a whole (organization, style, grammar, and so on are not graded separately), Your readers will first determine how thoroughly and meaningfully you responded to the three writing tasks. They'll note whether you offered appropriate illustrations or examples and how well you tied your thoughts into a unified whole. In addition, they'll consider how well you organized your paragraphs individually and collectively. They'll also look for varied sentence structure and word choice. This does not mean your readers want convoluted sentences or big "dictionary" words; they *do* want the kind of lively writing that comes with active *thinking*.

Question:

I'm lousy at grammar and punctuation. Will those kinds of errors count for very much?

Answer:

Your readers know you are writing with limited time and expect a certain number of mistakes in writing mechanics (grammar, spelling, etc.). A few scattered mistakes of this kind *do not* carry much weight. However, a series of such mistakes can mar your work's overall impression. So while you shouldn't be overly concerned with mistakes of this nature, don't ignore this area of the essay if it is a particularly weak one for you. If you're concerned to improve your grammar, punctuation, and sentence structure skills, see Part III for a thorough review of writing mechanics.

TEACHER TIP

There's no score for mechanics of language. However, if you make enough grammar, spelling, word choice or punctuation mistakes, the essay becomes disjointed and difficult for the readers to quickly read and assess, and that could lower your score.

Question:
In writing my essays, do I have to follow a certain format?

Answer:
Many students think they have to write a standard five-paragraph essay—an introductory paragraph, three body paragraphs, and a conclusion—the kind often taught in high schools. There is *no* set format. As long as you address all three writing tasks, you can do so in whatever order and form you choose. However, since you will be scored partly on the essay's unity, giving the reader a sense of a definite beginning, middle, and end will be an advantage.

Question:
My typing is terrible. Will this count against me?

Answer:
Yes and no. Typos turn out to be spelling errors, and though spelling is not a scorable criterion, too many errors make it difficult for the reader to review your essay quickly. Moreover, spelling errors can indicate a more serious communication problem.

TEACHER TIP

The two keys to a good score on the essay are to follow directions and write with clarity. Clarity requires using the right word—not the biggest word—to convey what you mean. In other words, the readers will prefer you write "people" instead of "Homo sapiens."

Question:
Do I need to throw around a lot of big, impressive-sounding words in order to do well?

Answer:
Some test-prep companies advise students to memorize impressive-sounding words and work them into each essay. That's cynical and silly. People who have to memorize impressive words probably don't have much practice using them—so the words stick out and look awkward. Besides, the best essays make their points simply, concisely, and straightforwardly. While a large vocabulary can allow you more precision with ideas, it's not essential. Don't use fancy words just to impress a reader. What your readers want is *clarity*. Better to stick to the words you know than run the risk of a malapropism.

Question: What if I want to delete a word or phrase...can I?

Answer:
Yes. You have basic word-processing functions on the computer. These include Delete and Insert. However, there are no spell, grammar, or style checks.

THE KAPLAN APPROACH

To most writers, the process of essay writing is one filled with starts and stops. As a writer drafting an essay thinks about the topic from several angles, he comes up with ideas that must be refined, rephrased, or thrown out. He might compose several introductory paragraphs before finding the right tack or be halfway through writing when a better idea comes to mind, requiring a major revision. This is the natural way for most people to compose.

But there is nothing natural about a timed essay test.

There is no time here to let your thoughts flow in their natural cyclic way, yet it is essential to hash out and refine your ideas. What to do?

What you need is a method to speed up the writing process and make it more efficient. We suggest you use a proven method that will help you take good advantage of each one of those 30 minutes. The purpose of the method is to provide you with a clearly defined track on which to move through the writing process, performing what needs to be done in as little time as possible. It consists of five steps:

TEACHER TIP

Every MCAT reader knows that you could have written a better essay if you'd had more time and that this is a first draft. But a first draft is not the same as a rough draft. The essay has to be much better written and organized than that.

THE KAPLAN FIVE-STEP METHOD

Step 1: Read and Annotate
Step 2: Prewrite Each Task
Step 3: Clarify Main Idea and Plan
Step 4: Write
Step 5: Proofread

Though they represent only about five minutes of your time, steps 1 to 3 are the most important. It is during the prewriting that you will do the hashing out, refining, and organizing of ideas required for a first-draft process.

In the rest of this book you'll have ample opportunity to practice the five-step approach. You'll become familiar with how each step relates to the whole. In time, you'll find yourself going through the steps in your own way—making them a natural part of your essay writing. As you do so, you'll find they take less and less time. Experienced Kaplan students can produce well-reasoned essays on the toughest topics within the 30-minute time limit.

TEACHER TIP

As with prepping for all sections of the MCAT, practice is the key. For the essay portion, writing several essays is, of course, excellent practice. But if you practice even just prewriting, you'll go a long way toward feeling confident in your writing.

CHAPTER 6

BUILDING YOUR ESSAY

DATABASES

It's true that you won't know ahead of time what essay prompts will appear on the exam, or even the general topics. But that doesn't mean you shouldn't come to the essay prepared. For unprepared students, the most challenging aspect of the MCAT Writing Sample is having to develop in such a short timeframe relevant ideas and examples that can be synthesized in sufficient depth. The most effective way to establish depth in your essay is to use poignant examples, which clarify ideas and help support a thesis. So how can you come up with examples under such time constraints?

The natural solution is to go into the exam with pre-thought-out examples, which we call *databases*. Databases are events, scenarios, or situations which are applicable to a wide variety of topics. The best databases are those that you know very well or have impacted you in some meaningful way: things that you enjoy talking about or have moved you, or things that you know extremely well. The ideas for your databases can come from current events, personal experiences, the arts, government, or even your own hobbies. Because the writing sample is a test of your ability to communicate and *not* the level of your outside knowledge, the sophistication of your ideas will not affect your score. Therefore, hypothetical examples are fine, as long as they are communicated well.

Teacher Tip

Having pre-thought-out databases eliminates the two scariest aspects of writing the MCAT essay; timing and coming up with ideas. When you already have some ideas in mind, the time you need to write is vastly reduced.

For each database, ask yourself: What happened? Why? Who was involved? What were the results? Why was it important? Say you took a philosophy of science class last semester, in which you did very well and have fresh in your mind. You may want to develop a database on the scientific revolution. Now, *what* happened? Many revolutionary scientific theories, including a paradigm shift from a geocentric view of the universe to a heliocentric view, Newtonian physics, and the development of the scientific method for conducting experimentation. *Why* did it happen? A proliferation of knowledge assisted by the invention of the printing press a few decades earlier, and response to the Aristotelian-dominated view of the way science was conducted. *Who*? Many players contributed to the movement:

TEACHER TIP

You don't need lots of information in your databases. You have neither the time nor the need to mention everything you know about a topic. You're writing a relatively short, contained essay, not a school thesis.

the Catholic Church, Galileo, Newton, Copernicus, Kepler, and Bacon, to name just a few. Why was it important? It forever changed the way people viewed the universe and their relation to it, as well as the way science is conducted. *Results*? Specifically, a major worldview shift occurred in that society moved from an Aristotelian perspective (that is, with everything in the universe having a distinct purpose) to a Newtonian paradigm (a mechanistic and empirical universe). This also had a profound effect on the way people viewed religion and the hierarchy of the Catholic Church.

Note how this database could be applied to a variety of prompts in many of the 10 writing sample categories shown on page 50.

You may be thinking to yourself: What if I don't know anything about the scientific revolution? Not a problem. Let's see how you could use a personal experience just as effectively. Let's say you happened to love playing Little League baseball or softball as a child. A lot of life lessons are learned playing team sports, so it's a good database. Why? You wanted to gain experience working collaboratively with your peers, staying healthy, aspirations of becoming a professional one day. Who? You and your peers. Why was it important? Personal growth. It allowed you to cope with losing and showed you the benefit of working hard to improve yourself. In addition, you learned how to deal with conflict with others, as well as personal internal conflict.

Even though your particular database may not be appropriate for the given prompt, at least you will have many ideas already prepared, which you can use as a jumping-off point to think of other ideas. It is a good practice to have three or four databases prepared for Test Day, and you should practice using them in the essays for your full-length exam.

PREWRITING—STEPS 1–3

As a refresher, here are the tasks you are asked to accomplish in your essay:

Task 1: Provide your interpretation or explanation of the statement.

Task 2: Offer a concrete example (hypothetical or actual) that illustrates a point of view directly opposite to the one expressed in the statement.

Task 3: Explain how the conflict between the viewpoint expressed in the statement and the viewpoint you described for task 2 might be resolved.

And here is your Kaplan Five-Step Method:

Step 1: Read and Annotate
Step 2: Prewrite Each Task
Step 3: Clarify Main Idea and Plan
Step 4: Write
Step 5: Proofread

Your ability to write is directly linked to your ability to think analytically and logically. You might have a wonderful command of the English language, but if you can't get your thoughts organized and your ideas clear in your mind, your essay will be a jumbled mess. Since you don't have time to write a sloppy first draft and then revise it, you must do the basic part of refining your ideas *before* starting to write. In other words, you must *prewrite*.

Teacher Tip

It's not possible to think carefully and write well at the same time. Thinking comes first, and that's the goal of the prewrite.

The prewriting steps clarify what work you must get done before you are ready to write. Also, they help you get that work done efficiently. At first, you should practice these steps in sequence to familiarize yourself thoroughly with what prewriting involves. But as you get to know them, you'll probably find it more natural to jump around from one step to another rather than to work in a linear way.

For instance, you'll find that as you do Step 1 (Read and Annotate), ideas for any one of the other prewriting steps may well start popping into your mind. Task 2 (thinking of an opposing example) often helps to clarify your ideas about the statement's meaning (Task 1). Clarifying a main idea (Step 3) helps to focus all of your ideas for Steps 2 and 3. And so on. Once you learn the process, don't feel you must perfect each step before moving on to the next. Going back and refining your ideas as you move through the prewriting process will allow you to build a set of ideas that fit together into a coherent whole.

TEACHER TIP

Taking notes for the essay is similar to taking notes for a passage map. Be brief, don't worry about spelling or grammar, and use whatever shorthand is best for you.

TAKING NOTES

It is essential to take notes on your scratch paper during the prewriting process. Only a very extraordinary person can keep straight all of the ideas generated during prewriting. But note taking is a difficult thing to teach since each person must develop her own style. No one but you is going to read your notes; they don't need to be clear or comprehensible to anyone else. The trick is to develop a style that you can read and understand but that lets you abbreviate your ideas as much as possible. You don't want to waste time writing out whole sentences, but you must be able to make sense of your notes when you work on your essay. This takes practice.

TEACHER TIP

You don't have to write your notes in order of the tasks. If task 3, criterion, comes to you first, write that one before you write notes for tasks 1 and 2.

STRATEGY

As you take your notes, categorize them according to the three tasks given in the essay instructions. Divide your note-taking page into three areas and number them, one for each task. Ideas that explain or illustrate the statement (the first task) get jotted down in area #1, ideas that explore the opposing view (the second task) go in area #2, etc. This method will automatically order your thoughts, even if you are not coming up with them in an orderly way.

TEACHER TIP

Prewriting is really a time-saver. After you prewrite and organize your ideas, the essay is essentially written. All you have to do is put those ideas into sentences and paragraphs.

ALL THREE STEPS IN JUST FIVE MINUTES?

As we discuss the prewriting process here, it may seem too time-consuming a process for a 30-minute essay. Don't worry. At first, the steps take explaining and practice, but once you understand the process, you'll be able to work efficiently. You'll discover that the five minutes you spend prewriting will speed up the writing process.

Most Common Prewriting Mistakes

- The student fails to pay close attention to the meaning of the statement and/or the instructions.
- The student rushes into writing, hoping to figure things out while composing the essay.
- The student is immediately struck by an idea that addresses the second or third task (the easier ones) and starts writing without prewriting the first task.

Most Common Symptoms of Poor Prewriting

- The essay doesn't thoroughly fulfill all of the tasks in the instructions.
- The essay has no clear main idea.
- The essay is poorly organized.

- The first paragraph or two are vague and pointless.
- All of the best ideas are jammed in at the end of the essay.
- The essay is incomplete: The student was "cut short" by the time limit and was unable to respond to all parts of the instructions.

Prewriting can be the single most important way of helping your final essay achieve clarity, order, and authority. Now let's look at the steps one by one.

STEP 1: READ AND ANNOTATE

PURPOSE: To clarify for yourself what the statement says and what the instructions require.
PROCESS: Read the statement and instructions carefully.

Annotate the statement: Mark any words or phrases that:

- are easy to miss but are crucial to a good understanding of the statement.
- are ambiguous or confusing.
- refer to vague or abstract concepts (e.g., "freedom," "happiness," etc.) that need clarification.

Annotate the instructions: Number the tasks and mark any words that will help you remember exactly what it is you're supposed to do.

Good communication requires more than just speaking or writing clearly—it requires paying attention to what you're being asked to communicate about. And that means paying attention to what the given statement and instructions say. An essay that doesn't relate clearly and directly to the idea expressed in the statement or that doesn't fulfill the specific tasks put forth in the instructions is unlikely to receive more than a grade of 3.

Why Bother Annotating?

Especially with limits of time, it's easy to waste the first few minutes with anxious worrying or nervous, unstructured thinking. Writing down key words on your scratch paper puts your mind in gear. It helps you focus on what needs to be done and forces you to concentrate on this important first step.

Example of Step 1

Here is an example of one way this essay topic might be annotated. On her scratch paper, the student had written words which she felt

TEACHER TIP

Reading the prompt may sound obvious, but you don't want to just read, you want to read carefully and for a real understanding of the prompt and its implications.

TEACHER TIP

MCAT prompts are purposefully general so they can be approached from any number of angles. You'll decide how you approach the prompt when you annotate and think about multiple meaning of the words, and which meaning(s) you'll use.

required more careful thought, and noted each task to help her zero in on exactly what she needed to do.

Consider this statement:
True leadership leads by example rather than by command.

Sample scratch paper:
leadership, example, command
1. explain, 2. counterexample, 3. determinant

STEP 2: PREWRITE EACH TASK

Task 1

PURPOSE: To develop depth and clarity in your interpretation of the statement.

PROCESS:

- Clarify/define/interpret abstract, ambiguous, or pivotal words.
- Ask yourself questions to get beyond the superficial meaning of the statement.
- Come up with databases that can serve as examples for a wide variety of prompts.

The statement in the essay assignment will not be simply factual or self-evident. So, in order to explain what the statement means, you'll have to develop some ideas about the words or concepts within. Imagine having to explain it to your 15-year-old sister so that she really grasped the idea.

Take, for instance, the following statement: The United States is a free country. This statement is used in many different contexts. Yet, if you asked 20 people what they thought about the statement, you'd get 20 different responses. So how do you explain to your sister why this is not just a simple statement of fact or opinion? You try to give an explanation of its deeper meaning. For one thing, there's a good deal of history behind the statement. The belief that the people of this country should be "free" to pursue their individual goals began with the first European settlers who came here in search of freedom from religious and economic oppression. But there's also the philosophical question, What is freedom? Much controversy revolves around this question. In fact, many people feel this country is "free" only for a privileged few. And so on. Thus, what might seem like a simple cliché is actually a very complex tangle of ideas and implications.

TEACHER TIP

Almost all MCAT prompts have multiple layers of meaning, depending on how you interpret the words.

Obviously, you can't go into depth on all these subjects in a 30-minute essay, but to explain the statement with any clarity you must consider these issues, narrow them down, and put your ideas together to make the best interpretation you can. The MCAT essay readers are looking for a thorough exploration of the topic.

TEACHER TIP

Asking yourself questions about the prompt will help you see it from different viewpoints.

Here is a sampling of some of the many questions you can ask yourself as you "explore" a statement:

- What are some situations (hypothetical or real) which illustrate what this statement is saying?
- Are there any specific words in the statement that need clarifying before you can discuss the meaning of the statement as a whole?
- What is the historical background of the idea(s) in the statement? (Have the ideas been around for a long or a short time? Why? Where did they come from?)
- What is the philosophical background of the statement? (Are there some basic beliefs or assumptions on which this statement depends?)
- What people are concerned with this statement today and why are they concerned with it?
- Does this statement mean different things to different people? If so, what are these different meanings? What meaning do you give it and why?

But with all of these possible directions to go in, how do you streamline your ideas? Here's one useful approach:

STRATEGY:

Before trying to define the statement, think up one or two *illustrations* of it. This will give you something concrete to consider and will help you identify what areas you need to explore with this particular topic.

The MCAT Writing Sample topic will likely strike you as at least partly true. Even if you disagree with the statement in a general way, you'll probably be able to think of *some* situation that illustrates how it could be true. This kind of illustration will help you figure out the *meaning* of the statement (and if you want, you can use the example in your essay).

TEACHER TIP

Look carefully at the instructions; you'll see that your opinion is not required for any task. It could even be counterproductive by taking your focus away from the task at hand.

Don't Let a Strong Personal Reaction to the Statement Ruin Your Essay.

Having a strong reaction to a statement can fool you into rushing headlong into writing. But by doing that, you run the risk of ignoring the instructions. Don't let your strong opinion take over.

REMEMBER: The first task asks you to explain what you think the statement means. You can talk about ideas that oppose the statement when you address the second task.

You Don't Have to Take a Stand.

You are not being tested on your opinions or your morals. The purpose of the assignment is to test your ability to think and to write. The directions won't ask you to agree or disagree with the statement. Nothing asks you to form an opinion about the prompt. You will stay on target if you follow directions and do not insert a point of view. If you feel you must state your opinion, do so at the end of the third task, after all other tasks are fully completed.

TEACHER TIP

Remember, the directions for task 1 require only an explanation. The example deepens the explanation, but don't write the example without the explanation. That won't complete the task.

Example

Presented below is the same essay topic shown in step 1, but here, the student's prewriting notes for task 1 have been added. These notes are just one student's response; naturally, there are many possible responses.

Consider the following statement:

True leadership leads by example rather than by command.

Sample scratch paper:

leadership, example, command

1. explain, 2. counterexample, 3. determinant

1. *By example—*
    Alexander
    Gandhi
    Agassiz
    Clara B.
    —had a special gift...... so people compelled to follow

This student first gets down to business by thinking up several examples of leaders who lead by example. With these in mind, she can generalize more clearly about the kind of leader who leads by example.

Task 2

PURPOSE: To further explore the meaning of the statement by examining a situation that represents an opposing point of view.

PROCESS: Think up one or more specific situations that demonstrate a way in which the statement is not true.

Of the three tasks, this one is the easiest for most students because it is so specific. Thinking up specific examples is a lot easier than defining abstract ideas. Furthermore, it's almost always easier to find a flaw in something than it is to explain what's true about it.

Once they learn to handle the prewriting process, many students find that it helps to work a bit on the second task before tackling the first. In any case, working on the second task is very likely to help you develop and clarify your ideas about a statement.

That the second task is helpful in clarifying ideas is no coincidence. The three tasks provided for you by the MCAT test-makers follow a standard method of argument. The tasks, if you follow them, actually help you write a good essay. So follow them.

STRATEGY

Don't try to write or outline the essay in your head while you're prewriting the three tasks. Do the tasks first. They'll help you develop a set of ideas on which you can build an essay. If you try to compose your essay before you're ready, you will only waste time.

Even If You Agree Completely with the Statement, You Can Come up with an Opposing Example.

The creators of the MCAT Writing Sample purposely pick statements that are sufficiently complex to have more than one side. If you are having trouble thinking of a good illustration, imagine a person who actively disagrees with the statement—what illustrations would he provide?

TEACHER TIP

You're not being asked for a personal opinion. Avoid the word "I" and write your ideas with a focus on completing the task rather than on stating your opinion.

STRATEGY:

Don't waste time struggling to think of an example from history or current events. If you can't think of a real-life example, make up a hypothetical one. You are not being tested on your knowledge of history, politics, or any other area.

If You Disagree with the Statement, the Second Task Allows You to Air Your Views.

If you have a strong reaction against a statement, it's difficult not to launch right away into an explanation of that reaction. But your ideas will sound much more level-headed if you clarify the statement's meaning with neutrality before talking about how it is wrong. Task 2 (as well as task 3) gives you a place to express an opposing opinion, so save your criticisms for that task. The result will be a set of logical prewriting notes rather than a jumble of reactions.

It's Okay to Discuss More than One Example, But Don't Spread Yourself Too Thin.

Sometimes students come up with several ways in which a statement isn't true. Should this happen to you, focus on limited examples. You may want to illustrate that the statement is untrue with a single example or with several examples—either way is fine. What's important is to make sure that all the examples work together to illustrate the same general idea. You don't want to tackle more than one opposing idea. You don't have the time, and your essay is likely to lose focus.

TEACHER TIP

There are no points to be gained for unique, creative, or brilliant ideas. However, there are points for depth. One good example, with details to add depth, is better than several superficial examples.

Example

Here is the same essay topic shown previously, but here the student's notes for task 2 have been added.

TEACHER TIP

Many students write a lovely example for task 2 but neglect to show the relevance of the example to the prompt and task. Always connect the example to both prompt and counterexample task.

Consider this statement:

True leadership leads by example rather than by command.

Sample scratch paper:

leadership, example, command

1. explain, 2. counterexample, 3. determinant

1. *By example—*
   Alexander
   Gandhi
   Agassiz
   Clara B.
   —had a special gift ...... so people compelled to follow

2. *By command—*
   When people confused/defeated/need a common goal
   leader takes charge
   nations, businesses, etc.

From the notes responding to the second task, we see that our student has developed the idea that leadership by command is appropriate in a certain kind of situation.

Task 3

PURPOSE: To find a way to resolve the conflict between the statement given in the essay topic and the opposing situation(s) you thought of for task 2.

PROCESS: Read the instructions for task 3 carefully. Look back at the ideas you generated for tasks 1 and 2. Develop your response based on these ideas.

The third task follows naturally from tasks 1 and 2. If you think of an idea and then think of an opposition to that idea, it's only natural to try to reach some kind of resolution of the conflict. In fact, many students find that a resolution to the conflict just comes to them, before they even really think about the third task. That's fine. You often have your best ideas when your thoughts get rolling. Nonetheless, do take the time to read the instructions regarding task 3.

Teacher Tip

When you first read the task, if your initial reaction is "well, that depends," just finish the sentence to yourself. What does that depend on? Whatever you come up with is the criterion you can use for task 3.

STRATEGY:

The instructions for task 3 are likely to give you a specific approach to resolving the conflict. This approach will make your job more specific and therefore easier. Be sure to check back to the wording of the instructions for this task.

What If You Can't Think of a Good Way to Resolve the Conflict?

This task tests your ability to look at a general problem (the conflict) and, using your powers of judgment and evaluation, to come up with a way of handling the problem. Kaplan's standard criteria are very helpful here because, like databases, they are pre-thought-out and can apply to a variety of situations. The criteria are survival/safety, time, size/demographics, and education. It's a good idea to try them out as you write your practice essays. Of course, you can also use your own good judgment to develop criteria. If you determine that there's no easy or problem-free solution, then write what you think is the best solution. You are not expected to solve the problems of the world in this essay.

Teacher Tip

Task 3 is often the hardest for MCAT essay writers. Just remember that this task is neither a summary nor a statement of opinion. The directions require you to resolve the conflict between tasks 1 and 2. They do not ask you to take a side.

You Don't Have to Resolve the Conflict in Support of, or in Opposition to, the Statement.

Remember, your readers don't care whether you agree or disagree with the statement. Use your own judgment to resolve the conflict in a way that makes sense to you. Just be sure to explain your reasoning. Your reasoning is what counts, not your particular stance on the conflict.

TEACHER TIP

Jot down your ideas in any way you want. It's the ideas and organization that count in a prewrite, not the structure of how you write your thoughts down.

Example

Here is the same essay topic shown previously. Here, the student's prewriting notes responding to task 3 have been added.

Consider this statement:

True leadership leads by example rather than by command.

Scratch paper:

leadership, example, command

1. explain, 2. counterexample, 3. determinant

1. *By example—*
   Alexander
   Gandhi
   Agassiz
   Clara B.
   —had a special gift . . . . . . people compelled to follow

2. *By command—*
   When people confused/defeated/need a common goal
   leader takes charge
   nations, businesses, etc.

3. *Followers shared a common vision*
   If no shared vision . . . command is needed.

The notes responding to the third task show that the student reviewed her notes and compared the kind of leadership she considered in task 1 with the kind she considered in task 2. She apparently found a clear point of contrast between her two ideas. In one type of leadership, the followers share a common vision; in the other, they do not. As a result, she can define what determines when leadership should be by example or by command.

STEP 3: CLARIFY MAIN IDEA AND PLAN

PURPOSE: To do final organization and clarification of ideas. To take a mental "breath" before beginning to write.

PROCESS: Take a quick moment to look back over your notes in light of the ideas you have reached in prewriting task 3. Make sure your ideas are consistent. Cross out those that no longer belong. Decide in what order your essay will address the three tasks.

Though it sounds like a lot to do, this step is actually the quickest of them all. If you have prewritten all three tasks and have clarified to yourself which ideas accompany which task, then most of your prewriting work is done.

You Already Have a Main Idea

Many people find it difficult to identify a main idea. But if you have prewritten the third task, you have everything you need. You have reached a conclusion, an idea toward which all your other ideas lead. Treat this as your main idea.

Take a quick look over the rest of your notes to eliminate or clarify any ideas that don't relate to your main idea. Then, plan how you're going to order the ideas in your essay and you'll be ready to write.

In Fact, You Already Have a Plan, too!

Although the test-makers say that you can structure your essay any way you'd like, there is one obvious and simple structure which will help make writing the essay easier. The three tasks, in the order in which they are given, supply you with a straightforward approach that makes good sense.

STRATEGY: Use the Basic Essay Format Provided By the Three Tasks

First Part of Essay—Address the first task: This gives you the perfect opportunity to introduce the topic to be discussed and clarify its meaning. Establishing the basics in this way is essential for any argument to be clear.

Second Part of Essay—Provide an opposing idea to the one expressed in the statement: This lets you look at the statement from a different angle. Doing this lets you further develop your essay, delving more deeply into the nature of the statement and expanding on your ideas.

Third Part of Essay—Resolve the conflict between the statement and the opposing idea: This lets you synthesize your ideas into a focused conclusion—a natural ending to your discussion.

TEACHER TIP

Decide which ideas and examples you're going to use; you probably won't need to use them all. Choose the ones most relevant to the prompt and which you can write best.

TEACHER TIP

You don't need a fancy general introduction. Just get right into the explanation and example for task 1, the counterexample for task 2, and the determinant for task 3. MCAT readers want to see that you've fully completed all tasks.

TEACHER TIP

Keep your eyes on the prize. As you review your prewrite ideas and determine which ones and what order to use, refer to the prompt. You must write on-topic, so remind yourself of what the topic is.

What do the Prewriting Notes for Step 3 Look Like?

Usually they are invisible, since most of step 3 is done simply by looking over your notes and clarifying how your main idea will be the focus of the essay. You might cross out a phrase, add a word or two, draw an arrow between two ideas—whatever you need for that final mental preparation before actually writing.

Final Prewriting Reminder

Keep your notes in order by categorizing them according to the task they address: three tasks, three bunches of notes. You don't have to *think* of them in order, just record them in the fashion we suggest and you'll have an effective outline to help you through your essay.

STEP 4: WRITE

PURPOSE: Write a complete essay that addresses all three tasks in approximately 23 minutes.
PROCESS: Using your prewriting notes for guidance, compose a straightforward essay that thoroughly explains your response to each of the three tasks.

TEACHER TIP

Write clearly and effectively. The reader will not appreciate a sentence such as "Excessive utilization of multisyllabic verbiage obfuscates the thematic intent." Sure it's grammatically correct, but there's nothing clear about this sentence.

Writing an essay can truly be fun if you have sufficiently clarified your basic ideas beforehand. If you have a good general sense of what you want to say, you can let your mind roll along without fear of getting seriously off track or losing your focus. This is the time when you will get your best ideas—when you become creative.

But Don't Let the Writing Carry You Away—Stick to the Tasks.

If the statement or some related idea inspires you to write an essay all your own, or only obliquely related to the topic, squelch that inspiration. You don't have time to fool around with experimental first drafts. If you want to produce a good essay and fulfill the three tasks, be conservative.

TEACHER TIP

You're not being graded against other essays but against the scoring rubric. Follow the tasks, write well and in detail, and you'll get a good score.

Does It Seem Unoriginal or Constrained to Follow the Tasks?

Follow them anyway. That's the requirement of the MCAT Writing Sample.

TEACHER TIP

You don't have to make sure each paragraph has the same number of lines, but you do want a balanced essay, so give each task a similar amount of attention.

Does the Length of the Essay Matter?

Typed essays tend to look shorter than handwritten ones because of the smaller fonts that they produce. Don't let this fool you into thinking that your essay is too short; what really matters is whether your essay is complete, well-written, and in-depth. A well-written essay means a well-thought-out essay in which ideas are explained, illustrated, and developed until the implications are clear. Just filling up pages with blather, so it *looks* as if you are thinking, won't get you anywhere.

Following the Tasks will Help You Produce a Unified Essay.
Unity in an essay means that all of the ideas focus on a common topic, and that they all lead to a central idea. If you fulfill each of the three tasks, you will probably achieve unity: The tasks should all relate to each other, and lead from first to second to third in a logical manner.

TEACHER TIP

Unity is also achieved by using examples on equal levels of importance. If you're writing about world peace in task 1, don't use a soap-opera example in task 2. You can even use the same example for both tasks if you can see it from the two sides.

STEP 5: PROOFREAD

Save about two minutes to proofread your essay, but don't nitpick mistakes. What you're really trying to correct are any mistakes which make it difficult for the MCAT readers to quickly read and understand your essay. Don't worry about whether the sentence needs a comma or a semicolon, but do rewrite the sentence if during your proofread you have a hard time understanding it. Check for omitted words, especially toward the end when you're writing fast. But keep in mind that it's too late to rewrite whole paragraphs and add new ideas. Your prewrite should have taken care of that! Even if you come up with a great new idea while you're writing, stick to your prewrite. If you abandon it, you're essentially trying to write and think at the same time, and that leads to confusing writing and organization.

TEACHER TIP

If you're not sure you're using the correct word or spelling it right, choose another word. Though a nice writing style is important, you're not being scored on the breadth of your vocabulary.

Practice typing to avoid typographical errors. Indent each paragraph, or leave one blank line between paragraphs, since paragraph breaks make your essay look well-planned, and they visually indicate to the reader that you are addressing all tasks.

SOME COMMON TRANSITION WORDS AND PHRASES

Using transition words is an important technique for achieving coherence and unity. These words provide signals to the reader about how your argument is structured; she should be able to guess at the direction in which you are going simply by looking at your transition words and phrases.

For Contrast:
although
however
counterevidence suggests
still
on the other hand
despite
otherwise
but
yet
though

For conclusion
in conclusion
therefore
if this is true, then
hence
finally
in sum
consequently

For comparison
likewise
similarly
just as... so

For continuing argument
also
moreover
further (more)
besides
in addition
not only... but also
this (argument)
that (attitude)
these (attempts)

To introduce examples
for instance
consider the case of
one reason for this is
another reason for this is
one example of this is
another example of this is

To introduce one idea and then suggest a better alternative:
certainly... yet
granted... however
undoubtedly... but
to be sure... nonetheless
obviously... nevertheless
admittedly... still

TEACHER TIP

Do you see how these transition words are important not only in writing your essay, but also in understanding and mapping the Verbal Reasoning passages?

SAMPLE ESSAYS

Essays #1 and #2 below are responses to the essay topic shown for Examples of Steps 1 through 3. The prewriting notes shown in those earlier examples were written in preparation for Essay #1.

ESSAY #1

Even though we might all disagree about the precise definition of the word "leadership," we could probably agree that, as one Supreme Court justice once wrote of pornography, we can recognize it when we see it. Through the lens of history, leadership can often seem mysteriously compelling, a kind of divine gift. In the story of Alexander the Great, legend and history combine to hand down the image of the brave, determined young man who fought more fiercely than his troops, proving by his own example that a band of Macedonians could indeed endure great hardship and overcome better-equipped adversaries in their conquest of the known world.

But we must not assume that leadership is only seen on the battlefield. It was by humble but powerful example that Gandhi taught his people that passive resistance could drive out their British oppressors. Thus, no matter what the field of endeavor, it is usually the case that great leaders seem to lead by setting an example. The person who truly leads does so by showing, rather than telling, his followers how success is achieved. Brave actions compel others to follow.

TEACHER TIP

Though the explanation of the prompt does not come until the end of paragraph 2, it's definitely there. Thus, task 1 is completed. By the way, you don't need two paragraphs for task 1. A single paragraph will do.

Yet these famous instances of successful leadership all benefit from a circumstance that does not always apply when strong leadership is needed. Those who followed Alexander and Gandhi were already united in purpose. By contrast, when a group is so diverse that common ground cannot be found, or when there is chaos instead of a shared goal, leadership can only succeed when the leader commands, using his authority to bring people together. During the Great Depression of 1929, President Franklin Roosevelt faced a divided Congress, unwilling to take the drastic steps needed to boost the country's economy and help people in dire need. Thus Roosevelt issued a number of executive orders, by-passing Congress and mandating bank closures, safety nets for destitute citizens, and the like. Roosevelt led by authority, not example, because the needs of the divided country required it.

TEACHER TIP

Task 2 requires a clear counter-example. Note how writing about Roosevelt fits the bill. Nice transition words, too, yes?

Thus, when members of a group are united in common purpose, a leader, such as Alexander or Gandhi, need only spur the group on by example. The group is already poised for action, needing only a charismatic leader to show people the way and assure them that, though it may take time, success is in sight. However, when a group threatens to fall apart because the common vision has been lost, a leader such as Roosevelt must take charge, order people to work together and insure that the shared goal can be attained. Only after the work begins to take shape can the leader relax his command and lead by example.

TEACHER TIP

The determinant comes right up front, where it should be. In this case, what determines when the prompt is true or not is if the group has a shared goal.

EVALUATION AND DISCUSSION OF ESSAY #1

TEACHER TIP

All three tasks are successfully completed. That's the bottom line for a score of 4 or above.

Holistic Score: 6

Each of the three writing tasks is addressed separately in a response that is unified by a steady focus on the topic. All three tasks are addressed in a thorough way, demonstrating complexity of thought.

Paragraphs 1 and 2 address the first task in some depth. Paragraph 1 opens with an attention-getting, yet relevant comparison to a famous comment about pornography. The author then goes on to provide two examples that work together to clarify the meaning of the statement. A clear explanation is stated at the end of paragraph 2. Paragraph 3 provides an appropriate counter-example, specific to the task, with good transition and key phrases which indicate that this paragraph is in opposition to the first two. Paragraph 3 states the criterion under which the prompt is true, then supports this determinant with references to previous examples, thus providing unity to the essay.

TEACHER TIP

Don't add new examples to task 3. Refer to your previous examples instead, as this writer did. New examples open up the essay to new ideas, thus don't provide the unity you need at the end.

The first sentence of paragraph 4 addreses the second task by describing a set of characteristics that make leading by command the best method. Although this discussion does not contain actual examples as in paragraphs 1 and 2, the characteristics described are specific and thorough enough to make the author's point clear.

The author's effective use of transitions (e.g., yet, therefore, however) creates a smooth progression of ideas. The transitional sentences beginning paragraphs 2 and 3 establish a clear relationship between the paragraphs.

STRATEGY:

Variety in sentence structure and length keeps your writing from sounding monotonous or mechanical; it also adds sophistication.

ESSAY #2

True leadership leads rather than commands. Where commands are given, followers do what they are told, but only what they are told, and only when they are told. When people are led by example they do as they are shown, not only when they are shown, but on their own as well. This is not to say that commanders do not get things done with their groups. Armies are run by commanders instead of leaders, because they want not soldiers who will work and think on their own, but who will do as they are told when they are told. But commanding is not the same as leadership.

True leaders lead by example rather than by command because leadership is different from command. In situations apart from the military, where it is preferable to have followers who think and act for themselves, leadership by example is a far more effective motivator and guiding force. Workers who are browbeaten into submission are far less motivated than workers encouraged to work steadily at their own pace, with their own ideas. Workers commanded to perform a duty a certain way are less productive than workers guided and trained to think cleverly and creatively about their tasks.

Commanding and leadership are two different things whose results are quite often similar, but also often not, depending on the situation. Leadership leads by example, not by command, because of its very nature. When leadership commands, it ceases to be leadership.

TEACHER TIP

What a confusing essay! The author seems to have mixed up all his ideas and neglected to complete all tasks.

EVALUATION AND DISCUSSION OF ESSAY #2

Holistic Score: 3

This essay contains the beginnings of some interesting ideas and is written in language that is quite clear and straightforward. It does not focus, however, on providing a thorough explanation of the statement and its implications.

Nor does it fulfill all three tasks. In fact, only the first task is addressed, in a response that is poorly developed and organized. All three paragraphs work in some way to reinforce the statement that true leadership leads by example. Paragraphs 1 and 2 provide us with partial development of the idea by stating that people led by example can think for themselves and that workers who think for themselves perform better than those who do not. Although both of these ideas are interesting, they lack the necessary development. The author never clarifies why leading by example creates followers who can think for themselves. And he never pulls his ideas together into a coherent explanation of the meaning of the statement.

The author's main purpose in this essay seems to have been to establish that leadership and command are two different things. Yet he never

TEACHER TIP

Take another look at essay #1 alongside this second essay. Describe to yourself the differences between the two so you can better understand what you should and should not do in your own essays.

makes clear what his purpose is in establishing this difference, nor does he use this difference to reach any conclusion. He simply restates the difference in each paragraph. The result is an excessive repetition of ideas.

It seems, therefore, that this author paid little attention to the tasks listed in the essay topic. Nonetheless, the paper receives a score of 3 rather than 2 for two reasons: 1) it succeeds in sustaining a focus on the topic provided without significant digression or distortion, and 2) the quality of language demonstrates adequate control of mechanics, sentence structure, and vocabulary.

In all likelihood, this author could have produced a significantly better essay had he paid closer attention to the precise requirements of the tasks. By prewriting, he would have had the chance to get himself on the right track before starting to write. By thinking about each task in turn, he would have had the opportunity to form a more fully developed sequence of ideas. By addressing each task in turn, he would have produced paragraphs with a single, logical purpose.

STRATEGY:

To achieve unified paragraphs, address one task per paragraph. This will help ensure that the ideas in each paragraph all share a common focus.

CHAPTER 7

USAGE AND STYLE

You've learned how to analyze an essay topic, organize your thoughts, and outline an essay. Once you have an overall idea of what you want to say in your essay, you can start thinking about how to say it. The writing process is about producing clearly developed and well-organized essays. We'll now look at specific aspects of producing clear expository prose. The best strategy here is to study this section and work the exercises in short, manageable blocks, interspersed with the study of other subjects in preparation for the MCAT.

TEACHER TIP

Good writing is important not only for your MCAT essay but also for your med school application essay. These writing tips are useful for good speech as well. You're going to have a med school interview, and if you're well-spoken, it says a lot of positive things about you.

Remember the writer's mantra: INTENT = CLARITY. Between the two comes the absolute necessity to *think*, which is what you're doing in your prewrite. Studies have shown that a writer's style improves dramatically when she knows what she's going to say. The message: Try not to generate too much anxiety over your writing style. Your goal here isn't to become a Hemingway, but only to produce solid, 30-minute, first-draft essays about general topics.

Most important, *keep it simple*. This applies to word choice, sentence structure, and argument. Obsession about how to spell a word can throw off your flow of thought. The more complicated (and wordy) your sentences, the more likely they'll be plagued by errors. The more convoluted your argument, the more likely you'll get bogged down in convoluted sentence structure. Recall that *simple* does not mean *simplistic*. A clear, straightforward approach can be sophisticated.

Many students mistakenly believe that their essays will be "downgraded" for such mechanical errors as misplaced commas, poor choice of words, misspellings, faulty grammar, and so on. Occasional problems of this type won't dramatically affect your score. The test-readers understand that you are writing first-draft essays. They will *not* be taking points off for such errors, provided you don't have a demonstrable pattern of such errors. If the essays are littered with misspellings and incorrect usage, then a more serious communication problem is indicated.

The idea is, don't worry excessively about writing mechanics but do try to train yourself out of poor habits. And do proofread your essays for obvious errors. Your objective in taking the MCAT is admission to medical school, and to achieve that, you should probably give the medical schools what they want. They don't expect eloquence in a 30-minute assignment, but they do expect effectiveness.

To help you achieve this effectiveness in your essay, we offer three broad objectives:

Be **CONCISE**
Be **FORCEFUL**
Be **CORRECT**

An effective essay is concise; it wastes no words. An effective essay is forceful; it makes its point. And an effective essay is correct; it conforms to the generally accepted rules of grammar and form.

The following pages break down the three objectives of **CONCISION, FORCEFULNESS**, and **CORRECTNESS** into 23 specific principles. Don't panic! You'll find many of them familiar. And besides, we'll give you many opportunities to practice.

Use your time wisely. Don't do all the examples if you're confident that you know the point. Move on, spending extra time on those that give you trouble.

Principles 1 to 4 focus on concision, **principles 5 to 11** focus on forcefulness, and **principles 12 to 23** focus on correctness. As you might expect, however, the objectives are interrelated. A forceful sentence is usually not verbose, and correct sentences tend to be more forceful than incorrect ones.

The principles of concise and forceful writing are generally not as rigid as the principles of grammatically correct writing. Concision and forcefulness are matters of art and personal style as well as common sense and tradition. But if you are going to disregard a principle, we hope you'll do so sparingly and out of educated choice. Sticking to the principles of standard English should produce a concise, forceful, and correct essay.

BE CONCISE

The goal of being concise is to learn to make every word you use count toward developing your ideas. That way, you're helping your reader to stay focused. Being concise means getting rid of the distractions.

PRINCIPLE 1. AVOID JUNK PHRASES

Do not use several words when one word will do. Junk phrases are like junk food: they add only fat, no muscle. Many people make the mistake of writing *at the present time* or *at this point in time* instead of the simpler *now*, or *take into consideration* instead of simply *consider*, in an attempt to make their prose seem more scholarly or more formal. It doesn't work. Their prose ends up seeming inflated and pretentious. Writing junk phrases is a waste of words, a waste of limited time, and a distraction from the point of the essay.

> **TEACHER TIP**
> Junk phrases seem to make people feel that they're saying something in a more important, intelligent way. The opposite is true. Just like using lots of big, confusing words, junk phrases add words that just gunk up the sentence.

JUNKY: I am of the opinion that the aforementioned managers should be advised that they will be evaluated with regard to the utilization of responsive organizational software for the purpose of devising a responsive network of customers.
CONCISE: We should tell the managers that we will evaluate their use of flexible computerized databases to develop a customer's network.

EXERCISE FOR PRINCIPLE 1: JUNK PHRASES

Improve the following sentences by omitting or replacing junk phrases. All answers to the exercises in Chapter 7 can be found at the back of the book.

1. The agency is not prepared to undertake expansion at this point in time.
2. In view of the fact that John has prepared with much care for this presentation, it would be a good idea to award him with the project.
3. The airline has a problem with always having arrivals that come at least an hour late, despite the fact that the leaders of the airline promise that promptness is a goal that has a high priority for all the employees involved.
4. In spite of the fact that she only has a little bit of experience in photography right now, she will probably do well in the future because she has a great deal of motivation to succeed in her chosen profession.
5. The United States is not in a position to spend more money to alleviate the suffering of the people of other countries considering the problems of its own citizens.

6. Although not untactful, George is a man who says exactly what he believes.
7. Accuracy is a subject that has great importance to English teachers and company presidents alike.
8. The reason why humans kill each other is that they experience fear of those whom they do not understand.
9. Ms. Miller speaks with a high degree of intelligence with regard to many aspects of modern philosophy.
10. The best of all possible leaders is one who listens and inspires simultaneously.

TEACHER TIP

When you're redundant, you're just repeating yourself. In other words, you're saying the same thing twice. And how's that for a redundancy?

PRINCIPLE 2. DO NOT BE REDUNDANT

Redundancy means that the writer needlessly repeats an idea because he fails to realize the scope of a word or phrase that has already been used; for example, "a beginner lacking experience." (The word *beginner* implies lack of experience.) You can eliminate redundant words or phrases without changing the meaning of the sentence. Watch out for words that add nothing to the sense of the sentence.

REDUNDANT	CONCISE
refer back	refer
few in number	few
small-sized	small
grouped together	grouped
in my own personal opinion	in my opinion
end result	result
serious crisis	crisis
new initiatives	initiatives

TEACHER TIP

Whenever you write a sentence and then follow it up with "in other words" or "by that I mean to say," you know you haven't explained the thought clearly in the initial sentence.

Redundancy often results from carelessness, but you can easily eliminate redundant elements in the proofreading stage.

EXERCISE FOR PRINCIPLE 2: REDUNDANCY

Repair the following sentences by marking out redundant elements.

1. All these problems have combined together to create a serious crisis.
2. A staff that large in size needs an effective supervisor who can get the job done.
3. He knows how to follow directions and he knows how to do what he is told.

4. The writer's technical skill and ability do not mask his poor plot line.
5. That monument continues to remain a significant tourist attraction.
6. The recent trend lately of spending on credit has created a more impoverished middle class.
7. Those who can follow directions are few in number.
8. She has deliberately chosen to change careers.
9. Such dialogue opens up many doors to compromise.
10. The ultimate conclusion is that environmental and economic concerns are intertwined.

PRINCIPLE 3. AVOID NEEDLESS QUALIFICATION

Since the object of your essay is to convince your reader, you'll want to adopt a reasonable tone. In most MCAT essays there's no single, clear-cut "answer," so you should not overstate your case. Occasional use of such modifiers as *fairly, rather, somewhat, relatively* and of such expressions as *seems to be, a little,* and *a certain amount of* will let the reader know you are reasonable, but using such modifiers too often weakens your argument. Excessive qualification makes you sound hesitant; like junk phrases, they add bulk without adding substance.

TEACHER TIP

Don't be shy in your MCAT writing; just come right out and say what you want. Don't write, "A possible counterexample might be . . ." The reader isn't interested in what "might be" but rather in what you clearly write.

WORDY: This rather serious breach of etiquette may possibly shake the very foundations of the corporate world.
CONCISE: This serious breach of etiquette may shake the foundations of the corporate world.

Just as bad is the overuse of the word *very*. Some writers use this intensifying adverb before almost every adjective in an attempt to be more forceful. If you need to add emphasis, look for a stronger adjective (or verb) instead.

WEAK: Novak is a very good pianist.
STRONG: Novak is a virtuoso pianist.
STRONG: Novak plays beautifully.

And don't try to modify words that are already absolute.

INCORRECT	CORRECT
more unique	unique
the very worst	the worst
completely full	full

TEACHER TIP

Don't worry that the reader may disagree with what you write, or be offended by strong, clear statements. MCAT readers are trained to be objective and they don't much care what you use for examples or criteria, as long as they're appropriate and well-done.

EXERCISE FOR PRINCIPLE 3: EXCESSIVE QUALIFICATION

Although reasonable qualification benefits an essay, an excessive amount of it debilitates your argument. Though the amount of qualification always varies according to context, eliminate qualification in the sentences below.

1. She is a fairly excellent teacher.
2. Ferrara seems to be sort of a slow worker.
3. There are very many reasons technology has not permeated all countries equally.
4. It is rather important to pay attention to all the details of a murder trial as well as to the "larger picture."
5. You yourself are the very best person to decide what you should do for a living.
6. It is possible that the author overstates his case somewhat.
7. The president perhaps should use a certain amount of diplomacy before he resorts to force.
8. In Italy I found about the best food I have ever eaten.
9. Needless to say, children should be taught to cooperate at home and in school.
10. The travel agent does not recommend the trip to Tripoli, since it is possible that one may be hurt.

TEACHER TIP

Every sentence you write should move the essay along. "Water-treading" sentences are just a lot of junk words strung together, and you already know to avoid junk words.

PRINCIPLE 4. DO NOT USE "WATER-TREADING" SENTENCES

This principle suggests several things:

- Do not write a sentence that gets you nowhere.
- Do not ask a question only to answer it (unless you have hit upon a brilliant exception!).
- Do not merely copy the essay's directions.
- Do not write a whole sentence only to announce that you're changing the subject.

If you have something to say, say it without preamble. If you need to smooth over a change of subject, do so with a transitional word or phrase rather than a meaningless sentence. If proofreading reveals unintentional wasted sentences, neatly cross them out.

WORDY: Which idea of the author's is more in line with what I believe? This is a very interesting . . .
CONCISE: The author's statement closely mirrors reality.

The author of the wordy example above is just treading water: wasting words and limited time and getting nowhere. Get to the point quickly and stay there.

BE FORCEFUL

PRINCIPLE 5. AVOID NEEDLESS SELF-REFERENCE

You do not need to make repeated references to yourself in your essay. There is no need to keep reminding your reader that what you are writing is your opinion; your reader does not expect you to be expounding someone else's opinion. Avoid such unnecessary phrases as I believe, I feel, and in my opinion. Self-reference is generally superfluous and therefore detracts from your essay's concision. Self-reference also detracts from the forcefulness of your essay by constantly reminding your reader that you are expressing an opinion. Practice expressing self-confidence in your writing: your opinion is legitimate and deserves to be stated.

WEAK: I am of the opinion that air pollution is a more serious problem than the government has led us to believe.
FORCEFUL: Air pollution is a more serious problem than the government has led us to believe.

Self-reference is another form of qualifying what you say—a very obvious form. Sometimes, toning down your statement is appropriate, perhaps necessary. Using qualifiers like *probably* and *perhaps* can be effective if you do it sparingly. One or two self-references in an essay might even be appropriate. Being forceful and unreasonable is certainly not a winning combination. You must practice walking the middle ground between overstatement and wishy-washy qualification. Practicing different approaches to stating your opinion is the only sure way to improve your writing.

EXERCISE FOR PRINCIPLE 5: NEEDLESS SELF-REFERENCE

1. I feel we ought to pay teachers more than we pay senators.
2. The author, in my personal opinion, is stuck in the past.
3. I do not think this argument can be generalized to most business owners.
4. My own experience shows me that food is the best social lubricant.
5. I doubt more people would vote even if they had more information about candidates.

Teacher Tip

How many ways can you think of to write "I agree" without using "I?" For instance, "Writing correctly on the MCAT essay is, without a doubt, an important component of a good score." Didn't you just agree about the importance of good writing without saying "I agree?" Good for you.

6. Although I am no expert, I do not think privacy should be valued more than social concerns.
7. My guess is that most people want to do good work, but many are bored or frustrated with their jobs.
8. I must emphasize that I am not saying the author does not have a point.
9. If I were a college president, I would implement several specific reforms to combat apathy.
10. It is my belief that either alternative would prove disastrous.

PRINCIPLE 6. AVOID THE PASSIVE VOICE

Using the passive voice is another way writers avoid accountability. Put verbs in the active voice whenever possible. In the active voice, the subject performs the action (we should do it...). In the passive voice, the subject is the receiver of the action and is often only implied (it should be done...).

You should avoid the passive voice **EXCEPT** in the following cases:

> When you don't know who performed the action (The letter was opened before I received it.)
> When you prefer not to refer directly to the person who performs the action (An error has been made in computing this data.)

TEACHER TIP

Though you don't want to write your entire essay in the passive voice, switching occasionally from the active to the passive voice can create an interesting writing style. Just don't overdo it.

PASSIVE: The estimate of this year's tax revenues was prepared by the General Accounting Office.
ACTIVE: The General Accounting Office prepared the estimate of this year's tax revenues.

To change from the passive to the active voice, ask yourself WHO or WHAT is performing the action. In the case above, the General Accounting Office is performing the action. Therefore, the GAO should be the subject of the sentence. Your prewriting, especially the game plan in which you began to outline ideas for sentences, should give you an idea of the purpose. Take a few seconds to find out what your sentence is going to do before you ask it to perform.

EXERCISE FOR PRINCIPLE 6: UNDESIRABLE PASSIVES

Repair the following sentences by fixing undesirable passives.

1. The Spanish-American War was fought by brave but misguided men.

2. The bill was passed in time, but it was not signed by the president until the time for action had passed.
3. Advice is usually requested by those who need it least; it is not sought out by the truly lost and ignorant.
4. That building should be relocated where it can be appreciated by the citizens.
5. Garbage collectors should be generously rewarded for their dirty, smelly labors.
6. The conditions of the contract agreement were ironed out minutes before the strike deadline.
7. The minutes of the City Council meeting should be taken by the city clerk.
8. With sugar, water, or salt, many ailments contracted in less-developed countries could be treated.
9. Test results were distributed with no concern for confidentiality.
10. The report was compiled by a number of field anthropologists and marriage experts.

PRINCIPLE 7. AVOID WEAK OPENINGS

Try not to begin a sentence with *There is, There are,* or *It is.* That's a roundabout way of getting to the main point and it usually indicates that you're trying to distance yourself from the position you are taking.

TEACHER TIP

"It" is a pronoun and requires an antecedent (the word it replaces). Starting a sentence with *it* means you're starting off a sentence by referring to something which hasn't been written yet. That's not effective writing.

EXERCISE FOR PRINCIPLE 7: WEAK OPENINGS

Repair the following sentences by changing the weak openings.

1. It would be unwise for businesses to ignore the illiteracy problem.
2. It can be seen that in many fields experience is more important than training.
3. There are several reasons why this plane is obsolete.
4. It would be of no use to fight a drug war without waging a battle against demand for illicit substances.
5. There are many strong points in the candidate's favor; intelligence, unfortunately, is not among them.
6. It is difficult to justify building a more handsome prison.
7. It has been decided that we, as a society, can tolerate homelessness.
8. There seems to be little doubt that Americans like watching television better than conversing.

9. It is clear that cats make better pets than mice.
10. It is obvious that intelligence is a product of environment and heredity.

PRINCIPLE 8. AVOID VAGUE LANGUAGE

TEACHER TIP

One of the vaguest, least informative words in the English language is "thing." If you were asked to take that *thing* off the table, would you know what to remove? Nope. Be more specific.

Choose specific, descriptive words. The key is to choose your words, not let them flow uncontrolled from your pencil. Vague language weakens your writing because it forces the reader to guess what you mean. You'll find that the essay topic will supply you with an abundance of specifics; your argument will be more forceful if you replace vague phrases with the particular facts at hand.

WEAK: Jose is highly educated.
FORCEFUL: Jose has a master's degree in business administration.

WEAK: She is a great communicator.
FORCEFUL: She speaks persuasively.

Sometimes, to be more specific and concrete, you'll have to use more words than you might with vague language. This principle does not conflict with the general objective of concision. Being concise means eliminating unnecessary words; avoiding vagueness will sometimes mean adding necessary words.

PRINCIPLE 9. AVOID CLICHÉS

TEACHER TIP

Clichés are, by definition, phrases so overused that they've lost their meaning. Why would you try to explain something with a meaningless phrase?

Clichés are expressions that may once have seemed colorful and powerful but now seem dull and lifeless because of overuse. When working under a deadline, you can easily let trite phrases slip into your writing. Clichés are often vague, even meaningless in the context of a sentence. Keep them out of your essay.

WEAK: Performance in a crisis is the acid test for a leader.
FORCEFUL: Performance in a crisis is the best indicator of a leader's abilities.

Putting a cliché in quotation marks in order to indicate your distance from the clichés does not strengthen the sentence; if anything, it merely calls attention to the weakness. If you are going to use a cliché, ask yourself whether the reader will truly understand your point and whether the cliché reflects exactly what you mean.

EXERCISE FOR PRINCIPLE 9: CLICHÉS

Make the following sentences more forceful by replacing clichés.

1. Beyond the shadow of a doubt Jefferson was a great leader.
2. I have a sneaking suspicion that families spend less time together than they did 15 years ago.
3. The pizza delivery man arrived in the sequestered jury's hour of need.
4. Trying to find the employee responsible for this embarrassing information leak is like trying to find a needle in a haystack.
5. Both strategies would be expensive and completely ineffective, so it's six of one and half a dozen of the other.
6. The military is putting all its eggs in one basket by relying so heavily on nuclear missiles for the nation's defense.
7. Older doctors should be required to update their techniques, but you can't teach an old dog new tricks.
8. You have to take this new fad with a grain of salt.
9. The politician reminds me of Abraham Lincoln: he's like a diamond in the rough.
10. A ballpark estimate of the number of fans in the stadium would be 120,000.

PRINCIPLE 10. AVOID JARGON

Jargon includes two categories of words that you should avoid. First is the specialized vocabulary of a group, such as doctors, lawyers, or baseball coaches. Second is the overly inflated and complex language that burdens many students' essays. You will not impress anyone with big words that do not fit the tone or context of your essay, especially if they're misused.

If you aren't certain of a word's meaning or appropriateness, leave it out. An appropriate vocabulary, even if simple, will add impact to your argument. One proofreading technique is to ask yourself as you come across words you are unsure of, "Would a reader in a different field be able to understand what these words mean?" If you aren't sure, select different words that are clearer.

WEAK: The international banks are cognizant of the new law's significance.
FORCEFUL: The international banks are aware of the new law's significance.

TEACHER TIP

If you must use a specialized word or phrase, be sure to add a short definition.

WEAK: The new law would negatively impact each of the nations involved.
FORCEFUL: The new law would hurt each of the nations involved. ("Impact" is also used to mean *affect* or *benefit*.)

The following are commonly used jargon words:

prioritize	target (*v.*)
parameter (boundary, limit)	originate (start, begin)
optimize	blindside
user-friendly (responsive, flexible, easy-to-understand)	facilitate (help, speed up)
utilize (use)	downside
finalize (end, complete)	bottom line
input/output	viable
conceptualize (imagine, think)	time frame
mutually beneficial	dialogue
maximize	alternatives (choices)
assistance	ongoing (continuing)
designate	

EXERCISE FOR PRINCIPLE 10: JARGON

Replace the jargon in the following sentences with more appropriate language.

1. We anticipate utilizing hundreds of paper clips in the foreseeable future.
2. The research-oriented person should not be hired for a people-oriented position.
3. Educationwise, our school children have been neglected.
4. Foreign diplomats should always interface with local leaders.
5. Pursuant to your being claimed as a dependent on the returns of another taxpayer or resident wage earner, you may not consider yourself exempt if your current nonwage income exceeds 500 dollars or if your non-wage income combined with current wage income amounts to or exceeds 500 dollars.
6. There is considerable evidentiary support for the assertion that Vienna sausages are good for you.
7. With reference to the poem, I submit that the second and third stanzas connote a certain despair.

8. Allow me to elucidate my position: this horse is the epitome, the very quintessence of equine excellence.
9. In the case of the recent railway disaster, it is clear that governmental regulatory agencies obfuscated in the preparation of materials for release to the public through both the electronic and print media.
10. Having been blindsided by innumerable unforeseen crises, this office has not been able to prepare for the aforementioned exigencies.

PRINCIPLE 11. VARY SENTENCES IN LENGTH AND STRUCTURE

Even when writing is clear and correct it can be tedious if sentences are all similar in length and structure. Take the following passage:

> The author suggests that a conflict exists between devoting limited resources to many people who would be affected positively or to a needy few for whom the effects would be less impressive. This conflict underlies many political arguments in the United States today about education, welfare, health care, and other issues that are costly and complex. We should direct resources where they will have the broadest impact if taxpayers are willing to devote only a limited portion of their income to the "general welfare" of the American people.

TEACHER TIP

Watch out for paragraphs that consist of one long sentence. They always become confusing and awkward.

Each sentence, taken singly, is adequate stylistically and grammatically, but the passage lacks force because the same construction is repeated in each sentence. Each sentence is more than 25 words long. All of the sentences begin with the subject (*the author*, *this conflict*, *we*).

Monotonous sentence construction makes the content seem flat and suggests that the writer may lack imagination. Your ideas will make more of an impact if you break up a series of long, complicated sentences by occasionally inserting a short and simple one. Usually you can do this by cutting one long, convoluted sentence into two shorter sentences. Changing the length of a sentence usually necessitates changing its structure as well, but if you concentrate on length, it will often be easier to restructure a sentence. You can also create dependent clauses for variation.

Now compare the passage above with the following revised version:

> According to the author, a conflict exists between devoting limited resources to many people who would be affected positively or to a needy few for whom the effects would be less impressive. This conflict underlies many political arguments in the United States today. People fight

about how to distribute resources for education, welfare, health care, and other issues that are costly and complex. But taxpayers are willing to devote only a limited portion of their income to the "general welfare" of the American people. As long as this is true, we should direct those resources where they will have the broadest impact.

The two passages contain the same information, often use the same phrasing, and are roughly the same length, yet the second passage is more interesting and persuasive. Sentence length ranges from 11 to 32 words, and structure is varied by the use of dependent clauses.

BE CORRECT

TEACHER TIP

This is all about grammar. You probably know most of the rules of written English, even if you don't always use them correctly. Here's your chance to brush up. The grammar words used in this section are defined on page 121.

Correctness is perhaps the most difficult objective for writers to achieve. The complex rules of English usage can leave you more than a bit confused. The most important lesson you can take from this section is how to organize your thoughts into a strong, well-supported argument. Style and grammar are important but secondary concerns. Many of the rules of English usage are designed to force the writer to stick with one structure or usage in a sentence or even an essay.

Do the exercises and then compare your answers to ours, making sure you understand what each error was. Proofread your practice essays in the Essay Practice Section; later, return to your practice essays and edit them. Better yet, ask a friend to edit them, paying special attention to correctness. Remember, 30 minutes is not enough time to achieve perfection. Luckily, your readers will not expect perfection. So just think of this section as helping you to improve the details of good writing. If it begins to overwhelm you, stop and take a break. The brain needs time to absorb all this information.

As you work through this section on the form of the English language, you'll come across a few technical words that describe particular word functions in a sentence. You will not be expected to know the exact definitions of these terms, only to understand their function so you can recognize errors. A list of definitions is provided at the end of this chapter with examples of each of these parts of speech. You will also find basic explanations throughout the text.

TEACHER TIP

"One" is a nice, neutral pronoun, but it can't be used in the same sentence as "you" or "we." Decide on which pronoun to use and stick with it, at least for that sentence.

PRINCIPLE 12. DO NOT SHIFT NARRATIVE VOICE

Principle 5 above advised you to avoid needless self-reference. Since you are asked to write an explanatory essay, however, an occasional self-reference may be appropriate. You may even call yourself "I" if you want, as long as you keep the number of first-person pronouns to a minimum. Less egocentric ways of referring to the narrator include "we" and "one." If these more formal ways of writing seem stilted, stay with "I."

I suggest that individuals best cherish principles of free speech when such principles are challenged.
We can see . . .
One must admit . . .

The method of self-reference you select is called the *narrative voice* of your essay. Any of the above narrative voices are acceptable. Whichever one you choose, be careful not to shift narrative voice throughout. If you use *I* in the first sentence, don't use *we* in a later sentence.

INCORRECT: I suggest that individuals best cherish principles of free speech when such principles are challenged. We can see how a free society can get too complacent when free speech is taken for granted.

It is likewise wrong to shift from *you* to *one*:

INCORRECT: You can readily see how politicians have a vested interest in pleasing powerful interest groups, though one should not generalize about this tendency.

To correct each of the above sentences, you need to change one pronoun to agree with the other:

CORRECT: "We can readily see..." (to agree with "though we should not generalize...")
CORRECT: "I can readily see..." (to agree with "though I would not generalize...")
CORRECT: "One can readily see..."(to agree with "though one should not generalize...")

EXERCISE FOR PRINCIPLE 12: SHIFTING NARRATIVE VOICE

Rewrite these sentences to give them consistent points of view.

1. I am disgusted with the waste we tolerate in this country. One cannot simply stand by without adding to such waste: living here makes you wasteful.

2. You must take care not to take these grammar rules too seriously, since one can often become bogged down in details and forget why he is writing at all.
3. We all must take a stand against waste in this country; how else will one be able to look oneself in the mirror?

TEACHER TIP

Subject/verb mistakes are some of the most common on MCAT essays, but they're completely avoidable by considering, Is the subject is singular or plural?

PRINCIPLE 13. BE SURE THAT THE VERB AGREES WITH THE SUBJECT

Singular and plural subjects take different forms of the verb in the present tense. Usually the difference lies in the presence or absence of a final *-s* (he becomes and they become), but sometimes the difference is more radical (he is, they are). If you're a native speaker of English, you can usually trust your ear to give you the correct verb form, but certain situations cause difficulty: when the subject and verb are separated by a number of words, when the subject is an indefinite pronoun, and when the subject consists of more than one noun.

A verb must agree with its subject in number regardless of intervening phrases. Don't let the words that come between the subject and verb confuse you as to the number (singular or plural) of the subject. Usually one word can be pinpointed as the grammatical subject of the sentence, and so the verb—no matter how far removed—must agree with that subject in number.

INCORRECT: The joys of climbing mountains, especially if one is a novice climber without the proper equipment, escapes me.
CORRECT: The joys of climbing mountains, especially if one is a novice climber without the proper equipment, escape me.

INCORRECT: A group of jockeys who have already finished the first race and who wish to have their pictures taken are blocking my view of the horses.
CORRECT: A group of jockeys who have already finished the first race and who wish to have their pictures taken is blocking my view of the horses. (The long prepositional phrase beginning with the preposition "of" qualifies the noun group. The subject of the sentence is the noun group, which takes a singular verb "is").

In both examples, the phrases and clauses between subject and verb do not affect the grammatical relationship between subject and verb. A plural intervening phrase doesn't change a singular subject into a plural one.

Look out for prepositional phrases intervening between subject and verb!

Here is a list of some of the most common prepositions:

in	about
out	to
up	from
down	by
over	onto
under	before
between	after
off	through
on	despite
behind	concerning
of	against
with	

Also, watch out for collective nouns like *group*—such nouns are often plural in meaning but are nevertheless grammatically singular. The word *number* takes a singular verb when preceded by *the* and a plural verb when preceded by *a*:

CORRECT: A *number* of fans *hope* for a mere glimpse of his handsome face; unfortunately, they are rarely satisfied with a mere glimpse.
CORRECT: The *number* of fans who catch a glimpse of his handsome face *seems* to grow exponentially each time the tabloids write a story of his seclusion.

- **A subject that consists of two or more nouns connected by *and* takes the plural form of the verb.**

CORRECT: *Karl*, who is expert in cooking Hunan spicy duck, and George, who is expert in eating Hunan spicy duck, have combined their expertise to start a new restaurant.

- **When the subject consists of two or more nouns connected by *or* or *nor*, the verb agrees with the CLOSEST noun.**

CORRECT: Either the senators or the president is misinformed.
CORRECT: Either the president or the senators are misinformed.

TEACHER TIP

When you write long, involved sentences with lots of modifying phrases between subject and verb, subject/verb agreement mistakes are bound to happen. Long, rambling sentences are a bad idea anyway because they lend themselves to both grammar and comprehension confusion.

TEACHER TIP

Either and *each* are always singular words. They both include the unwritten, though understood, additional word *one*. Think of "either one" or "each one."

There are some connecting phrases that look as though they should make a group of words into a plural but actually do not.

The only connecting word that can make a series of singular nouns into a plural subject is *and*. In particular, the following connecting words and phrases do NOT result in a plural subject:

along with   besides   together with   as well as   in addition to

INCORRECT: The president, along with the secretary of state and the director of the CIA, are misinformed.
CORRECT: The president, along with the secretary of state and the director of the CIA, is misinformed.

If a sentence that is grammatically correct still sounds awkward, you should probably rephrase your thought.

TEACHER TIP

An awkward sentence may be grammatically correct but will end up being confusing and difficult to read. Perfect grammar does not always a smooth sentence make.

LESS AWKWARD: Along with the secretary of state and the director of the CIA, the president is misinformed.

A note on the subjunctive: After verbs such as *recommend, require, suggest, ask, demand*, and *insist*, and after expressions of requirement, suggestion, and demand (*I demand that*), use the subjunctive form of the verb. The subjunctive form is used after such expressions as *I want to*________________ ."

TEACHER TIP

The subjective voice never takes additional words such as *should* or *must*. Thus the second example can never be written, "It is essential that the reader must understand what you are trying to say." That would also be redundant: *essential* and *must* mean the same thing.

CORRECT: I recommend that the chocolate cake *be* reinstated on your menu.
CORRECT: It is essential that the reader *understand* what you are trying to say.

EXERCISE FOR PRINCIPLE 13: SUBJECT-VERB AGREEMENT

Repair the incorrect verbs.

1. The logical structure of his complicated and rather tortuous arguments are always the same.
2. The majority of the organization's members is over 60 years old.
3. Both the young child and her grandfather was depressed for months after discovering that the oldest ice cream parlor in the city had closed its doors forever.
4. Hartz brought the blueprints and model that was still on the table instead of the ones that Mackenzie had returned to the cabinet.

5. A case of bananas have been sent to the local distributor in compensation for the fruit that was damaged in transit.
6. A total of 50 editors read each article, a process that takes at least a week, sometimes six months.
7. Neither the shipping clerk who packed the equipment nor the truckers who transported it admits responsibility for the dented circuit box.
8. Either Georgette or Robespierre are going to be asked to dinner by the madcap Calvin. I dread the results in either case.
9. I can never decide whether to eat an orange or a Belgian chocolate; each of them have their wondrous qualities.
10. Everyone in the United States, as well as the Canadians, expect the timber agreement to fall through.

PRINCIPLE 14. BEWARE OF FAULTY PARALLELISM

Faulty parallelism results from not seeing the structure of the sentence you are constructing. Matching constructions must be expressed in parallel form. It is often rhetorically effective to use a particular construction several times in succession, in order to provide emphasis. The technique is called parallel construction, and it is effective only when used sparingly. If your sentences are varied, a parallel construction will stand out. If your sentences are already repetitive, a parallel structure will further obscure your meaning. Look at the following sentence:

As a leader, Lincoln inspired a nation to throw off the chains of slavery; *as a philosopher*, he proclaimed the greatness of the little man; *as a human being*, he served as a timeless example of humility.

The repetition of the construction provides a strong sense of rhythm and organization to the sentence, and it alerts the reader to yet another aspect of Lincoln's character.

Writers often use a parallel structure for dissimilar items.

INCORRECT: They are sturdy, attractive, and cost only a dollar each. ("They are" makes sense before the adjectives *sturdy* and *attractive*, but makes no sense before "cost only a dollar each.")
CORRECT: They are sturdy and attractive, and they cost only a dollar each.

TEACHER TIP

Parallel structure simply means that items in a list must be in the same grammatical form—all verbs or all nouns. Pay attention to this when writing out a list.

Parallel constructions must be expressed in parallel grammatical form. In other words, each segment of the parallel must be in similar form to the other segments: all nouns, all infinitives, all gerunds, all prepositional phrases, or all clauses.

INCORRECT: All business students should learn word processing, accounting, and how to program computers.
CORRECT: All business students should learn word processing, accounting, and computer programming.

This principle applies to any words that might begin each item in a series: prepositions (*in, on, by, with,* etc.), articles (*the, a, an*), helping verbs (*had, has, would,* etc.) and possessives (*his, her, our,* etc.). Either repeat the word before every element in a series or include it only in the first item. Anything else violates the rules of parallelism.

TEACHER TIP

The way you write the third (and following) item in the list must be in the same form that you wrote the second.

In effect, your treatment of the *second* element of the series determines the form of all subsequent elements:

INCORRECT: He invested his money in stocks, in real estate, and a home for retired performers.
CORRECT: He invested his money in stocks, in real estate, and in a home for retired performers.
CORRECT: He invested his money in stocks, real estate, and a home for retired performers.

When proofreading, check that each item in the series agrees with the word or phrase that begins the series. In the above example, *invested his money* is the common phrase that each item shares. You would read, "He invested his money in real estate, *invested his money in stocks*, and *invested his money* in a home for retired performers."

A number of constructions call for you to express ideas in parallel form. These constructions include:

X is as ________ as Y.
X is more ________ than Y.
X is less ________ than Y.
Both X and Y...
Either X or Y...
Neither X nor Y...
Not only X but also Y...

X and Y can stand for as little as one word or as much as a whole clause, but whatever the case, the grammatical structure of X and Y must be identical.

INCORRECT: The view from this apartment is not nearly as spectacular as from that mountain lodge.
CORRECT: The view from this apartment is not nearly as spectacular as the one from that mountain lodge.

TEACHER TIP

Comparisons have to be parallel, too. You can't write, "Golden Retrievers are popular guide dogs because their dispositions are nicer than other breeds." That sentence incorrectly compares "dispositions" to "other breeds." You want to compare "breeds" to "breeds": Golden Retrievers are popular guide dogs because their dispositions are nicer than those of other breeds."

EXERCISE FOR PRINCIPLE 14: PARALLELISM

Correct the faulty parallelism in the following sentences.

1. This organization will not tolerate the consumption, trafficking, or promoting the use of drugs.
2. The dancer taught her understudy how to move, how to dress, and how to work with choreographers and deal with professional competition.
3. The student's knowledge of chemistry is as extensive as what the professor knows.
4. They should not allow that man either to supervise the project or assist another supervisor, since he has proven himself to be thoroughly incompetent.
5. Either the balloon business will have to expand or declare bankruptcy.
6. Before Gertrude begins to design the set, as well as hiring laborers to help her construct it, she should consult the director.
7. Merrill based his confidence on the futures market, the bond market, and on the strength of the president's popularity.
8. The grocery baggers were ready, able, and were quite determined to do a great job.
9. The requirements for a business degree are not as stringent as a law degree.
10. Not only did we sail, fish, and canoe that day, but also visited the quaint town on the island across the bay.

PRINCIPLE 15. BE SURE THAT PRONOUNS REFER CLEARLY AND PROPERLY TO THEIR ANTECEDENTS

A pronoun is a word that replaces a noun in a sentence. Every time you write a pronoun—*he, him, his, she, her, it, its, they, their, that,* and *which*—be sure there can be no doubt about which noun that pronoun

TEACHER TIP

Misuse of pronouns is possibly the most common grammar problem in essays and certainly in regular, spoken English. How many times have you heard someone say "They say it's a good movie." Who's "they?"

refers to (the antecedent). Careless use of pronouns (a common mistake) can obscure your intended meaning.

AMBIGUOUS: The teacher told the student he was lazy. (Does *he* refer to *teacher* or *student*?)
AMBIGUOUS: Sara knows more about history than Irina because she learned it from her father. (Does *she* refer to *Sara* or *Irina*?)

You can usually rearrange a sentence to avoid ambiguous pronoun reference.

CLEAR: The student was lazy, and the teacher told him so.
CLEAR: The teacher considered himself lazy and told the student so.
CLEAR: Since Sara learned history from her father, she knows more than Irina does.
CLEAR: Because Irina learned history from her father, she knows less about it than Sara does.

TEACHER TIP

Proper grammar usage is important for the MCAT essay but imperative for the med school application. Submitting a cogent, well-written application essay will increase your odds of being accepted to med school.

If you're worried that a pronoun reference will be ambiguous, rewrite the sentence so that there's no doubt. Don't be afraid to repeat the antecedent (the noun that the pronoun refers to) if necessary:

AMBIGUOUS: I would rather settle in Phoenix than in Albuquerque, although it lacks wonderful restaurants.

CLEAR: I would rather settle in Phoenix than in Albuquerque, although Phoenix lacks wonderful restaurants.

A reader must be able to pinpoint the pronoun's antecedent. Even if you think the reader will know what you mean, do not use a pronoun without a clear and appropriate antecedent.

INCORRECT: When you are painting, be sure not to get it on the floor. (*It* could refer only to the noun *paint*; pronouns cannot refer to implied nouns.)
CORRECT: When you are painting, be sure not to get any paint on the floor.

Avoid using *this*, *that*, *it*, or *which* to refer to a whole phrase, sentence, or idea. Even when these pronouns are placed very close to their intended antecedent, the references may still be unclear.

UNCLEAR: U.S. consumers use larger amounts of nonrecyclable diapers every year. This will someday turn the earth into a giant trashcan.
CLEAR: U.S. consumers use larger amounts of nonrecyclable diapers every year. This ever-growing mass of waste products will someday turn the earth into a giant trashcan. (Try not to begin a sentence with *that* or *this* unless accompanying a noun.)

UNCLEAR: The salesman spoke loudly, swayed back and forth, and tapped the table nervously, which made his customers extremely nervous.
CLEAR: The salesman spoke loudly, swayed back and forth, and tapped the table nervously, mannerisms which made his customers extremely nervous.

Also, unless you are talking about the weather, avoid beginning a sentence with *it*. (See principle 7: Avoid weak openings.)

WEAK: It is difficult to distinguish between the rights of criminals and those of victims.
BETTER: Distinguishing between the rights of criminals and those of victims is difficult.

TEACHER TIP

Some nouns and pronouns are singular in one context and plural in another, depending on the number of the antecedent.

A few of the indefinite pronouns that can be singular or plural are *some*, *all*, *most*, *any*, and *none*. When using one of these words as the subject, check to see whether the antecedent is singular or plural.

CORRECT: He was unable to finish his work last night. *Some remains* to be done today. *None* of it is easy. (Read: *Some* of his work *remains*; *none* of his work *is*)
CORRECT: His *superiors* have been following his progress. *Some are* more impressed than others. *None are* overwhelmed. (Read: *Some* of his superiors *are*; *none* of his superiors *are*)

Other indefinite pronouns are invariable in number:

SINGULAR

anybody	everybody	somebody	either	one
anyone	everyone	someone	neither	each
anything	every one	some one	no one	

(Just remember that *-body, -one*, and *-thing* pronouns are singular.)

TEACHER TIP

Despite a writer's best intentions, the use of "he/she" usually goes wrong. For one thing, it takes twice as long to write as does using a single pronoun. For another, the writer often drops this form later and reverts to "he" or "she," making the usage inconsistent. You can be sure that the MCAT reader doesn't care which gender pronoun you use.

PLURAL

both	few	many	several

A related problem has arisen recently because of concern over using gender-specific words in non-gender-specific situations. Writers might substitute the traditional generic singular pronoun *he* with the plural form *they*. But other methods exist to avoid using *he* as a generic pronoun.

INCORRECT: The author makes a strong statement about the individual: each person must protect their individuality if one wants to remain individual.
CORRECT: The author makes a strong statement about individualism: people must protect their individuality if they want to remain individuals.

When sentences contain a relative clause (one that begins with the relative pronoun *who, whom, that*, or *which*), it's easy to become confused about which pronoun to use. A useful technique is to turn the clause into a question.

CORRECT: Those people, whom I have been calling all day, never returned my call.
CORRECT: Those people, who have been calling all day, are harassing me.

In the first sentence, you would mentally ask, "I have been calling *who* or *whom*?" Answer your question, substituting a pronoun: "I have been calling *them*." In the second sentence, you would ask, "*Who* or *whom* has been calling all day?" Answer your question, substituting a pronoun: "*They* have been calling all day." If you use *her, him, them,* or *us* to answer the question, the appropriate relative pronoun is *whom*. If you use *she, he, they*, or *we* to answer the question, the appropriate relative pronoun is *who*.

That and *which* are often used interchangeably, but as a rule, *that* is a defining, or restrictive, pronoun, while *which* is a non-defining, or non-restrictive pronoun. Usually, this can be translated into a simple rule of thumb: If the relative clause is set off with commas (i.e., the clause is not crucial to the meaning of the sentence), use *which*. If the relative clause is not set off by commas (i.e., the clause is crucial to the meaning of the sentence), use *that*. (See principle 19: Use commas correctly when you punctuate.)

CORRECT: The movie, which was released two years behind schedule, was one of the few that were real box office hits this spring.

EXERCISE FOR PRINCIPLE 15: FAULTY PRONOUN REFERENCE

Repair the faulty pronoun references in the following sentences.

1. Clausen's dog won first place at the show because he was well bred.
2. The critic's review made the novel a commercial success. He is now a rich man.
3. The military advisor was more conventional than his commander, but he was a superior strategist.
4. Bertha telephoned her friends in California before going home for the night, which she had not done in weeks.
5. Although John hoped and prayed for the job, it did no good. He called him the next morning; they had hired someone else.
6. You must pay attention when fishing—otherwise, you might lose it.
7. Zolsta Karmagi is the better musician, but he had more formal training.
8. The director wanted to give the lead part to her, but the star, his girlfriend, disagreed and insisted that she was better qualified for the job.
9. Zalmen showed us his credentials, but Koenig refused to answer our inquiries.
10. A retirement community offers more activities than a private dwelling does, but it is cheaper.

PRINCIPLE 16. BE SURE THAT MODIFICATION IS CLEAR

In English, the position of the word within a sentence often establishes the word's relationship to other words in the sentence. This is especially true with modifying phrases. Modifiers, like pronouns, are generally connected to the nearest word that agrees with the modifier in person and number. If a modifier is placed too far from the word it modifies, the meaning may be lost or obscured. Notice how ambiguous the following sentences are when the modifying phrases are misplaced.

AMBIGUOUS: Gary and Martha sat talking about the movie in the office.
CLEAR: Gary and Martha sat in the office talking about the movie.

Avoid ambiguity by placing modifiers as close as possible to the words they are intended to modify.

TEACHER TIP

Modifiers are adjectives and adverbs, either single words or phrases. Their only function is to tell you more about something in the sentence, so they need to be as close as possible to that "something."

TEACHER TIP

Think of a traffic report with these words: "Traffic is only backed up on the 405 freeway." "Only" is a modifier and here it incorrectly modifies "backed up." It's supposed to indicate that traffic is backed up *only* on the freeway. The correct sentence is" Traffic is backed up only on the 405 freeway."

AMBIGUOUS: They wondered how much the house was really worth when they bought it.
CLEAR: When they bought the house, they wondered how much it was really worth.

Modifiers can refer to words that either precede or follow them. Ambiguity can also result when a modifier is squeezed between two possible referents and the reader has no way of knowing which is the intended referent:

AMBIGUOUS: The dentist instructed him regularly to brush his teeth.
CLEAR: The dentist instructed him to brush his teeth regularly.

Be sure that the modifier is closest to the intended referent and that there is no other possible referent on the other side of the modifier. If when proofreading your essay you find a misplaced modifier, just enclose it in parentheses and draw an arrow to its proper place in the sentence.

AMBIGUOUS: Tom said in the car he had a map of New Jersey.
CLEAR: Tom said he had a map of New Jersey in the car.

All the ambiguous sentences above are examples of misplaced modifiers: modifiers whose placement makes the intended reference unclear. In addition to misplaced modifiers, watch for dangling modifiers: modifiers whose intended referents are not even present.

INCORRECT: Coming out of context, Peter was startled by Julia's perceptiveness.

The modifying phrase *coming out of context* is probably not intended to refer to *Peter*, but if not, then to whom or what? *Julia? Perceptiveness?* None of these makes sense as the referent of *coming out of context*. What came out of context was more likely a *statement* or *remark*. The sentence is incorrect because there is no word or phrase that can be pinpointed as the referent of the opening modifying phrase. Rearrangement and rewording solved the problem.

CORRECT: Julia's remark, coming out of context, startled Peter with its perceptiveness.

EXERCISE FOR PRINCIPLE 16: FAULTY MODIFICATION

Repair the faulty modification in the following sentences.

1. Bentley advised him quickly to make up his mind.
2. I agree with the author's statements in principle.
3. Coming out of the woodwork, he was surprised to see termites.
4. The governor's conference met to discuss racial unrest in the auditorium.
5. Hernandez said in her office she had all the necessary documents.
6. All of his friends were not able to come, but he decided that he preferred small parties anyway.
7. Margolis remembered she had to place a telephone call when she got home.
8. George told Suzette he did not like to discuss politics as they walked through the museum.
9. Having worked in publishing for 10 years, Stokely's résumé shows that he is well qualified.
10. Without experience in community service, holding political office would be a farce.

PRINCIPLE 17. AVOID SLANG AND COLLOQUIALISMS

Conversational speech is filled with slang and colloquial expressions but these should be avoided in the formal expository writing appropriate for the MCAT. In fact, such informal language might even confuse your reader, since slang and colloquialisms are not universally understood. Even worse, such informality on paper may give readers the impression that you are poorly educated or arrogant.

TEACHER TIP

Slang and colloquialisms often come into style, stay a while, and then go out of favor. Thus you may be using words which just aren't used anymore. Not only do the words sound odd, they won't make sense to the reader because they're no longer common usage. Dig, cool cat?

INCORRECT: He is really into gardening.
CORRECT: He enjoys gardening.

INCORRECT: She plays a wicked game of tennis.
CORRECT: She excels in tennis.

INCORRECT: Myra has got to go to Memphis for a week.
CORRECT: Myra must go to Memphis for a week.

INCORRECT: Joan has been doing science for eight years now.
CORRECT: Joan has been a scientist for eight years now.

INCORRECT: The blackened salmon's been one of the restaurant's most popular entrees.
CORRECT: The blackened salmon has been one of the restaurant's most popular entrees.

TEACHER TIP

An MCAT essay is not an academic thesis, thus it needn't be that formal. But neither should it be too informal or colloquial. Avoid expressions such as, "Let's take a look at a good example." It's too chatty—and completely unnecessary. Rather than introducing the example, just give the example.

The English language has such a rich vocabulary that you should never have to resort to using a colloquialism to make a point. With a little thought you will find the right word. Using informal language is risky; play it safe by sticking to standard usage.

EXERCISE FOR PRINCIPLE 17: SLANG AND COLLOQUIALISMS

Replace the informal elements of the following sentences with more appropriate terms.

1. Cynthia Larson sure knows her stuff.
2. The crowd was really into watching the fire-eating juggler, but then the dancing horse grabbed their attention.
3. As soon as the personnel department checks out his résumé, I am sure we will hear gales of laughter issuing from the office.
4. Having something funny to say seems awfully important in our culture.
5. The chef had a nice way with salmon: his sauce was simple but the effect was sublime.
6. Normal human beings can't cope with repeated humiliation.
7. The world hasn't got much time to stop polluting; soon, we all will have to wear face masks.
8. If you want a good cheesecake, you must make a top-notch crust.
9. International organizations should try and cooperate on global issues like hunger and party decorations.
10. The environmentalists aren't in it for the prestige; they really care about protecting the yellow-throated hornswoggler.

TEACHER TIP

Sentence fragments are a common problem. They often slip in when the writer is introducing an example separate from what the example refers to. "Many brilliant minds have worked on the problem. For example, Einstein." That last phrase is not a full sentence.

PRINCIPLE 18. DO NOT WRITE SENTENCE FRAGMENTS OR RUN-ON SENTENCES

A sentence fragment has no independent clause; a run-on sentence has two or more independent clauses that are improperly connected. As you edit your practice essays, check your sentence constructions, noting any tendency toward fragments or run-on sentences.

Sentence Fragments

Every sentence in formal expository writing must have an independent clause: a clause that contains a subject and a predicate and does not begin with a subordinate conjunction such as:

after	if	than	whenever
although	in order that	though	where
as	provided that	unless	whether
because	since	until	while
before	so that		

When you proofread your essays, make sure that every sentence has at least one independent clause.

TEACHER TIP

Complete sentences need only two parts: subject and verb. Make sure you have both before you end a phrase with a period.

INCORRECT: Global warming. That is what the scientists and journalists are worried about this month.
CORRECT: Global warming *is* the cause of concern for scientists and journalists this month.

INCORRECT: Seattle is a wonderful place to live. Having mountains, ocean, and forests all within easy driving distance. If you can ignore the rain.
CORRECT: Seattle is a wonderful place to live, with mountains, ocean, and forests all within easy driving distance, but it certainly does rain often.

INCORRECT: Why do I think the author's position is preposterous? Because he makes generalizations that I know are rarely true.
CORRECT: I think the author's position is preposterous because he makes generalizations that I know are rarely true.

Beginning single-clause sentences with coordinate conjunctions—*and, but, or, nor,* and *for*—is acceptable in moderation, though some readers may object to beginning a sentence with *and.*)

CORRECT: Most people would agree that indigent patients should receive wonderful health care. But every treatment has its price.

Run-On Sentences

Time pressure may also cause you to write two or more sentences as one. When you proofread your essays, watch out for independent clauses that are not joined with any punctuation at all or are only joined with a comma.

TEACHER TIP

Since run-on sentences can be corrected in three ways, it would be nice to vary the way you do this. Different punctuation provides interesting sentence structure and style.

INCORRECT: Current insurance practices are unfair they discriminate against the people who need insurance most.
INCORRECT: Current insurance practices are unfair, they discriminate against the people who need insurance most.

You can repair run-on sentences in any one of three ways. First, you could use a period to make separate sentences of the independent clauses.

CORRECT: Current insurance practices are unfair. They discriminate against the people who need insurance most.

Second, you could use a semicolon. A semicolon is a weak period: it separates independent clauses but signals to the reader that the ideas in the clauses are related.

CORRECT: Current insurance practices are unfair; they discriminate against the people who need insurance most.

The third way to repair a run-on sentence is usually the most effective. Use a conjunction to turn an independent clause into a dependent one and to elucidate how the clauses are related.

CORRECT: Current insurance practices are unfair, in that they discriminate against the people who need insurance most.

One common way to end up with a run-on sentence is to try to use transitional adverbs like *however, nevertheless, furthermore, likewise*, and *therefore* as conjunctions.

INCORRECT: Current insurance practices are discriminatory, furthermore they make insurance too expensive for the poor.
CORRECT: Current insurance practices are discriminatory. Furthermore, they make insurance too expensive for the poor.

INCORRECT: Current insurance practices are discriminatory, however they make insurance too expensive for the poor.
CORRECT: Current insurance practices are discriminatory; however, they make insurance too expensive for the poor.

EXERCISE FOR PRINCIPLE 18: SENTENCE FRAGMENTS AND RUN-ON SENTENCES

Repair the following by eliminating sentence fragments and run-on sentences.

1. The private academy has all the programs Angie will need. Except that the sports program has been phased out.
2. Leadership ability. This is the elusive quality that our current government employees have yet to capture.
3. Antonio just joined the athletic club staff this year but Barry has been with us since 1975, therefore we would expect Barry to be more skilled with the weight-lifting equipment. What a surprise to find Barry pinned beneath a barbell on the weight-lifting bench with Antonio struggling to lift the 300-pound weight from poor Barry's chest.
4. However much she tries to act like a Southern belle, she cannot hide her roots. The daughter of a Yankee fisherman, taciturn and always polite.
5. There is always time to invest in property ownership. After one has established oneself in the business world, however.
6. Sentence fragments are often used in casual conversation, however they should not be used in written English under normal circumstances.
7. A documentary film, which at least has an aura of reality and truth, and which in this case is very well produced, however there is less overall impact than a personal biography, particularly one of someone the public knows and likes.
8. After living for many years alone, the decision to move into a retirement community, despite the many restrictions entailed, was a difficult one—made all the more difficult by the seeming impossibility of finding one that met all Mrs. Casey's needs, which is why the decision took a long time.

PRINCIPLE 19. USE COMMAS CORRECTLY WHEN YOU PUNCTUATE

Use commas to separate items in a series. If three or more items are listed in a series, separate them with commas; the final comma—the one that precedes the word *and*—is optional.

CORRECT: My recipe for buttermilk biscuits contains flour, baking soda, salt, shortening, and buttermilk.

TEACHER TIP

Punctuation is just a visual way to tell the reader when to breathe and "lower the voice." A comma says, "take a short breath but don't stop; this is really a single sentence." Read the sentence to yourself. If you take a quick pause between phrases, that's where you put a comma. If you read it all in one breath, you don't.

CORRECT: My recipe for chocolate cake contains flour, baking soda, sugar, eggs, milk and chocolate.

Do not place commas before the first element of a series or after the last element.

INCORRECT: My investment advisor recommended that I construct a portfolio of, stocks, bonds, commodities futures, and precious metals.
INCORRECT: The elephants, tigers, and dancing bears, were the highlights of the circus parade.

Use commas to separate two or more adjectives before a noun; do not use a comma after the last adjective in the series.

CORRECT: I can't believe you sat through that long, dull, uninspired movie three times.
INCORRECT: The manatee is a round, blubbery, bewhiskered, creature whose continued presence in American waters is endangered by careless boaters.

Use commas to set off parenthetical clauses and phrases. (A parenthetical expression is one that is not necessary to the main idea of the sentence.)

CORRECT: Gordon, who is a writer by profession, bakes an excellent cheesecake.

The main idea is that Gordon bakes an excellent cheesecake. The intervening clause merely serves to identify Gordon; thus, it should be set off with commas.

CORRECT: The newspaper that has the most insipid editorials is the Daily Times.
CORRECT: The newspaper, which has the most insipid editorials of any I have read, won numerous awards last week.

In the first of these examples the clause beginning with *that* defines which paper the author is discussing. In the second example, the main point is that the newspaper won numerous awards, the intervening clause beginning with *which* identifies the paper.

Use commas after introductory participial or prepositional phrases.

CORRECT: Having watered his petunias every day during the drought, Harold was very disappointed when his garden was destroyed by insects.
CORRECT: After the banquet, Harold and Martha went dancing.

Use commas to separate independent clauses (clauses that could stand alone as complete sentences) connected by a coordinate conjunction such as *and, but, not, yet,* etc.

CORRECT: Susan's old car has been belching blue smoke from the tail-pipe for two weeks, but it has not broken down yet.
CORRECT: Zachariah's pet frog eats 50 flies a day, yet it has never gotten indigestion.

Make sure the comma separates two independent clauses, each containing its own subject and verb. It is incorrect to use a comma to separate the two parts of a compound verb.

INCORRECT: Barbara went to the grocery store, and bought two quarts of milk.
INCORRECT: Zachariah's pet frog eats 50 flies a day, and never gets indigestion.

TEACHER TIP

Read these sentences to yourself. Do you take a breath between the clauses? No? Then the comma shouldn't be there.

EXERCISE FOR PRINCIPLE 19: COMMAS

Correct the punctuation errors in the following sentences.

1. Peter wants me to bring records games candy and soda to his party.
2. I need, lumber, nails, a hammer and a saw to build the shelf.
3. It takes a friendly energetic person to be a successful salesman.
4. I was shocked to discover that a large, modern, glass-sheathed, office building had replaced my old school.
5. The country club, a cluster of ivy-covered whitewashed buildings was the site of the president's first speech.
6. As we entered the park, a police officer clad in a crisp, well-starched uniform directed us to the theater.
7. Pushing through the panicked crowd the security guards frantically searched for the suspect.
8. Despite careful analysis of the advantages and disadvantages of each proposal Harry found it hard to reach a decision.

Teacher Tip

Think about how you would read the sentences below. Do you take a breath between clauses? Yes. Is it a short or long breath? Well, it's longer than a comma but shorter than a period. OK, that's the place to use a semicolon.

PRINCIPLE 20. USE SEMICOLONS CORRECTLY WHEN YOU PUNCTUATE

Use a semicolon instead of a coordinate conjunction such as *and, or*, or *but* to link two closely related independent clauses.

CORRECT: Whooping cranes are an endangered species; there are only 50 whooping cranes in New Jersey today.
CORRECT: Whooping cranes are an endangered species, and they are unlikely to survive if we continue to pollute.
INCORRECT: Whooping cranes are an endangered species; and they are unlikely to survive if we continue to pollute.

Use a semicolon between independent clauses connected by words like *therefore, nevertheless,* and *moreover.*

CORRECT: The staff meeting has been postponed until next Thursday; therefore, I will be unable to get approval for my project until then.
CORRECT: Farm prices have been falling rapidly for two years; nevertheless, the traditional American farm is not in danger of disappearing.

EXERCISE FOR PRINCIPLE 20: SEMICOLONS

1. Morgan has five years' experience in karate; but Thompson has even more.
2. Very few students wanted to take the class in physics, only the professor's kindness kept it from being canceled.
3. You should always be prepared when you go on a camping trip, however you must avoid carrying unnecessary weight.

Teacher Tip

If a comma means "take a short breath" and a semi-colon means "take a longer breath," a colon means "take a good breath—a list follows and you need to read it all without gasping."

PRINCIPLE 21. USE THE COLON CORRECTLY WHEN YOU PUNCTUATE

In formal writing the colon is used only as a means of signaling that what follows is a list, definition, explanation, or concise summary of what has gone before. The colon usually follows an independent clause, and it will frequently be accompanied by a reinforcing expression like *the following, as follows,* or *namely,* or by an explicit demonstrative like *this.*

CORRECT: Your instructions are as follows: read the passage carefully, answer the questions on the last page, and turn over your answer sheet.
CORRECT: This is what I found in the refrigerator: a moldy lime, half a bottle of stale soda, and a jar of peanut butter.

CORRECT: The biggest problem with America today is apathy: the corrosive element that will destroy our democracy.

Be careful not to separate a verb from its direct object with a colon.

INCORRECT: I want: a slice of pizza and a small green salad.
CORRECT: This is what I want: a slice of pizza and a small green salad. (The colon serves to announce that a list is forthcoming.)
CORRECT: I don't want much for lunch: just a slice of pizza and a small green salad. (Here, what follows the colon defines what "don't want much" means.)

Context will occasionally make clear that a second independent clause is closely linked to its predecessor, even without an explicit expression like those used above. Here, too, a colon is appropriate, although a period will always be correct as well.

CORRECT: We were aghast: the "charming country inn" that had been advertised in such glowing terms proved to be a leaking cabin full of mosquitoes.
CORRECT: We were aghast. The "charming country inn" that had been advertised in such glowing terms proved to be a leaking cabin full of mosquitoes.

EXERCISE FOR PRINCIPLE 21: COLONS

Repair the following sentences with colons as appropriate.

1. I am sick and tired of: your whining, your complaining, your nagging, your teasing, and most of all, your barbed comments.
2. The chef has created a masterpiece, the pasta is delicate yet firm, the mustard greens are fresh, and the medallions of veal are melting in my mouth.
3. In order to write a good essay, you must: get plenty of sleep, eat a good breakfast, and practice until you drop.

PRINCIPLE 22. USE HYPHENS AND DASHES CORRECTLY WHEN YOU PUNCTUATE

Use the hyphen to separate a word at the end of a line.

Use the hyphen with the compound numbers twenty-one to ninety-nine, and with fractions used as adjectives.

TEACHER TIP

If you must separate a word at the end of a line, be sure it's separated at a syllable. You can write "may-be," separating the word between syllables, but not "ma-ybe," which doesn't look like a word at all.

CORRECT: Sixty-five students constituted a majority.
CORRECT: A two-thirds vote was necessary to carry the measure.

Use the hyphen with the prefixes *ex, all,* and *self* and with the suffix *elect.*

CORRECT: The constitution protects against self-incrimination.
CORRECT: The President-elect was invited to chair the meeting.

Use the hyphen with a compound adjective when it comes *before* the word it modifies, but not when it comes after the word it modifies. In other words, if you're using two adjectives to modify the same noun, put a hyphen between the adjectives. That makes a well-punctuated sentence.

CORRECT: The no-holds-barred argument continued into the night.
CORRECT: The argument continued with no holds barred.

Use the hyphen with any prefix used before a proper noun or adjective.

CORRECT: His pro-African sentiments were heartily applauded.
CORRECT: They believed that his activities were un-American.

Use a hyphen to separate component parts of a word in order to avoid confusion with other words or to avoid the use of a double vowel.

CORRECT: The sculptor was able to re-form the clay after the dog knocked over the bust.
CORRECT: They had to be reintroduced, since it had been so long since they last met.

Use the dash to indicate an abrupt change of thought. In general, however, formal writing is best when you think out what you want to say in advance and avoid abrupt changes of thought. Though the dash indicates a new thought, the thought is closely related to what came before. It's just another way of modifying a phrase.

CORRECT: The inheritance must cover the entire cost of the proposal—Gail has no other money to invest.
CORRECT: To get a high score—and who doesn't want to get a high score—you need to devote yourself to prolonged and concentrated study.

EXERCISE FOR PRINCIPLE 22: HYPHENS AND DASHES

Repair the following sentences with hyphens and dashes as appropriate.

1. The child was able to count from 1 to ninety nine.
2. The adults only movie was banned from commercial TV.
3. It was the first time she had seen a movie that was for adults-only.
4. John and his ex wife remained on friendly terms.
5. A two thirds majority would be needed to pass the budget reforms.
6. The house, and it was the most dilapidated house that I had ever seen was a bargain because the land was so valuable.

PRINCIPLE 23. USE THE APOSTROPHE CORRECTLY WHEN YOU PUNCTUATE

Use the apostrophe with contracted forms of verbs to indicate that one or more letters have been eliminated in writing (just as sounds have been eliminated or shortened in speaking).

FULL FORMS	CONTRACTED
you are	you're
it is	it's
you have	you've
the boy is	the boy's
Harry has	Harry's
we would	we'd
was not	wasn't

TEACHER TIP

Know the difference between "its" and " it's." Many people don't, but these are basic spelling rules. Poor spelling has no place in an MCAT student's adult writing.

One of the most common errors involving use of the apostrophe is using it in the contraction *you're* or *it's* to indicate the possessive form of *you* or *it*. When you write *you're*, ask yourself whether you mean *you are*. If not, the correct word is *your*. Similarly, are you sure you mean *it is*? If not, use the possessive form *its*.

INCORRECT: You're chest of drawers is ugly.
CORRECT: Your chest of drawers is ugly.
INCORRECT: The dog hurt it's paw.
CORRECT: The dog hurt its paw.

Use the apostrophe to indicate the possessive form of a noun.

NOT POSSESSIVE

the boy	Harry	the children	the boys

POSSESSIVE

the boy's	Harry's	the children's	the boys'

Note: The word *boy's* could have one of three meanings:

- The boy's an expert at chess. (The boy is . . .)
- The boy's left for the day. (The boy has . . .)
- The boy's face was covered with pie. (possessive: the face of the boy)

The word *boys'* can have only one meaning: a plural possessive (the . . . of the boys).

CORRECT: I caught a glimpse of the fox's red tail as the hunters sped by. (The *'s* ending indicates that one fox is the owner of the tail.)
CORRECT: Ms. Fox's office is on the first floor. (One person possesses the office.)
CORRECT: The Foxes' apartment has a wonderful view. (There are several people named Fox living in the same apartment. First you must form the plural, then add the apostrophe to indicate possession.)

The apostrophe indicates possession only with nouns; in the case of pronouns, there are separate possessives for each person and number.

- my, mine
- our, ours
- your, yours
- his, his
- their, theirs
- her, hers
- its, its

The exception is the neutral "one," which forms its possessive by adding an apostrophe and an s.

EXERCISES FOR PRINCIPLE 23: APOSTROPHES

Insert or delete appropriate apostrophes as needed in the following sentences or change the possessive word if incorrect.

1. The Presidents limousine had a flat tire.
2. You're tickets for the show will be at the box office.
3. The opportunity to change ones lifestyle does not come often.
4. The desks' surface was immaculate, but it's drawers were messy.
5. The cat on the bed is hers'.

LIST OF COMMONLY MISUSED WORDS

This list includes common diction errors and common idiomatic errors. A diction error results from use of a word whose meaning does not fit in a particular context. Often the word that is needed and the word that is misused sound or look alike (e.g., affect/effect).

Idioms are established and accepted expressions. An idiomatic error usually involves use of the wrong preposition (*different than* versus *different from*).

accept/except	To *accept* is to willingly receive; to *except* is to omit or exclude. **Example:** Peter was *accepted* by the college because, if you *except* his failing grades in two courses, his academic record is excellent. **NOTE:** *Except* is usually used as a preposition meaning "with the exception of. **Example**: I'll be home every day except Friday, when I have a dance class.
adapt/adopt	To *adapt* is to change something to make it suitable for a certain purpose; to *adopt* is to make something one's own. **Example:** *To Have and Have Not* was adapted for the screen by William Faulkner. **Example:** The Robinsons have *adopted* a baby.
affect/effect	To *affect* is to influence or change; to *effect* is to cause or to make (something) happen. **Examples:** The size of the harvest was *affected* by the lack of rainfall. The medicine Allen took *effected* a rapid recovery. **NOTE:** *Effect* is usually used as a noun meaning "influence." **Example:** The illegible signs on this road have a bad *effect* on safety.
allusion/ delusion/illusion	An *allusion* is an indirect reference; a *delusion* is something that is falsely believed; an *illusion* is a false, misleading, or deceptive appearance. **Examples:** Mr. Harmon fills his talk with *allusions* to literature and art to create the *illusion* that he is very learned. He has *delusions* that he is quite a scholar.

among/between	In most cases, you should use *between* for two items and *among* for more than two. There are exceptions, however; *among* tends to be used for less definite or exact relationships. **Examples:** The competition *between* Anne and Fred has grown more intense. He is always at his best *among* strangers. BUT: Plant the trees *between* the road, the wall, and the fence.
amount/number	*Amount* should be used to refer to a singular or non-countable word; *number* should be used to refer to a countable quantity. **Examples:** The *amount* of cloth on the bolt was enough for several suits. I was not sure of the *number* of yards of cloth on the bolt.
another/ the other	*Another* refers to any other; *the other* is more specific; it refers to one particular other. **Examples:** Put *another* log on the fire (any one). Put *the other* log on the fire (the last one). The men were passing the pipe from one to the other (two men, back and forth). They passed the pipe from one to *another* (three or more).
as/like	*Like* is a preposition; it introduces a prepositional phrase. Remember, a phrase is a group of words that does not contain a subject and verb; *as,* when functioning as a conjunction, introduces a subordinate clause. Remember, a clause is a part of a sentence containing a subject and verb. **Examples:** She sings *like* an angel. She sings as an angel sings.
as . . . as . . .	The idiom is *as . . . . as. . . .* **Example:** That suit is as expensive as (NOT *than*) this one.
assure/ensure/ insure	To *ensure* is to make certain, safe, or secure; to *insure* is to provide for financial payment in case of loss; to *assure* is to inform positively. **Example:** Mr. Green *assured* his mother-in-law that he had *insured* his life for $30,000 to *ensure* that his wife would not suffer poverty if he died.

because	To say "the reason is *because* . . . " is considered ungrammatical in formal English. Use *that* instead. **Examples:** The reason I'm late is that my car refused to start. OR: I'm late *because* my car refused to start.
beside/besides	*Beside* means "next to" something; *besides* means "in addition to." **Examples:** She sat *beside* me at the basketball game. *Besides* the basketball team, there were only three other people in the gym.
between . . . and . . .	The idiom is *between . . . and . . .* **Example:** Call *between* five *and* (NOT *to*) six o'clock. He chose *between* meat *and* (NOT *or*) fish.
criteria/data	These are *plural* nouns that are often mistakenly used as singular nouns. **Examples:** One *criterion* (not *criteria*) for employment in this company is a willingness to work with surly people. The recently collected *data prove* (NOT *proves*) our original hypothesis was correct.
different from	*Different* is usually used with the preposition *from,* usually not with *than.* **Example:** Frank's attitude is *different from* Charlie's. **NOTE:** Remember that you say *differ from*, never *differ than. Differ* can also be used with *with.* **Example:** On that issue, I *differ with* you.
each other/ one another	In formal writing, *each other* is used to refer to two things, and *one another* is used for three or more. **Examples:** Len and Amy love each other. Those three theories contradict one another.
eminent/ imminent/ immanent	*Eminent* means prominent or outstanding; *imminent* means likely to happen soon, impending; *immanent* means existing within, intrinsic. **Examples:** The whole school was excited about the *imminent* arrival of the *eminent* scientist. Scrooge was characterized by *immanent* selfishness.

fewer/less	Use *fewer* before a plural noun, *less* before a singular one. **Examples:** This amazing product contains *less* fat, *less* salt, and *fewer* calories.
if/whether	*If* is used in conditional clauses. **Examples:** *If* I have the money, I will go. I do not know *whether* to go. (Nothing is conditional in this sentence.)
imply/infer	To *imply* is to state or indicate indirectly; to *infer* is to deduce or conclude. Authors and speakers *imply;* readers and listeners *infer.* **Examples:** Pete sarcastically *implied* that he was angry. Joe *inferred* from Mary's dejected look that she had failed the exam.
ingenious/ ingenuous	*Ingenious* means intelligent, clever, or resourceful; *ingenuous* means innocent, naive, or simple. **Examples:** The thief entered the bank vault by means of an *ingenious* magnetic device. Alice is so *ingenuous* that she refuses to believe anyone would deliberately do harm.
irregardless	The correct word is *regardless,* regardless of the context.
its/it's	*It's* is a contraction of it is; *its* is a possessive pronoun meaning something belongs to it. **Examples:** *It's* obvious that something is wrong with that dog; *it's* whining and chewing its paw. (Hint: During proofreading, if you have written *it's*, ask yourself, "Does this mean *it is* in the sentence?" If so, write out *it is*. If not, remove the apostrophe.)
maybe	Don't use *maybe* to modify an adjective or other adverb. **Example:** That is a potentially (NOT *maybe a*) dangerous thing to do.
neither . . . nor	The correlative conjunction is neither . . . nor, not neither . . . or. **Example:** He is *neither* strong *nor* flexible.

	NOTE: Avoid the redundancy caused by *neither . . . nor* following a negative. **Example:** Unnoticed by Debby or Sue (not *neither* Debby *nor* Sue), Naomi left.
not only . . . but (also)	If you use *not only,* it must be followed by *but;* the word *also* is optional. The words following *not only* must be parallel to the words following *but also.* **Example:** The book is not only fascinating, but also instructive.
number	*The number* should be followed by a singular verb; *a number* by a plural. **Examples:** *The number* of errors in his statement is astounding. *A number* of us are going camping.
regard as	*Regard as* is the correct idiom; *regard to be* is wrong. **Example:** I regard you *as* (NOT *to be*) a close friend.
to be able	Do not use a form of *to be able* preceding the passive form of an infinitive. **Example:** My old television cannot (NOT *is not able to*) be repaired. **NOTE:** *Is not able to* is wrong because it implies the TV lacks ability; it's the TV repairer who lacks ability. **Example:** He *is not able to* repair the TV.
when/where	Do not use *when* or *where* in a definition, or where *that* would be more appropriate. **Examples:** A convention is a meeting of people with something in common. (NOT *a convention is where a number of people . . .*). A diagram is a sketch *that* illustrates (NOT *is when a sketch is made to illustrate . . .*) the parts of something. I read *that* (NOT *where*) you had to leave town. Also, do not use *where* when you mean *when,* and vice versa. **Example:** She moved to New York in 1970, *when* (NOT *where*) she left for college.
that/which	These two words are used interchangeably, though rules govern when to use each of them appropriately. (See Principle 15.)

their/they're/ there — *Their* is a possessive pronoun meaning something belonging to them; *they're* is a contraction of *they are*; *there* means *that place* (among other things)
Examples: *They're* placing *their* bets over *there* at the race track, but *there's* no chance they will win *their* money back.

DEFINITIONS

subject — Who or what the sentence is about.
Example: The author embraces an idealistic philosophy. (Who or what embraces? *The author* embraces.)

verb — The part of the sentence that expresses an action or state of being of the subject.
Example: The author embraces an idealistic philosophy. (The author is what or does what? The author *embraces.*)

---

sentence — A group of words that expresses a complete thought; it must contain a SUBJECT and a VERB.
Example: DOGS BARK.
Example: The EXPLORERS SLEPT in a tent.

sentence fragment — A group of words that purports to be a sentence but lacks either a subject or a verb or some element necessary to make the sentence a complete thought.
Example: Shrimp and cod on sale at the fish market. (This "sentence" lacks a verb.)

run-on sentence — Two or more complete sentences connected with just a comma or with no punctuation at all.
Example: Sushi bores me, on the other hand teriyaki is one of my favorite dishes.

---

clause — A group of words that contains a subject and a verb.

phrase — A group of words that does not have a subject and a verb.
Example: Considering the weather, I think I'll stay indoors.
Considering the weather = clause
I think I'll stay indoors = phrase

relative clause	A clause beginning with a relative pronoun—*who, whom, that,* or *which.* The pronoun relates the information in the clause to the noun immediately preceding it. **Example:** This group, *which* has made a vocation of proving other people wrong, offers nothing positive to the world. **Example:** Those people, *whom* I have been calling all day, never returned my phone calls.
subordinate conjunction	A word or phrase that connects a dependent clause to a main, or independent, clause. **Example:** *Although* scientists argue that wearing a helmet reduces the risk of dying in a motorcycle accident, many riders choose to ride without a helmet.
participle	A word usually ending in *-ing* or *-ed.* They look like verbs but are used as adjectives. They are often found in modifying phrases. **Example:** The *pouring* rain depresses me. **Example:** *Looking* through the window, I watch the rain pouring into the gutters. (*Looking through the window* is a participial phrase modifying *I.*)
preposition	Word used to show the relationship of a *noun* or *pronoun* to another part of the sentence. **Example:** The author suggests that man cannot live *by* bread alone.
prepositional phrase	A phrase beginning with a preposition. Be careful with subject-verb agreement when a prepositional phrase intervenes. (In this sentence, *with subject-verb agreement* is a prepositional phrase.) **Example:** A group *of six German men* is taking the train to Belgium this afternoon.
Modifier	A word or phrase that qualifies the meaning of another word by making it more definite. A modifier can be a word (an adjective or an adverb) or a phrase (participial, adverbial, adjectival, or prepositional). The modifier should be placed as near as possible to the thing being modified. A modifying phrase that begins a sentence refers to the noun or subjective case pronoun immediately following the phrase.

referent	The word or phrase to which the modifier refers.
misplaced modifier	A modifier that seems to modify the wrong part of a sentence. **Example:** Misplaced modifier: She served cookies to the ladies *arranged on her best china.* Correctly placed modifier: She served cookies *arranged on her best china* to the ladies. (It is the cookies that are on the china, not the ladies.)
noun	A word that names a person, place, thing, event, or idea. **Example:** *Tolerance* is a *virtue* that few *people,* not even *Diane,* discuss these *days.*
antecedent	The noun to which a pronoun refers. **Example:** *Tolerance* is not discussed these days; *it* demands too much hard work to be a popular virtue.
adverb	A word that modifies a verb, an adjective, or another adverb. **Example:** She *lovingly* patted her dog on the head, before throwing him a very fine bone.
adjective or adjectival phrase	A word or phrase that modifies or describes a noun or pronoun. (You can ask, "What kind of ______ is it?") **Example:** One *excellent* example of bureaucratic ineptitude is the fact that I received my *office* fan in January. (What kind of example is it? It is an *excellent* example.) **Example:** The cheesecake, *which won the prize at the county fair for three consecutive years,* turned out to be an import from a New York bakery. (The underlined phrase describes the noun *cheesecake.*)

Part III
Verbal Reasoning and Essay Practice Sections

This section features three 40-question Verbal Reasoning practice sections with detailed answer explanations and four essay prompts with sample student essays and reader evaluations.

To help you see the Kaplan strategies in action, we have walked you through mapping and analysis of the first three passages in Verbal Reasoning Practice Section 1.

Follow along with your instructor to see the key words and phrases in each of the first three passages, the mapping techniques used, and how you can use the question type and the answer choices to lead you to the right answers. Then, for the remainder of section 1 and then all of sections 2 and 3, you're on your own!

Before taking each practice section or writing your essay, find a quiet place where you can work without interruption.

Good luck!

VERBAL REASONING PRACTICE SECTION 1

Time—60 minutes

DIRECTIONS: There are seven passages in this Verbal Reasoning test. Each passage is followed by several questions. After reading a passage, select the one best answer to each question. If you are not certain of an answer, eliminate the alternatives that you know to be incorrect and then select an answer from the remaining alternatives. Indicate your selection by blackening the corresponding circle on your answer sheet.

PASSAGE 1 (QUESTIONS 1–5)

Gautier was indeed a poet and a strongly representative one—a French poet in his limitations even more than in his gifts; and he remains an interesting example of the manner in which, even when the former are surprisingly great, a happy application of the latter may produce the most delightful works. Completeness on his own scale is to our mind the idea he most instantly suggests. Such as his finished task now presents him, *he is almost sole of his kind.* He has had imitators who have imitated everything but his spontaneity and his temper; and as they have therefore failed to equal him we doubt whether the literature of our day presents a genius so naturally perfect. We say this with no desire to transfer Gautier to a higher pedestal than he has fairly earned—a poor service, for the pedestal sometimes sadly dwarfs the figure. His great merit was that he *understood himself so perfectly and handled himself so skillfully.* Even more than Alfred de Musset (with whom the speech had a shade of mock-modesty) he might have said that, if his glass was not large, as least it was all his own glass.

TEACHER TIP

NOTE: We've used italics to indicate the important sentences in the paragraph.

TEACHER TIP

Map of Paragraph 1: **Gautier was a flawed poet, but was nevertheless unique and talented.** This is all you need to map the entire paragraph. Don't worry about what words you use to map; there's no such thing as a perfect map. Just use the words that make sense to you.

TEACHER TIP

To compare or not to compare? Who knows? Just recognize that it's something the author is dealing with.

There are a host of reasons why we should not compare Gautier with such a poet as Browning; and yet there are several why we should. If we do so, with all proper reserva-tions, we may wonder whether we are the richer, or, at all events, the better entertained, as a poet's readers should before all things be, by the clear, undiluted strain of Gautier's minor key, or by the vast, grossly commingled volume of utterance. It is idle at all times to point a moral. *But if there are sermons in stones, there are profitable reflections to be made even on Théophile Gautier; notably this one—that a man's supreme use in the world is to master his intellectual instrument and play it in perfection.*

Teacher Tip

Map of Paragraph 2: **Gautier was able to be uniquely himself in his poetry.** Compare with others? The question asked at the end of this paragraph map (compare?) indicates that the reader knows there's a comparison being written about but isn't sure exactly what the author is saying. Just noting the words, with the question mark, means "there's something in here about a comparison but I don't understand it." That's perfectly okay.

He brought to his task a sort of pagan bonhomie which makes most of the descriptive and pictorial poets seem, by contrast, a group of shivering ascetics or muddled metaphysicians. He excels them by *his magnificent good temper and the unquestioning serenity of his enjoyment of the great spectacle of nature and art.* His world was all material, and its outlying darkness hardly more suggestive, morally, than a velvet canopy studded with silver nails. To close his eyes and turn his back on it must have seemed to him the end of all things; death, for him, must have been as the sullen dropping of a stone into a well. His observation was so penetrating and his descriptive instinct so unerring, that one might have fancied grave nature, in a fit of coquetry, or tired of receiving but half-justice, had determined to construct a genius with senses of a finer strain than the mass of human family.

Teacher Tip

Pagan bonhomie? What does that mean? It's such a unique phrase that you should probably note it in the map even if you don't understand it.

Teacher Tip

Map of Paragraph 3: **Gautier was interested in life and nature.** Good temper? Pagan bonhomie? Here are phrases with question marks again. Remember, even though you've put them into a map, you don't have to really understand them unless there's a question on them. If there is, you'll go back to the passage anyway, so you get another shot at understanding the words.

1. In the passage, the author suggests that the French poet Théophile Gautier's talents included all of the following EXCEPT:

A. an innovative and unique artistic view of nature.

B. the ability to quickly and immediately compose poetry.

C. extensive training in rhetorical and literary techniques.

D. a strong understanding of his world and himself.

TEACHER TIP

This is a scattered detail question so you're going to have to look carefully at your map to determine which paragraph each answer is in. Then be even more careful researching the paragraphs.

TEACHER TIP

With an "everything except" question, it's easier to look for the three answers which are in the paragraph rather than the one that isn't. How can you find something that isn't there?

2. For what purpose can it reasonably be concluded does the author reference other writers in this passage, including Musset and Browning?

A. To prove that Gautier, as a poet, was unique among his contemporaries

B. To show that Gautier's poetry was representative of French lyricism at the time

C. To criticize Gautier's limited talent and creativity

D. To refute the idea that Gautier's colleagues could easily imitate his style

TEACHER TIP

This function question is really asking why the author refers to other poets.

3. Which of the following, if true, would most weaken the author's conclusion that Gautier's artistic gifts more than compensated for his creative limitations?

A. Gautier's poems are still studied more frequently than any of his prose writing.

B. Close study of Gautier's life has revealed that he frequently collaborated with other writers.

C. During the early 1800s, Gautier's primary success came from his critical reviews of art.

D. Numerous later writers acknowledged Gautier's work as an influence on their writing.

TEACHER TIP

This is a lovely question because the testmaker has given you the author's point of view: Gautier's gifts compensated for his limitations. To weaken this, just find some evidence that says no, the gifts don't compensate.

4. As used in the passage, the words "pagan bonhomie" (in the first sentence of the last paragraph) refer to:

   A. Gautier's extravagant and debauched lifestyle as revealed through his poetry.
   B. the unique descriptions of nature that are essential to Gautier's work.
   C. Gautier's lack of modesty and his desire for lasting notoriety.
   D. a particular attitude towards the world that set Gautier apart from his contemporaries.

Teacher Tip

Didn't you just know that you'd get a question on this? But don't worry. This time you don't have to figure out what it means, you just have to choose from four possibilities. Your map mentioned nature and good temper. Look for an answer that has something to do with those attributes.

5. Without regard for what other critics of the genre might purport, according to the passage, what is the primary reaction a reader should have to poetry?

   A. Poetry should produce a strong emotional response within the reader.
   B. A reader should enjoy and be entertained by poetry.
   C. Readers should learn a moral, social, or political lesson from poetry.
   D. Poetry should provide readers with ideas that are relevant to their own lives.

Teacher Tip

You didn't map anything about readers' reactions to poetry, so how will you find them? Quickly scan the passage for reference to those reactions—you'll find it in paragraph 2. When you're scanning for a word, phrase or idea, be sure to start from the top. If you start scanning from the middle of the passage (and many people do) you'll miss anything above the middle, and the answer you want could be at the very beginning.

PASSAGE 2 (QUESTIONS 6–12)

The study of the analog position of mental representation has many fascinating branches which help illuminate the inner workings of our minds and how we perceive images in our mind's eye. This theory points to the link between the time it takes to solve mental problems and their complexity.

In a now-famous study, Stephen Kosslyn asked subjects to imagine an animal, such as a rabbit, next to either an elephant or a fly. When the image was formed, Kosslyn would ask whether or not the target animal had a particular attribute. For example, Kosslyn

Teacher Tip

This time there are no italicized sentences, so see if you can identify the important ideas in each paragraph and put them in your map.

Teacher Tip

Map for Paragraph 1: **Intro analog position idea—how long it takes to solve problems depends on their complexity.**

might say, “elephant, rabbit,” and then “leg.” He found that it took subjects longer to answer when the target animal was next to the large animal than when it was next to the small animal. Kosslyn interpreted this to mean that subjects had to zoom in on the image to detect the particular feature. Just as one has difficulty seeing details on small objects, so the subjects could not simply mentally “see” details on the smaller object in their mental image.

Second, Kosslyn and colleagues demonstrated that the time it takes to scan between two points depends on the distance between the two points [in a memorized image]. In one experiment, subjects memorized an array of letters separated by different distances. Kosslyn found that the farther apart the letters were from each other, the longer it took to answer questions about one of the letters. One of the principal hypotheses of the analog position of mental representation, which is the idea that mental processing requires one to move sequentially through all intervening steps to solve a problem, is that mental images have regular properties. In a similar experiment, Kosslyn had subjects memorize pictures of objects like a plane or a motorboat. Then he had them focus on one part of the object (e.g., the motor) and move to another (e.g., the anchor).

He found that the time it took to determine whether the second part was present depended on the distance between the two parts in the memorized picture. In one of his more famous experiments of this type, Kosslyn and colleagues had subjects memorize the location of various objects (such as a hut or a tree) on a fictional map. Subjects were

TEACHER TIP

Map for Paragraph 2: **Kosslyn's 1st experiment—mind's reaction to relative sizes of mental images.**

TEACHER TIP

Always jot down names not only because they make excellent clues as to where to find things in the passage, but also because many questions refer not to theories or studies themselves but to the names of the people involved.

TEACHER TIP

Map for Paragraph 3: **K's 2nd experiment—longer distances of mental images=longer time to answer questions.**

then told to focus on one object and then scan the image to determine whether another object was or was not on the map. The amount of time it took to locate objects that were present on the memorized map was linearly related to the distance between the objects.

TEACHER TIP

Map for Paragraph 4: **more of 2nd experiment re: distance in mental images. Same result.**

Using a completely different paradigm, Shepard and Feng tested the amount of time that it would take for subjects to specify whether two arrows on unfolded blocks matched up. They found a linear relationship between the number of folds between the arrows and the time it took to make this judgment, suggesting that subjects went through a discrete series of organized steps in order to solve this problem.

TEACHER TIP

Map for Paragraph 5: **Shep/Feng study with folds and arrow. To solve, need to think through a series of steps.**

The final type of experiment showing that mental images have regular properties is perhaps the most famous: mental rotation experiments. In 1971, Shepard and Metzler tested subjects' abilities to make complex figure comparisons. They presented subjects with a three-dimensional "standard" figure and a comparison figure which was either identical to the standard figure or its mirror image; the comparison stimulus was rotated, either clockwise or into the third dimension. Shepard and Metzler found that the time needed to judge whether the comparison stimulus was identical or a mirror image depended directly on the size of the angle between the target orientation and the orientation of the standard.

TEACHER TIP

Map for Paragraph 6:- **4th experiment. Shep/Metzler. Time needed to mentally compare figures depends on how similar those figures initially look.**

6. According to the way it is presented by the author in the passage, the analog position of mental representation argues that:

   A. mental processing requires one to go sequentially through all intervening steps to solve a problem.
   B. one typically uses short cuts to solve mental problems.
   C. it should take longer to solve more complex problems.
   D. most problems are not able to be solved by people without help.

TEACHER TIP

This is a straightforward detail question (the words "according to" tell you that) and should immediately send you back to the map and passage to research the detail.

7. According to the scanning experiments mentioned in the passage, it should take longer to scan longer distances because the subjects:

   A. believe that there is no relationship between distance and time.
   B. have to keep time with a metronome set up by the experimenter.
   C. form a mental picture of the scene and go through all the intervening positions in the picture.
   D. are tricked by the experimenter into taking a longer time.

8. Which of the following conclusions not presented in the passage might be an alternate explanation for the map experiments described by the author?

   A. Subjects forget where the objects are.
   B. Subjects know that it should take longer to move longer distances and so answer accordingly.
   C. Subjects consult actual maps for the distances and this takes them more time the greater the distance.
   D. It takes subjects longer to start scanning longer distances and so it ultimately takes them longer to finish.

TEACHER TIP

Don't get nervous when you see an unusually worded question. For the most part, all questions on the MCAT will fall into one or another of the question catagories you learned about earlier. Consider which category this would fall into, then check it out with the explanation.

9. According to the passage, why does Kosslyn say it takes longer to identify attributes of objects when they are next to a bigger object than when they are next to a smaller object?

A. Because one scans objects in order of size from larger to smaller

B. Because the larger object covers the smaller object and one must move it out of the way

C. Because large and small objects have all the same features and so interfere with each other

D. Because one must "zoom in" to see parts of the smaller object when it is next to a larger object

TEACHER TIP

There are lots of detail questions with this passage, aren't there? That's because the passage is fact-, rather than author-driven. Since there's no real author opinion—the author is neutral, as the purpose verb "describe" indicates—most questions will relate to the facts in the passage instead.

10. If it were the case that subjects simply respond as the experimenters encourage them to do, based on information in the passage one would expect:

A. that the pattern of results would be just as they are.

B. that there would be a non-linear relationship between distance and reaction time.

C. that the relationship between distance and reaction time is constant.

D. that one could create any relationship between distance and reaction time.

11. Based on the passage, which of the following patterns of results would contradict the analog position?

I. It takes longer to scan longer distances.

II. There is no relationship between scanning time and distance.

III. It takes less time to scan longer distances.

A. I only

B. II and III

C. I and III

D. I, II, and III

TEACHER TIP

There are two ways to do this Roman-numeral question. You can simply start with one of the Roman-numeral answers and check it out with the passage, or you can look at A, B, C, and D and see if any one Roman numeral shows up most. Start with that last one.

12. Other researchers have found that subjects can alter the amount of time it takes to scan images based on the instructions they are given. What implications does this have for the analog view?

A. It implies that the analog view is more likely to be correct since subjects are scanning as they believe they should.
B. It implies that the analog view is more likely to be correct since subjects do not have control over the rate at which they scan.
C. It implies that the analog view is less likely to be correct because subjects might be scanning as they believe they should.
D. It implies that the analog view is more likely to be correct since subjects can control the rate at which they scan.

PASSAGE 3 (QUESTIONS 13–18)

Never accept anything as true that you do not clearly know to be so; that is, carefully avoid jumping to conclusions, and include nothing in judgments, other than what presents itself so clearly and distinctly to the spirit that you would never have any occasion to doubt it. Then, divide each of the difficulties being examined into as many parts as can be created and would be required to better resolve them. Order your thoughts, by starting with the simplest ideas, which are the easiest to comprehend, to advance little by little, by degrees, up to the most complex ideas, even believing that an order exists among those which do not naturally follow one another. And last, always make deductions so complete, and reviews so general, so as to be assured of omitting nothing.

When I was younger, I had studied a bit—in the field of philosophy, logic, and in the field of math, geometric analysis and algebra—the three arts or sciences that seemed as though

TEACHER TIP

The full map for this passage is at the very end. Start to work out your maps on their own without step-by-step guidance, then check to see how on-point you are!

they should contribute something to my methodological approach.

But while examining these fields, I noticed that, in logic, syllogisms and the bulk of other logical theorems serve only to explain to others the things that one already knows, or even to speak without judgment of things that one doesn't know, rather than to teach others anything; and, although logic contains, in effect, many true and just precepts, there are yet among these so many others mixed in, which are superfluous or refutable, that it is almost sickening to separate one from the other.

As for geometric analysis and modern algebra, in addition to the fact that they don't treat anything except abstract ideas, which seem to be of no use whatsoever, geometry is always so restricted to the consideration of figures that it can't stretch the intellect without exhausting the imagination; and algebra subjects one to certain rules and numbers, so that it has become a confused and obscure art that troubles the spirit rather than a science that cultivates it.

All of this made me think that it was necessary to look for some other methodological approach which, comprising the advantages of these three, was at the same time exempt from their defaults. And, just as the multitude of laws often provides rationalization for vice, such that any State is better ruled if, having but a few vices, it closely monitors them, thus likewise, instead of following the great number of precepts which compose logic, I thought that I would have enough with the four preceding, as long as I made a firm and constant resolution never—not even once—to neglect my adherence to them.

TEACHER TIP

Mapping the Passage:

Paragraph 1: **discusses the four principles of thought.** *There's no need to detail the four principles.* Your map will tell you where to go if you need to review them

Paragraph 2: **author's background and problems with logic**

Paragraph 3: **More of above.**

Paragraph 4: **author's problems with geometric analysis and algebra.**

Paragraph 5: **author's desire to find a new way of thinking. Mentions four principles of thought.**

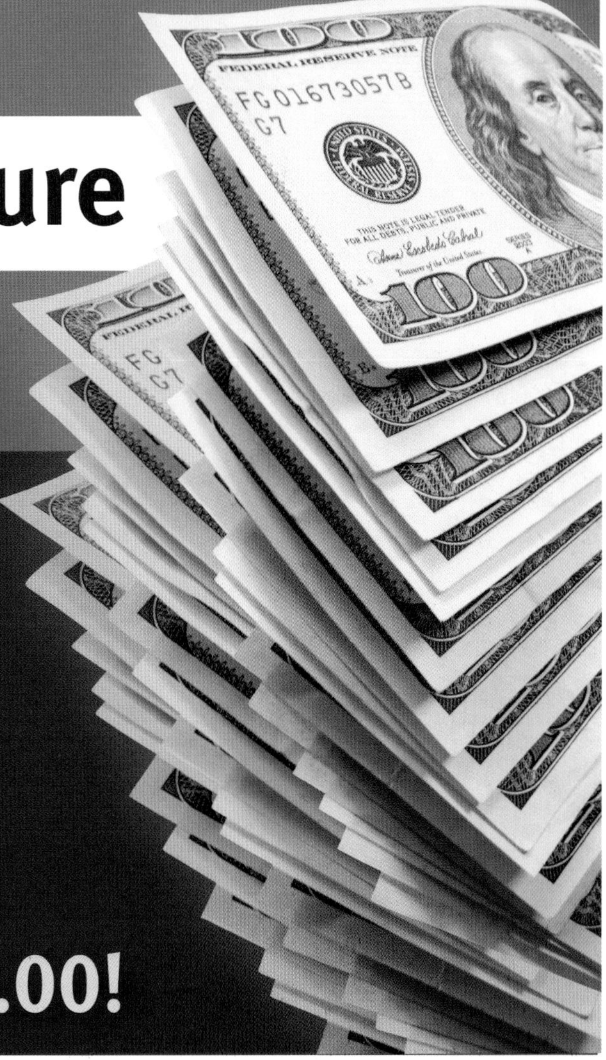

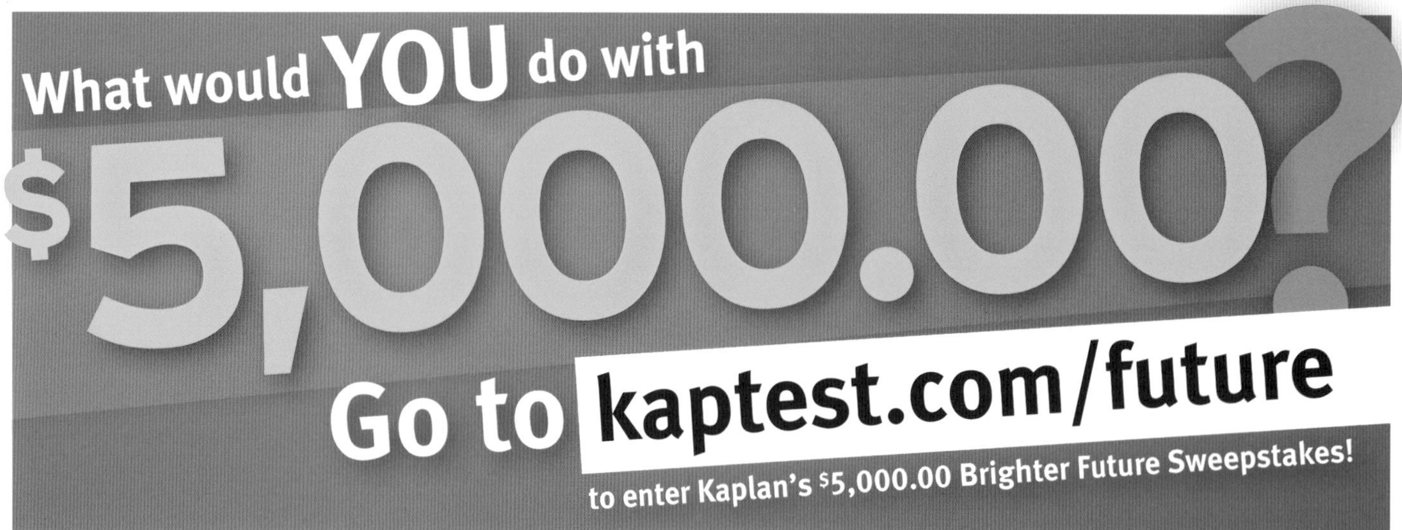
What would YOU do with
$5,000.00?
Go to kaptest.com/future
to enter Kaplan's $5,000.00 Brighter Future Sweepstakes!

Kaplan $5,000 Brighter Future Sweepstakes 2009 Complete and Official Rules

1. NO PURCHASE IS NECESSARY TO ENTER OR WIN. A PURCHASE WILL NOT INCREASE YOUR CHANCES OF WINNING.
2. PROMOTION PERIOD. The "Kaplan $5,000 Brighter Future Sweepstakes" ("Sweepstakes") commences at 6:59 A.M. EST on April 1, 2009 and ends at 11:59 P.M. EST on March 31, 2010. Entry forms can be found online at kaptest.com/brighterfuturesweeps. All online entries must be received by March 31, 2010 at 11:59 P.M. EST.
3. ELIGIBILITY. This Sweepstakes is open to legal residents of the 50 United States and the District of Columbia and Canada (excluding the Province of Quebec) who are sixteen (16) years of age or older as of April 1, 2009. Officers, directors, representatives and employees of Kaplan (from here on called "Sponsor"), its parent, affiliates or subsidiaries, or their respective advertising, promotion, publicity, production, and judging agencies and their immediate families and household members are not eligible to enter.
4. TO ENTER. To enter simply go to kaptest.com/brighterfuturesweeps and fill-out the online entry form between April 1, 2009 and March 31, 2010.
As part of your entry, you will be asked to provide your first and last name, email address, permanent address and phone number, parent or legal guardian name if under eighteen (18), and the name of your undergraduate school.

LIMIT ONE ENTRY PER PERSON AND EMAIL ADDRESS. Multiple entries will be disqualified. Entries are void if they contain typographical, printing or other errors. Entries generated by a script, macro or other automated means are void. Entries that are mutilated, altered, incomplete, mechanically reproduced, tampered with, illegible, inaccurate, forged, irregular in any way, or otherwise not in compliance with these Official Rules are also void. All entries become the property of the Sponsor and will not be returned to the entrant. Sponsor and those working on its behalf will not be responsible for lost, late, misdirected or damaged mail or email or for Internet, network, computer hardware and software, phone or other technical errors, malfunctions and delays that may occur. Entries will be deemed to have been submitted by the authorized account holder of the email account from which the entry is made. The authorized account holder is the natural person to whom an email address is assigned by an Internet access provider, online service provider or other organization (e.g. business, educational institution, etc.) responsible for assigning email addresses for the domain associated with the submitted email address. By entering or accepting a prize in this Sweepstakes, entrants agree to be bound by the decisions of the judges, the Sponsor and these Official Rules and to comply with all applicable federal, state and local laws and regulations. Odds of winning depend on the number of eligible entries received.
5. WINNER SELECTION. Two (2) winners will be selected for the First Prize; two (2) winners for the Second Prize, five (5) winners for the Third Prize, five (5) winners for Fourth Prize, five (5) winners for the Fifth Prize, and 25 winners for the Sixth Prize from all eligible entries received in a random drawing to be held on or about May 11, 2010. The drawing will be conducted by an independent judge whose decisions shall be final and binding in all regards. Participants need not be present to win. Please note that if the entrant selected as the winner resides in Canada, he/she will have to correctly answer a timed, test-prep question in order to be confirmed as the winner and claim the prize.
6. WINNER NOTIFICATION AND VALIDATION. Winners of the drawing will be notified by mail within 10 days after the drawing. An Affidavit of Eligibility and Compliance with these Official Rules and a Liability and (unless prohibited) Publicity Release must be executed and returned by the potential winner within twenty-one (21) days after prize notification is sent. If the winner is under eighteen (18) years of age, the prize will be awarded to the winner's parent or legal guardian who will be required to execute an affidavit. Failure of the potential winner to complete, sign and return any requested documents within such period or the return of any prize notification or prize as undeliverable may result in disqualification and selection of an alternate winner in Sponsor's sole discretion. You are not a winner unless your submissions are validated.

In the event that a winner chooses not to accept his or her prize, does not respond to winner notification within the time period noted on the notification or does not return a completed Affidavit of Eligibility and Compliance with these Official Rules and a Liability and (unless prohibited) Publicity Release within twenty-one (21) days after prize notification is sent, the prize may be forfeited and an alternate winner selected in Sponsor's sole discretion.
7. PRIZES.
- First Prize: Two (2) winners will be selected to win $5,000.00 USD.
- Second Prize: Two (2) winners will be selected to win $1,000.00 USD.
- Third Prize: Five (5) winners will be selected to win their choice of a Free Kaplan SAT, ACT, GMAT, GRE, LSAT, MCAT, DAT, OAT, or PCAT Classroom Course (retail value up to $1,899).
- Fourth Prize: Five (5) winners will be selected to win their choice of Ten (10) Free Hours of GMAT, GRE, LSAT, MCAT, DAT, OAT, PCAT Private Tutoring (retail value of $1,500), or Ten (10) Free Hours of SAT, ACT, PSAT Premier Tutoring (retail value of $2,000).
- Fifth Prize: Five (5) winners will be selected to win their choice of Three (3) Free Hours of Admissions Consulting for Precollege (retail value of $450) or three (3) Free Hours of Business School, Law School, Grad School or Med School Admissions Consulting (retail value of $729).
- Sixth Prize: Twenty-five (25) winners will be selected to win $100.00 USD.

For winners of the Third and Fourth Prizes, the winner must redeem the course at Kaplan locations in the US offering them and have completed the program before December 31, 2012.

Prizes are not transferable. No substitution of prizes for cash or other goods and services is permitted, except Sponsor reserves the right in its sole discretion to substitute any prize with a prize of comparable value. Any applicable taxes or fees are the winner's sole responsibility. All prizes must be redeemed within 21 days of notice of award and course prizes used by December 31, 2012.
8. GENERAL CONDITIONS. By entering the Sweepstakes or accepting the Sweepstakes prize, winner accepts all the conditions, restrictions, requirements and/or regulations required by the Sponsor in connection with the Sweepstakes. Unless otherwise prohibited by law, acceptance of a prize constitutes permission to use winner's name, picture, likeness, address (city and state) and biographical information for advertising and publicity purposes for this and/or similar promotions, without prior approval or compensation. Acceptance of a prize constitutes a waiver of any claim to royalties, rights or remuneration for said use. Winner agrees to release and hold harmless the Sponsor, its parent, affiliates and subsidiaries, and each of their respective directors, officers, employees, agents, and successors from any and all claims, damages, injury, death, loss or other liability that may arise from winner's participation in the Sweepstakes or the awarding, acceptance, possession, use or misuse of the prize. Sponsor reserves the right in its sole discretion to modify or cancel all or any portions of the Sweepstakes because of technical errors or malfunctions, viruses, hackers, or for other reasons beyond Sponsor's control that impair or corrupt the Sweepstakes in any manner. In such event, Sponsor shall award prizes at random from among the eligible entries received up to the time of the impairment or corruption. Sponsor also reserves the right in its sole discretion to disqualify any entrant who fails to comply with these Official Rules, who attempts to enter the Sweepstakes in any manner or through any means other than as described in these Official Rules, or who attempts to disrupt the Sweepstakes or the kaptest.com website or to circumvent any of these Official Rules.
9. WINNERS' LIST. Starting August 15, 2010, a winners' list may be obtained by sending a self-addressed, stamped envelope to: "$5,000 Kaplan Brighter Future Sweepstakes" Winners' List, Kaplan Test Prep and Admissions Marketing Department, 1440 Broadway, 8th Floor New York, NY 10018. All winners' list requests must be received by December 1, 2010.
10. USE OF ENTRANT AND WINNER INFORMATION. The information that you provide in connection with the Sweepstakes may be used for Sponsor's and select Corporate Partners' purposes to send you information about Sponsor's and its Corporate Partners' products and services. If you would like your name removed from Sponsor's mailing list or if you do not wish to receive information from Sponsor or its Corporate Partners, write to:

Direct Marketing Department
Attn: Kaplan Brighter Future Sweepstakes Opt Out
1440 Broadway
8th Floor
New York NY 10018

11. SPONSOR. The Sponsor of this Sweepstakes is: Kaplan Test Prep and Admissions and Kaplan Publishing, 1440 Broadway, 8th Floor New York, NY 10018.
12. THIS SWEEPSTAKES IS VOID WHERE PROHIBITED, TAXED OR OTHERWISE RESTRICTED BY LAW.

13. As presented within the context of the passage, the first precept of the author's methodological approach is based on the assumption that:

A. true comprehension depends primarily on rational comprehension and analysis.
B. theories can be accepted as true if they are perceived intellectually and instinctively.
C. relying solely on intellectual prowess is a valid way of determining the validity of a theory.
D. scholars must study philosophy and mathematics in order to understand abstract ideas.

14. Which of the following best expresses the author's attitude toward the existence of vice in a State?

A. National vices should be considered equivalent to deductive flaws in logic.
B. Vices can be justified or excused through legal channels.
C. An effective government must eradicate all vices in its rulers and citizens.
D. Certain vices may be unavoidable, but can be kept under control through careful observation.

15. According to the passage, which of the following statements are true about geometry?

I. Geometric analysis is not useful for a logical methodology.
II. Geometry focuses too narrowly on shapes and lines.
III. Geometry is largely visual, so comprehension requires both intellect and imagination.

A. II only
B. I and II
C. I, II, and III
D. III only

16. The author takes time in the passage to describe his study of philosophy and mathematics in an effort to:

A. justify his precepts as being validly based on personal knowledge and experience.
B. demonstrate the relationship between logic, geometry, and algebra.
C. provide a scholarly model for his readers so that they can expand their study of logic.
D. refute prior logicians' theories and indicate their flaws.

17. The author would be LEAST likely to agree with which of the following statements?

A. Logic is an inappropriate field of research for young scholars.
B. A scholar should always treat the subject of his or her study in its entirety.
C. Orderly study is based on the principle that a whole is the sum of its parts.
D. Teaching is one of the motivations for studying abstract ideas and theories.

Teacher Tip

The author would be most likely to disagree with anything contrary to what says he agrees with. Look over your map for a quick refresher on his ideas, then make a prediction before going to the answers.

18. Based on the point of view taken by the author in the passage, the author's primary concern in developing his method is:

A. objective examination of prior methodologies.
B. thorough grounding in a variety of academic disciplines.
C. consistent adherence to his principles.
D. extensive research in the natural sciences.

PASSAGE 4 (QUESTIONS 19–23)

With the collapse of the "dotcom" bubble in 2001 and the new trend towards outsourcing information technology labor demands, it becomes imperative to analyze the state of the economy which has brought us to this place. With the explosion of the technology industry in the late 1990s, the U.S. ushered in the so-called "new economy." Based largely on speculation and a "cash-in" mentality, the new economy bustled along until the bottom fell out and it came crashing back to earth. But what set the stage for this collapse to happen was put into motion years earlier.

The growth of productivity is defined as the rate of growth in product less the rate of growth in the labor used in production. Productivity can be affected by factors such as: amount of capital invested in production, methods used in production, educational or demographic composition of the labor force, business climate, global competition, and cost of environmental and safety regulations. Capital investment was booming in the U.S. in the post-1995 period, nearing a historic peak as a percentage of the U.S. gross domestic product. Furthermore, that part of capital invested in information technology, including computers, software, and communications equipment, rose to more than fifty times what it had been in 1975. Because of its high gross rate of return in improving methods of production, capital investment in information technology should have a particularly large impact on overall productivity.

For the past five years the big news for the U.S. economy has been a noticeable productivity growth spurt, which many have attributed to new information and communication technologies. The rate of growth in U.S. productivity had not been so high since the period extending from the end of World War II through the 1960s. In the early 1970s, productivity growth dropped suddenly. Apart from normal cyclical movements low productivity growth continued until the mid-1990s. Then, performance of the U.S. economy accelerated to a truly extraordinary level. From 1995 to 1999 real gross domestic product grew at an average rate of about 4 percent per year, and the rate of growth in labor productivity returned to the pre-1970 rate of increase.

The revolution in technology is, at least in some sense, a worldwide phenomenon. Therefore, one would expect the recent trend in the rate of growth in productivity in the U.S. to be shared by other developed countries. However, marked differences exist. Although the U.S. had the lowest rate of overall productivity growth in the 1981-95 period, in the post-1995 period the U.S. rate of productivity rose to third among the countries, behind only Ireland and Australia. In several other developed countries, including France, Italy, Japan, the United Kingdom, the Netherlands, and Spain, overall productivity growth slowed quite sharply. The questions then arise: Why are these trends in productivity growth so different; and does this difference illuminate anything about the role of the new technologies? Regression analysis of the rate of growth in productivity in each of these countries in the late 1990s, both as a function of the country's share of spending devoted to information technology and as a function of its number of internet servers, reveals a positive correlation that passes the test for statistical significance. Therefore, with due deference to the problems of international comparison, the data appears to reinforce the view that utilization of the new technologies has been important in raising productivity in the U.S. in recent years.

19. According to the passage, a resurgence in productivity occurred in:

I. the U.S. in the late 1990s.
II. Ireland in the late 1990s.
III. developed countries other than the U.S. in the 1981-95 period.

A. I only
B. II only
C. III only
D. I, II, and III

20. In concluding that utilization of new technologies has been important in raising productivity in the U.S. in recent years the author assumes all of the following EXCEPT:

A. other factors affecting productivity did not become significantly more favorable in this period.
B. the revolution in technology is a worldwide phenomenon.
C. amount of spending on information technology and number of internet servers are valid measures of utilization of new technologies in production.
D. the share of spending devoted to information technology and the number of internet servers are a cause of productivity growth.

21. If the passage were to continue, the next topic the author would discuss would most probably be:

A. what factors caused the drop in the growth of U.S. productivity in the early 1970s.
B. what factors prevented the productivity growth spurt in the U.S. from continuing.
C. the relative importance of other factors in fostering productivity growth in the U.S.
D. why different developed countries invested different shares of total spending on capital investment in new technologies.

22. If given the opportunity to rebut all of the following comments, with respect to the change in productivity growth in the U.S. in the late 1990s, the author would most probably agree with which of the following statements?

A. This change is typical of the type of change that is a natural part of the tendency of economies to cycle through periods of higher and lower growth.
B. This particular change is more remarkable than other changes that have occurred in the last half-century and, therefore, warrants a particular explanation.
C. The factors that caused this change should be identified so that they may be fostered in countries that are not experiencing strong productivity growth.
D. Investment in information and communication technologies has played a significant role in fostering the productivity gains in the U.S.

23. In paragraph 2, the author is primarily concerned with:

A. defining productivity and identifying the types of factors that can affect its growth.
B. noting a correlation between a peak in capital investment and a peak in the growth of productivity.
C. emphasizing the impact of the amount of capital invested on the degree of improvement in methods used for production.
D. introducing a explanation that will then be tested by further investigation.

PASSAGE 5 (QUESTIONS 24–30)

Should the soft spring breath of kindly appreciation warm the current chilly atmosphere, flowers of greater luxuriance and beauty would soon blossom forth, to beautify and enrich our literature. If these anticipations are not realized, it will not be because there is anything in our country that is uncongenial to poetry. If we are deprived of many of the advantages of older countries, our youthful country provides ample compensation not only in the ways in which nature unveils her most majestic forms to exalt and inspire, but also in our unshackled freedom of thought and broad spheres of action. Despite the unpropitious circumstances that exist, some true poetry has been written in our country, and represents an earnest hope of better things for the future and basis to hope that it will not always be winter with our native poetry.

Whenever things are discovered that are new, in the records of creation, in the relations of phenomenon, in the mind's operations, or in forms of thought and imagery, some record in the finer forms of literature will always be demanded. There is probably no country in the world, making equal pretensions to natural intelligence and progress in education, where the claims of native literature are so little felt, and where every effort in poetry has been met with so much coldness and indifference, as in ours.

The common method of accounting for this, by the fact almost everyone is engaged in the pursuit of the necessities of life, and that few possess the wealth and leisure necessary to enable devotion of time or thought to the study of poetry and kindred subjects, is by no means satisfactory. This state of things is doubtless unfavorable to the growth of poetry; but there are other causes less palpable, which exert a more subtle but still powerful antagonism. Nothing so seriously militates against the growth of our native poetry as the false conceptions that prevail respecting the nature of poetry.

Stemming either from a natural incapacity for appreciating the truths which find their highest embodiment in poetry or from familiarity only with more widely available, but lower forms, such notions conceive of poetry as fanciful, contrived, contrary to reason, or lacking the justification of any claim to practical utility. These attitudes, which admittedly may have some origin in the imperfection that even the most partial must confess to finding in our native poetry, nevertheless also can have the effect of discouraging native writers of undoubted genius from the sustained application to their craft that is essential to artistic excellence.

Poetry, like Truth, will unveil her beauty and dispense her honors only to those who love her with a deep and reverential affection. There are many who are not gifted with the power of giving expression to the deeper sensibilities who nevertheless experience them throbbing in their hearts. To them poetry appeals. But where this tongue-less poetry of the heart has no existence, or exists in a very feeble degree, the conditions for appreciating poetic excellence are wanting. Let no one, therefore, speak of disregard for poetry as if it indicated superiority.

Rather, it is an imperfection to be endured as a misfortune. Despite prevailing misconceptions, there always remain at least a few who appreciate fine literature. Why do these not provide sufficient nourishment for our native artists? Here, we must acknowledge the difficulty that so many of us, as emigrants from the Old Country, cling to memories of the lands we have left, and that this throws a charm around literary efforts originating in our former home, and it is indisputable that the productions of our young country suffer by comparison.

24. The passage asserts that which of the following are reasons for the indifference toward native poetry that the author finds in his country?

I. There has been insufficient edification of most of the population.
II. The highest achievements of native poets do not rise to the level achieved by poets of the immigrants' homeland.
III. Nostalgic feelings orient readers toward the literature of their former home.

A. I and II only
B. II and III only
C. I and III only
D. I, II, and III

25. An important contrast is made throughout the passage. The author developed this contrast between:

A. the subtle and the palpable.
B. false claims and real facts.
C. the appreciable and the insignificant.
D. the practical and the impractical.

26. Suppose that the passage does not stand on its own, but is excerpted from an introduction to a book. This book would most likely be:

A. a textbook on the techniques for writing good poetry.
B. a volume comparing the poetry of two countries.
C. a volume of recent native poetry.
D. a volume of essays on poetry and criticism.

27. In the sentence, "But where this tongue-less poetry of the heart has no existence, or exists in a very feeble degree, the conditions for appreciating poetic excellence are wanting," in the passage, the author most probably uses the phrase "tongue-less poetry of the heart" in order to:

A. emphasize that poetry is more commonly experienced through reading, rather by being heard.
B. emphasize a defect that exists in those who devalue poetry.
C. emphasize that appreciation of poetry is not limited to those who can write it.
D. express compassion for those who lack the gift of writing poetry.

28. The author probably considers which of the following "unpropitious circumstances" (line 13) most essential to explaining the state of native poetry?

A. Lack of available resources for the study of poetry
B. Failure of native poets to devote themselves to learning their craft
C. Prevalent misconceptions about poetry
D. Nostalgia of emigrants for their home country

29. Which of the following statements, made by poets about the creative process, is closest to the opinions expressed in the passage about what constitutes "true" poetry?

A. "Like a piece of ice on a hot stove the poem must ride on its own melting. A poem may be worked over once it is in being, but may not be worried into being."
B. "My method is simple: not to bother about poetry. It must come of its own accord. Merely whispering its name drives it away."
C. "If there's room for poets in this world... their sole work is to represent the age, their own age, not Charlemagne's."
D. "The only way of expressing emotion in the form of art is by finding an 'objective correlative'; in other words, a set of objects, a situation, a chain of events which shall be the formula of that particular emotion; such that when the external facts, which must terminate in sensory experience, are given, the emotion is immediately evoked."

30. By "native literature" the author most probably means:

A. literature written by the aboriginal people of his home country.
B. literature written by people who make his country their home.
C. literature written by people born in his country.
D. literature produced in and reflecting the circumstances and environment of his country.

PASSAGE 6 (QUESTIONS 31–35)

Without entering now into the *why*, let me observe that the printer may always ascertain when the dash of the manuscript is properly and when improperly employed, by bearing in mind that this point represents *a second thought—an emendation*. In using it just above I have exemplified its use. The words "an emendation" are, speaking with reference to grammatical construction, put in *ap*position with the words "a second thought." Having written these latter words, I reflected whether it would not be possible to render their meaning more distinct by certain other words.

Now, instead of erasing the phrase "a second thought," which is of *some* use, which *partially* conveys the idea intended—which advances me a *step toward* my full purpose—I suffer it to remain, and merely put a dash between it and the phrase "an emendation." The dash gives the reader a choice between two, or among three or more expressions, one of which may be more forcible than another, but all of which help out the idea.

It stands, in general, for the words "or, *to make my meaning more distinct*." This force *it has* and this force no other point can have; since all other points have well-understood uses quite different from this. Therefore, the dash *cannot* be dispensed with. It has its phases its variation of the force described; but the one principle that of second thought or emendation will be found at the bottom of all. That punctuation is important all agree; but how few comprehend the extent of its importance! The writer who neglects punctuation, or mispunctuates, is liable to be misunderstood; this, according to the popular idea, is the sum of the evils arising from heedlessness or ignorance. It does not seem to be known that, even where the sense is perfectly clear, a sentence may be deprived of half its force its spirit its point by improper punctuation. For the want of merely a comma, it often occurs that an axiom appears a paradox, or that a sarcasm is converted into a sermonoid. There is *no* treatise on the topic and there is no topic on which a treatise is more needed.

There seems to exist a vulgar notion that the subject is one of pure conventionality, and cannot be brought within the limits of intelligible and consistent *rule*. And yet, if fairly looked in the face, the whole matter is so plain that its *rationale* may be read as we run. If not anticipated, I shall, hereafter, make an attempt at a magazine paper on "The Philosophy of Point." In the meantime let me say a word more of *the dash*.

Every writer for the press, who has any sense of the accurate, must have been frequently mortified and vexed at the distortion of his sentences by the printer's now general substitution of a semicolon, or comma, for the dash in the manuscript. The total or nearly total disuse of the latter point, has been brought about by the revulsion consequent upon its excessive employment about twenty years ago. The Byronic poets were *all* dash.

31. According to the arguments presented in the passage by the author, which of the following are true about the dash?

I. It is often replaced by printers.
II. It is overused by some writers.
III. It serves a unique, necessary function.

A. I and II only
B. II and III only
C. I and III only
D. I, II, and III

32. According to the passage, the newspapers' printers' practice of replacing dashes in authors' manuscripts with other punctuation marks is due to:

A. the overuse of the dash by authors during the period closely preceding writing of the passage.
B. the widespread ignorance of the importance of punctuation.
C. the fact that the dash serves no function that is not better served by other punctuation marks.
D. the fact that authors seldom have second thoughts about their work.

33. The passage indicates that if given the chance to respond to the following claims, the author is LEAST likely to agree with which of the following statements?

A. There is a single ideal way in which any thought can be expressed.
B. The rules of punctuation are simple and rational.
C. Punctuation helps to convey the writer's intended meaning and tone.
D. Most people do not understand the correct use of punctuation.

34. The author most likely mentions his intention to write an article entitled "The Philosophy of Point" in order to:

A. remind the reader that grammar is a branch of philosophy.
B. indicate the possibility of explaining correct punctuation concisely.
C. furnish his own credentials as an expert on punctuation.
D. emend his statement about punctuation.

35. According to the passage, which of the following is true of the relationship between words or phrases separated by a dash?

A. Each word or phrase partially conveys the author's meaning.
B. The second word or phrase renders the first one superfluous.
C. The first word or phrase states the main topic, and the second states the sub-topic.
D. The two words or phrases pertain to separate topics.

PASSAGE 7 (QUESTIONS 36–40)

Let us consider whether women as a group have unique, politically relevant characteristics, whether they have special interests to which a representative could or should respond. Can we argue that women as a group share particular social, economic, or political problems that do not closely match those of other groups, or that they share a particular viewpoint on the solution to political problems? Framing the working definition of "representable interests" in this fashion does not mean that the problems or issues are exclusively those of the specified interest group, any more than we can make the same argument about other types of groups more widely accepted as interest groups.

The fact that there is a labor interest group, for example, reflects the existence of other groups such as the business establishment, consumers, and government, which in a larger sense share labor's concerns, but often have viewpoints on the nature of, or solutions to, the problems which conflict with those of labor.

Nor does our working definition of an interest group mean that all of the potential members of that group are consciously allied, or that there is a clear and obvious answer to any given problem articulated by the entire group that differs substantially from answers articulated by others. Research in various fields of social science provides evidence that women do have a distinct position and a shared set of problems that characterize a special interest.

Many of these distinctions are located in the institution in which women and men are probably most often assumed to have common interests, the family. Much has been made of the "sharing" or "democratic" model of the modern family, but whatever democratization has taken place, it has not come close to erasing the division of labor and, indeed, stratification, by sex. Time-use studies show that women spend about the same amount of time on and do the same proportion of housework and child care now as women did at the turn of the century. To say that women are in a different social position from that of men and therefore have unique interests to be represented is not, however, the same as saying that women are conscious of these differences, that they define themselves as having special interests requiring representation, or that men and women as groups now disagree on policy issues in which women might have a special interest.

Studies of public opinion on the status and roles of women show relatively few significant differences between the sexes, and do not reveal women to be consistently more feminist than men. On the other hand, law and public policy continue to create and reinforce differences between women and men in property and contract matters, economic opportunity, protection from violence, control over fertility and child care, educational opportunities, and civic rights and obligations. The indicators generally used to describe differences in socioeconomic position also show that the politically relevant situations of women and men are different. Women in almost all countries have less education than men, and where they achieve equivalent levels of education, segregation by field and therefore skills and market value remains.

36. Which of the following would the author be most likely to consider a necessary characteristic of a group having "representable interests" (paragraph 1)?

A. The problems of the group are unique to its members.

B. The group's proposed solutions to their problems differ radically from those proposed by other groups.

C. Members of the group are not already represented as individuals.

D. Members of the group tend to have similar opinions about the handling of particular political problems.

37. It can be inferred from the passage that which of the following statements is true of men and women as groups?

A. In public opinion polls on women's issues, men's responses do not differ in a consistent way from those of women.
B. Developments in recent years have given men more control over child care issues.
C. Women are becoming more aware of their differences from men than in the past.
D. Men do not wish to recognize the special interests of women.

38. According to the passage, which of the following experiences do modern women have most nearly in common with women who lived in 1900?

A. They are represented only as individuals and not as a group.
B. They spend about the same amount of time on housework.
C. They experience significant discrimination in employment.
D. The proportion of women among those designated as representatives is lower than among the represented.

39. Based on the passage, of the following issues the author is most concerned about the problem of:

A. the history of women's demands for representation as a group.
B. recent changes in the status of women in society.
C. opposing views concerning women's awareness of their own special interests.
D. the criteria that would justify group representation for women.

40. The passage offers the most support for concluding that which of the following is an important problem confronting women today?

A. Women are in a different socioeconomic position from that of men.
B. Men differ greatly from women in the answers they propose for women's problems.
C. Women do not qualify as an interest group, because they have not all banded together to pursue common goals
D. A lack of educational opportunities has inhibited women from voicing their concerns.

VERBAL REASONING PRACTICE SECTION 2

Time—60 minutes

DIRECTIONS: There are seven passages in this Verbal Reasoning test. Each passage is followed by several questions. After reading a passage, select the one best answer to each question. If you are not certain of an answer, eliminate the alternatives that you know to be incorrect and then select an answer from the remaining alternatives. Indicate your selection by blackening the corresponding circle on your answer sheet.

PASSAGE 1 (QUESTIONS 1–6)

The extent to which analysis of social phenomena is compatible with the scientific method is a hotly contested question. Among international relations scholars, historico-deductivist opponents of positivism claim that in the pursuit of objective depictions of the causes, course, and consequences of international phenomena the character and operation of which are purported to exist independently of the observer, positivists miss or dismiss the implicit attitudes, values, and ideologies embedded in their work, which personalize and subjectivize their conclusions. Positivism, these critics contend, attempts to impose on world politics a coherent facticity akin to that of the natural sciences, but to which the basic nature of world politics is indisposed. As Dougherty put it, "Aristotle warns in the *Nichomachaean* Ethics that the precision of an answer cannot exceed that of its question, but the positivists want clocks and necessity where there are really clouds and contingency."

For historico-deductivists, the problem of *a posteriori* overdetermination is a case in point. In the natural sciences, replicability and verifiability afford the findings of laboratory experimentation potentially nomothetic status. In international relations, however, such lawlike generalizations about cause and effect are rarely if ever possible, not only because events are unique, but also because of the multiplicity of potential causes. Whether World War I resulted from a disequilibrium in the international distribution of power, the ascendancy of government factions committed to aggression, or the accuracy of an assassin's bullet, is, ultimately, unknown. For opponents of positivism, it is better to recognize darkness than to pretend to see light.

While some leading positivists, most notably Pastore, admit as "knowledge" only the sum of all tested propositions, for most it is the very cloudlike nature of political phenomena that requires a clocklike approach. Conceding that their subject does not permit nomothetic propositions, the majority of positivists appear committed to Williams' more moderate rule: "The propensity to error should make us cautious, but not so desperate that we fear to come as close as possible to apodictic findings. We needn't grasp at the torch with eyes closed, fearing to be blinded."

Positivists point to the potential of scientific analysis to yield counterintuitive truths. A frequently cited example is Grotsky's study of the role of non-state actors in international trade. Published at a time when many scholars were convinced that multinational organizations had effectively "elbowed the traditional sovereign nation-state out of analytical existence in our field," Grotsky's research of the structure, timing, and variance of state expenditures on foreign direct investment effectively restored the state to its position as the dominant unit in international relations scholarship. Despite several efforts, historico-deductivists who had championed the new relevance of non-state actors have not, as yet, successfully refuted Grotsky's findings—a consideration that bodes well for those of us who believe that an end to this longstanding debate, which has produced much timely and relevant research, is not necessarily to be desired.

In addition to claiming that critics have mischaracterized their methodological commitments, positivists also contend that the historico-deductivist approach is subject to many of the same criticisms leveled against positivism. For example, on the twentieth anniversary of her seminal article depicting the Peloponnesian War as the archetypal case of power politics in action, Nash, perhaps the exemplar of the historico-deductivist school, revisited her earlier findings, only to conclude that the interaction between the Athenians and Spartans included significant instances of cooperation and reciprocity. Even as Nash's confederates praised the "illuminating evolution" in her thinking, many positivists questioned whether Nash's antipodal findings corresponded to a shift in her initial assumptions over time. The implication, of course, is that if positivists' commitments at the level of proto-theory color their eventual conclusions, then they are not alone in this regard.

1. According to information given in the passage, which of the following is true of *a posteriori* overdetermination?

I. It presents a challenge to scholars' ability to produce nomothetic statements about world politics.
II. It exemplifies the analytical confusion created by unique events that often have multiple effects.
III. It suggests that the historico-deductivism is better suited than is positivism to the study of international relations.

A. I only
B. III only
C. I and II only
D. II and III only

2. As used in lines 52–53, in the statement, "We needn't grasp at the torch with eyes closed, fearing to be blinded," the word "torch" refers to:

A. propensity to error.
B. nomothetic propositions.
C. political phenomena.
D. methodological commitments.

3. As described in the passage, historico-deductivist claims about the problem of *a posteriori* overdetermination in the study of political phenomena depend on the unstated assumption that:

   A. positivists' methodological commitments preclude positivists from providing a fully scientific account of the onset of World War I.
   B. complex social occurrences such as wars are ultimately insusceptible to scholarly analysis.
   C. replicability is a more severe obstacle than is verifiability to the scientific study of world politics.
   D. a causal claim that stipulates multiple indistinguishable causes for a certain effect is not likely to be a nomothetic proposition.

4. Which of the following would Dougherty be most likely to describe as "clocks and necessity where there are really clouds and contingency"?

   A. A historico-deductivist study of World War I
   B. A historico-deductivist study of the Peloponnesian War
   C. A positivist study of the nature of reciprocity in the relations among sovereign states
   D. A chemist's study of the behavior of a certain gas under conditions of standard temperature and pressure

5. The principle underlying which of the following is most analogous to "Williams's more moderate rule" (paragraph 3)?

   A. A student's estimation of her work is more important than either the grade awarded the work by the student's instructor or the opinion of the work expressed by the student's peers.
   B. The proficiency of an expert musician may reflect intelligence different in form from, but nonetheless equal in degree to, that of an accomplished painter or a pioneering physicist.
   C. If a worker were certain that he could never earn more than $50,000 per year, this in itself would not be a reason for him to refrain from trying to improve his lot at $20,000 per year.
   D. Hazardous road conditions constitute sufficient reason for a motorist to cancel her travel plans, even if the motorist is extremely reluctant to do so.

6. It can reasonably be inferred that the author of the passage is a:

   A. professor of history.
   B. professor of international relations.
   C. diplomat.
   D. journalist.

PASSAGE 2 (QUESTIONS 7–13)

After being formed deep within the earth, hydrocarbons migrate upwards, following a complex path of minute cracks and pore spaces, and will eventually reach the surface and be lost unless they encounter impermeable rocks (such as dense shale) through which they cannot travel. If the rock within which they are trapped is highly permeable (such as sandstone) the hydrocarbons can be extracted by drilling through the impermeable seal, and tapping into this permeable reservoir.

Our dependence, as a nation, and as a world, on fossil fuels is only increasing as the global population increases and our reliance on technology expands. There are few things that people in first-world countries do anymore that do not require an external power source of some kind. And in spite of the popularization of renewable sources of energy and nuclear energy, the chief source of power in the world is still derived from fossil fuels.

There are a number of different types of traps, but they can be divided into two broad categories. Structural traps are formed by deformation after the rocks have been formed, for example by folding or faulting. Stratigraphic traps are formed when the loose sediments that will eventually be turned into rocks were laid down. For example if the sea level rises and the permeable sands of a beach are covered with estuarine mud, the buried sediments will, under compression, become sandstone capped by impermeable siltstones, forming an ideal reservoir and trap.

By now the locations of all obvious reserves of oil and gas have been discovered. The need to expand oil and gas reserves therefore brings with it a need to find hydrocarbon reservoirs that are difficult to locate using current geological and geophysical means. To do so, geologists look for rock formations that constitute the seals and reservoirs within which hydrocarbons could be trapped.

Structural traps tend to be easier to locate and are the source of most of the known hydrocarbon reserves. Expanding our reserves therefore means locating more stratigraphically trapped hydrocarbons. The primary means of exploring for oil where there is no surface expression of the underlying geology is by seismology. When a seismic pulse transmitted into the earth encounters an interface where the density changes, typically the surface between two beds or an unconformity with velocity-density contrasts, some of the energy is reflected back upwards. A string of seismophones records these reflections and after extensive computation seismologists can build up a visual record of the intensity of each reflection and the time taken for it to reach the surface.

The primary limitation of the seismic method for locating stratigraphic traps is resolution: It is not possible to resolve features that are thinner than a seismic wavelet. The most common stratigraphic traps (with the possible exception of carbonate reservoirs) are in sandstone layers that are much thinner than a seismic wavelet. Seismic wavelets can be narrowed by increasing the frequency of the seismic pulse. However, high frequencies are selectively attenuated as the pulse travels through the earth, so there are limits to how much resolution can be improved by simply generating higher frequency pulses, or by filtering out the lower frequency components of the seismic source. Moreover, the density contrasts between oil-bearing sandstones and the shales that provide stratigraphic seals for the oil are often very small, so that the reflectivities, and hence the strength of the reflection, will be so low that the events may not be observable above background noise.

Recent developments such as zero-phase wavelet processing and multivariate analysis of reflection waveforms have decreased noise and increased resolution. In the future it is hoped that these techniques, and greater understanding of stratigraphy itself, will prove fruitful in expanding hydrocarbon reserves.

7. As opposed to other essays written on the same topic, it is likely that the primary purpose of this passage is to:

A. explain how hydrocarbons are formed and trapped within the earth.
B. detail how seismologists can locate hidden deposits of hydrocarbons.
C. contrast the relative difficulty of locating structural traps and stratigraphic traps.
D. discuss the formation of hydrocarbon reserves and how they can be located.

8. According to the passage, it is often difficult to distinguish reflections from the interface between oil-bearing sandstones and the shales that provide stratigraphic seals from background noise because:

A. high frequencies are attenuated as they travel through the earth.
B. there is little density contrast between the oil-bearing sandstone and the shales which provide stratigraphic seals.
C. the frequency of the seismic pulse is not high enough.
D. they are thinner than the seismic wavelet.

9. The example of a stratigraphic trap formed by a rise in sea level (paragraph 3) is brought up to make a certain point. It used by the author of the passage principally to:

A. contrast a typical stratigraphic trap with a typical structural trap.
B. explain why sandstones covered by siltstones make ideal reservoir and trap.
C. illustrate the point that stratigraphic traps are formed when sediments were laid down.
D. show why stratigraphic traps can be difficult to locate seismically.

10. According to the passage, all of the following are needed if oil is to be extracted from a reservoir EXCEPT:

A. an impermeable seal above the reservoir.
B. an original source of hydrocarbons below the reservoir.
C. high-density contrast between the reservoir rocks and the stratigraphic seal.
D. high permeability within the reservoir.

11. It can be inferred from the passage that, regardless of what angle the author may be trying to present, carbonate reservoirs are:

A. less dense than sandstone reservoirs.
B. easily located by seismology.
C. an important type of stratigraphic trap.
D. at least as thick as a seismic wavelet.

12. Based on the points made throughout the passage, which of the following best describes how the author views seismology as a tool in locating hydrocarbons?

A. Of limited effectiveness but showing promise
B. Intrinsically flawed
C. Effective and profitable
D. Theoretically useful but ineffectual in practice

13. Which of the following developments in seismic technique would the author view as the greatest aid in the detection of stratigraphic traps?

A. The discovery of a means of increasing the attenuation of high-frequency seismic wavelets within the earth
B. The development of a seismic source with an extremely high frequency that does not attenuate over distance
C. The development of a means of filtering all noise out of seismic sections
D. Further research into the origin of stratigraphic traps

PASSAGE 3 (QUESTIONS 14–19)

American culture changed forever in the latter part of the 20th century with the advent of pop music. Before the 1950s music defined its own circles, but, at best, only shaded the frame of popular American culture. The birth of rock-and-roll forever changed that as larger and larger numbers of youth came, not only to identify with the music they were listening to, but to identify themselves by that music.

We use pop songs to create for ourselves a particular sort of self-definition, a particular place in society. The pleasure that a pop song produces is a pleasure of identification: in responding to a song, we are drawn into affective and emotional alliances with the performers and with the performers' other fans. Thus, music, like sport, is clearly a setting in which people directly experience community, feel an immediate bond with other people, and articulate a collective pride.

At the same time, because of its qualities of abstractness, pop music is an individualizing form. Songs have a looseness of reference that makes them immediately accessible. They are open to appropriation for personal use in a way that other popular cultural forms (television soap operas, for example) are not—the latter are tied into meanings which we may reject.

This interplay between personal absorption into music and the sense that it is, nevertheless, something public, is what makes music so important in the cultural placing of the individual. Music also gives us a way of managing the relationship between our public and private emotional lives. Popular love songs are important because they give shape and voice to emotions that otherwise cannot be expressed without embarrassment or incoherence. Our most revealing declarations of feeling are often expressed in banal or boring language and so our culture has a supply of pop songs that say these things for us in interesting and involving ways.

Popular music also shapes popular memory, and organizes our sense of time. Clearly, one of the effects of all music, not just pop, is to focus our attention on the feeling of time, and intensify our experience of the present. One measure of good music is its "presence," its ability to "stop" time, to make us feel we are living within a moment, with no memory or anxiety about what has come before us, what will come after. It is this use of time that makes popular music so important in the social organization of youth. We invest most in popular music when we are teenagers and young adults—music ties into a particular kind of emotional turbulence, when issues of individual identity and social place, the control of public and private feelings, are at a premium. What this suggests, though, is not that young people need music, but that "youth" itself is defined by music. Youth is experienced, that is, as an intense presence, through an impatience for time to pass and a regret that it is doing so, in a series of speeding, physically insistent moments that have nostalgia coded into them.

14. While there are obviously many differences between the two, the author of the passage suggests that one similarity between popular and classical music is that both:

A. articulate a sense of community and collective pride.
B. give shape to inexpressible emotions.
C. emphasize the feeling of time.
D. define particular age groups.

15. It can be inferred from the passage that the author's attitude toward love songs in popular music is that of being:

A. bored by the banality of their language.
B. embarrassed by their emotional incoherence.
C. interested by their expressions of feeling.
D. unimpressed by their social function.

16. The author probably refers to sport in paragraph 2 primarily in order to:

A. draw a parallel.
B. establish a contrast.
C. challenge an assumption.
D. introduce a new idea.

17. Regardless of what the purpose of the passage is as a whole, in the last paragraph, the author is predominantly concerned with:

A. defining the experience of youth.
B. describing how popular music defines youth.
C. speculating about the organization of youth movements.
D. analyzing the relationship between music and time.

18. The author cites which one of the following in support of the argument that popular music creates our identity?

A. Pop songs are unpopular with older age groups.
B. Love songs shape our everyday language.
C. Pop songs become personalized like other cultural forms.
D. Popular music combines public and private experience.

19. In a debate on the importance of popular music in the social organization of youth, which of the following, if true, would most *weaken* the author's argument?

A. Popular songs often incorporate nostalgic lyrics.
B. Young people are ambivalent about the passage of time.
C. Older people are less interested in popular music than young people.
D. Pop songs focus our expectations on the future.

PASSAGE 4 (QUESTIONS 20–24)

Tracking seems to contradict the oft-stated assumption that "all kids can learn." If certain students are better in certain subjects, they must be allowed to excel in those areas and not be relegated to an inferior class simply because they have been tracked in another subject in which they don't excel. The major obstacle to eliminate tracking seems to be scheduling, and tracking has become, in many ways, a means to alleviate difficulties faced by administrators in scheduling their student body for classes.

Tracking has the ability to create divergent experiences, even in identical courses that are meant to be taught at the same level and speed. Administrators who support tracking generally assume that it promotes student achievement, citing that most students seem to learn best and develop the most confidence when they are grouped amongst classmates with similar capabilities. Yet, at least for the lower level tracks, this method of class assignment can encourage "dumbing down," or teaching to the lowest common denominator of ability within a particular class, rather than accommodating differences and pushing all students equally hard.

Tracking places different students in groups that are usually based on academic ability as demonstrated by their grades and as described in teacher reports. These tracks mean that a student will proceed through every school day with essentially the same group of peers, assigned to classes at a particular level of difficulty. Researcher R. Slavin notes that "students at various track levels experience school differently," depending on their track assignments. There are differences, for example, in how fast a class progresses through material, how talkative and energetic the classroom is, even how stressed or relaxed the teacher appears.

One of the major problems with tracking is that the level in which students are initially placed often determines not only where they remain throughout high school, but also the kinds of courses they are allowed to take. For example, schools that offer Advanced Placement (AP) courses often require that students take the honors-level version of the introductory course before enrolling in the AP course a year or two later. A student who is tracked into the "regular" introductory course, rather than the honors level, may not be able to take the AP course even after doing an exemplary job in the introductory course, simply because the honors course is offered a year earlier than the regular one—allowing honors-track students to complete enough other graduation requirements to have time for the AP course later on. And, even if the "regular"-track student could make it into the AP course, he or she would be at a disadvantage, because the introductory course couldn't cover key concepts when the teacher was compelled to slow down the class for the less able students.

20. If it were found that students who were tracked did better overall on standardized tests than those who were not tracked, this would most likely WEAKEN the author's argument that:

A. tracking has the ability to create a diversity of student experience in the classroom.
B. tracking encourages teaching to the lowest common denominator.
C. tracking allows administrators to overcome scheduling difficulties.
D. tracking allows students to learn best, as they are grouped with classmates with similar ability.

21. According specifically to the points laid out by the author in the various paragraphs of the passage, the main idea of the passage is that:

A. tracking should not be used by schools to try and promote student achievement.
B. tracking may be detrimental to many students' success in school.
C. teachers of tracked classes are often stressed and run their classes at a slow pace.
D. scheduling is a major problem for school administrators.

22. The author's argument that tracking contradicts the assumption that "all kids can learn" would be STRENGTHENED by which of the following findings?

I. Honors-track students almost always have AP classes on their transcripts, while regular-track students do not.
II. Students in tracked classes do significantly better on standardized tests.
III. Teachers of the lower math track in a school were unable to cover more than three-quarters of the textbook over the past few years, while their higher-track counterparts have consistently covered the entire book.

A. I only
B. III only
C. II and III
D. I and III

23. According to the arguments made in the passage, students may fall into a particular track because of all of the following conditions EXCEPT:

A. high grades.
B. learning difficulties.
C. honors-course enrollment.
D. how talkative and energetic they are.

24. If the author were to encounter a student in a class who was not doing the work because he or she claimed to be bored by the material, the author would most likely conclude that:

A. the student has been placed in a track that is too high.
B. the student is unmotivated and should be disciplined.
C. the student has been placed in a track that is too low.
D. the student should be in AP-level classes.

PASSAGE 5 (QUESTIONS 25–30)

This civil rights movement in the United States developed at the same time as the development of pluralist politics. And very much of the latter, especially in the northern urban area, was infused with a heavy dose of ethnicity. As blacks were coming out of slavery and going into courts, immigrant groups were coming out of Europe, passing through Ellis Island, and going into local political clubs and machines.

The politics of race has been mainly a struggle to restructure constitutional meaning and to establish certain legal claims. This emphasis was necessary precisely because the citizenship status of blacks was defined for a long period as quite different from that of whites. After the abolition of slavery, approximately 100 years ensued—into the 1960s—which were devoted essentially to interpreting the new *constitutional* status of the emancipated black citizens.

A "civil rights" movement developed that saw 95 years (1870-1965) devoted to establishing the privilege of blacks to vote unencumbered by racial barriers. The main arena was the court system. Congress and the presidency were not principal participants, because the political constituencies supporting their elections did not favor such participation. Civil rights advocates went to federal courts to challenge "grandfather clauses," white primaries, evasive voter registration practices, as well as economic intimidation. These important, tedious battles created a cadre of constitutional lawyers who became in a real sense the focal points of the civil rights struggle. Such was the situation in the famous Montgomery, Alabama bus boycott from 1955 to 1957, which began when Rosa Parks refused to abide by a municipal law requiring her to sit in the rear of the city bus, and ended when the U.S. Supreme Court in *Gayle v. Browder* said she did not have to do so.

But while the politics of race was characterized by a struggle for rights, the politics of plural-ethnicity was characterized by a struggle for resources. The latter was a struggle to capture and control public office and the ability to dispense patronage and divisible and indivisible benefits. Instead of nurturing and training lawyers and plaintiffs, plural-ethnicity focused on precinct captains and patronage. While the black racial political struggle utilized constitutional lawyers as sophisticated interpreters of new constitutional meaning, those focusing on ethnicity utilized lawyers to interpret immigration rules, obtain pushcart licenses, and negotiate the bureaucratic passage from alien to citizen. Both roles were fundamentally critical, but also fundamentally different. The point is the following: when the civil rights struggle evolved from rights to resources, as it certainly did beginning substantially in the 1960s, it took with it the orientation, language, and some of the tactics of the earlier struggle for constitutional rights.

25. According to the passage, how did the struggle for resources differ from the struggle for rights?

A. It focused on grass-roots activism instead of electoral power.
B. It emphasized control and political representation at a local level.
C. It was dedicated to effecting changes through election to national political positions.
D. It cooperated with newly arrived immigrant populations.

26. According to evidence put forth by the author of the passage, why was the executive branch of the government not targeted for civil rights participation in the 1950s?

A. Early activists had little political clout on a federal level at that time.
B. Federal policies banned lobbying of Congress by civil rights advocates.
C. Elected officials acted according to the expressed opinions of their voters.
D. No members of Congress were interested in enforcing new voting laws.

27. Paying particular attention to the thematic organization of the passage, which of the following statements best describes the structure of the passage?

A. Two historical developments are described and contrasted.
B. A historical movement is praised using two closely connected examples.
C. A general history of a struggle is presented, with a suggestion of how it will be resolved in the future.
D. Two different approaches to a problem are analyzed and then combined.

28. According to the author, prior to 1965 the civil rights movement on behalf of blacks was characterized by none of the following EXCEPT:

A. an emphasis on removing restrictions on black voting through court cases.
B. a struggle to overturn the decisions of constitutional lawyers.
C. the increasing ability of black voters to mobilize and elect black politicians to office.
D. frequent conflict between the Congress and Supreme Court over controversial issues.

29. In the passage, the author cites the Montgomery, Alabama bus boycott as an example of:

A. a crucial incident which marked the turn of the civil rights movement toward the goal of controlling resources.
B. an event important because it began the leadership career of Martin Luther King, Jr.
C. one of the better-known battles to assert the civil rights of blacks.
D. an event whose primary importance was its impact on the enforcement of constitutional rights.

30. According to the author, the "politics of plural-ethnicity" discussed in the fourth paragraph differed from the black civil rights movement before 1965 in all of the following ways EXCEPT that it:

A. concentrated more on elections as a way to achieve important goals.
B. initiated court cases for more sophisticated and theoretical reasons.
C. was more concerned with the dispensation and control of patronage benefits.
D. was more based on immigrant ethnicity in northern urban regions.

PASSAGE 6 (QUESTIONS 31–35)

The first great penal code in the Benthamite tradition, although never enacted, was prepared by an American, Edward Livingston, for the state of Louisiana in 1826. What led to the appearance of this draft code at this time in Louisiana? Many factors, doubtlessly, but conspicuously among them was the commitment of one man to the idea of codification. Livingston was a learned man, well read in Continental as well as English intellectual and social developments. He was captured by the ideas of Bentham and the ferment for legal reform and codification in revolutionary America and France. Earlier in his career as a U.S. Congressman, he sought a revision of the United States penal law. That his code was drafted for Louisiana may be due simply to the accident that led him to leave New York and to transplant his legal and public career there.

The modern codification tradition to which the Model Penal Code (1962) belongs has its roots in the new rationalism of the 18th-century Enlightenment, which saw reason as the instrument both for understanding and mastering the world. For law, reason provided a lodestar and an instrument for reform. The ideas of the Enlightenment took hold in England as well as the Continent and led to a powerful movement toward codification of law. But it was through the work of one man, Jeremy Bentham, that these ideas had their greatest influence on law reform. Bentham's thinking on codification of criminal law had a powerful influence on every codification effort in the English-speaking world in the 19th and 20th centuries, not excluding the Model Penal Code.

Within Bentham's legacy are such concepts as: law defined in advance with clarity and certainty to maximize its potential for guiding behavior; judicial discretion to make or change the law eliminated as productive of uncertainty and arbitrariness; the doctrines of the criminal law and the principles of punishment justified only by their service to the purpose of the criminal law to prevent crime; penalties proportioned to the offense; and refusal to punish where it would be "groundless, inefficacious, unprofitable, or needless."

The Penal Code, breathtaking in conception and achievement, included a Code of Procedure, a Code of Evidence, a Code of Reform and Prison Discipline, and a Code of Crimes and Punishments. Livingston's unassisted completion of this task within three years was one of those prodigious, virtuoso performances that is scarcely imaginable today. His Benthamite philosophy was manifested in many of the Code's provisions, notably those relating to the judicial function. Livingston distrusted judges no less than Bentham; consequently, common-law crimes, use of common-law terms, and all means through which judges might infuse their own moral views into the definition of crimes were outlawed. The object of the Code, to leave as little as possible to judicial creativity, is apparent in its preference for exhaustive and detailed specifications of rules. Other notable characteristics of the Code include its rejection of capital punishment, its moderation of punishments, its forceful protection of freedom of speech and the rights of the accused, the prominent place it gave to reform of the offender and its provision of means to accomplish it.

31. If the author read the following statements in an article on the topic of the development of the Penal Code, he would most likely agree with which of the following statements?

A. Edward Livingston's personal commitment to the codification of laws greatly influenced his colleagues, including Jeremy Bentham.

B. English and Continental lawmakers agreed wholeheartedly on the need for standardization of laws during the 18th and 19th centuries.

C. Developments in intellectual and philosophical thought during the Enlightenment were a major factor in leading to the establishment of the first penal codes.

D. The Benthamite concept of penal codes has been highly influential in theory, but rarely successful when written into law.

32. The author spends some time discussing Bentham's work on legal reform. Which of the following is NOT attributed by the author to Bentham's work on legal reform?

I. Making sure the punishment fits the crime

II. Outlawing unjust and arbitrary penalties

III. Legalization of capital punishment

A. II only

B. III only

C. I and III

D. I, II, and III

33. According to information put forth and argued by the author of the passage, which of the following was one of the primary reasons for the creation of Livingston's penal code?

A. Influence from previous codification efforts had finally spread from other parts of the country into Louisiana.
B. American legal figures were impressed by the legal systems in England and wished to emulate them.
C. Livingston was inspired by intellectual and social changes and progress from abroad.
D. Colleagues in the legal profession encouraged Livingston to develop a Penal Code based on the Benthamite tradition.

34. All of the following are strengths of Livingston's penal code EXCEPT:

A. specific protection of defendants' civil rights.
B. emphasis on reform rather than on punishment.
C. constraints on judicial discretion to modify rules and legal procedures.
D. successful implementation and expansion of his code.

35. Assuming that the author was correct and complete in his analysis of Livingston, one of the guiding motivations for Livingston's development of a penal code was:

A. to afford broader rights and less severe punishments to convicted criminals.
B. to decrease the possibility of judicial misinterpretation of laws.
C. to define penalties and crimes based on common-law terms.
D. to protect certain freedoms and civil rights of defendants.

PASSAGE 7 (QUESTIONS 36–40)

The recognition of exclusive chattels and estate has really harmed and obscured Individualism. It has led Individualism entirely astray. It has made gain, not growth, its aim, so that man has thought that the important thing is to have, and has not come to know that the important thing is to be. The true perfection of man lies, not in what man has, but in what man is.

This state has crushed true Individualism, and set up an Individualism that is false. It has debarred one part of the community from being individual by starving them. It has debarred the other part of the community from being individual by putting them on the wrong road and encumbering them. Indeed, so completely has man's personality been absorbed by his trinkets and entanglements that the law has always treated offenses against a man's property with far more severity than offenses against his person.

It is clear that no authoritarian socialism will do. For while under the present system a very large number of people can lead lives of a certain amount of freedom and expression and happiness, under an industrial barrack system, or a system of economic tyranny, nobody would be able to have any such freedom at all. It is to be regretted that a portion of our community should be practically in slavery, but to propose to solve the problem by enslaving the entire community is childish. Every man must be left quite free to choose his own work.

No form of compulsion must be exercised over him. If there is, his work will not be good for him, will not be good in itself, and will not be good for others. I hardly think that any socialist, nowadays, would seriously propose that an inspector should call every morning at each house to see that each citizen rose up and did manual labor for eight hours. Humanity has got beyond that stage, and reserves such a form of life for the people whom, in a very arbitrary manner, it chooses to call criminals.

Many of the socialistic views that I have come across seem to me to be tainted with ideas of authority, if not of actual compulsion. Of course, authority and compulsion are out of the question. All association must be quite voluntary. It is only in voluntary associations that man is fine. It may be asked how Individualism, which is now more or less dependent on the existence of private property for its development, will benefit by the abolition of such private property. The answer is very simple. It is true that, under existing conditions, a few men who have had private means of their own, such as Byron, Shelley, Browning, Victor Hugo, Baudelaire, and others, have been able to realize their personality, more or less completely.

Not one of these men ever did a single day's work for hire. They were relieved from poverty. They had an immense advantage. The question is whether it would be for the good of Individualism that such an advantage be taken away. Let us suppose that it is taken away. What happens then to Individualism? How will it benefit? Under the new conditions Individualism will be far freer, far finer, and far more intensified than it is now. I am not talking of the great imaginatively realized Individualism of such poets as I have mentioned, but of the great actual Individualism latent and potential in mankind generally.

36. The author of the passage most likely mentions Byron, Shelly, Browning, Hugo, and Baudelaire in an effort to:

A. give examples of the harmful effect of money on Individualism and art.
B. call attention to the rarity of artistic genius.
C. define what is meant by the phrase "realize their personality."
D. stress the importance of financial independence.

37. Which of the following would the author be most likely to consider an example of "enslaving the entire community"?

I. South Africa under apartheid, where rights of citizenship were denied to the Black majority, and granted in full only to the White minority
II. Cambodia under the Khmer Rouge, where the urban population was forcibly deported to the countryside to perform agricultural labor
III. Sweden under the Social Democrats, where all citizens pay high taxes to support extensive social programs

A. I only
B. II only
C. I and II
D. II and III

38. As used in the fourth paragraph of the passage, the phrase "the people whom, in a very arbitrary manner, it chooses to call criminals" implies which of the following?

A. All actions should be permitted.
B. Notions of justice are open to question.
C. No one would commit crimes in a Socialist society.
D. Criminals are better suited for mandatory labor than other people.

39. Suppose for a moment that Baudelaire was actually not wealthy, and often had to work to earn money. What relevance would this information have to the arguments posed by the author within the passage?

A. It would refute the author's claim that artists require independent wealth to create.
B. It would refute the author's claim that poets are people who can realize their own personality.
C. It would strengthen the author's claim that the acquisition of wealth leads Individualism astray.
D. The central thesis of the passage would remain equally valid

40. Based on the information in the passage, we can assume that the author is most likely to agree that:

A. most people who have sufficient private property are fully realized individuals.
B. even with sufficient private property, most people never realize their individuality.
C. artists are less likely than others to be dependent on private means to realize themselves.
D. no artists can realize themselves except with substantial private means.

VERBAL REASONING PRACTICE SECTION 3

Time—60 minutes

DIRECTIONS: There are seven passages in this Verbal Reasoning test. Each passage is followed by several questions. After reading a passage, select the one best answer to each question. If you are not certain of an answer, eliminate the alternatives that you know to be incorrect and then select an answer from the remaining alternatives. Indicate your selection by blackening the corresponding circle on your answer sheet.

PASSAGE 1 (QUESTIONS 1–7)

Suspicious as they are of American intentions, and bolstered by court rulings that seem to give them license to seek out and publish any and all government secrets, the media's distrust of our government, combined with their limited understanding of the world at large, damages our ability to design and conduct good policy in ways that the media rarely imagine.

The leak through which sensitive information flows from the government to the press is detrimental to policy insofar as it almost completely precludes the possibility of serious discussion. Leaders often say one thing in public and quite another thing in private conversation. The fear that anything they say, even in what is construed as a private forum, may appear in print, makes many people, whether our own government officials or the leaders of foreign countries, unwilling to speak their minds.

Must we be content with the restriction of our leaders' policy discussions to a handful of people who trust each other, thus limiting the richness and variety of ideas that could be brought forward through a larger group because of the nearly endemic nature of this problem? And along with the limiting of ideas, we have less reliable information to analyze. It is vitally important for the leaders of the United States to know the real state of affairs internationally, and this can occur only if foreign leaders feel free to speak their minds to our diplomats. This cannot occur when leaders are fearful of finding their private thoughts published in newspapers, and therefore do not share their real beliefs (let alone their secrets) unless they are certain that confidences will be respected.

Until recently, it looked as if the media had convinced the public that journalists were more reliable than the government; thus, many citizens came to believe that the media were the *best* sources of information. When the media challenged a governmental official, the public presumed that the official was in the wrong. However, this may be changing. With the passage of time, the media have lost luster. They—having grown large and powerful—provoke the same public skepticism that other large institutions in the society do. A series of media scandals has contributed to this. Many Americans have concluded that the media are no more credible than the government, and public opinion surveys reflect much ambivalence about the press.

While leaks are generally defended by media officials on the grounds of the public's "right to know," in reality they are part of the Washington political power game, as well as part of the policy process. The "leaker" may be currying favor with the media, or may be planting information to influence policy. In the first case, he is helping himself by enhancing the prestige of a journalist; in the second, he is using the media as a stage for his preferred policies. In either instance, it closes the circle: the leak begins with a political motive, is advanced by a politicized media, and continues because of politics. Although some of the journalists think *they* are doing the work, they are more often than not instruments of the process, not prime movers. The media must be held accountable for their activities, just like every other significant institution in our society, and the media must be forced to earn the public's trust.

1. Based on the information in the passage, with which of the following statements would the author most likely agree?

A. Keeping the public uninformed is warranted in certain situations.
B. The public has a right to know the real state of foreign affairs.
C. The fewer the number of people involved in policy discussions, the better.
D. Leaders give up their right to privacy when they are elected.

2. The passage suggests that press exposés of the private thoughts of foreign officials do NOT result in U.S. leaders having a better grasp of foreign affairs because:

A. U.S. leaders are already privy to the private thoughts of foreign leaders.
B. foreign officials begin to view their American counterparts as untrustworthy.
C. foreign officials do not reveal their secrets to the press.
D. the information that reaches the press about policy discussions is unreliable.

3. Imagine you are an opponent of the author and disagree with his conclusions. In an upcoming written rebuttal you want to address the author's best-supported claims first. For which of the following claims does the passage provide some supporting evidence or explanation?

A. The media rarely understand that their actions damage America's ability to conduct foreign policy.
B. Leaks can be an intentional part of the policy process.
C. Every significant institution in society besides the media is held accountable for their activities.
D. The media is suspicious of the intentions of the American government.

4. Implicit in the author's argument that leaks result in far more limited and unreliable policy discussions with foreign leaders is the idea that:

A. leaks should be considered breaches of trust and therefore immoral.
B. leaks have occurred throughout the history of politics.
C. foreign and U.S. leaders discussed policy without inhibition before the rise of the mass media.
D. leaders fear the public would react negatively if it knew the real state of affairs.

5. In the context of the fifth paragraph, the term "prime movers" (paragraph 5) would most accurately refer to:

A. U.S. officials who pass on sensitive information to the media.
B. journalists who are attempting to enhance their own prestige.
C. media executives who use their own journalists to further political causes.
D. the unwritten rules that govern the flow of leaked information in Washington.

6. Leaked information typically comes to journalists anonymously since the government official leaking the information fears reprisal. What relevance does this have to the passage?

A. It supports the claim that the leaker plants information to influence policy.
B. It supports the claim that journalists are more reliable than the government.
C. It weakens the claim that the media can be used as a stage for an official's preferred policies.
D. It weakens the claim that a leaker can curry favor with a journalist.

7. Based on the passage, when the media now challenge the actions of a public official, the public assumes that:

A. the official is wrong.
B. the media are always wrong.
C. the media may be wrong.
D. the official and the media may both be wrong.

PASSAGE 2 (QUESTIONS 8–13)

The person who, with inner conviction, loathes stealing, killing, and assault, may find himself performing these acts with relative ease when commanded by authority. Behavior that is unthinkable in an individual who is acting of his own volition may be executed without hesitation when carried out under orders. An act carried out under command is, psychologically, of a profoundly different character than spontaneous action.

The important task, from the standpoint of a psychological study of obedience, is to be able to take conceptions of authority and translate them into personal experience. It is one thing to talk in abstract terms about the respective rights of the individual and of authority; it is quite another to examine a moral choice in a real situation. We all know about the philosophic problems of freedom and authority. But in every case where the problem is not merely academic there is a real person who must obey or disobey authority. All musing prior to this moment is mere speculation, and all acts of disobedience are characterized by such a moment of decisive action.

When we move to the laboratory, the problem narrows: if an experimenter tells a subject to act with increasing severity against another person, under what conditions will the subject comply, and under what conditions will he disobey? The laboratory problem is vivid, intense, and real. It is not something apart from life, but carries to an extreme and very logical conclusion certain trends inherent in the ordinary functioning of the social world. The question arises as to whether there is any connection between what we have studied in the laboratory and the forms of obedience we have so often deplored throughout history. The differences in the two situations are, of course, enormous, yet the difference in scale, numbers, and political context may be relatively unimportant as long as certain essential features are retained.

To the degree that an absence of compulsion is present, obedience is colored by a cooperative mood; to the degree that the threat of force or punishment against the person is intimated, obedience is compelled by fear. The major problem for the individual is to recapture control of his own regnant processes once he has committed them to the purposes of others. The difficulty this entails represents the poignant and in some degree tragic element in the situation, for nothing is bleaker than the sight of a person striving yet not fully able to control his own behavior in a situation of consequence to him.

The essence of obedience is the fact that a person comes to view himself as the instrument for carrying out another's wishes, and he therefore no longer regards himself as culpable for his actions. Once this critical shift of viewpoint has occurred, all of the essential features of obedience—the adjustment of thought, the freedom to engage in cruel behavior, and the types of justification experienced by the person (essentially similar whether they occur in a psychological laboratory or on the battlefield)—follow. The question of generality, therefore, is not resolved by enumerating all of the manifest differences between the psychological laboratory and other situations, but by carefully constructing a situation that captures the essence of obedience—a situation in which a person gives himself over to authority and no longer views himself as the cause of his own actions.

8. Suppose that a pilot in the Rimland air force initially contests an order to bomb a city, but eventually agrees to carry it out willingly. How would this scenario affect the author's view of obedience to authority?

A. It would support the author's view.
B. It would contradict the author's view.
C. It would support the author's view only if it could be shown that the pilot had a history of carrying out orders that he did not initially support.
D. It would contradict the author's view only if it could be shown that the pilot had a history of refusing to carry out orders.

9. Which of the following would be considered "acts of disobedience" as this term is used in paragraph 2?

A. A nurse who administers a drug to a patient, even though the patient's doctor knows that the drug may kill the patient
B. An employee who refuses to work overtime, even though the employee's boss has told the employee that a certain project must be finished as soon as possible
C. A soldier who refuses to harm a civilian, even though the soldier's commanding officer has ordered that the civilian be shot as a spy
D. An engineer who certifies a building as safe, even though the engineer's construction company has not adhered to all government safety codes

10. In the context of the points being made by the author in the passage, the phrase "absence of compulsion" (paragraph 4) refers to:

A. the lack of punishment in psychological experiments.
B. obedience that is willingly given to one's superior.
C. the freedom to disobey the orders of those in authority.
D. one's ability to consider the moral implications of an act.

11. Which of the following findings would serve to most WEAKEN the author's claim in the passage about obedience to authority?

A. A study that concludes that most obedience to authority is motivated by fear
B. A study that demonstrates that most authority figures in government behave immorally
C. A study that shows that most people do not have strongly held ethical values
D. A study that asserts that people with a college education are less likely to obey authority figures than those with only a high school education are

12. For which of the following statements does the passage provide some explanation or evidence?

A. A laboratory experiment can be made to simulate real-world behavior.
B. The subject of obedience has not received the attention it deserves from the field of social psychology.
C. It is unfortunate that people are often not in full control of their own behavior.
D. People in positions of authority tend to have lower moral standards than people who are not in positions of authority.

13. Suppose that a person who is not in a position of authority kills a person who is in a position of authority. Would this information be relevant to the author's view of obedience to authority?

A. It would be relevant under any set of circumstances.
B. It would not be relevant under any set of circumstances.
C. It would be relevant under a certain set of circumstances.
D. It would be relevant only if the two had no prior relationship.

PASSAGE 3 (QUESTIONS 14–19)

Most diseases or conditions improve by themselves, are self-limiting, or even if fatal, seldom follow a strictly downward spiral. In each case, intervention can appear to be quite efficacious. This becomes all the more patent if you assume the point of view of a knowing practitioner of fraudulent medicine.

To take advantage of the natural ups and downs of any disease (as well as of any placebo effect), it's best to begin your treatment when the patient is getting worse. In this way, anything that happens can more easily be attributed to your wonderful and probably expensive intervention. If the patient improves, you take credit; if he remains stable, your treatment stopped his downward course. On the other hand, if the patient worsens, the dosage or intensity of the treatment was not great enough; if he dies, he delayed too long in coming to you.

In any case, the few instances in which your intervention is successful will likely be remembered (not so few, if the disease in question is self-limiting), while the vast majority of failures will be forgotten and buried. Chance provides more than enough variation to account for the sprinkling of successes that will occur with almost any treatment; indeed, it would be a miracle if there weren't any "miracle cures."

Even in outlandish cases, it's often difficult to refute conclusively some proposed cure or procedure. Consider a diet doctor who directs his patients to consume two whole pizzas, four birch beers, and two pieces of cheesecake for every breakfast, lunch, and dinner, and an entire box of fig bars with a quart of milk for a bedtime snack, claiming that other people have lost six pounds a week on such a regimen. When several patients follow his instructions for three weeks, they find they've gained about seven pounds each. Have the doctor's claims been refuted?

Not necessarily, since he might respond that a whole host of auxiliary understandings weren't met: the pizzas had too much sauce, or the dieters slept 16 hours a day, or the birch beer wasn't the right brand. Number and probability do, however, provide the basis for statistics, which, together with logic, constitutes the foundation of the scientific method, which will eventually sort matters out if anything can. However, just as the existence of pink does not undermine the distinction between red and white, and dawn doesn't indicate that day and night are really the same, this problematic fringe area doesn't negate the fundamental differences between science and its impostors.

The philosopher Willard Van Orman Quine ventures even further and maintains that experience never forces one to reject any particular belief. He views science as an integrated web of interconnecting hypotheses, procedures, and formalisms, and argues that any impact of the world on the web can be distributed in many different ways. If we're willing to make drastic enough changes in the rest of the web of our beliefs, the argument goes, we can hold to our belief in the efficacy of the above diet, or indeed in the validity of any pseudoscience.

14. In the context of the passage, its discussion of various medical conditions, and the particulars of those conditions, the term "self-limiting" (paragraph 2) refers to medical conditions that:

A. run a definite course that does not result in the patient's death.
B. impair the patient's ability to engage in everyday activities.
C. have a very high rate of mortality.
D. never shows improvement.

15. Suppose that in order to demonstrate the legitimacy of his work, a faith healer compiles a book of interviews of people who swear that he has cured them just by blessing them. The author would most likely respond by asserting that:

A. eyewitness testimony of emotional events tends to be unreliable.
B. the interviewees would have gotten better without the healer's intervention.
C. the ability to cure people does not justify shameless self-promotion.
D. the interviewees have been deluded into thinking that they have improved when they have not.

16. According to the passage, which of the following would best determine whether a practitioner's intervention is worthwhile or not?

A. Keeping a record of the time it takes for a patient to respond to the practitioner's treatment
B. Keeping a record of the number of patients the practitioner has treated successfully
C. Keeping a record of the dosage that the practitioner employs in his treatment
D. Keeping a record of both the successes and failures of the practitioner

17. Based on the information in the passage, which of the following opinions could most reasonably be ascribed to the author?

A. Too often nothing truly effective can be done to ameliorate the illness of a patient.
B. There is no way that pseudoscience will ever be eliminated.
C. Beliefs can be maintained even in the absence of strong supporting evidence.
D. Experience never forces one to reject any particular belief.

18. Doctors and scientists continue to debate whether certain types of alternative medicine are scientific or pseudoscientific. How is this information relevant to the passage?

A. It weakens the claim that one can hold onto whatever pet theory one fancies.
B. It weakens the claim that the scientific method is useful in sorting science from pseudoscience.
C. It strengthens the claim that there is a fundamental difference between medicine and science.
D. It strengthens the claim that science and pseudoscience cannot always be distinguished.

19. The author of the passage would most likely agree with an individual who argues that W.V.O. Quine's philosophical views are:

A. extreme, because some beliefs can be proven to be either true or false.
B. insightful, because any set of beliefs has to be as valid as any other.
C. flawed, because they do not explain why anyone would reject any belief.
D. bankrupt, because they do not apply to any particular situation.

PASSAGE 4 (QUESTIONS 20–24)

In the decades following World War II, American business had undisputed control of the world economy, producing goods of such high quality and low cost that foreign corporations were unable to compete. But in the mid-1960s the United States began to lose its advantage and by the 1980s, American corporations lagged behind the competition in many industries. In the computer chip industry, for example, American corporations had lost most of both domestic and foreign markets by the early 1980s.

The first analysts to examine the decline of American business blamed the U.S. government. They argued that stringent governmental restrictions on the behavior of American corporations, combined with the wholehearted support given to foreign firms by their governments, created an environment in which American products could not compete. Later analysts blamed predatory corporate raiders who bought corporations, not to make them more competitive in the face of foreign competition, but rather to sell off the most lucrative divisions for huge profits.

Still later, analysts blamed the American workforce, citing labor demands and poor productivity as the reasons American corporations have been unable to compete with Japanese and European firms. Finally, a few analysts even censured American consumers for their unpatriotic purchases of foreign goods. The blame actually lies with corporate management, which has made serious errors based on misconceptions about what it takes to be successful in the marketplace. These missteps involve labor costs, production choices, and growth strategies.

Even though labor costs typically account for less than 15% of a product's total cost, management has been quick to blame the costs of workers' wages for driving up prices, making American goods uncompetitive. As a result of attempts to minimize the cost of wages, American corporations have had trouble recruiting and retaining skilled workers.

The emphasis on cost minimization has also led to another blunder: an over-concentration on high technology products. Many foreign firms began by specializing in the mass production and sale of low technology products, gaining valuable experience and earning tremendous profits. Later, these corporations were able to break into high technology markets without much trouble; they simply applied their previous manufacturing experience and ample financial resources to the production of higher quality goods. American business has consistently ignored this very sensible approach.

The recent rash of corporate mergers and acquisitions in the United States has not helped the situation either. While American firms have neglected long-range planning and production, preferring instead to reap fast profits through mergers and acquisitions, foreign firms have been quick to exploit opportunities to ensure their domination over future markets by investing in the streamlining and modernization of their facilities.

20. The passage makes certain comparisons of American workers to Japanese workers. It suggests that compared to Japanese workers, American workers are often considered:

A. more content and more efficient.
B. more content but less efficient.
C. less content and less efficient.
D. less content but more efficient.

21. With which of the following general statements would the author most likely NOT agree?

A. American business has been hurt by the inability to plan for the long term.
B. Cutting production costs always leads to increased competitiveness.
C. American consumers are not the prime cause of the decline of American business.
D. Initial analysis of the decline of American business yielded only partially accurate conclusions.

22. Which of the following would most weaken the author's argument about the over-concentration of high-technology products?

A. Producing low-tech products is not as profitable as producing high-tech products.
B. Manufacturing high-tech products is a completely different process than manufacturing low-tech goods.
C. Most of the low-tech products purchased by Americans are made by foreign firms.
D. Most of the high-tech products purchased by Americans are made by foreign firms.

23. A reader of this passage is asked to decide whether or not she stands behind the author's arguments. Adopting the author's views as presented in the passage would most likely mean acknowledging that:

A. it should be the goal of American business to regain control of the market.
B. the major blunder of American businesses was to alienate the skilled workers.
C. the future of American business would appear to be hopeless.
D. the foreign market is more important for business survival than the domestic market.

24. The author of this passage would probably give his strongest support to which of the following actions by the corporate management of an American company?

A. Acquiring a smaller company in order to gain financial resources
B. Considering the option of paying the most highly skilled workers a higher wage
C. Imitating the general management strategy of foreign firms
D. Paying for television advertisements that will win back American consumers

PASSAGE 5 (QUESTIONS 25–30)

From the outset of his dramatic poem *Samson Agonistes* (1671), John Milton establishes and expands upon a hero/antihero dichotomy that has its roots in the Book of Judges. Samson is the "epic hero," a tragic figure who falls, despite tremendous personal strength. In prison, Samson's thoughts and words are melancholy and self-effacing. He compares his body to a vessel, tragically steered off course and consequently wrecked by his lust for Dalila.

The chorus of friends visiting him in prison does not allow their hero to take full blame, but placates him with the androcentric consolation: "wisest Men/Have err'd, and by bad women been deceiv'd." In this, the chorus' trope of woman-as-deceiver (and thus logical repository for blame) is much more simplified and essentialist than is Samson's view. While he clearly despises Dalila for leading him into such a trap ("That specious Monster, my accomplisht snare"), he also implicates himself in his capture.

Samson's confession of his culpability is, in a way, analogous to the scene in Milton's more widely read *Paradise Lost* in which Adam takes partial responsibility for the Fall. However, despite the similarities of the "falls" in *Samson Agonistes* and *Paradise Lost*, the overall gender relations in the two texts are not so simply analogous. Adam and Eve are co-creators of the Fall; Eve is not the deceiver but rather the deceived. She beseeches Adam to taste the fruit not out of malice or hope for worldly gain, but instead in an attempt to share the "wisdom" that she falsely believes she has acquired. Dalila, on the other hand, is much more cognizant of her deception; in fact, she revels in it as a means of gaining wealth and renown. She receives the forgiveness of neither her husband, Samson, nor her author, Milton. Samson may be aware of his culpability, but his anger toward and hatred of Dalila is not quelled by this self-awareness.

When Dalila first approaches Samson in the prison, she feigns contrition, telling Samson that she did not realize her deed would cause him so much agony—that she wishes to make amends for her "rash but more unfortunate misdeed." It is, however, difficult to believe that someone heretofore positioned as the deceiver would do anything *but* deceive. Samson rebukes her, regretting the lust that drew him to her side; he no longer wishes to be "entangl'd with a posynous bosom snake." This imagery calls to mind not only the deadly asp of another femme fatale, Cleopatra, but also Satan as the serpent in the Garden. This identification links Dalila more explicitly with the serpent than with Eve. Eve and Dalila, though both responsible to some degree for a "fall," are, in Milton's eyes, two very different women

It is interesting to note that, while Milton avoids the fallacy of overt stereotyping, by describing Dalila as a certain "type" of woman, Dalila herself *employs* essentialism to relieve herself of some culpability and ingratiate herself with Samson. She attempts to pass off her treachery as common to all women, saying, "it was a weakness/In me, but incident to all our sex." She uses antifeminist rhetoric to exonerate herself in the same way Samson used it to incriminate her. In both instances, the fallacy of sexual essentialism is clear.

When Samson rejects her advances, Dalila quickly reverts to the cold persona that the reader has come to expect. She gloats over the downfall of the great Samson and her "public marks of honor and reward" self-aggrandizing glee that certainly does not endear Dalila to Samson, to Milton, or to the reader, but does reemphasize her cleverness and power.

25. The primary purpose of this passage is to:

A. provide a detailed comparative study of gender roles in two of Milton's dramatic poems, *Samson Agonistes* and *Paradise Lost*.
B. examine the motivations and actions of a sometimes oversimplified character.
C. advocate a feminist reading of the character of Dalila in *Samson Agonistes*.
D. compare and contrast Milton's version of the Samson and Dalila story with that found in the biblical book of Judges.

26. The passage suggests that which of the following is NOT a tactic employed by Dalila in order to manipulate Samson?

A. Appropriating patriarchal stereotypes in order to further her argument
B. Deceiving under the guise of romantic and sexual interest
C. Arguing the superiority of the female intellect to the male
D. Giving false apologies in order to win back Samson's trust

27. The author most likely mentions the serpent (Paragraph 4) in order to:

A. make a comparison between Milton's portrayal of Dalila and Shakespeare's portrayal of Cleopatra.
B. remind the reader of the similar dichotomy between Adam/Eve and Samson/Dalila.
C. emphasize Milton's view of Dalila by comparing her to a creature traditionally associated with deception.
D. differentiate between the asp in the story of Cleopatra and the serpent of biblical tradition.

28. According to the passage, *Samson Agonistes* and *Paradise Lost* share all of the following characteristics EXCEPT:

A. the "fall" of a male character as the result of a decision made by a female character.
B. a similar gender hierarchy in which the woman wields the power of deception.
C. an acceptance of culpability by the male character.
D. the literary expansion of a biblical story.

29. Which of the following, if true, would be LEAST consistent with the author's claim that Milton views Eve and Dalila as two clearly different "types" of women?

A. The introduction of textual evidence that proves Samson's punishment was as devastating as Adam's
B. Evidence from *Paradise Lost* that proves Eve made Adam taste the fruit so that she might have some amount of power over him
C. The introduction of evidence that, in the Judges version of the story, Samson was neither as intelligent nor as self-reflective as he is in Milton's retelling
D. The introduction of evidence that, at the beginning of both the Judges story and *Samson Agonistes*, Dalila was in love with Samson

30. It can be reasonably inferred that the author of this passage is:

A. a biblical scholar doing comparative research on the similarities and differences between an Old Testament story and a literary retelling.
B. a feminist scholar researching examples of feminist characters in English literature.
C. a historian researching societal attitudes toward strong female figures.
D. a literary scholar exploring the personality and motivations of a significant female character.

PASSAGE 6 (QUESTIONS 31–35)

The planned expansion of the North Atlantic Treaty Organization (NATO) into Eastern Europe has been compared by one sour critic to the behavior of a couple in a crumbling marriage, who instead of going to a marriage counselor try to save their relationship by having a baby, or possibly even several babies. NATO itself is in the middle of a very confused debate about its identity and role, and partly as a result it is difficult to detect any honest, coherent discussion in the West of the necessity for expansion and of how it will affect relations with Russia, the security of the Ukraine and the Baltic States, and the peaceful integration of Ukraine into Europe.

The official Western line at present is that NATO expansion is meant to "strengthen European security," but not against Russia or against feared Russian aggression. Nevertheless, all public discussion in Poland—and much of it in the United States—has been conducted in terms of the need to contain a presumed Russian threat and to prevent Russia from exerting influence on its neighbors, influence that is automatically viewed as illegitimate and threatening to the West.

The overwhelming majority of Russian politicians, including most liberals, now believe it is necessary that most of the former Soviet Union excluding the Baltic States be within a Russian sphere of influence. They see this not as imperialism but as a justifiable defense of Russian interests against a multiplicity of potential threats (radical Islam, future Turkish expansionism), of Russian populations outside Russia, and of areas in which Russia has long maintained a cultural presence—Ukraine, for example. This does not necessarily involve demands for hegemony over Russia's neighbors, but it certainly implies the exclusion of any other bloc's or superpower's military presence. In justification, Russians point to the Monroe Doctrine and to the French sphere of influence in Africa. Most educated Russians now view Western criticism as mere hypocrisy masking Western aggrandizement.

The attitude of the entire Russian political establishment to the expansion issue is now strongly and unanimously negative, though the government hopes for the moment to continue exerting influence against expansion by cooperating with NATO—hence its agreement to join the Partnership for Peace. The reasons for Russian opposition are these: NATO expansion is seen as a betrayal of clear though implicit promises made by the West in 1990-91, and a sign that the West regards Russia not as an ally but as a defeated enemy. Russians point out that Moscow agreed to withdraw troops from the former East Germany following unification after NATO promised not to station its troops there.

Now NATO is planning to leapfrog over eastern Germany and end up 500 miles closer to Russia, in Poland. Western arguments that the 1990 promise to Mikhail Gorbachev referred only to East Germany, not to the rest of Eastern Europe, though strictly speaking correct, are not unnaturally viewed by Russians as purely Jesuitical.

Russian officials say that the NATO expansion would lead to a reversal of the previous pro-Western policy of the Yeltsin and Gorbachev governments. Also, Russians fear that NATO expansion will ultimately mean the inclusion of the Baltic States and Ukraine within NATO's sphere of influence, if not in NATO itself—and thus the loss of any Russian influence over these states and the stationing of NATO troops within striking distance of the Russian heartland. The West's inability publicly to rule out the possible future incorporation of any country in NATO makes it very difficult to assuage Russian fears.

31. In the context of the analogy in the first paragraph, the couple is to the baby as:

A. NATO is to Russia.
B. Russia and NATO together are to an Eastern European country.
C. NATO is to an Eastern European country.
D. Eastern Europe is to NATO.

32. If the author of this passage were asked in an interview about his feeling regarding potential action that NATO might take with regard to the passage, he would probably give his greatest support to which of the following actions by NATO?

A. Admitting officially that NATO expansion is meant to contain the Russian threat
B. Halting expansion once Poland has been absorbed into NATO
C. Stating publicly that Ukraine will never be included in NATO's sphere of influence
D. Reconsidering plans to establish a presence in Eastern Europe

33. Judging from the passage, the "clear though implicit promises" made by the West to Russia in 1990-91 were promises that:

A. the West would allow Russia to station troops in Poland.
B. the West would not station troops in any East European country.
C. the West would withdraw its troops from East Germany following unification.
D. the West would leapfrog over East Germany into Poland.

34. Based on the passage, which of the following could be considered true beliefs of the majority of Western diplomats?

I. Any expansion of Russia's influence on its neighbors would endanger the West.
II. Ukraine is not in any danger of being absorbed by NATO.
III. Russia would not be justified in regaining control of former Soviet territories.

A. II only
B. II and III
C. I and III
D. I, II, and III

35. Based on the passage, which of the following could one most reasonably expect of a country that is attempting to expand its sphere of influence?

A. A complete cessation of communication with potential enemies
B. A declaration that the purpose of expansion is greater security
C. A stubborn refusal to admit defeat when it has in fact been suffered
D. A prolonged period of careful planning and diplomatic negotiation

PASSAGE 7 (QUESTIONS 36–40)

The original Hellenistic community was idealized, the Greeks' own golden dream—a community never achieved but only imagined by the Macedonian Alexander, who was possessed of the true faith of all converts to a larger vision. The evolving system of city-states had produced not only unity with a healthy diversity, but also narrow rivalries. No Hellenic empire arose, only scores of squabbling cities pursuing bitter feuds born of ancient wrongs and existing ambitions. It was civil strife made possible by isolation from the great armies and ambitions of Asia.

Greek history could arguably begin in July of 776 B.C., the First Olympiad, and end with Theodosus's ban on the games in 393 A.D. Before this there had been a long era of two tribes, the Dorians and Ionians, scarcely distinguishable to the alien eye, but distinctly separate in their own eyes until 776. After Theodosus' ban most of the Mediterranean world was Greek-like, in fact, but the central core had been rendered impotent by diffusion.

During the eventful Greek millennium, the Olympics reflected not the high ideals of Hellenes but rather the mean reality of the times. Its founders had created a monster, games that twisted the strategists' aspirations to unity to fit the unpleasant reality of the Hellenistic world. The games not only mirrored the central practices of the Greek world that reformers would deny, they also imposed the flaws of that world. Like the atomic theory of the Greek philosophers, the Greek gamers' theories were far removed from reality; they were elegant, consistent, logical, and irrelevant.

Part religious ritual, part game rite, in the five-day Olympic Games, various athletes came together under the banner of their cities; winning became paramount, imposing defeat a delight. As Greek society evolved, so, too, did the games, but rarely as a unifying force. Athletes supposedly competing for the laurel of accomplishment in the name of idealism found that dried olive leaves changed to gold. Each local polis (city-state) sought not to contribute to the grandeur of Greece, but to achieve its own glory. As in the real world, in the games no Greek could trust another, and each envied rivals' victories. The Olympic spirit was not one of communal bliss but bitter lasting competition institutionalized in games.

36. In the context of the passage, the phrase "dried olive leaves changed to gold" (Paragraph 4) refers to:

A. the peace achieved by Greek city-states during Olympic years.

B. the benefits that athletes could expect to derive from Olympic victories.

C. the political unification of Dorian and Ionian tribes in 776 B.C.

D. the spread of Greek culture during the period from 776 B.C. to 393 A.D.

37. For which of the following statements does the passage provide some evidence or explanation?

I. Alexander united ancient Greece through a series of military conquests.

II. The divisions among Greek city-states were reflected in the Olympics.

III. The Olympic Games could not have occurred without a city-state system.

A. II only
B. III only
C. I and II
D. II and III

38. Suppose that a Greek wrestler had just won the Olympic wrestling contest. Which of the following rewards would he have been LEAST likely to receive?

A. A sense of pleasure in defeating an opponent
B. A grant of land from his own city-state
C. A political office in his own city-state
D. A monetary prize from another city-state

39. Which of the following, if true, would most STRENGTHEN the author's claims about the Olympic Games in ancient Greece?

A. Contested outcomes of Olympic events sometimes caused wars between city-states.
B. The Olympic Games began long before Alexander united all of the city-states.
C. Most city-states regularly applauded the Olympic victories of athletes from other city-states.
D. Each city-state was only allowed to send one athlete per Olympic event.

40. The statement: "The Olympic spirit was not one of communal bliss but bitter lasting competition institutionalized in games" (paragraph 4) indicates that the author believes that:

A. the Greeks were more internally divided than other Mediterranean civilizations.
B. the Greek millennium was a period of constant warfare.
C. the Olympic Games did not serve a beneficial national purpose.
D. the First Olympiad in 776 B.C. began the decline of Greek civilization.

ESSAY PRACTICE SECTION

This section provides you with essay-writing practice. The topics here resemble those you'll like see on Test Day, so you'll want to practice the Five-Step Method you learned in chapter 6.

> **TEACHER TIP**
> The Kaplan Method for prewriting and writing the MCAT essay is time-tested and proven. Though you might be able to write a good essay without it, you'd have to re-invent the wheel.

Practice is vital for this section of the MCAT. There is simply no substitute for testing yourself under test conditions. Make sure not to allow yourself any extra minutes to complete an essay, and don't look at the topic in advance. You should type your essays on the computer.

The first part of the chapter provides four essay topics, and the second part provides sample essay responses. These sample essays have been evaluated using the MCAT-style holistic grading technique discussed earlier. We have also included a "reactions" page after each essay where the student writer provides his first reactions to the challenges of the exam.

> **TEACHER TIP**
> Don't forget to develop databases and practice prewriting, too.

For each of the four essays, spend (a strict) 30 minutes. On the real exam, you'll have to write two essays back-to-back so you may want to do the same here. By having two one-hour sittings, you'll test yourself under conditions as realistic as possible. Alternatively, you may want to take four single-topic practice tests. That method would give you the chance to critique each essay before trying the next.

DEVELOP YOUR CRITICAL SKILLS

After you have completed an essay (or two), turn to the sample essays for an evaluation. First, try to form your *own* opinion regarding the sample essay's merits. Pretend you are a professional MCAT reader and grade the essay using the MCAT criteria discussed in chapter 5. Then look at how our readers evaluated the essay. Doing this will help you develop your own critical skills, a crucial step to becoming a good writer.

> **TEACHER TIP**
> Do NOT look at the sample responses before you write on the topic! That would defeat the purpose of this exercise.

The "reactions" comments from student writers should prove useful to you as well. They offer good insight into how your peers coped with this demanding assignment.

TEACHER TIP

Whomever you ask to critique your essay should be familiar with the unique requirements of an MCAT essay. If the reader is not MCAT-aware, she should read only for grammar, word choice, sentence structure, and style.

HAVE YOUR ESSAY CRITIQUED

Another way to critique your own work is to ask someone else's opinion. If you know someone else taking the MCAT, it might be a good idea to swap essays. Or you can give your work to someone whose writing skills you respect: a friend, teacher, or family member. If you do so, tell them about the nature of the assignment and about the time limit. Make sure that your readers understand the special requirements of the MCAT so they can have a better context of what they're reading.

Whatever the comments are which come back to you, take the suggestions with a cool head and objectivity. Your evaluators are not trying to tear you down when they point out areas of needed improvement.

TEACHER TIP

Since you'll be taking your MCAT in a room with others who have different start times, break times, and end times, you'll have to learn how to concentrate amidst a room of distractions.

REMEMBER THE FIVE STEPS

When judging your own essays' merits, think about your performance in terms of the five steps. Could your initial approach to the topic be better? Did you skip or skimp on any of the prewriting steps? Did you do all the prewriting steps but fail to finish your essay or leave time to proofread? If so, you probably need to practice the prewriting steps more. The goal is to accomplish them in five minutes.

TAKE THE PRACTICE TESTS SERIOUSLY

- Give yourself 30 minutes; don't allow yourself "extra" minutes to finish that last paragraph. You won't get extras on the day of the test.
- Take each practice test under test-like conditions. You should have total peace and quiet in which to write. Take notes on scratch paper and type the final essay on the computer, just as you will do on Test Day.
- Use the Five-Step Method. You can become comfortable with this efficient method only by practicing it. If you are not clear about any part of it, go back to refresh your memory.

PRACTICE ESSAY QUESTIONS

Observe the time limit. Use the lined pages that follow each question for your prewriting notes. Type the essays on a computer.

Time Limit: Each essay should take no longer than 30 minutes.

QUESTION 1

Consider the following statement:

The best kind of education encourages students to question authority.

Write a unified essay in which you accomplish the following tasks. Explain what you think the above statement means. Describe a specific situation in which encouraging students to question authority is not the best kind of education. Discuss what you think determines when students should be encouraged to question authority.

Scratch paper

Scratch paper

Scratch paper

Scratch paper

Scratch paper

QUESTION 2

Consider this statement:

Violence is never a real solution to a political crisis.

Write a unified essay in which you accomplish the following tasks. Explain what you think the above statement means. Describe a specific situation in which violence could be considered a real solution to a political crisis. Discuss what you think determines when violence is justified in solving such a crisis.

Scratch paper

Scratch paper

Scratch paper

Scratch paper

Scratch paper

QUESTION 3

Consider this statement:

To be effective, government officials must have completely crime-free pasts.

Write a unified essay in which you accomplish the following tasks. Explain what you think the above statement means. Describe a specific situation in which a government official who once committed a crime could still perform effectively. Discuss what you believe determines when a criminal past would not interfere with a government official's effectiveness.

Scratch paper

Scratch paper

Scratch paper

Scratch paper

Scratch paper

QUESTION 4

Consider this statement:

> **The government should fund scientific research only when it has a direct application to societal problems.**

Write a unified essay in which you accomplish the following tasks. Explain what you think the above statement means. Describe a specific situation in which the government should fund scientific research that does not have a direct application to societal problems. Discuss what you think determines whether or not the government should fund scientific research that has no direct application to societal problems.

Scratch paper

Scratch paper

Scratch paper

Scratch paper

Scratch paper

Answers and Explanations

CHAPTER 7: USAGE AND STYLE

The answers below are sample answers only. There are many possible ways to say something correctly and well. You'll find your own voice the more you write.

ANSWERS TO EXERCISE 1: JUNK PHRASES

1. The agency is not prepared to expand now.
2. Since John has prepared for this presentation so carefully, we should award him the project.
3. Flights are always at least an hour late on this airline, though its leaders promise that promptness is a high priority for all its employees.
4. Although she is inexperienced in photography, she will probably succeed because she is motivated.
5. The United States cannot spend more money to alleviate other countries' suffering when its own citizens suffer.
6. Although tactful, George says exactly what he believes.
7. Accuracy is important to English teachers and company presidents alike.
8. Humans kill each other because they fear those whom they do not understand.
9. Ms. Miller speaks intelligently about many aspects of modern philosophy.
10. The best leader listens and inspires simultaneously.

ANSWERS TO EXERCISE 2: REDUNDANCY

1. All these problems have combined to create a crisis.
2. A staff that large needs an effective supervisor.
3. He knows how to follow directions.
4. The writer's technical skill does not mask his poor plot line.
5. That monument remains a significant tourist attraction.

6. The recent trend of spending on credit has created a more impoverished middle class.
7. Few people can follow directions.
8. She has chosen to change careers.
9. Such dialogue opens many doors to compromise.
10. The conclusion is that environmental and economic concerns are intertwined.

ANSWERS TO EXERCISE 3: EXCESSIVE QUALIFICATION

1. She is a good teacher.
2. Ferrara is a slow worker.
3. There are many reasons technology has not permeated all countries equally.
4. In a murder trial, it is important to pay attention to all the details as well as to the "larger picture."
5. You are the best person to decide what you should do for a living.
6. The author overstates his case.
7. The president should use diplomacy before he resorts to force.
8. In Italy I found the best food I have ever eaten.
9. Children should be taught to cooperate at home and in school. (If there's no need to say it, don't!)
10. The travel agent said not to go to Tripoli, since one may be hurt. (Saying "it is possible that one may be hurt" is an example of redundant qualification since both *possible* and *may* indicate uncertainty.)

ANSWERS TO EXERCISE 5: NEEDLESS SELF-REFERENCE

1. We ought to pay teachers more than we pay senators.
2. The author is stuck in the past.
3. This argument cannot be generalized to most business owners.
4. Food is perhaps the best social lubricant.
5. More people would not vote even if they had more information about candidates.
6. Privacy should not be valued more than social concerns.
7. Most people want to do good work, but many are bored or frustrated with their jobs.
8. The author has a point.

9. College presidents should implement several specific reforms to combat apathy.
10. Either alternative would prove disastrous.

ANSWERS TO EXERCISE 6: UNDESIRABLE PASSIVES

1. Brave but misguided men fought the Spanish-American War.
2. Congress passed the bill in time, but the president did not sign it until the time for action had passed.
3. Those who need advice least usually request it; the truly lost and ignorant do not seek it at all.
4. We should relocate that building where citizens can appreciate it.
5. City government should generously reward garbage collectors for their dirty, smelly labors.
6. Negotiators ironed out the conditions of the contract agreement minutes before the strike deadline.
7. The city clerk should take the minutes of the City Council meeting.
8. With sugar, water, or salt, doctors can treat many of the ailments that citizens of less-developed countries contract.
9. The teacher distributed test results with no concern for confidentiality.
10. A number of field anthropologists and marriage experts compiled the report.

ANSWERS TO EXERCISE 7: WEAK OPENINGS

1. Businesses cannot ignore the illiteracy problem without suffering.
2. Experience is more important than training in many fields.
3. This plane is obsolete for several reasons.
4. The government cannot fight a drug war effectively without waging a battle against the demand for illicit substances.
5. The candidate has many strong points; intelligence, unfortunately, is not among them.
6. The city cannot justify building a more handsome prison.
7. We, as a society, have decided to tolerate homelessness.
8. Americans must like watching television better than conversing.
9. Cats make better pets than mice.
10. Intelligence is a product of environment and heredity.

ANSWERS TO EXERCISE 9: CLICHÉS

1. Jefferson was certainly a great leader.
2. Families probably spend less time together than they did 15 years ago.
3. The pizza delivery man arrived just when the sequestered jury most needed him.
4. Trying to find the employee responsible for this embarrassing information leak may be impossible.
5. Both strategies would be expensive and completely ineffective: they have an equal chance of failing.
6. The military should diversify its defense rather than rely so heavily on nuclear missiles.
7. Older doctors should be required to update their techniques, but many seem resistant to changes in technology.
8. You need not take this new fad very seriously; it will surely pass.
9. The politician reminds me of Abraham Lincoln with his rough appearance and warm heart.
10. I estimate that 120,000 fans were in the stadium. (Even when a cliché is used in its original context, it sounds old.)

ANSWERS TO EXERCISE 10: JARGON

1. We expect to use hundreds of paper clips in the next two months.
2. A person who likes research should not be hired for a position that requires someone to interact with customers all day.
3. Our schoolchildren's education has been neglected.
4. Foreign diplomats should always talk to local leaders.
5. If someone claims you as a dependent on a tax return, you may still have to pay taxes on your income in excess of 500 dollars.
6. Two recent studies suggest that Vienna sausages are good for you.
7. When the poet wrote the second and third stanzas, he must have felt despair.
8. This is a fine horse.
9. Government regulatory agencies were not honest in their press releases about the recent railway accident.
10. Having spent our time responding to many unexpected problems this month, we have not been able to prepare for these longer-term needs.

TEACHER TIP

Train your ear to be aware of correct and incorrect spoken and written English. Listen to people talking and try to catch the common mistakes we all make. Don't correct your friends out loud, of course (or you won't have many friends left), but make a mental note of incorrect English. Then determine to use spoken and written English correctly. It will serve you well in all your communication from now on.

ANSWERS TO EXERCISE 12: SHIFTING NARRATIVE VOICE

1. I am disgusted with the waste we tolerate in this country. People cannot simply stand by without adding to such waste: living here makes all of us wasteful.
2. You must take care not to take these grammar rules too seriously, since you can often become bogged down in details and forget why you are writing at all. (Or use *one* consistently.)
3. We all must take a stand against waste in this country; else how will we be able to look ourselves in the mirror? (When using *we*, you must make sure to use the plural form of verbs and pronouns.)

ANSWERS TO EXERCISE 13: SUBJECT-VERB AGREEMENT

1. The logical *structure* of his complicated and rather tortuous arguments *is* always the same.
2. The *majority* of the organization's members *are* over 60 years old.
3. *Both* the young child and her grandfather were depressed for months after discovering that the oldest ice-cream parlor in the city had closed its doors forever.
4. Hartz brought the *blueprints and model* that *were* still on the table instead of the ones that Mackenzie had returned to the cabinet. (The restrictive phrase beginning with *that* defines the noun phrase *blueprints and model.*)
5. A *case* of bananas *has* been sent to the local distributor in compensation for the fruit that was damaged in transit.
6. A *total* of 50 editors *reads* each article, a process that takes at least a week, sometimes six months.
7. Neither the shipping clerk who packed the equipment nor the *truckers* who transported it *admit* responsibility for the dented circuit box.
8. Either Georgette or *Robespierre* is going to be asked to dinner by the madcap Calvin. I dread the results in either case.
9. I can never decide whether to eat an orange or a Belgian chocolate; *each* of them *has* its wondrous qualities. (Note that you must also change the possessive pronoun to the singular form.)
10. *Everyone* in the United States, as well as in Canada, *expects* the timber agreement to fall through.

ANSWERS TO EXERCISE 14: PARALLELISM

1. This organization will not tolerate the consumption, trafficking, or promotion of drugs.
2. The dancer taught her understudy how to move, dress, work with choreographers, and deal with professional competition.
3. *The student's knowledge* of chemistry is as extensive as *the professor's knowledge.*
4. They should not allow that man *either to supervise* the project *or to assist* another supervisor, since he has proven himself to be thoroughly incompetent.
5. The balloon business will have to either expand or declare bankruptcy.
6. Before Gertrude begins to design the set, as well as to hire laborers to help her construct it, she should consult the director.
7. Merrill based his confidence on the futures market, the bond market, and the strength of the president's popularity.
8. The grocery baggers were ready, able, and quite determined to do a great job.
9. The *requirements for a business degree* are not as stringent as *those for a law degree.*
10. *Not only* did we sail, fish, and canoe that day, *but also* we visited the quaint town on the island across the bay.

ANSWERS TO EXERCISE 15: FAULTY PRONOUN REFERENCE

1. The structure of the sentence might leave us wondering whether Clausen or his dog was well bred. Instead, use the impersonal *it.*

   Rewrite: Clausen's dog won first place at the show because it was well bred.
2. *He* is probably meant to refer to the author of the book reviewed by the critic, but the context makes *he* appear to refer to *the critic,* who could be an author as well as a critic.

   Rewrite: The critic's review made the novel a commercial success, and the novelist is now a rich man.
3. We cannot tell from the context whether the military advisor or his superior was the superior strategist.

   Rewrite: The military advisor was more conventional than his commander, but the advisor was a superior strategist.

4. *Which* is the problem here: We do not know whether Bertha had not spent the night at home in weeks or whether she had not telephoned her friends in weeks.

   Rewrite: Because she had not telephoned her California friends in weeks, Bertha called them before she went home for the night.

5. Referring to some ambiguous *they* without identifying who *they* are beforehand is incorrect.

   Rewrite: John wanted the job badly, but when he called the employer the next morning he found that the company had hired someone else.

6. We don't know exactly what *it* is, but we can assume that *it* is a fish.

   Rewrite: You must pay attention when fishing, or you might lose your catch.

7. We do not know whether *he* refers to Zolsta or to the unnamed lesser musician.

   Rewrite: Zolsta Karmagi is the better musician, but Sven Wonderup had more formal training.

8. This sentence is extremely confusing because the reference of the two pronouns (*her, she*) is unclear. Who are *all* these women?

   Rewrite: The director wanted to give the lead part to another woman, but the star, his girlfriend, disagreed and insisted that she, the star of so many fine productions, was better qualified for the job.

9. Whose credentials? Zalmen's or Koenig's?

   Rewrite: Zalmen showed us his credentials, and was allowed into the press conference, but Koenig refused to answer our inquiries and was turned away.

10. Which is cheaper, the private dwelling or the retirement community? The pronoun *it* has no clear antecedent.

    Rewrite: A retirement community offers more activities than a private dwelling does, but a private dwelling is cheaper.

ANSWERS FOR EXERCISE 16: FAULTY MODIFICATION

1. *Quickly* is sandwiched between two verbs, and it could refer to either one.

   Rewrite: Bentley advised him to make up his mind quickly.

2. *In principle* probably modifies *agreed,* but its placement makes it appear to modify *statement.*

   Rewrite: I agree in principle with the author's statements.

3. Termites are probably coming out of the woodwork, not the man, but an introductory modifying phrase always refers to the grammatical subject of the sentence.

   Rewrite: He was surprised to see termites coming out of the woodwork.

4. Was the racial unrest in the auditorium, or was the conference merely held there?

   Rewrite: The governor's conference met in the auditorium to discuss racial unrest.

5. Did she say it in her office? Were the documents in her office? Or both?

   Rewrite: Hernandez said that she had all the necessary documents in her office.

6. If none of his friends came, it must have been a small party indeed.

   Rewrite: Not all of his friends were able to come, but he decided that he preferred small parties anyway.

7. Did she remember when she got home? Or did she have to call when she got home?

   Rewrite: When she got home, Margolis remembered she had to place a telephone call.

8. Either he didn't like discussing politics in the museum, or he didn't like discussing it at all.

   Rewrite: As they walked through the museum, George told Suzette he did not like to discuss politics.

9. Was it Stokely's résumé that worked in publishing for 10 years?

   Rewrite: Stokely, who has worked in publishing for 10 years, appears from his résumé to be well qualified.

10. It is the person holding the job, not the job itself, that requires experience in community service.

    Rewrite: A politician without experience in community service would fail to serve his constituents.

ANSWERS TO EXERCISE 17: SLANG AND COLLOQUIALISMS

1. Cynthia Larson is surely an expert. (It may go without saying that *knows her stuff* is a slang expression, but the substitution of *sure* for *surely* may be more difficult to identify as an error. *Sure* is an adjective, *surely* is an adverb, and an adverb is needed in this case, since the word is meant to modify *knows*.)

2. The crowd was absorbed in watching the fire-eating juggler, but then the dancing horse caught their attention.
3. As soon as the personnel department tries to verify his résumé, I am sure we will hear gales of laughter issuing from the office.
4. Having something funny to say seems to be very important in our culture.
5. The chef is skillful with salmon: his sauce was simple but the effect was sublime.
6. Normal human beings cannot tolerate repeated humiliation.
7. The world does not have much time to stop polluting; soon, we all will have to wear face masks. (*Hasn't got* is both a contraction and an example of the colloquial substitution of *have got* for *have.*)
8. If you want a good cheesecake, you must make a superb crust.
9. International organizations should try to cooperate on global issues like hunger and party decorations.
10. The environmentalists are not involved in the project for prestige; they truly care about protecting the yellow-throated hornswoggler.

ANSWERS TO EXERCISE 18: SENTENCE FRAGMENTS AND RUN-ON SENTENCES

1. In this context, *except* is a conjunction, and as such makes the clause to which it is attached a dependent one.

   Rewrite: The private academy has all the programs Angie will need, except that the sports program has been phased out.
2. *Leadership ability* is a sentence fragment, since it has no predicate.

   Rewrite: Leadership ability: this is the elusive quality that our current government employees have yet to capture.
3. Here we have both a run-on sentence (two independent clauses linked by *therefore* and a comma) and a sentence fragment ("What a surprise to find . . ." contains no subject or predicate).

   Rewrite: Antonio just joined the athletic club staff this year, but Barry has been with us since 1975; therefore, we would expect Barry to be more skilled with the weight-lifting equipment. It was quite a surprise to find Barry pinned beneath a barbell on the weight-lifting bench with Antonio struggling to lift the 300-pound weight from poor Barry's chest
4. *The daughter of a Yankee fisherman* is a sentence fragment, since the group of words contains no verb. Rewrite: However much she tries to

act like a Southern belle, she cannot hide her roots. She will always be the daughter of a Yankee fisherman, taciturn and ever polite.

5. The conjunction *after* makes the second group of words a sentence fragment.

   Rewrite: There is always time to invest in property ownership after one has established oneself in the business world, however.

6. Since transitional words like *however* do not subordinate a clause, this is a run-on sentence. You could either change the first comma to a semicolon or separate the clauses with a period.

   Rewrite: Sentence fragments are often used in casual conversation. They should not, however, be used in written English under normal circumstances.

7. The trouble here is that the sentence is made up of dependent clauses with no independent clauses to serve as a base.

   Rewrite: A truthful, well-produced documentary film has less impact than a biographical film about someone well-liked by the public.

8. This sentence must be broken down into two or more sentences.

   Rewrite: After living alone for many years, Mrs. Casey had difficulty making the decision to move into a retirement community. Many restrictions were entailed, and none of the homes met all Mrs. Casey's needs. For all these reasons, the decision took a long time.

ANSWERS FOR EXERCISE 19: COMMAS

1. Peter wants me to bring records, games, candy, and soda to his party.
2. I need lumber, nails, a hammer, and a saw to build the shelf.
3. It takes a friendly, energetic person to be a successful salesman.
4. I was shocked to discover that a large, modern, glass-sheathed office building had replaced my old school.
5. The country club, a cluster of ivy-covered whitewashed buildings, was the site of the president's first speech.
6. As we entered the park, a police officer, clad in a crisp, well-starched uniform, directed us to the theater.
7. Pushing through the panicked crowd, the security guards frantically searched for the suspect.
8. Despite careful analysis of the advantages and disadvantages of each proposal, Harry found it hard to reach a decision.

ANSWERS FOR EXERCISE 20: SEMICOLONS

1. Morgan has five years' experience in karate, but Thompson has even more.
2. Very few students wanted to take the class in physics; only the professor's kindness kept it from being canceled.
3. You should always be prepared when you go on a camping trip; however, you must avoid carrying unnecessary weight.

EXERCISE FOR PRINCIPLE 21: COLONS

1. I am sick and tired of your whining, your complaining, your nagging, your teasing, and most of all, your barbed comments.
2. The chef has created a masterpiece: the pasta is delicate yet firm, the mustard greens are fresh, and the medallions of veal are melting in my mouth.
3. In order to write a good essay, you must do the following: get plenty of sleep, eat a good breakfast, and practice until you drop.

ANSWERS TO EXERCISE 22: HYPHENS AND DASHES

1. The child was able to count from one to ninety-nine.
2. The adults-only movie was banned from commercial TV.
3. It was the first time she had seen a movie that was for adults only.
4. John and his ex-wife remained on friendly terms.
5. A two-thirds majority would be needed to pass the budget reforms.
6. The house—and it was the most dilapidated house that I had ever seen—was a bargain because the land was so valuable.

ANSWERS TO EXERCISE 23: APOSTROPHES

1. The President's limousine had a flat tire.
2. Your tickets for the show will be at the box office.
3. The opportunity to change one's lifestyle does not come often.
4. The desk's surface was immaculate, but its drawers were messy.
5. The cat on the bed is hers.

VERBAL REASONING PRACTICE SET 1

ANSWER KEY

1. D	15. B	29. A
2. A	16. A	30. D
3. B	17. B	31. D
4. D	18. C	32. A
5. B	19. A	33. A
6. A	20. B	34. B
7. C	21. B	35. A
8. B	22. D	36. D
9. D	23. D	37. A
10. D	24. C	38. B
11. B	25. A	39. D
12. C	26. C	40. A
13. B	27. C	
14. D	28. C	

EXPLANATIONS

Passage 1

Topic and Scope: An argument that Gautier was a flawed but good poet, true to himself

1. D

The presence of "suggests" in the question indicates that you'll probably be looking for inferences or paraphrases from the text. Since the question is an "All...EXCEPT" structure, use your map and the text to eliminate choices which fit with the passage or look for a choice that contradicts or falls outside what the author argues. (C) fits the latter: the passage doesn't discuss Gautier's educational background, and therefore nothing can be inferred about it. Strategy Point: When a question is set up in such a way that three answer choices are statements with which the author would agree, the correct answer will either contradict the author or be off-scope. While answer choices that contradict are much more common, be aware of the other type as well. (A) is an opposite; this is discussed in paragraph 3; Gautier's treatment of nature is, according to the author, "of a finer strain than the mass of human family." (B) is an opposite; it follows from the author's discussion of Gautier's "spontaneity" in paragraph 1. Finally, (D) is an opposite. This can be inferred from paragraphs 2 and 3, where the author discusses Gautier's self-understanding and keen observation of Nature.

2. A

Why does the author mention other poets? Evaluate the examples in the passage individually. At the end of paragraph 1 the author compares Gautier to Musset to say that Gautier was even more unique than was Musset; for Gautier, "Even more than Alfred de Musset. . . . if his glass was not large, at least it was all his own glass." When comparing Gautier to Browning in paragraph 2, the author argues that it's possible to be more entertained by Gautier than Browning, then goes on to say that "a man's supreme use in the world is to master his intellectual instrument . . ." which again suggests Gautier's uniqueness. The author suggests in paragraph 1 that Gautier was unique when he says he was never fully imitated. Finally, in the last paragraph, the author argues that Gautier "excels" other descriptive poets by his personal qualities, which yet again emphasizes uniqueness. Therefore there is overwhelming evidence for (A)! (B) is faulty use of detail. Though the author suggests this in the first sentence, it has nothing to do with Gautier's comparison to other poets, since French lyricism isn't mentioned again in the passage. (C) is opposite; the author is very positive about Gautier. Though limitations are mentioned, the author focuses more on his exceptional creativity. (D) is faulty use of detail. Though the author argues in the first paragraph that others have tried and failed to imitate Gautier completely, there's no claim that Gautier's colleagues *could* easily imitate his style to refute in the first place.

TEACHER TIP

Notice that two wrong answer choices are faulty use of detail traps. People fall for FUD answers if they don't research carefully to make sure that the detail they choose really answers the question asked.

3. B

Break the question down a bit before predicting. What are Gautier's artistic gifts? Mainly his uniqueness, ability to entertain, and powers of observation. If these were the things which overcame his limitations as a poet, you can predict that the right answer will somehow diminish these qualities. (B) does that. If Gautier collaborated with other writers, then he wasn't particularly unique, and at least one quality that the author uses to justify Gautier's limitations doesn't exist. Strategy Point: An argument can be weakened by attacking its evidences, assumptions, or conclusions. (A) is out of scope. The study of Gautier's poems has no impact on Gautier's value as a poet by itself since it doesn't impact the author's evidence or conclusion. (C), again, is out of scope. Even if this were true, Gautier's reviews wouldn't have any effect on the value of his poems. (D) too is out of scope. Though this would indicate that the writers who were influenced by Gautier were less unique, it does nothing to harm Gautier's own uniqueness.

TEACHER TIP

(B) really was tempting, wasn't it? But go back to the paragraph and you'll see that it's mostly about Gautier, the man, and not about what's essential to his work.

4. D

Review the phrase in context. "Pagan bonhomie" apparently makes the other descriptive poets seem not-so-descriptive. Keep reading. Why does he dwarf these poets? Among other things, because of "his magnificent good temper and the unquestioning serenity of his enjoyment of the great spectacle of nature and art." Pagan bonhomie must therefore be some sort of view of life in general that the other poets don't share. While (B) is tempting, (D) comes closer to capturing the author's overall point that Gautier's *attitude* set him apart, not just his descriptions of nature alone. (A) is out of scope. The author never claims that Gautier had this sort of lifestyle. Eliminate this choice immediately for its negativity. (B) is faulty use of detail. Though Gautier did have unique descriptions of nature, the author's more concerned with pointing out the difference in his overall personality. (C) is out of scope: another choice far too negative for the author's tone. The author never suggests that Gautier lacked modesty, and in fact argues the opposite at the end of the last paragraph.

TEACHER TIP

This was a pretty easy question. Yes, MCAT questions can be easy; take advantage of every question with an obvious answer. The more you understand the MCAT test-maker and how he makes this test, the more you'll find "gifts'" like this.

5. B

Where does the author discuss the reader's reaction to poetry? It's buried in paragraph 2; the author says, "...we may wonder whether we are...the better entertained, as a poet's readers should before all things be...." Therefore, the author believes that the first role of poetry is to bring enjoyment. (B) says the same. (A) is out of scope. Though this might be true, the author never discusses this. (C) is out of scope. As above, the author never discusses poetry and moral lessons. Though the author discusses a "moral" in paragraph 2, it's not a moral in poetry, but rather a lesson to be learned from Gautier in general. (D) is out of scope. Though it may be true, the author never argues that this is the case.

Passage 2

Topic and Scope: Description of the experiments and results of analog mental imaging

6. A

This question simply asks you to summarize the hypothesis described in paragraph 3. The fastest way to predict here it to read the text. The analog position is "the idea that mental processing requires one to go sequentially through all intervening steps to solve a problem." (A) repeats this almost word-for-word. (B) is opposite. This contradicts the argument that mental processing has to proceed step-by-step. (C) is faulty use of detail. Don't get sidetracked by the information in paragraph 1. This follows from the analog position, as supported by the experiments in the passage, but it's not the analog position itself. (D) is out of scope. There's no support for this statement in the passage.

TEACHER TIP

Do you see how the first sentence of the explanation asks another question? It's a good idea to reword the question itself and ask yourself exactly what you need to do. That way you're sure to understand what's required to find the right answer.

7. C

What reason would the analog position give for the fact that it takes longer to scan long distances in a mental image? Review the relevant parts of the passage, paragraph 2 in particular. The experiment suggests that people are building a mental map since the map is "fictional". Because the analog position suggests that one has to go through steps to solve a problem, it would be reasonable to infer that it takes longer to scan long distances because those doing the scanning are "looking" at all the intervening space in between the two given objects. (C) summarizes this. (A) is out of scope. There's nothing to suggest that those in the experiment don't believe that this relationship exists. The experiment is concerned with their mental images rather than their opinions. (B) is out of scope. There's no evidence for this in the passage. (D) is out of scope. As above, there's simply no support for this in the passage.

8. B

An unusual question. What would an alternate explanation do to the conclusions drawn from the experiment? It would weaken it, and this question can therefore be treated as a classic "weaken" question. Look for evidence that would weaken the passage's conclusions. (B) does this: if subjects change their answer based on what they think the answer should be, the argument that they take longer because they're referring to a mental map is weakened. (A) is distortion. This choice contradicts the basis of the experiment. Since subjects in the experiments had to memorize the positions of the objects, subjects who forgot the positions wouldn't be part of the experiment's focus. (C) is out of scope. The experiment is designed to deal only with "fictional" maps, and so any explanation that involves real maps would be implausible. (D) is out of scope. The passage states that response times depend on distance, but there's no reason to believe that it would take longer to begin scanning longer distances as opposed to shorter ones.

9. D

Where is Kosslyn mentioned? In paragraphs 2 and 3. Since the question mentions big and small objects, focus on the experiment described in paragraph 2. Review the text to determine why Kosslyn believes it takes longer to identify small objects next to large ones: Kosslyn believes "subjects had to zoom in on the image to detect the particular feature."

(D) says the same. (A) is out of scope. This isn't suggested in the passage. (B) is out of scope. Kosslyn's experiment says nothing about this either. (C) is out of scope. This is also unsupported by the passage.

TEACHER TIP

This incorporation question kept you within the realm of the experiments in the passage, but most will put you into entirely new situations. Nevertheless, all correct answers to incorporation questions are just as firmly based on the passage as are answers to main idea or detail questions.

10. D

Though it's not immediately obvious, this is an incorporation question because you're given new information and asked how it will affect the passage. What would be the case if subjects simply responded in the way they thought the experimenters wanted them to? Predict: the experiment wouldn't prove anything except the experimenters' own biases. (D) restates this: whatever relationship the experimenters want, they'll get. (A) is out of scope. Though this might be true, it misses the point that the results would be invalid because the experimenters could engineer any result they wanted. (B) is opposite. It would make more sense that the subjects would show a *linear* relationship, since the experimenters, in keeping with the analog model, were expecting that. (C) is out of scope. As with (A), even though this constant relationship might be reflected, it misses the point that *any* relationship is possible if the subjects are simply following the experimenters' lead.

TEACHER TIP

If you had started with Roman numeral III, which appears three times in the answer choices, you would have eliminated it and had your answer immediately: A, the only answer which doesn't include III.

11. B

Paraphrase the analog position before answering this to make evaluation easier: solving a problem requires step-by-step thought, and mental images have properties that can be tested. Start with statement I, which restates the conclusion of an experiment *supporting* the analog hypothesis. Since you're looking for statements that *contradict* it, eliminate (A), (C), and (D). Only (B) is left, and there's no need to evaluate the other remaining choices. Statements II and III contradict statement I and the conclusions of the map experiments, and are therefore valid elements of the correct answer. (A), (C), and (D) are opposite.

12. C

Another incorporation question which asks you to take new evidence and determine how it would affect the passage. Predict the result again: If subjects change their responses based on what they think "should" happen, then the results of the experiment should be called into question, as the subjects are simply reflecting experimental bias. (C) captures this. Strategy Point: The same point will often be tested repeatedly throughout a passage's questions. Don't reinvent the wheel! Use your previous work to save time and to maximize your points. (A) is opposite; if subjects are scanning in the way they think they should, the experiment is more likely revealing experimental bias than the actual mental images it sets out to describe. (B) is opposite; a lack of subject control over scanning contradicts the information in the question anyhow, since it's stated explicitly that subjects *can* alter the time they spend scanning. (D) is opposite; it suggests that the analog model would be strengthened. Even if subjects can control the rate at which they scan, as the question suggests, the analog model would still be weakened by this conscious response.

Passage 3

Topic and Scope: The development of a particular method of thought

Strategy Point: Passages written in the first person are rare. When they appear, keep an eye out for a potentially strong authorial opinion. There's no need to write out a full sentence for Purpose. Just read backwards, starting from Purpose, and you'll have the complete description of the passage.

13. B

Review the author's first precept in paragraph 1: Don't accept anything as true unless it's known to be true. Be sure to look through the rest of the (short) paragraph for evidence and support. The author's first precept depends on the assumption that the author's perception of truth is valid. (B) restates this. If in doubt, try the denial test: if theories *can't* be accepted as true by being perceived intellectually, then the author's attempt to know what is true in this way is unworkable. (A) is opposite. The author argues that he'll only believe what *he* perceives to be true, which means that knowing the truth is ultimately a subjective process. (A) argues that comprehension is ultimately based on rational analysis rather than personal knowledge, which the author rejects. (C) is opposite. As above, the author believes that it's necessary to rely on personal opinion in addition to pure intellect. (D) is distortion. Though the author argues that these disciplines are used for understanding abstract ideas, there's no argument that these things *must* be studied to understand abstract ideas. Even if this were true, it wouldn't have an impact on the author's argument in paragraph 1.

TEACHER TIP

The denial test is useful for assumption questions. You simply put the answer choice in the negative—deny it—and if that makes the author's argument fall apart, it's the necessary assumption. For example, if you denied answer D—scholars DO NOT need to study...—would that affect the argument in any way? No, because the author doesn't mention this one way or the other. But what if B were denied? The theory would fall apart since it would undermine the author's ideas. Thus B is a necessary assumption, and the correct answer.

14. D

Where does the author mention vice in a State? Go back to review the example in paragraph 5. The author says that a "State is better ruled if, having but a few vices, it closely monitors them..." Paraphrase: it's best to keep a close eye on the few flaws present. (D) restates this point. Strategy

Point: Questions and answers that follow complicated paragraphs will often make you earn the points by paraphrasing points in the passage. Get in the habit of restating difficult points in simpler words when predicting answers. (A) is out of scope. The author never makes a comparison between vices and logic. (B) is faulty use of detail. The author argues that many laws can rationalize vices, which is exactly why it's better to stick to just a few rules. This answer captures only the author's introduction to the main point: it's better to have a few rules that are always followed. (C) is distortion. The author argues that it's best to have a few vices, but never suggests it's advisable or even possible to get rid of all vice.

15. B

Another detail question. Focus your work in this question on paragraph 4, where geometry is discussed. First tackle statement II, which appears in three choices. The author argues that geometry is "so restricted to the consideration of figures" that it ends up being limited. Statement II paraphrases this, eliminate (D). Statement I states that geometric analysis isn't useful for logical analysis. The author argues that geometry not only deals too much with figures, but also doesn't "treat anything except abstract ideas, which seem to be of no use whatsoever," suggesting that it's not useful for logic. Statement III, however, contradicts the author's point that geometry stretches the intellect at the expense of the imagination. (B) catches the legitimate statements. (A), (C), and (D) are opposite.

TEACHER TIP

Did you remember that an evaluation question just asks "why?" Think of it that way and the answer becomes easy to predict and match.

16. A

An evaluation question. Why does the author describe his former study of philosophy and mathematics? Predict: He wants to show that they weren't useful by themselves, and that he needed new precepts that combined all their advantages (paragraph 5). Look for an answer choice that ties into this. (A) is reasonable. If the author wanted to create a new system based on the old ones, he'd mention his studies in the other fields in order to show that he had the necessary background to form these new ideas. (B) is distortion. Though the author wants to combine parts of these fields, he's not concerned with discussing their relationship to each other so much as with describing how they fit into his new way of thinking. (C) is opposite. The author argues in paragraph 3 that the study of logic by itself is pointless, so he wouldn't want to help readers expand their study of logic. (D) is distortion. Though the author does argue in paragraph 3 that much logic is flawed, he mentions his own study not so much as to refute specific theories but rather to describe his new method of thinking.

17. B

Since you have no information in the question to narrow your focus, you can be reasonably sure that the right answer will be something with which the author generally disagrees. The shortcomings of the old systems and the four precepts make up the meat of the passage, so look for something that conflicts with the author's negative view of traditional methods of thought and his positive view of his own precepts. (B) does the latter. The second precept argues that difficulties should be broken up into many small pieces that can be individually evaluated; (B) argues that subjects should *never* be broken up. The author would clearly disagree. Strategy Point: In questions that ask you to find a statement with which author disagrees, it is often much faster to find a choice that conflicts with the main points than to eliminate the three choices with which he would agree. (A) is opposite. This follows from the author's argument in paragraph 3 that logic isn't particularly useful. (C) is opposite. This is simply the opposite of the correct answer choice. The author would agree that it's possible to understand a big problem by breaking it down in to smaller problems. (D) is opposite. The author argues in paragraph 3 that logical theorems "serve only to explain to others the things that one already knows…" which suggests that the author is concerned with teaching abstract ideas in addition to simply learning them.

18. C

Where does the author discuss the reasoning behind his method? paragraph 5 is concerned almost entirely with this. The author argues that it was enough for him to have four principles as long as he was sure "never-not even once-to neglect my adherence to them." (C) is a close paraphrase of this particular concern about consistency. (A) is distortion. Though the other methodologies played a role in the author's new system, he doesn't suggest that his *primary* concern is the examination of these old systems. He's more concerned with having a few simple principles. (B) is distortion. As above, though the author suggests that he has this thorough grounding, he believes that it's better to have simple principles that are always followed. (D) is out of scope. The natural sciences aren't mentioned at all in the passage.

Passage 4

Topic and Scope: The role of information technology in a recent spike in American productivity

Mapping the Passage:

Paragraph 1 gives background about the dotcom boom and asks what the precursors to the condition were.

Paragraph 2 describes a productivity spike and the possible explanation some have given for the spike: information technology.

Paragraph 3 defines productivity growth and suggests that heavy investment in information technology should have led to an increase in productivity.

Paragraph 4 discusses productivity and technology investment in other countries, and concludes that the data supports the argument that information technology was important to American productivity gains.

19. A

What is a resurgence? It's a rise to previous levels; if it were just a rise, it would be a surge, but not a *re*-surgence. Only the United States has enough data in the passage to infer a resurgence from: the author says at the end of paragraph 2 that "the rate of growth in labor productivity returned to the pre-1970 rate of increase." While other nations are mentioned, their previous levels aren't mentioned. Therefore, statement I must fit, while the other ones don't.

20. B

An assumption question, but in an "All... EXCEPT" format that's rare for this type. Remember that an assumption is an unstated belief bridging evidence and conclusion. The conclusion is given: the author believes that information technology has raised American productivity. What is the evidence? Review the map: The author uses data on technology investment in the U.S. and other developed nations. Look for a choice that is *not* necessary to connect these. (B) fits for a few reasons. Perhaps most obviously, it's explicitly stated: the author says at the beginning of paragraph 4," The revolution in technology is...a worldwide phenomenon." Since an assumption is unstated, (B) must not be an assumption essential to the argument. Furthermore, using the denial test (which here you want to fail!), if this weren't true and the revolution *weren't* a worldwide phenomenon, it would do nothing to diminish the impact of information technology within the United States. Strategy Point: The Denial Test can be used to test whether an assumption is necessary to an argument. If it is, denying the assumption will cause the argument to fall apart. If the argument holds up even when the assumption is denied, the assumption isn't critical to the argument. (A) is opposite. The author must assume that other factors aren't significant; if they were, then the author couldn't make the argument that information technology is the major factor responsible for the surge in productivity. (B) is opposite. The author uses these measures when discussing levels of technology investment in paragraph 4. If these weren't valid measures, the author's point in mentioning them would be moot. (D) is opposite. If the author believes that these are valid measures of information technology and concludes that information technology was responsible for the productivity gains, an assumption must be that those measures were themselves responsible for the gain, as this choice suggests.

21. B

Review the topic and scope of the passage: the author is concerned with information technology's role in boosting American productivity in the recent past. Look for an answer choice that sticks as closely as possible to topic and scope. (B) does this: It's reasonable to guess that the author would continue the paragraph by talking about the next stage of these trends in the same topic and scope: information technology and its effect on productivity. (A) is out of scope. The author discusses the 1970s in paragraph 3, but only as background to discuss the current productivity spurt. It's more reasonable to think that the author will continue by talking about the future trajectory of the productivity gains. (C) is out of scope. The author doesn't mention any other possible causes for the increase in productivity and believes that information technology is the primary cause, and so it's unlikely that there would be a drastic shift that discussed other causes. (D) is out of scope. The author only discusses other countries to shed light on *American* productivity gains. Going into greater depth regarding other countries would veer out of scope.

22. D

This odd wording means that you can ignore the entire "rebut" portion of the question stem. You're just looking for the statement with which the author would agree. An inference question: Predict by reviewing the author's main point about U.S. productivity growth in the late '90s. The author believes that it was the result of heavy investment in information technology. (D) says the same, simply summarizing the author's main point. (A) is opposite. The author believes, as argued in paragraph 3, that this particular surge in productivity was "extraordinary," and therefore by definition *not* typical. (B) is out of scope. The author doesn't discuss other changes, which could encompass any number of subjects, and so there's no way to compare how the author feels about this particular change relative to others, or whether it merits a particular explanation. (C) is out of scope. A classic case of confusing description with prescription: while the author explains a possible cause for the productivity gain, there's no discussion of what should be done with this information.

23. D

An evaluation question: Predict by reviewing your map of paragraph 2. The author's main intent is to define productivity growth, and to suggest that the investment in information technology should have led to a growth in productivity. (D) most closely describes the author's purpose of providing a possible explanation, and suggests that the explanation is given with the intent of following it up with further evidence, which the author does in fact provide in paragraph 4. (A) is faulty use of detail. Though (A) might be tempting because the author does define productivity and identify the factors that can affect its growth, this choice neglects the second half of the paragraph, which provides an explanation for a growth in productivity. (B) is distortion. The author describes a correlation between investment and productivity, but doesn't describe peaks in either. (C) is distortion. As above, while the author proposes a broad correlation between investment and productivity, there's no specific discussion of how much investment is required for a certain amount of productivity.

Passage 5

Topic and Scope: The state of poetry in the author's country

Mapping the Passage:

Paragraph 1 says that some native "true poetry" has been written and that greater attention to poetry will produce benefits.

Paragraphs 2 and 3 describe the country's indifference to poetry, an explanation, and the author's rebuttal to the explanation.

Paragraph 4 describes the false conceptions that discourage native poets from writing quality poetry.

Paragraph 5 argues that poetry should be more appreciated.

Paragraph 6 argues that the country's immigrant population causes "Old Word" poetry to be valued over native poetry.

Strategy Point: Save clearly difficult passages until the end of the test, and don't get bogged down. Even the most difficult of passages will have manageable questions.

24. C

A detail question: Review your map to get a feel for the reasons the author gives for the country's indifference to poetry. Statement I is difficult to decipher in that it requires knowledge of what "edification" means. If you don't know, guess or move on to the next Roman numeral. "Edification" means instruction or enlightenment, and the author does in fact argue that the country's population is unenlightened, as described at the end of paragraph 2 and the beginning of paragraph 3. Statement II may be tempting from a quick review of paragraph 6, but distorts the author's argument. The author argues that *in spite* of the new country's quality poetry, immigrants read Old World poetry because of nostalgia. The issue isn't quality, but homesickness. There's no need to evaluate statement III at this point unless you skipped statement I. Statement III is correct for the same reasons as II: immigrants are reading their homeland's poetry because of nostalgia. Strategy Point: If you didn't know what "edification" meant, you could have skipped the choice and still gotten the right answer with certainty after evaluating the other two! Use the setup of Roman numeral questions to your advantage. (A), (B), and (D) are opposite.

25. A

This is a difficult question. One option is to use elimination. Predict a basic contrast in the passage: The author believes that poetry is all sorts of good, but that people don't appreciate it as much as they should. Why is poetry not appreciated in the country the author discusses? The author argues that people don't understand poetry as well as they should. Something palpable is easily accessible, and something subtle isn't. Even if you didn't know the definition of palpable, you could guess that since the choices are presented as contrasts it means the opposite of subtle. This contrast fits in with the author's general argument made throughout the passage that people simply lack a grasp of poetry's finer points. This claim is made in paragraph 3, when the author says that poetry isn't accepted for "other causes less palpable." In paragraph 4 the author argues that those who don't appreciate poetry are either incapable of doing so or are more familiar with "widely available, but lower forms," which again suggests a contrast between the subtle and the less so. In paragraph 5 the author argues that only those who pay careful attention to poetry appreciate it, and in paragraph 1 the author contrasts a "chilly atmosphere" with a more subtle spring breath. (A) is therefore correct as a contrast made throughout the passage, while the other choices are made only in certain parts of the author's argument. (B) is faulty use of detail. The author makes this distinction at the end of paragraph 3, but doesn't mention it throughout the rest of the passage. (C) is faulty use of detail. The author implies in paragraph 6 that some who do not appreciate poetry consider it insignificant, but doesn't make the claim again. (D) is faulty use of detail; the author suggests that those who don't appreciate poetry fail to do so because they consider poetry impractical.

26. C

What scope of poetry is the author concerned with? Predict: The author wants to discuss the state of poetry in one particular country. (C) makes the most sense; it's the only answer choice that would justify this focus on the poetry of a single country. (A) is out of scope. The author is less concerned with instructing people how to *write* poetry than he is with *appreciating* poetry. (B) is out of scope. Though the author compares Old World and New World poetry in paragraph 6, it's not the focus of the passage. (D) is out of scope; this doesn't include the author's focus on a particular country, which is an integral part of the passage.

27. C

Review the line in context. The author defines the phrase in the lines above when saying that there are "men who are not gifted with the power of giving expression...who nevertheless experience the throbbing in their hearts." Paraphrase: Some people can't write it, but they can still appreciate it. (C) says the same. (A) is out of scope. The author is distinguishing between those who can and cannot create, not between ways of communicating poetry. (B) is out of scope. The author is describing those who *do* value poetry. (D) is distortion. The author speaks about people who lack the gift of writing poetry but doesn't express sympathy toward them. The point is to show that appreciation can exist even when the person can't write poetry.

28. C

Review the phrase in the context of the structure around it. The author has just finished listing all the reasons why poetry isn't properly appreciated, and then says that some true poetry has been written "despite the unpropitious circumstances that exist." It's reasonable to guess that these circumstances are those things that keep true poetry from being written. The author argues in the paragraphs above that this is primarily due to misconceptions about poetry or a lack of understanding. (C) fits. (A) is faulty use of detail. This is an argument made in paragraph 3, but it's one that the author considers "by no means satisfactory." (B) is faulty use of detail. The author argues that this does happen, both immediately after this phrase and at the end of paragraph 4, but as the result rather than the cause. Native poets don't devote themselves to their craft *because* of misunderstandings about poetry. (D) is faulty use of detail. Though the author mentions this as one reason for the lack of poetry, it's not the main reason, and the author seems to treat this reason with some forgiveness. It therefore likely wouldn't fall under the negative "unpropitious circumstances" that the author discusses.

29. A

An application question. Predict by reviewing what the author considers true poetry to be. The author argues in paragraph 4 that it's *not* "fanciful or contrived," but that it requires "sustained application to...craft that is essential for artistic excellence." Look for an answer choice that fits with this idea of poetry. (A) most closely fits, describing poetry that can be edited and made better, but that can't be artificially contrived from the start. (B) is opposite. Though the author believes that poetry must be uncontrived, it's also made clear that good poetry requires a lot of work to perfect. This answer choice suggests the opposite. (C) is out of scope. The author discusses poetry that is tied to a particular country, but says nothing about poetry tied to a particular time. (D) is opposite. This description of poetry would likely be something the author would label as contrived, and therefore more in keeping with misconceptions of poetry than with what "true" poetry is.

30. D

What is the author describing when discussing "native literature"? The author argues that poets within the country should produce more literature for the people in the country. The author clearly believes that immigrants can be part of this native literature since the country is described as "young" and the author describes himself as part of a group of "emigrants from the Old Country." Furthermore, the author focuses in paragraph 1 on what true poetry should be by discussing the nature of the country itself rather than the nature of the poets. (D) therefore most closely fits with what the author is trying to convey. (A) is out of scope. The author is concerned with poetry that comes from and concerns a specific country, but there's no indication that only aboriginal poetry can be considered native. (B) is distortion. Though this might be an important part of native poetry, the author is more interested in poetry that takes on the characteristics of the country rather than poetry written by any particular group of people. (C) is distortion. As above, the author is concerned with a national poetry rather than the specific origin of the poets themselves.

Passage 6

Topic and Scope: The use of punctuation, and in particular, the dash

Mapping the Passage:

Paragraphs 1-3 explain the main use of the dash: to present multiple expressions describing the same idea.

Paragraph 4 argues that punctuation is extremely important to the meaning of language.

Paragraph 5 suggests that the topic of punctuation has not been sufficiently explored.

Paragraph 6 introduces the dash and notes that it has gone out of style in the press.

31. D

A detail question in Roman numeral format: target the last three paragraphs, all of which deal exclusively with the dash. Condition I is stated directly in paragraph 6: the author describes "the printer's now general substitution... for the dash." Condition II follows closely afterward; the author argues that this backlash against the dash came as a result of "its excessive employment about 20 years ago." III can be inferred from the author's general argument, and also the point that the dash is necessary and "*cannot* be dispensed with." (D) includes all three statements.

32. A

Use your work from the previous question to help yourself on this question. Conditions II and III above together deal with the reason why printers have gotten in the habit of removing dashes. Review paragraph 5: The dash-censoring "has been brought about by the revulsion consequent upon its excessive employment about 20 years ago." In other words, writers used it too much, so now it's kaput. (A) says the same. (B) is faulty use of detail. Though the author mentions this in paragraph 4, a totally different reason is given for why printers dislike the dash. (C) is opposite. The author argues vehemently in the next paragraph that the dash *does* serve a purpose that other punctuation can't replace. (D) is out of scope. Authorial second-guessing is never mentioned in the passage.

33. A

You're looking for a right answer that *isn't* a valid inference. Since there's not much information to go on in the question, the answer will probably have something to do with the author's main points. Predict: Punctuation is important, and the dash is unique—it allows multiple expressions of the same thought, something that other punctuation can't accomplish. (A) immediately recommends itself. (B) is opposite. The author argues in paragraph 5 that it's a "vulgar notion" to think that punctuation doesn't follow simple rules. Therefore, the author certainly believes that it does. (C) is opposite. This sums up the author's argument in paragraph 4. (D) is opposite. This also follows from the author's suggestion that "few comprehend the extent" of punctuation's importance.

34. B

Where is "The Philosophy of Point" mentioned? Go back to paragraph 5 and review your map: The author wants to argue that writing can follow clear and consistent rules. It's a good bet, then, that the author mentions the article in order to reinforce this point. (B) says the same, suggesting that the article would be the author's attempt to explain exactly what the rules of punctuation are. (A) is distortion. Though the author puts the word "philosophy" in the title, there's no suggestion that there's anything philosophical about grammar. (C) is out of scope. The author never suggests that the purpose of the proposed magazine article would be to reinforce his credentials. (D) is distortion. Though the author wants to expand on his statement that punctuation follows simple rules, he's not interested in emending—that is, modifying—his argument about punctuation.

35. A

A detail question. What does the author argue about different expressions separated by a dash? Predict: The main point of the dash is to separate multiple thoughts that together get at the meaning—"which *partially* convey the idea intended." (A) says the same. (B) opposite. The author argues that each phrase partially conveys the author's idea—each expression is useful. (C) is opposite. Each expression approaches the main thought partially, and so there's no subdivision of purpose as this answer choice suggests. (D) is opposite. The author states that each expression conveys the *same* idea.

Passage 7

Topic and Scope: The question of whether women should be represented as their own political group

Mapping the Passage:

Paragraphs 1-3 provide the author's definition of a legitimate political interest group.

Paragraph 4 cites research supporting the idea that women as a group fit this definition. The author provides evidence on the amount of housework and childcare.

Paragraph 5 argues that despite these differences, women may not be generally conscious of them and then goes on to cites further evidence in support the idea fit the definition of a political interest group.

36. D

Go back to paragraphs 1 and 2, where the author discusses the criteria for representable interests. The author implies in paragraph 1 that groups with representable interests "share a particular viewpoint on the solution to political problems." (D) paraphrases this. (A) is opposite. The author states in paragraph 1 that the problems *don't* need to be "exclusively those of the specified interest group." (B) is opposite. The end of paragraph 3 states that a legitimate political group doesn't need to have a view "that differs substantially from answers articulated by others." (C) is distortion. The author distinguishes between individual and group representation in the first sentence, but doesn't suggest that members of a group can't be represented individually.

37. A

The author discusses differences between men and women in paragraphs 3-5, so focus your search there. The author suggests that notwithstanding all the differences between men and women, there's no evidence that "men and women as groups now disagree on policy issues in which women might have a special interest." (A) follows logically from this. (B) is distortion. While the author argues in paragraph 5 that differences in childcare are being reinforced, there's no indication that they're doing so in such a way that gives more control to men. (C) is opposite. The author argues in paragraph 5 that women aren't particularly aware of their differences with men. (D) is distortion. The author suggests that men and women aren't that aware of the differences, but this doesn't imply that men are unwilling to do so.

38. B

Where does the author mention the year 1900? Though it's not specifically stated, author mentions the turn of the century in paragraph 4. Review the context: evidence shows that women spend about the same amount of time working around the house as they did around 1900. (B) matches up. (A) is distortion. This distorts the point made in the first sentence. There's no point of comparison on this point with the turn of the century. (C) is out of scope. This is never mentioned in the context of the turn of the century. (D) is out of scope—another choice that has no relation to the turn of the century.

39. D

Predict by reviewing the author's purpose in writing the passage. The author wants to discuss whether women constitute a politically representative group; (D) summarizes this. (A) is out of scope. The author only discusses history in passing, and only to support arguments in favor of the main focus: political representation for women. (B) is distortion. Though the author alludes to the changing status of women in paragraph 5, it's again less a concern than the appropriateness of political representation. (C) is out of scope. The author never mentions opposing views.

40. A

Most of the support that the author provides is in the form of evidence listed in paragraphs 3-5; keep this in mind when evaluating the answer choices. Socioeconomic position is discussed in paragraph 5. The author suggests that the socioeconomic status of women and men is different, and provides a list of evidence supporting this at the beginning of the paragraph. (B) is opposite. This contradicts the author's suggestion in paragraph 5 that women and men have few differences in their degree of feminism. (C) is opposite. The author argues in paragraph 3 that it's not necessary that the members of an interest group be "consciously allied." (D) is out of scope. The author never suggests that a lack of education is getting in the way of voicing concerns.

VERBAL REASONING PRACTICE SET 2

ANSWER KEY

1. A	15. C	29. D
2. B	16. A	30. B
3. D	17. B	31. C
4. C	18. D	32. B
5. C	19. D	33. C
6. B	20. B	34. D
7. D	21. B	35. B
8. B	22. D	36. D
9. C	23. D	37. B
10. C	24. C	38. B
11. D	25. B	39. D
12. A	26. C	40. B
13. B	27. A	
14. C	28. A	

EXPLANATIONS

Passage 1

Topic and Scope: Critiques of the positivist approach to studying international relations and the positivist response

Mapping the Passage:

Paragraph 1 notes the conflict between historico-deductivists and positivists and describes the former's main critique of positivism: it tries to be completely objective in a field where complete objectivity is impossible.

Paragraph 2 provides an example: the causes of World War I can't be precisely pinned down.

Paragraph 3 presents one of the positivists' defenses: they don't pretend to be completely objective, but it's still best to be as objective as possible.

Paragraph 4 presents a second defense: positivism can lead to unexpected conclusions. The author also argues that the conflict between the two groups is good for research.

Paragraph 5 presents a third defense of positivism: even if positivists are biased, historico-deductivists are too.

1. A

A tough question full of tough words. Since *a posteriori* is in italics, it's easy to spot. Go back to paragraph to review what this is. Immediately after the phrase the passage says that in natural sciences, lab experiments can have "nomothetic status." What must this mean? Paraphrase: Probably that the findings are assumed to be definitely true. Read on: there's a "however" keyword that contrasts international relations with science, saying that "such lawlike generalizations about cause and effect are rarely if ever possible." Therefore, nomothetic status must involve "lawlike generalizations," and *a posteriori* overgeneralization must *challenge* positivists' attempts to do this because the historico-deductivists consider it a "case in point." Statement I says the same, and so (B) and (D) can be eliminated. Statement II is false because the example of World War II talks about *causes*, not effects. Though there's no need to evaluate statement III at this point, quickly confirm: there's no suggestion that historico-deductivism is exempt from the problem of *a posteriori* overdetermination, so that by itself doesn't suggest that the historico-positivist approach is inherently better. (A) must be correct.

2. B

Read the word "torch" in context. The sentence in which the word appears immediately follows the positivists' "moderate rule" which says that "the propensity to error should make us cautious, but not so desperate that we fear to come as close as possible to apodictic findings." Paraphrase, keeping the main positivist idea of a scientific approach in mind: just because we can't eliminate error doesn't mean that we shouldn't try to work scientifically. What does the "torch" that the positivists want to grasp represent, then? Predict: the conclusions that they think they'll find. Three choices can be eliminated, leaving you with (B). You know that (B) must be true in any case from the mention of nomothetic propositions in paragraph 2: they're described as absolute scientific findings, exactly the sort of thing that the positivists want. Strategy Point: Pay close attention whenever a rule or definition is mentioned. The MCAT loves to test you on things, which are clearly defined, but in a difficult context. (A) has a faulty use of detail. The positivists acknowledge that error can't be eliminated, but that they can still grasp the "torch": the scientific certainty that they're after. (C) is a distortion. The positivists aren't trying to grasp political phenomena; they're trying to grasp an *understanding* of political phenomena. (D) is distortion. As above, positivists don't want to get a handle on methodological commitments; they want to use methodology in order to get to the "torch" of understanding.

3. D

Go back to paragraph 2 to review. Historico-deductivists believe that *a posteriori* overdetermination presents some sort of problem for positivists trying to find nomothetic propositions. They also believe that nomothetic propositions, the "lawlike generalizations" used in science, aren't applicable to the study of international relations because one event can have many possible causes. What assumption is necessary to bridge these two beliefs? Predict: Nomothetic propositions can't explain events by relying on multiple causes. If they could, there presumably wouldn't be a problem with applying them to international relations. (D) Paraphrases this. (A) has a faulty use of detail. While historico-deductivists probably do believe this, it's not an assumption. Try denying it: even if they didn't believe this, or if they believed that positivists *could* provide a fully scientific account of World War I, their argument about overdetermination wouldn't necessarily fall apart. (B) is a distortion. The historico-deductivists probably believe that complex events aren't susceptible to the scientific analysis that the positivists are trying to use, but they must believe that they can be analyzed somehow; they'd be out of work otherwise! (C) is out of scope. The passage suggests no distinction between replicability and verifiability. Since both of these are part of the scientific method, it's an irrelevant distinction.

4. C

Where is Dougherty mentioned? Go back to the end of paragraph 1. Immediately above the quote in the question is the argument that "the precision of an answer cannot exceed that of its question." The implication is that positivists want certainty where there isn't any. Tie it back into the metaphor: the "clocks and necessity" represent the certainty positivist's want, while the "clouds and contingency" represent that uncertainty that actually exists. Only one answer choice deals with a positivist study, and it's a study of international relations, which the critics of positivists believe is full of uncertainty. (C) must be correct. (A) and (B) are out of scope. A historico-deductivist study wouldn't be looking for "clocks and necessity" since the approach of the historico-deductivists is fuzzier than that of the positivists. (D) is also out of scope. While the chemist *would* probably be looking for "clocks and necessity," there's reason to believe, especially from the discussion in paragraph 2, that historico-deductivists would acknowledge natural science as a field where this precision is justified.

5. C

Review the "moderate rule" from the lines mentioned question 3. Paraphrase the rule: the likelihood of error should make positivists cautious, but not so cautious that they give up trying to find scientific explanations as best as they can. Look for a situation that matches with this: (C) fits. Just because a worker can't earn a lot of money doesn't mean he shouldn't try to earn as much as he can. (A) is out of scope. The principle behind this seems to be that the opinion of someone who creates a work is more important than that of anyone else judging the work, which is irrelevant to Williams' rule. (B) is also out of scope. This principle behind this is most likely that different kinds of intelligence can be equal, which has nothing to do Williams' principle of trying to do the best one individually can. (D) is an opposite. If anything, this is the opposite of what Williams suggests. The principle behind this situation seems to suggest that one should hold back from acting because of possible dangers, while Williams says that one should do as much as one can.

6. B

A quick scan of the answer choices shows a variety of professions. Who would be most likely to write a passage about a disagreement over how to study international relations? Predict: someone who studied international relations. (B) immediately recommends itself. (A) is a distortion. Though history is mentioned frequently in the passage, it's always in the context of international relations. The author argues that the debate is "among international relations scholars," so a history professor would be less likely to write about it than an international relations professor. (C) is also a distortion. While diplomats are *involved* in international relations, they're not necessarily dedicated to the *study* of it. A professor of international relations would be more likely to be interested in the academic side of the topic. (D) is out of scope. There's no reason to think that a journalist would be concerned with an academic debate about the study of international relations.

Passage 2

Topic and Scope: The formation and location of hydrocarbon reserves

Mapping the Passage:

Paragraph 1 explains how hydrocarbons form in pockets underground.

Paragraph 2 gives some background for our global dependence on fossil fuels.

Paragraph 3 describes the two types of hydrocarbon traps: structural traps and stratigraphic traps.

Paragraph 4 notes that new sources of hydrocarbons will come from reserves that are difficult to locate, and describes generally how reserves are located and extracted.

Paragraph 5 notes that most new oil will be found in stratigraphic traps and outlines the method for finding oil when surface geology doesn't help: seismic exploration.

Paragraph 6 describes the limitations to seismic exploration of stratigraphic traps.

Paragraph 7 notes recent developments in refining seismic exploration, and raises hope that discovery of stratigraphic traps will be easier in the future.

7. D

A global question: predict with topic, scope, and purpose. The author discusses how hydrocarbon reserves are formed (especially in paragraphs 1 and 3) and how they can be located (throughout the passage, but especially in the second half of the passage). (D) repeats this nearly word-forword. (A), (B), and (C) have a faulty use of detail. Choice (A) says nothing about the location of reserves, which the passage spends significant time on. The passage discusses seismic exploration, but it also discusses the formation of hydrocarbons before this. And the author argues in paragraph 5 that stratigraphic traps are harder to locate than structural traps, but this isn't itself the main idea of the passage; the author mentions this in order to explain the method for discovering stratigraphic traps.

8. B

This is a detail question; "According to the passage..." tips you off. Where are difficulties mentioned? Go back to paragraph 6. The last sentence of paragraph 6 states what the question does, that it's difficult to distinguish reflections between the two materials. The beginning of the sentence gives the reason: "the density contrasts between oil-bearing sandstones and the shales that provide stratigraphic seals for the oil are often very small." (B) says the same. (A) has a faulty use of detail. While the author mentions this in the same paragraph, it's used in the context of how resolution can be improved, not why it's difficult to distinguish between the sandstone and shale. (C) also has a faulty use of detail. This is part of the "primary limitation with the seismic method" that the author discusses towards the beginning of the paragraph, not the direct cause of the particular problem in the question. (D) is out of scope. Thinness has to do with the primary limitation of the method, not the specific problem mentioned in the question.

9. C

An evaluation question; review the lines in context. The author provides the example immediately after defining how stratigraphic traps are forming by stating "For example..." (note the keyword!). Predict the use: the author is simply giving an example of how the traps are formed. (C) says the same. (A) is out of scope. The author doesn't provide any contrast to structural traps in the example. (B) is faulty use of detail. The author does explain this, but only in order to explain how stratigraphic traps are formed. This is another part of the example rather than the point of the example. (D) is out of scope. This isn't mentioned until paragraph 6.

10. C

A scattered detail question. Either eliminate wrong answer choices or look for a choice that sticks out as correct. (C) should jump out; since not all traps are stratigraphic, it wouldn't make sense for the author to have said that oil couldn't be extracted without a density contrast between reservoir rocks and a stratigraphic seal. (A) is opposite. The author states in paragraph 1 that "hydrocarbons...will eventually reach the surface and be lost unless they encounter impermeable rocks." (B) is opposite. The author ties oil reserves to hydrocarbons in paragraphs 1 and 4, so it's reasonable to believe that it's not possible to get oil if an original source of hydrocarbons isn't present. (D) is opposite; the text states that drilling can't happen unless hydrocarbons are trapped within permeable rocks.

11. D

Where are carbonate reservoirs mentioned? Review the beginning of paragraph 6: "the most common stratigraphic traps (with the possible exception of carbonate reservoirs) are in sandstone layers that are much thinner than a seismic wavelet." What's the implication? Predict: carbonate reservoirs are in layers that *aren't* much thinner than a seismic wavelet. (D) comes close to this. (A) is out of scope. Density has nothing to do with the thickness of the layer, which is what we're concerned with in this part of the passage. (B) is out of scope. While carbonate layers might be *easier* to find than other stratigraphic traps because of their relative thickness, the author gives no indication that they're in fact *easy* to find. (C) is out of scope. The author says nothing about the importance or lack thereof of carbonate traps.

12. A

What is the author's opinion of seismology? The author discusses why seismology isn't a great way to find stratigraphic traps in paragraph 6, and raises the hope that seismology will become more effective in the future in paragraph 7. Paraphrase: Seismology has its problems, but will hopefully improve in the future. (A) says the same. (B) is distortion. Though seismology has limitations, there's no indication that it's intrinsically flawed. If it were, the author wouldn't argue for its improvement. (C) is distortion. The author believes that seismology has promise, but spends a significant part of the passage explaining why seismology *isn't* extremely effective. Nothing at all is said about profitability, so this choice is out of scope also. (D) is distortion. The author doesn't discuss the theory of seismology, instead focusing exclusively on the practical method and its limitations. Further, the author suggests that seismology is *ineffective* for only stratigraphic exploration, not completely ineffectual.

13. B

What sort of development would improve seismic exploration the most? Predict: something that overcame the seismic method's primary limitation. The author states in paragraph 6 that the primary limitation is resolution, and that the wavelets are too large to be useful in discovering stratigraphic traps. Therefore, something that allowed for higher resolution would be a major development, and if it overcame the problem of attenuation that the author mentioned, it would sidestep the current problems with high frequencies. (B) fits. (A) is opposite. While it would be good for the frequency to increase, increasing the *attenuation* of the wavelength only exacerbates the problem with high frequencies that the author mentions. (C) is distortion. While this would be an improvement, since the author mentions a problem associated with this in the paragraph, it wouldn't be as big an improvement as something that overcame the "principal limitation" of seismology. (D) is distortion. As above, while further research might be helpful in other ways, it wouldn't be as helpful as a practical way to overcome the main problems with seismology.

Passage 3

Topic and Scope: The three social functions of popular music

Mapping the Passage:

Paragraph 1 discusses the advent of pop music and the birth of Rock-and-Roll.

Paragraphs 2 and 3 discuss popular music's function of creating identity.

Paragraph 4 discusses its function in the management of feelings.

Paragraph 5 discusses its third function, organizing time, and notes that this is particularly important to the definition of youth.

14. C

Where is classical music mentioned in the passage? It isn't! How could we figure out anything about classical music, then? Predict: by relating it to music in general. The author notes in paragraph 5 "one of the effects of all music, not just pop, is to focus our attention on the feeling of time, and intensify our experience of the present." Therefore, both pop music and classical music must focus attention on time, since this is a general quality of music. (C) says the same. Strategy Point: Don't panic when a question throws a curve ball in the form of an unfamiliar situation or terminology that's not in the passage. If it's in a question, it can be related back to the passage; you just need to figure out how. (A) is faulty use of detail. This is a social function of pop music, but the author doesn't suggest that it's a function of music in general. (B) is faulty use of detail. The author uses this phrasing in describing "popular love songs", but again gives no indication that it's a function of music in general. (D) is faulty use of detail. The author argues in paragraph 5 that pop music defines what youth is, but doesn't argue a similar function for music in general.

15. C

A question about the author's tone. Scan the answer choices and note that only (C) is positive. Is the author's tone positive? Go back to paragraph 4: the author says that the love songs "give shape and voice to emotions that otherwise cannot be expressed without embarrassment or incoherence." The author also notes that the songs express feeling "for us in interesting and involving ways." The author is positive, and therefore (C) is correct. (A) is opposite. The author argues that love songs are the antidotes to banal language by expressing the same ideas in interesting ways. (B) is opposite. The author argues that our own expressions of feeling can be emotionally incoherent and that love songs help to compensate for this. (D) is opposite. The author clearly believes that popular love songs have an important social function: the management of feelings. Strategy Point: Identifying the author's tone (positive, negative, or neutral) helps narrow down answer choices with a quick vertical scan.

16. A

Why does the author discuss sports in paragraph 2? Go back to review: the author says that "music, like sport, is clearly a setting in which people directly experience community . . . " Sport is used as an example of a case in which something similar happens, or, in other words, a parallel. (A) says the same. (B) is opposite. The author says that music is like sport: "like," indicates a parallel, not a contrast. (C) is out of scope. There's no assumption mentioned that could be challenged. (D) is opposite. The mention of sport is used to elaborate on the *same* idea, not to introduce a new one.

17. B

What does the author do in the last paragraph? Predict from your map: The author describes the third function of popular music, the organization of time, and its relevance to the definition of youth. (B) captures the author's focus on youth. Strategy Point: Watch out for answer choices that take familiar wording and rearrange it into nonsensical, contradictory, or irrelevant answer choices. Familiar wording should be used to figure out what part of the passage to review, not to answer the question from the familiarity alone! (A) is distortion. The author briefly discusses the experience of youth, but only in the context of how youth relates to popular music, which this choice leaves out entirely. (C) is out of scope. This choice tries to capitalize on words familiar from the passage: "organization" and "youth." *Time* is organized, and youth is defined through popular music, but nothing at all is said about the organization of youth movements. (D) is faulty use of detail. Though the author does discuss the relationship between music and time, it's done so in the context of how it relates to youth, a topic that this choice completely omits.

18. D

Where is the creation of identity discussed? Go back to paragraph 2. Review the author's main points: pop music helps us "directly experience community" and at the same time has an "individualizing" effect. The author uses these ideas to show how identity is created through pop music. (D) paraphrases the idea that pop music operates on the communal and individual levels. (A) is out of scope. Though the author says in paragraph 5 that young people are most concerned with pop music, this doesn't mean it's unpopular with the older set. In any case, it's irrelevant to the author's point about identity, which is restricted to paragraph 2. (B) is faulty use of detail. The author makes this point in paragraph 4, but to support the idea that pop music helps to manage feelings, not to support pop music's role of creating identity. (C) is opposite. The author says that pop songs are "open to appropriation for personal use in a way that other popular cultural forms... are not." Pop music is therefore *unique* in this way.

19. D

Why does the author believe that popular music is important for social organization in youth? Go back to review the relevant text. The author makes the assertion in paragraph 5, and immediately above says that it's because good music has the ability to stop time, with "no memory or anxiety about what has come before us, what will come after." What would weaken this? Predict: something that said that good music *doesn't* stop time. (D) does just this. (A) is opposite. This would support the author's argument at the end of the passage that the moments associated with youth "have nostalgia coded into them" without necessarily weakening the author's point about forgetting the past. (B) is opposite. This would support, and in fact paraphrases, the author's argument that "youth is experienced...through an impatience for time to pass and a regret that it is doing so." (C) is opposite. This would also support the author's argument about youth, and in particular, the author's claim that "we invest most in popular music when we are teenagers and young adults."

Passage 4

Topic and Scope: The advantages and disadvantages of tracking

Purpose: To argue that tracking leads to differing educational experiences and puts lower-level students at a disadvantage

Mapping the Passage:

Paragraph 1 argues that tracking contradicts the philosophy that all can learn, and suggests that scheduling issues make tracking attractive to administrators.

Paragraph 2 responds to the argument that tracking improves learning by stating that tracking can "dumb down" lower-level tracks.

Paragraph 3 defines tracking and states that tracking affects the school experience.

Paragraph 4 notes a major problem with tracking: inability for some students in lower tracks to get into higher-level classes later.

20. B

An incorporation question. How would the author's argument be affected if tracked students did better than their non-tracked counterparts? The question tells you that the argument would be weakened, so you just need to find an answer choice summarizing an argument the author makes against tracking on the basis of performance. (B) is just such a choice: the author argues in paragraph 2 that tracking encourages "dumbing down." (A) is faulty use of detail. The author does argue this at the beginning of paragraph 2, but the statement isn't made in order to argue directly that tracking hurts academic performance. Therefore, it wouldn't be weakened by evidence that indicates higher performance. (C) is faulty use of detail. The author makes this point in paragraph 1, but this is an advantage of tracking, and one of the reasons it sticks around. Test scores—good or bad—would have no effect on this argument. (D) is faulty use of detail. This argument, found in paragraph 2, is presented as a belief of proponents of tracking. This is not the *author's* argument, as the author suggests that "dumbing down" is a likely outcome.

21. B

A main-idea question. Predict using topic, scope, and purpose. The author argues that tracking in schools leads to disadvantages for the students. Thus, he or she is not in favor of tracking. Focus in on the global choices, (A) and (B). Of the two, (A) oversteps the scope of the passage. Only (B) accurately encompasses what the author is arguing. (A) is out of scope. The author never actually argues that tracking should be eliminated; only that it has some negative consequences. (C) is faulty use of detail. Stress level is mentioned at the end of paragraph 3, but this is not the author's main point of the passage. (D) is faulty use of detail. Scheduling is mentioned at the end of paragraph 1, but this is not the author's main point of the passage.

22. D

Review the argument referenced by the question (it's at the beginning of paragraph 1). Why does the author believe this is the case? Paraphrase the argument: if students are assigned to a lower track, the school is assuming that they're unable to perform at a higher level, and so they might be held back when the teacher has to slow down the class. Look for evidence that would support this, starting with statement III, which appears in three out of the four choices. Statement III would strengthen the author's argument: lower-track classes that couldn't finish the work they were given would be an example of exactly what the author is discussing at the end of paragraph 4. Eliminate (A). Statement I also supports the author's argument, echoing the argument at the end of paragraph 4 that lower-track students find it hard to take AP courses. Only (D) remains, and there's no need to check statement II; that statement would *weaken* the author's argument. Strategy Point: Some questions will very clearly reward you for attention to structure rather than detail. In this question, very relevant information was in the paragraph above the lines quoted. Catching the keywords that tip this off will allow you to answer this question very quickly, since the correct Roman numerals are simply details from that paragraph.

23. D

A scattered-detail question. Either eliminate or look for a choice that seems foreign. While the first three are mentioned as criteria for tracking in the passage, (D) isn't. While the author notes in paragraph 3 that "there are differences...in...how talkative and energetic the classroom is" depending on tracking, there's no suggestion that students are tracked *based* on how talkative or energetic they are individually. (A) is opposite. The author mentions grades as a criterion in the opening lines of paragraph 3. (B) is opposite. The author cites "academic ability" as a criterion for tracking in paragraph 3. (C) is opposite. The author discusses the way students get locked in to higher tracks (i.e., AP courses) with honors courses (paragraph 4).

24. C

An application question. The trick to many application questions is simply remembering that the author believes his own argument. How would the author respond to a situation in which a student underachieves because of boredom in a way that would strengthen the author's argument? Predict:

He'd argue that the student was put in a track that isn't sufficiently challenging, a problem discussed at the end of paragraph 4. (C) rewards the careful prediction. (A) is opposite. The author doesn't address the possibility that students might be tracked too high; he's far more concerned with the "dumbing down" of classrooms. (B) is out of scope. There's nothing in the passage to suggest that the author considers lack of motivation in students a particular problem. (D) is distortion. Though the author might agree that the student should be in a higher track, the higher track doesn't necessarily need to include AP classes, which represent a very specific situation mentioned in paragraph 4.

Passage 5

Topic and Scope: The evolution of the civil rights movement and its relation to pluralist politics

Purpose: To compare and contrast the methods used to advance the civil rights movements with those used in pluralist politics

Passage Map:

Paragraph 1 points out that the civil rights movement came about at the same time as pluralist politics, as new immigrants banded together and joined organizations.

Paragraph 2 introduces the importance of constitutional interpretation to race politics.

Paragraph 3 describe the way that the civil rights movement fought for legal and constitutional legitimacy for blacks primarily through the court system.

Paragraph 4 contrasts the tactics of the civil rights movement with those of immigrants engaging in pluralist politics: the former worked for rights through the courts, while the latter worked for resources through politics.

25. B

A detail question that focuses on the main contrast in paragraph 4. Predict: the movement for rights worked through the courts, while the movement for resources worked through politics. Only (B) and (C) incorporate this idea of politics, and of these, only (B) focuses on the local politics that the author suggests when discussing "local clubs and machines" and "precinct captains and patronage." (A) is opposite. The author argues that the fight for resources *did* involve electoral power. (C) is distortion. While this choice does include a focus on politics, it specifically mentions national politics, when the author discusses "local political clubs and machines." (D) is faulty use of detail. It was the newly arrived immigrant population that struggled for resources, so it doesn't make sense to say immigrants "cooperated" with themselves.

26. C

Review the author's discussion of the executive branch, which appears in paragraph 3. The author argues that the presidency and Congress didn't get involved "because the political constituencies supporting their elections did not favor such participation." Paraphrase: The President didn't help with the civil rights movement because it was politically unpopular. (C) paraphrases this. (A) is out of scope. The national clout of activists isn't discussed, and the author is clear that the executive branch didn't act out of concern for voters. (B) is out of scope. Lobbying isn't discussed, and the author is clear that members of the legislative branch failed to act because of their voters. (D) is out of scope. The author never indicates this. In addition, this answer choice is a bit extreme.

27. A

A rare question asking about the structure of the whole passage; use your map to help you build a prediction. Paragraphs 2 and 3 describe attempts to gain rights through the courts, while paragraph 4 contrasts this effort with attempts to gain resources through politics. (A), though lacking in specifics, closely matches the structure of the prediction. Strategy Point: When evaluating the structure of a passage or paragraph, begin broadly, check the answers, and refine your prediction as needed. Most evaluation questions have straightforward answers; too much complexity in your prediction will waste time and make the right answer tougher to spot. (B) is out of scope. The author doesn't praise the movements and describes two completely different movements, not a single movement with two examples. (C) is out of scope. The author gives a general history of one struggle, but gives no indication of how it will play out in the future. This choice also leaves out the political struggle for resources discussed in paragraph 4. (D) is distortion. The author discusses two different approaches, but they're two different approaches to *different* problems, not the same problem.

28. A

Notice the unusual wording of this question. We are looking for a statement that characterizes the civil rights movement. This is a detail question, so start by finding where 1965 is mentioned in the passage. The author says in paragraph 3 that "a 'civil rights' movement developed that saw ninety-five years (1870-1965) devoted to establishing the privilege of Blacks to vote unencumbered by racial barriers." Paraphrase: Before 1965, the civil rights movement was primarily interested in the right to vote freely. Choice (A) fits the bill. (B) is opposite. The author argues that the movement "created a cadre of constitutional lawyers who became in a real sense the focal points of the civil rights struggle." In other words, the author likely believes that constitutional lawyers were the ones struggling to overturn unjust decisions, not the other way around. (C) is faulty use of detail. This characterizes the civil rights movement using the language the author reserves for the struggle for *resources* in paragraph 4. (D) is out of scope. The author never discusses any such conflict.

29. D

Congress kept a hands-off approach to the civil rights movement anyway. Review the lines describing the boycott: it started in response to the actions of Rosa Parks. The Supreme Court case vindicating Rosa Parks provided an example of civil disobedience that led to a change in law, which seems to be a good description of the author's mention of the boycott also. Looking for a choice that fits turns up choice (D), which simply focuses a little more on rights in general rather than the specific change in law. (A) is distortion. The author says at the end of paragraph 4 that the civil rights movement did eventually move from rights to resources, but says that it was an *evolution*, not something marked by a sudden turning point. In any case, the case of Rosa Parks represents a struggle for rights rather than resources. (B) is out of scope. Martin Luther King, Jr. isn't mentioned in the passage; this choice tries to play on your outside knowledge. Remember to stick only to what is said and necessarily implied by the passage! (C) is out of scope. As above, though it may very well be one of the better-known battles, the author doesn't suggest anywhere that this is the case, and the example isn't making this point.

30. B

A scattered-detail question. Since the question deals with the main contrast in the passage, review the basics: the civil rights movement fought for rights through the courts, while the movement of "plural ethnicity" fought for resources through politics. While three answer choices fit with the summary and with details from paragraphs 1 and 4, (B) suggests that the second movement used the courts to advance its ends, while the author says that this was a trait of the *civil rights* movement. Strategy Point: In scattered detail questions such as this, be on the lookout for an answer that contradicts the author's point of view or distorts a detail from another part of the passage. (A) is the author's main characterization of the movement in paragraph 4: politics instead of courts. (C) paraphrases the author's point that "plural-ethnicity focused on precinct captains and patronage." (D) is opposite. In paragraph 1 the author discusses immigrants "passing through Ellis Island, and going into local political clubs and machines," which suggests that most of the action was in northern cities.

Passage 6

Topic and Scope: Description of the influence that Livingston and Bentham had on the modern penal code

Passage Map:

Paragraph 1 introduces Livingston's penal code, and his background.

Paragraph 2 describes the intellectual tradition leading to the Model Penal Code, and in particular the influence of Jeremy Bentham.

Paragraph 3 lists the concepts within Bentham's legacy.

Paragraph 4 describes the details of Livingston's penal code.

31. C

A broad-inference question; review the author's main ideas: the author spends the passage discussing the traditions and people that led to the modern penal code. Choice (C) paraphrases this closely, echoing the author's points at the beginning of paragraph 2. (A) is out of scope. The author never suggests that Livingston influenced his colleagues, and reverses the order of influence between Livingston and Bentham, who preceded Livingston. (B) is distortion. The author says in paragraph 2 that there was a "powerful movement toward codification of law" in both of these places, but doesn't mention lawmakers specifically, nor is it suggested that they agreed wholeheartedly. (D) is out of scope. The author speaks very highly of the Benthamite codes, and so there's no reason to believe that he thinks that they aren't successful in practice. The answer is also off scope in that the author never discusses the practical application of the code.

32. B

Where will things attributed to Bentham's work be found? Predict: probably in the monster of a sentence that is paragraph 3, which starts out, "Within Bentham's legacy are such concepts as:" Statements I and II are mentioned in the list, but statement III is not and runs counter to Livingston's prohibition of capital punishment in his code, which was presumably borrowed from Bentham's ideas. (B) must be correct.

33. C

Where are the reasons for Livingston's creation of his penal code described? Review paragraph 1. The author says that "many factors" were responsible, and then describes Livingston's commitment to the idea. Choice (C) paraphrases the author's point that Livingston "was captured by the ideas of Bentham and the ferment for legal reform and codification in revolutionary America and France." (A) is distortion. The author describes Livingston's code as "the first great penal code in the Benthamite tradition," which suggests that the idea hadn't spread to Louisiana from other parts of the country, but originated in the country with Livingston. (B) is out of scope. Since Livingston's code was the first of its kind, it couldn't have come about as an attempt to emulate the legal system of another country. (D) is out of scope. The author emphasizes that the code came about as "the commitment of one man to the idea of codification," and states in paragraph 4 that Livingston's creation of the code was "unassisted," which suggests that Livingston's colleagues had nothing to do with the effort.

34. D

A scattered-detail question, though not too scattered since you know that the strengths of Livingston's code are mentioned in the second half of paragraph 4. All are mentioned except (D), which is specifically contradicted in paragraph 1 by the author's note that Livingston's code was "never enacted." (A) is opposite. The author notes that protection of "the rights of the accused" is part of Livingston's code. (B) is opposite. The author also mentions "the prominent place [Livingston's code] gave to reform." (C) is opposite. The author notes that "Livingston distrusted judges no less than Bentham" and notes that the point of the code was "to leave as little as possible to judicial creativity."

35. B

Why did Livingston want to create the code? The author gives several reasons, so review the basics in paragraphs 1 and 4 and look for an answer that fits. (B) echoes the point in paragraph 4 that the point of the code was "to leave as little as possible to judicial creativity," and notes that "all means through which judges might infuse their own moral views into the definition of crimes were outlawed." (A) is faulty use of detail. While these were characteristics of the code, there's no indication that it was one of the guiding motivations, while the author states explicitly that reigning judges in was *the* object of the code. (C) is opposite. The author notes that "use of common-law terms" was outlawed in Livingston's code. (D) is faulty use of detail. Though these are also described as characteristics of the code, like (A), they're not explicitly mentioned as reasons for creating the code.

Passage 7

Topic and Scope: An argument for the abolishment of private property in order to foster individualism

Mapping the Passage:

Paragraphs 1 and 2 explain how private property has harmed individualism.

Paragraphs 3 and 4 argue that socialism cannot be compulsory.

Paragraph 5 argues that while most socialists don't advocate compulsory socialism, authority is still overemphasized.

Paragraphs 5 and 6 tie individualism and private property together, and gives examples of people who were able to achieve individualism through wealth; and paragraph 6 argues that individualism will benefit from the elimination of personal property.

36. D

Where are these individuals mentioned? Look over your map of paragraph 5. These were all individuals who were able to maximize their individuality because they were so rich that they didn't have to work. Only (A) and (D) involve money, and (D) alone fits with the author's overall point in the paragraph. (A) is opposite. While this choice does talk about money, and while the author's overall point is that property should be abolished, in this paragraph the author is giving examples of artists who had an "immense advantage" by being rich. Money therefore must be *helpful* to individualism. (B) is out of scope. While the author might believe that genius is rare, the scope of the paragraph is on money and its advantages to individualism. (C) is distortion. The author does define this; it's simply individualism. The focus of the paragraph is on money, however.

37. B

Where does the author use the phrase mentioned in the question? It's mentioned in paragraph 4, where the author is arguing against compulsory socialism. Look for choices that exemplify compulsory socialism. Start with statement II, which appears in three choices: In this example, part of the population is forced to perform a certain type of labor, which certainly would qualify as compulsory socialism. Look at statement I: No socialism is suggested in this example, only segregation. Statement III represents socialism, but there's no suggestion that it's *compulsory* socialism. (B) must be correct.

38. B

Find the phrase mentioned in the question: it's in paragraph 4. Review the context: The author argues that "humanity has got beyond" enforced manual labor, and that it saves that for the criminals. He also mentions that criminals are labeled such "in a very arbitrary manner." What does this imply about the author's opinions toward society and criminals? He seems to think that the notion of criminality that society has isn't necessarily just. (B) paraphrases this. (A) is distortion. Though the author thinks that the label of "criminal" might be arbitrary and that people shouldn't be forced to work, this doesn't mean that *all* actions should be permitted. (C) is out of scope. The author never suggests this. (D) is distortion. Though society seems to think that this is true, the author doesn't necessarily agree, especially since he considers ideas of criminality to be very arbitrary.

39. D

What is Baudelaire used as an example of? Someone who was able to cultivate his genius because he didn't have to hold down a day job. If Baudelaire *did* have to work, this would weaken the author's idea of wealth as an advantage to attaining individuality. However, since he's one of six examples, it wouldn't weaken it all that much; the author would have plenty to fall back on. The only "weakeners" in the choices are outright refutations, which is far too strong an effect on the argument. It's clear that this information contradicting the author wouldn't strengthen the argument, though, so only (D) is left: The author's main points might not have as much evidence as they did, but there's still plenty for them to remain valid. (A) is distortion. As described above, it would only ever so slightly weaken it. (B) is out of scope. Even if Baudelaire did have to work, he could still be a poet who recognized his own personality. (C) is opposite. Baudelaire doesn't tie into this part of the argument, but if he was an individualist and did have to work for private property, the author's argument would be weakened.

40. B

An inference question without any hint as to specifics, which means that the answer will probably tie into the author's main idea. Predict it: Compulsory socialism is bad, but private property should be eliminated because it gets in the way of individuality. (B) fits most closely. The author believes that only a few people are able to achieve individuality with the help of wealth, but that "mankind generally" is a different matter. (A) is distortion. While the author mentions a few artists who were, he argues just that: that only a few have been able to achieve individuality with wealth. (C) is opposite. The author only mentions artists who *were* dependent on private means to achieve their individuality. (D) is distortion. Though the author believes that some artists had an advantage because of their private means, there's no indication that this is the only way that self-realization can occur.

VERBAL REASONING PRACTICE SET 3

ANSWER KEY

1. A	15. B	29. B
2. B	16. D	30. D
3. B	17. C	31. C
4. D	18. D	32. D
5. A	19. A	33. B
6. D	20. C	34. C
7. C	21. B	35. B
8. A	22. B	36. B
9. C	23. A	37. A
10. B	24. C	38. D
11. C	25. B	39. A
12. A	26. C	40. C
13. C	27. C	
14. A	28. B	

EXPLANATIONS

Passage 1

Topic and Scope: Negative effects that media "leaks" have on foreign policy and the media's credibility

Mapping the Passage:

Paragraph 1 argues that the media's suspicion of government and lack of knowledge about the world harm government policy.

Paragraphs 2 and 3 introduce the concept of the "leak" and explain why it's bad for foreign policy.

Paragraph 4 states that the media was trusted by the public until recently, as it is now met with skepticism.

Paragraph 5 argues that leaks are usually part of a power grab and that the media is a pawn in the game.

1. A

Review the author's main arguments before looking for an answer choice that he's likely to agree with. (A) recalls the author's point in paragraph 2: "Leaders often say one thing in public and something quite different in private conversation..." The author explains why this occurs (fear of media leaks) and clearly opposes such leaks. Therefore, the author must agree with (A)'s contention that keeping the public in the dark is sometimes warranted. (B) is opposite. This is the opposite of (A); for the same reasons that (A) is a valid inference, (B) isn't. (C) is opposite. The author argues in paragraph 3 that policy benefits from a "richness and variety of ideas." (D) is opposite. The author's point in decrying leaks is that privacy is a necessary component of leadership.

2. B

Scan back in the passage to find the author's mention of foreign officials. The author argues in paragraph 2 that foreign officials fear leaks and are less inclined to speak their minds if they think that their private thoughts will be revealed. So it makes sense that foreign policy would be harmed because the foreign leaders would be less likely to confide in American officials. (B) summarizes this point. (A) is distortion. While this may or may not be true, the author is arguing that it certainly won't be true if leaks continue. (C) is out of scope. The author doesn't suggest that foreign officials would do this in the first place, so it's an irrelevant hypothetical. (D) is out of scope. This isn't relevant to leaks of foreign officials' thoughts.

3. B

Review the author's main points before looking for an answer choice that is both a claim made in the passage *and* supported by evidence. This question is harder than some of the same type because *all* the answer choices are claims made by the passage. However, three claims are simply made, with no support. (B) alone is a claim made (in paragraph 5) and supported by explanation that makes up the bulk of the paragraph. Strategy Point: When looking for a claim supported by evidence, search for an answer choice that summarizes an entire paragraph. Claims not supported by evidence will usually be secondary claims that don't directly tie into the main points of the passage. (A) is faulty use of detail. While this claim is made in paragraph 1 when the author says that the media cause "damage...in ways they rarely imagine," it's given no support before the author moves on to discussing leaks. (C) is faulty use of detail. The author makes this claim in the end of the last paragraph, but provides no support. (D) is faulty use of detail. This is a claim made in paragraph 1, again without support.

4. D

Review the author's argument in paragraph 2 that leaks harm discussions with foreign leaders. What is the author assuming in this argument? The author argues that foreign leaders don't want their private thoughts to be made public; he must also therefore assume that leaders have some sort of reason for not wanting their views to be made public. (D) provides a possible reason. If unclear, use the denial test: if leaders didn't have this fear, what would be their motivation for hiding their personal views? (A) is distortion. The author dislikes leaks, but never argues that they're immoral. This is extreme. (B) is distortion. There's no evidence that leaks have occurred throughout history. (C) is out of scope. The author never suggests that there were no barriers to discussion before the press, only that there are far more barriers now that the press is in the habit of leaking these discussions.

5. A

Go back to the context to review what the author is saying: he's arguing that journalists are used as tools rather than being the ones in charge. Therefore, the "prime mover" must refer to whoever *is* in charge, which the author suggests is the official doing the leaking. (A) says just this. (B) is opposite. The author says just the opposite: the journalists *aren't* the prime mover. (C) is out of scope. Media executives aren't mentioned in the situation at all. (D) is out of scope. The author refers to the primer movers as the officials angling for power, not abstract rules that govern leaks.

6. D

How do anonymous leaks affect the author's argument? Use your work from the last question: Paragraph 5 argues that officials use leaks as a way of either currying favor with the media or planting information to influence policy. How does anonymity affect each of these? While it would have no effect on the policy aspect, it would negate the possibility of currying favor. Therefore, if most leaks are anonymous, the author's argument about favor-currying must be weakened. (A) is out of scope. As explained above, anonymity would have no effect on this motivation. (B) is out of scope. It would have no bearing on the issue of reliability, and the author argues that this isn't the case anyhow. (C) is opposite. As explained above, the policy aspect isn't affected by anonymity.

7. C

Go back to paragraph 4 to review what the public thinks of the media. The author says that in the past, the public always assumed the media was right when it challenged the government, but that "this may be changing." Therefore, the public *might* now consider the possibility that the media, rather than the government, is wrong. While the wrong answer choices distort this, (C) rewards careful and methodical thought. (A) is distortion. The author argued that the public generally thought this in the past, but that it's not necessarily the case anymore.

(B) is distortion. The author suggests that the public might believe that the media is wrong, but never says that the media's *always* considered wrong in a showdown with government. (D) is distortion. The author argues that in the past, the public generally thought officials under challenge were in the wrong; that isn't necessarily the case anymore.

Passage 2

Topic and Scope: The psychological ramifications of obedience to authority versus control over one's own actions

Mapping the Passage:

Paragraph 1 states that when so ordered by authority, people do things they otherwise wouldn't.

Paragraph 2 argues that psychological studies have to take into account the practical aspects of obedience in addition to theoretical ideas.

Paragraph 3 suggests that laboratory-tested obedience effectively highlights these practical aspects.

Paragraph 4 says that obedience is influenced by fear and the desire to cooperate, and that the individual obeying has trouble controlling his own behavior.

Paragraph 5 expands on the point in paragraph 4: the laboratory can effectively simulate real-world conditions that lead to obedience.

8. A

The situation involves someone who doesn't want to do something presumably against his morality, but who finally does it because he's ordered to. How does this fit in with the author's argument? It matches closely with the point made in paragraph 1 that because an authority tells them to do so, people will do things they don't really want to. Therefore, the author's argument is supported without qualification. (B) is opposite. For the reasons described above, the pilot's actions would support the author's argument. (C) is out of scope. While the author's argument would be supported, there's no reason to believe this would be the case only if the pilot had a history of obeying orders he disliked. This example, even if isolated, is enough by itself to support the author's argument. (D) is opposite. For the reasons described above, the author's argument would be supported.

9. C

Review the phrase in context: who is defying what? The author seems to be referring to a general case in which someone defies an order he doesn't want to obey, presumably for moral reasons. Looking for a situation that reflects this turns up (C): someone is disobeying an authority on principled grounds. The other choices do not explicitly defying orders at all. (A) is opposite. There's no defiance of orders. (B) has no *direct* defiance of orders here. The employee wasn't ordered to work overtime, but rather simply to finish the project as soon as possible. There's also no element of principle in this situation. (D), too, has no orders being defied.

10. B

Review the lines in context. The author argues that this "absence of compulsion" goes hand in hand with a "cooperative mood," which suggests that the phrase means the person is obeying on his or her own free will. (B) says the same. (A) is out of scope. While fear is mentioned as a factor later in the passage, it doesn't tie into this phrase, nor is there any indication that psychological experiments do lack punishment. (C) is distortion. While the person who has an absence of compulsion presumably is free to disobey, the phrase is more concerned with those who *do* obey, though free to refuse. (D) is out of scope. Moral implications aren't discussed or hinted at anywhere near this phrase.

11. C

What is the author's main argument about obedience? People do things they don't want to do because they feel compelled to by authority. Look for something that challenges this point: If (C) is true, the author's point about not wanting to do things, most clearly expressed in paragraph 1, makes no sense. If people have no strong ethical values, then bad actions wouldn't necessarily be against their will. (A) is opposite. This would support the author's point about fear made in the last paragraph. (B) opposite. This would support the author's idea that authority is often used to advance immoral aims. (D) is out of scope. This is an irrelevant distinction; the author doesn't say anything about which segments of society would be more or less willing to obey authority.

12. A

Keep the author's major point in mind while reviewing the choices. Choice (A) is the subject of paragraph 3. While (A) has a few paragraphs' worth of support, the other choices reflect claims either made but not supported or not made at all. (B) is out of scope. The passage does not comment on this. (C) is faulty use of detail. The author inserts this at the end of paragraph 4, again without support. (D) is out of scope. This claim isn't made at all in the passage. Though it must sometimes be true if people are forced to act against their morals, it's impossible to generalize to authority figures.

13. C

How would someone who is not an authority killing an authority figure affect the author's argument? It would probably weaken the author's argument that obedience is usually an overriding factor in decision-making *if* the authority figure had authority over the other. They could be working on two totally separate chains of command. Therefore, the situation will have relevance *only* if there's an authoritarian relationship between them. (C) states this broadly. (A), (B), and (D) are opposite.

Passage 3

Topic and Scope: Pseudoscience and the difficulties involved in refuting it, using the example of medical quackery

Mapping the Passage:

Paragraph 1 introduces the idea that most diseases go away on their own and that this information can be misused by unscrupulous individuals.

Paragraphs 2 and 3 explain the reasons why pseudoscience and medicine often go together and why pseudoscientists are successful in convincing others of their claims.

Paragraphs 4 and 5 give an example of the difficulties in refuting claims of pseudoscience and in distinguishing between real and pseudoscience (offering a metaphor to show that the distinction is real).

Paragraph 6 continues by giving one philosopher's reasons for why people believe false claims.

Strategy Points: Follow arguments through carefully—they sometimes lead in directions other than what you'd anticipate. When an author gives examples or metaphors, be sure to understand why they're given, i.e., how they support the author's point.

14. A

Research the text in the passage. The author uses the term "self-limiting" to discuss diseases that more or less keep themselves in check. (A) matches perfectly. (B) misinterprets what the "self" is (it is the disease, not the patient). (C) is opposite. If the disease ends with the patient's death, it's not doing much self-limiting! (D) is distortion. If the disease is self-limiting, the author says, any treatment will likely seem to be successful, which means that there must be natural improvement.

15. B

This question is simply asking how the author would respond to a medical charlatan, which is essentially the scope of the passage's first half. Some pseudoscience works because the body naturally improves. Look for the predictable answer choice: the "cure" didn't do the trick, the body's natural tendency to heal itself did so. (B) jumps out with this prediction in mind. (A) is never discussed. (C) is opposite. The author would never agree in the first place that the healer had the ability to cure people. (D) is opposite. The author's big point is that people usually heal on their own.

16. D

What does the author say is needed to evaluate scientific claims? "Statistics... with logic." Combine this with the author's argument that people usually only remember successes to zero in on the answer. (D) catches it all. (A) is out of scope. Measuring time of response does nothing to distinguish between treatments that work and those that don't. (B) is distortion. The author argues that people only remember the successes. Therefore, the failures must be recorded as well for accuracy. (C) is out of scope. Dosages have no necessary link to success, particularly if the success has nothing to do with the treatment!

17. C

An inference question: jump to the answer choices. While each of the wrong answer choices can be knocked out quickly as not necessarily following from what the author is arguing, (C) is essentially a paraphrase of the argument made in paragraph 5. (A) is distortion. Though quackery might not be effective, that doesn't mean that as a general rule *nothing* can be done. (B) is distortion. While Quine argues this in paragraph 6, it's not the view of the author. Note that at the beginning of paragraph 6 the author points out that Quine goes "even farther" than he. (D) is distortion. Quine again. It's crucial to distinguish between what Quine believes and what the author does. Strategy point: Be sure to distinguish the author's own opinion from opinions of other people to whom the author refers.

18. D

A quick scan of the answer choices shows that this is a weaken/strengthen question. Where does the author talk about distinguishing between science and pseudoscience? Target the final paragraph and summarize the argument: there is a difference, but it's sometimes tough to tell. A debate over whether a type of medicine is one or the other would support the idea that the line is fuzzy. (D) rewards the careful logic. (A) is out of scope—a weakener, for one, and without relevance to the question, to boot. (B) is distortion. The author *does* believe that the scientific method is useful for distinguishing, but acknowledges that there's a fuzzy middle ground. An example of that middle ground will do nothing to weaken the author's argument. (C) is out of scope.

19. A

Go back to the passage to research the structure. In paragraph 5 the author makes a claim, and opens paragraph 6 by saying that Quine goes "even farther." Therefore he is probably "extreme." (A) matches, with the extra confirmation in the second half: the author *does* believe that some beliefs can be proven as scientific or not, while Quine doesn't. (B) is opposite. The author would strongly disagree with the idea that all beliefs are equally valid. (C) is out of scope. While the author would consider Quine flawed, there's nothing in the passage dealing with the reason listed afterwards. (D) is out of scope. "Bankrupt" is far too extreme a word, and there's no reason to believe that Quine's views couldn't apply to a situation.

Passage 4

Topic and Scope: American business lags behind the competition because management has alienated workers, concentrated on high-tech products, and neglected long-range planning.

Mapping the Passage:

Paragraph 1 outlines the decline of American business.

Paragraphs 2 and 3 list reasons that analysts have given for the decline and introduce the author's own theory for American business problems: incompetent management.

Paragraph 4 lists management's problems with labor.

Paragraph 5 explains the problem with America's fixation on high-tech products.

Paragraph 6 uses mergers to show that corporations lack long-range planning.

Strategy Points: Some passages will consist of a "laundry list" of recommendations, criticisms, or facts, with very little competing opinion. Work efficiently through the passage to identify the main ideas, knowing that much of the time will be spent on the questions.

20. C

A quick scan of the answer choices shows that you have to compare the workers of the two nations on two criteria: contentedness and efficiency. Search for a part of the passage that touches on this. Paragraph 3 is the only one that cites Japan, and mentions that analysts consider American workers less productive and less content. (C) it is.

21. B

An inference question; make sure that you're clear on the main points of the author's argument. The author will agree with three, but will disagree with the correct answer. The three wrong answers could be easily eliminated, leading to (B). However, you can also reason that since management has suffered by cutting labor costs, cost-cutting doesn't always result in lowered prices. (A) is opposite. The author does believe this (paragraph 6). (C) is opposite. The author only briefly mentions that "a few analysts even censured American consumers for their unpatriotic purchases of foreign goods" but then says that the real blame "lies with corporate management" (paragraph 3). Therefore the author agrees. (D) is opposite. This is the focus of paragraphs 2 and 3.

22. B

Paraphrase the author's argument about high technology: it's better to start out with low-tech, get experience, and then ramp up to high-tech. Search the answer choices for something that would contradict this. (B) clearly does; if the processes are completely different, why start with low-tech? (A) is quite possibly true, but it wouldn't affect the author's chain of reasoning. (C) is out of scope. Though it might be true, it doesn't harm the author's argument. (D) strengthens the idea that starting out low-tech makes the high-tech business easier.

23. A

This is just a fancy way of asking what the author would agree with, and therefore a question requiring a deduction. Keep the author's main points in mind while determining whether an answer choice has to follow from them. If the author believes that America has stumbled by losing market share, it follows that regaining that control would be a good thing. If the author didn't believe this, there would have been no real reason to make his argument. (A) it is. (B) is distortion. While business has had trouble keeping skilled workers, there's no reason to believe either that they were alienated or that this was the major blunder. (C) is distortion. Bleak, but not hopeless. Approach extreme answer choices, especially on inference questions, with extreme skepticism. (D) is out of scope.

24. C

We're looking for a business action that would presumably fix one or more of the problems that the author sees in American business. While (C) offers no detailed prescriptions, we know that the author believes foreign models of management to be superior. If American business followed their lead, the author would probably give his support. (A) is opposite. The author attacks this strategy in paragraph 6. (B) is distortion. The author does argue that businesses should stop trying to minimize wages, but says nothing about wage fairness between groups of workers, only wage fairness as a whole. In fact, the author would probably say that more money should be funneled to lower-skilled workers making low-tech products. (D) is out of scope. There's nothing to suggest that the author would agree with this strategy, especially given the fact that he considers the American business model rotten at the core. Simple advertising won't cut it.

Passage 5

Topic and Scope: Description of the character of Dalila in Milton's *Samson Agonistes* and the effects that her decisions have on Samson

Mapping The Passage:

Paragraph 1: Introduces the poem and discusses the hero/antihero dichotomy present between Samson and Dalila, although it is not yet clear that Dalila will be the focus of the passage.

Paragraph 2: Introduces the chorus of visiting friends, who try to convince Samson that he is blameless; then, Samson explains his culpability.

Paragraph 3: Compares *Samson Agonistes* and *Paradise Lost*, but delineates the differences between the characters of Eve and Dalila.

Paragraph 4: Examines Dalila's motives and explains Milton's comparison of her character to the serpent in the Garden of Eden.

Paragraph 5: Discusses Dalila's employment of antifeminist rhetoric in order to make her argument.

Paragraph 6: Reemphasizes the strength of Dalila's character.

25. B

In paragraph 1, Dalila is introduced as the character who is to be most closely studied, choice (B). (A) is distortion. *Paradise Lost* is discussed, but only for the span of one paragraph; the passage is not a thorough comparison of *Paradise Lost* and *Samson Agonistes*. (C) is opposite. We're told in paragraph 5 that Dalila employs sexual essentialism and antifeminist rhetoric. (D) is distortion. While the biblical book of Judges is mentioned, it is included merely as a reference point for the original Samson and Dalila story, and is not discussed at length nor compared to Milton's version.

26. C

Dalila employs all of these tactics except for arguing the superiority of the female intellect to the male. (A) is opposite. In paragraph 5, the author discusses Dalila's appropriation of patriarchal stereotypes. (B) opposite. In paragraph 1, we learn that Samson felt he had been ensnared by his lust for Dalila. (D) is opposite. We see Dalila apologize to Samson in paragraph 4.

27. C

In paragraph 4, the author references the serpent in order to emphasize how strongly Milton felt about Dalila's deceptive nature; thus, (C) is correct. (A) is faulty use of detail. While the author mentions Cleopatra and the asp, this is only to give a nod to a common association, and not necessarily the association that Milton intended. (B) is distortion.

In mentioning the serpent in such close affiliation with Dalila, the author is making the point that Milton associated Dalila more with the serpent than with Eve. (D) is faulty use of detail. While the asp in the story of Cleopatra is mentioned, there's no real comparison of it to the serpent of biblical tradition.

28. B

All of the answer choices are valid comparisons except for (B). As discussed in paragraph 3, Eve beseeches Adam to taste the fruit not out of deception, but out of an honest desire for him to gain the knowledge that she believes she has gained. (A) is opposite. Both Adam and Samson experience a "fall" because of a decision made by a female character. (C) is opposite. To differing degrees, both Adam and Samson accept the blame for their situation. (D) is opposite. Both stories are expansions upon biblical passages.

29. B

None of the answer choices would adequately challenge the author's claim that Milton views Eve and Dalila as two clearly different "types" of women except for (B). If Eve made Adam taste the fruit so that she could gain power over him, she would fit the same mold of the deceptive and treacherous woman that Dalila does. (A) is out of scope. Even if Samson's punishment was equal to Adam's, this does not have any bearing on the personalities of Eve and Dalila. (C) is out of scope in the same way: Even if Milton has given his Samson a few more positive characteristics than are granted to the biblical Samson, this has no effect on the way Dalila treats him or on the way Eve treats Adam. (D) is out of scope. Even if Dalila was once genuinely in love with Samson, this has no real bearing on her later decision to betray and deceive him, and it doesn't bring her closer in personality type to Eve.

30. D

The best inference is that the author of this passage is a literary scholar. (A) is distortion. The passage does not include enough comparisons between *Samson Agonistes* and the Old Testament story to conclude that the author is a biblical scholar. (B) is opposite. Because Dalila uses antifeminist rhetoric, she would most likely not be included in research of feminist characters. (C) is distortion. Nowhere does the author mention general societal attitudes toward figures such as Dalila.

Passage 6

Topic and Scope: An argument that the expansion of NATO into Eastern Europe will create diplomatic problems with Russia

Mapping the Passage:

Paragraph 1 argues that the expansion of NATO reflects internal problems and may create a diplomatic crisis with Russia.

Paragraph 2 states that the perceived, if not official, purpose of NATO is to combat Russian aggression.

Paragraphs 3 and 4 argue why Russians feel they have a right to exert influence over former Soviet states.

Paragraphs 5 and 6 point out that Russia strongly opposes NATO expansion and provide one reason for Russian opposition: a betrayal of previous unstated promises not to expand.

Paragraph 7 gives another reason: potential encroachment on Russia's sphere of influence, which it views as necessary for its self-defense.

31. C

Go back to the first paragraph to review the analogy. NATO itself is compared to the couple; its new members are compared to the baby. Choice (C) matches the prediction. (A) is out of scope. The author describes NATO as adversarial towards Russia, which couples (hopefully!) wouldn't be toward a baby. (B) is out of scope. The couple refers to NATO alone. (D) confuses the pieces of the analogy.

32. D

Review what the author wants NATO to do: avoid threatening Russia's sphere of influence, and keep implicit promises. The final sentence of the passage laments the "West's inability...to rule out" incorporating "any country" into NATO. Therefore the author would support reconsidering the West's position, choice (D). (A) is distortion. While the author wouldn't mind this, it doesn't solve the main problems of NATO expansion. (B) is distortion. Though the author wouldn't argue against this, it's already far beyond what the author would want in terms of expansion. (C) is distortion. Though the author wouldn't consider this unwelcome, it would be far better to declare *all* countries in Russia's sphere of influence out-of-bounds for NATO.

33. B

Where does the author mention these promises? Go back to paragraph 5. In the second half of the paragraph, the author argues that promises to stay out of East Germany were in spirit the same as promises to stay out of Eastern Europe. (B) rewards the habit of reading in context. (A) is never mentioned in the paragraph. (C) is distortion. *Russia* withdrew its troops, not the West. (D) is opposite. The author argues that the promises implied just the opposite.

34. C

Take a moment to separate what the author argues the diplomats say from what he believes they *mean*. The author believes that NATO's true goal is to contain Russia, even if it's not said outright. Look for choices that fit with this, reading back in the passage as needed. Statement III would fit this view: the West would consider this unjust aggression. Eliminate (A). Statement I fits with the author's opinion of the unstated goal of NATO: to contain a threatening Russia. However, NATO clearly desires "the peaceful integration of Ukraine into Europe" (paragraph 1) and therefore most likely believes that the Ukraine will eventually become part of NATO (as Russia fears, paragraph 7). Eliminate statement II and (C) is your answer.

35. B

Consider spheres of influence in the context of the passage. Both NATO and Russia want to expand their spheres of influence. What do the two have in common in doing so? The author argues that both claim to be doing so in the name of national security. (B) rewards the prediction instantly. (A), (C), and (D) are out of scope.

Passage 7

Topic and Scope: The disunity and turmoil of the Greek Hellenic period, using the Olympic Games as an example and metaphor

Mapping the Passage:

Paragraph 1 argues that in reality the Hellenic period was tumultuous, not the idealized community that Alexander desired.

Paragraph 2 gives a time frame for Greek civilization and the Olympic Games.

Paragraph 3 argues that the Games reflected Greek culture, but not positively.

Paragraph 4 argues that the Games reinforced disunity instead of promoting the unity originally intended.

36. B

Go back to review the phrase in context. The author argues at the end of the paragraph that "the winner's spoils were political and economic gain." The phrase must therefore mean that athletes were in it to win for the money. (B) broadens this only slightly. (A) is out of scope. The phrase is referring to athletes, but the author would probably argue that peace did not in fact increase during Olympic years. (C) refers to a detail in paragraph 2, which has nothing to do with the phrase. Similarly, (D) has no thing to do with the phrase.

37. A

Take a moment to remind yourself of the author's main point about the Games and look at the layout of the choices before trying to answer. Statement II is the most frequent, so hit that first. Statement II is basically the author's main argument, and the passage itself is explanation and example for this. Eliminate (B). Statement I offers a point not made by the passage: the author argues that Alexander never truly unified Greece (and he offers no evidence for this). Eliminate (C). The author never makes the claim in statement III, so (D) can be eliminated. (A) alone is left.

38. D

Paragraph 4 discusses the rewards associated with victory; take a second to read it quickly before looking for an answer choice that doesn't match. While the wrong answer choices are all perks awarded by an athlete's home city, (D) jumps out as a sign of cooperation and friendship between city-states, which the author would argue didn't exist. (A) is opposite. The author argues that "imposing defeat [was] a delight." (B) would fit with the economic value the author says was associated with winning. (C) would be a tangible perk of winning.

39. A

Review the author's main point about the Games in Greece: they made the disunity between the city-states even worse than it already was. Look for a fact that would reinforce this point: (A) is an example of disunity specifically triggered by the Games themselves. (B) would have no effect on the author's argument that the Games fostered competition. (C) is opposite. This would *weaken* the author's claim that city-states were at each other's throats during the games. (D) is out of scope. The number of athletes would probably have little effect on how the city-states regarded each other.

40. C

Review the phrase in context; it reinforces the author's main point that the Games made a bad situation worse. Looking for a similar point leads to (C). The author clearly believes that the Games made the Greeks' warlike tensions worse than they already were. (A) is out of scope. The author doesn't discuss the divisions in other civilizations. (B) is distortion. The author argues that the Greeks were constantly divided, but doesn't claim that they were always at war as a result. (D) is opposite. The author argues in paragraph 2 that this marked the *beginning* of Greek history, and so surely couldn't also represent the point of decline.

ESSAY PRACTICE STUDENT RESPONSES AND EXPLANATIONS

The following pages contain student essays written in response to the questions provided in the previous section. Read each response only after you have first attempted to write on the question yourself.

Remember the tasks at hand on the Essay portion of the MCAT:

> **Task 1: Provide your interpretation or explanation of the statement.**
>
> **Task 2: Offer a concrete example (hypothetical or actual) that illustrates a point of view directly opposite to the one expressed in the statement.**
>
> **Task 3: Explain how the conflict between the viewpoint expressed in the statement and the viewpoint you described for task 2 might be resolved.**

STUDENT'S ESSAY IN RESPONSE TO QUESTION 1

Education that consists of just memorizing details and facts is hardly education at all. True education demands active participation of both teacher and student. In true education, the roles of the student and the teacher are somewhat flexible: the teacher can learn from the student as well as the student learn from the teacher. By actively participating, instead of taking for granted the truth of everything the teacher says, the student thinks about the issues more thoroughly. Rather than just parroting the views of the teacher, the student by questioning authority develops views that are his own, and also learns a way to think critically about future issues. He learns how to think rather than what to think. This gives him intellectual freedom and a framework for thinking that he can use throughout his life.

But there are moments when the best kind of education does not encourage students to question authority. For instance, education in the hard sciences requires an acceptance of basic formulas and theorems if the student is to make any progress at all. A basic foundation must be laid before the challenges can begin. In other words, questioning authority must take place within the proper sequence. If the student is unable to accept the teacher's authority at least partially, then he will find himself unable to learn from the teacher at all. Questioning authority should develop out of a mutual trust and if such questioning comes about prior to the establishment of such a trust, a student will do his education a real injury. To begin by questioning the teacher's authority, without first having a solid foundation of knowledge, would be counterproductive and tend to impede learning.

In determining when education that encourages students to question authority is the best, we must consider two main factors. First, what type of education is in question? If we are dealing with the physical sciences, a basic groundwork must be agreed upon before questioning authority can begin. Second, to what degree is the authority being questioned? If the authority is seen as totally questionable, the validity of the authority as an authority will be destroyed.

It is important to remember that when a student is taught to question authority he must be also taught to question his own authority as well as that of a teacher or textbook. The purpose of questioning authority is not to teach the student to place himself in the role of the authority figure while totally disregarding the teacher. In such a situation the learning process will fail miserably. The purpose of questioning authority is to examine and analyze ideas before accepting them as true. When a student learns to do this with his own ideas as well as with others', he will truly have received the best education.

STUDENT'S SELF-EVALUATION

In general, I feel good about this essay. I managed my time well and stuck to my prewriting main idea and defense. I also benefited from keeping track of the time and pacing myself accordingly.

TEACHER TIP

A more specific example, such as physics, couldn't hurt. Nevertheless, the writer's counterexample is clear and appropriate.

I felt a bit nervous about using the example of the hard sciences in paragraph 2. Perhaps that wasn't specific enough. Perhaps I'd have done better to use just one of the sciences—like physics—and thus avoid potential problems of over-generalization.

Reader's Evaluation of Student's Response to Question 1

Holistic Score: 6

This paper presents a thorough and thoughtful response to all three writing tasks, focusing clearly on the issue defined by the given statement. Paragraphs 1 and 2 address the first and second tasks, respectively; paragraphs 3 and 4 address the third task.

The discussion in each of the paragraphs is organized around a unifying idea and is presented coherently and logically. Furthermore, the paragraphs relate well to each other. For example, the transitional phrase, "But there are moments" (paragraph 2, sentence one), effectively guides the reader from the discussion in paragraph 1 to the new idea to be discussed in paragraph 2. The use of such transitional phrases occurs throughout the essay, creating a smooth and coherent argument. General statements are given an appropriate amount of specific explanation and/or illustration (paragraph 4).

Paragraph 1 introduces the topic with a straightforward clarification of the statement's meaning (sentences 1 to 3), and then continues with some analysis of the statement's meaning as it relates to the benefits of an education that questions authority (sentences 4 through 6). Paragraph 2's first sentence is a clear topic sentence, leading to the counterexample of education in the hard sciences. The bulk of paragraph 2 explores the implications of a student's premature questioning. The discussion is abstract—since it quickly leaves the specifics of the example behind—but precisely argued. It amply satisfies the requirement of the second task; it also paves the way for paragraph 3's examination of the two factors that should be taken into account in resolving the conflict between the ideas in the preceding two paragraphs. Paragraph 4 extends this discussion by introducing the related idea that students should question their own authority. These last two paragraphs amply discuss the third task: The author has explored the grounds for questioning authority, the problems associated with premature or unrestricted questioning, and the need for self-questioning.

The discussion in each of the paragraphs is organized around a unifying idea and is presented coherently and logically. Furthermore, the paragraphs relate well to each other. For example, the transitional phrase, "But there are moments" (paragraph 2, sentence 1), effectively guides the reader from the discussion in paragraph 1 to the new idea to be discussed in paragraph 2. The use of such transitional phrases

Teacher Tip

This is, indeed, a level 6 essay, though the last paragraph is not really necessary. The writer could have saved some time by writing only the really important, concluding sentences of the paragraph. So she could have combined the last two sentences of paragraph 4 with the end of paragraph 3. If you have timing problems, don't force yourself to write an extra concluding paragraph; just make sure you've written everything you want to say and ended with a solid, if short, conclusion.

occurs throughout the essay, creating a smooth and coherent argument. General statements are given an appropriate amount of specific explanation and/or illustration (paragraph 4, for instance).

The language is clear and effective throughout. The essay also provides variety in sentence structure (e.g., sentences 4, 5, and 6 of the first paragraph).

STUDENT'S ESSAY IN RESPONSE TO QUESTION 2

In a political crisis, violence is often the first reaction in trying to reach a solution, much as a tantrum is the first reaction when a child fails to get his way. Yet if anything is to be resolved, violence in itself is not a solution. While violence may have an immediate effect on a crisis, it does not solve the crisis. It may control the situation temporarily, but the roots are still there and may flare up once the violence has passed.

Certainly there are situations where violence seems justified. Terrorists' acts of violence must sometimes be curtailed with violence when negotiations have failed. Similarly, defense from offensive military maneuvers. But violence in and of itself is not a full solution. The bombing of Hiroshima was seen by some as the only solution to a long and bloody war. Yet this act of violence in a violent political crisis has left terrible scars on all of humanity, and further development of nuclear weapons has led to deeper political crises, crises too dangerous to the entire planet to be resolved by violence.

Yet violence, like an occasional tantrum, does get attention and does often begin a series of events that lead to a solution. The storming of the Bastille did lead—after years of violence and terror in France—to freedom from the aristocracy. And storming the beaches at Normandy did save Europe from Nazi rule.

Violence in itself is not a real solution to a political crisis, but it can be an effective step in reaching a solution. On that ground alone, one can say that it is justifiable. Nonetheless, violence in itself can lead to a bigger crisis. But violence can play a vital part as an intermediate step toward a real resolution of hostilities.

STUDENT'S SELF-EVALUATION

> I guess the main problem with this essay is that it got kind of repetitive. By the time I got around to really focusing on the third task, I felt I had said everything I had to say on the subject. As a result, I'm not happy with my final paragraph since it doesn't say much of substance. I wish I had focused more directly on each task.

TEACHER TIP

The main problem with this essay is organization and clarity. Repetition is just a symptom of the real diagnosis.

Reader's Evaluation of Student's Response to Question 2

Holistic Score: 4

This essay addresses the first and second tasks in paragraphs 1, 2, and 3. In paragraph 4, the third task is addressed as well.

The essay is confusingly organized and does not adequately respond to the third task; it is for these two reasons that it did not receive a score of 5. On the other hand, its use of relevant and interpreted examples raised it from a score of 3.

While paragraphs 1 and 4 are organized around central ideas, the remainder of the essay is confusingly put together. Paragraph 2's first sentence, for instance, seems as if it is introducing a paragraph that will take up the second task, but the rest of the paragraph reverts to a discussion of task 1.

The essay addresses the third task in the final paragraph—introducing the notion that violence can be an "intermediate step" in solving a political crisis—however, the essay presents no clear analysis of what constitutes justified use of violence in such circumstances. Instead, the author repeats the idea that violence can make bad things worse.

The essay's allusions to the Hiroshima catastrophe, the storming of the Bastille, and the invasion at Normandy create a solid sense of specificity. If the essay were better organized, such examples would gain more force. Furthermore, the essay lacks clear transitions (between paragraphs 3 and 4, for example); the author could improve the overall flow of the argument by creating more substantive links between major groups of ideas.

Though generally clear, the language at times lacks vigor (the repeated use of the word *violence,* for instance). Sentence structure does show some variety (paragraph 3, for example), though there are occasional

TEACHER TIP

It's pretty obvious why this essay doesn't score 5, but the real question is why it doesn't score 3. It could well be because the reader doesn't see the criterion clearly called for in task 3. Just because violence can be an effective step in reaching a solution (as the writer states) doesn't mean that this is the criterion. The criterion would be clearer if she had written: "whether or not violence is solution to a crisis depends on whether or not it will be an intermediate step which leads to resolution."

problems in sentence construction (e.g., the third sentence in paragraph 2 is missing a verb and predicate, and therefore constitutes a sentence fragment).

STUDENT'S ESSAY IN RESPONSE TO QUESTION 3

Of his own free will, no one would elect a known criminal to an important government post. In a free society, we like to have government leaders who honor and support the laws that we have made to protect the people and to keep the society smoothly running. When we find that a candidate or officeholder has not upheld the law in his earlier life, we doubt that he will do so in office. Hence, to be an effective politician, one must have a completely crime-free past.

Electing leaders with "clean records" must be kept in mind. We would not elect a known gangster or an individual with a long record of hideous or outrageous crimes or even a person accused of taking bribes because we fear that such individuals would continue such actions in office. Yet certainly one or two small spots on one's record in one's youth when for many years he has been "crime-free" cannot be considered reason enough not to elect an otherwise fine candidate. Certainly we would not want Al Capone or Charles Manson as our Senators, but even if John Kennedy had swiped an apple when he was ten years old or had a parking infraction at twenty, he would have still been one of our greatest leaders.

Having crime-free officials is a ideal, but there is a difference between <u>completely</u> crime-free and <u>generally</u> crime-free pasts. An effective official is more than merely one who has never committed a major crime. After all, Capone would probably be a more effective leader (in some ways) than many of the presidents we have had in the U.S. simply because he knew how to run a big organization and get things done quickly. Of course, his style of power is not how we would like to have things done in a free society, but it was effective.

The question of crime-free or not crime-free hinges on what we mean by "effective." In a free democracy, we like our leaders to be nearly crime-free, but we can see that it is nearly impossible to have officials who are completely crime-free.

STUDENT'S SELF-EVALUATION

I could have spent more time planning this essay. I started writing almost immediately because I felt I knew exactly what I wanted to say. But halfway in, I felt a bit lost. I also wondered whether my use of "we" to make general remarks about society was appropriate.

TEACHER TIP

Oops... the writer didn't prewrite. You won't end up with a cogent, well-organized essay without a prewrite.

Reader's Evaluation of Student's Response to Question 3

Holistic Score: 4

This essay accomplished all three writing tasks: paragraph 1 discusses the first task, paragraph 2 discusses the second, and paragraphs 3 and 4 discuss the third. Despite this relatively clear organization, however, the discussion lacks the depth of a level 5 essay.

TEACHER TIP

Remember step 1 of the Kaplan method, read and annotate? Annotate means define, even if it's only to yourself. The definition of "effective" should have gone in paragraph 1 and would have been part of task 1's instruction: explain.

Paragraph 1 introduces the topic by examining the meaning of the statement. The paragraph's ideas are well organized, but the writer does not closely analyze certain key terms, such as *effective* or *completely*. Doing so would have improved the essay's general clarity and sharpened its argument. Paragraph 1, in addition, ends somewhat too abruptly. Sentence 3 raises the issue of people doubting tainted candidates, but this is not linked to the next sentence's assertion that effectiveness requires a politician to have a completely crime-free past.

TEACHER TIP

It's a good idea to refer to previous examples to add depth in task 3. Thus the reader could have again pointed to Al Capone and John Kennedy to support what she means by "nearly" or "completely" crime-free.

Paragraph 2 describes a counterexample—the case of people having a slightly tarnished record, such as Kennedy—but spends too much time arguing that career criminals would not be trusted. Hence the paragraph does not elucidate the meaning of the counterexample as much as it could have. In addition, the writer's failure to specify what "completely crime-free" means causes a lack of depth in this paragraph.

This last conceptual weakness carries over into paragraphs 3 and 4, which examine the grounds for effectiveness by discussing the difference between degrees of criminality. The example of Capone in paragraph 3 directly addresses the third task, but the discussion borders on the simplistic. The final paragraph's first sentence makes a good point, but the essay never clarifies what "effectiveness" entails. Hence, the conclusion lacks clarity.

This paper would be most improved by a clarification of the author's main ideas. The last paragraph is headed in a productive direction since its extension would logically take up the definition of *effective*.

Yet this attempt is not enough and it comes too late to add direction to the preceding discussion.

The writing shows a basic control of vocabulary and sentence structure, but transitions could be more effectively used. The first sentence of paragraph 2, for example, does not effectively lead into the main topic of paragraph 2, nor does it link this paragraph to the preceding one. Similarly, paragraph 3 could be better tied to the discussion in paragraph 2; the phrase "having crime-free officials is a great idea" does not adequately make the necessary transition.

STUDENT'S ESSAY IN RESPONSE TO QUESTION 4

The statement "The government should restrict its funding of scientific research to programs with a direct application to societal problems" is defined by me as follows: no monies shall be allocated to commercial, military, or other programs not of benefit on some humanistic level.

In the case of space research, many would say that no funding should be given, in that this research is either pure adventurism or only of military or theoretical importance. But I believe that space research should be funded for two reasons: 1) it represents a solution other than population control for the problem of global overcrowding and 2) it advances many helpful technologies such as food preservation, fuel conservation, and computer applications.

The criteria used to determine whether or not government funds should be used for any individual research project are difficult to put boundaries on. But I will outline some parameters here.

Programs should not concern military issues. The funding of such programs is the responsibility of the Defense Department and are a different issue altogether. For nonmilitary research, researchers should be required to describe, in layman's terms, what their project is, what its history has been and what they think its future will be. There should be a board with as fair a cross-section of the people as possible to decide on funding. And there should be a set of regulations to add weight to research that does have a more direct application to immediate social problems.

STUDENT'S SELF-EVALUATION

> I think that when tested I get too hung up on trying to use fancy language and then lose track of my own thoughts. I think my ideas would flow better if I could get them clearer before I jump into building a sentence, but the time pressure makes me too nervous.
>
> Answering the third task seemed the hardest to me. I felt as if I had to start all over again and write a whole new essay.

TEACHER TIP

A whole new essay would have had at least a chance of scoring better, but it's too late for that. Learn what you did wrong in one practice essay and correct it in the next. By the time you get to the real MCAT essays, you'll know how to write good ones.

Reader's Evaluation of Student's Response to Question 4

Holistic Score: 3

This paper addresses all three tasks, focuses consistently on the given topic, presents paragraphs that are unified around a central topic, and contains a clear organization of ideas. Furthermore, the ideas are all substantial enough to be appropriate for an assignment of this kind. None of the ideas is sufficiently developed, however, and as a result, the paper is simplistic.

Paragraph 1 addresses the first task but merely rephrases the statement in different words. No attempt is made to expand our understanding of its meaning by explaining why or in what way it is valid.

TEACHER TIP

Don't include in your essay the precise text which appears in the exam prompt; that won't constitute an explanation.

Paragraph 2 addresses the second task by offering an example in which scientific research without direct application to societal problems deserves funding. The author provides a bit more explanation here than in paragraph 1, but it is still insufficient. Vague phrases such as "pure adventurism" and "theoretical importance" are left unexplained. More importantly, the author's defense for why space research should be supported is one-sided. Since paragraph 1 gives us no insight into why someone would oppose such research, the argument in paragraph 2 for supporting the research lacks a relevant context.

Paragraph 3 responds to the third task, but the ideas presented have little relation to the ideas in paragraph 2. Therefore, though the paper is unified in its focus on the statement provided, it lacks coherency—the ideas do not relate to each other.

TEACHER TIP

Paragraph 3 is useless. The author is simply stating that task 3 is hard but she'll attempt to answer it. What purpose does that paragraph serve? Don't introduce what you're going to do; just do it.

The language of the essay is quite clear, on the whole, and the ideas are expressed without difficulty. In addition, variety in sentence length adds some energy to the style (see first two sentences of paragraph 4).

TEACHER TIP

Criterion is in neither paragraph 3 nor paragraph 4. Paragraph 3, as already noted, is irrelevant. Paragraph 4 is full of the author's prescriptions about what should and should not happen, but it's personal opinion, not a determinant for the conditions under which the prompt is true and not true. Task 3 is not complete, thus the essay can score no higher than 3.

The most significant improvements to be made in this essay involve a more thorough exploration of ideas and a greater emphasis on the relationship between those ideas. The first place to work on improving these weaknesses is in the prewriting process. Asking questions will help expand the explanation of a topic (the first task). Looking back over the first and second tasks' prewriting notes (task 3) will help develop a central idea that will create a coherent relationship between all the ideas in the essay.

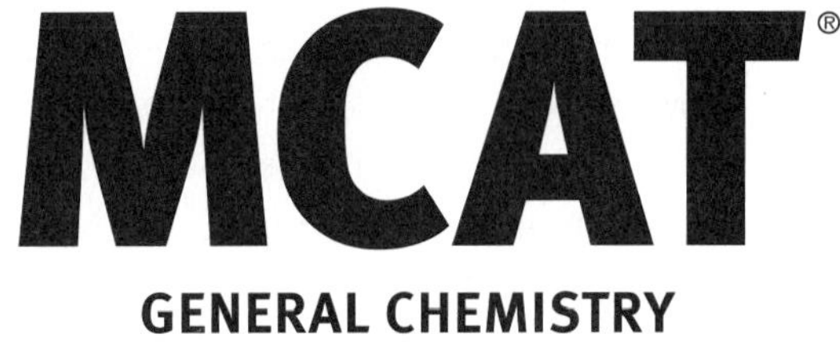

GENERAL CHEMISTRY

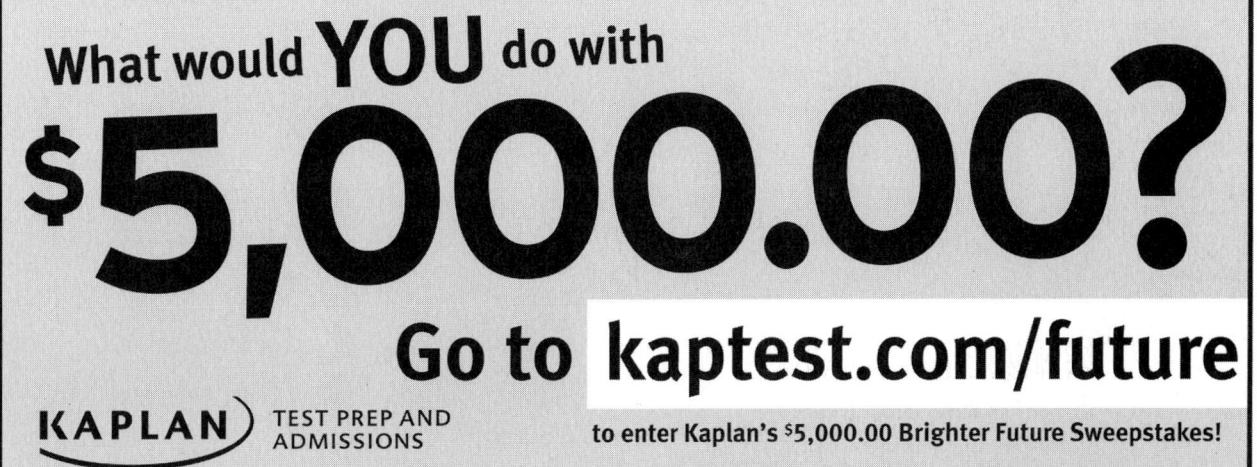

2009–2010 EDITION

Related Titles

Kaplan MCAT Biology 2009-2010
Kaplan MCAT Organic Chemistry 2009-2010
Kaplan MCAT Physics 2009-2010
Kaplan MCAT Verbal Reasoning and Writing 2009-2010

MCAT®

GENERAL CHEMISTRY

2009–2010 EDITION

The Staff of Kaplan

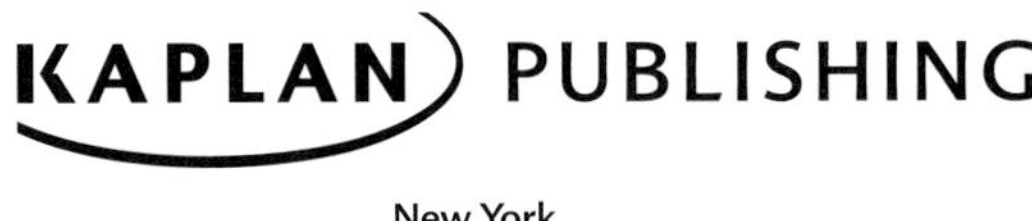

New York

Published by Kaplan Publishing, a division of Kaplan, Inc.
1 Liberty Plaza, 24th Floor
New York, NY 10006

Printed in the United States of America

10 9 8 7 6 5 4 3 2 1

ISBN: 978-1-4277-9873-2

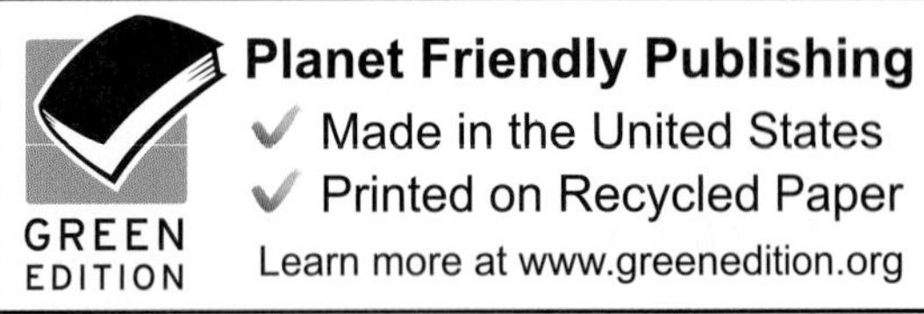

- Manufacturing books in the United States ensures compliance with strict environmental laws and eliminates the need for international freight shipping, a major contributor to global air pollution. Printing on recycled paper helps minimize our consumption of trees, water and fossil fuels.
- Trees Saved: 57 • Air Emissions Eliminated: 4,586 pounds
- Water Saved: 20,233 gallons • Solid Waste Eliminated: 1,990 pounds

Contents

How to Use this Book

Kaplan MCAT General Chemistry, along with the other four books in our MCAT subject review series, brings the Kaplan classroom experience right into your home!

Kaplan has been preparing premeds for the MCAT for more than 40 years in our comprehensive courses. In the past 15 years alone, we've helped over 400,000 students prepare for this important exam and improve their chances of medical school admission.

TEACHER TIPS

Think of Kaplan's five MCAT subject books as having a private Kaplan teacher right by your side! We've created a team of the **top MCAT teachers in the country,** who have read through these comprehensive guides. In the sidebars of every page, they offer the same tips, advice, and test day insight that they offer in their Kaplan classroom.

Pay close attention to **Teacher Tip** sidebars like this:

> **TEACHER TIP**
> Know the shorthand notation for cells; it might not be spelled on out on the exam.

When you see them, you know what you're getting the same insight and knowledge that students in Kaplan MCAT classrooms across the country receive.

HIGH-YIELD MCAT REVIEW

At the end of several chapters, you'll find a special **High-Yield Questions** spread. These questions tackle the most frequently tested topics found on the MCAT. For each type of problem, you will be provided with a stepwise technique for solving the question and key directional points on how to solve for the MCAT specifically.

Included on each spread are two icons: the first, a sideways hand pointing toward equations, notes equations that you should memorize for the MCAT. The second, an open hand, indicates where in a problem you can stop without doing further calculation.

At the end of each topic you will find a "Takeaways" box, which gives a concise summary of the problem-solving approach, and a "Things to watch out for" box, which points out any caveats to the approach discussed above that usually lead to wrong answer choices. Finally, there is a "Similar Questions" box at the end so you can test your ability to apply the stepwise technique to analogous questions. You can find the answers in the Answers and Explanations section of this book.

We're confident that this guide, and our award-wining Kaplan teachers, can help you achieve your goals of MCAT success and admission into medical school!

Good luck!

EXPERT KAPLAN MCAT TEAM

Marilyn Engle

MCAT Master Teacher; Teacher Trainer; Kaplan National Teacher of the Year, 2006; Westwood Teacher of the Year, 2007; Westwood Trainer of the Year, 2007; Encino Trainer of the Tear, 2005

John Michael Linick

MCAT Teacher; Boulder Teacher of the Year, 2007; Summer Intensive Program Faculty Member

Dr. Glen Pearlstein

MCAT Master Teacher; Teacher Trainer; Westwood Teacher of the Year, 2006

Matthew B. Wilkinson

MCAT Teacher; Teacher Trainer; Lone Star Trainer of the Year, 2007

Introduction to the MCAT

THE MCAT

The Medical College Admission Test, affectionately known as the MCAT, is different from any other test you've encountered in your academic career. It's not like the knowledge-based exams from high school and college, whose emphasis was on memorizing and regurgitating information. Medical schools can assess your academic prowess by looking at your transcript. The MCAT isn't even like other standardized tests you may have taken, where the focus was on proving your general skills.

TEST TIP

The MCAT places more weight on your thought process. However you must have a strong hold of the required core knowledge. The MCAT may not be a perfect gauge of your abilities, but it is a relatively objective way to compare you with students from different backgrounds and undergraduate institutions.

Medical schools use MCAT scores to assess whether you possess the foundation upon which to build a successful medical career. Though you certainly need to know the content to do well, the stress is on thought process, because the MCAT is above all else a thinking test. That's why it emphasizes reasoning, critical and analytical thinking, reading comprehension, data analysis, writing, and problem-solving skills.

The MCAT's power comes from its use as an indicator of your abilities. Good scores can open doors. Your power comes from preparation and mindset, because the key to MCAT success is knowing what you're up against. That's where this section of this book comes in. We'll explain the philosophy behind the test, review the sections one by one, show you sample questions, share some of Kaplan's proven methods, and clue you in to what the test makers are really after. You'll get a handle on the process, find a confident new perspective, and achieve your highest possible scores.

ABOUT THE MCAT

Information about the MCAT CBT is included below. For the latest information about the MCAT, visit www.kaptest.com/mcat.

MCAT CBT

Format	U.S.—All administrations on computer International—Most on computer with limited paper and pencil in a few isolated areas
Essay Grading	One human and one computer grader
Breaks	Optional break between each section
Length of MCAT Day	Approximately 5.5 hours
Test Dates	Multiple dates in January, April, May, June, July, August, and September Total of 24 administrations each year.
Delivery of Results	Within 30 days. If scores are delayed notification will be posted online at www.aamc.org/mcat Electronic and paper
Security	Government-issued ID Electronic thumbprint Electronic signature verification
Testing Centers	Small computer testing sites

PLANNING FOR THE TEST

As you look toward your preparation for the MCAT consider the following advice:

Complete your core course requirements as soon as possible. Take a strategic eye to your schedule and get core requirements out of the way now.

Take the MCAT once. The MCAT is a notoriously grueling standardized exam that requires extensive preparation. It is longer than the graduate admissions exams for business school (GMAT, 3½ hours), law school (LSAT, 3¼ hours) and graduate school (GRE, 2½ hours). You do not want to take it twice. Plan and prepare accordingly.

KAPLAN EXCLUSIVE

Go online and sign up for a local Kaplan Pre-Med Edge event to get the latest information on the test.

THE ROLE OF THE MCAT IN ADMISSIONS

More and more people are applying to medical school and more and more people are taking the MCAT. It's important for you to recognize that while a high MCAT score is a critical component in getting admitted to top med schools, it's not the only factor. Medical school admissions officers weigh grades, interviews, MCAT scores, level of involvement in extracurricular activities, as well as personal essays.

In a Kaplan survey of 130 pre-med advisors, 84 percent called the interview a "very important" part of the admissions process, followed closely by college grades (83%) and MCAT scores (76%). Kaplan's college admissions consulting practice works with students on all these issues so they can position themselves as strongly as possible. In addition, the AAMC has made it clear that scores will continue to be valid for three years, and that the scoring of the computer-based MCAT will not differ from that of the paper and pencil version.

REGISTRATION

The only way to register for the MCAT is online. The registration site is: www.aamc.org/mcat.

You will be able to access the site approximately six months before your test date. Payment must be made by MasterCard or Visa.

Go to www.aamc.org/mcat/registration.htm and download *MCAT Essentials* for information about registration, fees, test administration, and preparation. For other questions, contact:

MCAT Care Team
Association of American Medical Colleges
Section for Applicant Assessment Services
2450 N. St., NW
Washington, DC 20037
www.aamc.org/mcat
Email: mcat@aamc.org

You will want to take the MCAT in the year prior to your planned start date. For example, if you want to start medical school in Fall 2010, you will need to take the MCAT and apply in 2009. Don't drag your feet gathering information. You'll need time not only to prepare and practice for the test, but also to get all your registration work done.

TEST TIP

The MCAT should be viewed just like any other part of your application: as an opportunity to show the medical schools who you are and what you can do. Take control of your MCAT experience.

ANATOMY OF THE MCAT

Before mastering strategies, you need to know exactly what you're dealing with on the MCAT. Let's start with the basics: The MCAT is, among other things, an endurance test.

If you can't approach it with confidence and stamina, you'll quickly lose your composure. That's why it's so important that you take control of the test.

The MCAT consists of four timed sections: Physical Sciences, Verbal Reasoning, Writing Sample, and Biological Sciences. Later in this section we'll take an in-depth look at each MCAT section, including sample question types and specific test-smart hints, but here's a general overview, reflecting the order of the test sections and number of questions in each.

Physical Sciences

Time	70 minutes
Format	• 52 multiple-choice questions: approximately 7–9 passages with 4–8 questions each • approximately 10 stand-alone questions (not passage-based)
What it tests	basic general chemistry concepts, basic physics concepts, analytical reasoning, data interpretation

Verbal Reasoning

Time	60 minutes
Format	• 40 multiple-choice questions: approximately 7 passages with 5–7 questions each
What it tests	critical reading

Writing Sample

Time	60 minutes
Format	• 2 essay questions (30 minutes per essay)
What it tests	critical thinking, intellectual organization, written communication skills

Biological Sciences

Time	70 minutes
Format	• 52 multiple-choice questions: approximately 7–9 passages with 4–8 questions each • approximately 10 stand-alone questions (not passage-based)
What it tests	basic biology concepts, basic organic chemistry concepts, analytical reasoning, data interpretation

TEST TIP

There's no penalty for a wrong answer on the MCAT, so NEVER LEAVE ANY QUESTION BLANK, even if you only have time for a wild guess.

The sections of the test always appear in the same order:

Physical Sciences
[optional 10-minute break]
Verbal Reasoning
[optional 10-minute break]
Writing Sample
[optional 10-minute break]
Biological Sciences

SCORING

Each MCAT section receives its own score. Physical Sciences, Verbal Reasoning, and Biological Sciences are each scored on a scale ranging from 1–15, with 15 as the highest. The Writing Sample essays are scored alphabetically on a scale ranging from J to T, with T as the highest. The two essays are each evaluated by two official readers, so four critiques combine to make the alphabetical score.

TEST TIP

The percentile figure tells you how many other test takers scored at or below your level. In other words, a percentile figure of 80 means that 80 percent did as well or worse than you did, and that only 20 percent did better.

The number of multiple-choice questions that you answer correctly per section is your "raw score." Your raw score will then be converted to yield the "scaled score"—the one that will fall somewhere in that 1–15 range. These scaled scores are what are reported to medical schools as your MCAT scores. All multiple-choice questions are worth the same amount—one raw point—and *there's no penalty for guessing*. That means that *you should always select an answer for every question, whether you get to that question or not!* This is an important piece of advice, so pay it heed. Never let time run out on any section without selecting an answer for every question.

Your score report will tell you—and your potential medical schools—not only your scaled scores, but also the national mean score for each section, standard deviation, national scoring profile for each section, and your percentile ranking.

WHAT'S A GOOD SCORE?

There's no such thing as a cut-and-dry "good score." Much depends on the strength of the rest of your application (if your transcript is first rate, the pressure to strut your stuff on the MCAT isn't as intense) and on where you want to go to school (different schools have different score expectations). Here are a few interesting statistics:

For each MCAT administration, the average scaled scores are approximately 8s for Physical Sciences, Verbal Reasoning, and Biological Sciences, and N for the Writing Sample. You need scores of at least 10–11s to be considered competitive by most medical schools, and if you're aiming for the top you've got to do even better, and score 12s and above.

You don't have to be perfect to do well. For instance, on the AAMC's Practice Test 5R, you could get as many as 10 questions wrong in Verbal Reasoning, 17 in Physical Sciences, and 16 in Biological Sciences and still score in the 80th percentile. To score in the 90th percentile, you could get as many as 7 wrong in Verbal Reasoning, 12 in Physical Sciences, and 12 in Biological Sciences. Even students who receive perfect scaled scores usually get a handful of questions wrong.

It's important to maximize your performance on every question. Just a few questions one way or the other can make a big difference in your scaled score. Here's a look at recent score profiles so you can get an idea of the shape of a typical score distribution.

Physical Sciences

Scaled Score	Percent Achieving Score	Percentile Rank Range
15	0.1	99.9–99.9
14	1.2	98.7–99.8
13	2.5	96.2–98.6
12	5.1	91.1–96.1
11	7.2	83.9–91.0
10	12.1	71.8–83.8
9	12.9	58.9–71.1
8	16.5	42.4–58.5
7	16.7	25.7–42.3
6	13.0	12.7–25.6
5	7.9	04.8–12.6
4	3.3	01.5–04.7
3	1.3	00.2–01.4
2	0.1	00.1–00.1
1	0.0	00.0–00.0

Scaled Score
Mean = 8.1
Standard Deviation = 2.32

Verbal Reasoning

Scaled Score	Percent Achieving Score	Percentile Rank Range
15	0.1	99.9–99.9
14	0.2	99.7–99.8
13	1.8	97.9–99.6
12	3.6	94.3–97.8
11	10.5	83.8–94.2
10	15.6	68.2–83.7
9	17.2	51.0–68.1
8	15.4	35.6–50.9
7	10.3	25.3–35.5
6	10.9	14.4–25.2
5	6.9	07.5–14.3
4	3.9	03.6–07.4
3	2.0	01.6–03.5
2	0.5	00.1–01.5
1	0.0	00.0–00.0

Scaled Score
Mean = 8.0
Standard Deviation = 2.43

TEST TIP

The raw score of each administration is converted to a scaled score. The conversion varies with administrations. Hence, the same raw score will not always give you the same scaled score.

Writing Sample		
Scaled Score	Percent Achieving Score	Percentile Rank Range
T	0.5	99.9–99.9
S	2.8	94.7–99.8
R	7.2	96.0–99.3
Q	14.2	91.0–95.9
P	9.7	81.2–90.9
O	17.9	64.0–81.1
N	14.7	47.1–63.9
M	18.8	30.4–47.0
L	9.5	21.2–30.3
K	3.6	13.5–21.1
J	1.2	06.8–13.4
		02.9–06.7
		00.9–02.8
		00.2–00.8
		00.0–00.1
75th Percentile = Q 50th Percentile = O 25th Percentile = M		

Biological Sciences		
Scaled Score	Percent Achieving Score	Percentile Rank Range
15	0.1	99.9–99.9
14	1.2	98.7–99.8
13	2.5	96.2–98.6
12	5.1	91.1–96.1
11	7.2	83.9–91.0
10	12.1	71.8–83.8
9	12.9	58.9–71.1
8	16.5	42.4–58.5
7	16.7	25.7–42.3
6	13.0	12.7–25.6
5	7.9	04.8–12.6
4	3.3	01.5–04.7
3	1.3	00.2–01.4
2	0.1	00.1–00.1
1	0.0	00.0–00.0
Scaled Score Mean = 8.2 Standard Deviation = 2.39		

WHAT THE MCAT REALLY TESTS

It's important to grasp not only the nuts and bolts of the MCAT, so you'll know *what* to do on Test Day, but also the underlying principles of the test so you'll know *why* you're doing what you're doing on Test Day. We'll cover the straightforward MCAT facts later. Now it's time to examine the heart and soul of the MCAT, to see what it's really about.

THE MYTH

Most people preparing for the MCAT fall prey to the myth that the MCAT is a straightforward science test. They think something like this:

> *"It covers the four years of science I had to take in school: biology, chemistry, physics, and organic chemistry. It even has equations. OK, so it has Verbal Reasoning and Writing, but those sections are just to see if we're literate, right? The important stuff is the science. After all, we're going to be doctors."*

Well, here's the little secret no one seems to want you to know: The MCAT is not just a science test; it's also a thinking test. This means that the test is designed to let you demonstrate your thought process, not only your thought content.

The implications are vast. Once you shift your test-taking paradigm to match the MCAT modus operandi, you'll find a new level of confidence and control over the test. You'll begin to work with the nature of the MCAT rather than against it. You'll be more efficient and insightful as you prepare for the test, and you'll be more relaxed on Test Day. In fact, you'll be able to see the MCAT for what it is rather than for what it's dressed up to be. We want your Test Day to feel like a visit with a familiar friend instead of an awkward blind date.

THE ZEN OF MCAT

Medical schools do not need to rely on the MCAT to see what you already know. Admission committees can measure your subject-area proficiency using your undergraduate coursework and grades. Schools are most interested in the potential of your mind.

In recent years, many medical schools have shifted pedagogic focus away from an information-heavy curriculum to a concept-based curriculum. There is currently more emphasis placed on problem solving, holistic thinking, and cross-disciplinary study. Be careful not to dismiss this important point, figuring you'll wait to worry about academic trends until you're actually in medical school. This trend affects you right now, because it's reflected in the MCAT. Every good tool matches its task. In this case the tool is the test, used to measure you and other candidates, and the task is to quantify how likely it is that you'll succeed in medical school.

Your intellectual potential—how skillfully you annex new territory into your mental boundaries, how quickly you build "thought highways" between ideas, how confidently and creatively you solve problems—is far more important to admission committees than your ability to recite Young's modulus for every material known to man. The schools assume they can expand your knowledge base. They choose applicants carefully because expansive knowledge is not enough to succeed in medical school or in the profession. There's something more. It's this "something more" that the MCAT is trying to measure.

Every section on the MCAT tests essentially the same higher-order thinking skills: analytical reasoning, abstract thinking, and problem solving.

Most test takers get trapped into thinking they are being tested strictly about biology, chemistry, and so on. Thus, they approach each section with a new outlook on what's expected. This constant mental gear-shifting can be exhausting, not to mention counterproductive. Instead of perceiving the test as parsed into radically different sections, you need to maintain your focus on the underlying nature of the test: It's designed to test your thinking skills, not your information-recall skills. Each test section thus presents a variation on the same theme.

TEST TIP

Don't think of the sections of the MCAT as unrelated timed pieces. Each is a variation on the same theme, because the underlying purpose of each section and of the test as a whole is to evaluate your thinking skills. Memorizing formulas won't boost your score. Understanding fundamental scientific principles will.

WHAT ABOUT THE SCIENCE?

With this perspective, you may be left asking these questions: "What about the science? What about the content? Don't I need to know the basics?" The answer is a resounding "Yes!" You must be fluent in the different languages of the test. You cannot do well on the MCAT if you don't know the basics of physics, general chemistry, biology, and organic chemistry. We recommend that you take one year each of biology, general chemistry, organic chemistry, and physics before taking the MCAT, and that you review the content in this book thoroughly. Knowing these basics is just the beginning of doing well on the MCAT. That's a shock to most test takers. They presume that once they recall or relearn their undergraduate science, they are ready to do battle against the MCAT. Wrong! They merely have directions to the battlefield. They lack what they need to beat the test: a copy of the test maker's battle plan!

You won't be drilled on facts and formulas on the MCAT. You'll need to demonstrate ability to reason based on ideas and concepts. The science questions are painted with a broad brush, testing your general understanding.

TAKE CONTROL: THE MCAT MINDSET

TEST TIP

Those perfectionist tendencies that make you a good student and a good medical-school candidate may work against you in MCAT Land. If you get stuck on a question or passage, move on. Perfectionism is for medical school—not the MCAT. You don't need to understand every word of a passage before you go on to the questions—what's tripping you up may not even be relevant to what you'll be asked.

In addition to being a thinking test, as we've stressed, the MCAT is a standardized test. As such, it has its own consistent patterns and idiosyncrasies that can actually work in your favor. This is the key to why test preparation works. You have the opportunity to familiarize yourself with those consistent peculiarities, to adopt the proper test-taking mindset.

The following are some overriding principles of the MCAT mindset that will be covered in depth in the chapters to come:

- Read actively and critically.
- Translate prose into your own words.

- Save the toughest questions for last.
- Know the test and its components inside and out.
- Do MCAT-style problems in each topic area after you've reviewed it.
- Allow your confidence to build on itself.
- Take full-length practice tests a week or two before the test to break down the mystique of the real experience.
- Learn from your mistakes—get the most out of your practice tests.
- Look at the MCAT as a challenge, the first step in your medical career, rather than as an arbitrary obstacle.

That's what the MCAT mindset boils down to: Taking control. Being proactive. Being on top of the testing experience so that you can get as many points as you can as quickly and as easily as possible. Keep this in mind as you read and work through the material in this book and, of course, as you face the challenge on Test Day.

Now that you have a better idea of what the MCAT is all about, let's take a tour of the individual test sections. Although the underlying skills being tested are similar, each MCAT section requires that you call into play a different domain of knowledge. So, though we encourage you to think of the MCAT as a holistic and unified test, we also recognize that the test is segmented by discipline and that there are characteristics unique to each section. In the overviews, we'll review sample questions and answers and discuss section-specific strategies. For each of the sections—Verbal Reasoning, Physical/Biological Sciences, and the Writing Sample—we'll present you with the following:

- **The Big Picture**
  You'll get a clear view of the section and familiarize yourself with what it's really evaluating.
- **A Closer Look**
  You'll explore the types of questions that will appear and master the strategies you'll need to deal with them successfully.
- **Highlights**
  The key approaches to each section are outlined, for reinforcement and quick review.

TEST EXPERTISE

The first year of medical school is a frenzied experience for most students. In order to meet the requirements of a rigorous work schedule, students either learn to prioritize and budget their time or else fall hopelessly behind. It's no surprise, then, that the MCAT, the test specifically designed to predict success in the first year of medical school, is a high-speed, time-intensive test. It demands excellent time-management skills as well as that sine qua non of the successful physician—grace under pressure.

It's one thing to answer a Verbal Reasoning question correctly; it's quite another to answer several correctly in a limited time frame. The same goes for Physical and Biological Sciences—it's a whole new ballgame once you move from doing an individual passage at your leisure to handling a full section under actual timed conditions. You also need to budget your time for the Writing Sample, but this section isn't as time sensitive. When it comes to the multiple-choice sections, time pressure is a factor that affects virtually every test taker.

TEST TIP

For complete MCAT success, you've got to get as many correct answers as possible in the time you're allotted. Knowing the strategies is not enough. You have to perfect your time-management skills so that you get a chance to use those strategies on as many questions as possible.

So when you're comfortable with the content of the test, your next challenge will be to take it to the next level—test expertise—which will enable you to manage the all-important time element of the test.

THE FIVE BASIC PRINCIPLES OF TEST EXPERTISE

On some tests, if a question seems particularly difficult you'll spend significantly more time on it, as you'll probably be given more points for correctly answering a hard question. Not so on the MCAT. Remember, every MCAT question, no matter how hard, is worth a single point. There's no partial credit or "A" for effort, and because there are so many questions to do in so little time, you'd be a fool to spend 10 minutes getting a point for a hard question and then not have time to get a couple of quick points from three easy questions later in the section.

TEST TIP

In order to meet the stringent time requirements of the MCAT, you have to cultivate the following elements of test expertise:

- Feel free to skip questions.
- Learn to recognize and seek out questions you can do.
- Use a process of answer elimination.
- Remain calm.
- Keep track of time.

Given this combination—limited time, all questions equal in weight—you've got to develop a way of handling the test sections to make sure you get as many points as you can as quickly and easily as you can. Here are the principles that will help you do that:

1. FEEL FREE TO SKIP AROUND

One of the most valuable strategies to help you finish the sections in time is to learn to recognize and deal first with the questions that are easier and more familiar to you. That means you must temporarily skip those that promise to be difficult and time-consuming, if you feel comfortable doing so. You can always come back to these at the end, and if you run out of time, you're much better off not getting to questions you may have had difficulty with, rather than not getting to potentially feasible material. Of course, because there's no guessing penalty, always put an answer to every question on the test, whether you get to it or not. (It's not practical to skip passages, so do those in order.)

This strategy is difficult for most test takers; we're conditioned to do things in order, but give it a try when you practice. Remember, if you do the test in the exact order given, you're letting the test makers control you. You control how you take this test. On the other hand, if skipping around goes against your moral fiber and makes you a nervous wreck—don't do it. Just be mindful of the clock, and don't get bogged down with the tough questions.

2. LEARN TO RECOGNIZE AND SEEK OUT QUESTIONS YOU CAN DO

Another thing to remember about managing the test sections is that MCAT questions and passages, unlike items on the SAT and other standardized tests, are not presented in order of difficulty. There's no rule that says you have to work through the sections in any particular order; in fact, the test makers scatter the easy and difficult questions throughout the section, in effect rewarding those who actually get to the end. Don't lose sight of what you're being tested for along with your reading and thinking skills: efficiency and cleverness.

Don't waste time on questions you can't do. We know that skipping a possibly tough question is easier said than done; we all have the natural instinct to plow through test sections in their given order, but it just doesn't pay off on the MCAT. The computer won't be impressed if you get the toughest question right. If you dig in your heels on a tough question, refusing to move on until you've cracked it, well, you're letting your ego get in the way of your test score. A test section (not to mention life itself) is too short to waste on lost causes.

TEST TIP

Every question is worth exactly one point, but questions vary dramatically in difficulty level. Given a shortage of time, work on easy questions and then move on to the hard ones.

3. USE A PROCESS OF ANSWER ELIMINATION

Using a process of elimination is another way to answer questions both quickly and effectively. There are two ways to get all the answers right on the MCAT. You either know all the right answers, or you know all the wrong answers. Because there are three times as many wrong answers, you should be able to eliminate some if not all of them. By doing so you either get to the correct response or increase your chances of guessing the correct response. You start out with a 25 percent chance of picking the right answer, and with each eliminated answer your odds go up. Eliminate one, and you'll have a 33⅓ percent chance of picking the right one, eliminate two, and you'll have a 50 percent chance, and, of course, eliminate three, and you'll have a 100 percent chance. Increase your efficiency by actually crossing out the wrong choices on the screen using the strikethrough feature. Remember to look for wrong-answer traps when you're eliminating. Some answers are designed to seduce you by distorting the correct answer.

TEST TIP

Don't let your ego sabotage your score. It isn't easy for some of us to give up on a tough, time-consuming question, but sometimes it's better to say "uncle." Remember, there's no point of honor at stake here, but there are MCAT points at stake.

4. REMAIN CALM

It's imperative that you remain calm and composed while working through a section. You can't allow yourself to become so rattled by one hard reading passage that it throws off your performance on the rest of the section. Expect to find at least one killer passage in every section, but remember, you won't be the only one to have trouble with it. The test is curved to take the tough material into account. Having trouble with a difficult question isn't going to ruin your score—but getting upset about it and letting it throw you off track will. When you understand that part of the test maker's goal is to reward those who keep their composure, you'll recognize the importance of not panicking when you run into challenging material.

5. KEEP TRACK OF TIME

Of course, the last thing you want to happen is to have time called on a particular section before you've gotten to half the questions. Therefore, it's essential that you pace yourself, keeping in mind the general guidelines for how long to spend on any individual question or passage. Have a sense of how long you have to do each question, so you know when you're exceeding the limit and should start to move faster.

So, when working on a section, always remember to keep track of time. Don't spend a wildly disproportionate amount of time on any one question or group of questions. Also, give yourself 30 seconds or so at the end of each section to fill in answers for any questions you haven't gotten to.

SECTION-SPECIFIC PACING

Let's now look at the section-specific timing requirements and some tips for meeting them. Keep in mind that the times per question or passage are only averages; there are bound to be some that take less time and some that take more. Try to stay balanced. Remember, too, that every question is of equal worth, so don't get hung up on any one. Think about it: If a question is so hard that it takes you a long time to answer it, chances are you may get it wrong anyway. In that case, you'd have nothing to show for your extra time but a lower score.

VERBAL REASONING

Allow yourself approximately eight to ten minutes per passage and respective questions. It may sound like a lot of time, but it goes quickly. Keep in mind that some passages are longer than others. On average, give yourself about three or four minutes to read and then four to six minutes for the questions.

TEST TIP

For Verbal Reasoning, here are some of the important time techniques to remember:

- Spend eight to ten minutes per passage
- Allow about three to four minutes to read and four to six minutes for the questions

PHYSICAL AND BIOLOGICAL SCIENCES

Averaging over each section, you'll have about one minute and 20 seconds per question. Some questions, of course, will take more time, some less. A science passage plus accompanying questions should take about eight to nine minutes, depending on how many questions there are. Stand-alone questions can take anywhere from a few seconds to a minute or more. Again, the rule is to do your best work first. Also, don't feel that you have to understand everything in a passage before you go on to the questions. You may not need that deep an understanding to answer questions, because a lot of information may be extraneous. You should overcome your perfectionism and use your time wisely.

TEST TIP

Some suggestions for maximizing your time on the science sections:

- Spend about eight to nine minutes per passage
- Maximize points by doing the questions you can do first
- Don't waste valuable time trying to understand extraneous material

WRITING SAMPLE

You have exactly 30 minutes for each essay. As mentioned in discussion of the seven-step approach to this section, you should allow approximately five minutes to prewrite the essay, 23 minutes to write the essay, and two minutes to proofread. It's important that you budget your time, so you don't get cut off.

COMPUTER-BASED TESTING STRATEGIES

ARRIVE AT THE TESTING CENTER EARLY

Get to the testing center early to jump-start your brain. However, if they allow you to begin your test early, decline.

USE THE MOUSE TO YOUR ADVANTAGE

If you are right-handed, practice using the mouse with your left hand for Test Day. This way, you'll increase speed by keeping the pencil in your right hand to write on your scratch paper. If you are left-handed, use your right hand for the mouse.

KNOW THE TUTORIAL BEFORE TEST DAY

You will save time on Test Day by knowing exactly how the test will work. Click through any tutorial pages and save time.

PRACTICE WITH SCRATCH PAPER

Going forward, always practice using scratch paper when solving questions because this is how you will do it on Test Day. Never write directly on a written test.

GET NEW SCRATCH PAPER

Between sections, get a new piece of scratch paper even if you only used part of the old one. This will maximize the available space for each section and minimize the likelihood of you running out of paper to write on.

REMEMBER YOU CAN ALWAYS GO BACK

Just because you finish a passage or move on, remember you can come back to questions about which you are uncertain. You have the "marking" option to your advantage. However, as a general rule minimize the amount of questions you mark or skip.

MARK INCOMPLETE WORK

If you need to go back to a question, clearly mark the work you've done on the scratch paper with the question number. This way, you will be able to find your work easily when you come back to tackle the question.

LOOK AWAY AT TIMES

Taking the test on computer leads to faster eye-muscle fatigue. Use the Kaplan strategy of looking at a distant object at regular intervals. This will keep you fresher at the end of the test.

PRACTICE ON THE COMPUTER

This is the most critical aspect of adapting to computer-based testing. Like anything else, in order to perform well on computer-based tests you must practice. Spend time reading passages and answering questions on the computer. You often will have to scroll when reading passages.

Part I
Subject Review

CHAPTER 1

ATOMIC STRUCTURE

Chemistry is the study of the nature and behavior of matter. The **atom** is the basic building block of matter, representing the smallest unit of a chemical element. An atom in turn is composed of subatomic particles called **protons, neutrons,** and **electrons.** The protons and neutrons in an atom form the **nucleus,** the core of the atom. The electrons exist outside the nucleus in characteristic regions of space called **orbitals.** All atoms of an **element** show similar chemical properties and cannot be further broken down by chemical means.

TEACHER TIP

The building blocks of the atom are also the building blocks of knowledge for the General Chemistry on the MCAT. Understand these interactions well.

SUBATOMIC PARTICLES

A. PROTONS

Protons carry a single positive charge and have a mass of approximately one **atomic mass unit** or amu. The **atomic number** (Z) of an element equals the number of protons found in an atom of that element. All atoms of a given element have the same atomic number.

B. NEUTRONS

Neutrons carry no charge and have a mass only slightly larger than that of protons. Different **isotopes** of one element have different numbers of neutrons but the same number of protons. The **mass number** of an atom is equal to the total number of protons and neutrons. The convention ${}^{A}_{Z}X$ is used to show both the atomic number and mass number of an X atom, where Z is the atomic number and A is the mass number.

C. ELECTRONS

Electrons carry a charge equal in magnitude but opposite in sign to that of protons. An electron has a very small mass, approximately 1/1,837th the mass of a proton or neutron, which is negligible for most purposes. The electrons farthest from the nucleus are known as **valence electrons.** The farther the valence electrons are from the nucleus, the weaker the attractive force of the positively charged nucleus and the more likely the valence electrons are to be influenced by other atoms. Generally, the

TEACHER TIP

The valence, or outer, electrons are very important to us in both General and Organic Chemistry. Knowing how tightly held those electrons are will allow us to understand many of an atom's properties and interactions with other atoms.

valence electrons and their activity determine the reactivity of an atom. In a neutral atom, the number of electrons is equal to the number of protons. A positive or negative charge on an atom is due to a loss or gain of electrons; the result is called an **ion.**

Some basic features of the three subatomic particles are shown in the table below.

Table 1.1

Subatomic Particle	Symbol	Relative Mass	Charge	Location
Proton	${}^{1}_{1}H$	1	+1	Nucleus
Neutron	${}^{1}_{0}n$	1	0	Nucleus
Electron	e	0	−1	Electron Orbitals

Example: Determine the number of protons, neutrons, and electrons in a nickel-58 atom and in a nickel-60 2+ cation.

Solution: ${}^{58}Ni$ has an atomic number of 28 and a mass number of 58. Therefore, ${}^{58}Ni$ will have 28 protons, 28 electrons, and 58 – 28, or 30, neutrons.

In the ${}^{60}Ni^{2+}$ species, the number of protons is the same as in the neutral ${}^{58}Ni$ atom. However, ${}^{60}Ni^{2+}$ has a positive charge because it has lost two electrons and thus, Ni^{2+} will have 26 electrons. Also the mass number is 2 units higher than for the ${}^{58}Ni$ atom, and this difference in mass must be due to 2 extra neutrons, thus it has a total of 32 neutrons.

MCAT SYNOPSIS

- Atomic number (Z) = number of protons
- Mass number (A) = number of protons and number of neutrons
- In a neutral atom, number of protons = number of electrons

ATOMIC WEIGHTS AND ISOTOPES

A. ATOMIC WEIGHTS

The atomic mass of an atom is the relative mass of that atom compared with the mass of a carbon-12 atom, which is used as a standard with an assigned mass of 12.000. Atomic masses are expressed in terms of atomic mass units (amu), with one amu defined as exactly one-twelfth the mass of the carbon-12 atom, approximately 1.66×10^{-24} grams (g). A more common convention used to define the mass of an atom is **atomic weight.** The atomic weight is the weight in grams of one mole (mol) of a given element and is expressed in terms of g/mol. A mole is a unit used to count particles and is represented by **Avogadro's number,** 6.022×10^{23} particles. For example, the atomic weight of carbon is 12.0 g/mol, which means that 6.022×10^{23} carbon atoms weigh 12.0 g (see chapter 4, Compounds and Stoichiometry).

TEACHER TIP

Celebrate Science! Mole Day is celebrated at 6:02 on October 23rd (6:02 on 10/23) because of Avogadro's number (6.02×10^{23}). We will revisit this number in chapter 4 when we discuss moles in more detail.

B. ISOTOPES

For a given element, multiple species of atoms with the same number of protons (same atomic number) but different numbers of neutrons (different mass numbers) exist; these are called **isotopes** of the element. Isotopes are referred to either by the convention described above or, more commonly, by the name of the element followed by the mass number. For example, carbon-12 ($^{12}_{6}C$) is a carbon atom with 6 protons and 6 neutrons, while carbon-14 ($^{14}_{6}C$) is a carbon atom with 6 protons and 8 neutrons. Because isotopes have the same number of protons and electrons, they generally exhibit the same chemical properties.

In nature, almost all elements exist as a collection of two or more isotopes, and these isotopes are usually present in the same proportions in any sample of a naturally occurring element. The presence of these isotopes accounts for the fact that the accepted atomic weight for most elements is not a whole number. The masses listed in the periodic table are weighted averages that account for the relative abundance of various isotopes.

MCAT SYNOPSIS

Bromine is listed in the periodic table as having a mass of 79.9 amu. This is an average of the two naturally occurring isotopes, bromine-79 and bromine-81, which occur in almost equal proportions. There are no bromine atoms with an actual mass of 79.9 amu.

Example: Element Q consists of three different isotopes, A, B, and C. Isotope A has an atomic mass of 40.00 amu and accounts for 60.00 percent of naturally occurring Q. The atomic mass of isotope B is 44.00 amu and accounts for 25.00 percent of Q. Finally, isotope C has an atomic mass of 41.00 amu and a natural abundance of 15.00 percent. What is the atomic weight of element Q?

Solution: $0.60(40 \text{ amu}) + 0.25(44 \text{ amu}) + 0.15(41 \text{ amu}) = 24.00 \text{ amu} + 11.00 \text{ amu} + 6.15 \text{ amu} = 41.15 \text{ amu}$

The atomic weight of element Q is 41.15 g/mol.

BOHR'S MODEL OF THE HYDROGEN ATOM

In 1911, Ernest Rutherford provided experimental evidence that an atom has a dense, positively charged nucleus that accounts for only a small portion of the volume of the atom. In 1900, Max Planck developed the first

quantum theory, proposing that energy emitted as electromagnetic radiation from matter comes in discrete bundles called **quanta.** The energy value of a quantum is given by the equation $E = hf$ where h is a proportionality constant known as **Planck's constant,** equal to 6.626×10^{-34} J•s, and f (sometimes designated υ) is the **frequency** of the radiation.

A. THE BOHR MODEL

In 1913, Niels Bohr used the work of Rutherford and Planck to develop his model of the electronic structure of the hydrogen atom. Starting from Rutherford's findings, Bohr assumed that the hydrogen atom consisted of a central proton around which an electron travelled in a circular orbit, and that the centripetal force acting on the electron as it revolved around the nucleus was the electrical force between the positively charged proton and the negatively charged electron.

Bohr's model used the quantum theory of Planck in conjunction with concepts from classical physics. In classical mechanics, an object, such as an electron, revolving in a circle may assume an infinite number of values for its radius and velocity. Therefore, the angular momentum ($L = mvr$) and kinetic energy ($KE = mv^2/2$) can take on any value. However, by incorporating Planck's quantum theory into his model, Bohr placed conditions on the value of the angular momentum. Like Planck's energy, the angular momentum of an electron is quantized according to the following equation:

$$\text{angular momentum} = nh/2\pi$$

where h is Planck's constant and n is a quantum number that can be any positive integer. As h, 2, and π are constants, the angular momentum changes only in discrete amounts with respect to the quantum number, n. Bohr then equated the allowed values of the angular momentum to the energy of the electron. He obtained the following equation:

$$E = -R_H/n^2$$

where R_H is an experimentally determined constant (known as the Rydberg constant) equal to 2.18×10^{-18} J/electron. Therefore, like angular momentum, the energy of the electron changes in discrete amounts with respect to the quantum number.

A value of zero energy was assigned to the state in which the proton and electron were separated completely, meaning that there was no attractive force between them. Therefore, the electron in any of its quantized states in the atom would have a negative energy as a result of the attractive

TEACHER TIP

When you see a formula in your review or on Test Day, focus on ratios and relationships rather than the equation as a whole. This simplifies your "calculations" to a conceptual understanding and oftentimes still gets you the right answer.

TEACHER TIP

At first glance it may not be clear that the energy (E) is directly proportional to the principle quantum number (n). Take note of the negative charge, which causes the values to approach zero from a greater negative value as n increases (thereby increasing the energy). On Test Day, be sure to consider where the variable appears in the fraction *and* negative signs when determining proportionality.

forces between the electron and proton. This explains the negative sign in the previous equation for energy.

B. APPLICATIONS OF THE BOHR MODEL

In his model of the structure of hydrogen, Bohr postulated that an electron can exist only in certain fixed energy states. In terms of quantum theory, the energy of an electron is **quantized.** Using this model, certain generalizations concerning the characteristics of electrons can be made. The energy of the electron is related to its orbital radius: the smaller the radius, the lower the energy state of the electron. The smallest orbit (radius) an electron can have corresponds to $n = 1$, which is the ground state of the hydrogen electron. At the **ground state** level, the electron is in its lowest energy state. The Bohr model is also used to explain the atomic emission spectrum and atomic absorption spectrum of hydrogen, and is helpful in interpretation of the spectra of other atoms.

MCAT SYNOPSIS

Note that all systems tend toward minimal energy, thus atoms of any element will generally exist in the ground state unless subjected to extremely high temperatures or irradiation.

1. Atomic Emission Spectra

At room temperature, the majority of atoms in a sample are in the ground state. However, electrons can be excited to higher energy levels, by heat or other energy, to yield the excited state of the atom. Because the lifetime of the excited state is brief, the electrons will return rapidly to the ground state, emitting energy in the form of photons. The electromagnetic energy of these photons may be determined using the following equation:

$$E = hc/\lambda$$

where h is Planck's constant, c is the velocity of light (3×10^8 m/s), and λ is the wavelength of the radiation.

BRIDGE

$E = hf$ for photons in physics. This also holds true here since we know that $C = f\lambda$. This is based on the formula $V = f\lambda$ for photons.

The different electrons in an atom will be excited to different energy levels. When these electrons return to their ground states, each will emit a photon with a wavelength characteristic of the specific transition it undergoes. The quantized energies of light emitted under these conditions do not produce a continuous spectrum (as expected from classical physics). Rather, the spectrum is composed of light at specific frequencies and is thus known as a line spectrum, where each line on the emission spectrum corresponds to a specific electronic transition. Because each element can have its electrons excited to different distinct energy levels, each one possesses a unique **atomic emission spectrum,** which can be used as a fingerprint for the element. One particular application of atomic emissions spectroscopy is in the analysis of stars; while a physical sample cannot be taken, the light

MCAT FAVORITE

Emissions from electrons in molecules or atoms dropping from an excited state to a ground state give rise to fluorescence. We see the color of the light being emitted.

from a star can be resolved into its component wavelengths, which are then matched to the known line spectra of the elements.

The Bohr model of the hydrogen atom explained the atomic emission spectrum of hydrogen, which is the simplest emission spectrum among all the elements. The group of hydrogen emission lines corresponding to transitions from upper levels $n > 2$ to $n = 2$ is known as the **Balmer series** (4 wavelengths in the visible region), while the group corresponding to transitions between upper levels $n > 1$ to $n = 1$ is known as the **Lyman series** (higher energy transitions, occur in the UV region).

When the energy of each frequency of light observed in the emission spectrum of hydrogen was calculated according to Planck's quantum theory, the values obtained closely matched those expected from energy level transitions in the Bohr model. That is, the energy associated with a change in the quantum number from an initial value n_i to a final value n_f is equal to the energy of Planck's emitted photon. Thus:

$$E = hc/\lambda = -R_H[1/(n_i)^2 - 1/(n_f)^2]$$

and the energy of the emitted photon corresponds to the precise difference in energy between the higher-energy initial state and the lower-energy final state.

MCAT Favorite

Absorption is the basis for the color of compounds. We see the color of the light that is NOT absorbed by the compound.

2. Atomic Absorption Spectra

When an electron is excited to a higher energy level, it must absorb energy. The energy absorbed as an electron jumps from an orbital of low energy to one of higher energy is characteristic of that transition. This means that the excitation of electrons in a particular element results in energy absorptions at specific wavelengths. Thus, in addition to an emission spectrum, every element possesses a characteristic **absorption spectrum.** Not surprisingly, the wavelengths of absorption correspond directly to the wavelengths of emission since the energy difference between levels remains unchanged. Absorption spectra can thus be used in the identification of elements present in a gas phase sample.

MCAT Synopsis

Note that the magnitude of ΔE is the same for absorption or emission between any two energy levels. The sign of ΔE indicates whether the energy goes in or out, and therefore, whether the electron is going to an excited state (absorption) or to the ground state (emission), respectively.

QUANTUM MECHANICAL MODEL OF ATOMS

While the concepts put forth by Bohr offered a reasonable explanation for the structure of the hydrogen atom and ions containing only one electron (such as He^{1+} and Li^{2+}), they did not explain the structures of atoms containing more than one electron. This is because Bohr's model does not take into consideration the repulsion between multiple electrons surrounding one nucleus. Modern quantum mechanics has led to a more rigorous and generalized study of the electronic structure of atoms. The most important difference between the Bohr model and modern quantum mechanical models is that Bohr's assumption that electrons follow a circular orbit at a fixed distance from the nucleus is no longer considered valid. Rather, electrons are described as being in a state of rapid motion within regions of space around the nucleus, called **orbitals.** An orbital is a representation of the probability of finding an electron within a given region. In the current quantum mechanical description of electrons, pinpointing the exact location of an electron at any given point in time is impossible. This idea is best described by the **Heisenberg uncertainty principle,** which states that it is impossible to determine, with perfect accuracy, the momentum and the position of an electron simultaneously. This means that if the momentum of the electron is being measured accurately, its position will change, and vice versa.

A. QUANTUM NUMBERS

Modern atomic theory states that any electron in an atom can be completely described by four **quantum numbers:** n, ℓ, m_ℓ, and m_s. Further, according to the **Pauli exclusion principle,** no two electrons in a given atom can possess the same set of four quantum numbers. The position and energy of an electron described by its quantum numbers is known as its **energy state.** The value of n limits the values of ℓ, which in turn limits the values of m_ℓ. The values of the quantum numbers qualitatively give information about the orbitals: n about the size, ℓ about the shape, and m_ℓ about the orientation of the orbital. All four quantum numbers are discussed below.

1. Principal Quantum Number

The first quantum number is commonly known as the **principal quantum number** and is denoted by the letter n. This is the quantum number used in Bohr's model that can theoretically take on any positive integer value. The larger the integer value of n, the higher the energy level and radius of the electron's orbit. The maximum number of electrons in energy level n (electron shell n) is $2n^2$. The difference in energy between adjacent shells decreases as the distance from the nucleus increases, since it is related to the expression $1/n_2^2 - 1/n_1^2$. For example, the energy difference between the third and fourth shells, $n = 3$ to $n = 4$, is less than that between the second and third shells, $n = 2$ to $n = 3$.

TEACHER TIP

A larger integer value of the principal quantum number indicates a larger radius and higher energy. This is similar to gravitational potential energy, where the higher the object is above the earth, the higher its potential energy.

2. Azimuthal Quantum Number

The second quantum number is called the **azimuthal (angular momentum) quantum number** and is designated by the letter ℓ.

MCAT SYNOPSIS

For any principal quantum number n, there will be n possible values for ℓ.

The second quantum number refers to the **subshells** or **sublevels** that occur within each principal energy level. For any given n, the value of ℓ can be any integer in the range of 0 to $n - 1$. The four subshells corresponding to $\ell = 0, 1, 2$, and 3 are known as the s, p, d, and f subshells, respectively. The maximum number of electrons that can exist within a subshell is given by the equation $4\ell + 2$. The greater the value of ℓ, the greater the energy of the subshell. However, the energies of subshells from different principal energy levels may overlap. For example, the 4s subshell will have a lower energy than the 3d subshell because its average distance from the nucleus is smaller (see Figure 1.1).

MCAT Synopsis

For any value of ℓ there will be $2\ell + 1$ possible values for m_ℓ. For any n, this produces n^2 possible values of m_ℓ, i.e., n^2 orbitals (see table below).

3. Magnetic Quantum Number

The third quantum number is the **magnetic quantum number** and is designated m_ℓ. An orbital is a specific region within a subshell that may contain no more than two electrons. The magnetic quantum number specifies the particular orbital within a subshell where an electron is highly likely to be found at a given point in time. The possible values of m_ℓ are all integers from ℓ to $-\ell$, including 0. Therefore, the s subshell, where there is one possible value of m_ℓ (0), will contain 1 orbital; likewise, the p subshell will contain 3 orbitals, the d subshell will contain 5 orbitals, and the f subshell will contain 7 orbitals. The shape and energy of each orbital are dependent upon the subshell in which the orbital is found. For example, a p subshell has three possible m_ℓ values (−1, 0, +1). The three dumbbell-shaped orbitals are oriented in space around the nucleus along the x, y, and z axes and are often referred to as p_x, p_y, and p_z.

MCAT Synopsis

For any value of n there will be a maximum of $2n^2$ electrons, i.e., two per orbital.

4. Spin Quantum Number

The fourth quantum number is also called the **spin quantum number** and is denoted by ms. The spin of a particle is its intrinsic angular momentum and is a characteristic of a particle, like its charge. In classical mechanics an object spinning about its axis has an angular momentum; however, this does not apply to the electron. Classical analogies often are inapplicable in the quantum world. In any case, the two spin orientations are designated $+\frac{1}{2}$ and $-\frac{1}{2}$. Whenever two electrons are in the same orbital, they must have opposite spins. Electrons in different orbitals with the same ms values are said to have **parallel** spins.

The quantum numbers for the orbitals in the second principal energy level, with their maximum number of electrons noted in parentheses, are shown in Table 1.2. Electrons with opposite spins in the same orbital are often referred to as paired.

Table 1.2

n	2(8)			
ℓ	0(2)	1(6)		
M_ℓ	0(2)	+1(2)	0(2)	−1(2)
M_s	$+\frac{1}{2}, -\frac{1}{2}$	$+\frac{1}{2}, -\frac{1}{2}$	$+\frac{1}{2}, -\frac{1}{2}$	$+\frac{1}{2}, -\frac{1}{2}$

B. ELECTRON CONFIGURATION AND ORBITAL FILLING

For a given atom or ion, the pattern by which subshells are filled and the number of electrons within each principal level and subshell are designated by an **electron configuration.** In electron configuration notation, the first number denotes the principal energy level, the letter designates the subshell, and the superscript gives the number of electrons in that subshell. For example, $2p^4$ indicates that there are four electrons in the second (p) subshell of the second principal energy level.

TEACHER TIP

The shorthand used to describe the electron configuration is derived *directly* from the quantum numbers.

When writing the electron configuration of an atom, it is necessary to remember the order in which subshells are filled. Subshells are filled from lowest to highest energy, and each subshell will fill completely before electrons begin to enter the next one. The $(n + \ell)$ rule is used to rank subshells by increasing energy. This rule states that the lower the values of the first and second quantum numbers, the lower the energy of the subshell. If two subshells possess the same $(n + \ell)$ value, the subshell with the lower n value has a lower energy and will fill first. The order in which the subshells fill is shown in the following chart.

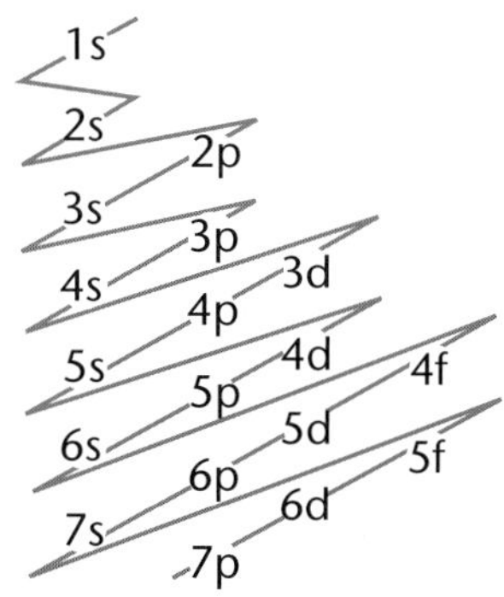

Figure 1.1

TEACHER TIP

Remember this chart for Test Day—being able to recreate it quickly on your scratch paper may save you time and get you that higher score!

Example: Which will fill first, the 3d subshell or the 4s subshell?

Solution: For 3d, $n = 3$ and $\ell = 2$, so $(n + \ell) = 5$. For 4s, $n = 4$ and $\ell = 0$, so $(n + \ell) = 4$. Therefore, the 4s subshell has lower energy and will fill first. This can also be determined from the chart by examination.

To determine which subshells are filled, you must know the number of electrons in the atom. In the case of uncharged atoms, the number of electrons equals the atomic number. If the atom is charged, the number of electrons is equal to the atomic number plus the extra electrons if the atom is negative, or the atomic number minus the electrons if the atom is positive.

TEACHER TIP

Hund's rule is like sitting down on a bus: Everyone wants an empty seat but we have to start pairing up after all the seats are half-filled.

In subshells that contain more than one orbital, such as the 2p subshell with its 3 orbitals, the orbitals will fill according to **Hund's rule.** Hund's rule states that within a given subshell, orbitals are filled such that there are a maximum number of half-filled orbitals with parallel spins. Electrons "prefer" empty orbitals to half-filled ones because a pairing energy must be overcome for two electrons carrying repulsive negative charges to exist in the same orbital.

Example: What are the written electron configurations for nitrogen (N) and iron (Fe) according to Hund's rule?

TEACHER TIP

Half- and fully-filled orbitals have lower energy than intermediate states. We will see this again when we talk about the transition metals.

Solution: Nitrogen has an atomic number of 7, thus its electron configuration is $1s^2\ 2s^2\ 2p^3$. According to Hund's rule, the two s-orbitals will fill completely, while the three p-orbitals will each contain one electron, all with parallel spins.

↑↓	↑↓	↑ ↑ ↑
$1s^2$	$2s^2$	$2p^3$

Iron has an atomic number of 26, and its 4s subshell fills before the 3d. Using Hund's rule, the electron configuraton will be:

↑↓	↑↓	↑↓ ↑↓ ↑↓	↑↓	↑↓ ↑↓ ↑↓	↑↓ ↑ ↑ ↑ ↑	↑↓
$1s^2$	$2s^2$	$2p^6$	$3s^2$	$3p^6$	$3d^6$	$4s^2$

Iron's electron configuration is written as $1s^2\ 2s^2\ 2p^6\ 3s^2\ 3p^6\ 3d^6\ 4s^2$. Subshells may be listed either in the order in which they fill (e.g., 4s before 3d) or with subshells of the same principal quantum number grouped together, as shown here. Both methods are correct.

The presence of paired or unpaired electrons affects the chemical and magnetic properties of an atom or molecule. If the material has unpaired electrons, a magnetic field will align the spins of these electrons and weakly attract the atom. These materials are said to be **paramagnetic.** Materials that have no unpaired electrons and are slightly repelled by a magnetic field are said to be **diamagnetic.**

Teacher Tip

Paramagnetic means that a magnetic field will cause *parallel* spins in unpaired electrons, and will therefore cause an attraction.

C. VALENCE ELECTRONS

The valence electrons of an atom are those electrons that are in its outer energy shell *or* that are available for bonding. For elements in Groups IA and IIA, only the outermost s electrons are valence electrons. For elements in Groups IIIA through VIIIA, the outermost s and p electrons in the highest energy shell are valence electrons. For transition elements, the valence electrons are those in the outermost s subshell and in the d subshell of the next-to-outermost energy shell. For the inner transition elements, the valence electrons are those in the *s* subshell of the outermost energy shell, the d subshell of the next-to-outermost energy shell, and the f subshell of the energy shell two levels below the outermost shell.

Teacher Tip

The valence electron configuration of an atom helps us understand its properties, and can be ascertained from the Periodic Table (the only "cheat sheet" you will have on Test Day).

IIIA–VIIA elements beyond Period II might, under some circumstances, accept electrons into their empty d subshell, which gives them more than 8 valence electrons (see Exceptions to the Octet Rule in chapter 3).

Example: Which are the valence electrons of elemental iron, elemental selenium, and the sulfur atom in a sulfate ion?

Solution: Iron has 8 valence electrons: 2 in its 4s subshell and 6 in its 3d subshell.

Selenium has 6 valence electrons: 2 in its 4s subshell and 4 in its 4p subshell. Selenium's 3d electrons are not part of its valence shell.

Sulfur in a sulfate ion has 12 valence electrons: its original 6 plus 6 more from the oxygens to which it is bonded. Sulfur's 3s and 3p subshells can contain only 8 of these 12 electrons; the other 4 electrons have entered the sulfur atom's 3d subshell, which in elemental sulfur is empty (see Figure 3.1).

PRACTICE QUESTIONS

1. The image below illustrates the charged surface of an unknown substance at a certain point in time. Each arrow represents an individual dipole moment, reflecting the overall orientation of electron charge density at that point on the surface. The individual dipole moments in each parallelogram all have the same magnitude and direction.

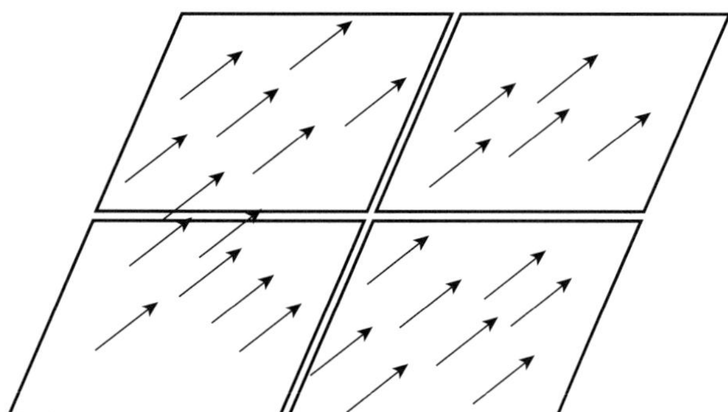

Which of the following terms best describes the magnetic properties of this substance?

A. Ferromagnetic
B. Paramagnetic
C. Diamagnetic
D. There is not enough information to determine the magnetic properties of the material.

2. Which of the following is the correct electron configuration for Zn^{2+}?

A. $1s^22s^22p^63s^23p^64s^03d^{10}$
B. $1s^22s^22p^63s^23p^64s^23d^8$
C. $1s^22s^22p^63s^23p^64s^23d^{10}$
D. $1s^22s^22p^63s^23p^64s^03d^8$

3. Which of the following quantum number sets describes a possible element?

A. $n = 2; l = 2; m_l = 1; m_s = +\frac{1}{2}$
B. $n = 2; l = 1; m_l = -1; m_s = +\frac{1}{2}$
C. $n = 2; l = 0; m_l = -1; m_s = -\frac{1}{2}$
D. $n = 2 ; l = 0; m_l = 1; m_s = -\frac{1}{2}$

4. What is the maximum number of electrons allowed in a single atomic energy level in terms of the principal quantum number n?

A. 2n
B. 2n + 2
C. $2n^2$
D. $2n^2 + 2$

5. Which of the following equations describes the maximum number of electrons that can fill a subshell?

A. 2l + 2
B. 4l + 2
C. $2l^2$
D. $2l^2 + 2$

6. Which of the following substances is most likely to be diamagnetic?

A. Hydrogen
B. Iron
C. Cobalt
D. Sulfur

7. An electron returns from an excited state to its ground state, emitting a photon at $\lambda = 500$ nm. If this process were repeated such that a mole of these photons were emitted, what would be the magnitude of the energy change?

A. 3.98×10^{-19} J
B. 3.98×10^{-21} J
C. 2.39×10^{5} J
D. 2.39×10^{3} J

8. Suppose an electron falls from n = 4 to its ground state, n = 1. Which of the following effects is most likely?

A. A photon is absorbed.
B. A photon is emitted.
C. The electron gains velocity.
D. The electron loses velocity.

9. Which of the following compounds is NOT a possible isotope of carbon?

A. ^{6}C
B. ^{12}C
C. ^{13}C
D. ^{14}C

10. According to the Heisenberg uncertainty principle, which of the following properties of a particle can an observer measure simultaneously?

I. Position
II. Momentum
III. Velocity

A. I and II
B. I and III
C. II and III
D. I, II, and III

11. Orbitals like the one pictured below are characteristic of which of the following shells?

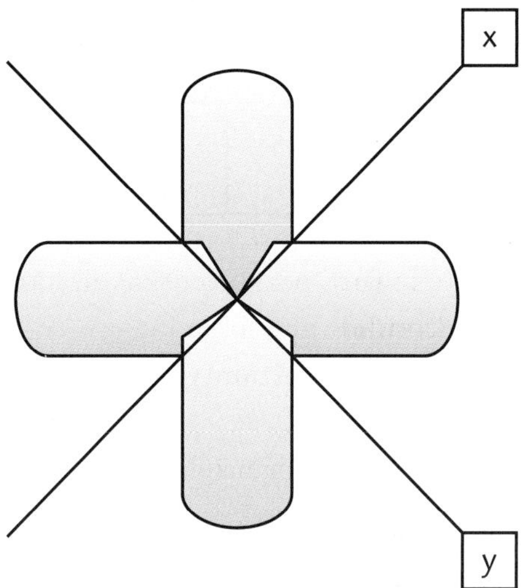

A. s
B. p
C. d
D. f

12. Which of the following electronic transitions would result in the greatest gain in energy for a single hydrogen electron, assuming that its ground state is n = 1?

A. An electron moves from n = 6 to n = 2.
B. An electron moves from n = 2 to n = 6.
C. An electron moves from n = 3 to n = 4.
D. An electron moves from n = 4 to n = 3.

13. Suppose a chemical species fills its orbitals as shown below. Which of the following laws of atomic physics could this compound be said to obey?

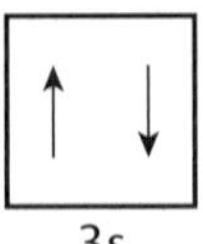

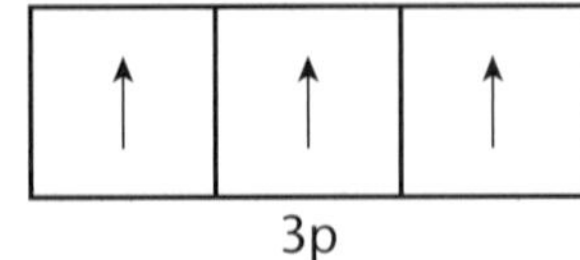

A. Hund's rule
B. Heisenberg uncertainty principle
C. Bohr model
D. Pauli exclusion principle

14. Which of the following correctly places the theories of atomic structure in proper chronological order, from the oldest theory to the most recent?

I. Bohr model
II. Rutherford model
III. Thomson model

A. I, II, III
B. I, III, II
C. III, II, I
D. II, III, I

15. How many total electrons are in a ^{133}Cs cation?

A. 54
B. 55
C. 78
D. 133

16. The atomic mass of hydrogen is 1.008 amu. What is the percent composition of hydrogen by isotope, assuming that hydrogen's only isotopes are ^{1}H and ^{2}D?

A. 92% H, 8% D
B. 99.2% H, 0.8% D
C. 99.92% H, 0.08% D
D. 99.992% H, 0.008% D

17. Consider the following two sets of quantum numbers, which describe two different electrons in the same atom. Which of the following best describes these two electrons?

n	l	m_l	m_s
1	1	1	+½
2	1	−1	+½

A. Parallel
B. Opposite
C. Antiparallel
D. Paired

18. The electron configuration $1s^2 2s^2 2p^6 3s^2 3p^6 4s^1 3d^5$ can describe several different transition metals. Which of the following species is represented by this configuration?

A. Cr
B. Mn^+
C. Fe^{2+}
D. Co^{3+}

19. Which of the following statements is NOT true of an electron's ground state?

A. The electron is at its lowest possible energy level.
B. The electron is in a quantized energy level.
C. The electron is traveling along its smallest possible orbital radius.
D. The electron is static.

20. Which of the following experimental conditions would NOT excite an electron out of the ground state?

A. Radiation
B. High temperature
C. High pressure
D. None of the above

Periodic Table of the Elements

Group**

Period	1 IA 1A	2 IIA 2A	3 IIIB 3B	4 IVB 4B	5 VB 5B	6 VIB 6B	7 VIIB 7B	8 -------	9 VIII -- ------- 8 -------	10 -----	11 IB 1B	12 IIB 2B	13 IIIA 3A	14 IVA 4A	15 VA 5A	16 VIA 6Λ	17 VIIA 7Λ	18 vIIIA 8A
1	1 H 1.008																	2 He 4.003
2	3 Li 6.941	4 Be 9.012											5 B 10.81	6 C 12.01	7 N 14.01	8 O 16.00	9 F 19.00	10 Ne 20.18
3	11 Na 22.99	12 Mg 24.31											13 Al 26.98	14 Si 28.09	15 P 30.97	16 S 32.07	17 Cl 35.45	18 Ar 39.95
4	19 K 39.10	20 Ca 40.08	21 Sc 44.96	22 Ti 47.88	23 V 50.94	24 Cr 52.00	25 Mn 54.94	26 Fe 55.85	27 Co 58.47	28 Ni 58.69	29 Cu 63.55	30 Zn 65.39	31 Ga 69.72	32 Ge 72.59	33 As 74.92	34 Se 78.96	35 Br 79.90	36 Kr 83.80
5	37 Rb 85.47	38 Sr 87.62	39 Y 88.91	40 Zr 91.22	41 Nb 92.91	42 Mo 95.94	43 Tc (98)	44 Ru 101.1	45 Rh 102.9	46 Pd 106.4	47 Ag 107.9	48 Cd 112.4	49 In 114.8	50 Sn 118.7	51 Sb 121.8	52 Te 127.6	53 I 126.9	54 Xe 131.3
6	55 Cs 132.9	56 Ba 137.3	57 La* 138.9	72 Hf 178.5	73 Ta 180.9	74 W 183.9	75 Re 186.2	76 Os 190.2	77 Ir 190.2	78 Pt 195.1	79 Au 197.0	80 Hg 200.5	81 Tl 204.4	82 Pb 207.2	83 Bi 209.0	84 Po (210)	85 At (210)	86 Rn (222)
7	87 Fr (223)	88 Ra (226)	89 Ac~ (227)	104 Rf (257)	105 Db (260)	106 Sg (263)	107 Bh (262)	108 Hs (265)	109 Mt (266)	110 --- ()	111 --- ()	112 --- ()		114 --- ()		116 --- ()		118 --- ()

Lanthanide Series*	58 Ce 140.1	59 Pr 140.9	60 Nd 144.2	61 Pm (147)	62 Sm 150.4	63 Eu 152.0	64 Gd 157.3	65 Tb 158.9	66 Dy 162.5	67 Ho 164.9	68 Er 167.3	69 Tm 168.9	70 Yb 173.0	71 Lu 175.0
Actinide Series~	90 Th 232.0	91 Pa (231)	92 U (238)	93 Np (237)	94 Pu (242)	95 Am (243)	96 Cm (247)	97 Bk (247)	98 Cf (249)	99 Es (254)	100 Fm (253)	101 Md (256)	102 No (254)	103 Lr (257)

CHAPTER 2

THE PERIODIC TABLE

In 1869, the Russian chemist Dmitri Mendeleev published the first version of his periodic table, in which he showed that ordering the elements according to atomic weight produced a pattern in which similar properties periodically recurred. This table was later revised, using the work of the physicist Henry Moseley, to organize the elements on the basis of increasing atomic number. Using this revised table, the properties of certain elements that had not yet been discovered were predicted: A number of these predictions were later borne out by experimentation. The substance of this work is summarized in the **periodic law,** which states that the chemical properties of the elements are dependent, in a systematic way, upon their atomic numbers.

MCAT Favorite

Don't memorize the periodic table because you have access to it on Test Day. Do know about its configuration and trends.

In the periodic table used today, the elements are arranged in **periods** (rows) and **groups** (columns). There are seven periods, representing the principal quantum numbers $n = 1$ to $n = 7$, and each period is filled sequentially. Groups represent elements that have the same electronic configuration in their **valence,** or outermost shell, and share similar chemical properties. The electrons in the outermost shell are called **valence electrons.** They are involved in chemical bonding and determine the chemical reactivity and properties of the element. The Roman numeral above each group represents the number of valence electrons. There are two sets of groups, designated A and B. The A elements are the **representative elements,** which have either s- or p-sublevels as their outermost orbitals. The B elements are the **nonrepresentative elements,** including the **transition elements,** which have partly filled d sublevels, and the **lanthanide** and **actinide series,** which have partly filled f-sublevels. The electron configuration for the valence electrons is given by the Roman numeral and letter designations. For example, an element in Group VA will have a valence electron configuration of s^2p^3 ($2 + 3 = 5$ valence electrons).

PERIODIC PROPERTIES OF THE ELEMENTS

The properties of the elements exhibit certain trends, which can be explained in terms of the position of the element in the periodic table, or in terms of the electron configuration of the element. All elements seek to gain or lose valence electrons so as to achieve the stable octet formation possessed by the **inert** or **noble gases** of Group VIII. Two other important trends exist within the periodic table. First, as one goes from left to right across a period, electrons are added one at a time; the electrons of the outermost shell experience an increasing amount of nuclear attraction, becoming closer and more tightly bound to the nucleus. Second, as one goes down a given column, the outermost electrons become less tightly bound to the nucleus. This is because the number of filled principal energy levels (which shield the outermost electrons from attraction by the nucleus) increases downward within each group. These trends help explain elemental properties such as atomic radius, ionization potential, electron affinity, and electronegativity.

A. ATOMIC RADII

Teacher Tip

The further an electron and proton get from one another, the easier it is to pull them apart. This helps us understand all the trends with respect to the radius.

The **atomic radius** of an element is equal to one-half the distance between the centers of two atoms of that element that are just touching each other. In general, the atomic radius decreases across a period from left to right and increases down a given group; The atoms with the largest atomic radii will be located at the bottom of groups, and in Group I.

As one moves from left to right across a period, electrons are added one at a time to the outer energy shell. Electrons within a shell cannot shield one another from the attractive pull of protons. Therefore, because the number of protons is also increasing, producing a greater positive charge attracting the valence electrons, the effective nuclear charge increases steadily across a period. This causes the atomic radius to decrease.

As one moves down a group of the periodic table, the number of electrons and filled electron shells will increase, but the number of valence electrons will remain the same. Thus, the outermost electrons in a given group will feel the same amount of effective nuclear charge, but electrons will be found farther from the nucleus as the number of filled energy shells increases. Thus, the atomic radii will increase.

B. IONIZATION ENERGY

The **ionization energy** (IE), or **ionization potential,** is the energy required to completely remove an electron from a gaseous atom or ion. Removing an electron from an atom always requires an input of energy (is endothermic; see chapter 6, Thermodynamics). The closer and more tightly bound an electron is to the nucleus, the more difficult it will be to remove, and the higher the ionization energy will be. The **first ionization energy** is the energy required to remove one valence electron from the parent atom, the **second ionization energy** is the energy needed to remove a second valence electron from the univalent ion to form the divalent ion, and so on. Successive ionization energies grow increasingly large; i.e., the second ionization energy is always greater than the first ionization energy. For example:

$$Mg(g) \longrightarrow Mg^{+}(g) + e^{-} \text{ First Ionization Energy} + 7.646 \text{ eV}$$

$$Mg^{+}(g) \longrightarrow Mg^{2+}(g) + e^{-} \text{ Second Ionization Energy} + 15.035 \text{ eV}$$

Ionization energy increases from left to right across a period as the atomic radius decreases. Moving down a group, the ionization energy decreases as the atomic radius increases. Group I elements have low ionization energies because the loss of an electron results in the formation of a stable octet.

MCAT STRATEGY

To recall the various trends, remember this: Cesium (Cs) is the largest, most metallic, and least electronegative of all naturally occurring elements. It also has the smallest ionization energy and the least exothermic electron affinity.

C. ELECTRON AFFINITY

Electron affinity is the energy change that occurs when an electron is added to a gaseous atom, and it represents the ease with which the atom can accept an electron. The stronger the attractive pull of the nucleus for electrons **(effective nuclear charge, or Z_{eff})**, the greater the electron affinity will be. In discussing electron affinities, two sign conventions are used. The more common one states that a positive electron affinity value represents energy release when an electron is added to an atom; the other states that a negative electron affinity represents a release of energy. In this discussion, the first convention will be used.

MCAT STRATEGY

In contrast to cesium, fluorine (F) is the smallest, most electronegative element. It also has the largest ionization energy and most exothermic electron affinity.

Generalizations can be made about the electron affinities of particular groups in the periodic table. For example, the Group IIA elements, or **alkaline earths,** have low electron affinity values. These elements are relatively stable because their s subshell is filled. Group VIIA elements, or **halogens,** have high electron affinities because the addition of an electron to the atom results in a completely filled shell, which represents a stable electron configuration. Achieving the stable octet involves a release of energy, and the strong attraction of the nucleus for the electron leads to a high energy change. The Group VIII elements, or **noble gases,** have electron affinities on the order of zero, because they already possess a stable octet and cannot readily accept an electron. Elements of other groups generally have low values of electron affinity.

MCAT Synopsis

Electronegativity might better be called "nuclear positivity." It is a result of the nucleus' attraction for electrons, that is, the Z_{eff} perceived by the electrons in a bond.

MCAT Tip

L → R
Atomic radius ↓
Ionization energy ↑
Electron affinity ↑
Electronegativity ↑

Top → bottom
Atomic radius ↑
Ionization energy ↓
Electron affinity ↓
Electronegativity ↓

Note: Atomic radius is always opposite the other trends.

MCAT Synopsis

The effective nuclear charge, Z_{eff} can explain all periodic trends as well as chemical properties.

D. ELECTRONEGATIVITY

Electronegativity is a measure of the attraction an atom has for electrons in a chemical bond. The greater the electronegativity of an atom, the greater its attraction for bonding electrons. Electronegativity values are not determined directly. The most common electronegativity scale is the Pauling electronegativity scale, with values ranging from 0.7 for the most electropositive elements, like cesium, to 4 for the most electronegative element fluorine. Electronegativities are related to ionization energies: Elements with low ionization energies will have low electronegativities because their nuclei do not attract electrons strongly, while elements with high ionization energies will have high electronegativities because of the strong pull their nuclei have on electrons. Therefore, electronegativity increases from left to right across periods. In any group, the electronegativity decreases as the atomic number increases, as a result of the increased distance between the valence electrons and the nucleus, i.e., greater atomic radius.

TYPES OF ELEMENTS

The elements of the periodic table may be classified into three categories: **metals,** located on the left side and in the middle of the periodic table; **nonmetals,** located on the right side of the table; and **metalloids (semimetals),** found along a diagonal line between the other two.

A. METALS

Metals are shiny solids (except for mercury) at room temperature, and generally have high melting points and densities. Metals have the characteristic ability to be deformed without breaking. The ability of a metal to be hammered into shapes is called **malleability** and the ability to be drawn into wires is called **ductility.** Many of the characteristic properties of metals, such as large atomic radius, low ionization energy, and low electronegativity, are due to the fact that the few electrons in the valence shell of a metal atom can easily be removed. Because the valence electrons can move freely, metals are good conductors of heat and electricity. Group IA and IIA represent the most reactive metals and will be discussed. The transition elements, also discussed later, are metals that have partially filled d orbitals.

B. NONMETALS

Nonmetals are generally brittle in the solid state and show little or no metallic luster. They have high ionization energies and electronegativities, and are usually poor conductors of heat and electricity. Most nonmetals share the ability to gain electrons easily, but otherwise they display a wide range of chemical behaviors and reactivities. The nonmetals are located on the upper-right side of the periodic table; they are separated from the metals by a line cutting diagonally through the region of the periodic table containing elements with partially filled p orbitals.

C. METALLOIDS

The metalloids or semimetals are found along the line between the metals and nonmetals in the periodic table, and their properties vary considerably. Their densities, boiling points, and melting points fluctuate widely. The electronegativities and ionization energies of metalloids lie between those of metals and nonmetals; therefore, these elements possess characteristics of both those classes. For example, silicon has a metallic luster, yet it is brittle and is not an efficient conductor. The reactivity of metalloids is dependent upon the element with which they are reacting. For example, boron (B) behaves as a nonmetal when reacting with sodium (Na) and as a metal when reacting with fluorine (F). The elements classified as metalloids are boron, silicon, germanium, arsenic, antimony, and tellurium.

MCAT SYNOPSIS

Metalloids are intermediate in properties between metals and nonmetals. Such properties include electrical conductivity, thus semimetals tend to make good semiconductors.

THE CHEMISTRY OF GROUPS

A. ALKALI METALS

The **alkali metals** are the elements of Group IA. They possess most of the physical properties common to metals, yet their densities are lower than those of other metals. The alkali metals have only one loosely bound electron in their outermost shell, giving them the largest atomic radii of all the elements in their respective periods. Their metallic properties and high reactivity are determined by the fact that they have low ionization energies; thus they easily lose their valence electron to form univalent cations. Alkali metals have low electronegativities and react very readily with nonmetals, especially halogens.

TEACHER TIP

These two groups of compounds are both metallic in nature because they both lose electrons easily from the s-orbital of their valence shell.

B. ALKALINE EARTHS

The **alkaline earths** are the elements of Group IIA, which also possess many characteristically metallic properties. Like the alkali metals, these properties are dependent upon the ease with which they lose electrons. The alkaline earths have two electrons in their outer shell and thus have smaller atomic radii than the alkali metals. However, the two valence electrons are not held very tightly by the nucleus, so they can be removed to form divalent cations. Alkaline earths have low electronegativities and low electron affinities.

C. HALOGENS

The **halogens,** Group VIIA, are highly reactive nonmetals with seven valence electrons (one short of the favored octet configuration). Halogens are highly variable in their physical properties. For instance, the halogens range from gaseous (F_2 and Cl_2) to liquid (Br_2) to solid (I_2) at room temperature. Their chemical properties are more uniform: The electronegativities of halogens are very high, and they are particularly reactive towards alkali metals and alkaline earths, which "want" to donate electrons to the halogens to form stable ionic crystals. Fluorine (F) has the highest electronegativity of all the elements.

D. NOBLE GASES

The **noble gases,** also called the **inert gases,** are found in Group VIII (also called Group 0). They are fairly nonreactive because they have a complete valence shell, which is an energetically favored arrangement. This gives them little or no tendency to gain or lose electrons, high ionization energies, and no real electronegativities. They possess low boiling points and are all gases at room temperature.

TEACHER TIP

Transition metals are seen in biological systems and are therefore seen on the MCAT. You don't need to memorize them but understand how the transition metals ionize and act.

E. TRANSITION ELEMENTS

The **transition elements,** Groups IB to VIIIB, are all considered metals; hence, they are also called the **transition metals.** These elements are very hard and have high melting points and boiling points. As one moves across a period, the five d-orbitals become progressively more filled. The d-electrons are held only loosely by the nucleus and are relatively mobile, contributing to the malleability and high electrical conductivity of these elements. Chemically, transition elements have low ionization energies and may exist in a variety of positively charged forms or **oxidation states.** This is because transition elements are capable of losing various numbers of electrons from the s- and d-orbitals of their valence shell. Theoretically, the transition metals in Group VIIIB could have eight different oxidation states, from +1 to +8; however, they typically do not exhibit so many. For instance, copper (Cu), in group IB, can exist in either the +1 or the +2 oxidation state, and manganese (Mn), in Group VIIB, occurs in the +2, +3, +4, +6, or +7 state. Because of this ability to attain positive oxidation states, transition metals form many different ionic and partially ionic compounds. The dissolved ions can form **complex ions** either with molecules of water **(hydration complexes)** or with nonmetals, forming highly colored solutions and compounds (e.g., $CuSO_4.5H_2O$), and this complexation may enhance the relatively low solubility of certain compounds (e.g., AgCl is insoluble in water, but quite soluble in aqueous ammonia due to the formation of the complex ion $[Ag(NH_3)_2]^+$). The formation of complexes causes the d-orbitals to be split into two energy sublevels. This enables many of the complexes to absorb certain frequencies of light—those containing the precise amount of energy required to raise electrons from the lower to the higher d-sublevel. The frequencies not absorbed—known as the subtraction frequencies—give the complexes their characteristic colors.

PRACTICE QUESTIONS

1. Lithium and sodium have similar chemical properties, such as the ability to form ionic bonds with chloride. Which of the following best explains this similarity?

   A. Both lithium and sodium ions are positively charged.
   B. Lithium and sodium are in the same group within the periodic table.
   C. Lithium and sodium are in the same period of the periodic table.
   D. Both lithium and sodium have low atomic weights.

2. Carbon and silicon, elements used as the basis of biologic life and synthetic computing, respectively, are often considered elements with similar chemical properties. Which of the following is true about the differences between the two elements?

   A. Carbon has a smaller atomic radius than silicon.
   B. Silicon has a smaller atomic radius than carbon.
   C. Carbon has fewer valence electrons than silicon.
   D. Silicon has fewer valence electrons than carbon.

3. One important property of any element is its atomic radius, because this can affect its chemical properties. Which of the following determines the length of an element's radius?

   I. The number of valence electrons
   II. The number of electron shells
   III. The number of neutrons in the nucleus

   A. I only
   B. III only
   C. I and II only
   D. I, II, and III

4. Ionization energy contributes to an atom's chemical reactivity. Which of the following would be an accurate ordering of ionization energies, from lowest ionization energy to highest?

   A. Be, first ionization energy → Be, second ionization energy → Li, first ionization energy
   B. Be, second ionization energy → Be, first ionization energy → Li, first ionization energy
   C. Li, first ionization energy → Be, first ionization energy → Be, second ionization energy
   D. Li, first ionization energy → Be, second ionization energy → Be, first ionization energy

5. Selenium is often an active component of scalp treatments for scalp dermatitis. What type of element is selenium?

   A. Metal
   B. Metalloid
   C. Halogen
   D. Nonmetal

6. The properties of atoms can be predicted, to some extent, by their location within the periodic table. Which of the following properties increases in the direction of the arrows shown below?

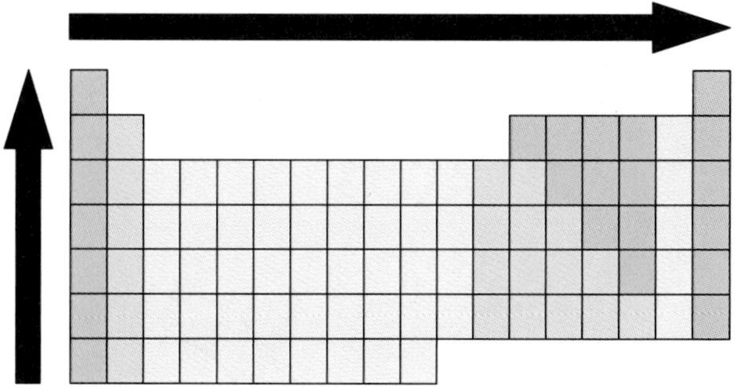

I. Electronegativity
II. Atomic radius
III. First ionization energy

A. I only
B. II only
C. I and III
D. I, II, and III

7. Metals are often used for making wires that conduct electricity. Which of the following properties of many metals is most important to making them good conductors?

A. Metals are malleable.
B. Metals have high electronegativity.
C. Metals have valence electrons that can move freely.
D. Metals have high melting points.

8. In the periodic table below, which of the following is an important property of the set of elements shaded?

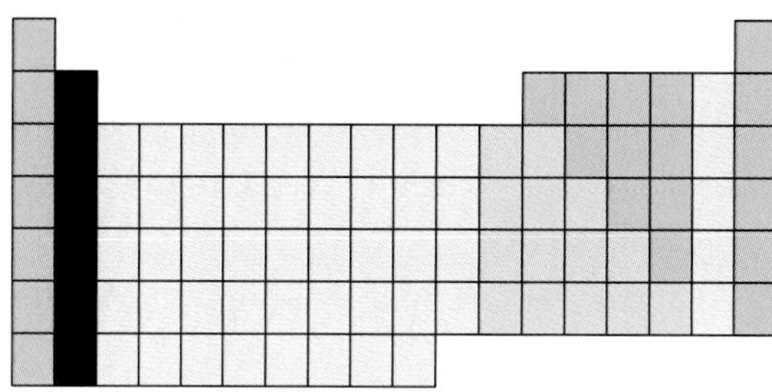

A. These elements are the best electrical conductors in the periodic table.
B. These elements form divalent cations.
C. The second ionization energy for these elements is lower than the first ionization energy.
D. The atomic radii of these elements decrease as one moves down the column.

9. Despite the fact that silicon and aluminum are adjacent in the periodic table, they react differently with 6M HCl, as demonstrated by the following reactions:[1] What best explains the difference in reactivity of silicon and aluminum?

$$Si + HCl \longrightarrow \text{No Reaction}$$

$$6Al + 6HCl \longrightarrow 3H_2 + 2AlCl_3$$

A. Silicon and aluminum are in different periods.
B. Silicon and aluminum are in different groups.
C. Silicon is a metalloid while aluminum is a metal.
D. Both silicon and aluminum are metalloids.

[1] www.chemicool.com/elements/aluminum.html; www.chemicool.com/elements/silicon.html

10. Which of the following is the correct order of groups in terms of increasing electronegativity?

A. Group VIIA → Group VIA → Group VA → Group IIA
B. Group 7 → Group 6 → Group 5 → Group 2
C. Group IIA → Group VA → Group VIA → Group VIIA
D. Group 2 → Group 5 → Group 6 → Group 7

11. When dissolved in water, what ion is most likely to form a complex ion with H_2O?

A. Na^+
B. Fe^{2+}
C. Cl^-
D. S^{2-}

12. How many valence electrons are present in elements in the third period?

A. 2
B. 3
C. The number decreases as the atomic number increases.
D. The number increases as the atomic number increases.

13. Which of the following elements has the highest electronegativity?

A. Mg
B. Cl
C. Li
D. I

14. Of the four atoms depicted below, which has the highest electron affinity?

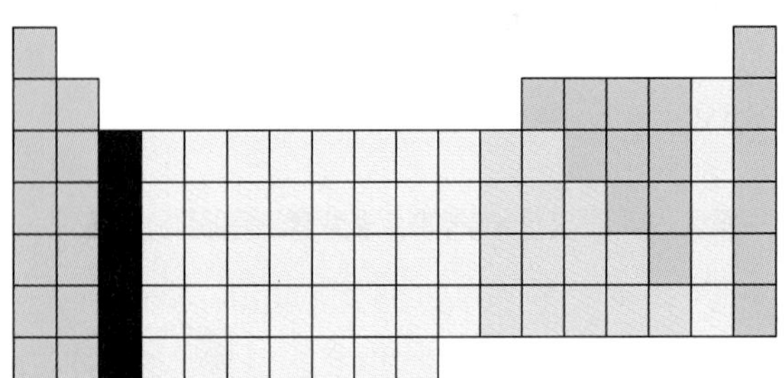

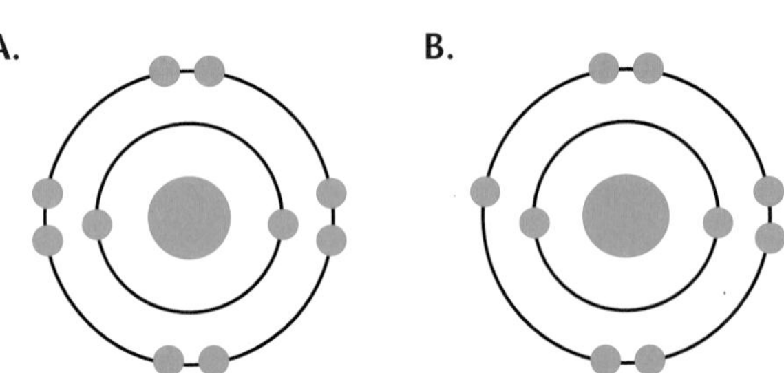

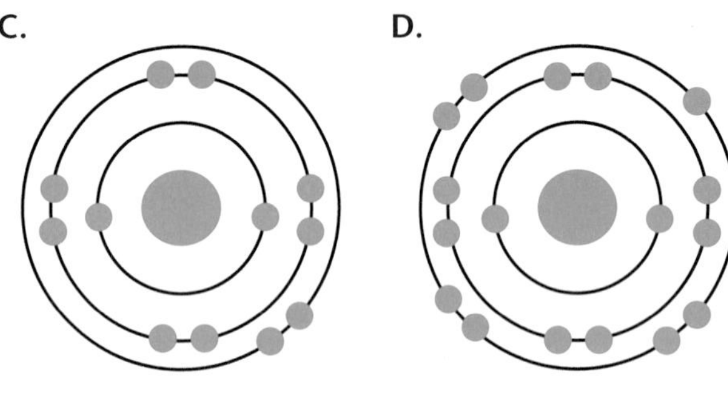

15. An atom with a large atomic radius

A. is likely to be on the right side of the periodic table.
B. is likely to have a high second ionization energy.
C. is likely to have low electronegativity.
D. is likely to form ionic bonds.

16. Which of the following atoms/ions has the largest effective nuclear charge?

A. Cl
B. Cl^-
C. K
D. K^+

17. Why do halogens often form ionic bonds with alkaline earth metals?

A. The alkaline earth metals have much higher electron affinity than the halogens.
B. By sharing electrons equally, the alkaline earth metals and halogens both form full octets.
C. Within the same row, the halogens have smaller atomic radii than the alkaline earth metals.
D. The halogens have much higher electron affinity than the alkaline earth metals.

18. What is the outermost orbital of elements in the third period?

A. s-orbital
B. p-orbital
C. d-orbital
D. f-orbital

19. A student undertakes the following experiment. In beaker A, the student places 500 mL of water and 0.500 g of AgBr. In beaker B, the student places 500 mL of ammonia and 0.500 g of AgBr. She notices that nearly none of the AgBr dissolves in beaker A, while it begins dissolving nearly immediately in beaker B. What best explains this phenomenon?

A. Formation of a hydration complex between silver and water
B. Ionic bonding between silver and ammonia
C. Hydrogen bonding of bromide with water
D. Formation of a complex between silver and ammonia

CHAPTER 3

BONDING AND CHEMICAL INTERACTIONS

The atoms of many elements can combine to form **molecules.** The atoms in most molecules are held together by strong attractive forces called **chemical bonds.** These bonds are formed via the interaction of the valence electrons of the combining atoms. The chemical and physical properties of the resulting molecules are often very different from their constituent elements. In addition to the very strong forces within a molecule, there are weaker intermolecular forces between molecules. These **intermolecular forces,** although weaker than the intramolecular chemical bonds, are of considerable importance in understanding the physical properties of many substances.

TEACHER TIP

Electronegativity (which we learned about in the last chapter) is a property that addresses how an individual atom acts within a bond and will help us understand the quality of the molecules formed from atoms with different electronegativities.

BONDING

Many molecules contain atoms bonded according to the **octet rule,** which states that an atom tends to bond with other atoms until it has eight electrons in its outermost shell, thereby forming a stable electron configuration similar to that of the Group VIII (noble gas) elements. **Exceptions** to this rule are as follows: **hydrogen,** which can have only two valence electrons (the configuration of He); **lithium** and **beryllium,** which bond to attain two and four valence electrons, respectively; **boron,** which bonds to attain six; and elements beyond the second row, such as phosphorus and sulfur, which can expand their octets to include more than eight electrons by incorporating d orbitals.

TEACHER TIP

Think of the octet rule as someone who wants to be a physician. An atom strives to be noble by gaining eight valence electrons the way a pre-med strives to be noble by graduating medical school!

When classifying chemical bonds, it is helpful to introduce two distinct types: **ionic bonds** and **covalent bonds.** In ionic bonding, an electron(s) from an atom with a smaller ionization energy is transferred to an atom with a greater electron affinity. This results in a positive and negative ion. These resulting ions are held together by electrostatic forces. In covalent bonding, an electron pair is shared between two atoms. In many cases, the bond is partially covalent and partially ionic; we call such bonds polar covalent bonds.

KAPLAN EXCLUSIVE

The *t* in cation looks like a plus sign: ca + ion.

IONIC BONDS

When two atoms with large differences in electronegativity react, there is a complete transfer of electrons from the less electronegative atom to the more electronegative atom. The atom that loses electrons becomes a positively charged ion, or **cation,** and the atom that gains electrons becomes a negatively charged ion, or **anion.** For this transfer to occur, the difference in electronegativity must be greater than 1.7. In general, the elements of Groups I and II (low electronegativities) bond ionically to elements of Group VII (high electronegativities). Hence, ionic bonds occur between metals and nonmetals. Elements of Groups I and II give up their electrons to achieve a noble gas configuration, while Group VII elements gain an electron to achieve the noble gas configuration. For example, $Na + Cl \longrightarrow Na^+ Cl^-$ (sodium chloride). The electrostatic force of attraction between the charged ions is called an **ionic** or **electrovalent bond.**

Ionic compounds have characteristic physical properties. They have high melting and boiling points due to the strong electrostatic forces between the ions. They can conduct electricity in the liquid and aqueous states, though not in the solid state. Ionic solids form crystal lattices consisting of infinite arrays of positive and negative ions in which the attractive forces between ions of opposite charge are maximized, while the repulsive forces between ions of like charge are minimized.

TEACHER TIP

Think of bonds as a tug of war between two atoms: when the difference in electronegativity is great (more than 1.7), then the "stronger" molecule wins all of the electrons and becomes the anion. When the values are close to equal, then there's a stalemate or a covalent bond with mostly equal sharing of electrons.

COVALENT BONDS

When two or more atoms with similar electronegativities interact, the energy required to form ions is greater than the energy that would be released upon the formation of an ionic bond (i.e., the process is not energetically favorable). However, because a complete transfer of electrons cannot occur, such atoms achieve a noble gas electron configuration by **sharing** electrons in a covalent bond. The binding force between the two atoms results from the attraction that each electron of the shared pair has for the two positive nuclei.

Covalent compounds contain discrete molecular units with weak intermolecular forces. Consequently, they are low-melting solids, and do not conduct electricity in the liquid or aqueous states.

A. PROPERTIES OF COVALENT BONDS

Atoms can share more than one pair of electrons. Two atoms sharing one, two, or three electron pairs are said to be joined by a **single, double,** or **triple covalent bond,** respectively. The number of shared electron pairs between two atoms is called the **bond order;** hence a single bond has a bond order of one, a double bond has a bond order of two, and a triple bond has a bond order of three.

A covalent bond can be characterized by two features: **bond length** and **bond energy.**

1. Bond Length

Bond length is the average distance between the two nuclei of the atoms involved in the bond. As the number of shared electron pairs increases, the two atoms are pulled closer together, leading to a decrease in bond length. Thus, for a given pair of atoms, a triple bond is shorter than a double bond, which is shorter than a single bond.

2. Bond Energy

Bond energy is the energy required to separate two bonded atoms. For a given pair of atoms, the strength of a bond (and therefore the bond energy) increases as the number of shared electron pairs increases. (Bond energy is further discussed in chapter 6, Thermodynamics.)

BRIDGE

We see a great example of covalent bonds in Organic Chemistry, and we can see here the inverse proportionality between bond length and strength.

	Bond length	Bond strength
C–C	longest	weakest
C=C	medium	medium
C≡C	shortest	strongest

B. COVALENT BOND NOTATION

The shared valence electrons of a covalent bond are called the **bonding electrons.** The valence electrons not involved in the covalent bond are called **nonbonding electrons.** The unshared electron pairs can also be called **lone electron pairs.** A convenient notation, called a **Lewis structure,** is used to represent the bonding and nonbonding electrons in a molecule, facilitating chemical "bookkeeping." The number of valence electrons attributed to a particular atom in the Lewis structure of a molecule is not necessarily the same as the number would be in the isolated atom, and the difference accounts for what is referred to as the **formal charge** of that atom. Often, more than one Lewis structure can be drawn for a molecule; this phenomenon is called **resonance.** Lewis structures, formal charge, and resonance are discussed in detail next.

1. Lewis Structures

A Lewis structure, or **Lewis dot symbol,** is the chemical symbol of an element surrounded by dots, each representing one of the s and/or

TEACHER TIP

When dealing with Lewis Dot structures, we only deal with the eight valence electrons (s- and p-orbitals of the outer shell) on each atom. Remember that some atoms can expand their octets by utilizing the d-orbitals in this outer shell, but this will take place only with atoms in period 3 or greater.

p-valence electrons of the atom. The Lewis symbols of the elements found in the second period of the periodic table are shown below.

Table 3.1

·Li	Lithium	·N· (with 2 dots above and 1 below)	Nitrogen
·Be·	Beryllium	·O: (with 2 dots above and 1 below)	Oxygen
·B· (with 1 dot above)	Boron	·F: (with 2 dots above and 2 below)	Fluorine
·C· (with 1 dot above and 1 below)	Carbon	:Ne: (with 2 dots above and 2 below)	Neon

Just as a Lewis symbol is used to represent the distribution of valence electrons in an atom, it can also be used to represent the distribution of valence electrons in a molecule. For example, the Lewis symbol of an F ion is :F̤̈:; the Lewis structure of an F_2 molecule is :F̤̈ — F̤̈:.

Certain steps must be followed in assigning a Lewis structure to a molecule. These steps are outlined below, using HCN as an example.

- Write the skeletal structure of the compound (i.e., the arrangement of atoms). In general, the least electronegative atom is the central atom. Hydrogen (always) and the halogens F, Cl, Br, and I (usually) occupy the end position.

  In HCN, H must occupy an end position. Of the remaining two atoms, C is the least electronegative, and therefore occupies the central position. The skeletal structure is as follows:

  H – C – N

- Count all the valence electrons of the atoms. The number of valence electrons of the molecule is the sum of the valence electrons of all atoms present:

  H has 1 valence electron;
  C has 4 valence electrons;
  N has 5 valence electrons; therefore,
  HCN has a total of 10 valence electrons.

- Draw single bonds between the central atom and the atoms surrounding it. Place an electron pair in each bond (bonding electron pair).

  H : C : N

  Each bond has two electrons, so 10 – 4 = 6 valence electrons remain.

- Complete the octets (eight valence electrons) of all atoms bonded to the central atom, using the remaining valence electrons still to be assigned. (Recall that H is an exception to the Octet rule because it can have only two valence electrons.) In this example H already has two valence electrons in its bond with C.

:H : C : N̤̈:

- Place any extra electrons on the central atom. If the central atom has less than an octet, try to write double or triple bonds between the central and surrounding atoms using the nonbonding, unshared lone electron pairs.

  The HCN structure above does not satisfy the Octet rule for C because C possesses only four valence electrons. Therefore, two lone electron pairs from the N atom must be moved to form two more bonds with C, creating a triple bond between C and N. Finally, bonds are drawn as lines rather than pairs of dots.

  $$H - C \equiv N:$$

  Now the Octet rule is satisfied for all three atoms, because C and N have eight valence electrons and H has two valence electrons.

2. Formal Charges

The number of electrons officially assigned to an atom in a Lewis structure does not always equal the number of valence electrons of the free atom. The difference between these two numbers is the **formal charge** of the atom. Formal charge can be calculated using the following formula:

$$\text{Formal charge} = V - \frac{1}{2} N_{\text{bonding}} - N_{\text{nonbonding}}$$

where V is the number of valence electrons in the free atom, N_{bonding} is the number of bonding electrons, and $N_{\text{nonbonding}}$ is the number of nonbonding electrons.

The formal charge of an ion or molecule equals the sum of the formal charges of the individual atoms comprising the ion or molecule.

Formal charge also contributes to stability. The lower the overall formal charge of the molecule, the more stable the molecule.

TEACHER TIP

Practicing with many molecules and remembering the "normal" amount of bonds on common central atoms will allow you to save time on Test Day from complicated equations like this. For example, the nitrogen atom here normally has three bonds and one lone pair. Here, it is sharing more than usual, so it will have a positive charge. If a molecule is selfish and is sharing less than usual, it will be negative (as we often see with oxygen atoms).

Example: Calculate the formal charge on the central N atom of $[NH_4]^+$.

Solution: The Lewis structure of $[NH_4]^+$ is

$$\left[\begin{array}{c} \text{H} \\ | \\ \text{H—N—H} \\ | \\ \text{H} \end{array}\right]$$

Nitrogen is in group VA; thus it has five valence electrons. In $[NH_4]^+$,

N has 4 bonds (i.e., eight bonding electrons and no nonbonding electrons).

So, $V = 5$; $N_{bonding} = 8$; $N_{nonbonding} = 0$

$$\text{Formal charge} = 5 - \frac{1}{2}(8) - 0 = +1$$

Thus, the formal charge on the N atom in $[NH_4]^+$ is +1.

Teacher Tip

Resonance is important when discussing aromatic compounds and carboxylic acids in Organic Chemistry. It allows for great stability by spreading electrons and negative charges over a larger area.

3. Resonance

For some molecules, two or more nonidentical Lewis structures can be drawn; these are called **resonance structures.** The molecule doesn't actually exist as either one of the resonance structures, but is rather a composite, or hybrid, of the two. For example, SO_2 has three resonance structures, two of which are minor: O = S – O and O – S = O. The actual molecule is a hybrid of these three structures (spectral data indicate that the two S–O bonds are identically equivalent). This phenomenon is known as resonance, and the actual structure of the molecule is called the **resonance hybrid.** Resonance structures are expressed with a double-headed arrow between them; thus,

$$\ddot{\underset{\cdot\cdot}{O}}=\ddot{S}=\ddot{\underset{\cdot\cdot}{O}} \longleftrightarrow \ddot{\underset{\cdot\cdot}{O}}=\ddot{S}-\ddot{\underset{\cdot\cdot}{O}}\!: \longleftrightarrow :\!\ddot{\underset{\cdot\cdot}{O}}-\ddot{S}=\ddot{\underset{\cdot\cdot}{O}}$$

represents the resonance structures of SO_2.

The last two resonance structures of sulfur dioxide shown above have equivalent energy or stability. Often, nonequivalent resonance structures may be written for a molecule. In these cases, the more stable the structure, the more that structure contributes to the character of the resonance hybrid. Conversely, the less stable the resonance structure, the less that structure contributes to the resonance hybrid.

It is the structure on the left of the diagram that is the most stable. Formal charges are often useful for qualitatively assessing the stability of a particular resonance structure; the following guidelines are used:

a. A Lewis structure with small or no formal charges is preferred over a Lewis structure with large formal charges.

b. A Lewis structure in which negative formal charges are placed on more electronegative atoms is more stable than one in which the formal charges are placed on less electronegative atoms.

Example: Write the resonance structures for $[NCO]^-$.

Solution: 1. C is the least electronegative of the three given atoms, N, C, and O. Therefore the C atom occupies the central position in the skeletal structure of $[NCO]^-$.

N C O

2. N has 5 valence electrons;
C has 4 valence electrons;
O has 6 valence electrons;
and the species itself has one negative charge.
Total valence electrons = 5 + 4 + 6 + 1 = 16

3. Draw single bonds between the central C atom and the surrounding atoms, N and O. Place a pair of electrons in each bond.

N : C : O

4. Complete the octets of N and O with the remaining 16 – 4 = 12 electrons.

$$:\underset{\cdot\cdot}{\ddot{N}}:C:\underset{\cdot\cdot}{\ddot{O}}:$$

5. The C octet is incomplete. There are three ways in which double and triple bonds can be formed to complete the C octet: two lone pairs from the O atom can be used to form a triple bond between the C and O atoms;

$$:\underset{\cdot\cdot}{\ddot{N}}-C\equiv O:$$

Teacher Tip

We spoke earlier in the book about how atoms strive for nobility. Here we can see that molecules strive to be like Switzerland. No, not cheesy—neutral! By spreading out charges amongst more than one atom, the charge gets closer to zero and therefore more stable.

or one lone electron pair can be taken from both the O and the N atoms to form two double bonds, one between N and C, and the other between O and C;

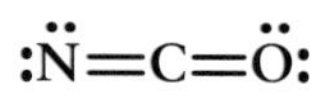

$$:\ddot{N}{=}C{=}\ddot{O}:$$

or two lone electron pairs can be taken from the N atom to form a triple bond between the C and N atoms.

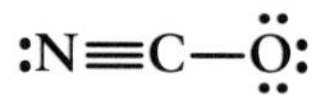

$$:N{\equiv}C{-}\ddot{\underset{..}{O}}:$$

These three are all resonance structures of $[NCO]^-$.

6. Assign formal charges to each atom of each resonance structure.

   The most stable structure is:

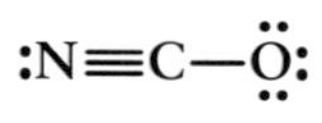

$$:N{\equiv}C{-}\ddot{\underset{..}{O}}:$$

   because the negative formal charge is on the most electronegative atom, O.

4. Exceptions to the Octet Rule

Atoms found in or beyond the third period can have more than 8 valence electrons, because some of the valence electrons may occupy *d* orbitals. These atoms can be assigned more than four bonds in Lewis structures. When drawing the Lewis structure of the sulfate ion, giving the sulfur 12 valence electrons permits three of the five atoms to be assigned a formal charge of zero. The sulfate ion can be drawn in six resonance forms, each with the two double bonds attached to a different combination of oxygen atoms.

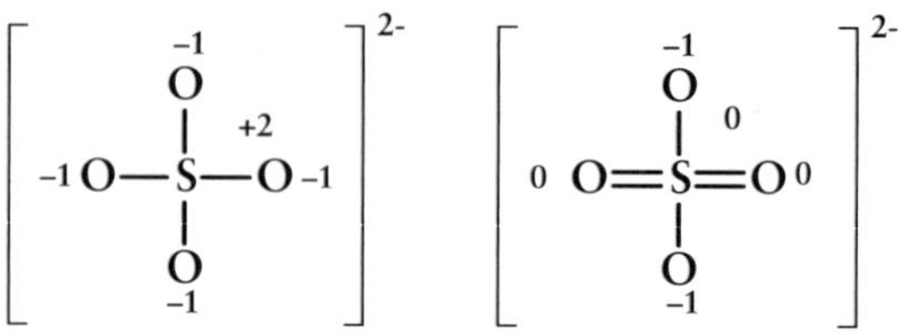

Note

As with all rules, the Octet "rule" has exceptions. It *always* applies to neutral atoms and anions of C, N, O, and F (which are common on the MCAT). It *often* (not always) applies to the halogens and other representative elements, but never applies to H, He, Li, Be, or neutral B and Al. Other notable exceptions are elements beyond period 3 because they have d orbitals (sulfur and phosphorous will be the most common examples seen on Test Day)

Figure 3.1

C. TYPES OF COVALENT BONDING

The nature of a covalent bond depends on the relative electronegativities of the atoms sharing the electron pairs. Covalent bonds are considered to be **polar** or **nonpolar** depending on the difference in electronegativities between the atoms.

1. Polar Covalent Bond

Polar covalent bonding occurs between atoms with small differences in electronegativity, generally in the range of 0.4 to 1.7 Pauling units. The bonding electron pair is not shared equally but pulled more toward the element with the higher electronegativity. As a result, the more electronegative atom acquires a partial negative charge, δ^-, and the less electronegative atom acquires a partial positive charge, δ^+, giving the molecule partially ionic character. For instance, the covalent bond in HCl is polar because the two atoms have a small difference in electronegativity (approximately 0.9). Chlorine, the more electronegative atom, attains a partial negative charge and hydrogen attains a partial positive charge. This difference in charge between the atoms is indicated by an arrow crossed (like a plus sign) at the positive end pointing to the negative end, as shown below:

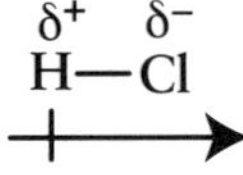

Figure 3.2

TEACHER TIP

Back to that tug of war from earlier, sometimes we can see the winner before the final flag. Here, the chlorine has the flag closer to its side (therefore, a partial negative charge), but it hasn't won the match yet.

A molecule that has such a separation of positive and negative charges is called a polar molecule. The **dipole moment** itself is a vector quantity μ, defined as the product of the charge magnitude (q) and the distance between the two partial charges (r):

$$\mu = qr$$

The dipole moment is denoted by an arrow pointing from the positive to the negative charge, and is measured in Debye units (coulomb-meters).

2. Nonpolar Covalent Bond

Nonpolar covalent bonding occurs between atoms that have the same electronegativities. The bonding electron pair is shared equally, with no separation of charge across the bond. Not surprisingly, nonpolar covalent bonds occur in diatomic molecules such as H_2, Cl_2, O_2, and N_2.

3. Coordinate Covalent Bond

In a coordinate covalent bond, the shared electron pair comes from the lone pair of one of the atoms in the molecule. Once such a bond forms, it is indistinguishable from any other covalent bond. Distinguishing such a bond is useful only in keeping track of the valence electrons and formal charges. Coordinate bonds are typically found in Lewis acid-base compounds (see chapter 10, Acids and Bases). A **Lewis acid** is a compound that can accept an electron pair to form a covalent bond; a **Lewis base** is a compound that can donate an electron pair to form a covalent bond. For example, in the reaction between borontrifluoride (BF_3) and ammonia (NH_3):

TEACHER TIP

In this figure, the nitrogen atom is sharing the electrons that are normally unpaired and so has a positive charge. The boron atom, which normally has an incomplete octet (only six electrons), has more than usual and therefore has a formal negative charge.

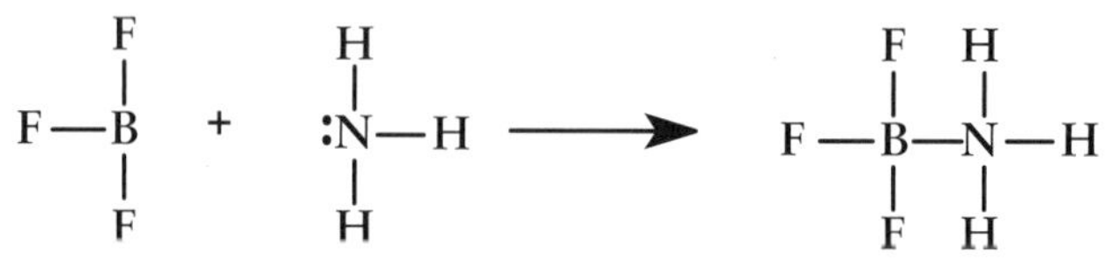

Lewis acid — Lewis base — Lewis acid–base compound

Figure 3.3

NH_3 donates a pair of electrons to form a coordinate covalent bond; thus, it acts as a Lewis base. BF_3 accepts this pair of electrons to form the coordinate covalent bond; thus, it acts as a Lewis acid.

D. GEOMETRY AND POLARITY OF COVALENT MOLECULES

1. The Valence Shell Electron-Pair Repulsion Theory

The valence shell electron-pair repulsion (VSEPR) theory uses Lewis structures to predict the molecular geometry of covalently bonded molecules. It states that the three-dimensional arrangement of atoms surrounding a central atom is determined by the repulsions between the bonding and the nonbonding electron pairs in the valence shell of the central atom. These electron pairs arrange themselves as far apart as possible, thereby minimizing repulsion.

The following steps are used to predict the geometrical structure of a molecule using the VSEPR theory.

- Draw the Lewis structure of the molecule.
- Count the total number of bonding and nonbonding electron pairs in the valence shell of the central atom.
- Arrange the electron pairs around the central atom so that they are as far apart from each other as possible. For example, the compound AX_2 has the Lewis structure, X : A : X. A has two bonding electron pairs in its valence shell. To make these electron pairs as far apart as possible, their geometric structure should be linear,

$$X - A - X$$

Valence electron arrangements are summarized in Table 3.2.

Table 3.2

Regions of Electron Density	Example	Geometric Arrangement of Electron Pairs Around the Central Atom	Shape	Angle between Electron Pairs
2	$BeCl_2$	X – A – X	linear	180°
3	BH_3		trigonal planar	120°
4	CH_4		tetrahedral	109.05°
5	PCl_5		trigonal bipyramidal	90°, 120°, 180°
6	SF_6		octahedral	90°, 180°

Example: Predict the geometry of NH_3.

Solution: 1. The Lewis structure of NH_3 is:

H—N—H (with H above N and a lone pair below N)

2. The central atom, N, has three bonding electron pairs and one nonbonding electron pair, for a total of four electron pairs.

3. The four electron pairs will be farthest apart when they occupy the corners of a tetrahedron. As one of the four electron pairs is a lone pair, the observed geometry is trigonal pyramidal.

TEACHER TIP

Know some of these shapes and angles on Test Day, particularly the tetrahedral shape because it is seen with carbon, nitrogen, and oxygen-common topics in both science sections of the MCAT.

TEACHER TIP

The shapes from Table 3.2 refer to *electronic geometry*, which is different from *molecular geometry*. In Figure 3.4, we see an ammonia molecule, which has a tetrahedral *electronic* structure but is considered to have a *molecular* structure that is trigonal pyramidal. Keep these clear on Test Day.

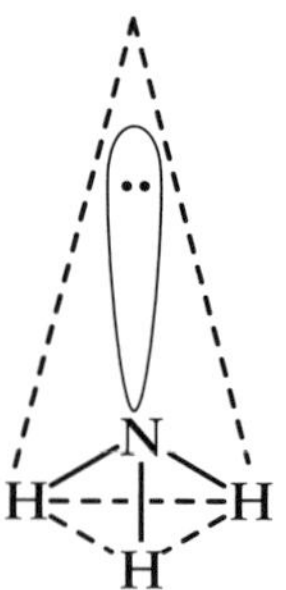

Figure 3.4

In describing the shape of a molecule, only the arrangement of atoms (not electrons) is considered. Even though the electron pairs are arranged tetrahedrally, the shape of NH_3 is pyramidal. It is not trigonal planar because the lone pair repels the three bonding electron pairs, causing them to move as far away as possible.

Example: Predict the geometry of CO_2.

Solution: The Lewis structure of CO_2 is $:\ddot{O}::C::\ddot{O}:$.

The double bond behaves just like a single bond for purposes of predicting molecular shape. This compound has two groups of electrons around the carbon. According to the VSEPR theory, the two sets of electrons will orient themselves 180° apart, on opposite sides of the carbon atom, minimizing electron repulsion. Therefore, the molecular structure of CO_2 is linear: $:\ddot{O}{=}C{=}\ddot{O}:$

MCAT SYNOPSIS

A molecule with polar bonds need not be polar: The bond dipole moments may cancel each other out, resulting in a nonpolar molecule. Although a molecule with polar bonds need not be polar, a polar molecule must have polar bonds.

2. Polarity of Molecules

A molecule with a net dipole moment is called polar, as previously mentioned, because it has positive and negative poles. The polarity of a molecule depends on the polarity of the constituent bonds and on the shape of the molecule. A molecule with nonpolar bonds is always nonpolar; a molecule with polar bonds may be polar or nonpolar depending on the orientation of the bond dipoles.

A molecule of two atoms bound by a polar bond must have a net dipole moment and therefore be polar. The two equal and opposite partial charges are localized at the ends of the molecule on the two atoms. A molecule consisting of more than two atoms bound with polar bonds may be either polar or nonpolar, because the overall dipole moment of a molecule is the vector sum of the individual bond dipole moments. If the molecule has a particular shape such that the bond dipole moments cancel each other, i.e., if the vector sum is zero, then the result is a nonpolar molecule. For instance, CCl_4 has four polar C–Cl bonds. According to the VSEPR theory, the shape of CCl_4 is tetrahedral. The four bond dipoles point to the vertices of the tetrahedron and cancel each other, resulting in a nonpolar molecule.

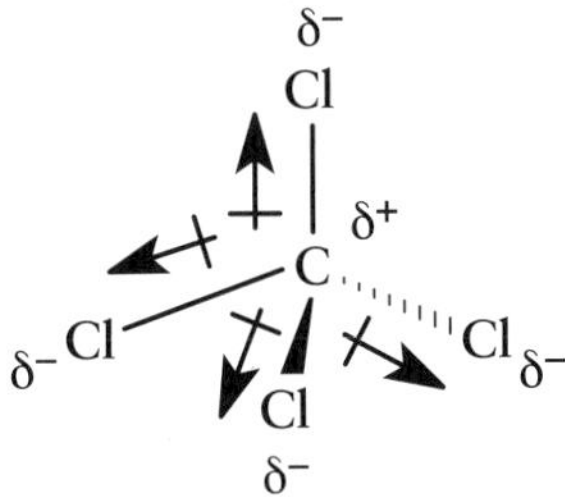

Figure 3.5. No Net Dipole Moment

However, if the orientation of the bond dipoles are such that they do not cancel out, the molecules will have a net dipole moment and therefore be polar. For instance, H_2O has two polar O–H bonds. According to the VSEPR model, its shape is angular. The two dipoles add together to give a net dipole moment to the molecule, making the H_2O molecule polar.

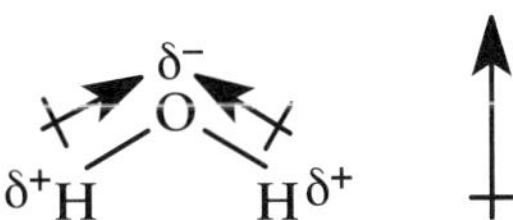

Figure 3.6. Net Dipole Moment

E. ATOMIC AND MOLECULAR ORBITALS

A description of the quantum numbers has already been given in chapter 1. The azimuthal quantum number ℓ describes the orbitals of each n shell. The shapes of these orbitals represent the probability of finding an electron at any given instant. When $\ell = 0$, the orbital is an s-orbital. s-orbitals are spherically symmetric. The 1s-orbital ($n = 1, \ell = 0$) is plotted on the following page.

FLASHBACK

Quantum numbers (chapter 1) revisited:

- For any value of n, there are n values of ℓ ($0 \rightarrow n - 1$).
- $\ell = 0 \rightarrow$ s
  $\ell = 1 \rightarrow$ p
  $\ell = 2 \rightarrow$ d
- For any value of ℓ, there are $2\ell + 1$ values of m_ℓ (number of orbitals); values themselves will range from $-\ell$ to ℓ.

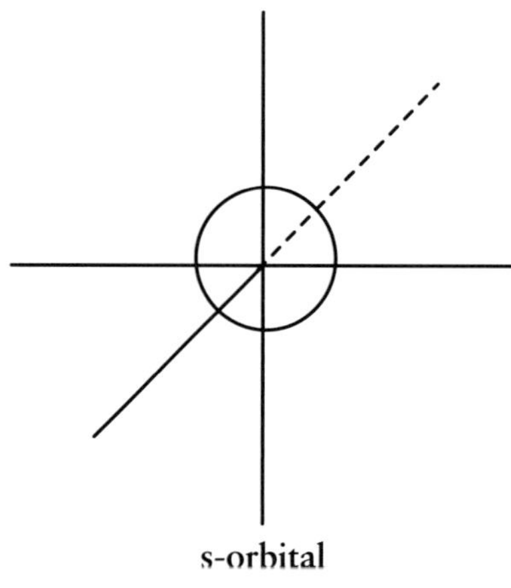

Figure 3.7

When $\ell = 1$, there are three possible orbitals (because the magnetic quantum number, m_ℓ may equal –1, 0, or 1). These are called p-orbitals and have a dumbbell shape. The three p-orbitals, designated p_x, p_y, and p_z, are oriented at right angles to each other; the p_x-orbital is plotted below.

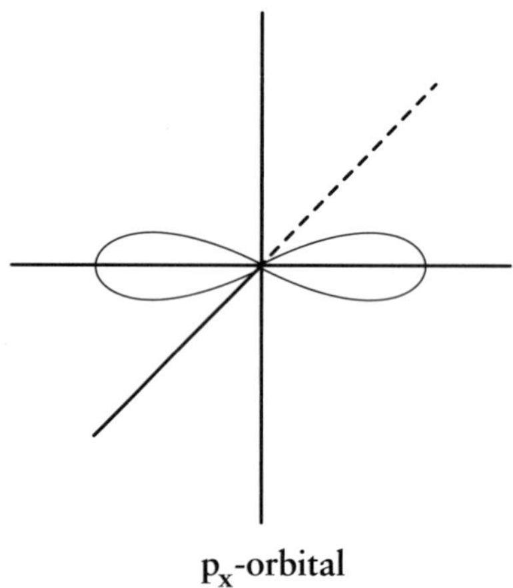

Figure 3.8

Plus and minus signs, determined from the mathematics of the wave function, are assigned to each lobe of the p-orbitals. The shapes of the five d-orbitals ($\ell = 2$, $m_\ell = -2, -1, 0, 1, 2$) and the seven f-orbitals ($\ell = 3$, $m_\ell = -3, -2, -1, 0, 1, 2, 3$) are more complex and need not be memorized.

BRIDGE

It is the pi bonds of alkenes, alkynes, aromatic compounds, and carboxylic acid derivates that lend the functionality so important in organic chemistry.

When two atoms bond to form a molecule, the atomic orbitals interact to form a **molecular orbital** that describes the probability of finding the bonding electrons. Molecular orbitals are obtained by adding the wave functions of the atomic orbitals. Qualitatively, this is described by the **overlap** of two atomic orbitals. If the signs of the two atomic orbitals are the same, a **bonding orbital** is formed. If the signs are different, an

antibonding orbital is formed. In addition, two different types of overlap are possible. When orbitals overlap head-to-head, the resulting bond is called a **sigma** (σ) bond. When the orbitals are parallel, a **pi** (π) bond is formed.

THE INTERMOLECULAR FORCES

The attractive forces that exist between molecules are collectively known as **intermolecular forces.** These include **dipole-dipole interactions, hydrogen bonding,** and **dispersion forces.** Dipole-dipole interactions and dispersion forces are often referred to as **van der Waals forces.**

MCAT SYNOPSIS

These intermolecular forces are the binding forces which keep a substance together in its solid or liquid state (see chapter 8). These same forces determine whether two substances are miscible or immiscible in the solution phase (see chapter 9).

1. Ion-Dipole Interactions

When dipoles are dissolved in solutions where ions are present, ions will arrange themselves with the opposite charged end of the dipole. For example, positive ions will be attracted to and bond with the negative end of the dipole and vice versa.

2. Dipole-Dipole Interactions

Polar molecules tend to orient themselves such that the positive region of one molecule is close to the negative region of another molecule. This arrangement is energetically favorable because an attractive dipole force is formed between the two molecules.

Dipole-dipole interactions are present in the solid and liquid phases but become negligible in the gas phase because the molecules are generally much farther apart. Polar species tend to have higher boiling points than nonpolar species of comparable molecular weight.

3. Hydrogen Bonding

Hydrogen bonding is a specific, unusually strong form of dipole-dipole interaction, which may be either intra- or intermolecular. When hydrogen is bound to a highly electronegative atom such as fluorine, oxygen, or nitrogen, the hydrogen atom carries little of the electron density of the covalent bond. This positively charged hydrogen atom interacts with the partial negative charge located on the electronegative atoms of nearby molecules. Substances that display hydrogen bonding tend to have unusually high boiling points compared with compounds of similar molecular formula that do not hydrogen bond. The difference derives from the energy required to break the hydrogen bonds. Hydrogen bonding is particularly important in the behavior of water, alcohols, amines, and carboxylic acids.

MCAT APPLICATION & REAL-WORLD CORRELATION

While van der Waals forces are the weakest of intermolecular attractions, when there are millions of these interactions like there are on the bottom of a gecko's foot due to many microfibers, there is an amazing power of adhesion that is demonstrated by the animal's ability to climb smooth vertical, even inverted, surfaces.

4. Dispersion Forces

The bonding electrons in covalent bonds may appear to be equally shared between two atoms, but at any particular point in time they will be located randomly throughout the orbital. This permits unequal sharing of electrons, causing rapid polarization and counterpolarization of the electron cloud and formation of short-lived dipoles. These dipoles interact with the electron clouds of neighboring molecules, inducing the formation of more dipoles. The attractive interactions of these short-lived dipoles are called dispersion or **London forces.**

Dispersion forces are generally weaker than other intermolecular forces. They do not extend over long distances and are therefore most important when molecules are close together. The strength of these interactions within a given substance depends directly on how easily the electrons in the molecules can move (i.e., be polarized). Large molecules in which the electrons are far from the nucleus are relatively easy to polarize and therefore possess greater dispersion forces. If it were not for dispersion forces, the noble gases would not liquefy at any temperature because no other intermolecular forces exist between the noble gas atoms. The low temperature at which the noble gases liquefy is to some extent indicative of the magnitude of dispersion forces between the atoms.

PRACTICE QUESTIONS

1. What is the character of the bond in carbon monoxide?

   A. Ionic
   B. Polar covalent
   C. Nonpolar covalent
   D. Coordinate covalent

2. Which of the following molecules has the oxygen atom with the most negative formal charge?

   A. H_2O
   B. CO_3^{2-}
   C. O_3
   D. CH_2O

3. Which of the following are the most important resonance structures for NO_2?

   I. $^{-}$O—N^{+}=O II. O=N^{+}—O^{-} III. $^{-}$O—N^{2+}—O^{-}

   A. I only
   B. II only
   C. I and II only
   D. I, II, and III

4. Order the following compounds shown from lowest to highest boiling point.

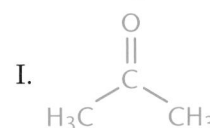

   I. H_3C–C(=O)–CH_3
   II. KCl
   III. Kr
   IV. Isopropyl alcohol

   A. I → II → IV → III
   B. III → IV → I → II
   C. II → IV → I → III
   D. I → IV → II → III

5. What should be changed in the following ClF4- Lewis configuration?

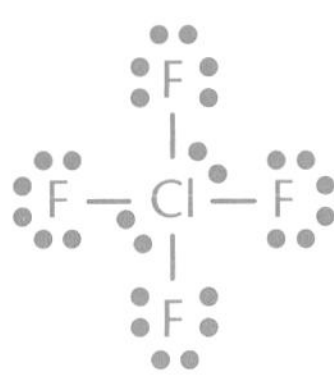

   A. The central chloride atom should have fewer electrons.
   B. The central chloride should carry an additional electron pair.
   C. The central chloride should carry a formal charge of –1.
   D. The central chloride should have a formal charge of –2.

6. Both CO_3^{2-} and ClF_3 have three atoms bonded to a central atom. How would one best explain why CO_3 has trigonal planar geometry, while ClF_3 is trigonal bipyramidal?

   A. CO_3 has multiple resonance structures, while ClF_3 does not.
   B. CO_3 has a charge of –2, while ClF_3 has no charge.
   C. ClF_3 has lone pairs on its central atom, while CO_3 has none.
   D. CO_3 has lone pairs on its central atom, while ClF_3 has none.

7. Which of the following has the largest dipole moment?

   A. HCN
   B. H_2O
   C. CCl_4
   D. SO_2

8. Despite the fact that both C_2H_2 and NCH contain triple bonds, the lengths of these triple bonds are not equal. Which of the following best explains this finding?

A. In C_2H_2, because the triple bond is between similar atoms, it is shorter in length.
B. The two molecules have different resonance structures.
C. Carbon is more electronegative than hydrogen.
D. Nitrogen is more electronegative than carbon.

9. Which of the following best explains the phenomenon of hydrogen bonding?

A. Hydrogen has a strong affinity for holding onto valence electrons.
B. Hydrogen can only hold two valence electrons.
C. Electronegative atoms disproportionately carry shared pairs when bonded to hydrogen.
D. Hydrogen bonds have ionic character.

10. Which of the following best describes the character of the bonds in a molecule of ammonium?

A. Three polar covalent bonds
B. Four polar covalent bonds
C. Two polar covalent bonds, one coordinate covalent bond
D. Three polar covalent bonds, one coordinate covalent bond

11. Although the Octet rule dictates much of molecular structure, some atoms can exceed the Octet rule and be surrounded by more than eight electrons. Some atoms can exceed the Octet rule because they

A. already have eight electrons in their outermost electron shell.
B. do so only when bonding with transition metals.
C. have f-orbitals in which extra electrons can reside.
D. have d-orbitals in which extra electrons can reside.

12. Noble gases can liquefy as a result of

A. van der Waals force.
B. ion-dipole interaction.
C. dispersion force.
D. dipole-dipole interaction.

13. What is correct electron configuration for elemental chromium?

A. [Ar] $3p^6$
B. [Ar] $3d^5$ $4s^1$
C. [Ar] $3d^6$
D. [Ar] $3d^4$ $4s^2$

14. In the structure shown below, which atoms have the most positive charge?

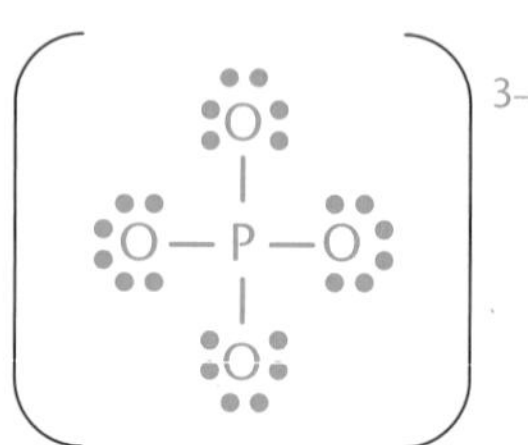

A. Phosphorous atom
B. All atoms equally
C. Four oxygens
D. Oxygen, at the peak of the trigonal pyramidal geometry

15. Which of the following is most characteristic of the bonding of $CaCl_2$?

A. Low melting point
B. No conduction of electricity in liquid state
C. No conduction of electricity in aqueous state
D. No conduction of electricity in solid state

16. The new bond formed in the reaction below is best called a(n)

$$H_2O + H^+ \longrightarrow \left[H{-}\underset{\displaystyle H}{\underset{|}{O}}{-}H \right]^+$$

A. polar covalent bond.
B. ionic bond.
C. coordinate covalent bond.
D. hydrogen bond.

17. Both BF_3 and NH_3 have three atoms bonded to the central atom. Which of the following best explains why the geometry of these two molecules is different?

A. BF_3 has three bonded atoms and no lone pairs, which makes its geometry trigonal pyramidal.
B. NH_3 is sp^3 hybridized, while BF_3 is sp^2 hybridized.
C. NH_3 has one lone pair.
D. BF_3 is nonpolar while NH_3 is polar.

18. Which of the following is a proper Lewis structure for $BeCl_2$?

A. :Cl — Be — Cl: (each Cl with three lone pairs; Be with two lone pairs)

B. :Cl — Be — Cl: (each Cl with three lone pairs)

C. Cl = Be = Cl (each Cl with two lone pairs)

D. :Cl = Be = Cl: (each Cl with three lone pairs)

19. Which of the following best describes an important property of bond energy?

A. Bond energy increases with increasing bond length.
B. The more shared electron pairs comprising a bond, the higher the energy of that bond.
C. Single bonds are more difficult to break than double bonds.
D. Bond energy and bond length are unrelated.

20. Which of the following is true about the polarity of molecules?

A. Polarity is dependent on the vector sum of dipole moments.
B. Polarity does not depend upon molecular geometry.
C. If a molecule is comprised of one or more polar bonds, the molecule is polar.
D. If a molecule is comprised of one or more nonpolar bonds, the molecule is nonpolar.

KEY CONCEPTS

Polarity

Molecular symmetry

Melting points

TAKEAWAYS

Forces that stabilize a molecule more in the solid state than in the liquid state will cause a molecule to have a higher melting point.

THINGS TO WATCH OUT FOR

Be careful not to confuse melting points with boiling points. Remember that in general, symmetry raises melting points, whereas branching lowers them.

SIMILAR QUESTIONS

1) For straight chain alkanes, which do you suppose have higher melting points: alkanes with an odd number of carbons, or those with an even number of alkanes?
2) Which molecule would you expect to melt higher, *n*–pentane or neopentane (2,2–dimethylpropane)? Why?
3) Between phenol (hydroxybenzene) and aniline (aminobenzene), which would melt higher and why?

MELTING POINTS

Arrange the following compounds in order of *increasing* melting point:

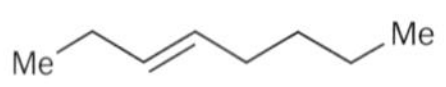

Me Me NH2 Me Me

1 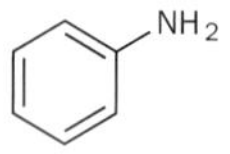 2 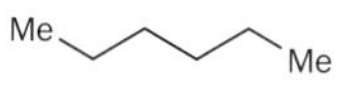 3

O Me NH Me Me

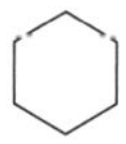

4 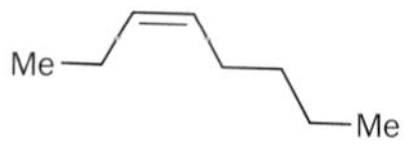 5 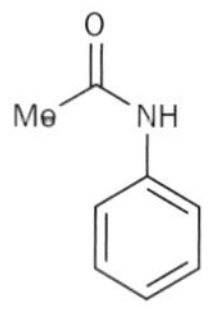 6

1) Separate the compounds by general polarity.

In this series, we can separate the compounds into three groups of two. The alkanes (**3** and **4**) will be the least polar, and therefore will melt the lowest; the alkenes (**1** and **5**) will be in the middle, and the aromatic compounds (**2** and **6**) will melt the highest.

---

2) Examine each grouping for trends in polarity and/or molecular symmetry.

For the lowest melting compounds, notice that cyclohexane has a higher degree of molecular symmetry than does *n*–hexane; this will cause it to melt significantly higher.

With the alkenes, the *trans* alkene has more symmetry than the *cis* alkene because the *cis* alkene has a rather large "kink" in the middle of the chain that prevents it from packing together as well in the crystal, and thus lowers its melting point.

Finally, acetanilide (**6**) is significantly more polar than aniline (**2**) because the amide carbonyl bond is highly polar, causing these molecules to stick together better and consequently raising their melting point.

Therefore, the ordering of the compounds' melting points is as follows:

3 < 4 < 5 < 1 < 2 < 6

Polarity affects melting point just as it does boiling points: more polar molecules melt higher because they tend to stick together better. Molecular symmetry also plays a more prominent role than with boiling point because another consideration is how well molecules pack or "fit together" in the crystal. The more symmetrical a molecule is, the better it packs in the crystal, just like symmetrical puzzle pieces in a jigsaw puzzle fit together better than asymmetrical pieces.

BOILING POINTS

Given the following five molecules, place them in order of increasing boiling point:

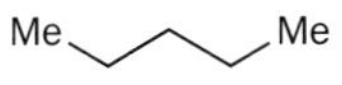

1 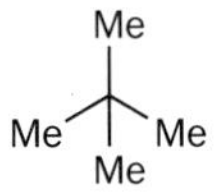 2 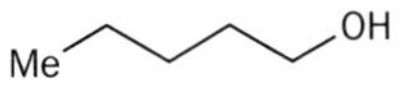 3

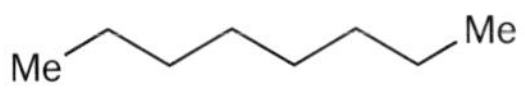

4 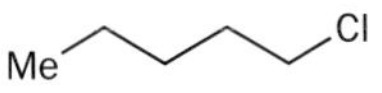 5

1) **Look for unusually heavy molecules.**
Remember that molecular weight is one of the key determinants of boiling point. Something that is extraordinarily heavy is going to be harder to boil than something that is lighter. In this case, all the molecules are in the same general range of molecular weight, so this factor won't help us place the molecules in order.

2) **Look for highly polar functional groups.**
Compounds **3** and **5** are going to have higher-than-usual boiling points. Between compounds **3** and **5**, compound **3** will boil higher because it has a more polar functional group, and also the alcohol is capable of hydrogen bonding. Compound **3** will have hydrogen bonds that are a stronger version of dipole–dipole interactions.

The other factor that affects boiling point is the presence of polar functional groups. These groups help *increase* boiling point because they increase the attractions of molecules for each other.

Remember: *Hydrogen bonding is the strongest type of intermolecular attraction.*

---

3) **Look for the effect of dispersion forces.**
Compound **4** will boil higher than **1**, **2**, and **5** because it is longer (eight carbons versus five, which increases its London Forces); therefore, there are more opportunities for it to attract other molecules of **4**.

Although **1**, **2**, and **5** all have the same surface area, the polar group on **5** gives it a higher boiling point than **1** and **2.**

KEY CONCEPTS

Boiling points

Intermolecular forces

Molecular symmetry

TAKEAWAYS

Remember that there are only two factors that affect relative boiling points between substances: *molecular weight* and *intermolecular forces.*

Things to Watch Out For

Be sure to consider the factors in the order presented here. For example, polarity is more important than size.

Remember: *Dispersion forces are the only kind of intermolecular attractions that cause* ***nonpolar*** *molecules to stick together.*

---

4) Look for trends in the symmetry of molecules.
In this case, pentane, **1**, will boil higher than neopentane, **2.** This is because neopentane is more symmetrical and therefore a more compact molecule; thus, it has a less effective surface area. You can determine this by imagining a "bubble" around each molecule. Neopentane could very easily fit into a spherically shaped bubble, whereas pentane would require an elongated, elliptical bubble with a greater surface area.

If neopentane has a smaller surface area, then there are less opportunities for it to engage in dispersion-type attractions with other molecules of neopentane, making it a lower boiling compound (the actual boiling points are 36.1°C for pentane and 9.4°C for neopentane).

Similar Questions

1) How could you easily alter the structure of compound 3 to lower its boiling point?
2) How could you easily alter the structure of compound 5 to raise its boiling point?

At this point, we're really splitting hairs. Notice that compounds **1** and **2** are merely constitutional isomers of one another. If two molecules have the same weight and are relatively nonpolar, *symmetry* is the factor that decides which one will boil higher.

---

5) Put it all together. Order the compounds as specified by the question.
The ordering of the boiling points will therefore be:

$$\mathbf{2 < 1 < 5 < 4 < 3}$$

CHAPTER 4

COMPOUNDS AND STOICHIOMETRY

A **compound** is a pure substance that is composed of two or more elements in a fixed proportion. Compounds can be broken down chemically to produce their constituent elements or other compounds. All elements, except for some of the noble gases, can react with other elements or compounds to form new compounds. These new compounds can react further to form yet different compounds.

MOLECULES AND MOLES

A **molecule** is a combination of two or more atoms held together by covalent bonds. It is the smallest unit of a compound displaying the properties of that compound. Molecules may contain two atoms of the same element, as in N_2 and O_2, or may be comprised of two or more different atoms, as in CO_2 and $SOCl_2$. Molecules are usually discussed in terms of molecular weights and moles.

MCAT Synopsis

Ionic compounds form from combinations of elements with large electronegativity differences (and far apart on the periodic table), such as sodium with chlorine. Molecular compounds form from the combination of elements of similar electronegativity (or close to each other on the periodic table), such as carbon with oxygen.

Ionic compounds do not form true molecules. In the solid state they can be considered to be a nearly infinite, three-dimensional array of the charged particles of which the compound is composed. Because no actual molecule exists, molecular weight becomes meaningless, and the term **formula weight** is used in its place.

A. MOLECULAR WEIGHT

Like atoms, molecules can be characterized by their weight. The molecular weight is the sum of the atomic weights (in amu) of the atoms in the molecule. Similarly, the formula weight of an ionic compound is found by adding the atomic weights according to the empirical formula of the substance.

Example: What is the molecular weight of $SOCl_2$?

Solution: To find the molecular weight of $SOCl_2$, add together the atomic weights of each of the atoms.

$$1\text{S} = 1 \times 32 \text{ amu} \quad = 32 \text{ amu}$$
$$1\text{O} = 1 \times 16 \text{ amu} \quad = 16 \text{ amu}$$

2Cl = 2 × 35.5 amu	=	<u>71 amu</u>
molecular weight	=	119 amu

MCAT SYNOPSIS

Here we mention Avogadro's number again and can see that the mole is just a unit of convenience, like the dozen is a convenient unit for eggs.

B. MOLE

A mole is defined as the amount of a substance that contains the same number of particles that are found in a 12.000 g sample of carbon-12. This quantity, **Avogadro's number,** is equal to 6.022×10^{23}. One mole of a compound has a mass in grams equal to the molecular weight of that compound in amu, and contains 6.022×10^{23} molecules of the compound. For example, 62 g of H_2CO_3 represents 1 mole of carbonic acid and contains 6.022×10^{23} H_2CO_3 molecules. The mass of 1 mole of a compound is called its **molar weight** or **molar mass,** and is usually expressed as g/mol. Therefore, the molar mass of H_2CO_3 is 62 g/mol.

The following formula is used to determine the number of moles that are present:

$$\text{mol} = \frac{\text{weight of sample (g)}}{\text{molar weight (g/mol)}}$$

Example: How many moles are in 9.52 g of $MgCl_2$?

Solution: First, find the molar mass of $MgCl_2$.

$1(24.31 \text{ g/mol}) + 2(35.45 \text{ g/mol}) = 95.21 \text{ g/mol}$

Now, solve for the number of moles.

$$\frac{9.52}{95.21 \text{ g/mol}} = 0.10 \text{ mol of } MgCl_2$$

C. EQUIVALENT WEIGHT

For some substances, it is useful to define a measure of reactive capacity. This expresses the fact that some molecules are more potent than others in performing certain reactions. An example of this is the ability of different acids to donate protons (H^+ ions) in solution (see chapter 10, Acids and Bases). For instance, one mole of HCl can donate one mol of hydrogen ions, while one mol of H_2SO_4 can donate two moles of hydrogen ions. This difference is expressed using the term **equivalent:** one mole of HCl contains one equivalent of hydrogen ions while one mol of H_2SO_4 contains two equivalents of hydrogen ions. To determine the number of equivalents a compound contains, a new measure of weight called **gram-equivalent weight (GEW)** was developed.

$$\text{equivalents} = \frac{\text{weight of compound}}{\text{gram equivalent weight}}$$

and

$$\text{gram equivalent weight} = \frac{\text{molar mass}}{n}$$

where n is usually either the number of hydrogens used per molecule of acid in a reaction, or the number of hydroxyl groups used per molecule of base in a reaction. This value is strictly dependent on reaction conditions. By using equivalents, it is possible to say that one equivalent of acid will neutralize one equivalent of base, a statement which may not necessarily be true when dealing with moles.

REPRESENTATION OF COMPOUNDS

A. LAW OF CONSTANT COMPOSITION

The **law of constant composition** states that any sample of a given compound will contain the same elements in the identical mass ratio. For instance, every sample of H_2O will contain two atoms of hydrogen for every atom of oxygen, or, in other words, one gram of hydrogen for every eight grams of oxygen.

B. EMPIRICAL AND MOLECULAR FORMULAS

There are two ways to express a formula for a compound. The **empirical formula** gives the simplest whole number ratio of the elements in the compound. The **molecular formula** gives the exact number of atoms of each element in the compound and is usually a multiple of the empirical formula. For example, the empirical formula for benzene is CH, while the molecular formula is C_6H_6. For some compounds, the empirical and molecular formulas are the same, as in the case of H_2O. An ionic compound, such as NaCl or $CaCO_3$, will have only an empirical formula.

C. PERCENT COMPOSITION

The percent composition by mass of an element is the weight percent of the element in a specific compound. To determine the percent composition of an element X in a compound, the following formula is used:

$$\%\ \text{composition} = \frac{\text{mass of} \times \text{in formula}}{\text{Formula weight of compound}} \times 100\%$$

The percent composition of an element may be determined using either the empirical or molecular formula. If the percent compositions are

TEACHER TIP

Percent composition questions are bound to appear on the MCAT. Be sure to know how to simplify them, thereby minimizing calculation errors on Test Day.

known, the empirical formula can be derived. It is possible to determine the molecular formula if both the percent compositions and molecular weight of the compound are known.

Example: What is the percent composition of chromium in $K_2Cr_2O_7$?

Solution: The formula weight of $K_2Cr_2O_7$ is:

$$2(39 \text{ g/mol}) + 2(52 \text{ g/mol}) + 7(16 \text{ g/mol}) = 294 \text{ g/mol}$$

$$\text{Percent composition of Cr} = \frac{2(52 \text{ g/mol})}{294 \text{ g/mol}} = 100$$

$$= 0.354 \times 100$$

$$= 35.4 \text{ percent}$$

Example: What are the empirical and molecular formulas of a compound that contains 40.9 percent carbon, 4.58 percent hydrogen, 54.52 percent oxygen, and has a molecular weight of 264 g/mol?

Method One: First, determine the number of moles of each element in the compound by assuming a 100-gram sample; this converts the percentage of each element present directly into grams of that element. Then convert grams to moles:

$$\#\text{mol of C} = \frac{40.9 \text{ g}}{12 \text{ g/mol}} = 3.41 \text{ mol}$$

$$\#\text{mol of H} = \frac{4.58 \text{ g}}{1 \text{ g/mol}} = 4.58 \text{ mol}$$

$$\#\text{mol of O} = \frac{54.52 \text{ g}}{16 \text{ g/mol}} = 3.41 \text{ mol}$$

Next, find the simplest whole number ratio of the elements by dividing the number of moles by the smallest number obtained in the previous step.

$$\text{C:} \frac{3.41}{3.41} = 1.00 \qquad \text{H:} \frac{4.58}{3.41} = 1.33 \qquad \text{O:} \frac{3.41}{3.41} = 1.00$$

Finally, the empirical formula is obtained by converting the numbers obtained into whole numbers (multiplying them by an integer value).

$$C_1H_{1.33}O_1 \times 3 = C_3H_4O_3$$

$C_3H_4O_3$ is the empirical formula. To determine the molecular formula, divide the molecular weight by the weight represented by the empirical formula. The resultant value is the number of empirical formula units in the molecular formula.

The empirical formula weight of $C_3H_4O_3$ is:

3(12 g/mol) + 4(1 g/mol) + 3(16 g/mol) = 88 g/mol

$$\frac{264 \text{ g/mol}}{88 \text{ g/mol}} = 3$$

$C_3H_4O_3 \times 3 = C_9H_{12}O_9$ is the molecular formula.

Method Two: When the molecular weight is given, it is generally easier to find the molecular formula first. This is accomplished by multiplying the molecular weight by the given percentages to find the grams of each element present in one mole of compound, then dividing by the respective atomic weights to find the mole ratio of the elements:

$$\# \text{ mol of C} = \frac{(0.409)(264) \text{ g}}{12 \text{ g/mol}} = 9 \text{ mol}$$

$$\# \text{ mol of H} = \frac{(0.458)(264) \text{ g}}{1 \text{ g/mol}} = 12 \text{ mol}$$

$$\# \text{ mol of O} = \frac{(0.5452)(264) \text{ g}}{16 \text{ g/mol}} = 9 \text{ mol}$$

Thus the molecular formula, $C_9H_{12}O_9$, is the direct result.

The empirical formula can now be found by reducing the subscript ratio to the simplest integral values.

MCAT SYNOPSIS

The molecular formula is either the same as the empirical formula or a multiple of it. To calculate the molecular formula, you need to know the mole ratio (this will give you the empirical formula) and the molecular weight (molecular wt. ÷ empirical formula wt. will give you the multiplier for the empirical formula → molecular formula conversion).

TYPES OF CHEMICAL REACTIONS

There are many ways in which elements and compounds can react to form other species; memorizing every reaction would be impossible, as well as unnecessary. However, nearly every inorganic reaction can be classified into at least one of four general categories.

MCAT SYNOPSIS

Combination reactions generally have more reactants than products.

$A + B \rightarrow C$

A. COMBINATION REACTIONS

Combination reactions are reactions in which two or more **reactants** form one **product.** The formation of sulfur dioxide by burning sulfur in air is an example of a combination reaction.

$$S(s) + O_2(g) \rightarrow SO_2(g)$$

MCAT Synopsis

Decomposition reactions generally have more product than reactants.
$C \rightarrow A + B$

B. DECOMPOSITION REACTIONS

A **decomposition reaction** is defined as one in which a compound breaks down into two or more substances, usually as a result of heating or electrolysis. An example of a decomposition reaction is the breakdown of mercury (II) oxide (the sign Δ represents the addition of heat).

$$2HgO(s) \xrightarrow{\Delta} 2Hg(l) + O_2(g)$$

MCAT Synopsis

Single displacement reactions are also known as redox reactions.

C. SINGLE DISPLACEMENT REACTIONS

Single displacement reactions occur when an atom (or ion) of one compound is replaced by an atom of another element. For example, zinc metal will displace copper ions in a copper sulfate solution to form zinc sulfate.

$$Zn(s) + CuSO_4(aq) \rightarrow Cu(s) + ZnSO_4(aq)$$

Single displacement reactions are often further classified as **redox** reactions. (These will be discussed in more detail in chapter 11, Redox Reactions and Electrochemistry.)

D. DOUBLE DISPLACEMENT REACTIONS

In double displacement reactions, also called **metathesis reactions,** elements from two different compounds displace each other to form two new compounds. This type of reaction occurs when one of the products is removed from the solution as a precipitate or gas, or when two of the original species combine to form a weak electrolyte that remains undissociated in solution. For example, when solutions of calcium chloride and silver nitrate are combined, insoluble silver chloride forms in a solution of calcium nitrate.

$$CaCl_2(aq) + 2\,AgNO_3(aq) \rightarrow Ca(NO_3)_2(aq) + 2\,AgCl(s)$$

NET IONIC EQUATIONS

Because reactions such as displacements often involve ions in solution, they can be written in ionic form. In the example where zinc is reacted with copper sulfate, the **ionic equation** would be:

$$Zn(s) + Cu^{2+}(aq) + SO_4^{2-}(aq) \rightarrow Cu(s) + Zn^{2+}(aq) + SO_4^{2-}(aq)$$

When displacement reactions occur, there are usually **spectator ions** that do not take part in the overall reaction but simply remain in solution throughout. The spectator ion in the equation above is sulfate, which does not undergo any transformation during the reaction. A **net ionic reaction** can be written showing only the species that actually participate in the reaction:

$$Zn(s) + Cu^{2+}(aq) \rightarrow Cu(s) + Zn^{2+}(aq)$$

Net ionic equations are important for demonstrating the actual reaction that occurs during a displacement reaction.

NEUTRALIZATION REACTIONS

Neutralization reactions are a specific type of double displacement that occur when an acid reacts with a base to produce a solution of a salt and water. For example, hydrochloric acid and sodium hydroxide will react to form sodium chloride and water.

$$HCl(aq) + NaOH(aq) \rightarrow NaCl(aq) + H_2O(\ell)$$

(This type of reaction will be discussed further in chapter 10, Acids and Bases.)

MCAT SYNOPSIS

Acids and bases (which we'll study later in Chapter 10) combine in neutralization reactions to produce salt and water.

BALANCING EQUATIONS

A. BALANCING EQUATIONS

Chemical equations express how much and which type of reactant must be used to obtain a given quantity of product. From the law of conservation of mass, the mass of the reactants in a reaction must be equal to the mass of the products. More specifically, chemical equations must be balanced so that there are the same number of atoms of each element in the products as there are in the reactants. **Stoichiometric coefficients** are used to indicate the number of moles of a given species involved in the reaction. For example, the reaction for the formation of water is:

$$2\ H_2(g) + O_2(g) \rightarrow 2\ H_2O(g)$$

The coefficients indicate that two moles of H_2 gas must be reacted with one mole of O_2 gas to produce two moles of water. In general, stoichiometric coefficients are given as whole numbers.

MCAT FAVORITE

You will rarely need to balance an equation on the MCAT. However, you need to recognize reactions that are or are not balanced.

Look at the:

1) charge of each side; and
2) number of atoms of each element.

MCAT SYNOPSIS

When balancing equations, focus on the least represented elements first, and work your way to the most represented element of the reaction (usually oxygen or hydrogen).

Example: Balance the following reaction.

$$C_4H_{10}(\ell) + O_2(g) \rightarrow CO_2(g) + H_2O(\ell)$$

Solution: First, balance the carbons in reactants and products.

$$C_4H_{10} + O_2 \rightarrow 4\ CO_2 + H_2O$$

Second, balance the hydrogens in reactant and products.

$$C_4H_{10} + O_2 \rightarrow 4\ CO_2 + 5\ H_2O$$

Third, balance the oxygens in the reactants and products.

$$2\ C_4H_{10} + 13\ O_2 \rightarrow 8\ CO_2 + 10\ H_2O$$

Finally, check that all of the elements, and the total charges, are balanced correctly. If there is a difference in total charge between the reactants and products, then the charge will also have to be balanced. (Instructions for balancing charge are found in chapter 11.)

TEACHER TIP

Because the MCAT is a critical-thinking exam, we see many application and analysis questions. It's likely you will see either a limiting reagent or yield question.

B. APPLICATIONS OF STOICHIOMETRY

Once an equation has been balanced, the ratio of moles of reactant to moles of product is known, and that information can be used to solve many types of stoichiometry problems. It is important to use proper units when solving such problems. If and when you are faced with doing the calculations, the units should cancel out, so that the units obtained in the answer represent those asked for in the problem.

Example: How many grams of calcium chloride are needed to prepare 72 g of silver chloride according to the following equation?

$$CaCl_2(aq) + 2AgNO_3(aq) \rightarrow Ca(NO_3)_2(aq) + 2AgCl(s)$$

Solution: Noting first that the equation is balanced, 1 mole of $CaCl_2$ yields 2 moles of AgCl when it is reacted with 2 moles of $AgNO_3$. The molar mass of $CaCl_2$ is 110 g, and the molar mass of AgCl is 144 g.

$$72\text{ g AgCl} \times \frac{1\text{ mol AgCl}}{144\text{ g AgCl}} \times \frac{1\text{ mol CaCl}_2}{2\text{ mol AgCl}} \times \frac{110\text{ g CaCl}_2}{1\text{ mol CaCl}_2}$$

Thus, 27.5 g of $CaCl_2$ are needed to produce 72 g of AgCl.

PAVLOV'S DOG

When the quantities of two reactants are given, you are dealing with a limiting reactant problem.

1. Limiting Reactants

When reactants are mixed, they are seldom added in the exact stoichiometric proportions as shown in the balanced equation. Therefore, in most reactions, one reactant will be consumed first. This reactant is known as the **limiting reactant** because it limits the amount of product that can be formed in the reaction. The reactant that remains after all of the limiting reagent is used is called the **excess reactant.**

Example: If 28 g of Fe react with 24 g of S to produce FeS, what would be the limiting reagent? How many grams of excess reagent would be present in the vessel at the end of the reaction?

The balanced equation is: $Fe + s \xrightarrow{\Delta} FeS$.

Solution: First, determine the number of moles for each reactant.

$$28 \text{ g Fe} \times \frac{1 \text{ mol Fe}}{56 \text{ g}} = 0.5 \text{ mol Fe}$$

$$24 \text{ g S} \times \frac{1 \text{ mol S}}{32 \text{ g}} = 0.75 \text{ mol S}$$

Because 1 mole of Fe is needed to react with 1 mole of S, and there are 0.5 moles Fe for every 0.75 moles S, the limiting reagent is Fe. Thus, 0.5 moles of Fe will react with 0.5 moles of S, leaving an excess of 0.25 moles of S in the vessel. The mass of the excess reagent will be:

$$\text{mass of S} = 0.25 \text{ mol S} \times \frac{32 \text{ g}}{1 \text{ mol S}}$$
$$= 8 \text{ g of S}$$

2. Yields

The **yield** of a reaction, which is the amount of product predicted or obtained when the reaction is carried out, can be determined or predicted from the balanced equation. There are three distinct ways of reporting yields. The **theoretical yield** is the amount of product that can be predicted from a balanced equation, assuming that all of the limiting reagent has been used, that no competing side reactions have occurred, and that all of the product has been collected. The theoretical yield is seldom obtained; therefore, chemists speak of the **actual yield,** which is the amount of product that is isolated from the reaction experimentally.

The term **percent yield** is used to express the relationship between the actual yield and the theoretical yield and is given by the following equation:

$$\text{percent yield} = \frac{\text{actual yield}}{\text{theoretical yield}} \times 100\%$$

Example: What is the percent yield for a reaction in which 27 g of Cu is produced by reacting 32.5 g of Zn in excess $CuSO_4$ solution?

Solution: The balanced equation is as follows:

$$Zn(s) + CuSO_4(aq) \rightarrow Cu(s) + ZnSO_4(aq)$$

Calculate the theoretical yield for Cu.

$$32.5 \text{ g Zn} \times \frac{1 \text{ mol Zn}}{65 \text{ g}} = 0.5 \text{ mol Zn}$$

$$0.5 \text{ mol Zn} \times \frac{1 \text{ mol Cu}}{1 \text{ mol Zn}} = 0.5 \text{ mol Cu}$$

$$0.5 \text{ mol Cu} \times \frac{64 \text{ g}}{1 \text{ mol Cu}} = 32 \text{ g Cu} = \text{theoretical yield}$$

Finally, determine the percent yield.

$$\frac{27 \text{ g}}{32 \text{ g}} \times 100\% = 84\%$$

MCAT SYNOPSIS

When we are given excess of one reagent on the MCAT, we know that the other reactant is the limiting reagent.

PRACTICE QUESTIONS

1. Ionic compounds are

   A. formed from molecules containing two or more atoms.
   B. formed from charged particles and are measured by molecular weight.
   C. formed from charged particles, which share electrons equally.
   D. three-dimensional arrays of charged particles.

2. Which of the following has a formula weight between 74 and 75 grams per mole?

   A. KCl
   B. $C_4H_{10}O$
   C. $[LiCl]_2$
   D. BF_3

3. Which of the following is the gram equivalent weight of H_2SO_4?

   A. 98.08 g/mol
   B. 49.04 g/mol
   C. 196.2 g/mol
   D. 147.1 g/mol

4. Which of the following molecules CANNOT be expressed by the empirical formula CH?

   A. Benzene
   B. Ethyne
   C. $H_2C=C=CH_2$
   D. [structure: vinyl group attached to benzene ring]

5. In which of the following compounds is the percent composition of carbon closest to 63?

   A. Acetone
   B. Ethanol
   C. C_3H_8
   D. Methanol

6. Calcium carbonate and aluminum nitrate react in solution, as demonstrated by the following reactants shown below. Which of the following answer choices best completes the equation?

   $CaCO_3(s) + Al(NO_3)_3(aq) \longrightarrow$ __________

   A. $3CaCO_3 + Al(NO_3)_3 \longrightarrow 3CaNO_3 + Al(CO_3)_3$
   B. $CaCO_3 + 2Al(NO_3)_3 \longrightarrow Ca(NO_3)_6 + Al_2CO_3$
   C. $2CaCO_3 + Al(NO_3)_3 \longrightarrow 2CaNO_3 + Al_2(CO_3)_3$
   D. $3CaCO_3 + 2Al(NO_3)_3 \longrightarrow 3Ca(NO_3)_2 + Al_2(CO_3)_3$

7. Single displacements are chemical reactions which

   A. typically have more reactants than products.
   B. typically have more products than reactants.
   C. are often redox reactions.
   D. typically have aqueous reactants and solid products.

8. What is the most accurate characterization of the following reaction shown below?

$Ca(OH)_2(aq) + H_2SO_4(aq) \longrightarrow CaSO_4(aq) + H_2O(l)$

A. Single displacement
B. Neutralization
C. Double displacement
D. Redox

9. In the following reaction, if 39.03 g of Na_2S is reacted with 113.3 g of $AgNO_3$, how much, if any, of either reagent will be left over once the reaction has gone to completion?

$Na_2S + 2\ AgNO_3 \longrightarrow Ag_2S + 2\ NaNO_3$

A. 41.37 g $AgNO_3$
B. 13.00 g Na_2S
C. 14.16 g Na_2S
D. 74.27 g $AgNO_3$

10. How would one calculate the mass of oxygen produced in the following reaction shown below, assuming it goes to completion?

$2\ KClO_3 \longrightarrow 2\ KCl + 3\ O_2$

A. $\dfrac{(\text{grams } KClO_3 \text{ consumed})(3 \text{ moles } O_2)(\text{molar mass } O_2)}{(\text{molar mass } KClO_3)(2 \text{ moles } KClO_3)}$

B. $\dfrac{(\text{grams } KClO_3 \text{ consumed})(\text{molar mass } O_2)}{(\text{molar mass } KClO_3)(2 \text{ moles } KClO_3)}$

C. $\dfrac{(\text{molar mass } KClO_3)(2 \text{ moles } KClO_3)}{(\text{grams } KClO_3 \text{ consumed})(\text{molar mass } O_2)}$

D. $\dfrac{(\text{grams } KClO_3 \text{ consumed})(3 \text{ moles } O_2)}{(\text{molar mass } KClO_3)(2 \text{ moles } KClO_3)(\text{molar mass } O_2)}$

11. Aluminum metal can be used to remove tarnish from silver when the two solid metals are placed in water, according to the following reaction. Which of the following describe this reaction?

$2\ AgO + 2\ Al \longrightarrow 3\ Ag + Al_2O_3$

I. Double displacement reaction
II. Single displacement reaction
III. Redox reaction
IV. Combination reaction

A. II only
B. IV only
C. II and III
D. I, II, and III

12. The following reaction is an example of the combustion of glucose to yield carbon dioxide, water, and heat. If 10 grams of glucose is reacted with excess oxygen, what is the approximate volume of liquid water that will be produced? Assume the density of water is similar to the density of water at room temperature.

$C_6H_{12}O_6 + 6\ O_2 \longrightarrow 6\ CO_2 + 6\ H_2O + \text{heat}$

A. 0.6 milliliters
B. 0.1 milliliters
C. 1 milliliter
D. 6 milliliters

13. Several samples of water are taken: one from the product of a combustion reaction, one from solid ice, and a final sample in the liquid phase. Which of the following would best explain why all three samples have the molecular formula H_2O?

A. Constant composition
B. Empirical formula
C. Percent composition
D. Steady-state

14. Which of the following reaction types generally have the same number of reactants and products?

I. Single displacement reaction
II. Double displacement reaction
III. Combination reaction

A. I only
B. II only
C. I and II
D. I, II, and III

15. Which of the following is the correct net ionic reaction for the reaction of copper with silver nitrate?

A. $Cu + AgNO_3 \longrightarrow Cu(NO_3)_2 + Ag$

B. $Cu + 2\ Ag^+ + NO_3^- \longrightarrow Cu^{2+} + 2\ NO_3^- + 2\ Ag^+$

C. $2\ Ag^+ + 2\ NO_3^- \longrightarrow 2\ NO_3^- + 2\ Ag$

D. $Cu + 2\ Ag^+ \longrightarrow Cu^{2+} + 2\ Ag$

16. In the process of photosynthesis, carbon dioxide and water are combined with energy to form glucose and oxygen, according to the equation shown below. What is the theoretical yield, in grams, of glucose if 30 grams of water is reacted with excess carbon dioxide and energy, in the balanced equation?

$$CO_2 + H_2O + \text{Energy} \longrightarrow C_6H_{12}O_6 + O_2$$

A. 50.02 grams glucose
B. 300.1 grams glucose
C. 30.03 grams glucose
D. 1801 grams glucose

17. One way to test for the presence of iron in solution is to add potassium thiocyanate to the solution. The resulting product is $FeSCN^{2+}$, which creates a dark red color in solution via the following net ionic equation shown below. How many grams of iron sulfate would be needed to produce 2 moles of $FeSCN^{2+}$?

$$Fe^{3+}(aq) + SCN^- \longrightarrow FeSCN^{2+}$$

A. 400 grams
B. 800 grams
C. 200 grams
D. 500 grams

CHAPTER 5

CHEMICAL KINETICS AND EQUILIBRIUM

When studying a chemical reaction, it is important to consider not only the chemical properties of the reactants, but also the **conditions** under which the reaction occurs, the **mechanism** by which it takes place, the rate at which it occurs, and the **equilibrium** (or steady state) toward which it proceeds.

CHEMICAL KINETICS

Chemical kinetics is the study of the rates of reactions, the effect of reaction conditions on these rates, and the mechanisms implied by such observations.

REACTION MECHANISMS

The **mechanism** of a reaction is the actual series of steps through which a chemical reaction occurs. Knowing the accepted mechanism of a reaction often helps to explain the reaction's rate, position of equilibrium, and thermodynamic characteristics (see chapter 6). Consider the reaction below:

TEACHER TIP

Mechanisms are proposed pathways for a reaction that must coincide with rate data information from experimental observation. This is also addressed in Organic Chemistry.

Overall reaction: $A_2 + 2\,B \rightarrow 2\,AB$

This equation seems to imply a mechanism in which two molecules of B collide with one molecule of A_2 to form two molecules of AB. But suppose instead that the reaction actually takes place in two steps.

Step 1:	$A_2 + B \rightarrow A_2B$	(Slow)
Step 2:	$A_2B + B \rightarrow 2\,AB$	(Fast)

Note that these two steps add up to the overall (net) reaction. A_2B, which does not appear in the overall reaction because it is neither a reactant nor a product, is called an **intermediate.** Reaction intermediates are often difficult to detect, but a proposed mechanism can be supported through kinetic experiments.

REAL-WORLD ANALOGY

The slowest step is rate determining because it holds up the whole process. An analogy is an assembly line where the rate of production is determined by the slowest person or step.

The slowest step in a proposed mechanism is called the **rate-determining step,** because the overall reaction cannot proceed faster than that step.

REACTION RATES

A. DEFINITION OF RATE

Consider a reaction 2A + B → C, in which one mole of C is produced from every two moles of A and one mole of B. The rate of this reaction may be described in terms of either the disappearance of reactants over time, or the appearance of products over time.

$$\text{rate} = \frac{\text{decrease in concentration of reactions}}{\text{time}} = \frac{\text{increase in concentration of products}}{\text{time}}$$

Because the concentration of a reactant decreases during the reaction, a minus sign is placed before a rate that is expressed in terms of reactants. For the reaction above, the rate of reaction with respect to A is $-\Delta[A]/\Delta t$, with respect to B is $-\Delta[B]/\Delta t$, and with respect to C is $\Delta[C]/\Delta t$. In this particular reaction, the three rates are not equal. According to the stoichiometry of the reaction, A is used up twice as fast as B ($-\frac{1}{2}\Delta[A]/\Delta t = -\Delta[B]/\Delta t$), and A is consumed twice as fast as C is produced ($-\frac{1}{2}\Delta[A]/\Delta t = \Delta[C]/\Delta t$). To show a standard rate of reaction in which the rates with respect to all substances are equal, the rate for each substance should be divided by its stoichiometric coefficient.

$$\text{rate} = -\frac{1}{2}\frac{\Delta[A]}{\Delta t} = -\frac{\Delta[B]}{\Delta t} = \frac{\Delta[C]}{\Delta t}$$

In general, for the reaction

$$a\,A + b\,B \rightarrow c\,C + d\,D,$$

$$\text{rate} = -\frac{1}{a}\frac{\Delta[A]}{\Delta t} = -\frac{1}{b}\frac{\Delta[B]}{\Delta t} = \frac{1}{c}\frac{\Delta[C]}{\Delta t} = \frac{1}{d}\frac{\Delta[D]}{\Delta t}$$

Rate is expressed in the units of moles per liter per second (mol/L × sec) or molarity per second (molarity/sec).

B. RATE LAW

For nearly all forward, irreversible reactions, the rate is proportional to the product of the concentrations of the reactants, each raised to some power. For the general reaction

$$a\,A + b\,B \rightarrow c\,C + d\,D$$

the rate is proportional to $[A]^x [B]^y$, that is:

$$rate = k [A]^x [B]^y$$

This expression is the **rate law** for the general reaction above, where k is the **rate constant.** Multiplying the units of k by the concentration factors raised to the appropriate powers gives the rate in units of concentration/time. The exponents x and y are called the **orders of reaction;** x is the order with respect to A and y is the order with respect to B. These exponents may be integers, fractions, or zero, and must be determined experimentally.

MCAT SYNOPSIS

The exponents in the rate law are not equal to the stoichiometric coefficients unless the reaction actually occurs via a single step mechanism. Also note that product concentrations never appear in a rate law. Many students confuse the rate law with the equilibrium expression.

It is important to note that the exponents of the rate law are *not* necessarily equal to the stoichiometric coefficients in the overall reaction equation. (The exponents *are* equal to the stoichiometric coefficients of the rate-determining step. If one of the reactants or products in this step is an intermediate not included in the overall reaction, then calculating the rate law in terms of the original reactants is more complex.)

MCAT FAVORITE

The stoichiometric coefficients for the overall reaction will most likely be different from those for the rate-determining step, and will therefore not be the same as the order of the reaction

The **overall order of a reaction** (or the **reaction order**) is defined as the sum of the exponents, here equal to x + y.

1. Experimental Determination of Rate Law

The values of k, x, and y in the rate law equation (rate = $k [A]^x [B]^y$) must be determined experimentally for a given reaction at a given temperature. The rate is usually measured as a function of the **initial concentrations** of the reactants, A and B.

Example: Given the data below, find the rate law for the following reaction at 300 K.

$$A + B \rightarrow C + D$$

Trial	$[A]_{initial}$(M)	$[B]_{initial}$(M)	$r_{initial}$(M/sec)
1	1.00	1.00	2.0
2	1.00	2.00	8.1
3	2.00	2.00	15.9

Solution: First, look for two trials in which the concentrations of all but one of the substances are held constant.

a) In trials 1 and 2, the concentration of A is kept constant while the concentration of B is doubled. The rate increases by a factor of 8.1/2.0, approximately 4. Write down the rate expression of the two trials.

MCAT FAVORITE

Traditionally, the MCAT has loved rate problems. With practice, you'll be able to do these quickly in your head with minimal paper and pencil calculations. Remember to look for pairs of reaction trials in which the concentration of only one species changes, while the other(s) remains constant.

Trial 1: $r_1 = k[A]^x [B]^y = k(1.00)^x (1.00)^y$

Trial 2: $r_2 = k[A]^x [B]^y = k(1.00)^x (2.00)^y$

Divide the second equation by the first.

$$\frac{r_2}{r_1} = \frac{8.1}{2.0} = \frac{k\,(1.00)^x\,(2.00)^y}{k\,(1.00)^x\,(1.00)^y} = (2.00)^y$$

$$4 = (2.00)^y$$

$$y = 2$$

b) In trials 2 and 3, the concentration of B is kept constant while the concentration of A is doubled; the rate is increased by a factor of 15.9/8.1, approximately 2. The rate expressions of the two trials are:

Trial 2: $r_2 = k(1.00)^x (2.00)^y$

Trial 3: $r_3 = k(2.00)^x (2.00)^y$

Divide the second equation by the first.

$$\frac{r_3}{r_2} = \frac{15.9}{8.1} = \frac{k\,(2.00)^x\,(2.00)^y}{k\,(1.00)^x\,(2.00)^y} = (2.00)^y$$

$$2 = (2.00)^y$$

$$x = 1$$

So $r = k[A]\,[B]^2$

The order of the reaction with respect to A is 1 and with respect to B is 2; the overall reaction order is 1 + 2 = 3.

To calculate k, substitute the values from any one of the above trials into the rate law, e.g.:

$$2.0\text{ M/sec} = k \times 1.00\text{ M} \times (1.00\text{ M})^2$$

$$k = 2.0\text{ M}^{-2}\text{ sec}^{-1}$$

Therefore, the rate law is $r = 2.0\text{ M}^{-2}\text{ sec}^{-1}\,[A][B]^2$.

MCAT SYNOPSIS

Temperature is the only factor that can change the rate of a zero-order reaction.

C. REACTION ORDERS

Chemical reactions are often classified on the basis of kinetics as zero-order, first-order, second-order, mixed-order, or higher-order reactions. The general reaction $a\,A + b\,B \rightarrow c\,C + d\,D$ will be used in the discussion next.

1. Zero-Order Reactions

A zero-order reaction has a constant rate, which is independent of the reactants' concentrations. Thus the rate law is: rate = k, where k has units of $Msec^{-1}$. An increase in temperature or a decrease in temperature is the only factor that can change the rate of a zero-order reaction.

2. First-Order Reactions

A first-order reaction (order = 1) has a rate proportional to the concentration of one reactant.

$$\text{rate} = k[A] \text{ or rate} = k[B]$$

First-order rate constants have units of sec^{-1}.

The classic example of a first-order reaction is the process of radioactive decay. The concentration of radioactive substance A at any time t can be expressed mathematically as

$$[A_t] = [A_o]\, e^{-kt}$$

where $[A_o]$ = initial concentration of A
$[A_t]$ = concentration of A at time t
k = rate constant
t = elapsed time

The half-life ($t_{1/2}$) of a reaction is the time needed for the concentration of the radioactive substance to decrease to one-half of its original value. Half-lives can be calculated from the rate law as follows:

$$t_{1/2} = \ln 2/k = 0.693/k$$

where k is the first order rate constant.

3. Second-Order Reactions

A second-order reaction (order = 2) has a rate proportional to the product of the concentration of two reactants, or to the square of the concentration of a single reactant; for example, rate = $k[A]^2$, rate = $k[B]^2$, or rate = $k[A][B]$. The units of second-order rate constants are $M^{-1}\ sec^{-1}$.

4. Higher-Order Reactions

A higher-order reaction has an order greater than 2.

5. Mixed-Order Reactions

A mixed-order reaction has a fractional order; e.g., rate = $k[A]^{1/3}$.

D. EFFICIENCY OF REACTIONS

1. Collision Theory of Chemical Kinetics

In order for a reaction to occur, molecules must collide with each other. The **collision theory of chemical kinetics** states that the rate of a reaction is proportional to the number of collisions per second between the reacting molecules.

Not all collisions, however, result in a chemical reaction. An **effective collision** (one that leads to the formation of products) occurs only if the molecules collide with correct orientation and sufficient force to break the existing bonds and form new ones. The minimum energy of collision necessary for a reaction to take place is called the **activation energy, E_a,** or the **energy barrier.** Only a fraction of colliding particles have enough kinetic energy to exceed the activation energy. This means that only a fraction of all collisions are effective. The rate of a reaction can therefore be expressed as:

$$\text{rate} = fZ$$

where Z is the total number of collisions occurring per second and f is the fraction of collisions that are effective.

TEACHER TIP

Because the transition state structure is at the highest energy state, it is only a theoretical structure and cannot be isolated. We can still use the proposed structures, however, to better understand the reactions in which they are involved.

2. Transition State Theory

When molecules collide with sufficient energy, they form a **transition state,** in which the old bonds are weakened and the new bonds are beginning to form. The transition state then dissociates into products, and the new bonds are fully formed. For a reaction $A_2 + B_2 \rightarrow 2\,AB$, the change along the reaction coordinate (a measure of the extent to which the reaction has progressed from reactants to products; see Figures 5.1 and 5.2) can be represented as follows:

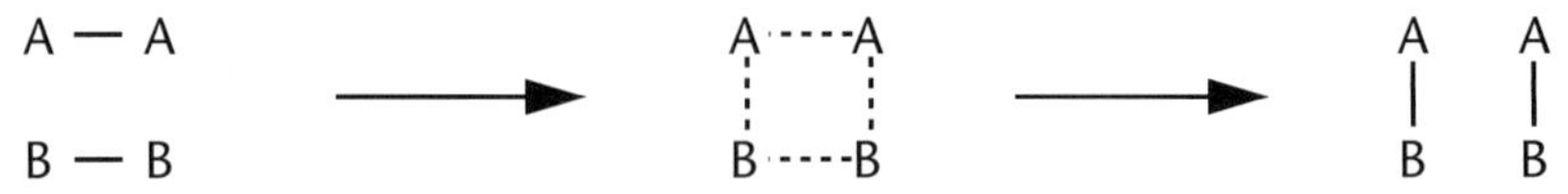

```
A — A                A····A              A   A
          ——→        :    :    ——→       |   |
B — B                B····B              B   B
```

Figure 5.1

The **transition state,** also called the **activated complex,** has greater energy than either the reactants or the products and is denoted by the symbol ‡. The activation energy is required to bring the reactants to this energy level. Once an activated complex is formed, it can either dissociate into the products or revert to reactants without any additional energy input. Transition states are distinguished from intermediates in that, existing as they do at energy maxima, transition states do not have a finite lifetime.

A **potential energy diagram** illustrates the relations among the activation energy, the heats of reaction, and the potential energy of the system. The most important factors in such diagrams are the *relative* energies of the products and reactants. The **enthalpy change** of the reaction (**ΔH**) is the difference between the potential energy of the products and the potential energy of the reactants (see chapter 6). A negative enthalpy change indicates an exothermic reaction (where heat is given off) and a positive enthalpy change indicates an endothermic reaction (where heat is absorbed). The activated complex exists at the top of the energy barrier. The difference in potential energies between the activated complex and the reactants is the activation energy of the forward reaction; the difference in potential energies between the activated complex and the products is the activation energy of the reverse reaction.

MCAT Synopsis

$-\Delta H$ = exothermic = heat given off
$+\Delta H$ = endothermic = heat absorbed

For example, consider the formation of HCl from H_2 and Cl_2. The following figure, which gives the energy profile of the reaction

$$H_2 + Cl_2 \rightleftarrows 2\ HCl$$

shows that the reaction is exothermic. The potential energy of the products is less than the potential energy of the reactants; heat is evolved, and the heat of reaction is negative.

MCAT Synopsis

Note that the potential energy of the product can be raised or lowered, thereby changing the value of ΔH, without affecting the value of E_{act} forward, i.e., kinetics and thermodynamics are separate considerations.

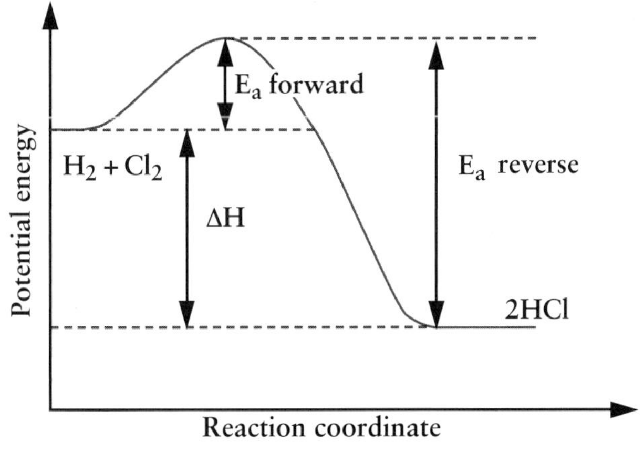

Figure 5.2

The thermodynamic properties of reactions are discussed further in chapter 6.

E. FACTORS AFFECTING REACTION RATE

The rate of a chemical reaction depends upon the individual species undergoing reaction, and upon the reaction environment. The rate of reaction will increase if either of the following occurs: an increase in the number of effective collisions, or a stabilization of the activated complex compared with the reactants.

TEACHER TIP

We know that, in many reactions, when we change the concentrations of reaction, the rate will generally increase. But be aware of the order of the reaction in each of the reactants before making this leap.

1. Reactant Concentrations

The greater the concentrations of the reactants (the more particles per unit volume), the greater will be the number of effective collisions per unit time, and therefore the reaction rate will increase for all but zero-order reactions. For reactions occurring in the gaseous state, the partial pressures of the reactants can serve as a measure of concentration (see chapter 7).

2. Temperature

For nearly all reactions, the reaction rate will increase as the temperature of the system increases. Because the temperature of a substance is a measure of the particles' average kinetic energy, increasing the temperature increases the average kinetic energy of the molecules. Consequently, the proportion of molecules having energies greater than E_a (thus capable of undergoing reaction) increases with higher temperature.

3. Medium

The rate of a reaction may also be affected by the medium in which it takes place. Certain reactions proceed more rapidly in aqueous solution, whereas other reactions may proceed more rapidly in benzene. The state of the medium (liquid, solid, or gas) can also have a significant effect.

4. Catalysts

Catalysts are substances that increase reaction rate without themselves being consumed; they do this by lowering the activation energy. Catalysts are important in biological systems and in industrial chemistry; enzymes are biological catalysts. Catalysts may increase the frequency of collision between the reactants, change the relative orientation of the reactants making a higher percentage of collisions effective, donate electron density to the reactants, or reduce intramolecular bonding within reactant molecules. Figure 5.3 compares the energy profiles of catalyzed and uncatalyzed reactions.

The energy barrier for the catalyzed reaction is much lower than the energy barrier for the uncatalyzed reaction. Note that the rates of both the forward and the reverse reactions are increased by catalysis, because E_a of the forward and reverse reactions are lowered by the same amount. Therefore, the presence of a catalyst causes the reaction to proceed more quickly toward equilibrium.

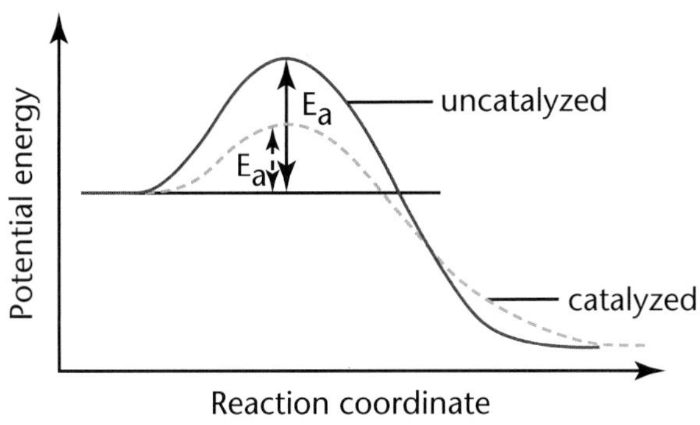

Figure 5.3

EQUILIBRIUM

THE DYNAMIC CONCEPT OF EQUILIBRIUM

So far, reaction rates have been discussed under the assumption that the reactions were **irreversible** (i.e., only proceeded in one direction), and that the reactions proceeded to completion. However, a **reversible** reaction often does not proceed to completion, because (by definition) the products can react to reform the reactants. This is particularly true of reactions occurring in closed systems, where products are not allowed to escape. When there is no **net** change in the concentrations of the products and reactants during a reversible chemical reaction, equilibrium exists. This is not to say that a reaction in equilibrium is static; change continues to occur in both the forward and reverse directions. Equilibrium can be thought of as a balance between the two reaction directions.

TEACHER TIP

Like homeostasis in Biology, equilibrium is a dynamic process that seeks to find balance in all systems. We can use this concept to our advantage in all four of the basic sciences. Remember that these are dynamic processes and are defined by no *net* change, or equal and opposite "forces" rather than a stagnant state.

Consider the following reaction:

$$A \rightleftarrows B$$

At equilibrium, the concentrations of A and B are constant, yet the reactions $A \rightarrow B$ and $B \rightarrow A$ continue to occur at equal rates.

LAW OF MASS ACTION

Consider the following *one-step* reaction:

$$2A \rightleftarrows B + C$$

Because the reaction occurs in one step, the rates of the forward and reverse reaction are given by:

$$\text{rate}_f = k_f[A]^2 \text{ and } \text{rate}_r = k_r[B][C]$$

When $rate_f = rate_r$, equilibrium is achieved. Because the rates are equal, it can be stated that

$$k_f[A]^2 = k_r[B][C] \text{ or } \frac{k_f}{k_r} = \frac{[B][C]}{[A]^2}$$

Because k_f and k_r are both constants, this equation may be rewritten:

$$K_c = \frac{[B][C]}{[A]^2} \text{ (see below for general equation)}$$

MCAT SYNOPSIS

For most purposes you will not need to distinguish between different K values. For dilute solutions, $K_{eq} \approx K_c$ and is calculated in terms of concentration.

where K_c is called the **equilibrium constant,** and the subscript c indicates that it is in terms of concentration (when dealing with gases, the equilibrium constant is referred to as K_p, and the subscript p indicates that it is in terms of pressure). For dilute solutions, K_c and K_{eq} are used interchangeably; the symbol K is also often used, although it is not completely correct to do so.

When the forward and reverse reaction rates are equal at equilibrium, the molar concentrations of the reactants and products usually are not equal. This means that the forward and reverse rate constants, k_f and k_r, are also usually unequal. For the *one-step* reaction described above:

$$k_f[A]^2 = k_r[B][C]$$

$$k_f = k_r \frac{[B][C]}{[A]^2}$$

In a reaction of more than one step, the equilibrium constant for the overall reaction is found by multiplying the equilibrium constants for each step of the reaction. When this is done, the equilibrium constant for the overall reaction is equal to the concentrations of products divided by reactants in the overall reaction, each raised to its stoichiometric coefficient.

The forward and reverse rate constants for any step n are designated k_n and k_{-n} respectively. For example, if the reaction

$$a\,A + b\,B \rightleftarrows c\,C + d\,D$$

occurs in three steps, then

$$K_c = \frac{k_1 k_2 k_3}{k_{-1} k_{-2} k_{-3}} \text{ will equal } \frac{[C]^c[D]^d}{[A]^a[B]^b}$$

This expression is known as the **Law of Mass Action.**

Example: What is the expression for the equilibrium constant for the following reaction?

$$3\ H_2\ (g) + N_2\ (g) \rightleftarrows 2\ NH_3\ (g)$$

Solution: $K_c = \dfrac{[NH_3]^2}{[H_2]^3[N_2]}$

The **reaction quotient,** Q, is a measure of the degree to which a reaction has gone to completion. Q_c is equal to

$$\frac{[C]^c[D]^d}{[A]^a[B]^b}$$

Q_c is a constant only at equilibrium, when it is equal to K_c.

PROPERTIES OF THE EQUILIBRIUM CONSTANT

The equilibrium constant, K_{eq}, has the following characteristics:

- Pure solids and liquids do not appear in the equilibrium constant expression.
- K_{eq} is characteristic of a given system at a given temperature.
- If the value of K_{eq} is very large compared to 1, an equilibrium mixture of reactants and products will contain very little of the reactants compared to the products.
- If the value of K_{eq} is very small compared to 1 (i.e., less than 0.1), an equilibrium mixture of reactants and products will contain very little of the products compared to the reactants.
- If the value of K_{eq} is close to 1, an equilibrium mixture of products and reactants will contain approximately equal amounts of reactants and products.

MCAT SYNOPSIS

Remember our earlier warning about an oft-confused issue dealing with reaction coefficients and rate laws? Well, here the coefficients *ARE* equal to the exponents in the equilibrium expression. On Test Day, if the reaction is balanced, then the equilibrium expression should just about write itself on your scratch paper.

LE CHÂTELIER'S PRINCIPLE

The French chemist Henry Louis Le Châtelier stated that a system to which a stress is applied tends to change so as to relieve the applied stress. This rule, known as **Le Châtelier's principle,** is used to determine the direction in which a reaction at equilibrium will proceed when subjected to a stress, such as a change in concentration, pressure, temperature, or volume.

A. CHANGES IN CONCENTRATION

Increasing the concentration of a species will tend to shift the equilibrium away from the species that is added to reestablish its equilibrium concentration, and vice versa. For example, in the reaction:

$$A + B \rightleftarrows C + D$$

if the concentration of A and/or B is increased, the equilibrium will shift toward (or favor production of) C and D. Conversely, if the concentration of C and/or D is increased, the equilibrium will shift away from the production of C and D, favoring production of A and B. Similarly, decreasing the concentration of a species will tend to shift the equilibrium toward the production of that species. For example, if A and/or B is removed from the above reaction, the equilibrium will shift so as to favor increasing concentration of A and B.

MCAT FAVORITE

LeChâtelier's principle applies to a wide variety of systems and as such, appears in many disguises in both MCAT science sections.

This effect is often used in industry to increase the yield of a useful product or drive a reaction to completion. If D were constantly removed from the above reaction, the net reaction would produce more D and concurrently more C. Likewise, using an excess of the least expensive reactant would help to drive the reaction forward.

B. CHANGE IN PRESSURE OR VOLUME

In a system at constant temperature, a change in pressure causes a change in volume, and vice versa. Because liquids and solids are practically incompressible, a change in the pressure or volume of systems involving only these phases has little or no effect on their equilibrium. Reactions involving gases, however, may be greatly affected by changes in pressure or volume, Because gases are highly compressible.

BRIDGE

Remember the equation:

$CO_2 + H_2O \rightarrow HCO_3^- + H^+$

In the tissues, there is a lot of CO_2 and the reaction shifts to the right. In the lungs, CO_2 is lost and the reaction shifts to the left. Note that blowing off CO_2 (hyperventilation) is used as a mechanism of dealing with acidosis (excess H^+).

Pressure and volume are inversely related. An increase in the pressure of a system will shift the equilibrium so as to decrease the number of moles of gas present. This reduces the volume of the system and relieves the stress of the increased pressure. Consider the following reaction:

$$N_2(g) + 3\ H_2(g) \rightleftarrows 2\ NH_3(g)$$

The left side of the reaction has four moles of gaseous molecules, whereas the right side has only two moles. When the pressure of this system is increased, the equilibrium will shift so that the side of the reaction producing fewer moles is favored. Because there are fewer moles on the right, the equilibrium will shift toward the right. Conversely, if the volume of the same system is increased, its pressure immediately decreases, which, according to Le Châtelier's principle, leads to a shift in the equilibrium to the left.

C. CHANGE IN TEMPERATURE

Changes in temperature also affect equilibrium. To predict this effect, heat may be considered as a product in an exothermic reaction and as a reactant in an endothermic reaction. Consider the following exothermic reaction:

$$A \rightleftarrows B + \text{heat}$$

If this system were placed in an ice bath, its temperature would decrease, driving the reaction to the right to replace the heat lost. Conversely, if the system were placed in a boiling-water bath, the reaction equilibrium would shift to the left because of the increased "concentration" of heat.

Not only does a temperature change alter the position of the equilibrium, it also alters the numerical value of the equilibrium constant. In contrast, changes in the concentration of a species in the reaction, in the pressure, or in the volume, will alter the position of the equilibrium without changing the numerical value of the equilibrium constant.

MCAT SYNOPSIS

$$A + B \rightleftarrows C + \text{heat}$$

will shift to Ⓡ	will shift to Ⓛ
• If more A or B is added	• If more C is added
• If C is taken away	• If A or B is taken away
• If pressure is applied or volume reduced (assuming A, B, and C gases)	• If pressure is reduced or volume increased (assuming A, B, and C gases)
• If temperature is reduced	• If temperature is increased

PRACTICE QUESTIONS

1. In a third-order reaction involving two reactants and two products, doubling the concentration of the first reactant causes the rate to increase by a factor of 2. If the concentration of the second reactant is cut in half, the rate of this reaction will

   A. increase by a factor of 2.
   B. increase by a factor of 4.
   C. decrease by a factor of 2.
   D. decrease by a factor of 4.

2. In a certain equilibrium process, the activation energy of the forward reaction is greater than the activation energy of the reverse reaction. What type of reaction is this?

   A. Endothermic
   B. Exothermic
   C. Spontaneous
   D. Nonspontaneous

3. The volume of a gas is increased without changing the overall number of molecules present in the system. For this system, which of the following statements is always true?

   A. Pressure decreases and temperature increases.
   B. Pressure decreases or temperature increases.
   C. If temperature decreases, then pressure decreases.
   D. If pressure decreases, then temperature decreases.

4. Carbonated beverages are produced by dissolving carbon dioxide in water to produce carbonic acid:

   $$CO_2(g) + H_2O(l) \rightleftarrows H_2CO_3(aq)$$

   When a bottle containing carbonated water is opened, the taste of the beverage gradually changes until all of the carbonation is lost. Which of the following statements best explains this phenomenon?

   A. The change in pressure and volume causes the reaction to shift to the left, thereby decreasing the amount of aqueous carbonic acid.
   B. The change in pressure and volume causes the reaction to shift to the right, thereby decreasing the amount of gaseous carbon dioxide.
   C. Carbonic acid reacts with environmental oxygen and nitrogen.
   D. Carbon dioxide reacts with environmental oxygen and nitrogen.

5. A certain chemical reaction is endothermic. It occurs spontaneously. Which of the following must be true for this reaction?

   I. $\Delta H > 0$
   II. $\Delta G < 0$
   III. $\Delta S > 0$

   A. I only
   B. I and II only
   C. II and III only
   D. I, II, and III

6. A certain ionic salt, A_3B, has a molar solubility of 10 M at a certain temperature. What is the K_{sp} of this salt at the same temperature?

A. 10^4
B. 3×10^4
C. 2.7×10^5
D. 8.1×105

7. Acetic acid dissociates in solution according to the equation, $CH_3COOH \Leftrightarrow CH_3COO^- + H^+$. If sodium acetate is added to a solution of acetic acid in excess water, what effect would be observed?

A. Decreased Ph
B. Increased Ph
C. Decreased pK_a
D. Increased pK_a

8. A certain chemical reaction follows the rate law, rate = k $[NO_2]$ $[Br_2]$. Which of the following statements describe the kinetics of this reaction?

I. The reaction is second-order.
II. The amount of NO_2 consumed is equal to the amount of Br_2 consumed.
III. The rate will not be affected by the addition of a compound other than NO_2 and Br_2.

A. I only
B. III only
C. I and II only
D. I, III, and III

9. The data in the following table is collected for the combustion of the theoretical compound XH_4: $XH_4 + 2O_2 \rightarrow XO_2 + 2H_2O$. What is the rate law for the reaction described?

Trial	$[XH_4]_{initial}$ (M)	$[O_2]_{initial}$ (M)	Rate (M/min)
1	0.6	0.6	12.4
2	0.6	2.4	49.9
3	1.2	2.4	198.3

A. Rate = k $[XH_4]$ $[O_2]$
B. Rate = k $[XH_4]$ $[O_2]^2$
C. Rate = k $[XH_4]^2$ $[O_2]$
D. Rate = k $[XH_4]^2$ $[O_2]^2$

10. A solution is prepared with an unknown concentration of a theoretical compound whose K_a is exactly 1. What is the pH of this solution?

A. Higher than 7
B. Exactly 7
C. Lower than 7
D. Impossible to determine

11. Which of the following actions does NOT affect the rate of a reaction?

A. Adding/subtracting heat
B. Increasing/decreasing activation energy
C. Increasing/decreasing concentration of reactants
D. Increasing/decreasing volume of reactants

12. In a sealed 1 L container, 1 mol of nitrogen gas reacts with 3 mol of hydrogen gas to form 0.05 mol of NH_3. Which of the following is closest to the K_{eq} of the reaction?

A. 0.0001
B. 0.001
C. 0.01
D. 0.1

FOR QUESTIONS 13–15, CONSIDER THE ENERGY DIAGRAM SHOWN BELOW.

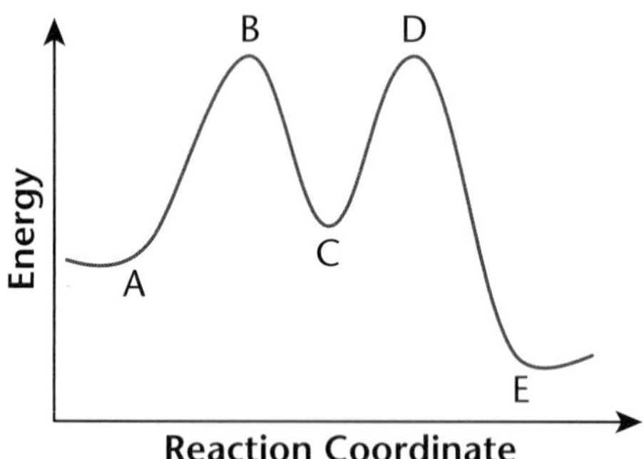

13. The overall reaction depicted by this energy diagram is

A. endothermic, because point B is higher than point A.
B. endothermic, because point C is higher than point A.
C. exothermic, because point D is higher than point E.
D. exothermic, because point A is higher than point E.

14. What process has the highest activation energy?

A. The first step of the forward reaction
B. The first step of the reverse reaction
C. The second step of the forward reaction
D. The second step of the reverse reaction

15. Which of the following components of the reaction mechanism will never be present in the reaction vessel when the reaction coordinate is at point B?

A. Reactants
B. Products
C. Intermediates
D. Catalysts

16. Consider the following two reactions. If K_{eq} for reaction 1 is equal to 0.1, what is K_{eq} for reaction 2?

$3A + 2B \leftrightharpoons 3C + 4D$ (Reaction 1)
$4D + 3C \leftrightharpoons 3A + 2B$ (Reaction 2)

A. 0.1
B. 1
C. 10
D. 100

17. Which of the following statements would best describe the experimental result if the temperature of the following theoretical reaction were decreased?

$A + B \leftrightharpoons C + D$ $\Delta H = -1.12$ kJ/mol

A. [C] + [D] would increase.
B. [A] + [B] would increase.
C. ΔH would increase.
D. ΔH would decrease.

18. Compound A has a K_a of approximately 10^{-4}. Which of the following compounds is most likely to react with a solution of compound A?

A. HNO_2
B. NO_2
C. NH_3
D. N_2O_5

19. The following system obeys second-order kinetics:

$2NO_2 \rightarrow NO_3 + NO$ (slow)
$NO_3 + CO \rightarrow NO_2 + CO2$ (fast)
What is the rate law for this reaction?

A. Rate = k $[NO_2]$ [CO]
B. Rate = k $[NO_2]^2$ [CO]
C. Rate = k $[NO_2]$ $[NO_3]$
D. Rate = k $[NO_2]^2$

20. The potential energy diagram below represents four different reactions. Assuming identical conditions, which of the reactions displayed proceeds the fastest?

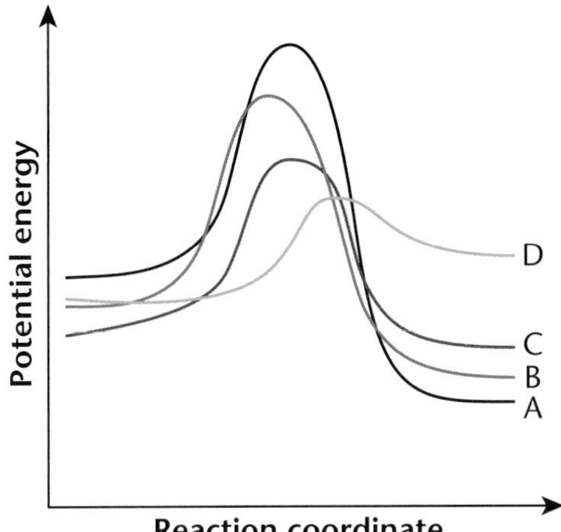

A. A
B. B
C. C
D. D

KEY CONCEPTS

Kinetics

Reaction mechanisms

Rate law

RATE LAW FROM EXPERIMENTAL RESULTS

Consider the nitration reaction of benzene, an example of electrophilic aromatic substitution:

HNO_2 + [benzene] ⟶ [nitrobenzene, NO_2]

The rate data below were collected with the nitration of benzene carried out at 298 K. From this information, determine the rate law for this reaction.

Trial	$[C_6H_6]$ (M)	$[HNO_2]$ (M)	Initial Rate ($M \cdot s^{-1}$)
1	1.01×10^{-3}	2×10^{-2}	5.96×10^{-6}
2	4.05×10^{-3}	2×10^{-2}	5.96×10^{-6}
3	3.02×10^{-3}	6.01×10^{-2}	5.4×10^{-5}

TAKEAWAYS

Remember that the rate constant k depends only on temperature.

A shortcut to determine order is to use the following relation when you find two trials where one reagent's concentration changes, but all other concentrations are constant:

Change in rate = (Proportional change in concentration)^x, where x = the order with respect to that reagent.

1) Write down the general form of the rate law.

Rate = $k[C_6H_6]^x[HNO_2]^y$

Remember: *The general form of the rate law must include a constant, k, that is multiplied by the concentrations of each of the reactants raised to a certain power.*

---

2) Determine the order of the reaction with respect to each reactant.

$$\frac{\text{Rate of trial 2}}{\text{Rate of trial 1}} = \frac{k[C_6H_6]_2^{\,x}[HNO_2]_2^{\,y}}{k[C_6H_6]_1^{\,x}[HNO_2]_1^{\,y}}$$

$$\frac{\text{Rate of trial 2}}{\text{Rate of trial 1}} = \left(\frac{k[C_6H_6]_2}{k[C_6H_6]_1}\right)^x \left(\frac{[HNO_2]_2}{[HNO_2]_1}\right)^y$$

$$\frac{5.96 \times 10^{-6}}{5.96 \times 10^{-6}} = \left(\frac{4.05 \times 10^{-3}}{1.01 \times 10^{-3}}\right)^x \left(\frac{2 \times 10^{-2}}{2 \times 10^{-2}}\right)^y$$

$$\frac{\text{Rate of trial 3}}{\text{Rate of trial 1}}=\left(\frac{[HNO_2]_3}{[HNO_2]_1}\right)^y$$

$$\left(\frac{5.4\times10^{-5}}{5.96\times10^{-6}}\right)=\left(\frac{6.01\times10^{-2}}{2.01\times10^{-2}}\right)^y$$

$$\left(\frac{54\times10^{-6}}{6\times10^{-6}}\right)=\left(\frac{6\times10^{-2}}{2\times10^{-2}}\right)^y$$

Choose two trials in which the concentration of one reagent is changing, but the other is not. Take the *ratio* of these two trials and set up an equation.

Cancel the rate constants because they are equal to each other. Collect terms raised to the same exponent together.

Plug and chug. Substitute numbers from the rate data table into the equation.

$1 = 4^x$

The term raised to the y power disappears because 1 raised to any power equals 1. The only way that 4^x can equal 1 is if $x = 0$.

To determine the order with respect to HNO_2, note that there are no two trials in which the concentration of benzene stays the same. However, this does not matter, because the reaction is zero order with respect to benzene.

Plug in numbers from the table as before.

Simplify the numbers to make them easy to handle. Note that 5.40×10^{-5} is the same thing as 54.0×10^{-6}.

$9 = 3^y$

The only way this equation can be true is if $y = 2$.

---

3) Write down the rate law with the correct orders.

Rate = $k[C_6H_6]^0[HNO_2]^2 = k[HNO_2]^2$

THINGS TO WATCH OUT FOR

Make sure that initially you select two trials where *one reagent's concentration* changes, but *all other concentrations are constant*. Otherwise, you won't come out with the correct rate law!

SIMILAR QUESTIONS

1) What is the value of the rate constant *k* for the original reaction above? What are its units?

2) Given the data below, determine the rate law for the reaction of pyridine with methyl iodide. Find the rate constant *k* for this reaction and its units. Use the rate law to determine what type of reaction this is.

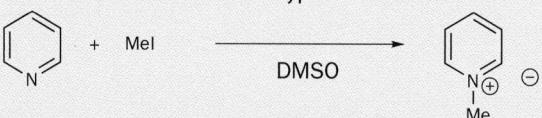

Trial	$[C_5H_5N]$ (M)	[MeI] (M)	Initial Rate (M s^{-1})
1	1×10^{-4}	1×10^{-4}	7.5×10^{-7}
2	2×10^{-4}	2×10^{-4}	3×10^{-6}
3	2×10^{-4}	4×10^{-4}	6×10^{-6}

3) Cerium(IV) is a common inorganic oxidant. Determine the rate law for the following reaction and compute the value of the rate constant *k* along with its units.

$Ce^{4+} + Fe^{2+} \rightarrow Ce^{3+} + Fe^{3+}$

Trial	$[Ce4^{+}]$ (M)	$[Fe^{2+}]$ (M)	Initial Rate (M s^{-1})
1	1.1×10^{-5}	1.8×10^{-5}	2×10^{-7}
2	1.1×10^{-5}	2.8×10^{-5}	3.1×10^{-7}
3	3.4×10^{-5}	2.8×10^{-5}	9.5×10^{-7}

RATE LAW FROM REACTION MECHANISMS

Often, changing the medium of a reaction can have a dramatic effect on its mechanism. In the gas phase, HCl reacts with propene according to the following reaction mechanism:

Step 1: $HCl + HCl \rightleftharpoons H_2Cl_2$ (fast, equilibrium)

Step 2: $HCl + CH_3CHCH_2 \rightleftharpoons CH_3CHClCH_3{}^*$ (fast, equilibrium)

Step 3: $CH_3CHClCH_3{}^* + H_2Cl_2 \rightarrow CH_3CHClCH_3 + 2\ HCl$ (slow)
where CH_3CHCH_2 is propene and $CH_3CHClCH_3{}^*$ represents an excited state of 2–chloropropane.
Based on these reaction steps, derive the rate law for this reaction.

1) Identify the slow step in the reaction and write down the rate law expression for that step.

Rate = $k_3[CH_3CHClCH_3{}^*][H_2Cl_2]$

---

2) If intermediates exist in the rate law from step 1, use prior steps to solve for their concentration and eliminate them from the rate law.

$k_1[HCl]^2 = k_{-1}[H_2Cl_2]$

$[H_2Cl_2] = \frac{k_1}{k_{-1}}[HCl]^2$

$k_2[HCl][CH_3CHCH_2] = k_{-2}[CH_3CHClCH_3{}^*]$

$[CH_3CHClCH_3{}^*] = \frac{k_2}{k_{-2}}[HCl][CH_3CHCH_2]$

$$\text{rate} = \left[k_3[\frac{k_2}{k_{-2}}[HCl][CH_3CHCH_2]][\frac{k_1}{k_{-1}}HCl]^2\right]$$

Here, we are taking advantage of the fact that step 1 of the mechanism is in equilibrium; therefore, the rates of the forward and reverse reactions are equal.

Solve for the concentration of H_2Cl_2, one of the intermediates from above.

Step 2 from the mechanism is also in equilibrium, so the rates of the forward and reverse reactions are equal.

Solve for the intermediate, as above.

KEY CONCEPTS

Equilibrium

Rate laws

Reaction mechanisms

TAKEAWAYS

With reaction mechanisms, the goal is to eliminate the concentrations of intermediates because they are usually high-energy species that exist only briefly.

SIMILAR QUESTIONS

1) What are the units of the rate in the original question? Based on this, what must the units of k_{obs} be for this reaction?
2) How does this rate law differ from the one that you might expect if this reaction were to be carried out in solution, instead of in the gas phase?
3) How would the key intermediates differ between this reaction in the gas phase and in solution?

THINGS TO WATCH OUT FOR

In this case, you may assume that the stoichiometric coefficients of each reactant are equal to the order. When you are presented with rate data, you *may not* make this assumption but must use the rate data to determine order.

Plug the concentrations into the rate law for the slow step.

Remember: *Intermediates are assumed to exist for only a brief period of time because they are produced in one step and consumed in another. Therefore, their concentration cannot be measured, and so they* ***must*** *be eliminated from the rate law.*

---

3) Combine constants and simplify the rate law.

$$\text{rate} = \left[\frac{k_1k_2k_3}{k_{-1}k_{-2}}\right][\text{HCl}][\text{CH}_3\text{CHCH}_2][\text{HCl}]^2]$$

$$\text{rate} = k_{obs}[\text{HCl}]^3[\text{CH}_3\text{CHCH}_2],$$

$$\text{where } k_{obs} = \frac{k_1k_2k_3}{k_{-1}k_{-2}}$$

Combine all of the constants and concentrations.

Remember: *A constant times a constant times a constant, and so on, is just another constant.*

CHAPTER 6

THERMOCHEMISTRY

All chemical reactions are accompanied by energy changes. Thermal, chemical, potential, and kinetic energies are all interconvertible, as they must obey the **Law of Conservation of Energy.** Energy changes determine whether reactions can occur and how easily they will do so, thus an understanding of **thermodynamics** is essential to an understanding of chemistry. In chemistry, thermodynamics help determine whether a chemical reaction is **spontaneous,** i.e., if under a given set of conditions it can occur, by itself, without outside assistance. A spontaneous reaction may or may not proceed to completion, depending upon the rate of the reaction, which is determined by chemical kinetics (see chapter 5).

The application of thermodynamics to chemical reactions is called **thermochemistry.** Several thermodynamic definitions are very useful in thermochemistry. A **system** is the particular part of the universe being studied; everything outside the system is considered the **surroundings** or **environment.** A system may be:

- **isolated**—when it cannot exchange energy or matter with the surroundings, as with an insulated bomb reactor;
- **closed**—when it can exchange energy but not matter with the surroundings, as with a steam radiator;
- **open**—when it can exchange both matter and energy with the surroundings, as with a pot of boiling water.

A system undergoes a **process** when one or more of its properties changes. A process is associated with a change of state. An **isothermal** process occurs when the temperature of the system remains constant; an **adiabatic** process occurs when no heat exchange occurs; and an **isobaric** process occurs when the pressure of the system remains constant. Isothermal and isobaric processes are common, because it is usually easy to control temperature and pressure.

MCAT SYNOPSIS

Remember that heat and temperature are different; heat is a specific form of energy that can leave or enter a system, while temperature is a measure of the average kinetic energy of the particles in a system.

HEAT

A. DEFINITION

Heat is a form of energy that can easily transfer to or from a system, the result of a temperature difference between the system and its surroundings; this transfer will occur spontaneously from a warmer system to a cooler system. According to convention, heat absorbed by a system (from its surroundings) is considered positive, while heat lost by a system (to its surroundings) is considered negative.

Heat change is the most common energy change in chemical processes. Reactions that absorb heat energy are said to be **endothermic,** while those that release heat energy are said to be **exothermic.** Heat is commonly measured in **calories (cal),** or **joules (J),** and more commonly in kcal or kJ (1 cal = 4.184 J).

MCAT SYNOPSIS

Endothermic is positive +
Exothermic is negative –

B. CALORIMETRY

Calorimetry measures heat changes. The terms **constant-volume calorimetry** and **constant-pressure calorimetry** are used to indicate the conditions under which the heat changes are measured. The heat (**q**) absorbed or released in a given process is calculated from the equation:

$$q = mc\Delta T$$

where m is the mass, c is the **specific heat.** Thermodynamics), and ΔT is the change in temperature.

KAPLAN EXCLUSIVE

Ever notice how the equation for heat spells out the name of the test you are preparing for?

Constant-Volume Calorimetry

In constant-volume calorimetry, the volume of the container holding the reacting mixture does not change during the course of the reaction. The heat of reaction is measured using a device called a bomb calorimeter. This apparatus consists of a steel bomb into which the reactants are placed. The bomb is immersed in an insulated container containing a known amount of water. The reactants are electrically ignited and heat is absorbed or evolved as the reaction proceeds. The heat of the reaction, q_{rxn}, can be determined as follows. Because no heat enters or leaves the system, the net heat change for the system is zero; therefore, the heat change for the reaction is compensated for by the heat change for the water and the bomb, which is easy to measure.

$$q_{system} = q_{rxn} + q_{water} + q_{steel} = 0$$

$$\text{Thus: } q_{rxn} = -(q_{water} + q_{steel}) = -(m_{water}\, c_{water}\, \Delta T + m_{steel}\, c_{steel}\, \Delta T)$$

MCAT FAVORITE

You can only calculate $q = mc\Delta T$ when there is no phase change.

Note that the overall system, as defined, is adiabatic, because no net heat gain or loss occurs. However, the heat exchange between the various components makes it possible to determine the heat of reaction.

STATES AND STATE FUNCTIONS

The state of a system is described by the macroscopic properties of the system. Examples of macroscopic properties include temperature (T), pressure (P), and volume (V). When the state of a system changes, the values of the properties also change. Properties whose magnitude depends only on the initial and final states of the system, and not on the path of the change (how the change was accomplished), are known as **state functions.** Pressure, temperature, and volume are important state functions. Other examples are **enthalpy (H), entropy (S), free energy (G)** (all discussed below), and **internal energy (E** or **U)**. Although independent of path, state functions are not necessarily independent of one another.

A set of **standard conditions** (25°C and 1 atm) is normally used for measuring the enthalpy, entropy, and free energy of a reaction. A substance in its most stable form under standard conditions is said to be in its **standard state.** Examples of substances in their standard states include hydrogen as $H_2(g)$, water as H_2O (ℓ), and salt as NaCl (*s*). The changes in enthalpy, entropy, and free energy that occur when a reaction takes place under standard conditions are called the **standard enthalpy, standard entropy,** and **standard free energy** changes respectively, and are symbolized by $\Delta H°$, $\Delta S°$, and $\Delta G°$.

MCAT SYNOPSIS

Standard conditions in thermodynamics must not be confused with standard temperature and pressure (STP) in gas law calculations. (See chapter 7.)

A. ENTHALPY

Most reactions in the lab occur under constant pressure (at 1 atm, in open containers). To express heat changes at constant pressure, chemists use the term **enthalpy (H).** The change in enthalpy (ΔH) of a process is equal to the heat absorbed or evolved by the system at constant pressure. The enthalpy of a process depends only on the enthalpies of the initial and final states, *not* on the path. Thus to find the enthalpy change of a reaction, ΔH_{rxn}, one must subtract the enthalpy of the reactants from the enthalpy of the products:

$$\Delta H_{rxn} = H_{products} - H_{reactants}$$

A positive ΔH corresponds to an endothermic process, and a negative ΔH corresponds to an exothermic process.

Unfortunately, it is not possible to measure H directly; only ΔH can be measured, and even then, only for certain fast and spontaneous processes. Thus several standard methods have been developed to calculate ΔH for any process.

1. Standard Heat of Formation

The enthalpy of formation of a compound, ΔH°_f, is the enthalpy change that would occur if one mole of a compound were formed directly from its elements in their standard states. Note that ΔH°_f of an element in its standard state is zero. The ΔH°_f of most known substances is tabulated.

2. Standard Heat of Reaction

The standard heat of a reaction, ΔH°_{rxn}, is the hypothetical enthalpy change that would occur if the reaction were carried out under standard conditions; i.e., when reactants in their standard states are converted to products in their standard states at 298K. It can be expressed as:

$$\Delta H^\circ_{rxn} = (\text{sum of } \Delta H^\circ_f \text{ of products}) - (\text{sum of } \Delta H^\circ_f \text{ of reactants})$$

Teacher Tip

The concept of state functions and the idea of path independence is important. Applying Hess's law is a common MCAT topic.

3. Hess's Law

Hess's law states that enthalpies of reactions are additive. When thermochemical equations (chemical equations for which energy changes are known) are added to give the net equation for a reaction, the corresponding heats of reaction are also added to give the net heat of reaction. Because enthalpy is a state function, the enthalpy of a reaction does not depend on the path taken but depends only on the initial and final states. For example, consider the reaction:

$$Br_2(\ell) \rightarrow Br_2(g) \quad \Delta H = (31 \text{ kJ/mol})(1 \text{ mol}) = 31 \text{ kJ}$$

The enthalpy change of the above reaction, called the **heat of vaporization, ΔH°_{vap},** will always be 31 kJ/mol provided that the same initial and final states, $Br_2(\ell)$ and $Br_2(g)$ respectively, exist at standard conditions. $Br_2(\ell)$ could instead be decomposed to Br atoms and then recombined to form $Br_2(g)$, but because the net reaction is the same, the change in enthalpy will always be the same.

$$\begin{array}{lll} Br_2(\ell) & \rightarrow 2\,Br(g) & \Delta H_1 \\ 2\,Br(g) & \rightarrow Br_2(g) & \Delta H_2 \\ \hline \end{array}$$
$$Br_2(\ell) \rightarrow Br_2(g) \ \Delta H = \Delta H_1 + \Delta H_2 = 31 \text{ kJ}$$

Example: Given the following thermochemical equations:

a) $C_3H_8(g) + 5\ O_2(g) \rightarrow 3\ CO_2(g) + 4\ H_2O(\ell)$ $\quad \Delta H_a = -2220.1$ kJ

b) C (*graphite*) + $O_2(g) \rightarrow CO_2(g)$ $\quad \Delta H_b = -393.5$ kJ

c) $H_2(g) + 1/2\ O_2(g) \rightarrow H_2O(l)$ $\quad \Delta H_c = -285.8$ kJ

Calculate ΔH for the reaction:

d) 3 C(*graphite*) + $4\ H_2(g) \rightarrow C_3H_8(g)$

Solution: Equations a, b, and c must be combined to obtain equation d. Because equation d contains only C, H_2, and C_3H_8, we must eliminate O_2, CO_2, and H_2O from the first three equations. Equation a is reversed to get C_3H_8 on the product side (this gives equation e).

Next, equation b is multiplied by 3 (this gives equation f) and c by 4 (this gives equation g). The following addition is done to obtain the required equation d: 3b + 4c + e.

e) $3\ CO_2(g) + 4\ H_2O(\ell) \rightarrow C_3H_8(g) + 5\ O_2(g)$ $\Delta H_e = 2220.1$ kJ

f) 3 × [C(*graphite*) + $O_2(g) \rightarrow CO_2(g)$] $\quad \Delta H_f = 3 \times -393.5$ kJ

g) $4 \times [H_2(g) + \frac{1}{2}O_2(g) \rightarrow H_2O(\ell)]$ $\quad \Delta H_g = 4 \times -285.8$ kJ

---

3 C(*graphite*) + $4\ H_2(g) \rightarrow C_3H_8(g)$ $\quad \Delta H_d = -103.6$ kJ

where $\Delta H_d = \Delta H_e + \Delta H_f + \Delta H_g$.

It is important to note that the reverse of any reaction has an enthalpy of the same magnitude as that of the forward reaction, but its sign is opposite.

4. Bond Dissociation Energy

Heats of reaction are related to changes in energy associated with the break down and formation of chemical bonds. **Bond energy,** or **bond dissociation energy,** is an average of the energy required to break a particular type of bond in one mole of gaseous molecules. It is tabulated as the positive value of the energy absorbed as the bonds are broken. For example:

$$H_2(g) \rightarrow 2H(g) \qquad \Delta H = 436 \text{ kJ}$$

A molecule of H_2 gas is cleaved to produce two gaseous, unassociated hydrogen atoms. For each mole of H_2 gas cleaved, roughly 436 kJ of energy is absorbed by the system. The reaction is therefore endothermic.

TEACHER TIP

Make sure to switch signs when you reverse the equation and to multiply by the correct stoichiometric coefficient when doing your calculation.

MCAT SYNOPSIS

Because it takes energy to pull two atoms apart, bond breakage is always endothermic. Bond formation is the reverse process, and thus must always be exothermic.

For bonds found in other than diatomic molecules, many compounds have been measured and the energy requirements averaged. For example, the C–H bond dissociation energy one would find in a table (415 kJ/mol) was compiled from measurements on thousands of different organic compounds.

Bond energies can be used to estimate enthalpies of reactions. The enthalpy change of a reaction is given by:

$$\Delta H_{rxn} = (\Delta H \text{ of bonds broken}) - (\Delta H \text{ of bonds formed})$$
$$= \text{total energy input} - \text{total energy released}$$

Example: Calculate the enthalpy change for the following reaction:

$$C(s) + 2\,H_2(g) \rightarrow CH_4(g) \qquad \Delta H = ?$$

Bond dissociation energies of H–H and C–H bonds are 436 kJ/mol and 415 kJ/mol, respectively.

$$\Delta H_f \text{ of } C(g) = 715 \text{ kJ/mol}$$

Solution: CH_4 is formed from free elements in their standard states (C in solid and H_2 in gaseous state).

Thus here, $\Delta H_{rxn} = \Delta H_f$

The reaction can be written in three steps:

a) $C(s) \rightarrow C(g)$ $\qquad \Delta H_1$
b) $2\,[H_2(g) \rightarrow 2\,H(g)]$ $\qquad 2\Delta H_2$
c) $C(g) + 4\,H(g) \rightarrow CH_4(g)$ $\qquad \Delta H_3$

and $\Delta H_f = [\Delta H_1 + 2\Delta H_2] + [\Delta H_3]$

$$\Delta H_1 = \Delta H_f C(g) = 715 \text{ kJ/mol},$$

ΔH_2 is the energy required to break the H–H bond of one mole of H_2. So:

$$\Delta H_2 = \text{bond energy of } H_2$$
$$= 436 \text{ kJ/mol}$$

ΔH_3 is the energy released when 4 C–H bonds are formed. So:

$$\Delta H_3 = -(4 \times \text{bond energy of C–H})$$
$$= -(4 \times 415 \text{ kJ/mol})$$
$$= -1{,}660 \text{ kJ/mol}$$

(**Note:** Because energy is released when bonds are formed, ΔH_3 is negative.)

Therefore:

$$\Delta H_{rxn} = \Delta H_f = [715 + 2(436)] - (1{,}660) \text{ kJ/mol} = -73 \text{ kJ/mol}$$

5. Heats of Combustion

One more type of standard enthalpy change which is often used is the standard heat of combustion, $\mathbf{\Delta H^\circ_{comb}}$. As stated earlier, a requirement for relatively easy measurement of ΔH is that the reaction be fast and spontaneous; combustion generally fits this description. The reactions used in the C_3H_8 (*g*) example previous were combustion reactions, and the corresponding values ΔH_a, ΔH_b, and ΔH_c were thus heats of combustion.

MCAT SYNOPSIS

Combustion of large carbohydrates yields large numbers of products. The larger the reactant, the more numerous the products.

B. ENTROPY

Entropy (S) is a measure of the disorder, or randomness, of a system. The units of entropy are energy/temperature, commonly J/K or cal/K. The greater the order in a system, the lower the entropy; the greater the disorder or randomness, the higher the entropy. At any given temperature, a solid will have lower entropy than a gas, because individual molecules in the gaseous state are moving randomly, while individual molecules in a solid are constrained in place. Entropy is a state function, so a change in entropy depends only on the initial and final states:

$$\Delta S = S_{final} - S_{initial}$$

A change in entropy is also given by:

$$\Delta S = \frac{q_{rev}}{T}$$

where q_{rev} is the heat added to the system undergoing a reversible process (a process that proceeds with infinitesimal changes in the system's conditions) and T is the absolute temperature.

MCAT SYNOPSIS

Entropy changes accompanying phase changes (see chapter 8) can be easily estimated, at least qualitatively. For example, freezing is accompanied by a decrease in entropy as the relatively disordered liquid becomes a well-ordered solid. Meanwhile, boiling is accompanied by a large increase in entropy as the liquid becomes a much more highly disordered gas. For any substance, sublimation will be the phase transition with the greatest entropy change.

A standard entropy change for a reaction, ΔS°, is calculated using the standard entropies of reactants and products:

$$\Delta S^\circ_{rxn} = (\text{sum of } S^\circ_{products}) - (\text{sum of } S^\circ_{reactants})$$

The second law of thermodynamics states that all spontaneous processes proceed such that the entropy of the system plus its surroundings (i.e., the entropy of the universe) increases:

$$\Delta S_{universe} = \Delta S_{system} + \Delta S_{surroundings} > 0$$

A system reaches its maximum entropy at **equilibrium,** a state in which no observable change takes place as time goes on. For a reversible process, $\Delta S_{universe}$ is zero:

$$\Delta S_{universe} = \Delta S_{system} + \Delta S_{surroundings} = 0$$

A system will spontaneously tend toward an equilibrium state if left alone.

C. GIBBS FREE ENERGY

1. Spontaneity of Reaction

The thermodynamic state function, **G** (known as the **Gibbs free energy**), combines the two factors which affect the spontaneity of a reaction—changes in enthalpy, ΔH, and changes in entropy, ΔS. The change in the free energy of a system, ΔG, represents the maximum amount of energy released by a process, occurring at constant temperature and pressure, that is available to perform useful work. ΔG is defined by the equation:

MCAT FAVORITE

$\Delta G = \Delta H - T\Delta S$

Memorize it.

$$\Delta G = \Delta H - T\Delta S$$

where T is the absolute temperature and $T\Delta S$ represents the total amount of heat absorbed by a system when its entropy increases reversibly.

MCAT FAVORITE

Recall that thermodynamics and kinetics are separate topic areas. When a reaction is thermodynamically spontaneous, it has no bearing on how fast it goes; it means only that it will proceed *eventually.*

In the equilibrium state, free energy is at a minimum. A process can occur spontaneously if the Gibbs function decreases, i.e., $\Delta G < 0$.

a) If ΔG is negative, the reaction is spontaneous.
b) If ΔG is positive, the reaction is not spontaneous.
c) If ΔG is zero, the system is in a state of equilibrium; thus, $\Delta G = 0$ and $\Delta H = T\Delta S$.

Because the temperature is always positive, i.e., in Kelvins, the effects of the signs of ΔH and ΔS and the effect of temperature on spontaneity can be summarized as follows:

MCAT FAVORITE

The only temperature-dependent states are when both ΔH and ΔS are either negative or positive.

ΔH	ΔS	Outcome
–	+	Spontaneous at all temperatures
+	–	Nonspontaneous at all temperatures
+	+	Spontaneous only at high temperatures
–	–	Spontaneous only at low temperatures

It is very important to note that the **rate** of a reaction depends on the **activation energy,** not the ΔG.

2. Standard Free Energy

Standard free energy, ΔG°, is defined as the ΔG of a process occurring at 25°C and 1 atm pressure, and for which the concentrations of any solutions involved are 1 M. The **standard free energy of formation** of a compound, $\Delta G°_f$, is the free-energy change that occurs when 1 mol of a compound in its standard state is formed from its elements in their standard states under standard conditions. The standard free energy of formation of any element in its most stable form (and, therefore, its standard state) is zero. The standard free energy of a reaction, $\Delta G°_{rxn}$, is the free-energy change that occurs when that reaction is carried out under standard state conditions; i.e., when the reactants in their standard states are converted to the products in their standard states, at standard conditions of T and P. For example: under standard conditions conversion of C (*diamond*) to C (*graphite*) is spontaneous. However, its rate is so slow that the rxn is never observed.

$$\Delta G°_{rxn} = (\text{sum of } \Delta G°_f \text{ of products}) - (\text{sum of } \Delta G°_f \text{ of reactants}).$$

MCAT SYNOPSIS

Note the similarity of this equation to Hess's law. Almost any state function could be substituted for ΔG here.

3. Reaction Quotient

$\Delta G°_{rxn}$ can also be derived from the equilibrium constant for the equation:

$$\Delta G° = -RT \ln K_{eq}$$

where K_{eq} is the equilibrium constant, R is the gas constant, and T is the temperature in K.

Once a reaction commences, however, the standard state conditions no longer hold. K_{eq} must be replaced by another parameter, the **reaction quotient (Q).** For the reaction, $a\,A + b\,B \rightleftarrows c\,C + d\,D$,

$$Q = \frac{[C]^c[D]^d}{[A]^a[D]^b}$$

TEACHER TIP

Note that the right side of this equation is the same as that for $K_{eq,}$ and rather than representing the reaction at equilibrium it represents a snapshot of the reaction at any time.

Likewise, ΔG must be used in place of ΔG°. The relationship between the two is as follows:

$$\Delta G = \Delta G° + RT \ln Q$$

where R is the gas constant and T is the temperature in K.

4. Examples

a. Vaporization of water at one atmosphere pressure

$$H_2O(\ell) + \text{heat} \rightarrow H_2O(g)$$

When water boils, hydrogen bonds (H-bonds) are broken. Energy is absorbed (the reaction is endothermic), and thus ΔH is positive. Entropy increases as the closely packed molecules of the liquid become the more randomly moving molecules of a gas; thus, $T\Delta S$ is also positive. Because ΔH and $T\Delta S$ are each positive, the reaction will proceed spontaneously only if $T\Delta S > \Delta H$. This is true only at temperatures above 100°C. Below 100°C, ΔG is positive and the water remains a liquid. At 100°C, $\Delta H = T\Delta S$ and $\Delta G = 0$: an equilibrium is established between water and water vapor. The opposite is true when water vapor condenses: H-bonds are formed, and energy is released; the reaction is exothermic (ΔH is negative) and entropy decreases, as a liquid is forming from a gas ($T\Delta S$ is negative). Condensation will be spontaneous only if $\Delta H < T\Delta S$. This is the case at temperatures below 100°C; above 100°C, $T\Delta S$ is more negative than H, ΔG is positive, and condensation is not spontaneous. Again, at 100°C, an equilibrium is established.

b. The combustion of C_6H_6 (benzene)

$$2\ C_6H_6(\ell) + 15\ O_2(g) \rightarrow 12\ CO_2(g) + 6\ H_2O(g) + \text{heat}$$

In this case, heat is released (ΔH is negative) as the benzene burns and the entropy is increased ($T\Delta S$ is positive), because two gases (18 moles total) have greater entropy than a gas and a liquid (15 moles gas and 2 liquid). ΔG is negative and the reaction is spontaneous.

PRACTICE QUESTIONS

1. Consider the cooling of an ideal gas in a closed system. This process is illustrated in the pressure-volume graph shown below. This process could be called which of the following?

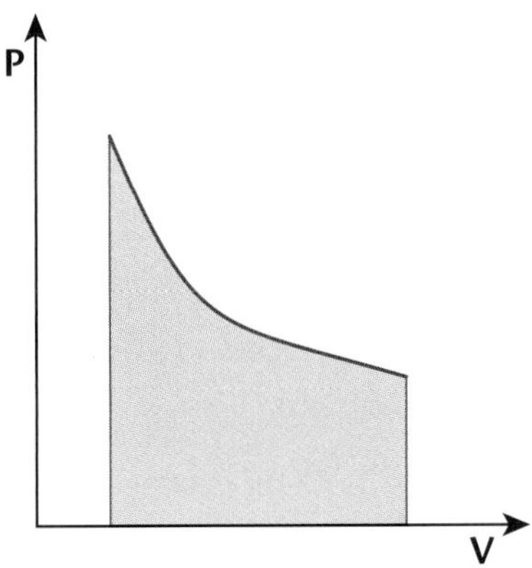

A. Adiabatic
B. Isobaric
C. Isothermal
D. None of the above

2. An ideal gas of volume 7 L undergoes an adiabatic expansion. The molar specific heat of this ideal gas at constant volume is 3 $Jmol^{-1}K^{-1}$. At constant pressure, its molar specific heat is 5 $Jmol^{-1}K^{-1}$. The structure of this ideal gas is

A. monatomic.
B. diatomic.
C. triatomic.
D. unable to be determined without more information.

3. A reaction has a positive entropy and enthalpy. What can be inferred about the progress of this reaction from this information?

A. The reaction is spontaneous.
B. The reaction is nonspontaneous.
C. The reaction is at equilibrium.
D. More information is required.

4. Pure sodium metal spontaneously combusts upon contact with room temperature water. What is true about the equilibrium constant of this combustion reaction at 25°C?

A. $K_{eq} < 1$
B. $K_{eq} > 1$
C. $K_{eq} = 1$
D. More information is required.

5. Which of the following processes has the most exothermic heat of reaction?

A. Combustion of ethane
B. Combustion of propane
C. Combustion of n-butane
D. Combustion of isobutane

6. Methanol reacts with acetic acid to form methyl acetate and water as shown below in the presence of an acid catalyst. What is the heat of formation of methyl acetate in kJ/mol?

$$CH_3OH\ (l) + CH_3COOH\ (aq) \longrightarrow CH_3COOCH_3\ (aq) + H_2O\ (l)$$

Type of Bond	Bond Disassociation Energy (kJ/mol)
C—C	348
C—H	413
C=O	805
O—H	464
C—O	360

A. –464 kJ/mol
B. +464 kJ/mol
C. –1,288 kJ/mol
D. +1,288 kJ/mol

7. At standard temperature and pressure, a chemical process is at equilibrium. What is the free energy of reaction (ΔG) for this process?

A. $\Delta G > 0$
B. $\Delta G < 0$
C. $\Delta G = 0$
D. More information is required.

8. For a certain chemical process, $\Delta G° = -4,955.14$ kJ/mol. What is the equilibrium constant K_{eq} for this reaction?

A. $K_{eq} = 0.13$
B. $K_{eq} = 7.4$
C. $K_{eq} = 8.9$
D. $K_{eq} = 100$

9. Consider the chemical reaction in the vessel depicted below. The reaction is:

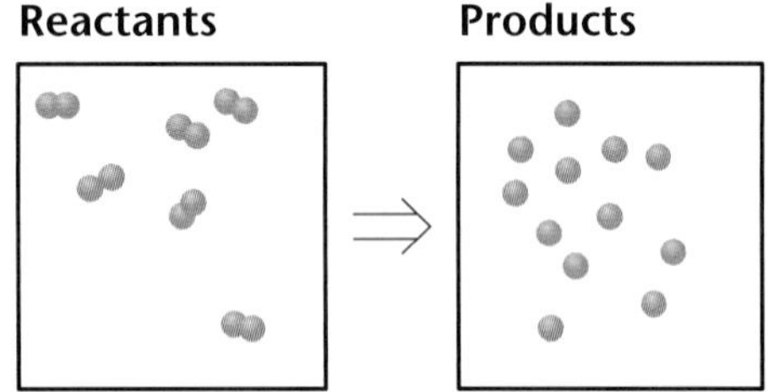

A. spontaneous.
B. nonspontaneous.
C. equilibrium.
D. unable to be determined without more information.

10. Suppose $\Delta G_{rxn}° = -2,000$ kJ/mol for a chemical reaction. At 300 K, what is the reaction quotient Q?

A. $\Delta G = -2,000$ kJ/mol + (300 K)(8.314 $Jmol^{-1}K^{-1}$)ln(Q).
B. $\Delta G = -2,000$ kJ/mol – (300 K)(8.314 $Jmol^{-1}K^{-1}$)ln(Q).
C. $\Delta G = -2,000$ kJ/mol + (300 K)(8.314 $Jmol^{-1}K^{-1}$)log(Q).
D. $\Delta G = -2,000$ kJ/mol – (300 K)(8.314 $Jmol^{-1}K^{-1}$)log(Q).

11. An ideal gas undergoes a reversible expansion at constant pressure.

Which of the following terms could describe this expansion?

I. Adiabatic
II. Isothermal
III. Isobaric

A. I only
B. I and II only
C. I and III only
D. I, II, and III

12. A chemical reaction has a negative enthalpy and negative entropy. Which of the following terms describes the energy of this reaction?

A. Exothermic
B. Endothermic
C. Endergonic
D. Exergonic

13. Consider the chemical reaction in the vessel pictured below. What can we say about the entropy of this reaction?

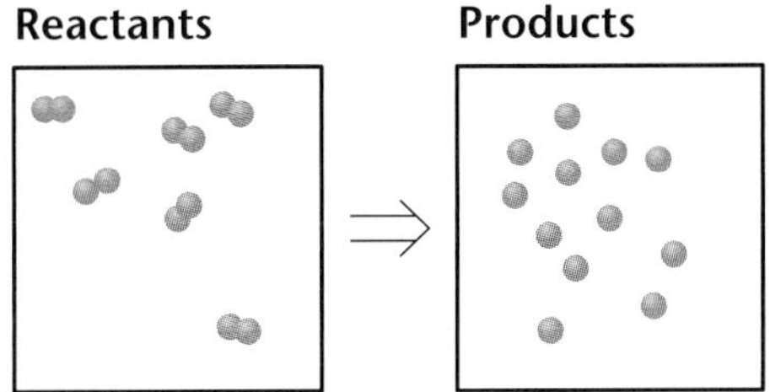

A. $\Delta S > 0$
B. $\Delta S < 0$
C. $\Delta S = 0$
D. More information is required to determine ΔS.

14. Which of the following statements is true of a spontaneous reaction?

A. $\Delta G > 0$ and $K_{eq} > 1$
B. $\Delta G > 0$ and $K_{eq} < 1$
C. $\Delta G < 0$ and $K_{eq} > 1$
D. $\Delta G < 0$ and $K_{eq} > 1$

15. Which of the following devices would be most appropriate to measure the heat capacity of a liquid?

A. Thermometer
B. Calorimeter
C. Barometer
D. Volumetric flask

16. Which of the following equations does not state a law of thermodynamics?

A. $\Delta E_{system} + \Delta E_{surroundings} = \Delta E_{universe}$
B. $\Delta S_{system} + \Delta S_{surroundings} = \Delta S_{universe}$
C. $\Delta H_{system} + \Delta H_{surroundings} = \Delta H_{universe}$
D. $S_{universe} = 0$ at $T = 0$ K

17. A reaction coordinate for a chemical reaction is displayed below. Which of the following terms describes the energy of this reaction?

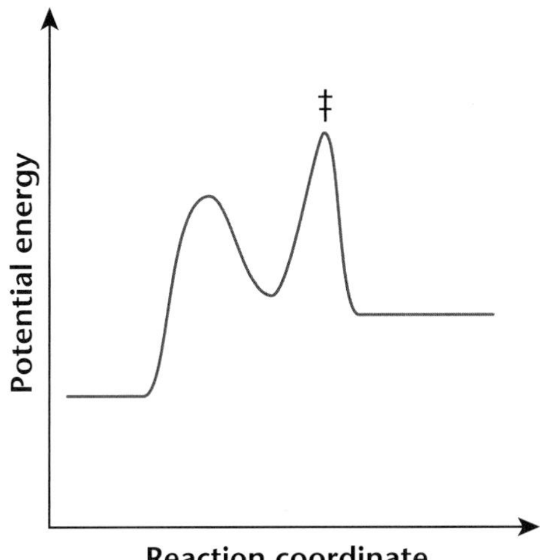

A. Endothermic
B. Exothermic
C. Endergonic
D. Exergonic

REACTION ENERGY PROFILES

KEY CONCEPTS

Thermodynamics

Kinetics

Reaction profiles

When chalcone (**A**) is subjected to reductive conditions with sodium borohydride, two products can result. The two products are the so-called "1,2–reduction" product (**B**), in which the carbonyl is reduced, and the "1,4–reduction" product (**C**), in which the conjugated alkene is reduced.

$$\left(R = 1.99\frac{\text{cal}}{\text{mol k}}\right)$$

C "1,4–reduction" $\xleftarrow{NaBH_4}$ A $\xrightarrow{NaBH_4}$ B "1,2–reduction"

TAKEAWAYS

The goal of a reaction profile is to give you information about energy *differences*. Make sure that you identify the important differences and their significances, as above.

The reaction profiles leading to each reduction product are both shown in the plot below.

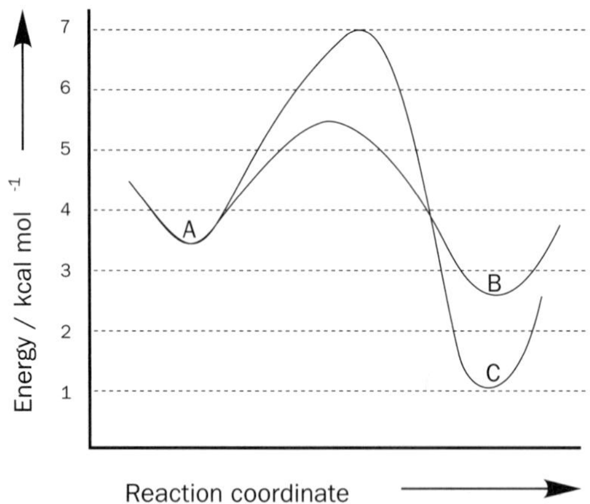

THINGS TO WATCH OUT FOR

Be careful to take note of the units of energy on the *y*-axis if you plan on doing any computations.

Based on the plot above, answer the following questions:

1) Which product is more thermodynamically stable? Which one forms faster?
2) Assume that **A** is in equilibrium with **C.** What will the ratio of **C** to **A** be at equilibrium?
3) How could the rate of the reaction of **A** to **C** be made closer to the rate of the reaction of **A** to **B**?
4) Which product would be favored if **A** were subjected to high temperatures for a long time? If **A** were subjected to low temperatures for only a brief period of time? Explain why for each situation.

1) Look at the energy differences between the starting material and the product(s) as well as the differences between the starting material and the transition state leading to each product.

Notice that the energy of **C** is lower than that of **B.** Therefore, it is the more thermodynamically stable product.

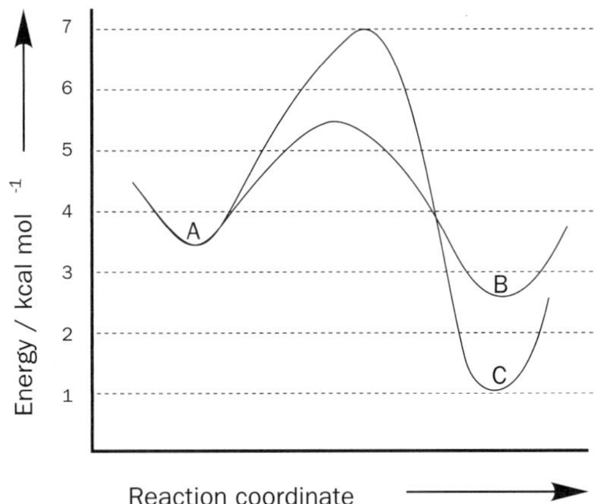

The rate of formation of each product is determined by the difference in energy between the starting material **A** and the top of the "hump" leading to each product. Because this distance is lower for the formation of **B,** it forms faster.

---

2) Note that the difference in energy between the starting material and the product(s) determines the ratio of products to reactants at equilibrium.

$\Delta G° = -RT \ln K_{eq}$

$K_{eq} = e^{\frac{-\Delta G°}{RT}}$

$K_{eq} = e^{\frac{-\Delta G°}{RT}} = e^{\frac{-(-2500)}{(2)(300)}} = e^{\frac{2500}{600}}$

$K_{eq} = e^4 = 81 = \frac{[C]}{[A]}$

This equation provides the relationship between K_{eq} and $\Delta G°$. We need to rearrange it to solve for K_{eq}.

Note that $\Delta G° \approx 1{,}000 - 3{,}500 = -2{,}500$ cal mol^{-1}, from the diagram, and $R =$ 1.99 cal (mol K)$^{-1} \approx 2$ cal (mol K)$^{-1}$, and $T = 298 \approx 300$ K.

Let's say 2,500/600 is about equal to 4, and $e = 2.7818 \approx 3$.

Note that a negative $\Delta G°$ gives more product than reactant, as you would expect for a spontaneous reaction.

---

3) Consider what role(s) the addition of a catalyst might play.

Remember: *A catalyst is something that speeds up a reaction and is not consumed during a reaction. If it speeds up a reaction, it lowers the "hump" in the reaction profile. So, we could increase the rate of formation of **C** by adding a catalyst to that reaction, making the rate closer to the rate of formation of **B**.*

---

4) Consider the effects of temperature on the reaction(s).

At high temperatures for long times, **A** has the energy to go back and forth over and over again between **B** and **C**. Then, over time, the lowest energy product **C** would predominate, just as rolling a ball down a hill would cause it to fall to the lowest location.

Between the two products, **B** will form much faster than **C** because its energy of activation (height of the "hump") is lower. At low temperatures, the products won't have the energy to go back over the hill to get to **A**, so the faster-forming product will predominate (i.e., **B**).

SIMILAR QUESTIONS

1) What would be the ratio of **B** to **A** at equilibrium?
2) If a catalyst were added to the reaction of **A** going to **C**, as in step 3 above, would the energies of **A** and **C** be changed as a result? Why or why not?
3) There are actually intermediates involved in the reactions producing both **B** and **C**. These intermediates are shown below. Sketch how each reaction profile would look, including the involvement of these intermediates. Be sure to indicate which intermediate is relatively more stable.

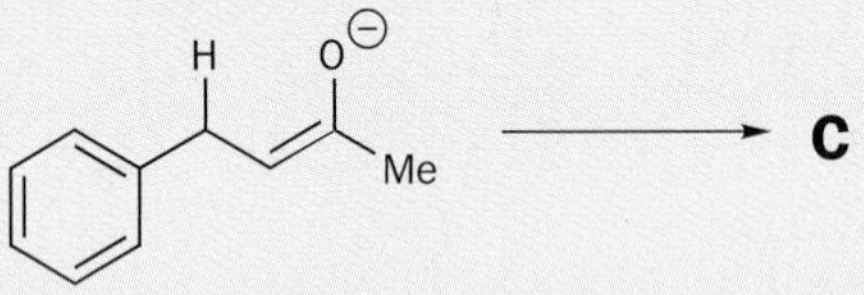

H O⊖ Me → **C**

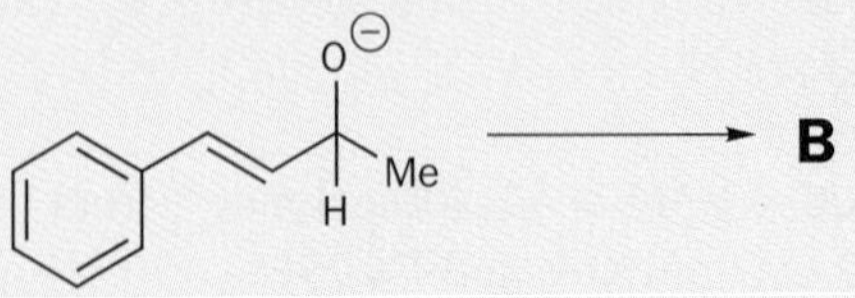

O⊖ Me H → **B**

THERMODYNAMIC EQUILIBRIUM

The reaction $2NO(g) + Cl_2(g) \rightarrow 2NOCl(g)$ adheres to the following thermodynamic data:

ΔH	–77.1 kJ/mol
ΔS	–121 J/K
ΔG	–44.0 kJ/mol
K_{eq}	1.54×10^7

Suppose that, in equilibrium, NO exerts 0.6 atm of pressure and Cl_2 adds 0.3 atm, find the partial pressure of NOCl in this equilibrium. Also, find the temperature at which the thermodynamic data in the table were reported. K_{eq} is related to K_p by the following equation: $K_p = K_{eq}(RT)^{\Delta n}$ where Δn is the change in number of moles of gas evolved as the reaction moves forward. (R = 8.314 J/K · mol)

1) Find the temperature at which the thermodynamic data is true.

☞ $\Delta G = \Delta H - T\Delta S$

(–44 kJ/mol) = (–77 kJ/mol) – T(–0.121 kJ/K × mol) → T = 273 K

Being able to work with the equation $\Delta G = \Delta H - T\Delta S$ is absolutely crucial for Test Day. Specifically concerning the data here, because both ΔH and ΔS are negative, the reaction will become "less spontaneous" as we increase temperature. This will help narrow down our answer choices on Test Day.

MCAT Pitfall: *Notice that not all of the state functions were given in the same unit! Had you blindly put in entropy without changing its units, you would have obtained a temperature near absolute zero (0 K). At absolute zero, molecules no longer move, and it is unlikely that this reaction would have such a high equilibrium constant.*

---

2) Find Δn.

For the equation:

$2NO(g) + Cl_2(g) \rightarrow 2NOCl(g)$

Δn = 2 – (2 + 1) = –1

3) Find K_p.

$K_p = K_{eq}(RT)^{\Delta n}$

$K_p = (1.54 \times 10^7)(18.314\ J/K{\cdot}mole)(273\ K)^{-1}$

= 6785

Use the temperature value from step 1.

KEY CONCEPTS

Thermochemistry

Gibbs free energy

Enthalpy

Entropy

Equilibrium constant, K_{eq}

Reaction quotient, Q

$\Delta G = \Delta H - T\Delta S$ (kJ/mol)

$\Delta G° = -RT \ln K_{eq}$ (kJ/mol)

$\Delta G = \Delta G° + RT \ln Q$ (kJ/mol)

TAKEAWAYS

Two equations should get you through nearly any thermochemistry question. Remember to round your numbers and to predict the ballpark for your answers wherever possible.

THINGS TO WATCH OUT FOR

Pay close attention to the units used.

You are not responsible for memorizing the equation. However, in the MCAT, you have to be able to use a brand new equation to solve for the answer.

---

4) Find the partial pressure.

$$K_p = \frac{(P^{eq}_{NOCl})^2}{(P^{eq}_{NO})^2\left(P^{eq}_{Cl_2}\right)}$$

$$6785 = \frac{(P^{eq}_{NOCl})^2}{(0.6)^2\cdot(0.3)}$$

$$733 = (P^{eq}_{NOCl})^2$$

$$27\text{ atm} = P^{eq}_{NOCl}$$

Plug in the given data into the reaction quotient.

SIMILAR QUESTIONS

1) If $K_{eq} = 7.4 \times 10^{-3}$ for $CH_4(g) + 2H_2O(g) \rightarrow CO_2(g) + 4H_2(g)$, which is more plentiful, the reactants or the products?
2) If pyrophosphoric acid ($H_4P_2O_7$) and arsenous acid (H_3AsO_3) have acid dissociation constants of 3×10^{-2} and 6.6×10^{-10}, respectively, at room temperature, find the Gibbs free energy of each dissociation reaction and determine if it is spontaneous. What does this mean for the ΔH and ΔS for these reactions?
3) A chemist is given three liquid-filled flasks, each labeled with generic thermodynamic data. She is told to put one in a cold room, to put one on a Bunsen burner, and to leave one on the benchtop—whatever conditions will best facilitate the reaction. If the flasks are labeled as follows, which flask goes where?

   A $\Delta H < 0, \Delta S > 0$

   E $\Delta H < 0, \Delta S < 0$

   P $\Delta H > 0, \Delta S > 0$

BOND ENTHALPY

An unknown compound containing only carbon and hydrogen is subjected to a combustion reaction in which 2,059 kJ of heat are released. If 3 moles of CO_2 and 4 moles of steam are produced for every mole of the unknown compound reacted, find the enthalpy for a single C–H bond.

Bond	Bond Dissociation Energy (kJ/mol)
O=O	497
C=O	805
O–H	464
C–C	347

KEY CONCEPTS

Hess's law:

$\Delta H_{rxn} = \Delta H_f$(products) – ΔH_f(reactants)(kJ/mol)

Enthalpy

Bond dissociation energy

Combustion

Stoichiometry

$\Delta H_{rxn} = \Delta H_b$ (reactants) – ΔH_b (products) (kJ/mol)

ΔH_{rxn} = total energy input – total energy released (kJ/mol)

1) Write a balanced equation for the reaction.

$C_3H_8 + 5O_2 \rightleftharpoons 3CO_2 + 4H_2O$

The question stem tells us a few things about the reaction: it is combustion, the carbon source has the generic structure C_xH_y, and the products include 10 oxygen atoms, 3 carbon atoms, and 8 H atoms. To balance the reaction, we'd need those atoms on the left side too. Thus, we find that our unknown sample is actually propane and that we need 5 O_2 molecules.

Remember: *For our purposes, it is completely acceptable to have a fractional coefficient in front of a diatomic molecule.* $2C_2H_4 + (7/2)O_2 \rightarrow 3H_2O + 2CO_2$ *is equivalent to* $4C_2H_4 + 7CO_2 \rightarrow 6H_2O + 4CO_2$.

---

2) Determine which bonds are broken and which are formed.

C_3H_8: 2 C–C bonds broken, 8 C–H bonds broken
$5O_2$: 5 O=O bonds broken
$3CO_2$: 6 C=O bonds formed
$4H_2O$: 8 O–H bonds formed

Combustion of C_3H_8 will break apart the carbon backbone and the C–H bonds. The carbon is in a straight chain (as opposed to cyclic or branched), so 2 C–C bonds and 8 C–H bonds are broken. For O_2, only one O=O bond is broken. However, we have 5 moles of this reactant, and thus we have 5 O=O bonds broken. Each molecule of carbon dioxide has 2 C=O bonds, but we have 3 moles of CO_2, so we have 6 C=O bonds formed. Similarly, 8 O–H bonds are formed in the 4 moles of water produced.

TAKEAWAYS

Consider the number of bonds before applying Hess's law. Make sure to take note of how many bonds are in a given molecule as well as how many stoichiometric equivalents of that molecule you have.

THINGS TO WATCH OUT FOR

There are a number of ways to set up the equation for ΔH_{rxn}. Whatever equation you use, keep your signs straight. Remember that forming bonds releases energy, whereas breaking bonds requires energy.

3) Apply Hess's law.

- $\Delta H_{rxn} = \Delta H_b$ (reactants) – ΔH_b (products)
- ΔH_{rxn} = total energy input – total energy released

$-2{,}059 = [2(347) + 8x + 5(497)] - [6(805) + 8(464)]$
$-2{,}059 = [3{,}179 + 8x] - [8{,}542]$
$-2{,}059 + 8{,}542 - 3{,}179 = 8x$
$x = 413$ kJ/mol

Bond dissociation energy is the energy required to break a particular type of bond in one mole of gaseous molecules. Bond energies can be used to estimate the enthalpy of reaction as given by the two equations above. When we start plugging in numbers, we are given all data except for C–H bond enthalpy. We solve for this variable (x in the above equations).

Remember: *The equation $\Delta H_{rxn} = \Delta H_b$ (reactants) – ΔH_b (products) is simply a restatement of Hess's Law. Bond enthalpy is for bond breaking and enthalpy of formation, of course, is for bond making. Changing ΔH_F to ΔH_b switches the signs and, thus, the order of the equation. Keep in mind that it can also be written as $\Delta H_{rxn} = \Delta H_b$ (bonds broken) + ΔH_b (bonds formed), but you must remember to make the bond enthalpies for the products negative because forming bonds releases energy.*

---

4) Use Avogadro's number.

$(413 \text{ kJ/mol}) \times [1 \text{ mol}/(6.022 \times 10^{23} \text{ molecules})]$
$= 6.86 \times 10^{-22}$ kJ/molecule

We see that 413 kJ are found in one mole of C–H bonds. One mole of a substance is equal to 6.022×10^{23} molecules. Here, we simply use that conversion factor. The result tells us that 6.86×10^{-22} kJ are stored in each C–H bond.

SIMILAR QUESTIONS

1) Ethanol metabolism in yeast consists of the conversion of ethanol (C_2H_5OH) to acetic acid (CH_3COOH). What is the enthalpy of the reaction if 0.1 mmol of ethanol is metabolized?
2) A second metabolic process involves the net production of 2 ATP and 2 NADH from 2 ADP and 2 NAD^+. If the conversion of these molecules is endothermic and adds 443.5 kJ to the overall enthalpy of the reaction, find the enthalpy for a "high-energy" phosphate bond.
3) Tristearin is oxidized in the body according to the following reaction: $2C_{57}H_{110}O_6 + 163O_2 \rightarrow 114CO_2 + 110H_2O$. If the standard enthalpy for this reaction is –34 MJ mol^{-1}, find the total enthalpy for the bonds in tristearin.

HEAT OF FORMATION

The heat of combustion of glucose ($C_6H_{12}O_6$) is –2,537.3 kJ/mol. If the $\Delta H°_f$ of CO_2(g) is –393.5 kJ/mol, and the $\Delta H°_f$ of H_2O(g) is –241.8 kJ/mol, what is the $\Delta H°_f$ of glucose?

KEY CONCEPTS

Hess's law:

$\Delta H_{rxn} = \Delta H_F$(products) – ΔH_F(reactants) (kJ/mol)

Heat of formation

Combustion

1) Write a balanced equation for the reaction.

Unbalanced reaction: $C_6H_{12}O_6 + O_2 \rightarrow CO_2 + H_2O$

Balanced reaction: $C_6H_{12}O_6 + 6\,O_2 \rightarrow 6\,CO_2 + 6\,H_2O$

The unbalanced reaction to the left is typical of all hydrocarbon combustion reactions. (Unless otherwise noted, presume that combustion of carbohydrates is with oxygen gas.) Begin by balancing the carbons on the left side (6 CO_2), then balance the hydrogens on the left side (12 H_2O), and conclude by balancing the oxygen gas on the right side (6 O_2).

Remember: *For our purposes, it is completely acceptable to have a fractional coefficient in front of a diatomic molecule.* $2C_2H_4 + (7/2)O_2 \rightarrow 3H_2O + 2CO_2$ *is equivalent to* $4C_2H_4 + 7CO_2 \rightarrow 6H_2O + 4CO_2$ *but the math is simpler for the former.*

---

2) Apply Hess's law.

$\Delta H_{rxn} = \Delta H_F$(products) – ΔH_F(reactants)

–2,537.3 = [6(–393.5) + 6(–241.8)] – [ΔH_F(glucose)]

Rearranging to solve for ΔH_F(glucose):

ΔH_f(glucose) = 2,537.3 + [6(–393.5) + 6(–241.8)]

ΔH_f(glucose) = 2,537.3 + [–2,361 + –1,450.8]

ΔH_f(glucose) = 2,537.3 + [–3,811.8]

$\Rightarrow \Delta H_f$(glucose) = –1274.5

The heat of formation is defined as the heat absorbed or released during the formation of a pure substance from the elements at a constant pressure. Therefore, by definition, diatomic gases like oxygen have a heat of formation of zero. A negative heat of formation means that heat is released to form the product, whereas a positive heat of formation means that heat is required to form the product. The overall combustion reaction of glucose releases 2,537.3 kJ/mol of heat.

TAKEAWAYS

Always identify the balanced equation for the reaction before you begin to apply Hess's law. There is a second way of thinking about Hess's law that may be applicable in some questions as well (see previous topic). The given information in the passage and/or question stem will dictate which equation to use. Finally, recall that enthalpy is a state function, and regardless of the path you take to get from the reactants to the products, the change in enthalpy will be the same.

THINGS TO WATCH OUT FOR

At least one of the wrong answer choices for thermochemistry questions will be a result from carelessness with signs. Organized scratchwork in a stepwise fashion will facilitate avoiding this problem, but perhaps more important is maintaining the ability to approximate the answer. Only experience (a.k.a. practice!) will breed such wisdom.

SIMILAR QUESTIONS

1) Given the ΔH_F of carbon dioxide and water, what other piece(s) of information must you have to calculate the ΔH_{comb} of ethane?
2) If the ΔH_F of acetylene is 226.6 kJ/mol, what is the ΔH_{comb} of acetylene?
3) If the ΔH_F of NaBr (s) is –359.9 kJ/mol, what is the sum of each ΔH_F of the following series of five reactions?

$$Na(s) \rightarrow Na(g) \rightarrow Na^+(g)$$
$$\frac{1}{2} Br_2(g) \rightarrow Br(g) \rightarrow Br^-(g)$$
$$Na^+(g) + Br^-(g) \rightarrow NaBr(s)$$

CHAPTER 7

THE GAS PHASE

Matter can exist in three different physical forms, called **phases** or **states: gas, liquid,** and **solid.** Liquids and solids will be discussed in chapter 8.

The gaseous phase, the subject of this chapter, is the simplest to understand, because all gases display similar behavior and follow similar laws regardless of their identity. The atoms or molecules in a gaseous sample move rapidly and are far apart from each other. In addition, only very weak intermolecular forces exist between gas particles; this results in certain characteristic physical properties, such as the ability to expand to fill any volume and to take on the shape of a container. Further, gases are easily, though not infinitely, compressible.

The state of a gaseous sample is generally defined by four variables: pressure (P), volume (V), temperature (T), and number of moles (n). Gas pressures are usually expressed in units of atmospheres (atm) or millimeters of mercury (mm Hg or torr), which are related as follows:

$$1 \text{ atm} = 760 \text{ mm Hg} = 760 \text{ torr}$$

Volume is generally expressed in liters (L) or milliliters (mL). The temperature of a gas is usually given in Kelvin (K, **not** °K). Gases are often discussed in terms of **standard temperature and pressure (STP),** which refers to conditions of 273.15 K (0°C) and 1 atm.

Note: It is important not to confuse **STP** with **standard conditions**—the two standards involve different temperatures and are used for different purposes. STP (0°C or 273 K) is generally used for gas law calculations; standard conditions (25°C or 298 K) is used when measuring standard enthalpy, entropy, Gibbs's free energy, and voltage.

MCAT FAVORITE

STP is different from standard state. Temperature at STP is 0°C, i.e., 273.15 K. Temperature at standard state is 25°C.

IDEAL GASES

When examining the behavior of gases under varying conditions of temperature and pressure, scientists speak of ideal gases. An ideal gas represents a hypothetical gas whose molecules have no intermolecular forces and occupy no volume. Although gases actually deviate from this idealized behavior, at relatively low pressures (atmospheric pressure) and high temperatures many gases behave in a nearly ideal fashion. Therefore, the assumptions used for ideal gases can be applied to real gases with reasonable accuracy.

MCAT FAVORITE

Boyle's law, a common topic on the exam, states that pressure and volume are inversely related. When one increases, the other decreases.

A. BOYLE'S LAW

Experimental studies performed by Robert Boyle in 1660 led to the formulation of Boyle's law. His work showed that for a given gaseous sample held at constant temperature (isothermal conditions), the volume of the gas is inversely proportional to its pressure:

$$PV = k \text{ or } P_1V_1 = P_2V_2$$

where k is a proportionality constant and the subscripts 1 and 2 represent two different sets of conditions. A plot of pressure versus volume for a gas is shown in Figure 7.1.

TEACHER TIP

Remembering the shape of the graph might help you recall the relationship on Test Day. Here we can see that as pressure increases, volume decreases, and vice versa.

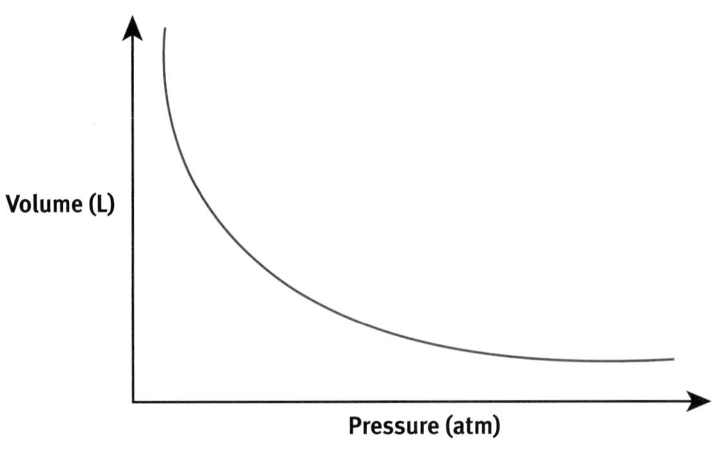

Figure 7.1

Example: Under isothermal conditions, what would be the volume of a 1 L sample of helium if its pressure is changed from 12 atm to 4 atm?

Solution:

$P_1 = 12$ atm $\quad P_2 = 4$ atm

$V_1 = 1$ L $\quad V_2 = X$

$$P_1V_1 = P_2V_2$$

$$12 \text{ atm } (1 \text{ L}) = 4 \text{ atm } (X)$$

$$\frac{12}{4}\text{L} = X$$

$$X = 3 \text{ L}$$

B. LAW OF CHARLES AND GAY-LUSSAC

The law of Charles and Gay-Lussac, or simply Charles's law, was developed during the early 19th century. The law states that at constant pressure, the volume of a gas is directly proportional to its absolute temperature. The absolute temperature is the temperature expressed in Kelvin, which can be calculated from the expression $T_K = T_{°C} + 273.15$.

MCAT FAVORITE

Charles's law, another common topic, states that volume and temperature are directly proportional. When one increases the other increases.

$$\frac{V}{T} = k \text{ or } \frac{V_1}{T_1} = \frac{V_2}{T_2}$$

where k is a constant and the subscripts 1 and 2 represent two different sets of conditions. A plot of temperature versus volume is shown in Figure 7.2.

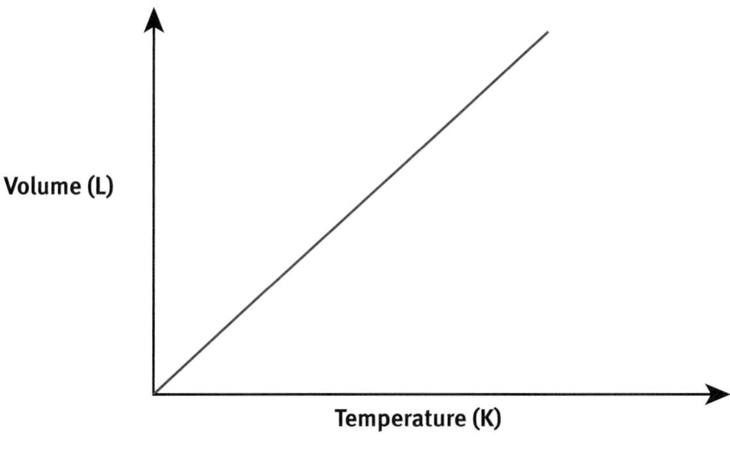

Figure 7.2

MCAT SYNOPSIS

While the temperature of 0K cannot be physically attained, curves such as this one were originally used to figure out its location.

Example: If the absolute temperature of 2 L of gas at constant pressure is changed from 283.15 K to 566.30 K, what would be the final volume?

Solution:

$T_1 = 283.15$ K $\qquad V_1 = 2$ L

$T_2 = 566.30$ K $\qquad V_2 = X$

$$\frac{V_1}{T_1} = \frac{V_2}{T_2}$$

$$\frac{2\text{L}}{283.15\text{ K}} = \frac{X}{566.30\text{ K}}$$

$$X = \frac{2\text{L}(566.30\text{ K})}{283.15\text{ K}}$$

$$X = 4\text{L}$$

C. AVOGADRO'S PRINCIPLE

In 1811, Amedeo Avogadro proposed that for all gases at a constant temperature and pressure, the volume of the gas will be directly proportional to the number of moles of gas present; therefore, all gases have the same number of moles in the same volume.

$$\frac{n}{V} = k \text{ or } \frac{n_1}{V_1} = \frac{n_2}{V_2}$$

The subscripts 1 and 2 once again apply to two different sets of conditions with the same temperature and pressure.

TEACHER TIP

On the MCAT you may not have to do as many calculations as you may think. With ideal gas law problems, you may find that the changes in conditions can be examined separately, and by using Boyle's and Charles's laws, you can arrive at an answer much more easily.

D. IDEAL GAS LAW

MCAT FAVORITE

PV = nRT

Memorize it.

The ideal gas law combines the relationships outlined in Boyle's law, Charles's law, and Avogadro's principle to yield an expression which can be used to predict the behavior of a gas. The ideal gas law shows the relationship among four variables that define a sample of gas—pressure (P), volume (V), temperature (T), and number of moles (n)—and is represented by the equation

$$PV = nRT$$

The constant R is known as the **gas constant.** Under STP conditions (273.15 K and 1 atmosphere), 1 mole of gas was shown to have a volume of 22.4 L. Substituting these values into the ideal gas equation gave R = 8.21×10^{-2} L • atm/(mol • K).

The gas constant may be expressed in many other units: another common value is 8.314 J/(K • mol), which is derived when SI units of pascals (for pressure) and cubic meters (for volume) are substituted into the ideal gas law. **When carrying out calculations based on the ideal gas law, it is important to choose a value of R that matches the units of the variables.**

Example: What volume would 12 g of helium occupy at 20°C and a pressure of 380 mm Hg?

Solution: The ideal gas law can be used, but first, all of the variables must be converted to yield units that will correspond to the expression of the gas constant as 0.0821 L • atm/(mol • K).

$$P = 380 \text{ mm Hg} \times \frac{1\text{atm}}{760 \text{ mm Hg}} = 0.5 \text{ atm}$$

$$T = 20°\text{C} + 273.15 = 293.15 \text{ K}$$

$$n = 12\text{g He} \times \frac{1 \text{ mol He}}{4.0 \text{ g}} = 3 \text{ mol He}$$

Substituting into the ideal gas equation:

$$PV = nRT$$

$$(0.5 \text{ atm})(V) = (3 \text{ mol})(0.0821 \text{ L} \bullet \text{atm}/(\text{mol} \bullet \text{K})(293.15 \text{ K})$$

$$V = 144.4 \text{ L}$$

In addition to standard calculations to determine the pressure, volume, or temperature of a gas, the ideal gas law may be used to determine the density and molar mass of the gas.

1. Density

Density is defined as the mass per unit volume of a substance and, for gases, is usually expressed in units of g/L. By rearrangement, the ideal gas equation can be used to calculate the density of a gas.

$$PV = nRT$$

$$\text{where} \quad n = \frac{m}{MM} \quad \frac{(\text{mass in g})}{(\text{molar mass})}$$

$$\text{therefore} \quad PV = \frac{m}{MM} \quad RT$$

$$\text{and} \quad d = \frac{m}{v} = \frac{P(MM)}{RT}$$

Another way to find the density of a gas is to start with the volume of a mole of gas at STP, 22.4 L, calculate the effect of pressure and temperature on the volume, and finally calculate the density by dividing the mass by the new volume. The following equation, derived from Boyle's and Charles's laws, is used to relate changes in the temperature, volume and pressure of a gas:

$$\frac{P_1V_1}{T_1} = \frac{P_2V_2}{T_2}$$

where the subscripts 1 and 2 refer to the two states of the gas (at STP and under the actual conditions). To calculate a change in volume, the equation is rearranged as follows.

$$V_2 = V_1\left(\frac{P_1}{P_2}\right)\left(\frac{T_2}{T_1}\right)$$

V_2 is then used to find the density of the gas under nonstandard conditions.

$$d = \frac{m}{V_2}$$

If you *visualize* how the changes in pressure and temperature affect the volume of the gas, you can check to be sure you have not accidentally confused the pressure or temperature value that belongs in the numerator with the one that belongs in the denominator.

Example: What is the density of HCl gas at 2 atm and 45°C?

Solution: At STP, a mole of gas occupies 22.4 liters. Because the increase in pressure to 2 atm decreases volume, 22.4 L must be multiplied by $\left(\frac{1\text{ atm}}{2\text{ atm}}\right)$. Because the increase in temperature increases volume, the temperature factor will be $\left(\frac{318\text{ K}}{273\text{ K}}\right)$.

$$V_2 = \left(\frac{22.4\text{ L}}{\text{mol}}\right)\left(\frac{1\text{ atm}}{2\text{ atm}}\right)\left(\frac{318\text{ K}}{273\text{ K}}\right) = 13.0\text{ L/mol}$$

$$d = \left(\frac{36\text{ g/mol}}{13.0\text{ L/mol}}\right) = 2.77\text{g/L}$$

2. Molar Mass

Sometimes the identity of a gas is unknown, and the molar mass (see chapter 4) must be determined in order to identify it. Using the equation for density derived from the ideal gas law, the molar mass of a gas can be determined experimentally as follows. The pressure and temperature of a gas contained in a bulb of a given volume are measured, and the weight of the bulb plus sample is found. Then, the bulb is evacuated, and the empty bulb is weighed. The weight of the bulb plus sample minus the weight of the bulb yields the weight of the sample. Finally, the density of the sample is determined by dividing the weight of the sample by the volume of the bulb. The density at STP is calculated. The molecular weight is then found by multiplying the number of grams per liter by 22.4 liters per mole.

Example: What is the molar mass of a 2 L sample of gas that weighs 8 g at a temperature of 15°C and a pressure of 1.5 atm?

$$d = \frac{8\text{ g}}{2\text{ L}} \text{ at } 15°\text{C and } 1.5\text{ atm}$$

$$V_{STP} = (2\text{L})\left(\frac{273\text{ K}}{288\text{ K}}\right)\left(\frac{1.5\text{ atm}}{1\text{ atm}}\right) = 2.84\text{ L}$$

$$\frac{8\text{ g}}{2.84\text{ L}} = 2.82\text{ g/L at STP}$$

$$\left(\frac{2.82\text{ g}}{\text{L}}\right)\left(\frac{22.4\text{ L}}{\text{mol}}\right) = 63.2\text{ g/mol}$$

DALTON'S LAW OF PARTIAL PRESSURES

When two or more gases are found in one vessel without chemical interaction, each gas will behave independently of the other(s). Therefore, the pressure exerted by each gas in the mixture will be equal to the pressure that gas would exert if it were the only one in the container. The pressure exerted by each individual gas is called the **partial pressure** of that gas. In 1801, John Dalton derived an expression, now known as **Dalton's Law of Partial Pressures,** which states that the total pressure of a gaseous mixture is equal to the sum of the partial pressures of the individual components. The equation is:

$$P_T = P_A + P_B + P_C + \ldots$$

The partial pressure of a gas is related to its mole fraction and can be determined using the following equations:

$$P_A = P_T X_A$$

where $$X_A = \frac{n_A \text{ (moles of A)}}{n_T \text{ (total moles)}}$$

Example: A vessel contains 0.75 mol of nitrogen, 0.20 mol of hydrogen, and 0.05 mol of fluorine at a total pressure of 2.5 atm. What is the partial pressure of each gas?

First calculate the mole fraction of each gas.

$$X_{N_2} = \frac{0.75 \text{ mol}}{1.0 \text{ mol}} = 0.75 \quad X_{H_2} = \frac{0.20 \text{ mol}}{1.0 \text{ mol}} = 0.20 \quad X_{F_2} = \frac{0.05 \text{ mol}}{1.0 \text{ mol}} = 0.05$$

Then calculate the partial pressure.

$$P_A = X_A P_T$$

$$P_{N_2} = (2.5 \text{ atm})(0.75) = 1.875 \text{ atm} \quad P_{H_2} = (2.5 \text{ atm})(0.20) = 0.5 \text{ atm} \quad P_{F_2} = (2.5 \text{ atm})(0.05) = 0.125 \text{ atm}$$

REAL GASES

In general, the ideal gas law is a good approximation of the behavior of real gases, but all real gases deviate from ideal gas behavior to some extent, particularly when the gas atoms or molecules are forced into close proximity under high pressure and at low temperature, so that molecular volume and intermolecular attractions become significant.

MCAT SYNOPSIS

At high temperature and low pressure, deviations from ideality are usually small; good approximations can still be made from the ideal gas law.

TEACHER TIP

All gases were created equal, so when more than one gas is in a container, each contributes to the whole as much as if it were the only gas. Add up all the pressures of the individual gases and you get the whole pressure of the system.

TEACHER TIP

Understanding when conditions are not ideal for gases will help you to understand how their behavior may deviate.

A. DEVIATIONS DUE TO PRESSURE

As the pressure of a gas increases, the particles are pushed closer and closer together. As the condensation pressure for a given temperature is approached, intermolecular attraction forces become more and more significant until the gas condenses into the liquid state (see Gas-Liquid Equilibrium in chapter 8).

At moderately high pressure (a few hundred atmospheres) a gas's volume is less than would be predicted by the ideal gas law, due to intermolecular attraction. At extremely high pressure the size of the particles becomes relatively large compared to the distance between them, and this causes the gas to take up a larger volume than would be predicted by the ideal gas law.

B. DEVIATIONS DUE TO TEMPERATURE

As the temperature of a gas is decreased, the average velocity of the gas molecules decreases, and the attractive intermolecular forces become increasingly significant. As the condensation temperature is approached for a given pressure, intermolecular attractions eventually cause the gas to condense to a liquid state (see Gas-Liquid Equilibrium in chapter 8).

As the temperature of a gas is reduced toward its condensation point (which is the same as its boiling point), intermolecular attraction causes the gas to have a smaller volume than would be predicted by the ideal gas law. The closer the temperature of a gas is to its boiling point, the less ideal is its behavior.

MCAT Synopsis

Note that if *a* and *b* are both zero, this reduces to the ideal gas law.

C. VAN DER WAALS EQUATION OF STATE

Several real gas equations, or gas laws, exist that attempt to correct for the deviations from ideality that occur when a gas does not closely follow the ideal gas law. The van der Waals equation is a case in point.

$$\left(P+\frac{n^2a}{V^2}\right)(V-nb)=nRT$$

In this equation, *a* and *b* are physical constants, experimentally determined for each gas. The *a* term corrects for the attractive forces between molecules, and as such will be small in value for a gas such as helium, larger for more polarizable gases such as Xe or N_2, and larger yet for polar molecules such as HCl or NH_3. The *b* term corrects for the volume of the molecules themselves. Larger values of *b* are thus found for larger molecules. Numerical values for *a* are generally much larger than those for *b*.

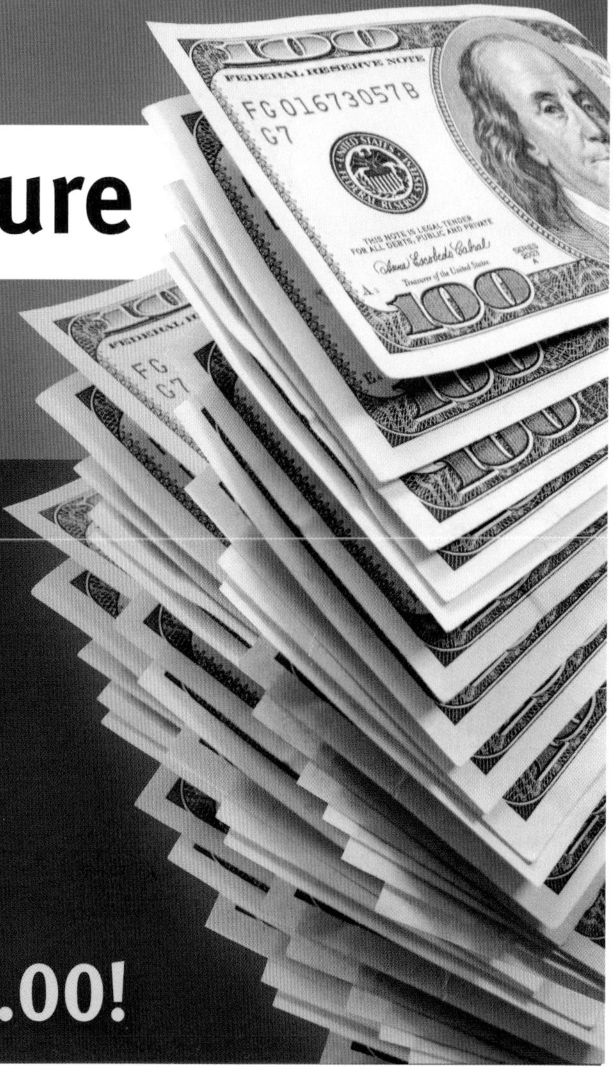

Example: Find the correction in pressure necessary for the deviation from ideality for 1 mole of ammonia in a 1 liter flask at 0°C. (For NH_3, a = 4.2, b = 0.037)

Solution: According to the ideal gas law,

$P = nRT/V = (1)(0.0821)(273)/(1) = 22.4$ atm, while according to the van der Waals equation,

$$P = \frac{nRT}{(V-nb)} - \frac{n^2a}{V^2} = \frac{(1)(0.821)(273)}{(1-0.037)} - \frac{1^2(4.2)}{1}$$

$$= 23.3 - 4.2 = 19.1 \text{ atm.}$$

The pressure is thus 3.3 atm less than would be predicted from the ideal gas law, or an error of 15 percent.

KINETIC MOLECULAR THEORY OF GASES

As indicated by the gas laws, all gases show similar physical characteristics and behavior. A theoretical model to explain the behavior of gases was developed during the second half of the 19th century. The combined efforts of Boltzmann, Maxwell, and others led to a simple explanation of gaseous molecular behavior based on the motion of individual molecules. This model is called the **Kinetic Molecular Theory of Gases.** Like the gas laws, this theory was developed in reference to ideal gases, although it can be applied with reasonable accuracy to real gases as well.

A. ASSUMPTIONS OF THE KINETIC MOLECULAR THEORY

1. Gases are made up of particles whose volumes are negligible compared to the container volume.
2. Gas atoms or molecules exhibit no intermolecular attractions or repulsions.
3. Gas particles are in continuous, random motion, undergoing collisions with other particles and the container walls.
4. Collisions between any two gas particles are elastic, meaning that there is no overall gain or loss of energy.
5. The average kinetic energy of gas particles is proportional to the absolute temperature of the gas, and is the same for all gases at a given temperature.

TEACHER TIP

The higher the temperature, the faster the molecules move. The larger the molecule, the slower it moves.

B. APPLICATIONS OF THE KINETIC MOLECULAR THEORY OF GASES

1. Average Molecular Speeds

According to the kinetic molecular theory of gases, the average kinetic energy of a gas particle is proportional to the absolute temperature of the gas:

$$KE = \frac{1}{2}mv^2 = \frac{3}{2}kt$$

where k is the Boltzmann constant. This equation also shows that the speed of a gas molecule is related to its absolute temperature. However, because of the large number of rapidly and randomly moving gas particles, the speed of an individual gas molecule is nearly impossible to define. Therefore, the speeds of gases are defined in terms of their average molecular speed ($\bar{c}$), which represents the mathematical average of all the speeds of the gas particles in the sample. This is given by the following equation:

$$\bar{c} = \left(\frac{3RT}{MM}\right)^{\frac{1}{2}} \quad \text{where R = gas constant}$$

MM = molecular mass

A **Maxwell-Boltzmann distribution curve** shows the distribution of speeds of gas particles at a given temperature. Figure 7.3 shows a distribution curve of molecular speeds at two temperatures, T_1 and T_2, where $T_2 > T_1$. Notice that the bell-shaped curve flattens and shifts to the right as the temperature increases, indicating that at higher temperatures more molecules are moving at high speeds.

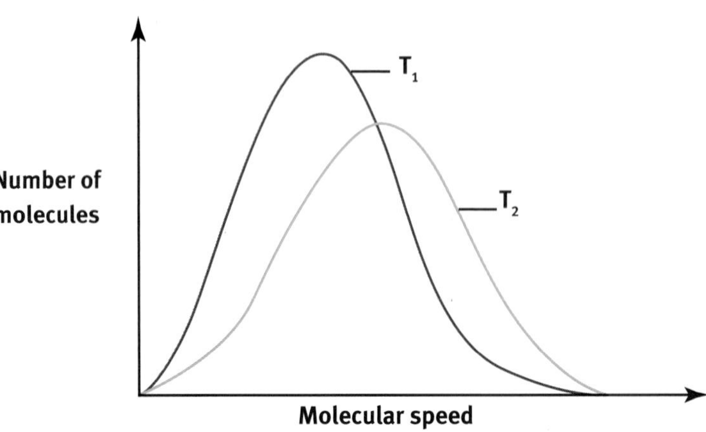

Figure 7.3

Example: What is the average speed of sulfur dioxide molecules at 37°C?

Solution: The gas constant R = 8.314 J/(K • mol) should be used and MM must be expressed in kg/mol.

$$\bar{c} = \left(\frac{3RT}{MM}\right)^{\frac{1}{2}}$$

$$\bar{c} = \left[\frac{3(8.314 \text{ J/K mol})(310.15 \text{ K})}{0.064 \text{ kg/mol}}\right]^{\frac{1}{2}}$$

$$\bar{c} = \sqrt{120871.3 \text{ J/kg}}$$

Use the conversion factor 1 J = 1 kg • m^2/s^2:

$$\bar{c} = \sqrt{120871.3 \text{ kg} \bullet \text{m}^2/\text{s}^2 \bullet \text{kg}}$$

$$\bar{c} = 347.7 \text{ m/s}$$

2. Graham's Law of Diffusion and Effusion

a. Diffusion

Diffusion occurs when gas molecules diffuse through a mixture. Diffusion accounts for the fact that an open bottle of perfume can quickly be smelled across a room. The kinetic molecular theory of gases predicted that heavier gas molecules diffuse more slowly than lighter ones because of their differing average speeds. In 1832, Thomas Graham showed mathematically that under isothermal and isobaric conditions, the rates at which two gases diffuse are inversely proportional to the square root of their molar masses. Thus:

$$\frac{r_1}{r_2} = \left(\frac{MM_2}{MM_1}\right)^{\frac{1}{2}} = \sqrt{\frac{MM_2}{MM_1}}$$

where r_1 and MM_1 represent the diffusion rate and molar mass of gas 1, and r_2 and MM_2 represent the diffusion rate and molar mass of gas 2.

TEACHER TIP

Diffusion is when gases mix with one another. Effusion is when a gas moves through a small hole under pressure. Both will be slower for larger molecules.

b. Effusion

Effusion is the flow of gas particles under pressure from one compartment to another through a small opening. Graham used the kinetic molecular theory of gases to show that for two gases at the same temperature, the rates of effusion are proportional to the average speeds. He then expressed the rates of effusion in terms of molar mass and found that the relationship is the same as that for diffusion:

$$\frac{r_1}{r_2} = \left(\frac{MM_2}{MM_1}\right)^{\frac{1}{2}}$$

PRACTICE QUESTIONS

1. The graph below shows a plot of PV versus P for 1 mol of ammonia gas. Experimental data was used to plot the line at pressures of 0.20 atm and above. The line was then extrapolated in order to determine the value of PV at zero pressure. Does the graph accurately describe the relationship between pressure and volume that would be seen for an ideal gas?

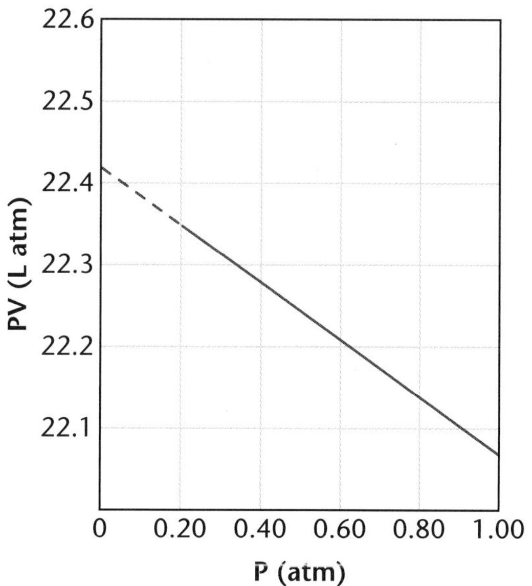

Graph of experimental results of PV versus V for 1 mol of ammonia gas. The data is extrapolated to zero pressure.

A. Yes, the graph describes an ideal gas because the value of PV at zero pressure is approximately 22.4 L.
B. Yes, the graph describes an ideal gas because the slope of the line is equal to –0.33 L.
C. No, the graph does not describe an ideal gas because as pressure increases the product of P and V deviates from 22.4L.
D. No, the graph does not describe an ideal gas because the line is not horizontal.

2. Based on the graph in the previous question and your knowledge of gases, what conditions would be least likely to result in ideal gas behavior?

A. High pressure and low temperature
B. Low temperature and large volume
C. High pressure and large volume
D. Low pressure and high temperature

3. Calculate the density of neon gas at STP in g L^{-1}. The molar mass of neon can be approximated to 20.18 g mol^{-1}.

A. 452.3 g L^{-1}
B. 226.0 g L^{-1}
C. 1.802 g L^{-1}
D. 0.9009 g L^{-1}

4. A leak of helium gas through a small hole occurs at a rate of 3.22×10^{-5} mol s^{-1}. Will a leak of neon gas at the same temperature and pressure occur at a slower or faster rate than helium? Will a leak of oxygen gas at the same temperature and pressure occur at a slower or faster rate than helium?

A. Neon will leak faster than helium; oxygen will leak slower than helium.
B. Neon will leak faster than helium; oxygen will leak slower than helium.
C. Neon will leak slower than helium; oxygen will leak slower than helium.
D. Neon will leak slower than helium; oxygen will leak faster than helium.

5. A manometer is open to the atmosphere. The pressure of the gas in the flask can be calculated by the difference in the mercury levels in the arms of the U-shaped tube. If the atmospheric pressure is equal to 760 torr, calculate the pressure in the flask shown in below.

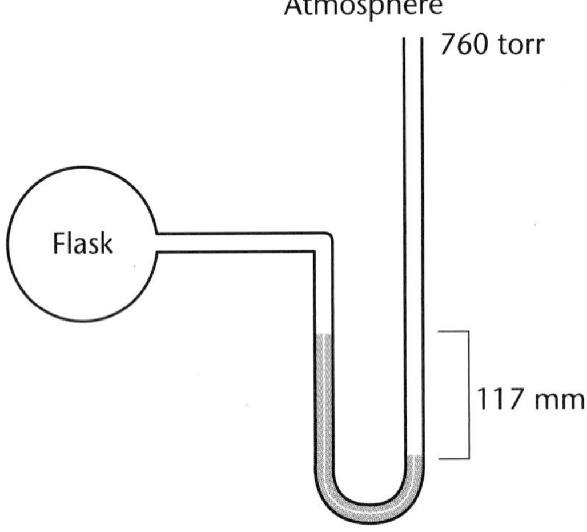

A. 117 mm Hg
B. 877 mm Hg
C. 643 mm Hg
D. 760 mm Hg

6. A hot-air balloon rises because

A. the air molecules move faster due to the high temperature. The molecules escape through the bottom of the balloon, which forces the balloon upward.
B. the higher temperature within the balloon creates a larger volume, which decreases the density of air inside the balloon, allowing it to rise.
C. the air molecules inside the balloon circulate to increase the upward force lifting the balloon.
D. the volume inside the increasing balloon increases as a result of the increasing number of air molecules entering through the bottom of the hole.

7. A 0.04 gram piece of magnesium is placed in a beaker of hydrochloric acid. Hydrogen gas is generated according to the following equation. The gas is collected over water at 25°C, and the pressure during the experiment reads 784 mm Hg. The gas displaces a volume of 100 mL. The vapor pressure of water at 25°C is approximately 24 mm Hg. How many moles of hydrogen are produced?

$$Mg_{(s)} + 2HCl_{(aq)} \rightarrow MgCl_{2(aq)} + H_{2(g)}$$

A. 4.22×10^{-3} moles hydrogen
B. 4.08×10^{-3} moles hydrogen
C. 3.11 moles hydrogen
D. 3.2 moles hydrogen

8. Which of the following properties are true of ideal gases?

I. No volume
II. No attractive forces between them
III. No mass

A. I only
B. I and II only
C. I and III only
D. I, II, and III

9. An 8.01 g sample of $NH_4NO_{3(s)}$ is placed into an evacuated 10 L flask and heated to 227°C. After the NH_4NO_3 totally decomposes, what is the approximate pressure in the flask?

$$NH_4NO_{3(s)} \rightarrow N_2O_{(g)} + H_2O_{(g)}$$

A. 0.6 atm
B. 0.41 atm
C. 1.23 atm
D. 0.672 atm

10. In the diagram below, what is the partial pressure of each gas if all of the stopcocks are opened? Assume that the volume in the connecting tubes is negligible.

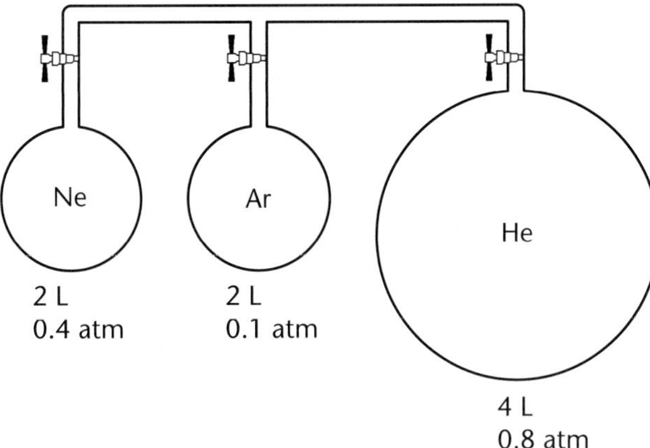

A. P_{Ne} = 0.1 atm; P_{Ar} = 0.25 atm; P_{He} = 0.25 atm
B. P_{Ne} = 0.025 atm; P_{Ar} = 0.4 atm; P_{He} = 0.1 atm
C. P_{Ne} = 0.2 atm; P_{Ar} = 0.1 atm; P_{He} = 0.4 atm
D. P_{Ne} = 0.1 atm; P_{Ar}= 0.025 atm; P_{He}= 0.4 atm

11. The kinetic molecular theory states that

A. the average kinetic energy of a molecule of gas is directly proportional to the temperature of the gas in Kelvin.
B. collisions between gas molecules are inelastic.
C. elastic collisions result in a loss of energy.
D. all gas molecules have the same kinetic energy.

12. Use the velocity distribution curves shown below to answer the question. The plots of two gases at STP are shown. One of the gases is 1 L of helium and the other is 1 L of bromine. Which plot corresponds to each gas and why?

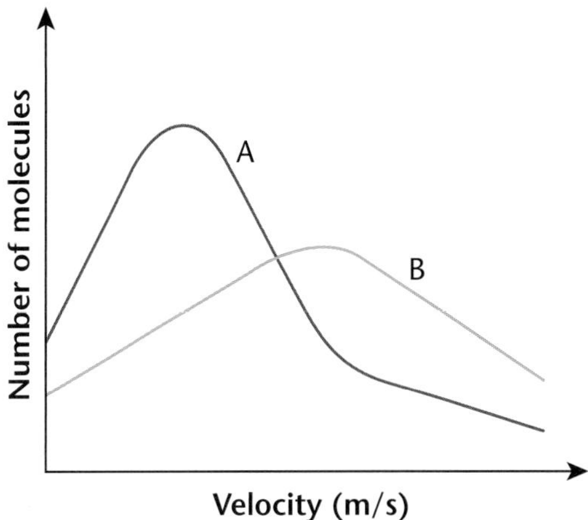

A. Curve A is helium and curve B is bromine because helium has a smaller molar mass than bromine.
B. Curve A is helium and curve B is bromine because the average kinetic energy of bromine is greater than the average kinetic energy of helium.
C. Curve A is bromine and curve B is helium because helium has a smaller molar mass than bromine.
D. Curve A is bromine and curve B is helium because the average kinetic energy of bromine is greater than the average kinetic energy of helium.

13. A balloon at standard temperature and pressure contains 0.2 moles of oxygen and 0.6 moles of nitrogen. What is the partial pressure of oxygen in the balloon?

A. 0.2 atm
B. 0.3 atm
C. 0.6 atm
D. 0.25 atm

14. The temperature at the center of the sun can be estimated based on the approximation that the gases at the center of the sun have an average molar mass equal to 2 g/mole. Approximate the temperature at the center of the sun using these additional values: the pressure equals 1.3×10^9 atm and the density at the center equals 1.2 g/cm^3.

A. 2.6×10^{7}°C
B. 2.6×10^{10}°C
C. 2.6×10^{4}°C
D. 2.6×10^{6}°C

15. Which of the following are true about the gaseous state of matter?

I. Gases are compressible.
II. Gases readily conduct electricity.
III. Gases assume the volume of their container.
IV. Gas particles exist as diatomic molecules.

A. I and II only
B. I and III only
C. I, III, and IV
D. I, II, III, and IV

16. A gas at a temperature of 27°C has a volume of 60 mL. What temperature change is needed to increase this gas to a volume of 90 mL?

A. Reduce temperature by 150°C
B. Increase temperature by 150°C
C. Reduce temperature by 40.5°C
D. Increase temperature by 40.5°C

17. Gases X and Y are contained in a moveable piston system. They are beneath the pistons in an enclosed space. They react completely to form gas XY, and the reaction is not reversible. What movement will the pistons exhibit during the reaction?

A. They will move up due to an increase in the volume of gas.
B. They will move up due to the energy given off by the reaction.
C. They will not move.
D. They will move down due to a decrease in the volume of gas.

18. A gaseous mixture contains nitrogen and helium and has a total pressure of 150 torr. The nitrogen particles comprise 80 percent of the gas and the helium particles make up the other 20 percent of the gas. What is the pressure exerted by each individual gas?

A. 100 torr nitrogen, 50 torr helium
B. 120 torr nitrogen, 30 torr helium
C. 30 torr nitrogen, 150 torr helium
D. 50 torr nitrogen, 100 torr helium

19. In which of the following situations is it impossible to predict how the pressure will change for the gas sample?

A. Gas is cooled at a constant volume
B. Gas is heated at a constant volume
C. Gas is heated and the volume is simultaneously increased
D. Gas is cooled and the volume is simultaneously increased

CHAPTER 8

PHASES AND PHASE CHANGES

When the attractive forces between molecules (i.e., van der Waals forces) overcome the kinetic energy that keeps them apart, the molecules move closer together such that they can no longer move about freely, entering the **liquid** or **solid** phase. Because of their smaller volume relative to gases, liquids and solids are often referred to as the **condensed phases.**

LIQUIDS

In a liquid, atoms or molecules are held close together with little space between them. As a result, liquids have definite volumes and cannot easily be expanded or compressed. However, the molecules can still move around and are in a state of relative disorder. Consequently, the liquid can change shape to fit its container, and its molecules are able to **diffuse** and **evaporate.**

Teacher Tip

Because the molecules in liquids and solids are much closer together than those in gases, intermolecular forces are very important and there is no such thing as "ideal" behavior. However, due to these forces, the behavior is predictable in other ways than the gases.

One of the most important properties of liquids is their ability to mix, both with each other and with other phases, to form **solutions** (see chapter 9). The degree to which two liquids can mix is called their **miscibility.** Oil and water are almost completely **immiscible;** that is, their molecules tend to repel each other due to their polarity difference. Oil and water normally form separate layers when mixed, with oil on top because it is less dense. Under extreme conditions, such as violent shaking, two immiscible liquids can form a fairly homogeneous mixture called an **emulsion.** Although they look like solutions, emulsions are actually mixtures of discrete particles too small to be seen distinctly.

SOLIDS

In a solid, the attractive forces between atoms, ions, or molecules are strong enough to hold them rigidly together; thus the particles' only motion is vibration about fixed positions, and the kinetic energy of solids is predominantly vibrational energy. As a result, solids have definite shapes and volumes.

A solid may be **crystalline** or **amorphous.** A crystalline solid, such as NaCl, possesses an ordered structure; its atoms exist in a specific three-dimensional geometric arrangement with repeating patterns of atoms, ions, or molecules. An amorphous solid, such as glass, has no ordered three-dimensional arrangement, although the molecules are also fixed in place.

Most solids are crystalline in structure. The two most common forms of crystals are **metallic** and **ionic** crystals.

Ionic solids are aggregates of positively and negatively charged ions; there are no discrete molecules. The physical properties of ionic solids include high melting points, high boiling points, and poor electrical conductivity in the solid phase. These properties are due to the compounds' strong electrostatic interactions, which also cause the ions to be relatively immobile. Ionic structures are given by empirical formulas that describe the ratio of atoms in the lowest possible whole numbers. For example, the empirical formula $BaCl_2$ gives the ratio of barium to chloride within the crystal.

TEACHER TIP

The crystal structures allow for a balance of both attractive and repulsive forces to minimize energy. The ionic solids often have extremely strong attractive forces as we saw in chapter 4, thereby causing extremely high meting points.

Metallic solids consist of metal atoms packed together as closely as possible. Metallic solids have high melting and boiling points as a result of their strong covalent attractions. Pure metallic structures (consisting of a single element) are usually described as layers of spheres of roughly similar radii.

The repeating units of crystals (both ionic and metallic) are represented by **unit cells.** There are many types of unit cells. We will now consider only the three cubic unit cells: **simple cubic, body-centered cubic,** and **face-centered cubic.**

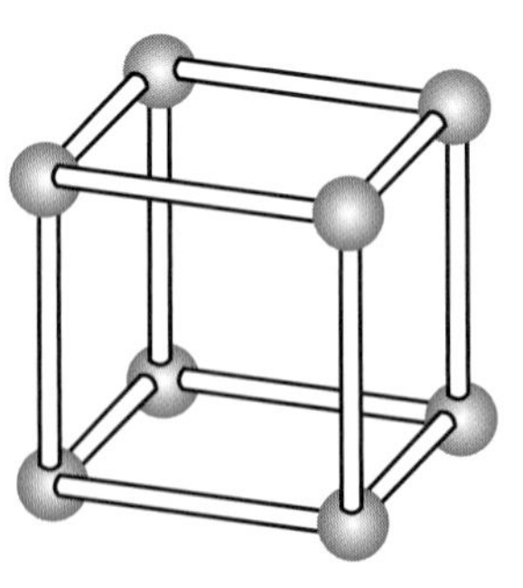

simple cubic

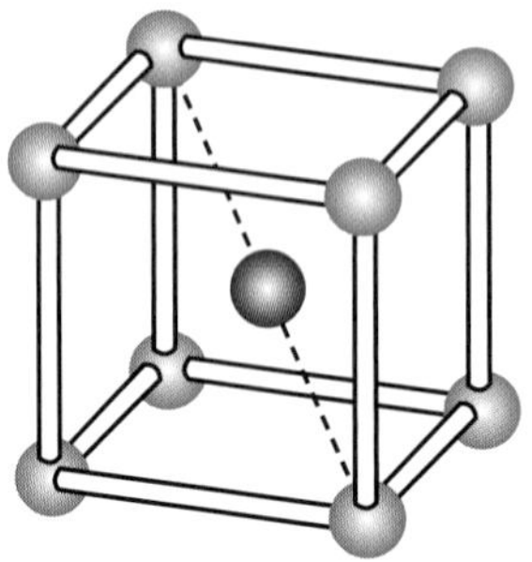

body-centered cubic

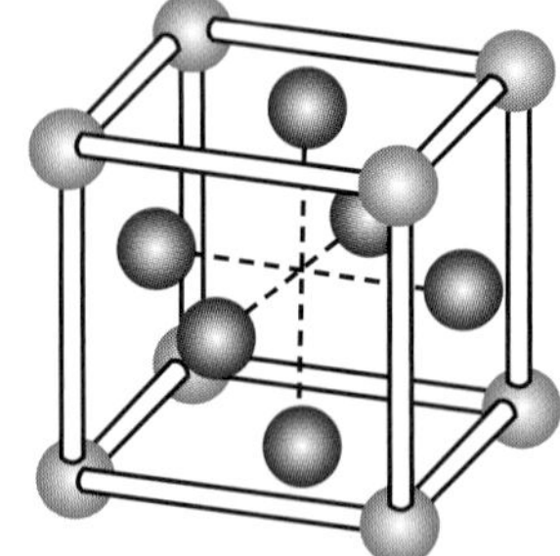

face-centered cubic

Figure 8.1

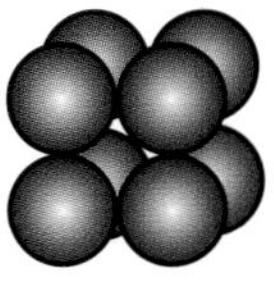

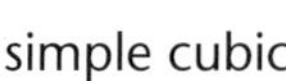

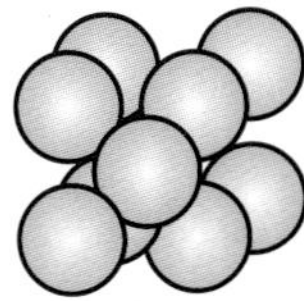

body-centered cubic

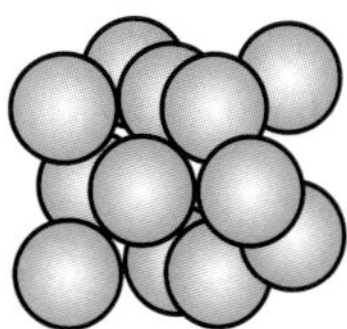

face-centered cubic

Figure 8.2

Atoms are represented as points, but are actually adjoining spheres. Each unit cell is surrounded by similar units. In the ionic unit cell, the spaces between points (anions) are filled with other ions (cations).

PHASE EQUILIBRIA

In an isolated system, phase changes (solid to liquid to gas) are reversible, and an equilibrium exists between phases. For example, at 1 atm and 0°C in an isolated system, an ice cube floating in water is in equilibrium. Some of the ice may absorb heat and melt, but an equal amount of water will release heat and freeze. Thus, the relative amounts of ice and water remain constant.

> **TEACHER TIP**
>
> As with all equilibriums, we know that the rates of the forward and reverse processes will be the same.

A. GAS-LIQUID EQUILIBRIUM

The temperature of a liquid is related to the average kinetic energy of the liquid molecules; however, the kinetic energy of the molecules will vary. A few molecules near the surface of the liquid may have enough energy to leave the liquid phase and escape into the gaseous phase. This process is known as **evaporation** (or **vaporization**). Each time the liquid loses a high-energy particle, the temperature of the remaining liquid decreases; thus, evaporation is a cooling process. Given enough kinetic energy, the liquid will completely evaporate.

If a cover is placed on a beaker of liquid, the escaping molecules are trapped above the solution. These molecules exert a countering pressure, which forces some of the gas back into the liquid phase; this process is called **condensation.** Atmospheric pressure acts on a liquid in a similar fashion as a solid lid. As evaporation and condensation proceed, an equilibrium is reached in which the rates of the two processes become equal. Once this equilibrium is reached, the pressure that the gas exerts over the liquid is called the **vapor pressure** of the liquid. Vapor pressure increases as temperature increases, because more molecules have sufficient kinetic energy to escape into the gas phase. The temperature at which the vapor pressure of the liquid equals the external pressure is called the **boiling point.**

B. LIQUID-SOLID EQUILIBRIUM

The liquid and solid phases can also coexist in equilibrium (e.g., the ice-water mixture previously discussed). Even though the atoms or molecules of a solid are confined to definite locations, each atom or molecule can undergo motions about some equilibrium position. These motions (vibrations) increase when heat is applied. If atoms or molecules in the solid phase absorb enough energy in this fashion, the solid's three-dimensional structure breaks down and the liquid phase begins. The transition from solid to liquid is called **fusion** or **melting.** The reverse process, from liquid to solid, is called **solidification, crystallization,** or **freezing.** The temperature at which these processes occur is called the **melting point** or **freezing point,** depending on the direction of the transition. Whereas pure crystals have distinct, very sharp melting points, amorphous solids, such as glass, tend to melt over a larger range of temperatures, due to their less-ordered molecular distribution.

C. GAS-SOLID EQUILIBRIUM

A third type of phase equilibrium is that between a gas and a solid. When a solid goes directly into the gas phase, the process is called **sublimation.** Dry ice (solid CO_2) sublimes; the absence of the liquid phase makes it a convenient refrigerant. The reverse transition, from the gaseous to the solid phase, is called **deposition.**

D. THE GIBBS FUNCTION

The thermodynamic criterion for each of the above equilibria is that the change in Gibbs free energy must equal zero; $\Delta G = 0$. For an equilibrium between a gas and a solid:

$$\Delta G = G(g) - G(s),$$
$$\text{so } G(g) = G(s) \text{ at equilibrium.}$$

The same is true of the Gibbs functions for the other two equilibria.

E. HEATING CURVES

When a compound is heated, the temperature rises until the melting or boiling points are reached. Then the temperature remains constant as the compound is converted to the next phase, i.e., liquid or gas, respectively. Once the entire sample is converted, then the temperature begins to rise again (Figure 8.3).

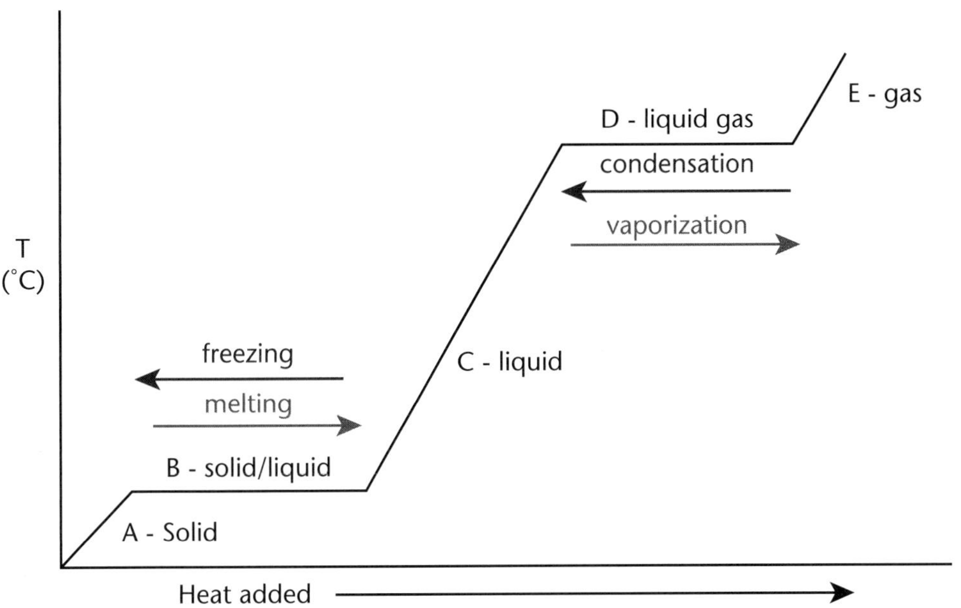

Figure 8.3: Heating Curves

PHASE DIAGRAMS

A. SINGLE COMPONENT

A standard **phase diagram** depicts the phases and phase equilibria of a substance at defined temperatures and pressures. In general, the gas phase is found at high temperature and low pressure; the solid phase at low temperature and high pressure; and the liquid phase is found at high temperature and high pressure. A typical phase diagram is shown in Figure 8.4.

MCAT SYNOPSIS

Every pure substance has a characteristic phase diagram.

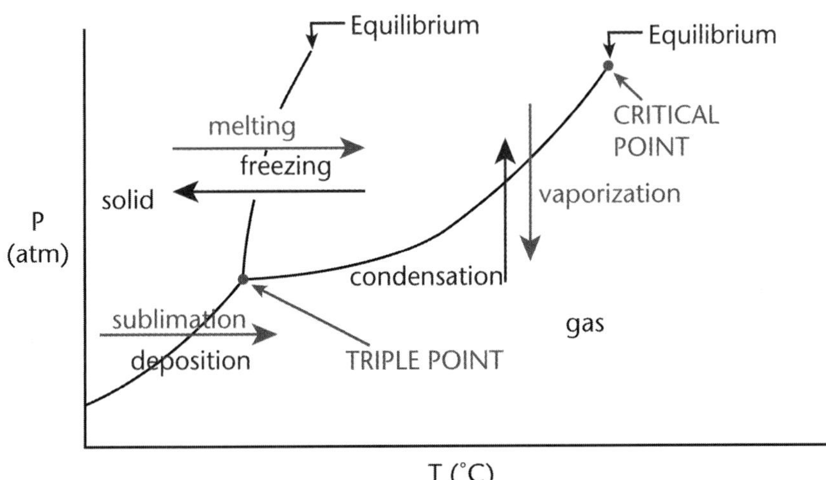

Figure 8.4: Gas-Liquid Equilibrium

MCAT FAVORITE

You should be able to identify and explain each area and every line of a phase diagram.

MCAT Synopsis

H_2O is a unique molecule because of its different properties, ice floats and ice skates flow smoothly over ice. This all "boils" down to the slope of the solid-liquid equilibrium line in its phase diagram. Because the density of ice is less than that of liquid H_2O, an increase in pressure (at a constant temperature) will actually melt ice (the opposite of the substance seen in Figure 8.4)

The three phases are demarcated by lines indicating the temperatures and pressures at which two phases are in equilibrium. Line A represents freezing/melting, line B evaporation/condensation, and line C sublimation/deposition. The intersection of the three lines is called the **triple point.** At this temperature and pressure, unique for a given substance, all three phases are in equilibrium. The point at B is known as the **critical point,** the temperature and pressure above which no distinction between liquid and gas is possible.

B. MULTIPLE COMPONENTS

The phase diagram for a mixture of two or more components (Figure 8.5) is complicated by the requirement that the composition of the mixture, as well as the temperature and pressure, must be specified. Consider a solution of two liquids, A and B. The vapor above the solution is a mixture of the vapors of A and B. The pressures exerted by vapor A and vapor B on the solution are the vapor pressures that each exerts above its individual liquid phase. **Raoult's law** (described later in this chapter) enables one to determine the relationship between the vapor pressure of vapor A and the concentration of liquid A in the solution.

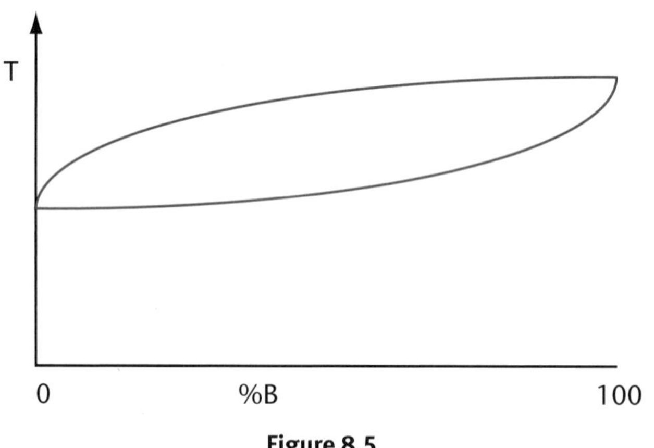

Figure 8.5

Curves such as this show the different compositions of the liquid phase and the vapor phase above a solution; the upper curve is that of the vapor while the lower curve is that of the liquid. It is this difference in composition that forms the basis of distillation, an important separation technique in organic chemistry.

COLLIGATIVE PROPERTIES

Colligative properties are physical properties derived solely from the number of particles present, not the nature of those particles. These properties are usually associated with dilute solutions (see chapter 9).

A. FREEZING-POINT DEPRESSION

Pure water (H_2O) freezes at 0°C; however, for every mole of solute particles dissolved in 1 L of water, the freezing point is lowered by 1.86°C. This is because the solute particles interfere with the process of crystal formation that occurs during freezing; the solute particles lower the temperature at which the molecules can align themselves into a crystalline structure.

The formula for calculating this **freezing-point depression** is:

$$\Delta T_f = K_f m$$

where ΔT_f is the freezing-point depression, K_f is a proportionality constant characteristic of a particular solvent, and m is the molality of the solution (mol solute/kg solvent; see chapter 9). The K_f for water—which you do not need to memorize for the MCAT—is 1.86°Cm^{-1}. Each solvent has its own characteristic K_f.

B. BOILING-POINT ELEVATION

A liquid boils when its vapor pressure equals the atmospheric pressure. If the vapor pressure of a solution is lower than that of the pure solvent, more energy (and consequently a higher temperature) will be required before its vapor pressure equals atmospheric pressure. The extent to which the boiling point of a solution is raised relative to that of the pure solvent is given by the following formula:

$$\Delta T_b = K_b m$$

where ΔT_b is the boiling-point elevation, K_b is a proportionality constant characteristic of a particular solvent, and m is the molality of the solution. The K_b for water is 0.51°Cm^{-1}.

REAL-WORLD ANALOGY

In cold climates, roads are often salted during snowstorms to decrease the freezing point of water, thereby lessening the formation of ice.

C. OSMOTIC PRESSURE

Consider a container separated into two compartments by a semipermeable membrane (which, by definition, selectively permits the passage of certain molecules). One compartment contains pure water, while the other contains water with dissolved solute. The membrane allows water but not solute to pass through. Because substances tend to flow, or **diffuse,** from higher to lower concentrations (which increases entropy), water will diffuse from the compartment containing pure water to the compartment containing the water-solute mixture. This net flow will cause the water level in the compartment containing the solution to rise above the level in the compartment containing pure water.

MCAT SYNOPSIS

Remember to always use Kelvin temperature if T is in an equation!.

MCAT FAVORITE

Water will move toward the chamber with either greater molarity or higher temperature (assuming that the molarity is the same).

Because the solute cannot pass through the membrane, the concentrations of solute in the two compartments can never be equal. However, the pressure exerted by the water level in the solute-containing compartment will eventually oppose the influx of water; thus, the water level will rise only to the point at which it exerts a sufficient pressure to counterbalance the tendency of water to flow across the membrane. This pressure is defined as the **osmotic pressure** (Π) of the solution, and is given by the formula:

$$\Pi = \mathbf{MRT}$$

where M is the molarity of the solution (see chapter 9), R is the ideal gas constant, and T is the temperature on the Kelvin scale. This equation clearly shows that molarity and osmotic pressure are directly proportional, i.e., as the concentration of the solution increases, the osmotic pressure also increases. Thus, the osmotic pressure depends only on the amount of solute, not its identity.

D. VAPOR-PRESSURE LOWERING (RAOULT'S LAW)

TEACHER TIP

Think of this in the same vein as boiling-point elevation: The lowering of a solution's vapor pressure would mean that we'd need a higher temperature to overcome atmospheric pressure, thereby raising the boiling point. These two concepts go hand-in-hand.

When solute B is added to pure solvent A, the vapor pressure of A above the solvent decreases (see Figure 8.4). If the vapor pressure of A above pure solvent A is designated by $P°_A$ and the vapor pressure of A above the solution containing B is P_A, the vapor pressure decreases as follows:

$$\Delta P = P°_A - P_A$$

In the late 1800s, the French chemist François Marie Raoult determined that this vapor pressure decrease is also equivalent to:

$$\Delta P = X_B P°_A$$

where X_B is the mole fraction of the solute B in solvent A. Since $X_B = 1 - X_A$ and $\Delta P = P°_A - P_A$, substitution into the above equation leads to the common form of Raoult's law:

$$P_A = X_A P°_A$$

Similarly, the expression for the vapor pressure of the solute in solution (assuming it is volatile) is given by:

$$P_B = X_B P°_B$$

Raoult's law holds only when the attraction between molecules of the different components of the mixture is equal to the attraction between the molecules of any one component in its pure state. When this condition does not hold, the relationship between mole fraction and vapor pressure will deviate from Raoult's law. Solutions that obey Raoult's law are called **ideal solutions.**

PRACTICE QUESTIONS

1. The phase diagram below illustrates what substance?

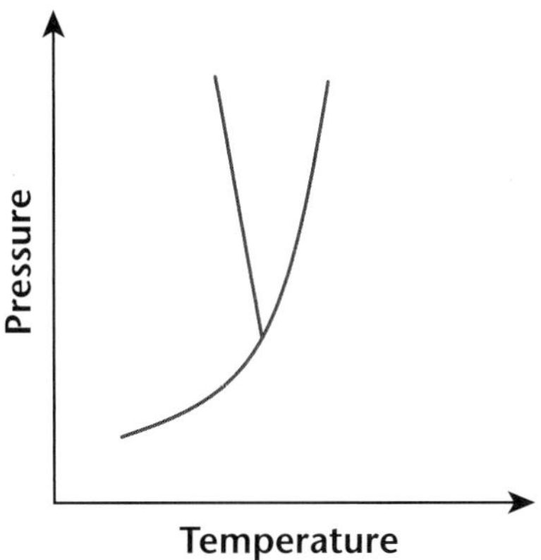

A. CO_2
B. NaCl
C. Ne
D. H_2O

2. Living cells are comprised of a significant amount of water. Which of the following best explains why frostbite—the result of freezing living tissue—is so harmful to living cells?

A. Water is very dense at 4° Celsius.
B. Water is not very dense at 4° Celsius.
C. Water is less dense at 0° Celsus than at 4° Celsius.
D. Water is more dense at 0° Celsius than at 4° Celsius.

3. What phase change occurs to the ice beneath an ice skater as pressure is applied by the skates?

A. Condensation
B. Crystallization
C. Deposition
D. Melting

4. Which of the following proportionalities best describes the relationship between intermolecular forces and heat of vaporization for a given substance?

A. Intermolecular forces are proportional to ΔH_{vap}.
B. Intermolecular forces are inversely proportional to $\Delta H_{vap.}$
C. The relationship between intermolecular forces and ΔH_{vap} cannot be generalized.
D. There is no relationship between intermolecular forces and ΔH_{vap}.

5. What molecule below is likely to have the highest melting point?

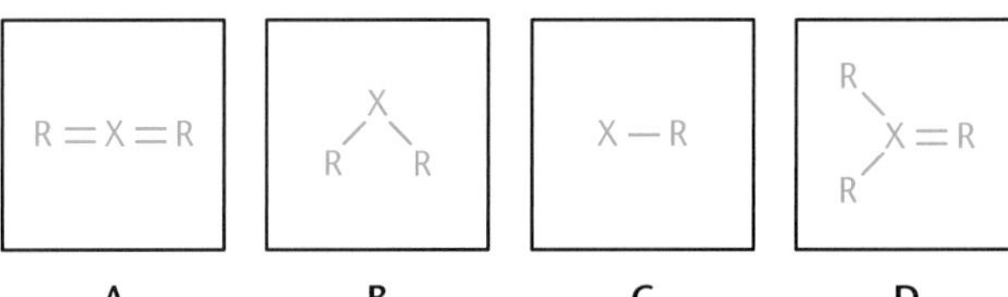

A. A
B. B
C. C
D. D

6. Which of the following physical conditions favor a gaseous state for most substances?

A. High pressure and high temperature
B. Low pressure and low temperature
C. High pressure and low temperature
D. Low pressure and high temperature

7. When ambient pressure increases, the heating/coiling curve for a substance will be shifted in which of the following directions?

A. Up
B. Down
C. Right
D. Left

8. Which of the following best explains the mechanism by which solute particles affect the melting point of ice?

A. Melting point elevates because the kinetic energy of the substance increases.
B. Melting point elevates because the kinetic energy of the substance decreases.
C. Melting point depresses because solute particles interfere with lattice formation.
D. Melting point depresses because solute particles enhance lattice formation.

9. A viscous substance is most likely to have a

A. low precipitation rate.
B. high heat of vaporization.
C. low heat of fusion.
D. high critical mass.

10. Fractional distillation of crude oil involves heating the oil at very high temperatures to the gaseous state, then allowing parts of the oil to condense at different temperatures. Which hydrocarbon component of crude oil would you predict is the last to vaporize?

A. Gasoline
B. Natural gas
C. Propane
D. Tar

11. In the figure below, what phase change is represented by the arrow?

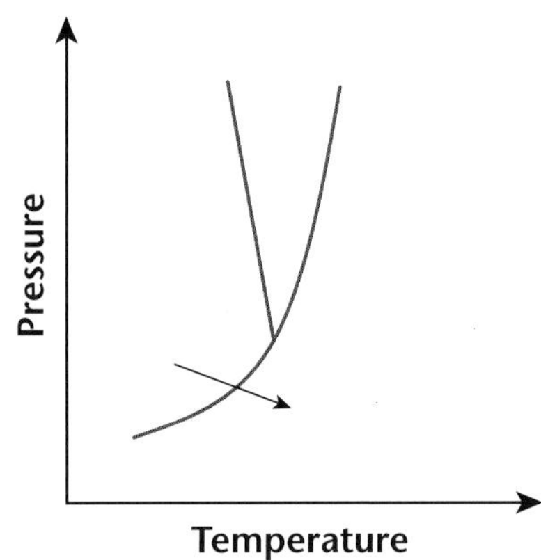

A. Condensation
B. Deposition
C. Sublimation
D. Vaporization

12. It is impossible to skate on dry ice because it has a

A. positive solid/liquid equilibrium line slope.
B. negative solid/liquid equilibrium line slope.
C. positive liquid/gas equilibrium line slope.
D. negative liquid/gas equilibrium line slope.

13. Which of the following best describes the chemical activity depicted by the region X on the heating/cooling curve for a substance shown below?

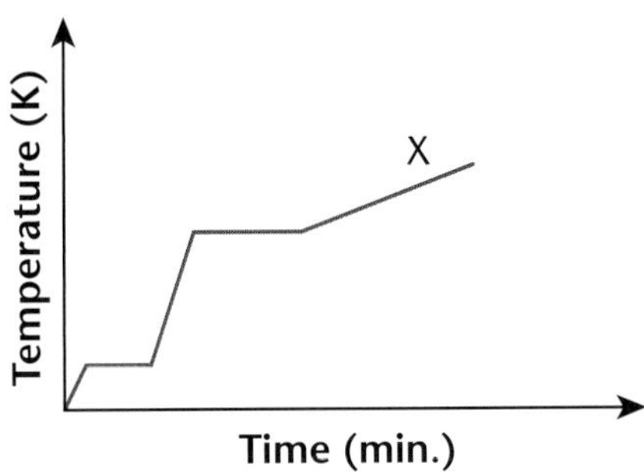

A. Average kinetic energy of the particles is changing.
B. Particles are locked in a lattice-like state.
C. Particles are in a liquid state.
D. Particle size is decreasing.

14. Which of the following statements best explains the effect of sweating on body temperature in animals?

A. Condensation of sweat leads to the gain of low-energy molecules.
B. Condensation of sweat leads to the loss of high-energy molecules.
C. Evaporation of sweat leads to the gain of low-energy molecules.
D. Evaporation of sweat leads to the loss of high-energy molecules.

15. Which of the following situations would most favor the change of water from a liquid to a solid?

I. Decreased solute concentration of a substance
II. Decreased temperature of a substance
III. Decreased pressure on a substance

A. I only
B. II only
C. I and II only
D. I, II, and III

16. A person feels warmer on a humid day compared with a very dry one, even though the temperature on both days is the same. On the humid day, the person is experiencing the process of

A. condensation.
B. evaporation.
C. transpiration.
D. sublimation.

17. Rain is a form of

A. condensation.
B. evaporation.
C. transpiration.
D. sublimation.

18. The heats of vaporization of four substances are given below. Which of these substances has the lowest boiling point?

Comparative Heats of Vaporization

Liquid	Heat Required (cal/g)
Chlorine	67.4
Ether	9.4
Carbon dioxide	72.2
Ammonia	295.0

A. Chlorine
B. Ether
C. Carbon dioxide
D. Ammonia

Key Concepts

Dalton's law

$P_A = X_A P_{Total}$ (atm)

Mole fraction

$$X_A = \frac{(\text{moles of } A)}{(\text{total \# of moles in container})}$$

PARTIAL PRESSURES

32 g of oxygen, 28 g of nitrogen, and 22 g of carbon dioxide are confined in a container with partial pressures of 2 atm, 2 atm and 1 atm respectively. A student added 57 g of a halogen gas to this container and observed that the total pressure increased by 3 atm. Can you identify this gas?

1) Determine the number of moles for each gas.

$MW_{oxygen} = 32$ g/mol
$MW_{nitrogen} = 28$ g/mol
$MW_{carbon\ dioxide} = 44$ g/mol

$$n = \frac{\text{mass}}{MW}$$

$n_{oxygen} = 1$ mole
$n_{nitrogen} = 1$ mole
$n_{carbon\ dioxide} = 0.5$ moles

This is a more complicated style of partial pressure question, yet the first step is still the basic one of identifying the number of moles for each gas.

Takeaways

Partial pressure questions will require manipulation of the formulas above, so the key is to always keep track of what is given to you and what the question is asking for.

---

2) Solve for the relevant variable.

$$P_A = X_A P_{Total}$$

$$X_A = \frac{P_A}{P_{Total}}$$

$$X_A = \frac{3}{8}$$

All partial pressure questions boil down to this formula. The relevant variable here is the mole fraction of the halogen gas. The partial pressure of the gas is 3 atm, and the total pressure is 8 atm.

---

3) Use the mole fraction X_A to solve for the number of moles and the MW of the halogen gas.

$$X_A = \frac{(\text{moles of } A)}{(\text{total \# of moles in container})}$$

\# moles of $A = (X_A)$(total # of moles)

$$n_A = \left(\frac{3}{8}\right)(2.5 + n_A)$$

$8n_A = 7.5 + 3n_A$
$5n_A = 7.5$
$n_A = 1.5$

Things to Watch Out For

Dalton's law assumes that the gases do not react with each other.

$$MW = \frac{57\text{ g}}{1.5\text{ mol}}$$
MW of 38 g/mol

The mole fraction of a substance is the number of moles of the substance as a fraction of the total number of moles in the container:

$$X_A = \frac{(\text{moles of } A)}{(\text{total \# of moles in container})}$$

Rearranging the formula, we have # moles of $A = (X_A)$(total # of moles). Note that the total number of moles is not known, but we can express it algebraically as $2.5 + n_A$, where n_A is defined as the number of moles of A.

This MW corresponds to F_2. Of course, on Test Day you will roughly round such that 60 g = 1.5 mole and look for the halogen gas using your calculated MW of 40 g/mol. Again, the only gas possible is F_2.

SIMILAR QUESTIONS

1) 64 g of oxygen, 14 g of nitrogen, and 66 g of carbon dioxide are confined in a container. If the total pressure is 10 atm, what is the partial pressure of each gas?
2) The partial pressure of nitrogen is 2 atm. If its mole fraction is 2/10 and the only other gas in the container is oxygen, how many moles of oxygen are in the container?
3) An unknown substance's mole fraction is 4/10. If its partial pressure is 5 atm, what is the sum pressure of all the other gases in the container?

CHAPTER 9

SOLUTIONS

Solutions are **homogeneous** (everywhere the same) mixtures of substances that combine to form a single phase, generally the liquid phase. Many important chemical reactions, both in the laboratory and in nature, take place in solution (including almost all reactions in living organisms).

NATURE OF SOLUTIONS

A solution consists of a **solute** (e.g., NaCl, NH_3, or $C_{12}H_{22}O_{11}$) dispersed (dissolved) in a **solvent** (e.g., H_2O or benzene). The solvent is the component of the solution whose phase remains the same after mixing. If the two substances are already in the same phase, the solvent is the component present in greater quantity. Solute molecules move about freely in the solvent and can interact with other molecules or ions; consequently, chemical reactions occur easily in solution.

A. SOLVATION

The interaction between solute and solvent molecules is known as **solvation** or **dissolution;** when water is the solvent, it is called **hydration** and the resulting solution is known as an **aqueous solution.** Solvation is possible when the attractive forces between solute and solvent are stronger than those between the solute particles. For example, when NaCl dissolves in water, its component ions dissociate from one another and become surrounded by water molecules. Because water is polar, ion-dipole interactions can occur between the Na^+ and Cl^- ions and the water molecules. For nonionic solutes, solvation involves van der Waals forces between the solute and solvent molecules. The general rule is that like dissolves like; ionic and polar solutes are soluble in polar solvents, and nonpolar solutes are soluble in nonpolar solvents.

B. SOLUBILITY

The **solubility** of a substance is the maximum amount of that substance that can be dissolved in a particular solvent at a particular temperature. When this maximum amount of solute has been added, the solution is

MCAT Synopsis

Note that "dilute" is a relative term.

in equilibrium and is said to be **saturated;** if more solute is added, it will not dissolve. For example, at 18°C, a maximum of 83 g of glucose ($C_6H_{12}O_6$) will dissolve in 100 mL of H_2O. Thus the solubility of glucose is 83 g/100 mL. If more glucose is added, it will remain in solid form, precipitating to the bottom of the container. A solution in which the proportion of solute to solvent is small is said to be **dilute,** and one in which the proportion is large is said to be **concentrated.**

TEACHER TIP

Because most solutions involve water as the solvent in the real world, they are commonly seen on the exam. The solubility rules are not bad to know but memorizing them all is excessive. Being able to apply them is more important. Know rules 1 and 2 for sure, and learn the more common insoluble exceptions (Pb^{2+} and Ag^+).

C. AQUEOUS SOLUTIONS

The most common class of solutions are the aqueous solutions, in which the solvent is water. The aqueous state is denoted by the symbol (*aq*). In discussing the chemistry of aqueous solutions, it is useful to know how soluble various salts are in water; this information is given by the solubility rules below.

1. All salts of alkali metals are water soluble.
2. All salts of the ammonium ion (NH_4^+) are water soluble.
3. All chlorides, bromides, and iodides are water soluble, with the exceptions of Ag^+, Pb^{2+}, and Hg_2^{2+}.
4. All salts of the sulfate ion (SO_4^{2-}) are water soluble, with the exceptions of Ca^{2+}, Sr^{2+}, Ba^{2+}, and Pb^{2+}.
5. All metal oxides are insoluble, with the exception of the alkali metals and CaO, SrO , and BaO, all of which hydrolyze to form solutions of the corresponding metal hydroxides.
6. All hydroxides are insoluble, with the exception of the alkali metals and Ca^{2+}, Sr^{2+}, and Ba^{2+}.
7. All carbonates (CO_3^{2-}), phosphates (PO_4^{3-}), sulfides (S^{2-}), and sulfites (SO_3^{2-}) are insoluble, with the exception of the alkali metals and ammonium.

IONS

Ionic solutions are of particular interest to chemists because certain important types of chemical interactions—acid-base reactions and oxidation-reduction reactions, for instance—take place in ionic solutions. Ions and their properties in solution will be introduced here; the chemical reactions mentioned are discussed in detail in chapter 10, Acids and Bases, and chapter 11, Redox Reactions and Electrochemistry.

A. CATIONS AND ANIONS

Ionic compounds are made up of **cations** and **anions,** where a cation is a positive ion and an anion is a negative ion. The nomenclature of ionic compounds is based on the names of the component ions.

1. For elements (usually metals) that can form more than one positive ion, the charge is indicated by a Roman numeral in parentheses following the name of the element.

   Fe^{2+} Iron (II) — Cu^{+} Copper (I)
   Fe^{3+} Iron (III) — Cu^{2+} Copper (II)

2. An older but still commonly used method is to add the endings **-ous** or **-ic** to the root of the Latin name of the element, to represent the ions with lesser or greater charge respectively.

   Fe^{2+} Ferrous — Cu^{+} Cuprous
   Fe^{3+} Ferric — Cu^{2+} Cupric

3. Monatomic anions are named by dropping the ending of the name of the element and adding **-ide.**

   H^{-} Hydride — S^{2-} Sulfide
   F^{-} Fluoride — N^{3-} Nitride
   O^{2-} Oxide — P^{3-} Phosphide

4. Many polyatomic anions contain oxygen and are therefore called **oxyanions**. When an element forms two oxyanions, the name of the one with less oxygen ends in **-ite** and the one with more oxygen ends in **-ate.**

   NO_2^{-} Nitrite — SO_3^{2-} Sulfite
   NO_3^{-} Nitrate — SO_4^{2-} Sulfate

5. When the series of oxyanions contains four oxyanions, prefixes are also used. **Hypo-** and **per-** are used to indicate less oxygen and more oxygen, respectively.

   ClO^{-} Hypochlorite
   ClO_2^{-} Chlorite
   ClO_3^{-} Chlorate
   ClO_4^{-} Perchlorate

6. Polyatomic anions often gain one or more H^+ ions to form anions of lower charge. The resulting ions are named by adding the word **hydrogen** or **dihydrogen** to the front of the anion's name. An older method uses the prefix **bi-** to indicate the addition of a single hydrogen ion.

   HCO_3^- Hydrogen carbonate or bicarbonate

   HSO_4^- Hydrogen sulfate or bisulfate

   $H_2PO_4^-$ Dihydrogen phosphate

B. ION CHARGES

Metals, which are found in the left part of the periodic table, generally form positive ions, whereas nonmetals, which are found in the right part of the periodic table, generally form negative ions. Note, however, the existence of anions that contain metallic elements, e.g., MnO_4^- (permanganate) and CrO_4^{2-} (chromate). All elements in a given group tend to form monatomic ions with the same charge. Thus ions of alkali metals (Group I) usually form cations with a single positive charge, the alkaline earth metals (Group II) form cations with a double positive charge, and the halides (Group VII) form anions with a single negative charge. Though other main group elements follow this trend, the intermediate electronegativity of such elements (making them less likely to form ionic compounds) and the transition from metallic to nonmetallic character complicates the picture.

MCAT SYNOPSIS

Oxyanions of transition metals like the MnO^{4-} and CrO_4^{2-} ions have an inordinately high oxidation number on the metal. As such, they tend to gain electrons in order to reduce this oxidation number, and thus make good oxidizing agents. (See chapter 11.)

C. ELECTROLYTES

The electrical conductivity of aqueous solutions is governed by the presence and concentration of ions in solution. Therefore, pure water does not conduct an electrical current well because the concentrations of hydrogen and hydroxide ions are very small. Solutes whose solutions are conductive are called **electrolytes.** A solute is considered a **strong electrolyte** if it dissociates completely into its constituent ions. Examples of strong electrolytes include ionic compounds, such as NaCl and KI, and molecular compounds with highly polar covalent bonds that dissociate into ions when dissolved, such as HCl in water. A **weak electrolyte,** on the other hand, ionizes or hydrolyzes incompletely in aqueous solution and only some of the solute is present in ionic form. Examples include acetic acid and other weak acids, ammonia and other weak bases, and $HgCl_2$. Many compounds do not ionize at all in aqueous solution, retaining their molecular structure in solution, which usually limits their solubility. These compounds are called nonelectrolytes and include many nonpolar gases and organic compounds, such as oxygen and sugar.

MCAT SYNOPSIS

Because electrolytes ionize in solution, they will produce a larger effect on colligative properties (see chapter 8) than one would expect from the given concentration.

CONCENTRATION

A. UNITS OF CONCENTRATION

Concentration denotes the amount of solute dissolved in a solvent. The concentration of a solution is most commonly expressed as **percent composition by mass, mole fraction, molarity, molality,** or **normality.**

TEACHER TIP

Know the different ways to express concentration.

1. Percent Composition by Mass

The percent composition by mass (percent) of a solution is the mass of the solute divided by the mass of the solution (solute plus solvent), multiplied by 100.

Example: What is the percent composition by mass of a salt water solution if 100 g of the solution contains 20 g of NaCl?

Solution:

$$\frac{20\text{g NaCl}}{100\text{ g}} \times 100 = 20\%\ \text{NaCl solution}$$

2. Mole Fraction

The mole fraction (**X**) of a compound is equal to the number of moles of the compound divided by the total number of moles of all species within the system. The sum of the mole fractions in a system will always equal 1.

Example: If 92 g of glycerol is mixed with 90 g of water, what will be the mole fractions of the two components? (MW of H_2O = 18; MW of $C_3H_8O_3$ = 92.)

Solution:

$$90\text{ g water} = 90\text{ g} \times \frac{1\text{ mol}}{18\text{ g}} = 5\text{ mol}$$

$$92\text{ g glycerol} = 92\text{ g} \times \frac{1\text{ mol}}{92\text{ g}} = 1\text{ mol}$$

$$\text{Total mol} = 5 + 1 = 6\text{ mol}$$

$$X_{\text{water}} = \frac{5\text{ mol}}{6\text{ mol}} = 0.833$$

$$X_{\text{glycerol}} = \frac{1\text{ mol}}{6\text{ mol}} = 0.167$$

$$X_{\text{water}} + X_{\text{glycerol}} = 0.833 + 0.167 = 1$$

MCAT SYNOPSIS

Note that for dilute solutions, the volume of the solution is approximately equal to the volume of solvent used.

3. Molarity

The molarity (**M**) of a solution is the number of moles of solute per liter of **solution.** Solution concentrations are usually expressed in terms of molarity. Molarity depends on the volume of the solution, not on the volume of solvent used to prepare the solution.

Example: If enough water is added to 11 g of $CaCl_2$ to make 100 mL of solution, what is the molarity of the solution?

Solution:

$$\frac{11\text{ g }CaCl_2}{110\text{ g }CaCl_2/\text{mol }CaCl_2} = 0.1\text{ mol }CaCl_2$$

$$100\text{ mL} \times \frac{1\text{L}}{1{,}000\text{ mL}} = 0.1\text{ L}$$

$$\text{molarity} = \frac{0.1\text{ mol}}{0.1\text{ L}} = 1\text{ M}$$

4. Molality

The molality (**m**) of a solution is the number of moles of solute per kilogram of **solvent**. For dilute aqueous solutions at 25°C the molality is approximately equal to the molarity, because the density of water at this temperature is 1 kilogram per liter. However, note that this is an approximation and true only for **dilute aqueous** solutions.

Example: If 10 g of NaOH are dissolved in 500 g of water, what is the molality of the solution?

Solution:

$$\frac{10\text{ g NaOH}}{40\text{ g NaOH/mol NaOH}} = 0.25\text{ mol NaOH}$$

$$500\text{ g} \times \frac{1\text{kg}}{1{,}000\text{ g}} = 0.5\text{ kg}$$

$$\text{molality} = \frac{0.25\text{ mol}}{0.5\text{ kg}} = 0.5\text{ mol/kg} = 0.50\text{ m}$$

MCAT SYNOPSIS

Normality is best thought of as "molarity of the stuff of interest" in the reaction.

5. Normality

The normality (**N**) of a solution is equal to the number of gram equivalent weights of solute per liter of solution. A gram equivalent weight, or equivalent, is a measure of the reactive capacity of a molecule (see chapter 4, Compounds and Stoichiometry).

To calculate the normality of a solution, we must know for what purpose the solution is being used, because it is the concentration of the reactive species with which we are concerned. Normality is unique among concentration units in that it is reaction dependent. For example, a 1 molar solution of sulfuric acid would be 2 normal for acid-base reactions (because each mole of sulfuric acid provides 2 moles of H^+ ions) but is only 1 normal for a sulfate precipitation reaction (because each mole of sulfuric acid only provides 1 mole of sulfate ions).

B. DILUTION

A solution is **diluted** when solvent is added to a solution of high concentration to produce a solution of lower concentration. The concentration of a solution after dilution can be conveniently determined using the equation below:

$$M_iV_i = M_fV_f$$

where M is molarity, V is volume, and the subscripts i and f refer to initial and final values, respectively.

MCAT FAVORITE

This equation is worthy of memorization. Note that it works for any units of concentration, not just molarity, if we replace the M with C for concentration.

Example: How many mL of a 5.5 M NaOH solution must be used to prepare 300 mL of a 1.2 M NaOH solution?

Solution:

$$5.5\ \text{M} \times V_i = 1.2\ \text{M} \times 0.3\ \text{L}$$

$$V_i = \frac{1.2\ \text{M} \times 0.3\ \text{L}}{5.5\ \text{M}}$$

$$V_i = 0.065\ \text{L} = 65\ \text{mL}$$

SOLUTION EQUILIBRIA

The process of solvation, like other reversible chemical and physical changes, tends toward an equilibrium. Immediately after solute has been introduced into a solvent, most of the change taking place is dissociation, because no dissolved solute is initially present. However, according to Le Châtelier's principle, as solute dissociates, the reverse reaction (precipitation of the solute) also begins to occur. Eventually an equilibrium is reached, with the rate of solute dissociation equal to the rate of precipitation, and the net concentration of the dissociated solute remains unchanged regardless of the amount of solute added.

An ionic solid introduced into a polar solvent dissociates into its component ions. The dissociation of such a solute in solution may be represented by

$$A_mB_n(s) \rightleftharpoons mA^{n+}(aq) + nB^{m-}(aq)$$

A. THE SOLUBILITY PRODUCT CONSTANT

A slightly soluble ionic solid exists in equilibrium with its saturated solution. In the case of AgCl, for example, the solution equilibrium is as follows:

$$AgCl(s) \rightleftharpoons Ag^{+}(aq) + Cl^{-}(aq)$$

The **ion product, I.P.,** of a compound in solution is defined as follows:

$$\text{I.P.} = [A^{n+}]^m[B^{m-}]^n$$

TEACHER TIP

K_{sp} is just a specialized form of K_{eq}, so we can use the same concepts we use for all equilibriums, including Le Châtelier's principle.

The same expression for a saturated solution at equilibrium defines the **solubility product constant, K_{sp}.**

$$K_{sp} = [A^{n+}]^m[B^{m-}]^n \text{ in a saturated solution}$$

MCAT SYNOPSIS

If the solution is supersaturated, $Q_{sp} > K_{sp}$, precipitation will occur.

If the solution is undersaturated $Q_{sp} < K_{sp}$, the solute will continue to dissolve.

If the solution is saturated, $Q_{sp} = K_{sp}$, then the solution is at equilibrium.

However, I.P. is defined with respect to initial concentrations and does not necessarily represent either an equilibrium or a saturated solution, while K_{sp} does; at any point other than at equilibrium, the ion product is often referred to as Q_{sp}.

Each salt has its own distinct K_{sp} at a given temperature. If at a given temperature a salt's I.P. is equal to its K_{sp}, the solution is saturated, and the rate at which the salt dissolves equals the rate at which it precipitates out of solution. If a salt's I.P. exceeds its K_{sp}, the solution is supersaturated (holding more salt than it should be able to at a given temperature) and unstable. If the supersaturated solution is disturbed by adding more salt, other solid particles, or jarring the solution by a sudden decrease in temperature, the solid salt will precipitate until I.P. equals the K_{sp}. If I.P. is less than K_{sp}, the solution is unsaturated and no precipitate will form.

Example: The solubility of $Fe(OH)_3$ in an aqueous solution was determined to be 4.5×10^{-10}mol/L. What is the value of the K_{sp} for $Fe(OH)_3$?

Solution: The molar solubility (the solubility of the compound in mol/L) is given as 4.5×10^{-10} M. The equilibrium concentration of each ion can be determined from the molar solubility and the balanced dissociation reaction of $Fe(OH)_3$. The dissociation reaction is:

$$Fe(OH)_3(s) \rightleftarrows Fe^{3+}(aq) + 3OH^-(aq)$$

Thus, for every mol of $Fe(OH)_3$ that dissociates, one mol of Fe^{3+} and three mol of OH^- are produced. Since the solubility is 4.5×10^{-10} M, the K_{sp} can be determined as follows:

$$K_{sp} = [Fe^{3+}][OH^-]^3$$

$[OH^-] = 3[Fe^{3+}]$; $[Fe^{3+}] = 4.5 \times 10^{-10}$ M

$$K_{sp} = [Fe^{3+}](3[Fe^{3+}])^3 = 27[Fe^{3+}]^4$$

$$K_{sp} = (4.5 \times 10^{-10})[3(4.5 \times 10^{-10})]^3 = 27(4.5 \times 10^{-10})^4$$

$$K_{sp} = 1.1 \times 10^{-36}$$

MCAT Synopsis

Every slightly soluble salt of general formula MX_3 will have $K_{sp} = 27x^4$, where x is the molar solubility.

Example: What are the concentrations of each of the ions in a saturated solution of $PbBr_2$, given that the K_{sp} of $PbBr_2$ is 2.1×10^{-6}? If 5 g of $PbBr_2$ are dissolved in water to make 1 L of solution at 25°C, would the solution be saturated, unsaturated, or supersaturated?

Solution: The first step is to write out the dissociation reaction:

$$PbBr_2(s) \rightleftarrows Pb^{2+}(aq) + 2Br^-(aq)$$

$$K_{sp} = [Pb^{2+}][Br^-]^2$$

Let x equal the concentration of Pb^{2+}. Then 2x equals the concentration of Br^- in the saturated solution at equilibrium (as $[Br^-]$ is 2 times $[Pb^{2+}]$).

$$(x)(2x)^2 = 4x^3$$

$$2.1 \times 10^{-6} = 4x^3$$

Solving for x, the concentration of Pb^{2+} in a saturated solution is 8.07×10^{-3} M and the concentration of Br^- (2x) is 1.61×10^{-2} M.

MCAT Synopsis

Every slightly soluble salt of general formula MX_2 will have $K_{sp} = 4x^3$, where x is the molar solubility.

Next, we convert 5 g of $PbBr_2$ into moles:

$$5 \text{ g} \times \frac{1 \text{ mol PbBr}_2}{367 \text{ g}} = 1.36 \times 10^{-2} \text{ mol}$$

1.36×10^{-2} mol of $PbBr_2$ is dissolved in 1 L of solution, so the concentration of the solution 1.36×10^{-2} M. Because this is higher than the concentration of a saturated solution, this solution would be supersaturated.

B. FACTORS AFFECTING SOLUBILITY

The solubility of a substance varies depending on the temperature of the solution, the solvent, and, in the case of a gas-phase solute, the pressure. Solubility is also affected by the addition of other substances to the solution.

The solubility of a salt is considerably reduced when it is dissolved in a solution that already contains one of its ions, rather than in a pure solvent. For example, if a salt such as CaF_2 is dissolved in a solution already containing Ca^{2+} ions, the dissociation equilibrium will shift toward the production of the solid salt. This reduction in solubility, called the **common ion effect,** is another example of Le Châtelier's principle.

Example: The K_{sp} of AgI in aqueous solution is 1×10^{-16} mol/L. If a 1×10^{-5} M solution of $AgNO_3$ is saturated with AgI, what will be the final concentration of the iodide ion?

Solution: The concentration of Ag^+ in the original $AgNO_3$ solution will be 1×10^{-5} mol/L. After AgI is added to saturation, the iodide concentration can be found by the formula:

$$1 \times 10^{-16} = [Ag^+][I^-]$$
$$= (1 \times 10^{-5})[I^-]$$
$$[I^-] = 1 \times 10^{-11} \text{ mol/L}$$

If the AgI had been dissolved in pure water, the concentration of both Ag^+ and I^- would have been 1×10^{-8} mol/L. The presence of the common ion, silver, at a concentration one thousand times higher than what it would normally be in a silver iodide solution, has reduced the iodide concentration to one thousandth of what it would have been otherwise. An additional 1×10^{-11} mol/L of silver will, of course, dissolve in solution along with the iodide ion, but this will not significantly affect the final silver concentration, which is much higher.

MCAT SYNOPSIS

Every slightly soluble salt of general formula MX will have $K_{sp} = x^2$, where x is the molar solubility.

PRACTICE QUESTIONS

1. An aqueous solution is prepared by mixing 70 grams of a solid into 100 grams of water. The solution has a boiling point of 101.11° C. What is the molar mass of the solute? (K_b = 0.512° C)

   A. 322.58 g/mol
   B. 32.26 g/mol
   C. 123.24 g/mol
   D. 233.59 g/mol

2. Which of the following phases of solvent and solute, respectively, can form a solution?

   I. Solid solvent, gaseous solute
   II. Solid solvent, solid solute
   III. Gaseous solvent, gaseous solute

   A. I and II only
   B. II and III only
   C. I and III only
   D. I, II, and III

3. Two organic liquids, below, are combined to form a solution. Based on the structures, will the solution closely obey Raoult's law?

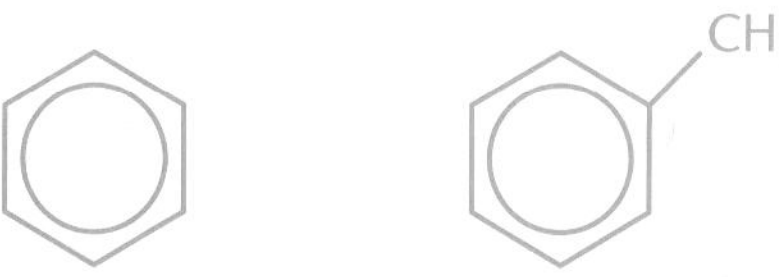

   A. Yes, the liquids differ due to the additional methyl group on toluene and therefore will not deviate from Raoult's law.
   B. Yes, the liquids are very similar and therefore will not deviate from Raoult's law.
   C. No, the liquids differ due to the additional methyl group on toluene and therefore will deviate from Raoult's law.
   D. No, the liquids both contain benzene rings which will interact with each other and cause deviation from Raoult's law.

4. The diagram below shows two arms separated by an impermeable membrane. If the membrane were replaced with a semipermeable one which allowed water molecules to move across, the level of liquid in the two branches would

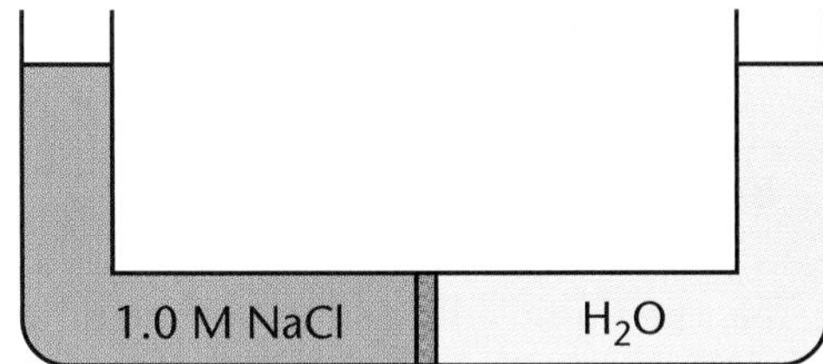

A. decrease on the right and increase on the left.
B. remain the same on both sides.
C. increase on the right and decrease on the left.
D. stay the same on the right and increase on the left.

5. The process of formation of a liquid solution can be better understood by breaking the process into three steps, below. The overall energy change to form a solution can be estimated by taking the sum of each of the three steps. Identify whether the steps are most likely to be endothermic or exothermic.

Step 1: Break up the solute into individual components.
Step 2: Make room for the solute in the solvent by overcoming intermolecular forces in the solvent.
Step 3: Allow solute-solvent interactions to occur to form the solution.

A. Endothermic, exothermic, endothermic
B. Exothermic, endothermic, endothermic
C. Exothermic, exothermic, endothermic
D. Endothermic, endothermic, exothermic

6. The entropy change when a solution forms can be expressed by the term $\Delta S°_{soln}$. When an ion dissolves and water molecules are ordered around it, the ordering would be expected to make a negative contribution to $\Delta S°_{soln}$. An ion that has more charge density will have a greater hydration effect, or ordering of water molecules. Based on this information, which of the following compounds will have the most negative $\Delta S°_{soln}$?

A. KCl
B. LiF
C. CaS
D. NaCl

7. A 0.01 M solution of a nonelectrolyte has an osmotic pressure of 15 mm Hg. What is the osmotic pressure of a 0.02 M solution of $Mg(NO_3)_2$? The temperature of both solutions is the same.

A. 15 mm Hg
B. 30 mm Hg
C. 45 mm Hg
D. 90 mm Hg

8. Vitamins A and C both have many functions in the body. They are essential for normal function, and deficiencies can lead to medical illness. While people can regularly consume large amounts of vitamin C and experience virtually no negative effects, those who consume large amounts of vitamin A can contract hypervitaminosis, an illness with various consequences. Which of the following best explains the differences between vitamins A and C?

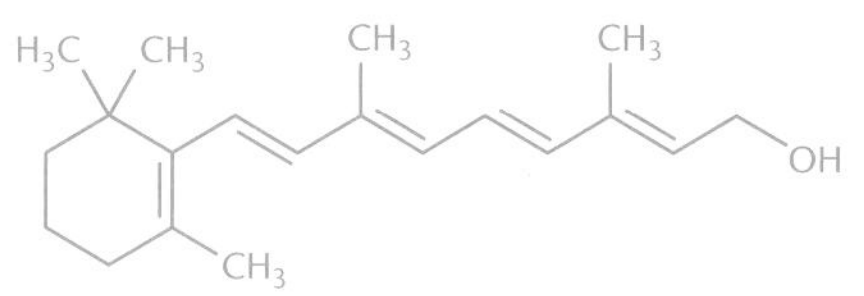

Vitamin A 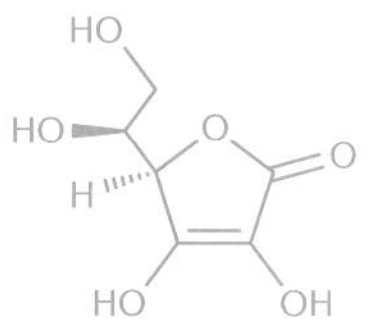　　Vitamin C

A. Vitamin A is hydrophobic and will not be excreted in the urine. Therefore, ingesting large amounts will be toxic. Vitamin C is hydrophilic and will be excreted. Therefore, large amounts will exit the body and cause no damage.
B. Vitamin A is a larger molecule than vitamin C and will accumulate much more rapidly due to its large size. Consumption of large amounts of vitamin A will be toxic to the body.
C. Vitamin A contains more methyl groups that are toxic to cells when large amounts of vitamin A are consumed.
D. Vitamin A's long carbon chain causes it to interact with lipids in membrane bilayers and disrupt the transport of other molecules. Therefore, large amounts of vitamin A will impede too much transport in the body and lead to illness.

9. A 3 gram sugar cube is dissolved in a cup of hot water at 80° C. The cup of water contains 300 mL of water. What is the mass percentage of sugar in the resulting solution? (Sugar = $C_{12}H_{22}O_{11}$, density of water at 80° C = 0.975 g/ml)

A. 0.52%
B. 1.02%
C. 1.52%
D. 2.02%

10. Which of the following combinations of liquids would be expected to have a vapor pressure higher than the vapor pressure predicted by Raoult's law?

A. Ethanol and hexane
B. Acetone and water
C. Isopropanol and methanol
D. Nitric acid and water

11. The salt KCl is dissolved in a beaker of water that you are holding. You can feel the solution cool as the KCl dissolves. You can conclude which of the following?

A. $\Delta S°_{soln}$ is large enough to overcome the unfavorable $\Delta H°_{soln}$.
B. KCl is mostly insoluble in water.
C. $\Delta S°_{soln}$ must be negative when KCl dissolves.
D. Boiling point depression will occur in this solution.

12. What will give the greatest increase in the boiling point of water when it is dissolved in 1 kg H_2O?

A. 0.4 mol calcium sulfate
B. 1 mol acetic acid
C. 0.25 mol iron(III) nitrate
D. 1.1 mol sucrose

13. At sea level and 25°C, the solubility of oxygen gas in water is 1.25×10^{-3} M. In a U.S. city that lies high above sea level, the atmospheric pressure is 0.8 atm. What is the solubility of oxygen in water there?

A. 1.05×10^{-3} M
B. 1.56×10^{-3} M
C. 1×10^{-3} M
D. 1.25×10^{-3} M

14. Lead is a dangerous element that exists in the environment in large quantities due to man-made pollution. Lead poisoning has many symptoms, including mental retardation in children. If a body of water is polluted with lead ions at 30 ppb (parts per billion), what is the concentration of lead in molarity? The density of water is 1 g/mL, ppb equals grams per 10^9 grams of solution.

A. 6.2×10^{-7} M Pb^{2+}
B. 1.4×10^{-10} M Pb^{2+}
C. 1.4×10^{-7} M Pb^{2+}
D. 6.2×10^{-6} M Pb^{2+}

15. Which of the following statements are correct?

I. NaF is an electrolyte.
II. Glucose is a nonelectrolyte.
III. CH_3OH is a weak electrolyte.
IV. CH_3CH_2COOH is a weak electrolyte.

A. III only
B. I and III only
C. I, II, and IV only
D. I, II, III, and IV

16. Which of the following is not a colligative property?

A. Boiling point elevation
B. Vapor pressure of a mixture
C. Osmotic pressure
D. Entropy of dissolution

17. The following equilibrium exists when AgBr is in solution. Calculate the solubility of AgBr in g/L in a solution of 0.001 M NaBr.

$$AgBr(s) \longleftrightarrow Ag^{+}(aq) + Br^{-}(aq)$$

$$Ksp = 7.7 \times 10^{-13}$$

A. 1.4×10^{-7} g/L
B. 7.7×10^{-10} g/L
C. 7.7×10^{-13} g/L
D. 2.8×10^{-7} g/L

18. When ammonia, NH_3, is a solvent, complex ions can form. For example, dissolving AgCl in NH_3 will result in the complex ion $Ag(NH_3)^{2+}$. What effect would you expect the formation of complex ions to have on the solubility of a compound like AgCl in NH_3?

A. The solubility of AgCl will increase because complex ion formation will cause more ions to exist in solution that interact with AgCl to cause it to dissociate.
B. The solubility of AgCl will increase because complex ion formation will consume Ag^+ molecules and cause the equilibrium to shift away from solid AgCl.
C. The solubility of AgCl will decrease because Ag^+ ions are in complexes and the Ag^+ ions that are not complexed will want to associate with Cl^- to form solid AgCl.
D. The solubility of AgCl will decrease because complex ion formation will consume Ag^+ molecules and cause the equilibrium to shift toward the solid AgCl.

19. Detergents are compounds that are dissolved in water. They are also able to dissolve hydrophobic stains such as oil and grease on clothing and other fabrics. Detergents can fulfill both hydrophilic and hydrophobic functions because they

A. contain a hydrophobic core molecule that is encased in a hydrophilic shell.
B. can ionize into two parts: one part is ionic and the other part is hydrophobic.
C. have two states: in water they are ionic, and in hydrophobic solvents they circularize to form a nonpolar ring structure.
D. have two functionally distinct parts: one side is a hydrophobic chain while the other side is a polar ionic end.

KEY CONCEPTS

Normality

Molarity

Oxidation and reduction

Concentration

NORMALITY AND MOLARITY

What volume of a 2 M solution of lithium aluminum hydride in ether is necessary to reduce 1 mole of methyl 5-cyanopentanoate to the corresponding amino alcohol? What if a 2 N (with respect to H^-) solution were used instead?

NC–(CH₂)₄–C(=O)OMe → 1) $LiAlH_4$ 2) H_3O^+ → H_2N–(CH₂)₆–OH

1) Determine the number of equivalents of reagent necessary to accomplish the desired transformation.

R–C(=O)OMe → (H^-) → R–C(=O)H → (H^-) → R–CH₂–OH

R–C≡N → (H^-) → R–CH=NH → (H^-) → R–CH₂–NH_2

TAKEAWAYS

The molecular formula of a molecule tells you how many equivalents of a desired reagent/atom are contained within the reagent. This is why it's important to balance reactions and draw Lewis structures correctly.

There are two functional groups that need to be reduced in the molecule, the nitrile and the ester.

The ester will require two moles of hydride to be reduced to the alcohol.

The nitrile will also require two moles of hydride because it proceeds through an imine intermediate.

THINGS TO WATCH OUT FOR

Be careful to distinguish between equivalents and moles. With molecules containing several equivalents of reagents, the number of equivalents and moles are not equal!

2) Compute the necessary volume of the given solution.

$$4 \text{ mol hydride} \times \left(\frac{1 \text{ mol LiAlH}_4}{4 \text{ mol hydride}}\right) = 1 \text{ mol LiAlH}_4$$

$$\frac{1 \text{ mol LiAlH}_4}{(2 \text{ mol LiAlH}_4\ \text{L}^{-1})} = 0.5 \text{ L}$$

$$\frac{1 \text{ mol LiAlH}_4}{(0.5 \text{ mol LiAlH}_4\ \text{L}^{-1})} = 2 \text{ L of 2 N solution}$$

Don't forget that one mole of lithium aluminum hydride contains four moles of hydride.

So, we'll need 500 mL of the 2 M solution.

With the 2 N solution, things get a little trickier. If the solution is 2 N with respect to H^-, that means that each liter of solution contains 2 moles of hydride, or 0.5 moles of $LiAlH_4$.

Remember: *Normality refers to equivalents per unit volume, not necessarily moles of compound per unit volume.*

SIMILAR QUESTIONS

1) Determine the volumes necessary for the same reaction as that in the initial question if 4 M and 4 N solutions of lithium aluminum hydride were used instead.
2) If the following molecule were subjected to $LiAlH_4$ reduction as well, what would the product be? How much of the 2 M solution would be necessary? The 2 N solution?

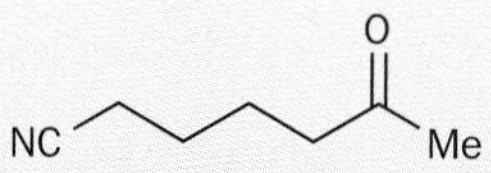

3) Diisobutylaluminum hydride (DIBAL) is a common alternate hydride reducing agent. Its structure is shown below. How much of a 2.5 M solution would be necessary to carry out the same reaction described above? A 2.5 N solution?

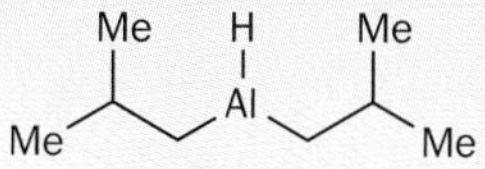

MOLAR SOLUBILITY

The molar solubility of iron(III) hydroxide in pure water at 25°C is 9.94×10^{-10} mol/L. How would the substance's molar solubility change if placed in an aqueous solution of pH 10.0 at 25°C?

1) Identify the balanced equation for the dissociation reaction.

The generic dissociation reaction may be expressed as:

$A_xB_y(s) \rightarrow xA^+(aq) + yB^-(aq)$

Plugging in for iron(III) hydroxide, the reaction expression is:

$Fe(OH)_3(s) \rightarrow Fe^{+3}(aq) + 3OH^-(aq)$

This step allows us to see how many moles of ions are added to the solution per mole dissolved.

---

2) Find the K_{sp} expression for the dissociation reaction.

☞ Generic: $K_{sp} = [xA^+]^x_{sat}\,[yB^-]^y_{sat}$

$Fe(OH)_3$: $K_{sp} = [Fe^{+3}]\,[OH^-]^3$

K_{sp} is merely an equilibrium constant just like K, and it is given the special name "solubility product" because it tells us how soluble a solid is.

Recall that the concentrations are those at equilibrium, thus the solution is saturated. A saturated solution contains the maximum concentration of dissolved solute.

Remember: *Like all K's, a substance's K_{sp} varies only with temperature.*

---

3) Calculate molar solubility of each product by assuming that you're starting with x mols of reactant.

x mol $Fe(OH)_3 \rightarrow x$ mol $Fe^{+3} + 3x$ mol OH^-

Use the balanced equation from step 1 to determine the appropriate coefficients. For each mole of iron hydroxide dissolved, four ions are created: one Fe^{+3} and three OH^-.

KEY CONCEPTS

pH

Molar solubility

Common Ion effect

Le Châtelier's principle

$K_{sp} = [A^+]^x_{sat}\,[B^-]^y_{sat}$

TAKEAWAYS

The value of K_{sp} does not change when a common ion is present; it is a constant that is dependent on temperature. The molar solubility of the salt, however, does change if a common ion is present. To find the change in molar solubility due to the common ion effect, you must find the K_{sp} of the substance first.

THINGS TO WATCH OUT FOR

Be careful when applying Le Châtelier's principle in cases of precipitation and solvation. For a solution at equilibrium (i.e., saturated), adding more solid would not shift the equilibrium to the right. More solid does not dissociate to raise the ion concentrations; the solid just piles up at the bottom.

4) Plug the molar solubility for each product into the K_{sp} equation:

$Fe(OH)_3$: $K_{sp} = [Fe^{+3}]\,[OH^-]^3$

$K_{sp} = [x]\,[3x]^3 = 27x^4$ ($x = 9.94 \times 10^{-10}$)

$K_{sp} = 27(9.94 \times 10^{-10})^4 = 2.64 \times 10^{-35}$

Simply plug in the coefficients from step 3 into the K_{sp} equation. The molar solubility, *x*, was given in the question stem. Thus, to calculate K_{sp}, plug in 9.94×10^{-10}. Now that we are armed with the K_{sp}, we can find the change in molar solubility due to the common ion.

---

5) If a common ion is present in a solution, it must also be accounted for in the K_{sp} equation:

$Fe(OH)_3$: $K_{sp} = [Fe^{+3}]\,[OH^-]^3$

$2.64 \times 10^{-35} = x(3x + 10^{-4})^3 \approx x(10^{-4})^3$

$2.64 \times 10^{-35} = x10^{-12}$

$x = 2.64 \times 10^{-23}$

A solution of pH 10.0 has an OH^- concentration of 10^{-4}. Although iron hydroxide will also contribute to the solution's total concentration of OH^-, its contribution will be negligible relative to the 10^{-4} already present in solution; thus, when plugging in for the $[OH^-]$, we can approximate that it equals 10^{-4}. For the pH 10.0 solution, the molar solubility is on the order of 10^{-23} mol/L, a steep decrease from the 10^{-9} in pure water. This is due to the common ion effect. Look at it from the perspective of Le Châtelier's principle: the addition of more OH^- will shift the reaction to the left, so that less iron hydroxide will dissociate.

SIMILAR QUESTIONS

1) Given a substance's K_{sp}, how would you solve for its molar solubility in pure water? What if a common ion were also present in solution?
2) Given a table listing substances and their solubility constants, how would you determine which substance was most soluble in pure water?
3) Given that the sulfate ion can react with acid to form hydrogen sulfate, how would the molar solubility of sulfate salts be affected by varying a solution's pH?

CHAPTER 10

ACIDS AND BASES

Many important reactions in chemical and biological systems involve two classes of compounds called **acids** and **bases.** Acids and bases cause color changes in certain compounds called **indicators,** which may be in solution or on paper. A particular common indicator is litmus paper, which turns red in acidic solution and blue in basic solution. A more extensive discussion of the chemical properties of acids and bases is outlined below.

DEFINITIONS

A. ARRHENIUS DEFINITION

The first definitions of acids and bases were formulated by Svante Arrhenius toward the end of the 19th century. Arrhenius defined an acid as a species that produces H^+ (a proton) in an aqueous solution, and a base as a species that produces OH^- (a hydroxide ion) in an aqueous solution. These definitions, though useful, fail to describe acidic and basic behavior in nonaqueous media.

TEACHER TIP

This is the most specific definition of acids and bases, and the least useful.

B. BRØNSTED-LOWRY DEFINITION

A more general definition of acids and bases was proposed independently by Johannes Brønsted and Thomas Lowry in 1923. A Brønsted-Lowry acid is a species that donates protons, while a Brønsted-Lowry base is a species that accepts protons. For example, NH_3 and Cl^- are both Brønsted-Lowry bases because they accept protons. However, they cannot be called Arrhenius bases because in aqueous solution they do not dissociate to form OH^-. The advantage of the Brønsted-Lowry concept of acids and bases is that it is not limited to aqueous solutions.

TEACHER TIP

This is the more general and most useful of the three definitions. It is all about the proton (H^+). It is seen frequently on the MCAT.

Brønsted-Lowry acids and bases always occur in pairs, called **conjugate acid-base pairs.** The two members of a conjugate pair are related by the transfer of a proton. For example, H_3O^+ is the conjugate acid of the base H_2O, and NO_2^- is the conjugate base of HNO_2.

$$H_3O^+(aq) \rightleftarrows H_2O(aq) + H^+(aq)$$

$$HNO_2(aq) \rightleftarrows NO_2^-(aq) + H^+(aq)$$

Teacher Tip

This is the most general and inclusive definition, and is sometimes seen on the MCAT.

C. LEWIS DEFINITION

At approximately the same time as Brønsted and Lowry, Gilbert Lewis also proposed definitions of acids and bases. Lewis defined an acid as an electron-pair acceptor, and a base as an electron-pair donor. Lewis's are the most inclusive definitions. Just as every Arrhenius acid is a Brønsted-Lowry acid, every Brønsted-Lowry acid is also a Lewis acid (and likewise for bases). However, the Lewis definition encompasses some species not included within the Brønsted-Lowry definition. For example, BCl_3 and $AlCl_3$ can each accept an electron pair and are therefore Lewis acids, despite their inability to donate protons.

NOMENCLATURE OF ARRHENIUS ACIDS

The name of an acid is related to the name of the parent anion (the anion that combines with H^+ to form the acid). Acids formed from anions whose names end in **-ide** have the prefix **hydro-** and the ending **-ic.**

F^-	Fluoride	HF	Hydrofluoric acid
Br^-	Bromide	HBr	Hydrobromic acid

MCAT Synopsis

Some exceptions to the rules exist. For instance, MnO_4^- is called permanganate even though there are no "manganate" or "manganite" ions.

Acids formed from oxyanions are called **oxyacids.** If the anion ends in **-ite** (less oxygen), then the acid will end with **-ous acid.** If the anion ends in **-ate** (more oxygen), then the acid will end with **-ic acid.** Prefixes in the names of the anions are retained. Some examples:

ClO^-	Hypochlorite	HClO	Hypochlorous acid
ClO_2^-	Chlorite	$HClO_2$	Chlorous acid
ClO_3^-	Chlorate	$HClO_3$	Chloric acid
ClO_4^-	Perchlorate	$HClO_4$	Perchloric acid
NO_2^-	Nitrite	HNO_2	Nitrous acid
NO_3^-	Nitrate	HNO_3	Nitric acid

PROPERTIES OF ACIDS AND BASES

MCAT Synopsis

Recall that a fundamental property of logarithms is that the log of a product is equal to the sum of the logs, i.e., $\log(xy) = \log x + \log y$.

A. HYDROGEN ION EQUILIBRIA (pH AND pOH)

Hydrogen ion concentration, $[H^+]$, is generally measured as **pH,** where:

$$pH = -\log[H^+] = \log(1/[H^+])$$

Likewise, hydroxide ion concentration, $[OH^-]$, is measured as **pOH** where:

$$pOH = -\log[OH^-] = \log(1/[OH^-])$$

In any aqueous solution, the H_2O solvent dissociates slightly:

$$H_2O(\ell) \rightleftarrows H^+(aq) + OH^-(aq)$$

This dissociation is an equilibrium reaction and is therefore described by a constant, **K_w, the water dissociation constant.**

$$K_w = [H^+][OH^-] = 10^{-14}$$

Rewriting this equation in logarithmic form gives:

$$pH + pOH = 14$$

In pure H_2O, $[H^+]$ is equal to $[OH^-]$, because for every mole of H_2O that dissociates, one mole of H^+ and one mole of OH^- are formed. A solution with equal concentrations of H^+ and OH^- is neutral, and has a pH of 7($-\log 10^{-7} = 7$). A pH below 7 indicates a relative excess of H^+ ions, and therefore an acidic solution; a pH above 7 indicates a relative excess of OH^- ions, and therefore a basic solution.

MCAT SYNOPSIS

Other important properties of logarithms include:

$\text{Log } x^n = n\text{Log } x$, and $\text{Log } 10^x = x$. From these two properties one can derive the particularly useful relationship: $-\text{Log } 10^{-x} = x$.

Math Note: Estimating p-Scale Values
A useful skill for various problems involving acids and bases, as well as their corresponding buffer solutions, is the ability to quickly convert pH, pOH, pK_a, and pK_b into nonlogarithmic form and vice versa.

When the original value is a power of 10, the operation is relatively simple; changing the sign on the exponent gives the corresponding p-scale value directly. For example:

If $[H^+] = 0.001$, or 10^{-3}, then pH = 3.

If $K_b = 1 \times 10^{-7}$, then $pK_b = 7$.

More difficulty arises (in the absence of a calculator) when the original value is not an exact power of 10; exact calculation would be excessively onerous, but a simple method of approximation exists. If the nonlogarithmic value is written in proper scientific notation, it will look like: $n \times 10^{-m}$, where n is a number between 1 and 10. The log of this product can be written as: $\log(n \times 10^{-m}) = -m + \log n$, and the negative log is thus $m - \log n$. Now, because n is a number between 1 and 10, its logarithm will be a fraction between 0 and 1, thus $m - \log n$ will be between $m - 1$ and m. Further, the larger n is, the larger the fraction log n will be, and therefore the closer to $m - 1$ our answer will be.

Example: If $Ka = 1.8 \times 10^{-5}$, then $pKa = 5 - \log 1.8$. Because 1.8 is small, its log will be small, and the answer will be closer to 5 than to 4. (The actual answer is 4.74.)

TEACHER TIP

Learning how to estimate is an important skill.

B. STRONG ACIDS AND BASES

Strong acids and bases are those that completely dissociate into their component ions in aqueous solution. For example, when NaOH is added to water, it dissociates completely:

$$NaOH(s) + \text{excess } H_2O(\ell) \rightarrow Na^+(aq) + OH^-(aq)$$

Hence, in a 1 M solution of NaOH, complete dissociation gives 1 mole of OH^- ions per liter of solution.

$$pH = 14 - (-\log[OH^-]) = 14 + \log[1] = 14$$

TEACHER TIP

Be sure to think about the answer and whether it makes sense. As seen here, a basic pH for an acidic solution should make you think about what might be wrong with your answer.

Virtually no undissociated NaOH remains. Note that the $[OH^-]$ contributed by the dissociation of H_2O is considered to be negligible in this case. The contribution of OH^- and H^+ ions from the dissociation of H_2O can be neglected only if the concentration of the acid or base is greater than 10^{-7} M. For example, the pH of a 1×10^{-8} M HCl solution (HCl is a strong acid) might appear to be 8, since $[-\log(1 \times 10^{-8})] = 8$. However, a pH of 8 is in the basic pH range, and an HCl solution is not basic. The discrepancy arises from the fact that at low HCl concentrations, H^+ from the dissociation of water does contribute significantly to the total $[H^+]$. The $[H^+]$ from the dissociation of water is less than 1×10^{-7} M due to the common ion effect. The total concentration of H^+ can be calculated from $K_w = (x + 1 \times 10^{-8})(x) = 1.0 \times 10^{-14}$, where $x = [H^+] = [OH^-]$ (both from the dissociation of water molecules).

MCAT FAVORITE

The K_w, like all equilibrium constants, will change if the temperature changes. This will change the pH scale. In other words, our pH scale of 1–14 is only valid at 25°C.

Solving for x gives $x = 9.5 \times 10^{-8}$ M,
so $[H^+]_{total} = (9.5 \times 10^{-8} + 1 \times 10^{-8})$ M $= 1.05 \times 10^{-7}$ M
and $pH = -\log(1.05 \times 10^{-7}) = 6.98$, slightly less than 7, as should be expected for a very dilute, yet acidic solution.

Strong acids commonly encountered in the laboratory include $HClO_4$ (perchloric acid), HNO_3 (nitric acid), H_2SO_4 (sulfuric acid), and HCl (hydrochloric acid). Commonly encountered strong bases include NaOH (sodium hydroxide), KOH (potassium hydroxide), and other soluble hydroxides of Group IA and IIA metals. Calculation of the pH and pOH of strong acids and bases assumes complete dissociation of the acid or base in solution: $[H^+]$ = normality of strong acid and $[OH^-]$ = normality of strong base.

C. WEAK ACIDS AND BASES

Weak acids and bases are those that only partially dissociate in aqueous solution. A weak monoprotic acid, HA, in aqueous solution will achieve the following equilibrium after dissociation (H_3O^+ is equivalent to H^+ in aqueous solution.):

$$HA(aq) + H_2O(\ell) \rightleftarrows H_3O^+(aq) + A^-(aq)$$

The **acid dissociation constant, K_a,** is a measure of the degree to which an acid dissociates.

$$K_a = \frac{[H_3O^+][A^-]}{[HA]}$$

The weaker the acid, the smaller the K_a. Note that K_a does not contain an expression for the pure liquid, water.

A weak monovalent base, BOH, undergoes dissociation to give B^+ and OH^-. The **base dissociation constant, K_b,** is a measure of the degree to which a base dissociates. The weaker the base, the smaller its K_b. For a monovalent base, K_b is defined as follows:

$$K_b = \frac{[B^+][OH^-]}{[BOH]}$$

A **conjugate acid** is defined as the acid formed when a base gains a proton. Similarly, a **conjugate base** is formed when an acid loses a proton. For example, in the HCO_3^-/CO_3^{2-} conjugate acid/base pair, CO_3^{2-} is the conjugate base and HCO_3^- is the conjugate acid:

$$HCO_3^-(aq) \rightleftarrows H^+(aq) + CO_3^{2-}(aq)$$

To find the K_a of the conjugate acid HCO_3^-, the reaction with water must be considered.

$$HCO_3^-(aq) + H_2O(\ell) \rightleftarrows H_3O^+(aq) + CO_3^{2-}(aq)$$

Likewise, for the K_b of CO_3^{2-}:

$$CO_3^{2-}(aq) + H_2O(\ell) \rightleftarrows HCO_3^-(aq) + OH^-(aq)$$

In a conjugate acid/base pair formed from a weak acid, the conjugate base is generally stronger than the conjugate acid. Thus, for HCO_3^- and CO_3^{2-}, the reaction of CO_3^{2-} (the conjugate base) in water to produce HCO_3^- (the conjugate acid) and OH^- occurs to a great extent (i.e., is more favorable) than the reverse reaction.

The equilibrium constants for these reactions are as follows:

$$K_a = \frac{[H^+]\left[CO_3^{2-}\right]}{\left[HCO_3^-\right]} \text{ and } K_b = \frac{\left[HCO_3^-\right][OH^-]}{\left[CO_3^{2-}\right]}$$

TEACHER TIP

Weak acids and bases are seen often on the exam. In Organic Chemistry, all carboxylic acids are considered to be weak bases.

TEACHER TIP

Be aware of the relationship between conjugate acids and bases: Taking a proton from a molecule will give you the conjugate base; putting on a proton will give you the conjugate acid!

Adding the two reactions shows that the net reaction is simply the dissociation of water:

$$H_2O(\ell) \rightleftarrows H^+(aq) + OH^-(aq)$$

Teacher Tip

We are dealing with an equilibrium process here, so we can apply these principles to those MCAT questions that address weak acids and bases.

The equilibrium constant for this net reaction is $K_w = [H^+][OH^-]$, which is the product of K_a and K_b. Thus, if the dissociation constant either for an acid or for its conjugate base is known, then the dissociation constant for the other can be determined, using the equation:

$$K_a \times K_b = K_w = 1 \times 10^{-14}$$

Thus K_a and K_b are inversely related. In other words, if K_a is large (the acid is strong), then K_b will be small (the conjugate base will be weak), and vice versa.

D. APPLICATIONS OF K_a AND K_b

To calculate the concentration of H^+ in a 2 M aqueous solution of acetic acid, CH_3COOH ($K_a = 1.8 \times 10^{-5}$) , first write the equilibrium reaction:

$$CH_3COOH(aq) \rightleftarrows H^+(aq) + CH_3COO^-(aq)$$

Next, write the expression for the acid dissociation constant:

$$K_a = \frac{[H^+][CH_3COO^-]}{[CH_3COOH]} = 1.8 \times 10^{-5}$$

Because acetic acid is a weak acid, the concentration of CH_3COOH at equilibrium is equal to its initial concentration, 2 M, less the amount dissociated, x. Likewise $[H^+] = [CH_3COO^-] = x$, because each molecule of CH_3COOH dissociates into one H^+ ion and one CH_3COO^- ion. Thus, the equation can be rewritten as follows:

$$K_a = \frac{[X][X]}{[2-X]} = 1.8 \times 10^{-5}$$

We can approximate that $2 - x \approx 2$ because acetic acid is a weak acid, and only slightly dissociates in water. This simplifies the calculation of x:

$$K_a = \frac{[X][X]}{[2.0]} = 1.8 \times 10^{-5}$$

$$X = 6 \times 10^{-3} M$$

Teacher Tip

This estimation makes life easy and will almost always get you to the correct answer on Test Day.

The fact that [x] is so much less than the initial concentration of acetic acid (2 M) validates the approximation; otherwise, it would have been necessary to solve for x using the quadratic formula. (A rule of thumb is that the approximation is valid as long as x is less than 5 percent of the initial concentration.)

SALT FORMATION

Acids and bases may react with each other, forming a salt and (often, but not always) water, in what is termed a **neutralization reaction** (see chapter 4). For example,

$$HA + BOH \rightarrow BA + H_2O$$

The salt may precipitate out or remain ionized in solution, depending on its solubility and the amount produced. Neutralization reactions generally go to completion. The reverse reaction, in which the salt ions react with water to give back the acid or base, is known as **hydrolysis.**

Four combinations of strong and weak acids and bases are possible:

1. strong acid + strong base: e.g., $HCl + NaOH \rightarrow NaCl + H_2O$
2. strong acid + weak base: e.g., $HCl + NH_3 \rightarrow NH_4Cl$
3. weak acid + strong base: e.g., $HClO + NaOH \rightarrow NaClO + H_2O$
4. weak acid + weak base: e.g., $HClO + NH_3 \rightleftarrows NH_4ClO$

TEACHER TIP

Remember the reaction types discussed in the Compounds and Stoichiometry chapter? Well, here is our neutralization reaction.

The products of a reaction between equal concentrations of a strong acid and a strong base are a salt and water. The acid and base neutralize each other, so the resulting solution is neutral (pH = 7), and the ions formed in the reaction do not react with water. The product of a reaction between a strong acid and a weak base is also a salt but usually no water is formed because weak bases are usually not hydroxides; however, in this case, the cation of the salt will react with the water solvent, reforming the weak base. This reaction constitutes hydrolysis. For example:

$$HCl(aq) + NH_3(aq) \rightleftarrows NH_4^+(aq) + Cl^-(aq) \text{ Reaction I}$$

$$NH_4^+(aq) + H_2O(aq) \rightleftarrows NH_3(aq) + H_3O^+(aq) \text{ Reaction II}$$

NH_4^+ is the conjugate acid of a weak base (NH_3), and is therefore stronger than the conjugate base (Cl^-) of the strong acid HCl. NH_4^+ will thus react with OH^-, reducing the concentration of OH^-. There will thus be an excess of H^+, which will lower the pH of the solution.

On the other hand, when a weak acid reacts with a strong base the solution is basic, due to the hydrolysis of the salt to reform the acid, with the concurrent formation of hydroxide ion from the hydrolyzed water molecules. The pH of a solution containing a weak acid and a weak base depends on the relative strengths of the reactants. For example, the acid HClO has a $K_a = 3.2 \times 10^{-8}$, and the base NH_3 has a $K_b = 1.8 \times 10^{-5}$.

Thus an aqueous solution of HClO and NH_3 is basic because K_a for HClO is less than K_b for NH_3.

POLYVALENCE AND NORMALITY

The relative acidity or basicity of an aqueous solution is determined by the relative concentrations of **acid** and **base equivalents.** An acid equivalent is equal to one mole of H^+ (or H_3O^+) ions; a base equivalent is equal to one mole of OH^- ions. Some acids and bases are polyvalent, that is, each mole of the acid or base liberates more than one acid or base equivalent. For example, the diprotic acid H_2SO_4 undergoes the following dissociation in water:

$$H_2SO_4(aq) \rightarrow H^+(aq) + HSO_4^-(aq)$$
$$HSO_4^-(aq) \rightleftarrows H^+(aq) + SO_4^{2-}(aq)$$

One mole of H_2SO_4 can thus produce two acid equivalents (two moles of H^+). The acidity or basicity of a solution depends upon the concentration of acidic or basic equivalents that can be liberated. The quantity of acidic or basic capacity is directly indicated by the solution's normality (see chapter 9, Solutions). Because each mole of H_3PO_4 can liberate three moles (equivalents) of H^+, a 2 M H_3PO_4 solution would be 6 N (6 normal).

FLASHBACK

Recall that we spoke about gram equivalent weights in the Compounds and Stoichiometry chapter, and about normality and all units of concentration in the Solutions chapter.

Another useful measurement is equivalent weight. For example, the gram molecular weight of H_2SO_4 is 98 g/mol. Because each mole liberates two acid equivalents, the gram equivalent weight of H_2SO_4 would be $\frac{98}{2} = 49g$; that is, the dissociation of 49 g of H_2SO_4 would release one acid equivalent. Common polyvalent acids include H_2SO_4, H_3PO_4, and H_2CO_3.

AMPHOTERIC SPECIES

An **amphoteric,** or **amphiprotic,** species is one that can act either as an acid or a base, depending on its chemical environment. In the Brønsted-Lowry sense, an amphoteric species can either gain or lose a proton. Water is the most common example. When water reacts with a base, it behaves as an acid:

$$H_2O + B^- \rightleftarrows HB + OH^-$$

When water reacts with an acid, it behaves as a base:

$$HA + H_2O \rightleftarrows H_3O^+ + A^-$$

The partially dissociated conjugate base of a polyprotic acid is usually amphoteric (e.g., HSO_4^- can either gain an H^+ to form H_2SO_4, or lose an H^+ to form SO_4^{2-}). The hydroxides of certain metals, e.g., Al, Zn, Pb, and Cr, are also amphoteric. Furthermore, species that can act as either oxidizing or reducing agents (see chapter 11, Redox Reactions and Electrochemistry) are considered to be amphoteric as well, because by accepting or donating electron pairs they act as Lewis acids or bases, respectively.

FLASHBACK

Le Châtelier's principle:

$HIN \rightleftarrows H^+ + IN^-$

(color 1) (color 2)

Adding H^+ shifts equilibrium to left. Adding OH^- removes H^+ and therefore shifts equilibrium to the right.

TITRATION AND BUFFERS

Titration is a procedure used to determine the molarity of an acid or base. This is accomplished by reacting a known volume of a solution of unknown concentration with a known volume of a solution of known concentration. When the number of acid equivalents equals the number of base equivalents added, or vice versa, the **equivalence point** is reached. It is important to emphasize that, while a strong acid/strong base titration will have an equivalence point at pH 7, the equivalence point **need not** always occur at pH 7. Also, when titrating polyprotic acids or bases, there are several equivalence points, as each different acidic or basic species is titrated separately (see Polyprotic Acids and Bases later in this chapter).

The equivalence point in a titration is estimated in two common ways: either by using a graphical method, plotting the pH of the solution as a function of added titrant by using a **pH meter** (e.g. Figure 10.1), or by watching for a color change of an added **indicator.** Indicators are weak organic acids or bases that have different colors in their undissociated and dissociated states. Indicators are used in low concentrations and therefore do not significantly alter the equivalence point. The point at which the indicator actually changes color is not the equivalence point but is called the end point. If the titration is performed well, the volume difference (and therefore the error) between the end point and the equivalence point is usually small and may be corrected for, or ignored.

MCAT SYNOPSIS

An easy way to calculate the volume added to reach the endpoint is by use of the formula: $V_AN_A = V_BN_B$, where V is for volume, N is for normality (see chapter 9), A is for acid, and B is for base.

A. STRONG ACID AND STRONG BASE

Consider the titration of 10 mL of a 0.1 N solution of HCl with a 0.1 N solution of NaOH. Plotting the pH of the reaction solution versus the quantity of NaOH added gives the following curve:

TEACHER TIP

Our tug-of-war analogy for a bond between two atoms can be recycled here for titrations. Whichever is stronger (our acid or our base) will determine the equivalence point for the titration. Here they are equal, so the equivalence point is at a neutral pH.

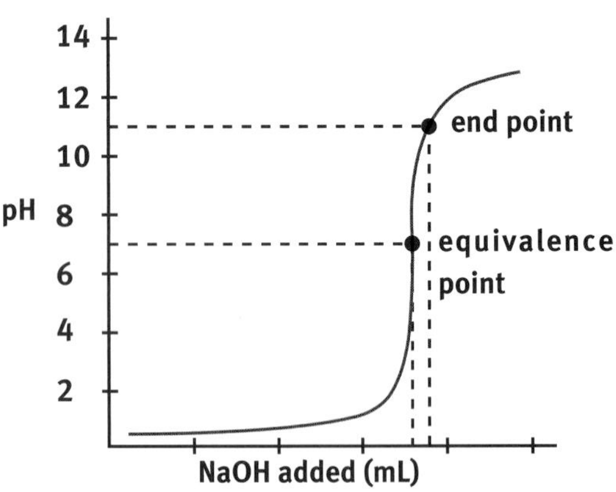

Figure 10.1. Titration of HCl with NaOH

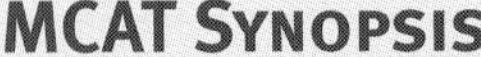

MCAT SYNOPSIS

Any monoprotic strong acid titrated with a strong base will give a similar curve. The pH of the equivalence point is 7.

Because HCl is a strong acid and NaOH is a strong base, the equivalence point of the titration will be at pH 7 and the solution will be neutral. Note that the endpoint shown is close to, but not exactly equal to, the equivalence point; selection of a better indicator, say one that changes colors at pH 8, would have given a better approximation.

In the early part of the curve (when little base has been added), the acidic species predominates, and so the addition of small amounts of base will not appreciably change either the $[OH^-]$ or the pH. Similarly, in the last part of the titration curve (when an excess of base has been added), the addition of small amounts of base will not change the $[OH^-]$ significantly, and the pH remains relatively constant. The addition of base most alters the concentrations of H^+ and OH^- near the equivalence point, and thus the pH changes most drastically in that region.

B. WEAK ACID AND STRONG BASE

Titration of a weak acid, HA, with a strong base produces the following titration curve:

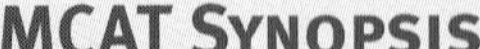

MCAT SYNOPSIS

Note that any monoprotic weak acid titrated with a strong base will give a similar curve. The pH of the equivalence point depends on the identity of the weak acid.

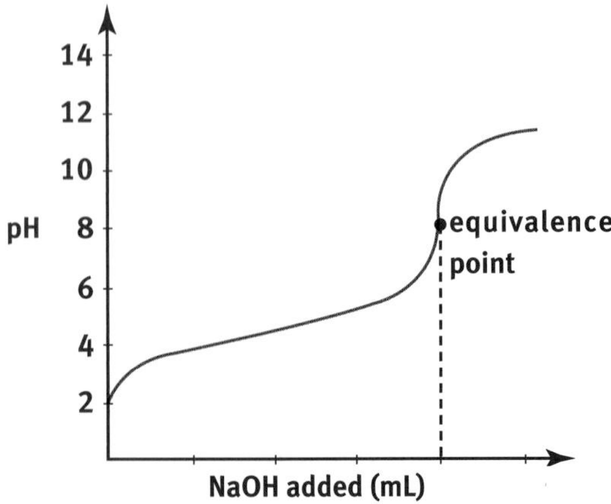

Figure 10.2. Titration of a Weak Acid, HA, with NaOH

Comparing Figure 10.2 with Figure 10.1 shows that the initial pH of the weak acid solution is greater than the initial pH of the strong acid solution. The pH changes most significantly early on in the titration, and the equivalence point is in the basic range.

C. BUFFERS

A **buffer solution** consists of a mixture of a weak acid and its salt (which consists of its conjugate base and a cation), or a mixture of a weak base and its salt (which consists of its conjugate acid and an anion). Two examples of buffers are: a solution of acetic acid (CH_3COOH) and its salt, sodium acetate ($CH_3COO^-Na^+$); and a solution of ammonia (NH_3) and its salt, ammonium chloride ($NH_4^+Cl^-$). Buffer solutions have the useful property of resisting changes in pH when small amounts of acid or base are added.

Consider a buffer solution of acetic acid and sodium acetate:

$$CH_3COOH \rightleftarrows H^+ + CH_3COO^-$$

When a small amount of NaOH is added to the buffer, the OH^- ions from the NaOH react with the H^+ ions present in the solution; subsequently, more acetic acid dissociates (equilibrium shifts to the right), restoring the $[H^+]$. Thus, an increase in $[OH^-]$ does not appreciably change pH. Likewise, when a small amount of HCl is added to the buffer, H^+ ions from the HCl react with the acetate ions to form acetic acid. Thus $[H^+]$ is kept relatively constant and the pH of the solution is relatively unchanged.

MCAT Synopsis

The Henderson-Hasselbalch equation is also useful in the creation of buffer solutions other than those formed during the course of a titration. By careful selection of the weak acid (or base) and its salt, a buffer at almost any pH can be produced.

The **Henderson-Hasselbalch equation** is used to estimate the pH of a solution in the buffer region where the concentrations of the species and its conjugate are present in approximately equal concentrations. For a weak acid buffer solution:

$$pH = pK_a + \log\frac{[\text{conjugate base}]}{[\text{weak acid}]}$$

Note that when [conjugate base] = [weak acid] (in a titration, halfway to the equivalent point) the pH = pK_a because the log 1 = 0. Likewise, for a weak base buffer solution:

$$pOH = pK_b + \log\frac{[\text{conjugate acid}]}{[\text{weak base}]}$$

and pOH = pK_b when [conjugate acid] = [weak base].

CLINICAL CORRELATE

Blood pH is maintained in a relatively small range (slightly above 7) by a bicarbonate buffer system. This homeostasis can be upset, leading to a condition known as acidosis.

D. POLYPROTIC ACIDS AND BASES

The titration curve for a polyprotic acid or base looks different from that for a monoprotic acid or base. Figure 10.3 shows the titration of Na_2CO_3 with HCl in which the polyprotic acid H_2CO_3 is the ultimate product.

In region I, little acid has been added and the predominant species is CO_3^{2-}. In region II, more acid has been added and the predominant species are CO_3^{2-} and HCO_3^-, in relatively equal concentrations. The flat part of the curve is the first buffer region, corresponding to the pK_a of HCO_3^- ($K_a = 5.6 \times 10^{-11}$ implies $pK_a = 10.25$).

Region III contains the equivalence point, at which all of the CO_3^{2-} is titrated to HCO_3^-. As the curve illustrates, a rapid change in pH occurs at the equivalence point; in the latter part of region III, the predominant species is HCO_3^-.

In region IV, the acid has neutralized approximately half of the HCO_3^-, and now H_2CO_3 and HCO_3^- are in roughly equal concentrations. This flat region is the second buffer region of the titration curve, corresponding to the pK_a of H_2CO_3 ($K_a = 4.3 \times 10^{-7}$ implies $pK_a - 6.37$). In region V, the equivalence point for the entire titration is reached, as all of the HCO_3^- is converted to H_2CO_3. Again, a rapid change in pH is observed near the equivalence point as acid is added.

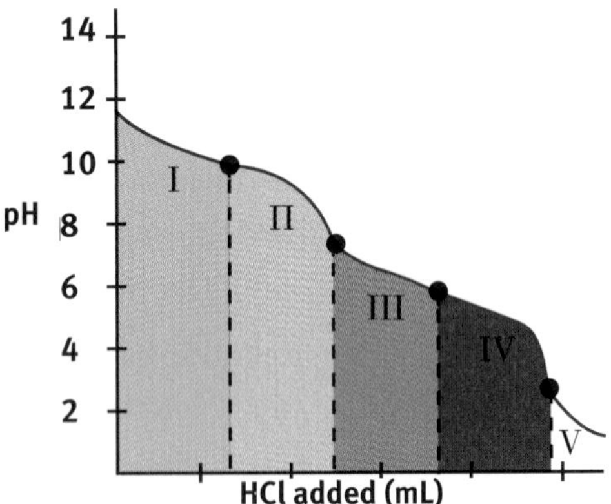

Figure 10.3. Titration of Na_2CO_3 with HCl

PRACTICE QUESTIONS

1. Which of the following is NOT a Brønsted-Lowry base?

A.
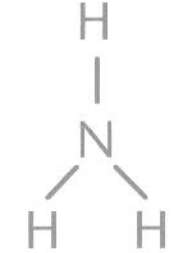

B. F^-

C.
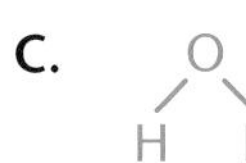

D.
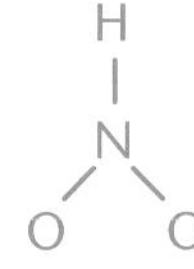

2. What is the pH of a solution containing 5 mM H_2S?

A. 1
B. 1.5
C. 2
D. 4

3. Which of the following is chloric acid?

A. $HClO_3$
B. ClO_3^-
C. $HClO_2$
D. HClO

4. Which of the following is the weakest base of those provided?

A. KOH
B. $Ca(OH)_2$
C. CH_3NH_2
D. NaH

5. The function of a buffer is to

A. speed up reactions between acids and bases.
B. resist changes in pH when small amounts of acid or base are added.
C. slow down reactions between acids and bases.
D. keep pH constant throughout an acid/base reaction.

6. What is the pH of the following solution shown below?

$pK_b = 3.45$	$[NH_4^+] = 70$ mM	$[NH_3] = 712$ mM

A. 4.45
B. 7.55
C. 9.55
D. 10.65

Questions 7–9 are based on the titration curve of acid X shown below:

Titration Curve of Weak Acid X

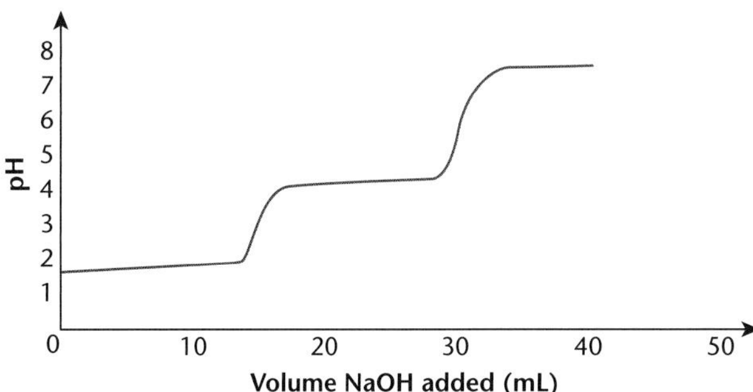

7. What is the approximate value of the first pK_a on the cuve above?

A. 1.9
B. 2.9
C. 3.8
D. 4.1

8. Where is the second equivalence point on the previous curve?

A. pH = 3
B. pH = 4.1
C. pH = 5.9
D. pH = 7.2

9. What is the approximate value of the second pK_a on the previous curve?

A. 3.6
B. 4.1
C. 5.5
D. 7.2

10. What is the approximate gram equivalent weight of phosphoric acid?

A. 25 g
B. 33 g
C. 49 g
D. 98 g

11. What is the $[H^+]$ of a 2M aqueous solution of a weak acid "HXO_2" with $K_a = 3.2 \times 10^{-5}$?

A. 8×10^{-3} M
B. 6.4×10^{-5} M
C. 1.3×10^{-4} M
D. 4×10^{-3} M

12. Which of the following is NOT true of an amphoteric species?

A. It can act as a base or an acid depending on its environment.
B. It can act as an oxidizing or reducing agent depending on its environment.
C. It is always protic.
D. It is always a nonpolar species.

13. What is the approximate pH of a 1.2×10^{-5} M aqueous solution of NaOH?

A. 4.85
B. 7.5
C. 9.15
D. 12.45

PH AND PK_a

What is the pH of the resulting solution if 4 g of sodium acetate (CH_3CO_2Na) is dissolved in 0.5 L of water? (The pK_a of acetic acid, CH_3CO_2H, is 4.74.)

1) Convert masses to concentrations.

Molecular weight of sodium acetate in g mol^{-1}: $23 + 2(12) + 3(1) + 2(16) = 82$

The concentration of a solution is usually expressed in units of moles per liter.

Choose numbers that are easy to work with, i.e., 80 g mol^{-1} instead of 82 g mol^{-1}. Remember, you won't have a calculator on Test Day! Moles of sodium acetate:

$$\frac{4\text{ g}}{80\text{ g mol}^{-1}} = \frac{1}{20}\text{ mol} = 0.05\text{ mol}.$$

$$\text{Concentration} = \frac{0.05\text{ mol}}{0.5\text{ L}} = 0.1\text{ M}$$

Remember: Moles, not grams, *are the "common currency" of chemistry problems dealing with reactions. Concentration, usually in units of moles per liter, is the essential quantity for these acid–base problems.*

---

2) Choose the constant that will make most sense for the reaction in question and compute its value.

$$-\log(K_a \times K_b) = -\log(10^{-14})$$
$$-\log K_a + -\log K_b = -\log 10^{-14} = 14$$
$$pK_a + pK_b = 14$$
$$pK_b = 14 - pK_a = 9$$
$$K_b = 10^{-pK_b} = 10^{-9}$$

Now we need to decide which constant we will use, K_a or K_b. Here's where a little common sense goes a long way. If you think about sodium acetate, you should realize that it is the conjugate base of acetic acid. Therefore, we need the value of K_b for sodium acetate. Even though we are given the pK_a of acetic acid, getting the K_b from this information is no sweat.

In water, $K_a \times K_b$ is always equal to K_w, or 10^{-14}. Take the negative logarithm of both sides.

Remember that $\log(a \times b) = \log a + \log b$ and that $\log 10^x = x$.

Don't forget that –log(whatever) = p(whatever). We will want to find K_b because sodium acetate is the conjugate base of acetic acid.

Plug in the pK_a from above (to make our lives easier, let's say $4.74 \approx 5$).

KEY CONCEPTS

Acids and bases

Chemical equilibrium

TAKEAWAYS

Keep in mind that K_b is nothing more than an *equilibrium constant* for the reaction of a base picking up a proton from water. So, all of the things that are true for K_{eq} are true for K_b, especially that K_{eq} only depends on temperature. At constant temperature, *it never changes* (as the name suggests), even if the concentrations of the species in solution change.

THINGS TO WATCH OUT FOR

Remember that the cardinal principle of handling computation on the MCAT is to *avoid it whenever possible* because it is so time consuming and drastically increases the chances of making a mistake. If you can't avoid doing computation, *choose numbers that are easy to work with*. So, for example, you wouldn't want to use 199.9999, you would just use 200.

Remember: *The p-scale is a hugely important value for acid-base problems. Remember that p(something) = –log(something).*

---

3) Write down the appropriate chemical reaction and set up a table.

Here we need to set up a table to reflect the data we've collected. This is the "putting it all together" step and is crucial.

Our table will be as follows:

	$H_2O\,(\ell)$ +	$CH_3CO_2^-(aq)$ →	$CH_3CO_2H\,(aq)$ +	$OH^-(aq)$
Initial	–	0.1	0	0
Change	–	$-x$	$+x$	$+x$
Equilibrium	–	$0.1-x$	x	x

Initial: The idea is that we're going to take some sodium acetate, dump it into water, and see what happens. Our initial row in the table shows the concentrations that we have before any reaction takes place. That means that we'll start with the amount of sodium acetate we computed, 0.1 M. There's no acetic acid or hydroxide because no reaction has happened yet.

Change: Here's where all the action happens. As our acetate reacts with water, the concentration is going to decrease by some amount. We don't know what that will be yet, so let's just call it x. If the acetate concentration goes *down* by x, the concentrations of acetic acid and hydroxide must go *up* by the same amount, so we put x's in their columns.

Equilibrium: This is the easy part. Just add up all of the columns above. Our completed table will look like the table at left.

Remember: Always, always, always *make sure that* ***any*** *chemical reaction you write down is* ***balanced.*** *This means to make sure that* ***mass*** *is balanced (the number of atoms on either side of the reaction) and that* ***charge*** *is balanced. Also, the concentration of pure liquids (e.g., water) and pure solids is never taken into account in equilibria.*

---

4) Plug the equilibrium concentrations from the table into the appropriate acidity or basicity expression.

$$K_b = \frac{[CH_3CO_2]_{eq}[OH^-]_{eq}}{[CH_3CO_2^-]_{eq}} = \frac{X\,X}{0.1-X} = \frac{X^2}{0.1-X} = 10^{-9}$$

We know that K_b is just the K_{eq} for the reaction in our table above. Plug in the numbers from the table.

---

5) Simplify the expression from step 4 and solve it.

$$\frac{x^2}{0.1} = 10^{-9}$$

$$x^2 = (0.1)(10^{-9}) = 10^{-10}$$

$$x = 10^{-5}$$

Let's make our lives easier (*and* save ourselves time on Test Day) by assuming that x is much, much smaller than 0.1, so that $0.1 - x \approx 0.1$.

Now why would we want to assume that x is very, very small? Well, remember that sodium acetate is a weak base because it has a K_b value. So, if it's a weak base, it won't react much with water, thus making x a very small number.

***Remember:** Don't forget to check the assumption we made to simplify our equation. Because $x = 10^{-5}$, which is indeed much less than 0.1 (by a factor of 10,000), our assumption holds.*

---

6) Answer the question.

$$-\log[OH^-] = -\log[10^{-5}] = 5 = pOH$$

$$pH = 14 - 5 = 9$$

This step is trickier than it sounds and is where many, many mistakes are committed. Here's where attention to detail counts. You don't want to slog through all of the work above and then mess up at the end, when 99 percent of the work is done!

Think about what you've solved for. What is x? Well, if we look at the table, we see that x is the concentration of hydroxide. So, if we take the negative log of the hydroxide ion concentration, we get the pOH.

Remember that pH + pOH = 14. The actual pH is 8.89. So, all of our assumptions and roundings didn't affect the answer much, but saved us a lot of time in computation!

***Remember:** Always ask yourself whether your final answer makes sense. The MCAT isn't a computation test, it's a test of critical thinking. Here, we have a base being dissolved in water, so at the end of the day, the pH better be above 7, which it is.*

SIMILAR QUESTIONS

1) What would be the pH if the initial concentration of sodium acetate in the opening question was halved? If it were doubled?
2) Compute the pH of the resulting solution if 0.1 mol of *pure NaOH* were added to 1 L of water. How does this pH compare to that of the solution with sodium acetate?
3) What would the pH of the solution be if just enough HCl were added to the solution in the original problem to consume all of the sodium acetate?

KEY CONCEPTS

Titration

Acids and bases

Equivalence point

Half-equivalence point

pH

TAKEAWAYS

Setting up the tables as shown makes quick work of titration pH questions. Remember to make approximations and use numbers that are easy to work with in order to minimize the computation necessary to get to the answer.

TITRATION

Hydrazoic acid, HN_3, is a highly toxic compound that can cause death in minutes if inhaled in concentrated form. 100 mL of 0.2 M aqueous solution of HN_3 (pK_a = 4.72) is to be titrated with a 0.5 M solution of NaOH.

a) What is the pH of the HN_3 solution before any NaOH is added?

b) The *half-equivalence* point of a titration is where half the titrant necessary to get to the equivalence point has been added. How much of the NaOH solution will be needed to get to the half-equivalence point? What is the pH at the half-equivalence point?

c) What is the pH at the equivalence point?

1) Determine the pH before the titration.

What you need to ask yourself in each stage of this problem is which species is present, H^+ or OH^-, and where is it coming from? Before the titration begins, we have H^+ around because, as the name of the compound suggests, hydrazoic acid is *acidic*. The major source of H^+ is from the hydrazoic acid itself, so we can set up a table as follows:

	$H_2O\,(\ell)$ +	$HN_3(aq)$ →	$H_3O^+(aq)$ +	$OH^-(aq)$
Initial	–	0.2	0	0
Change	–	$-x$	$+x$	$+x$
Equilibrium	–	$0.2-x$	x	x

$$K_a = \frac{[H_3O^+][N_3^-]}{[HN_3]} = \frac{X^2}{0.2-X} = \frac{X^2}{0.2} = 10^{-5}$$

$$X^2 = 2 \times 10^{-1} \times 10^{-5} = 2 \times 10^{-6}$$

$$\Rightarrow X = \sqrt{0.2 \times 10^{-6}} \approx 1.4 \times 10^{-3}$$

$$\Rightarrow [H_3O^+]_{eq} = 1.4 \times 10^{-3}$$

$$\Rightarrow pH = -\log[H_3O^+] = -\log(1.4 \times 10^{-3}) = 3 - \log(1.4)$$

$$2 < pH < 3$$

Plug in the concentrations from the table. We know the pK_a is around 5, so the K_a must be 10^{-5}. Whenever exponents or logarithms are involved, *use numbers that are easy to work with*. Make the approximation that $0.2 - x \approx 0.2$ because HN_3 is a weak acid.

If you must take a square root, try and get the power of 10 to be even to make matters simple. Remember from the table that x is the hydronium ion concentration.

Remember that $-\log[a \times 10^{-b}] = b - \log[a]$ = somewhere between $b - 1$ and b.

---

2) Find the equivalence point and half-equivalence point.

mol $HN_3 = 0.1\ L \times 0.2\ mol\ L^{-1} = 0.02$ mol HN_3

$$\frac{0.02\ \text{mol NaOH}}{0.5\ \text{mol L}^{-1}} = 0.04\ \text{L NaOH solution}$$

$$K_a = \frac{[H_3O^+][N_3^-]}{[HN_3]} = [H_3O^+] = [H_3O^+]$$

Compute the number of moles of HN_3 that you start with.

Each mole of HN_3 will react with one mole of OH^-. Therefore, the equivalence point is reached when 40 mL of the NaOH solution are added and the half-equivalence point is at 40/2 = 20 mL. We could go through the whole rigamarole of setting up another table to figure out the pH at the half-equivalence point, or we could use a little common sense to avoid computation. At the half-equivalence point, half of the HN_3 has been consumed and converted to N_3^-. Therefore, the HN_3 and N_3 concentrations are equal.

Because $[HN_3] = [N_3^-]$, $K_a = [H_3O^+]$, and $pH = pK_a = 4.72$.

Remember: *Whenever possible, avoid computation!*

---

3) Determine the reactive species at the equivalence point to find the pH.

$$K_b = \frac{K_w}{K_a} = \frac{10^{-14}}{10^{-5}} = 10^{-9}$$

Remember that $K_a \times K_b = K_w = 10^{-14}$. Now we can set up our table:

	$H_2O(\ell)$ +	$N_3(aq)^-$ →	$HN_3(aq)$ +	$OH^-(aq)$
Initial	–	0.15	0	0
Change	–	$-x$	$+x$	$+x$
Equilibrium	–	$0.15 - x$	x	x

Remember that the volume of our solution has increased by 40 mL, so the concentration of N_3^- is $\frac{0.02\ \text{mol}}{(0.1 + 0.04)\ \text{L}} \approx 0.15$ M.

$$K_b = \frac{[HN_3][OH^-]}{[N_3^-]} = \frac{X^2}{0.15 - X} = \frac{X^2}{0.15} = 10^{-9}$$

$$x^2 = 0.15 \times 10^{-9} = 0.15 \times 10^{-10} \approx 1.6 \times 10^{-10} \approx 160 \times 10^{-12}$$

$$\Rightarrow X = \sqrt{160 \times 10^{-12}} = 4\sqrt{10} \times 10^{-6} \approx 12 \times 10^{-6} = 1.2 \times 10^{-5}$$

$$\Rightarrow [OH^-]_{eq} = 1.2 \times 10^{-5}$$

$$\Rightarrow pOH = -\log([OH^-]) = -\log(1.2 \times 10^{-5}) = 5 - \log(1.2) \approx 5$$

$$\Rightarrow pH = 14 - pOH = 14 - 5 = 9$$

THINGS TO WATCH OUT FOR

Be careful in choosing whether you will use K_a or K_b to determine the pH. Make this decision based on whether the dominant species in solution is acidic or basic, respectively.

SIMILAR QUESTIONS

1) What is the pH after the equivalence point has been exceeded by 5 mL of the NaOH solution in the opening question?
2) What would be the pH if the same amount of NaOH solution necessary to get to the half-equivalence point in this titration were added to pure water? How does the pH of each situation compare? This demonstrates how weak acids can serve as *buffers*, solutions that resist changes in pH.
3) What would be the pH of a solution that was 0.2 M in HN_3 and 0.1 M in N_3^-?

At the equivalence point, all of the HN_3 has been consumed, leaving only N_3^- behind. Because N_3^- is a Brønsted–Lowry *base*, we need to worry about OH^-, not H_3O^+.

Make the approximation that $0.15 - x \approx 0.15$.

Here, let's say that 1.6 is close to 1.5 to make the square root computation trivial.

Note that pH + pOH = 14 in water. Remember to ask yourself whether or not a result makes sense. Here, because we have a basic species (N_3^-), the pH should be above 7, which it is.

CHAPTER 11

REDOX REACTIONS AND ELECTROCHEMISTRY

Electrochemistry is the study of the relationships between chemical reactions and electrical energy. **Electrochemical reactions** include spontaneous reactions that produce electrical energy, and nonspontaneous reactions that use electrical energy to produce a chemical change. Both types of reactions always involve a transfer of electrons with conservation of charge and mass.

OXIDATION-REDUCTION REACTIONS

A. OXIDATION AND REDUCTION

The law of conservation of charge states that an electrical charge can be neither created nor destroyed. Thus, an isolated loss or gain of electrons cannot occur; **oxidation** (loss of electrons) and **reduction** (gain of electrons) must occur simultaneously, resulting in an electron transfer called a **redox reaction.** An **oxidizing agent** causes another atom in a redox reaction to undergo oxidation, and is itself reduced. A **reducing agent** causes the other atom to be reduced, and is itself oxidized.

KAPLAN EXCLUSIVE

OIL RIG stands for "Oxidation Is Loss, Reduction Is Gain," of electrons that is.

Alternatively, reduction is just what it sounds like: reduction of charge.

B. ASSIGNING OXIDATION NUMBERS

It is important, of course, to know which atom is oxidized and which is reduced. **Oxidation numbers** are assigned to atoms in order to keep track of the redistribution of electrons during a chemical reaction. From the oxidation numbers of the reactants and products, it is possible to determine how many electrons are gained or lost by each atom. The oxidation number of an atom in a compound is assigned according to the following rules:

TEACHER TIP

Don't forget that you'll have the periodic table available on Test Day. Beware of transition metals but realize we can often figure their oxidation by default.

1. **The oxidation number of free elements is zero.** For example, the atoms in N_2, P_4, S_8, and He all have oxidation numbers of zero.
2. **The oxidation number for a monatomic ion is equal to the charge of the ion.** For example, the oxidation numbers for Na^+, Cu^{2+}, Fe^{3+}, Cl^-, and N^{3-} are +1, +2, +3, –1, and –3, respectively.
3. **The oxidation number of each Group IA element in a compound is +1. The oxidation number of each Group IIA element in a compound is +2.**

4. **The oxidation number of each Group VIIA element in a compound is –1, except when combined with an element of higher electronegativity.** For example, in HCl, the oxidation number of Cl is –1; in HOCl, however, the oxidation number of Cl is +1.
5. **The oxidation number of hydrogen is –1 in compounds with less electronegative elements than hydrogen (Groups IA and IIA.)** Examples include NaH and CaH_2.The more common oxidation number of hydrogen is +1.

MCAT SYNOPSIS

The conventions of formula writing put cation first and anion second. Thus NaH implies H^- while HCl implies H^+.

6. **In most compounds, the oxidation number of oxygen is –2.** This is not the case, however, in molecules such as OF_2. Here, because F is more electronegative than O, the oxidation number of oxygen is +2. Also, in peroxides such as BaO_2, the oxidation number of O is –1 instead of –2 because of the structure of the peroxide ion, $[O–O]^{2-}$. (Note that Ba, a group IIA element, can not be a +4 cation.)
7. **The sum of the oxidation numbers of all the atoms present in a neutral compound is zero. The sum of the oxidation numbers of the atoms present in a polyatomic ion is equal to the charge of the ion.** Thus, for SO_4^{2-}, the sum of the oxidation numbers must be –2.

Example: Assign oxidation numbers to the atoms in the following reaction in order to determine the oxidized and reduced species and the oxidizing and reducing agents.

$$SnCl_2 + PbCl_4 \rightarrow SnCl_4 + PbCl_2$$

Solution: All these species are neutral, so the oxidation numbers of each compound must add up to zero. In $SnCl_2$, because there are two chlorines present, and chlorine has an oxidation number of –1, Sn must have an oxidation number of +2. Similarly, the oxidation number of Sn in $SnCl_4$ is +4; the oxidation number of Pb is +4 in $PbCl_4$ and +2 in $PbCl_2$. Notice that the oxidation number of Sn goes from +2 to +4; it loses electrons and thus is oxidized, making it the reducing agent. Because the oxidation number of Pb has decreased from +4 to +2, it has gained electrons and been reduced. Pb is the oxidizing agent. The sum of the charges on both sides of the reaction is equal to zero, so charge has been conserved.

C. BALANCING REDOX REACTIONS

By assigning oxidation numbers to the reactants and products, one can determine how many moles of each species are required for conservation of charge and mass, which is necessary to balance the equation. To balance a redox reaction, both the net charge and the number of atoms must be equal on both sides of the equation. The most common method for balancing redox equations is the **half-reaction method,** also known as the **ion-electron method,** in which the equation is separated into two half-reactions—the oxidation part and the reduction part. Each half-reaction is balanced separately, and they are then added to give a balanced overall reaction. Consider a redox reaction between $KMnO_4$ and HI in an acidic solution.

$$MnO_4^- + I^- \rightarrow I_2 + Mn^{2+}$$

Step 1: Separate the two half-reactions.

$I^- \rightarrow I_2$

$MnO_4^- \rightarrow Mn^{2+}$

Step 2: Balance the atoms of each half-reaction. First, balance all atoms except H and O. Next, in an acidic solution, add H_2O to balance the O atoms and then add H^+ to balance the H atoms. (In a basic solution, use OH^- and H_2O to balance the O's and H's.)

To balance the iodine atoms, place a coefficient of 2 before the I^- ion.

$2\ I^- \rightarrow I_2$

For the permanganate half-reaction, Mn is already balanced. Next, balance the oxygens by adding $4H_2O$ to the right side.

$MnO_4^- \rightarrow Mn^{2+} + 4H_2O$

Finally, add H+ to the left side to balance the 4 H_2Os. These two half-reactions are now balanced.

$MnO_4^- + 8\ H^+ \rightarrow Mn^{2+} + 4H_2O$

Step 3: Balance the charges of each half-reaction. The reduction half-reaction must consume the same number of electrons as are supplied by the oxidation half. For the oxidation reaction, add 2 electrons to the right side of the reaction:

$2\ I^- \rightarrow I_2 + 2e^-$

For the reduction reaction, a charge of +2 must exist on both sides. Add 5 electrons to the left side of the reaction to accomplish this:

$5\ e^- + 8\ H^+ + MnO_4^- \rightarrow Mn^{2+} + 4\ H_2O$

TEACHER TIP

This type of methodical, step-by-step approach is great for the MCAT. Chances are you'll come up with your answer only halfway through the process.

Next, both half-reactions must have the same number of electrons so that they will cancel. Multiply the oxidation half by 5 and the reduction half by 2.

$5(2I^- \rightarrow I_2 + 2e^-)$
$2(5e^- + 8H^+ + MnO_4^- \rightarrow Mn^{2+} + 4\ H_2O)$

Step 4: Add the half-reactions:

$10\ I^- \rightarrow 5\ I_2 + 10\ e^-$
$16\ H^+ + 2\ MnO_4^- + 10\ e^- \rightarrow 2\ Mn^{2+} + 8\ H_2O$

The final equation is:

$10\ I^- + 10\ e^- + 16\ H^+ + 2\ MnO_4^- \rightarrow 5\ I_2 + 2\ Mn^{2+} + 10\ e^- + 8\ H_2O$

To get the overall equation, cancel out the electrons and any H_2Os, H^+s, or OH^-s that appear on both sides of the equation.

$10\ I^- + 16\ H^+ + 2\ MnO_4^- \rightarrow 5\ I_2 + 2\ Mn^{2+} + 8\ H_2O$

Step 5: Finally, confirm that mass and charge are balanced. There is a +4 net charge on each side of the reaction equation, and the atoms are stoichiometrically balanced.

ELECTROCHEMICAL CELLS

Electrochemical cells are contained systems in which a redox reaction occurs. There are two types of electrochemical cells, **galvanic cells** (also known as **voltaic cells**), and **electrolytic cells.** Spontaneous reactions occur in galvanic cells, and nonspontaneous reactions in electrolytic cells. Both types contain **electrodes** at which oxidation and reduction occur. For all electrochemical cells, the electrode at which oxidation occurs is called the **anode,** and the electrode where reduction occurs is called the **cathode.**

KAPLAN EXCLUSIVE

A way to remember which electrode is which is: AN OX and a RED CAT. Another easy way to remember this is by the spelling of the words: oxidAtion and reduCtion

A. GALVANIC CELLS

A redox reaction occurring in a **galvanic cell** has a negative ΔG and is therefore a **spontaneous reaction.** Galvanic cell reactions supply energy and are used to do work. This energy can be harnessed by placing the oxidation and reduction half-reactions in separate containers called **half-cells.** The half-cells are then connected by an apparatus that allows for the flow of electrons.

MCAT SYNOPSIS

Galvanic cells are commonly used as batteries; to be economically viable, batteries must be spontaneous!

A common example of a galvanic cell is the Daniell cell in Figure 11.1.

In the Daniell cell, a zinc bar is placed in an aqueous $ZnSO_4$ solution, and a copper bar is placed in an aqueous $CuSO_4$ solution. The anode of this cell is the zinc bar where Zn(*s*) is oxidized to $Zn^{2+}(aq)$. The cathode is the copper bar, and it is the site of the reduction of $Cu^{2+}(aq)$ to Cu(*s*). The half-cell reactions are written as follows:

$$Zn(s) \rightarrow Zn^{2+}(aq) + 2e^- \rightarrow \text{(anode)}$$
$$Cu^{2+}(aq) + 2e \rightarrow Cu(s) \rightarrow \text{(cathode)}$$

If the two half-cells were not separated, the Cu^{2+} ions would react directly with the zinc bar and no useful electrical work would be obtained. To complete the circuit, the two solutions must be connected. Without connection, the electrons from the zinc oxidation half reaction would not be able to get to the copper ions, thus a wire (or other conductor) is necessary. If only a wire were provided for this electron flow, the reaction would soon cease anyway because an excess negative charge would build up in the solution surrounding the cathode and an excess positive charge would build up in the solution surrounding the anode. This charge gradient is dissipated by the presence of a **salt bridge,** which permits the exchange of cations and anions. The salt bridge contains an inert electrolyte, usually KCl or NH_4NO_3, whose ions will not react with the electrodes or with the ions in solution. At the same time the anions from the salt bridge (e.g., Cl^-) diffuse from the salt bridge of the Daniell cell into the $ZnSO_4$ solution to balance out the charge of the newly created Zn^{2+} ions, the cations of the salt bridge (e.g., K^+) flow into the $CuSO_4$ solution to balance out the charge of the SO_4^{2-} ions left in solution when the Cu^{2+} ions deposit as copper metal.

MCAT FAVORITE

The purpose of the salt bridge is to exchange anions and cations to balance, i.e., dissipate, newly generated charges.

During the course of the reaction, electrons flow from the zinc bar (anode) through the wire and the voltmeter, toward the copper bar (cathode). The anions (Cl^-) flow externally (via the salt bridge) into the $ZnSO_4$, and the cations (K^+) flow into the $CuSO_4$. This flow depletes the salt bridge and, along with the finite quantity of Cu^{2+} in the solution, accounts for the relatively short lifetime of the cell.

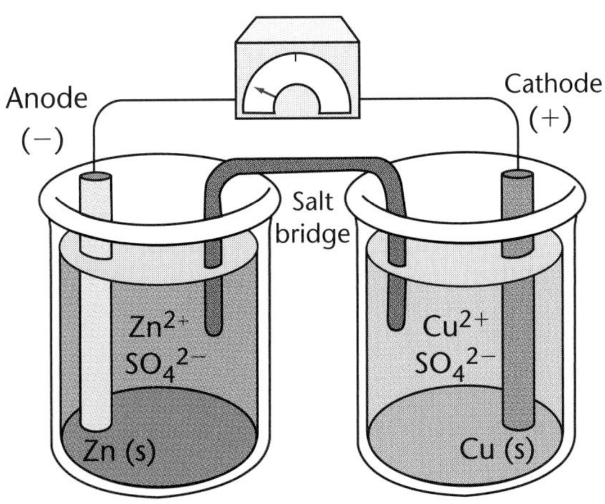

Figure 11.1: Daniell Cell

TEACHER TIP

Know the shorthand notation for cells; it might not be spelled on out on the exam.

A **cell diagram** is a shorthand notation representing the reactions in an electrochemical cell. A cell diagram for the Daniell cell is as follows:

$$Zn(s) \mid Zn^{2+}(x\text{M } SO_4^{2-}) \parallel Cu^{2+}(y\text{M } SO_4^{2-}) \mid Cu(s)$$

The following rules are used in constructing a cell diagram:

1. The reactants and products are always listed from left to right in the form:

   anode | anode solution || cathode solution | cathode

2. A single vertical line indicates a phase boundary.
3. A double vertical line indicates the presence of a salt bridge or some other type of barrier.

NOTE

$(1.6 \times 10^{-19})(6.022 \times 10^{23})$
$= 96{,}487$ C/mol e^-

This number is called **Faraday's constant,** and one **faraday (F)** is equivalent to the amount of charge contained in one mole of electrons (1 F = 96,487 coulombs, or J/V).

B. ELECTROLYTIC CELLS

A redox reaction occurring in an **electrolytic cell** has a positive ΔG and is therefore **nonspontaneous.** In **electrolysis,** electrical energy is required to induce reaction. The oxidation and reduction half-reactions are usually placed in one container.

An example of an electrolytic cell, in which molten NaCl is electrolyzed to form Cl_2 (*g*) and Na (ℓ), is shown in Figure 11.2.

In this cell, Na^+ ions migrate towards the cathode, where they are reduced to Na (ℓ). Similarly, Cl^- ions migrate towards the anode, where they are oxidized to Cl_2 (*g*). This cell is used in industry as the major means of sodium and chlorine production. Note that sodium is a liquid at the temperature of molten NaCl; it is also less dense than the molten salt, and thus is easily removed as it floats to the top of the reaction vessel.

TEACHER TIP

*An*ions are negatively charged and travel to the *an*ode. *Cat*ions are positively charged and travel to the *cat*hode. This is also helpful in electrophoresis, seen in purification and separation techniques in Organic Chemistry.

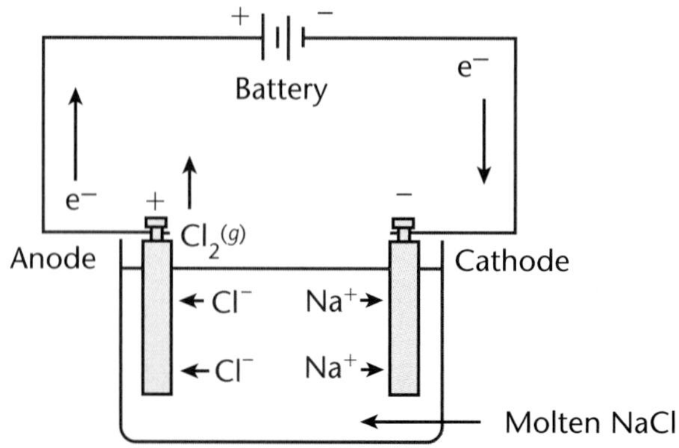

Figure 11.2: Example of an Electrolytic Cell

C. ELECTRODE CHARGE DESIGNATIONS

The anode of an **electrolytic cell** is considered **positive,** because it is attached to the positive pole of the battery and so attracts anions from the solution. The anode of a **galvanic cell,** on the other hand, is considered **negative** because the **spontaneous** oxidation reaction that takes place at the galvanic cell's anode is the original source of that cell's negative charge, i.e., is the source of electrons. In spite of this difference in designating charge, oxidation takes place at the anode in both types of cells, and electrons always flow through the wire from the anode to the cathode.

In a galvanic cell, charge is spontaneously created as electrons are released by the oxidizing species at the anode; because this is the source of electrons, the anode of a galvanic cell is considered the negative electrode.

In an electrolytic cell, electrons are forced through the cathode where they encounter the species that is to be reduced. Here it is the cathode that is providing electrons, and thus the cathode of an electrolytic cell is considered the negative electrode. Alternatively, one can think of the cathode as the electrode attached to the negative pole of the battery (or other power source) used for the electrolysis.

In either case, a simple mnemonic is that the CAThode attracts the CATions. In the Daniell cell, for example, the electrons created at the anode as the zinc oxidizes travel through the wire to the copper half cell where they attract copper (II) cations to the cathode.

One common topic in which this distinction arises is electrophoresis, a technique often used to separate amino acids based on their isoelectronic points, or pIs. The positively charged amino acids, i.e., those that are protonated at the pH of the solution, will migrate toward the cathode; negatively charged amino acids, i.e., those that are deprotonated at the solution pH, migrate instead toward the anode.

MCAT Synopsis

In an electrolytic cell, the anode is positive and the cathode is negative. In a galvanic cell, the anode is negative and the cathode is positive. However, in both types of cells, reduction occurs at the cathode and oxidation occurs at the anode.

REDUCTION POTENTIALS AND THE ELECTROMOTIVE FORCE

A. REDUCTION POTENTIALS

Sometimes when electrolysis is carried out in an aqueous solution, water rather than the solute is oxidized or reduced. For example, if an aqueous solution of NaCl is electrolyzed, water may be reduced at the cathode to

Teacher Tip

A reduction potential is exactly what it sounds like: It tells us how likely a compound is to be reduced. The higher the value, the more likely it is to be reduced.

produce $H_2(g)$ and OH^- ions, instead of Na^+ being reduced to Na(*s*), as occurs in the absence of water. The species in a reaction that will be oxidized or reduced can be determined from the **reduction potential** of each species, defined as the tendency of a species to acquire electrons and be reduced. Each species has its own intrinsic reduction potential; the more positive the potential, the greater the specie's tendency to be reduced.

A reduction potential is measured in volts (V) and is defined relative to the **standard hydrogen electrode (SHE),** which is arbitrarily given a potential of 0 volts. **Standard reduction potential, (E°),** is measured under **standard conditions:** 25°C, a 1 M concentration for each ion participating in the reaction, a partial pressure of 1 atm for each gas that is part of the reaction, and metals in their pure state. The relative reactivities of different half-cells can be compared to predict the direction of electron flow. A higher or more positive E° means a greater tendency for reduction to occur, while a lower E° means a greater tendency for oxidation to occur.

Example: Given the following half-reactions and E° values, determine which species would be oxidized and which would be reduced.

$Ag^+ + e \rightarrow Ag\ (s)$ E° = +0.8 V

$Tl^+ + e- \rightarrow Tl\ (s)$ E° = −0.34 V

Solution: Ag+ would be reduced to Ag(*s*) and Tl(*s*) would be oxidized to Tl^+, because Ag^+ has the higher E°. Therefore, the reaction equation would be:

$Ag^+ + Tl(s) \rightarrow Tl^+ + Ag(s)$

which is the sum of the two spontaneous half-reactions.

It should be noted that reduction and oxidation are opposite processes. Therefore, in order to obtain the oxidation potential of a given half-reaction, the reduction half-reaction and the sign of the reduction potential are both reversed. For instance, from the example above, the oxidation half reaction and oxidation potential of Tl(*s*) are:

$Tl(s) \rightarrow Tl^+ + e^-$ E° = +0.34 V

B. THE ELECTROMOTIVE FORCE

Standard reduction potentials are also used to calculate the **standard electromotive force** (**EMF or** $\mathbf{E°_{cell}}$) of a reaction, the difference in potential between two half-cells. The EMF of a reaction is determined by adding the standard reduction potential of the reduced species and the standard oxidation potential of the oxidized species. When adding standard potentials, *do not* multiply by the number of moles oxidized or reduced.

$$EMF = E^\circ_{red} + E^\circ_{ox} \qquad \text{(Equation 1)}$$

The standard EMF of a galvanic cell is positive, while the standard EMF of an electrolytic cell is negative.

TEACHER TIP

In this equation we must change the sign of the second value because it is an oxidation potential, the exact opposite of a reduction potential. This equation can also be written as $EMF = E^\circ_{cathode} - E^\circ_{anode}$ (using only reduction potential) and still get the same result.

Example: Given that the standard reduction potentials for Sm^{3+} and $[RhCl_6]^{3-}$ are –2.41 V and +0.44 V respectively, calculate the EMF of the following reaction:

$$Sm^{3+} + Rh + 6\ Cl^- \rightarrow [RhCl_6]^{3-} + Sm$$

Solution: First, determine the oxidation and reduction half-reactions. As written, the Rh is oxidized and the Sm^{3+} is reduced. Thus the Sm^{3+} reduction potential is used as is, while the reverse reaction for Rh, $[RhCl_6]^{3-} \rightarrow Rh + 6\ Cl^-$, applies and the oxidation potential of $[RhCl_6]^{3-}$ must be used. Then, using Equation 1, the EMF can be calculated to be (–2.41 V) + (–0.44 V) = –2.85 V. The cell is thus electrolytic as written. From this result, it is evident that the reaction would proceed spontaneously to the left, in which case the Sm would be oxidized while $[RhCl_6]^{3-}$ would be reduced.

THERMODYNAMICS OF REDOX REACTIONS

A. EMF AND GIBBS FREE ENERGY

The thermodynamic criterion for determining the spontaneity of a reaction is ΔG, Gibbs free energy, the maximum amount of useful work produced by a chemical reaction. In an electrochemical cell, the work done is dependent on the number of coulombs and the energy available. Thus, ΔG and EMF are related as follows:

$$\Delta G = -nFE_{cell} \qquad \text{(Equation 2)}$$

where n is the number of moles of electrons exchanged, F is Faraday's constant, and E_{cell} is the EMF of the cell. **Keep in mind that if Faraday's constant is expressed in coulombs (J/V), then ΔG must be expressed in J, not kJ.**

FLASHBACK

Recall that if ΔG is positive, the reaction is not spontaneous; if ΔG is negative, the reaction is spontaneous.

If the reaction takes place under standard conditions (25°C, 1 atm pressure, and all solutions at 1M concentration), then the ΔG is the standard Gibbs free energy and E_{cell} is the standard cell potential. The above equation then becomes:

$$\Delta G^\circ = -nFE^\circ_{cell} \qquad \text{(Equation 3)}$$

B. THE EFFECT OF CONCENTRATION ON EMF

Thus far, only the calculations for the EMF of cells in unit concentrations (all the ionic species present have a molarity of 1 and all gases are at a pressure of 1 atm) have been discussed. However, concentration does have an effect on the EMF of a cell: EMF varies with the changing concentrations of the species involved. It can also be determined by the use of the **Nernst equation:**

$$E_{cell} = E^\circ_{cell} - (RT/nF)(\ln Q)$$

Q is the reaction quotient for a given reaction. For example, in the following reaction:

$$a\,A + b\,B \rightarrow c\,C + d\,D$$

the reaction quotient would be:

$$Q = \frac{[C]^c[D]^d}{[A]^a[B]^b}$$

The EMF of a cell can be measured by a **voltmeter.** A **potentiometer** is a kind of voltmeter that draws no current, and gives a more accurate reading of the difference in potential between two electrodes.

C. EMF AND THE EQUILIBRIUM CONSTANT (K_{eq})

For reactions in solution, ΔG° can be determined in another manner, as follows:

$$\Delta G^\circ = -RT \ln K_{eq} \qquad \text{(Equation 4)}$$

where R is the gas constant 8.314 J/(K•mol), T is the temperature in K, and K_{eq} is the equilibrium constant for the reaction.

> **MCAT SYNOPSIS**
>
> If E°_{cell} is positive, then ln K is positive. This means that K must be greater than one, and that the equilibrium must lie toward the right, i.e., products are favored.

If Equations 3 and 4 are combined, then:

$$\Delta G^\circ = -nFE^\circ_{cell} = -RT \ln K_{eq}$$

or simply:

$$nFE^\circ_{cell} = RT \ln K_{eq} \qquad \text{(Equation 5)}$$

If the values for n, T, and K_{eq} are known, then the E°_{cell} for the redox reaction can be readily calculated.

PRACTICE QUESTIONS

1. An electrolytic cell is filled with water. Which of the following will move toward the cathode of such a cell?

I. H^+ ions
II. $O2^-$ ions
III. Electrons

A. I only
B. II only
C. I and III
D. I, II, and III

2. The anode of a certain galvanic cell is composed of copper. What metal from the data below can be used at the cathode?

Reaction	Reduction Potential
$Hg^{2+} + 2e^- \longrightarrow Hg$	+0.85 V
$Cu^+ + e^- \longrightarrow Cu$	+0.52 V
$Zn^{2+} + 2e^- \longrightarrow Zn$	−0.76 V
$Al^{3+} + 3e^- \longrightarrow Al$	−1.66 V

A. Hg
B. Al
C. Zn
D. None of the above

3. Considering the following equation, what species acts as an oxidizing agent?

$3Na(s) + H_3N(aq) \rightarrow Na_3N(s) + H_2(g)$

A. H^+
B. H_2N
C. Na
D. Na^+

4. How many electrons are involved in the following unbalanced reaction?

$Cr_2O_7^{2-} + H^+ + e^- \rightarrow 2Cr^{2+} + H_2O$

A. 2
B. 8
C. 12
D. 16

QUESTIONS 5 AND 6 REFER TO THE FOLLOWING HALF–REACTIONS:

$O_2 + 4H^+ + 4e^- \rightarrow 2H_2O + 1.23\text{ V}$ (Reaction 1)

$PbO_2 + 4H^+ + 2e^- \rightarrow Pb^{2+} + 2H_2O + 1.46\text{ V}$ (Reaction 2)

5. If the two half–reactions above combine to form a spontaneous system, what is the net balanced equation of the full reaction?

A. $2PbO_2 + 4H^+ \rightarrow Pb^{2+} + O_2 + 2H_2O$
B. $PbO_2 \rightarrow Pb^{2+} + O_2 + 2e^-$
C. $Pb^{2+} + O_2 + 2H_2O \rightarrow 2PbO_2 + 4H^+$
D. $Pb^{2+} + O_2 + 2e^- \rightarrow PbO_2$

6. Find the standard potential of the following reaction:

$Pb^{2+} + O_2 + 2H_2O \rightarrow 2PbO_2 + 4H^+$

A. +0.23 V
B. −0.23 V
C. −1.69 V
D. +2.69 V

7. A certain electrochemical cell produces elemental sodium from a solution of sodium chloride. How many electrons must be donated by the electric current?

A. 3
B. 2
C. 1
D. 0

8. Rusting occurs due to the oxidation–reduction reaction of iron with environmental oxygen:

$4Fe(s) + 3O_2(g) \rightarrow 2Fe_2O_3(s)$

Some metals, such as copper, are unlikely to react with oxygen. Which of the following best explains this observation?

A. Iron has a more positive reduction potential, making it more likely to donate electrons to oxygen.
B. Iron has a more positive reduction potential, making it more likely to accept electrons from oxygen.
C. Iron has a less positive reduction potential, making it more likely to donate electrons to oxygen.
D. Iron has a less positive reduction potential, making it more likely to accept electrons from oxygen.

9. Lithium aluminum hydride ($LiAlH_4$) is often used in laboratories because of its tendency to donate a hydride ion. Which of the following properties does $LiAlH_4$ exhibit?

A. Strong reducing agent
B. Strong oxidizing agent
C. Strong acid
D. Strong base

10. If the value of $E°_{cell}$ is known, what other data are needed to calculate ΔG?

A. Equilibrium constant
B. Reaction quotient
C. Temperature of the system
D. Number of moles of reactant

11. Which of the following compounds is least likely to be found in the salt bridge of a galvanic cell?

A. NaCl
B. SO_3
C. $MgSO_3$
D. NH_4NO_3

12. What is the oxidation number of chlorine in NaClO?

A. –1
B. 0
C. +1
D. +2

13. The following cell maintains a pH of 7. What is the ratio of the volume of hydrogen produced to the volume of oxygen produced?

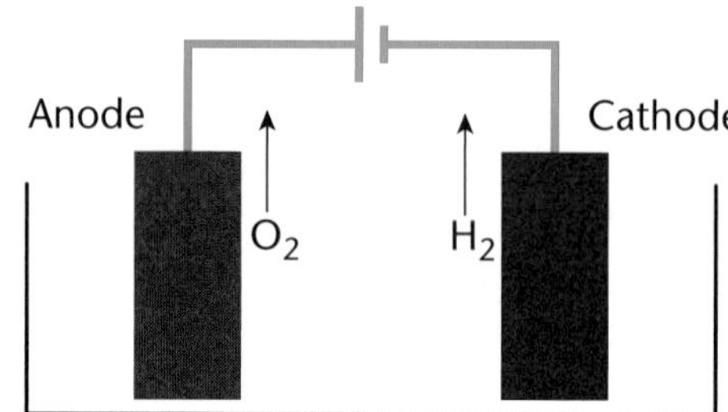

A. 2:1
B. 1:2
C. 1:1
D. 1:4

14. Which of the following is most likely to increase the rate of an electrolytic reaction?

A. Increasing the resistance in the circuit
B. Increasing the volume of electrolyte
C. Increasing the current
D. Increasing the pH

15. The following electronic configurations represent elements in their neutral form. Which element is the strongest oxidizing agent?

A. $1s^22s^2p^63s^2p^64s^2$
B. $1s^22s^2p^63s^2p^64s^23d^5$
C. $1s^22s^2p^63s^2p^64s^23d^{10}4p^1$
D. $1s^22s^2p^63s^2p^64s^23d^54p^5$

BALANCING REDOX REACTIONS

Balance the following reaction that takes place in basic solution.

$$ZrO(OH)_2(s) + SO_3^{2-}(aq) \rightleftharpoons Zr(s) + SO_4^{2-}(aq)$$

1) Separate the overall reaction into two half-reactions.

$ZrO(OH)_2 \rightleftharpoons Zr$

$SO_3^{2-} \rightleftharpoons SO_4^{2-}$

Break the reactions up by looking at atoms other than hydrogen and oxygen.

---

2) Balance the oxygens in each reaction by adding the necessary number of moles of water to the appropriate side.

$ZrO(OH)_2 \rightleftharpoons Zr(s) + 3\ H_2O$

$H_2O + SO_3^{2-} \rightleftharpoons SO_4^{2-}$

---

3) Balance hydrogen by adding the necessary number of H^+ ions to the appropriate side of each reaction.

$4\ H^+ + ZrO(OH)_2 \rightleftharpoons Zr + 3\ H_2O$

$H_2O + SO_3^{2-} \rightleftharpoons SO_4^{2-} + 2\ H^+$

---

4) If the reaction is carried out in basic solution, "neutralize" each equivalent of H^+ with one equivalent of OH^-.

$4\ OH^- + 4\ H^+ + ZrO(OH)_2 \rightleftharpoons Zr + 3\ H_2O + 4\ OH^-$

$2\ OH^- + H_2O + SO_3^{2-} \rightleftharpoons SO_4^{2-} + 2\ H^+ + 2\ OH^-$

$4\ H_2O + ZrO(OH)_2 \rightleftharpoons Zr + 3\ H_2O + 4\ OH^-$

$2\ OH^- + H_2O + SO_3^{2-} \rightleftharpoons SO_4^{2-} + 2\ H_2O$

Combine each mole of H^+ and OH^- into one mole of water and simplify each reaction.

Remember: *Don't forget to add OH^- to each side of both reactions!*

---

5) Balance the overall charge in each reaction using electrons.

$4\ e^- + 4\ H_2O + ZrO(OH)_2 \rightleftharpoons Zr + 3\ H_2O + 4\ OH^-$

$2\ OH^- + H_2O + SO_3^{2-} \rightleftharpoons SO_4^{2-} + 2\ H_2O + 2\ e^-$

The top equation has a total charge of 4^- on the right from the 4 moles of hydroxide, so 4 electrons need to be added to the left side of the equation. In the bottom equation, there is a total charge of 4^- on the left, 2^- from the 2 moles of hydroxide, and 2^- from the 2 moles of sulfite anion (SO_3^{2-}).

KEY CONCEPTS

Oxidation

Reduction

Balancing electrochemical half-reactions

TAKEAWAYS

Don't fall into the trap of simply balancing mass in these reactions. If oxidation and reduction are occurring, you must go through this procedure to balance the reaction.

THINGS TO WATCH OUT FOR

These kinds of problems can be extremely tedious. You must take extra care to avoid careless addition and subtraction errors!

Similar Questions

1) Which atom is being oxidized in the original equation? Which is being reduced? Identify the oxidizing and reducing agents.
2) A *disproportionation* is a redox reaction in which the same species is both *oxidized* and *reduced* during the course of the reaction. One such reaction is shown below. Balance the reaction, assuming that it takes place in acidic solution:

   $PbSO_4(s) \rightarrow Pb(s) + PbO_2(s) + SO_4^{2-}(aq)$
3) Dentists often use zinc amalgams to make temporary crowns for their patients. It is absolutely vital that they keep the zinc amalgam dry. Any exposure to water would cause pain to the patient and might even crack a tooth. The reaction of zinc metal with water is shown below:

   $Zn(s) + H_2O(\ell) \rightarrow Zn^{2+}(aq) + H_2(g)$

   Balance this reaction, assuming that it takes place in basic solution. Why would exposure to water cause the crown, and perhaps the tooth, to crack?

Remember: *Don't forget to account for all charges in this step, including the charge contributed by molecules other than H^+ and OH^-.*

---

6) Multiply each reaction by the necessary integer to ensure that equal numbers of electrons are present in each reaction.

$4\ e^- + 4\ H_2O + ZrO(OH)_2 \rightleftharpoons Zr + 3\ H_2O + 4\ OH^-$

$4\ OH^- + 2\ H_2O + 2\ SO_3^{2-} \rightleftharpoons 2\ SO_4^{2-} + 4\ H_2O + 4\ e^-$

Here, the lowest common multiple among the four electrons in the top reaction and the two in the bottom is four electrons, so we must multiply everything in the bottom reaction by 2.

---

7) Combine both reactions and simplify by eliminating redundant molecules on each side of the reaction.

$4\ e^- + 4\ H_2O(\ell) + ZrO(OH)_2(s) + 4\ OH^-(aq) + 2\ H_2O(\ell) + 2\ SO_3^{2-}(aq)$
$\rightleftharpoons Zr(s) + 3\ H_2O(\ell) + 4\ OH^-(aq) + 2\ SO_4^{2-}(aq) + 4\ H_2O(\ell) + 4\ e^-$

$4\ e^- + 6\ H_2O(\ell) + ZrO(OH)_2(s) + 4\ OH^-(aq) + 2\ SO_3^{2-}(aq)$
$\rightleftharpoons Zr(s) + 7\ H_2O(\ell) + 4\ OH^-(aq) + 2\ SO_4^{2-}(aq) + 4\ e^-$

$ZrO(OH)_2(s) + 2\ SO_3^{2-}(aq) \rightleftharpoons Zr(s) + 2\ SO_4^{2-}(aq) + H_2O(\ell)$

Combine common terms on each side of the net reaction.

Eliminate the redundant water molecules, as well as the electrons and excess hydroxide equivalents.

Check to make sure that the reaction is balanced, in terms of both *mass* (number of atoms on each side) and *overall charge*.

Remember: *This last step is* ***extremely important.*** *If mass and charge aren't balanced, then you made an error in one of the previous steps.*

ELECTROCHEMICAL CELLS

A galvanic cell is to be constructed using the $MnO_4^- \mid Mn^{2+}$ ($E°_{red}$ = 1.49 V) and $Zn^{2+} \mid Zn$ ($E°_{red}$ = –0.76 V) couples placed in an acidic solution. Assume that all potentials given are measured against the standard hydrogen electrode at 298 K and that all reagents are present in 1 M concentration (their standard states). What is the maximum possible work output of this cell per mole of reactant if it is used to run an electric motor for one hour at room temperature (298 K)? During this amount of time, how much Zn metal would be necessary to run the cell, given a current of 5 A?

KEY CONCEPTS

Oxidation/reduction

Electrochemical cells

Work

Stoichiometry

$E°_{cell} = E°_{cathode} - E°_{anode}$ (V)

$\Delta G° = -nFE°_{cell}$ (kJ/mol)

1) Determine which half-reaction is occurring at the anode and which is occurring at the cathode of the cell.

$MnO_4^-(aq) + 5\ e^- \rightarrow Mn^{2+}(aq)\ E°_{red} = 1.49$ V

$Zn^{2+}(aq) + 2\ e^- \rightarrow Zn(s)\ E°_{red} = -0.76$ V

Compare the standard reduction potentials for both reactions. The permanganate reduction potential is greater than the zinc potential, so it would prefer to be reduced and zinc-oxidized. Therefore, the zinc is being oxidized at the anode and the manganese is being reduced at the cathode.

Remember: ***O****xidation occurs at the* ***a****node. (Hint: they both start with a vowel.)*

TAKEAWAYS

Double-check your work when you balance the cell equation to make sure that you haven't made any arithmetic errors. One small addition or subtraction mistake can have drastic consequences!

---

2) Write a balanced reaction for the cell.

$MnO_4^- \rightarrow Mn^{2+}$

$8\ H^+ + MnO_4^- \rightarrow Mn^{2+} + 4\ H_2O$

$8\ H^+ + MnO_4^- + 5\ e^- \rightarrow Mn^{2+} + 4\ H_2O$

$Zn \rightarrow Zn^{2+} + 2\ e^-$

$16\ H^+ + 2\ MnO_4^- + 10\ e^- \rightarrow 2\ Mn^{2+} + 8\ H_2O$
$5\ Zn \rightarrow 5\ Zn^{2+} + 10\ e^-$

$16\ H^+(aq) + 2\ MnO_4^-(aq) + 5\ Zn(s) \rightarrow 2\ Mn^{2+}(aq) + 5\ Zn^{2+}(aq) + 8\ H_2O(\ell)$

Balance the reactions one at a time.

Balance oxygen with water, and then hydrogen with acid (H^+).

Balance overall charge with electrons.

This one is easy; all you have to do is balance electrons.

THINGS TO WATCH OUT FOR

Remember to balance the electron flow in order to figure out the maximum amount of work that the cell can perform.

SIMILAR QUESTIONS

1) How could you alter the cell setup to reverse the direction of current flow?
2) What would the cell potential be if Mn^{2+} and Zn^{2+} were at 2 M concentration and the MnO_4^- concentration remained at 1 M? Would changing the amount of zinc metal present in the cell change this potential? Why or why not?
3) Compute the minimum mass of potassium permanganate ($KMnO_4$) necessary to run the cell for the same amount of time as specified above.

To combine both equations, we need to multiply each by the appropriate integer to get to the lowest common multiple of 2 and 5, which is 10.

Now add the equations up to get the balanced cell equation, and you're golden.

---

3) Calculate the standard potential for the cell as a whole.

$E^\circ_{cell} = 1.49\text{ V} - (-0.76\text{ V}) = 2.25\text{ V}$

Use the equation $E^\circ_{cell} = E^\circ_{cathode} - E^\circ_{anode}$. Because the standard potential for the cell is positive, this confirms that this is a galvanic (or voltaic) cell—once you hook up the electrodes and immerse them in the designated solutions, current will start to flow on its own.

---

4) Compute ΔG° for the cell.

$\Delta G^\circ = -(10\text{ mol e}^-)(10^5\text{ C mol}^{-1})(2.25\text{ V}) = -2.25 \times 10^6\text{ J mol}^{-1}$

$\Rightarrow$ maximum work output per mole of reactant $= 2.25 \times 10^3\text{ KJ mol}^{-1}$

Use the equation $\Delta G^\circ = -nFE^\circ_{cell}$. The upper limit on the amount of work a reaction can perform is the same thing as ΔG°.

Remember: *Power is work over time, and 1 h = 3,600 s ≈ 4 × 10³ s.*

---

5) Use Faraday's constant to determine the number of moles of electrons transferred and to do any stoichiometric calculations.

$4 \times 10^3\text{ s }(5\text{ C s}^{-1})\ (10^{-5}\text{ mol e}^-\text{ C}^{-1}) = 0.2\text{ mol e}^-$

$$0.2\text{ mol e}^-\left(\frac{1\text{ mol Zn}}{2\text{ mol e}^-}\right) = 0.1\text{ mol Zn} \times (70\text{ g mol}^{-1}) = 7\text{ g Zn}$$

Remember that current is charge passing though a point per unit of time, and Faraday's constant tells us how many coulombs of charge make up one mole of electrons.

The balanced half-reaction is used to determine the necessary mole ratio.

THE NERNST EQUATION

A galvanic cell is created at 298 K using the following net reaction:

$$2\ H^+(aq) + Ca(s) \rightarrow Ca^{2+}(aq) + H_2(g)$$

Fluoride anions are added to the anode section of the cell only until precipitation is observed. Right at this point, the concentration of fluoride is 1.4×10^{-2} M, the pH is measured to be 0, the pressure of hydrogen gas is 1 atm, and the measured cell voltage is 2.96 V. Given this information, compute the K_{sp} of CaF_2 at 298 K.

Additional information:

$R = 8.314\ J\ (mol\ K)^{-1}$
$Ca^{2+}(aq) + 2\ e^- \rightarrow Ca(s) \quad E°_{red} = -2.76\ V$
$2\ H^+(aq) + 2\ e^- \rightarrow H_2(g) \quad E°_{red} = 0.00\ V$
$F = 96\ 485\ C\ mol^{-1}$

1) Write down the expression for the K_{sp}.

$CaF_2(s) \rightarrow Ca^{2+}(aq) + 2\ F^-(aq)$
$K_{eq} = [Ca^{2+}][F^-]^2 = K_{sp}$

The first part of this problem begins as with any other solubility problem: we need to right down the expression for the K_{sp}.

We're given the concentration of fluoride right when precipitation begins, so we can plug that right into the K_{sp} expression above. All we need is the concentration of Ca^{2+} ions, and we're golden.

---

2) Separate the net cell reaction into half reactions, and find $E°_{cell}$.

$Ca(s) \rightarrow Ca^{2+}(aq) + 2\ e^- \quad E° = 2.76\ V$
$2\ H^+(aq) + 2\ e^- \rightarrow H_{2\ (g)} \quad E° = 0\ V$
NET: $2\ H^+(aq) + Ca(s) \rightarrow Ca^{2+}(aq) + H_2(g)$
$E°_{cell} = 0.00\ V - (-2.76\ V) = 2.76\ V$

Now we know what the standard potential for the cell is. Our only problem is that, in the situation given in the problem, we are in *nonstandard conditions*, because the concentration of fluoride is not 1 M.

Remember: *Remember that* $E°_{cell} = E°_{cathode} - E°_{anode}$.

KEY CONCEPTS

Oxidation and reduction
Electrochemistry
Equilibrium
Solubility equilibria
Nernst equation
$E°_{cell} = E°_{cathode} - E°_{anode}$ (V)

TAKEAWAYS

Remember what the superscript "°" means: that a reaction is at standard conditions. This means that reagents are at 1 M or 1 atm, depending on their phase. If you are working with an electrochemical cell where the concentrations are nonstandard, you must apply the Nernst equation to determine what the effect on the cell voltage will be.

THINGS TO WATCH OUT FOR

Don't forget to check signs during problems that require computation. When logarithms and exponents are involved, one small sign error can have a massive impact on the answer!

SIMILAR QUESTIONS

1) If the K_{sp} of copper(I) bromide is 4.2×10^{-8}, compute the concentration of bromide necessary to cause precipitation in an electrochemical cell with the $Cu|Cu^+$ and $H^+|H_2$ couples. Assume the conditions are as follows: E°_{red} of $Cu^+ = 0.521$ V; pH = 0; $P_{H2\,(g)} = 1$ atm; $T = 298$ K; E_{cell} when precipitation begins = 0.82 V.
2) Compute the equilibrium constant at 298 K for the cell comprised of the Zn^{2+} | Zn ($E_{red}{}^\circ = -0.76$ V) and MnO_4^- | Mn^{2+} ($E_{red}{}^\circ = 1.49$ V) couples. Given this number, comment on the oxidizing ability of the permanganate anion.
3) A buffer solution is prepared that is 0.15 M in acetic acid and 0.05 M in sodium acetate. If oxidation is occuring at a platinum wire with 1 atm of H_2 bubbling over it that is submerged in the buffer solution, and the wire is connected to a standard Cu^{2+} | Cu half cell ($E_{red}{}^\circ = 0.34$ V), the measured cell voltage is 0.592 V. Based on this information, compute the pK_a of acetic acid.

3) Apply the Nernst equation.

$$E = E^\circ - \frac{RT}{nF} \ln Q$$

$$Q = \frac{[Ca^{2+}]Ph_{2(g)}}{[H^+]^2} = [Ca^{2+}]$$

$$E = E^\circ - \frac{RT}{nF} \ln [Ca^{2+}]$$

$$E - E^\circ = -\frac{RT}{nF} \ln [Ca^{2+}]$$

$$-\left(\frac{nF}{RT}\right)(E - E^\circ) = \ln [Ca^{2+}]$$

$$-\left(\frac{2\times 10^5}{8\times 300}\right)(2.96 - 2.76) = \ln [Ca^{2+}]$$

$$-\left(\frac{2\times 10^5}{8\times 300}\right)2\times 10^{-1} = \ln [Ca^{2+}]$$

$$-20 = \ln [Ca^{2+}]$$

$$-20 = 2.3 \log[Ca^{2+}]$$

$$-8 = \log[Ca^{2+}]$$

$$[Ca^{2+}] = 10^{-8}$$

The reaction quotient (Q) in this case is of the cell reaction. Recall that the pressure of hydrogen gas is 1 atmosphere. As the pH = 0, $[H^+] = 10^{-0} = 1.0$ M.

Rearrange the Nernst equation to solve for $\ln[Ca^{2+}]$.

Start plugging in numbers. Here, $n = 2$ mol e^-, from the cell equation; $F = 96{,}485 \approx 100{,}000$ C mol^{-1}; T = 298 ≈ 300 K; R ≈ 8 J (mol K)$^{-1}$; and 2.96 – 2.76 = 0.2 = 2×10^{-1} V.

Here, assume $-16.7 \approx -20$.

Recall that $\ln x = 2.3 \log x$. Assume that 2.3 ≈ 2.5 so that $-\frac{20}{2.5} \approx -8$.

Remember: *When you absolutely must do computation, choose numbers that are easy to work with.*

---

4) Plug the concentrations into the K_{sp} expression and solve.

$K_{sp} = [Ca^{2+}][F^-]^2$

$K_{sp} = (10^{-8})(10^{-2})^2 = 10^{-12}$

The "actual" value for the K_{sp} is 3.9×10^{-11}, so we are quite close.

Part II
Practice Sections

INSTRUCTIONS FOR TAKING THE PRACTICE SECTIONS

Before taking each Practice Section, find a quiet place where you can work uninterrupted. Take a maximum of 70 minutes per section (52 questions) to get accustomed to the length and scope.

Keep in mind that the actual MCAT will not feature a section made up of General Chemistry questions alone, but rather a Physical Sciences section made up of both General Chemistry and Physics questions. Use the following three sections to hone your General Chemistry skills.

Good luck!

PRACTICE SECTION 1

Time—70 minutes

QUESTIONS 1–52

Directions: Most of the questions in the following General Chemistry Practice Section are organized into groups, with a descriptive passage preceding each group of questions. Study the passage, then select the single-best answer to the question in each group. Some of the questions are not based on a descriptive passage; you must also select the best answer to these questions. If you are unsure of the best answer, eliminate the choices that you know are incorrect, then select an answer from the choices that remain.

Period	1 IA 1A	2 IIA 2A	3 IIIB 3B	4 IVB 4B	5 VB 5B	6 VIB 6B	7 VIIB 7B	8 -------	9 VIII -- 8	10 -----	11 IB 1B	12 IIB 2B	13 IIIA 3A	14 IVA 4A	15 VA 5A	16 VIA 6A	17 VIIA 7A	18 vIIIA 8A
1	1 H 1.008																	2 He 4.003
2	3 Li 6.941	4 Be 9.012											5 B 10.81	6 C 12.01	7 N 14.01	8 O 16.00	9 F 19.00	10 Ne 20.18
3	11 Na 22.99	12 Mg 24.31											13 Al 26.98	14 Si 28.09	15 P 30.97	16 S 32.07	17 Cl 35.45	18 Ar 39.95
4	19 K 39.10	20 Ca 40.08	21 Sc 44.96	22 Ti 47.88	23 V 50.94	24 Cr 52.00	25 Mn 54.94	26 Fe 55.85	27 Co 58.47	28 Ni 58.69	29 Cu 63.55	30 Zn 65.39	31 Ga 69.72	32 Ge 72.59	33 As 74.92	34 Se 78.96	35 Br 79.90	36 Kr 83.80
5	37 Rb 85.47	38 Sr 87.62	39 Y 88.91	40 Zr 91.22	41 Nb 92.91	42 Mo 95.94	43 Tc (98)	44 Ru 101.1	45 Rh 102.9	46 Pd 106.4	47 Ag 107.9	48 Cd 112.4	49 In 114.8	50 Sn 118.7	51 Sb 121.8	52 Te 127.6	53 I 126.9	54 Xe 131.3
6	55 Cs 132.9	56 Ba 137.3	57 La* 138.9	72 Hf 178.5	73 Ta 180.9	74 W 183.9	75 Re 186.2	76 Os 190.2	77 Ir 190.2	78 Pt 195.1	79 Au 197.0	80 Hg 200.5	81 Tl 204.4	82 Pb 207.2	83 Bi 209.0	84 Po (210)	85 At (210)	86 Rn (222)
7	87 Fr (223)	88 Ra (226)	89 Ac~ (227)	104 Rf (257)	105 Db (260)	106 Sg (263)	107 Bh (262)	108 Hs (265)	109 Mt (266)	110 --- ()	111 --- ()	112 --- ()		114 --- ()		116 --- ()		118 --- ()

Lanthanide Series*	58 Ce 140.1	59 Pr 140.9	60 Nd 144.2	61 Pm (147)	62 Sm 150.4	63 Eu 152.0	64 Gd 157.3	65 Tb 158.9	66 Dy 162.5	67 Ho 164.9	68 Er 167.3	69 Tm 168.9	70 Yb 173.0	71 Lu 175.0
Actinide Series~	90 Th 232.0	91 Pa (231)	92 U (238)	93 Np (237)	94 Pu (242)	95 Am (243)	96 Cm (247)	97 Bk (247)	98 Cf (249)	99 Es (254)	100 Fm (253)	101 Md (256)	102 No (254)	103 Lr (257)

PASSAGE I (QUESTIONS 1–9)

Acid rain is a meteorological phenomenon that is defined as any type of precipitation that is unusually acidic. Rain is naturally slightly acidic (pH = 5.2) due to the reaction of water with environmental CO_2 gas to produce carbonic acid. Experts agree that it is mainly a result of pollution, particularly sulfur and nitrogen compounds that react in the atmosphere to produce acids. These reactions are shown below:

$$SO_2 + OH\cdot \rightarrow HOSO_2\cdot$$
$$HOSO_2\cdot + O_2 \rightarrow HO_2\cdot + SO_3$$
$$SO_3 + H_2O \rightarrow H_2SO_4$$
$$NO_2 + OH\cdot \rightarrow HNO_3$$

A college chemistry student was studying outside one day, sipping on a glass of purified water with a pH of 7, when a sudden rainstorm occurred. Wanting to protect his books, he ran inside with them, leaving the glass out on the ledge of his deck. While studying inside, he reviewed the section on acids and bases and decided to run some tests on the glass of water outside, which had collected approximately 100 mL of rainwater mixed with 300 mL of purified water.

1. The acidity of rain is based on the acidity of the contaminating pollutants. Would H_2SO_4 or HNO_3 produce a more acidic rain?

   A. H_2SO_4, because it has a lower pK_a.
   B. HNO_3, because it has a lower pK_a.
   C. H_2SO_4, because it has a greater pK_a.
   D. HNO_3, because it has a greater pK_a.

2. What is the approximate concentration of H^+ in normal rain due to the reaction between $CO_{2(g)}$ and $H_2O_{(l)}$?

   A. 8×10^{-3} M
   B. 6×10^{-5} M
   C. 7×10^{-6} M
   D. 2×10^{-7} M

3. Under which of the following classifications of "acid" does H_2SO_4 fall?

   I. Arrhenius
   II. Brønsted-Lowry
   III. Lewis

   A. I only
   B. II only
   C. II and III only
   D. I, II, and III

4. Suppose a few drops of acid rain fell on an open cut in the student's hand. Would the bicarbonate (HCO_3^-) that exists in blood have any effect?

   A. Yes, bicarbonate will buffer by accepting a H^+ ion.
   B. Yes, bicarbonate will buffer by donating a H^+ ion.
   C. No, bicarbonate does not act as a buffer.
   D. There is not enough information in the passage to determine the correct answer.

5. If the rainwater that mixed with the pure water had original concentrations of $[H_2SO_4] = 2 \times 10^{-3}$ M, $[HNO_3] = 3.2 \times 10^{-3}$ M, what is the approximate final pH of the glass of water?

   A. 1.2
   B. 2.8
   C. 3.4
   D. 4.6

6. Which of the following is an incorrect pair of an acid and its conjugate base?

   A. $H_2SO_4 : HSO_4^-$
   B. $CH_3COOH : CH_3COO^-$
   C. $H_3O^+ : H_2O$
   D. $H_2CO_3 : CO_2$

7. With which of the following statements would the student most likely NOT agree?

A. Acid rain has increased in frequency and intensity over the past 150 years.
B. Radicals play an integral role in the development of acid rain.
C. Acid rain lessens the conductive capabilities of water.
D. Acid rain is dangerous to the environment even though rain is naturally acidic.

QUESTIONS 8–9 ARE BASED ON THE FOLLOWING TITRATION CURVE SHOWN BELOW:

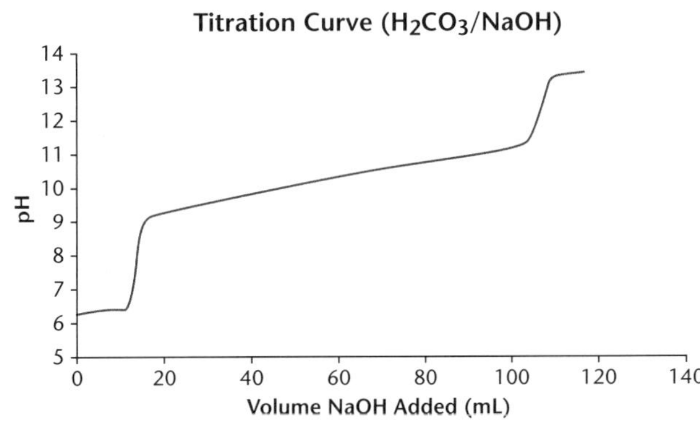

8. What is the approximate ratio of $pK_{a1} : pK_{a2}$ for H_2CO_3?

A. 9.0 : 13.0
B. 7.8 : 12.0
C. 6.3 : 10.3
D. 6.0 : 11.1

9. What is the approximate ratio of equivalence points for H_2CO_3?

A. 9.0 : 13.0
B. 7.8 : 12.0
C. 6.3 : 10.3
D. 6.0 : 11.1

PASSAGE II (QUESTIONS 10–17)

The specific heat of a substance, *c*, measures the amount of heat required to raise the temperature of the mass of substance by a specific number of degrees. In certain cases, the chemical literature reports specific heat in terms of moles. Specific heat differs from heat capacity, a measurement of the amount of heat required to change the temperature of an object by a specific number of degrees.

In SI units, specific heat indicates the number of joules of heat needed to raise the temperature of 1 gram of the substance by 1 degree Kelvin. The specific heat of water reported in the chemical literature is 4.184 $Jg^{-1}K^{-1}$. Specific heat can be measured by a calorimeter, a device that insulates a sample from atmospheric conditions in order to measure the change in the sample material's temperature over a set interval.

A student used a coffee cup calorimeter to compare the specific heat of water to the specific heat of a commercial fruit punch. The punch is made from a mixture of sugar water and powder flavoring. The student's coffee cup calorimeter used a stack of two foam coffee cups and a thermometer, which the student stuck through a hole in a plastic lid covering the top cup in the stack. Such calorimeters are inexpensive and accurate experimental substitutes for industrial bomb calorimeters, which hold samples at constant volume to measure water temperature changes under high-pressure conditions.

To calibrate the calorimeter, the student combined known quantities of hot and cold water in the coffee cup until the thermometer read a steady temperature, as described in Table 1.

	Hot Water	Cold Water
Volume	100 mL	100 mL
Start Temp	90°C	20°C
End Temp	54°C	54°C

Table 2 summarizes the specific heat data the student collected for the water and the fruit punch using the calibrated coffee cup setup.

Trial	1	2	3
Water (mL)	200 mL	200 mL	200 mL
Punch (g)	0 g	0 g	4 g
Sugar (g)	0 g	16 g	16 g
Start Temp	20.5°C	20.5°C	21°C
End Temp	89°C	91.5°C	91°C

10. Which of the following values reports the molar specific heat of water from the chemical literature?

A. 4.184 $Jmol^{-1}K^{-1}$
B. 75.31 $Jmol^{-1}K^{-1}$
C. 4184 $Jmol^{-1}K^{-1}$
D. 75310 $Jmol^{-1}K^{-1}$

11. What measurement is also an intrinsic property of fruit punch?

A. Mass
B. Heat
C. Enthalpy
D. Viscosity

12. What is the heat capacity of the student's coffee cup calorimeter?

A. 4.184 J/°C
B. 24.6 J/°C
C. 861 J/°C
D. 0.0246 J/°C

13. Suppose the student breaks his glass alcohol thermometer in the lab. The lab instructor's only available replacement is a mercury thermometer. How would this change to the experimental set-up affect the student's measurements?

A. The calorimeter would measure a higher specific heat.
B. The calorimeter would measure a lower specific heat.
C. The thermometer would give a less-precise specific heat measurement.
D. There would be no change to the specific heat measurement.

14. Which of the following rationales best explains why the student calibrated the coffee cup calorimeter before the experiment?

A. The coffee cup calorimeter can absorb heat.
B. The coffee cup calorimeter does not dry between uses.
C. The coffee cup calorimeter's thermometer does not produce precise values.
D. The coffee cup calorimeter contents do not always reach equilibrium.

15. Suppose the student decided to compare his sugar water measurements to those from a salt water sample, in which 16 g NaCl replace the 16 g table sugar in Trial 2. How would the specific heat of this salt water differ from that of sugar water?

A. The calorimeter would measure a lower specific heat.
B. The calorimeter would measure a higher specific heat.
C. The calorimeter would measure the same specific heat.
D. The calorimeter would decompose.

16. Which of the following experimental quantities must remain constant in Trial 1 in order for the student to obtain a specific heat for water close to the literature value?

I. Pressure
II. Mass
III. Heat

A. I only
B. I and III only
C. II and III only
D. I, II, and III

17. For which of the following laboratory measurements would a bomb calorimeter be more useful than a coffee cup calorimeter?

A. To measure the specific heat of salt water
B. To measure the specific heat of ethanol
C. To measure the specific heat of water vapor
D. To measure the specific heat of copper

QUESTIONS 18–21 ARE NOT BASED ON A DESCRIPTIVE PASSAGE.

18. Given the balanced equation, $Mg(s) + 2HCl(aq) \rightarrow MgCl_2(aq) + H_2(g)$, how many liters of hydrogen gas is produced at STP if 3 moles HCl are reacted with excess magnesium?

A. 1.2 L
B. 33.6 L
C. 2.4 L
D. 44.8 L

19. Increasing the temperature of a system at equilibrium favors the

A. exothermic reaction, decreasing its rate.
B. exothermic reaction, increasing its rate.
C. endothermic reaction, increasing its rate.
D. endothermic reaction, decreasing its rate.

20. Which type of radiation has neither mass nor charge?

A. Alpha
B. Beta
C. Gamma
D. Delta

21. Iron rusts more easily than aluminum or zinc because the latter two

A. form self-protective oxides.
B. form extremely reactive oxides.
C. are better reducing agents.
D. are good oxidizing agents.

PASSAGE III (QUESTIONS 22–29)

Product BD can be prepared by the following reaction mechanism, which is known to exhibit first-order kinetics with respect to each of the reactants:

1. AB(g) + C(g) $\leftrightharpoons$ A(g) + BC(aq)(fast)
2. BC(aq) + D(aq) + heat $\leftrightharpoons$ BCD(aq) (slow)
3. BCD(aq) + heat $\leftrightharpoons$ C(aq) + BD(aq) + heat(fast)

To determine the effect of heat on the overall reaction, a scientist mixed one equivalent each of compounds AB, C, and D with excess water in identical reaction flasks at five different temperatures. The scientist then recorded the rate of formation of the product at each temperature, as well as the final concentration of that product when the reaction reached equilibrium, shown in Table 1:

Temperature	Rate of Formation of BD	[BD] at Equilibrium
40°C	6.5 mmol/hr	37 mM
80°C	18.1 mmol/hr	965 mM
100°C	24.9 mmol/hr	1.16 M
120°C	31.2 mmol/hr	1.19 M
150°C	37.5 mmol/hr	1.21 M

The scientist ran a second experiment in which she omitted the equivalent of Compound C from the reaction mixture. The results of this second experiment are shown in Table 2:

Temperature	Rate of Formation of BD	[BD] at Equilibrium
40°C	0.02 mmol/hr	37 mM
80°C	0.13 mmol/hr	965 mM
100°C	0.47 mmol/hr	1.16 M
120°C	1.23 mmol/hr	1.19 M
150°C	29.3 mmol/hr	1.21 M

22. Compound C's most likely role in this reaction is to

A. donate an electron to Compound B.
B. accept an electron from Compound B.
C. decrease the amount of energy required for Compound D to bind with Compound B.
D. decrease the amount of energy required for Compound A to dissociate from Compound B.

23. Which of the following compounds could the scientist add to the initial reaction mixture to increase the yield of product BD?

A. Compound A
B. Compound B
C. Compound C
D. Compound D

24. Which of the following graphs best demonstrates the effect of temperature on the equilibrium constant of the reaction in the passage?

A. 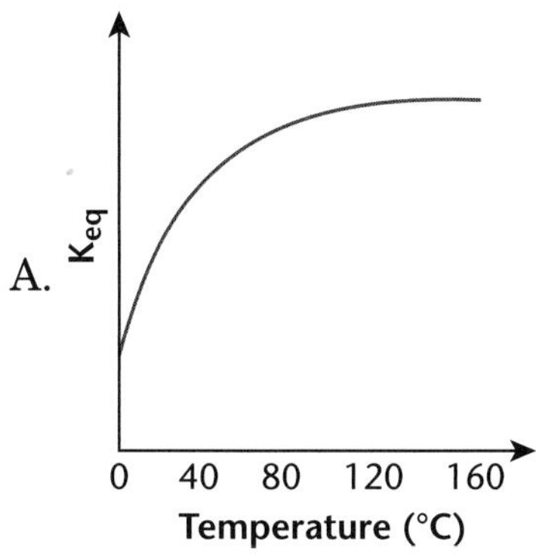

B. 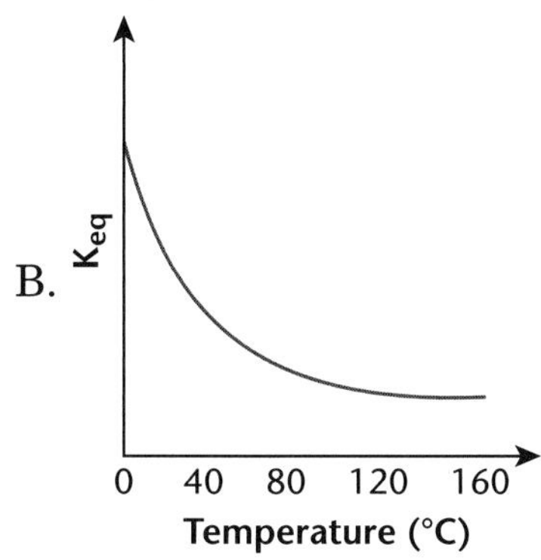

C. 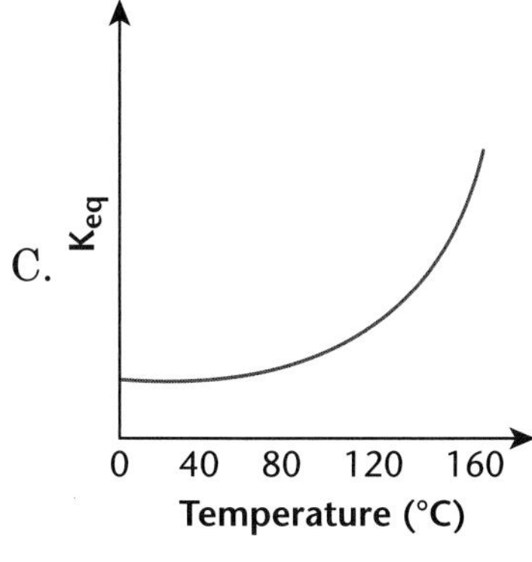

D. 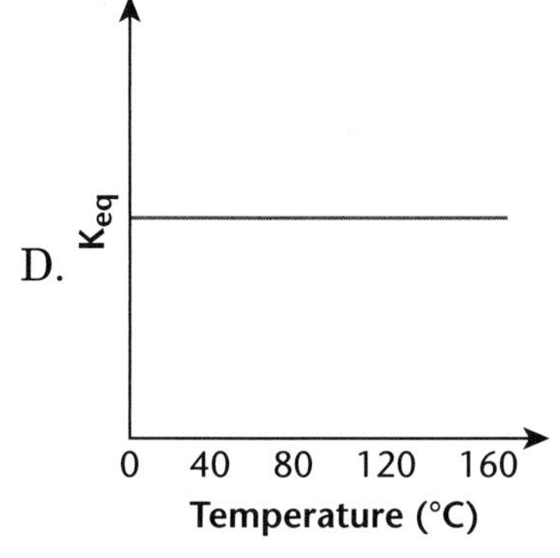

25. The scientist runs a third experiment in which she adds two equivalents of aqueous compound A to one equivalent each of compound BC and compound D at 80°C. What is the expected rate of formation of product BD under these conditions?

A. 9.1 mmol/hr
B. 18.1 mmol/hr
C. 36.2 mmol/hr
D. 54.3 mmol/hr

26. If no catalyst is present, what is the approximate minimum temperature range in which the reaction in the passage would immediately reach its activation energy?

A. 40–80°C
B. 80–100°C
C. 100–120°C
D. 120–150°C

27. What reaction type best describes step 1 of the reaction mechanism in the passage?

A. Double replacement
B. Single replacement
C. Combination
D. Decomposition

28. What step of the reaction mechanism from the passage would be affected most by a change in pressure?

A. Step 1
B. Step 2
C. Step 3
D. All steps to a roughly equal extent

29. Which of the following statements must be true for the overall reaction in the passage?

I. $\Delta H > 0$
II. $\Delta G > 0$
III. $\Delta S < 0$

A. I only
B. III only
C. I and II only
D. I, II, and III

PASSAGE IV (QUESTIONS 30–36)

A few years before Dmitri Mendeleev published the first rendition of the modern periodic table, the English chemist John Newlands suggested the concept of periodicity when he arranged all of the then-known elements by increasing atomic weights and found that every eighth element exhibited similar properties. He dubbed his principle the "Law of Octaves" and created a chart in which the elements would be organized into groups of seven. In this chart (below), the eighth element would appear immediately to the right of the previous element that shares its properties:

H	F	Cl	Co/Ni	Br	Pd	I	Pt/Ir
Li	Na	K	Cu	Rb	Ag	Cs	Tl
G	Mg	Ca	Zn	Sr	Cd	Ba/V	Pb
B	Al	Cr	Y	Ce/Le	U	Ta	Th
C	Si	Ti	In	Zn	Sn	W	Hg
N	P	Mn	As	Di/Mo	Sb	Nb	Bi
O	S	Fe	Se	Ro/Ru	Te	Au	Os

Newlands's discovery was initially dismissed as a coincidence. Soon afterward, Mendeleev created a more elaborate table that was eventually refined into the version that is common today. This table also arranged the elements by molecular weight, but refuted the idea of octaves. It was capable of accommodating the s-block (groups 1A and 2A), the p-block (groups 3A to 8A), the d-block (transition metals), and the f-block (lanthanoids and actinoids). In anticipation of the discovery of more elements, Mendeleev left several empty spaces in the table; for instance, he predicted the discovery of two elements with mass between 65 and 75 amu and a third element with mass between 40 and 50 amu.

30. Several of the atomic mass calculations were inaccurate during the time that periodicity was first discovered. Which of the following pairs of elements were arranged incorrectly by mass on Newlands's table?

A. Gold and platinum
B. Manganese and iron
C. Yttrium and indium
D. Tantalum and tungsten

31. Which of the following most strongly discredits the accuracy of the law of octaves?

A. The discovery of all of the naturally occurring elements in the s-block and the p-block.
B. The discovery of most of the naturally occurring elements in the d-block and the f-block.
C. J. J. Thomson's discovery of the electron.
D. Ernest Rutherford's discovery of the nucleus.

32. Mendeleev's table was modified several times after its initial publication. Which of the following findings did NOT require modification of the existing entries in the table?

I. A unique element is characterized by a specific number of protons.
II. Electrons are arranged in orbitals and energy levels.
III. The atomic mass of Gallium is approximately 70 amu.

A. II only
B. III only
C. II and III only
D. I, II, and III

33. Assuming that all known elements at the time were accounted for in Newland's table of elements, which of the following had not been discovered when Newlands published his table?

A. f-block elements
B. Halogens
C. Metalloids
D. Noble gases

34. Mendeleev predicted the existence of an element with atomic mass of 44. If his prediction were correct, which of the following properties would it exhibit?

A. Its atomic radius would be larger than calcium's atomic radius.
B. Its ionic radius would be larger than calcium's atomic radius.
C. It would lose an electron less readily than calcium would.
D. It would accept an electron less readily than calcium would.

35. What element on Newlands's table had the largest atomic radius?

A. Uranium
B. Cesium
C. Bismuth
D. Osmium

36. Which of the following, if true, would most strengthen the claim that Newlands should be credited as the inventor of the modern periodic table?

A. Although most scientists dismissed Newlands's theory, it was widely accepted within his home country of England.
B. Mendeleev approved of Newlands's work upon reading about it a few years after he formulated his own periodic table.
C. Mendeleev created his version of the periodic table in an attempt to refute Newlands's theory.
D. Newlands created a refined version of his system that was similar to Mendeleev's table, but failed to publish it before Mendeleev.

PASSAGE V (QUESTIONS 37–44)

A student inserts a sliding divider into a simple cylinder to perform a series of three experiments with an unknown gas. The gas exhibits ideal behavior. Before each experiment, the divider is reset so that $V_1 = V_2$ and the contents are at STP. The total volume of the cylinder is 2 L. The student's cylinder apparatus is illustrated below:

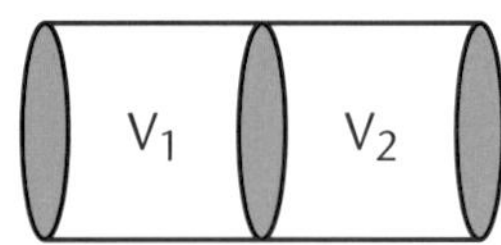

Experiment 1

The student increases the temperature of the gas in V_1 to 45°C while keeping the temperature of V_2 constant.

Experiment 2

The student uses mechanical force to move the central divider in the cylinder such that $3V_1 = V_2$. The temperature of the gas and the cylinder remains constant throughout this experiment.

Experiment 3

The student releases half of the molar contents of V_2, and does not change the molar contents of V_1.

While these experiments are being performed in near-ideal conditions (can be assumed to be ideal), an equation was derived in 1873 by Johannes van der Waals to account for the nonideal behavior of gases:

$$\left(p+\frac{a}{V^2}\right)(V-b)=kT$$

37. In Experiment 1, what is the final volume of 1 mol of gas in V_1?

A. 164*R* L
B. 318*R* L
C. 358*R* L
D. 403*R* L

38. Which of the following graphs most accurately illustrates the relationship between volume (V) and temperature (T) in experiment 1, assuming isobaric conditions?

A.

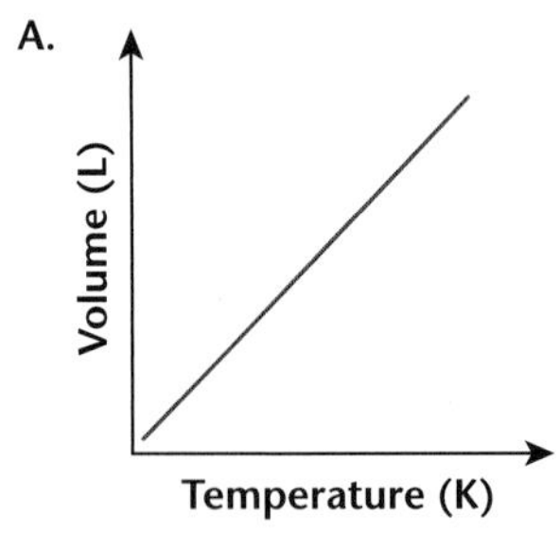

B.

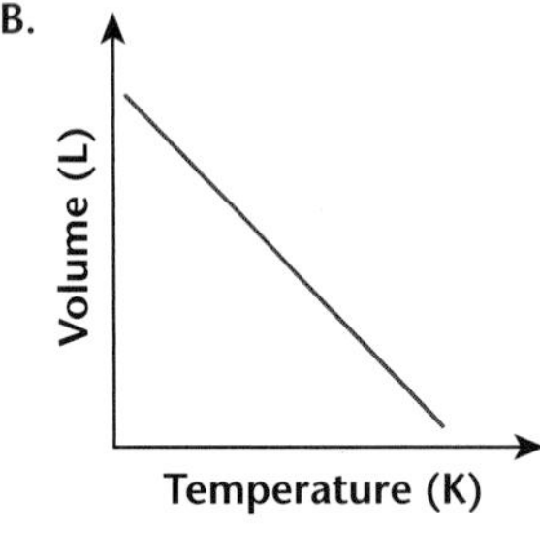

C.

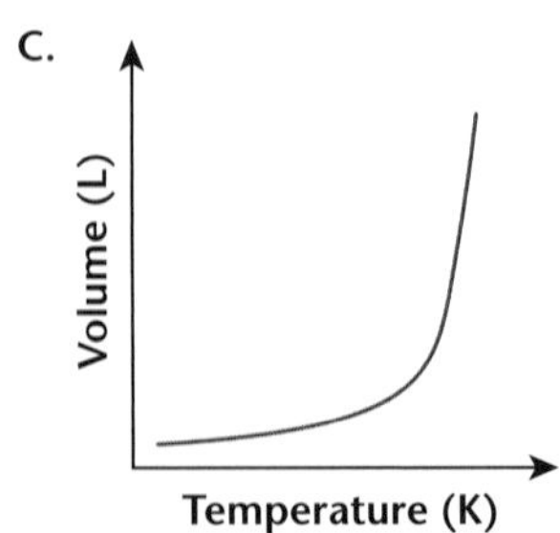

D.

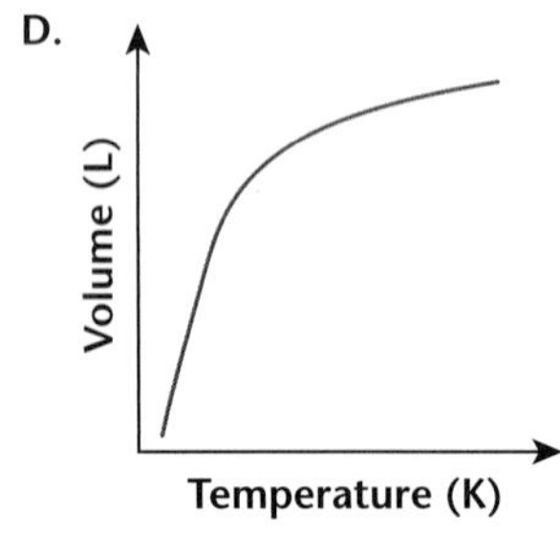

39. In experiment 2, what is the final pressure of the gas with volume V_1?

A. 0.5 atm
B. 1.5 atm
C. 2 atm
D. 3 atm

40. In the van der Waals equation for nonideal gas behavior, "a" corrects for

A. intermolecular repulsive forces.
B. the volume of the molecules themselves.
C. minute changes in atmospheric pressures.
D. intermolecular attractive forces.

41. What is the temperature of 64 g of pure O_2 gas in a 3 atm, 2L environment?

A. 1.5/*R* K
B. 2/*R* K
C. 3/*R* K
D. 6/*R* K

42. The student removes the partition, creating a cylinder with V = 2L. If there are 0.5 mol CO_2(g), 1.5 mol NO(g), and 1 mol Cl_2(g), in the cylinder, what is the partial pressure of the NO(g) at 300 K?

A. 115*R* atm
B. 225*R* atm
C. 375*R* atm
D. 450*R* atm

43. Under which of the following conditions do the contents of V_1 behave most like an ideal gas?

A. High temperature, low pressure
B. Low volume, high pressure
C. Low temperature, high volume
D. Low temperature, high pressure

44. Which of the following is the most likely result of experiment 3 after re-equilibration with the new molar concentrations?

A. V_1 will expand and V_2 will shrink.
B. P_2 will be greater than P_1.
C. Neither V nor P will change because they are unrelated to molar concentration.
D. P_1 will be greater than P_2.

PASSAGE VI (QUESTIONS 45–52)

Patients often use antacids to counteract potential adverse effects caused by an excess of stomach acid. Most antacids are weak bases whose primary function is to neutralize the hydrochloric acid in the stomach. Because of their simplicity, a wide variety of such drugs is available on the market; however, some are more effective than others. The drug typically reacts with the antacid to produce a conjugate acid and a conjugate base, as in the following examples:

Reaction 1

$Mg(OH)_2(s) + HCl(aq) \rightarrow MgCl_2(aq) + H_2O(l)$

Reaction 2

$Al_2(CO_3)_3(s) + 6HCl(aq) \rightarrow 2AlCl_3(aq) + 3H_2CO_3(aq)$

A student attempted to test the efficacy of various antacids by adding 1 gram of each drug to a beaker containing 100 mL of 0.1 M HCl. He noticed that stronger antacids tend to leave larger precipitates, so he determined that the strength of an antacid could be estimated by measuring the mass of the precipitate after complete neutralization and comparing it with the molecular weight of the reactant. His results were fairly accurate for magnesium salts, aluminum salts, and calcium salts (Group A); however, they disagreed with published results for sodium salts and potassium salts (Group B).

After inspecting the student's experimental setup, the professor pointed out a flaw in the student's reasoning. The student then decided to redesign his experiment; in the second setup, he chemically combined various quantities of antacid along with a standard amount of HCl and measured the pH of the resulting solutions. This time, he determined that an HCl sample was completely neutralized when its pH was equal to 7. The "overall efficacy" of each antacid was quantified as the number of moles of HCl that can be neutralized by one gram of antacid.

45. Which of the following does NOT describe reaction 1?

A. Double-displacement reaction
B. Neutralization reaction
C. Oxidation-reduction reaction
D. Acid-base reaction

46. What is the approximate percent composition of the cation in the conjugate base of the acid from reaction 1?

A. 10%
B. 25%
C. 75%
D. 90%

47. If the student tested each of the following antacids, which would yield the greatest overall efficacy?

A. $Al_2(CO_3)_3$
B. $Al(OH)_3$
C. $Al(HCO_3)_3$
D. $AlPO_4$

48. Which of the following is true about $NaHCO_3$ in the following reaction?

$NaHCO_3(s) + HCl(aq) \rightarrow NaCl(aq) + H_2CO_3(aq)$

A. Because one of the products of the reaction is an acid, $NaHCO_3$ does not function as an antacid.
B. Because one of the products of the reaction is a weaker acid than HCl, $NaHCO_3$ is capable of raising the pH of the stomach but cannot neutralize the acid completely.
C. Because H_2CO_3 decomposes into $H_2O(l)$ and $CO_2(g)$, $NaHCO_3$ is an effective antacid.
D. Because H_2CO_3 decomposes into $H_2O(l)$ and $CO_2(g)$, $NaHCO_3$ is capable of raising the pH of the stomach but cannot neutralize the acid completely.

49. Antacid AX reacts with HCl to yield a mixture with a pH of 5.4 according to the equation below. What is the limiting reagent?

$AX(s) + HCl(aq) \rightarrow ACl(aq) + HX(aq)$

A. HCl
B. Antacid
C. Conjugate base of HCl
D. Conjugate acid of antacid

50. When the student tested magnesium hydroxide with his first experimental setup, approximately how much antacid remained at the end of the reaction?

A. 750 mg
B. 500 mg
C. 200 mg
D. 300 mg

51. The student noticed that stronger antacids often leave larger precipitates when they are present as an excess reagent because a stronger antacid

A. neutralizes more acid, which subsequently produces a larger precipitate.
B. produces more product, which subsequently appears in the precipitate.
C. requires more of the reactant, higher quantities of unreacted material are usually present in the precipitate.
D. requires less of the reactant, so higher quantities of unreacted material are usually present in the precipitate.

52. Which of the following best explains why the student's initial results were correct for group A but incorrect for group B?

A. Group A contains very strong bases, while group B contains slightly weaker bases.
B. Group A contains compounds that dissociate into multiple ions, while group B contains compounds that dissociate into only two ions.
C. Group A contains compounds with insignificant solubility, while group B contains compounds with considerable solubility.
D. Group A contains cations with a +1 oxidation state, while group B contains cations with a +2 or +3 oxidation state.

PRACTICE SECTION 2

Time—70 minutes

QUESTIONS 1–52

Directions: Most of the questions in the following General Chemistry Practice Section are organized into groups, with a descriptive passage preceding each group of questions. Study the passage, then select the single-best answer to the question in each group. Some of the questions are not based on a descriptive passage; you must also select the best answer to these questions. In you are unsure of the best answer, eliminate the choices that you know are incorrect, then select an answer from the choices that remain.

Period	1 IA 1A	2 IIA 2A	3 IIIB 3B	4 IVB 4B	5 VB 5B	6 VIB 6B	7 VIIB 7B	8 -------	9 VIII -- ------- 8 -------	10 -----	11 IB 1B	12 IIB 2B	13 IIIA 3A	14 IVA 4A	15 VA 5A	16 VIA 6A	17 VIIA 7A	18 vIIIA 8A
1	1 H 1.008																	2 He 4.003
2	3 Li 6.941	4 Be 9.012											5 B 10.81	6 C 12.01	7 N 14.01	8 O 16.00	9 F 19.00	10 Ne 20.18
3	11 Na 22.99	12 Mg 24.31											13 Al 26.98	14 Si 28.09	15 P 30.97	16 S 32.07	17 Cl 35.45	18 Ar 39.95
4	19 K 39.10	20 Ca 40.08	21 Sc 44.96	22 Ti 47.88	23 V 50.94	24 Cr 52.00	25 Mn 54.94	26 Fe 55.85	27 Co 58.47	28 Ni 58.69	29 Cu 63.55	30 Zn 65.39	31 Ga 69.72	32 Ge 72.59	33 As 74.92	34 Se 78.96	35 Br 79.90	36 Kr 83.80
5	37 Rb 85.47	38 Sr 87.62	39 Y 88.91	40 Zr 91.22	41 Nb 92.91	42 Mo 95.94	43 Tc (98)	44 Ru 101.1	45 Rh 102.9	46 Pd 106.4	47 Ag 107.9	48 Cd 112.4	49 In 114.8	50 Sn 118.7	51 Sb 121.8	52 Te 127.6	53 I 126.9	54 Xe 131.3
6	55 Cs 132.9	56 Ba 137.3	57 La* 138.9	72 Hf 178.5	73 Ta 180.9	74 W 183.9	75 Re 186.2	76 Os 190.2	77 Ir 190.2	78 Pt 195.1	79 Au 197.0	80 Hg 200.5	81 Tl 204.4	82 Pb 207.2	83 Bi 209.0	84 Po (210)	85 At (210)	86 Rn (222)
7	87 Fr (223)	88 Ra (226)	89 Ac~ (227)	104 Rf (257)	105 Db (260)	106 Sg (263)	107 Bh (262)	108 Hs (265)	109 Mt (266)	110 --- ()	111 --- ()	112 --- ()		114 --- ()		116 --- ()		118 --- ()

Lanthanide Series*	58 Ce 140.1	59 Pr 140.9	60 Nd 144.2	61 Pm (147)	62 Sm 150.4	63 Eu 152.0	64 Gd 157.3	65 Tb 158.9	66 Dy 162.5	67 Ho 164.9	68 Er 167.3	69 Tm 168.9	70 Yb 173.0	71 Lu 175.0
Actinide Series~	90 Th 232.0	91 Pa (231)	92 U (238)	93 Np (237)	94 Pu (242)	95 Am (243)	96 Cm (247)	97 Bk (247)	98 Cf (249)	99 Es (254)	100 Fm (253)	101 Md (256)	102 No (254)	103 Lr (257)

PASSAGE I (QUESTIONS 1–9)

Swimming pools are filled with water containing a number of dissolved ions for the purpose of purification and maintenance of pH. One chemical that is added to pools, chlorine, is used to kill bacteria and harmful contaminants and can be added to pools in a number of ways. Calcium hypochlorite, $Ca(OCl)_2$, is an inorganic chlorinating agent that contributes chlorine and calcium ions to the water.

Other chemicals and materials in swimming pools can also contribute calcium ions to the water. The concentration of calcium and other ions must be closely monitored so that the water does not become saturated with a particular compound. The solubility product constant, termed K_{sp}, describes the amount of salt in moles that can be dissolved in one liter of solution to reach saturation. No more salt can dissolve after reaching the point of saturation.

Plaster that lines swimming pools is a form of hydrated calcium sulfate, $CaSO_4$. The calcium from chlorinating agents along with the calcium from plaster that lines swimming pools makes it necessary to monitor the concentrations of Ca^{2+} and SO_4^{2-} to make sure that saturation is not reached. The following equation describes the dissociation of calcium sulfate in water:

$$CaSO_4 \longleftrightarrow Ca^{2+} + SO_4^{2-}$$

The K_{sp} value for the discussed dissociation reaction can be calculated by determining the values of $[Ca^{2+}]$ and $[SO_4^{2-}]$ in a saturated solution. If the K_{sp} value is known, the ion concentrations in swimming pools can be used with the K_{sp} value to predict whether or not the levels are at or near saturation.

1. If the K_{sp} of $CaSO_4$ is calculated to be 4.93×10^{-5} at 25°C, what is the minimum amount of $CaSO_4$ that can be added to 3.75×10^5 L of water to create a saturated solution?

A. 2.63×10^3 grams
B. 3.58×10^5 grams
C. 7.16×10^5 grams
D. 2.52×10^3 grams

2. Which of the following compounds, when dissolved in water, has the highest concentration of calcium for one mole of the compound?

A. $CaCO_3$ ($K_{sp} = 4.8 \times 10^{-9}$)
B. CaF_2 ($K_{sp} = 3.9 \times 10^{-11}$)
C. $Ca_3(PO_4)_2$ ($K_{sp} = 1 \times 10^{-25}$)
D. $Ca(IO_3)_2$ ($K_{sp} = 6.47 \times 10^{-6}$)

3. The K_{sp} of $CaSO_4$ can be calculated by determining the concentration of a saturated solution of $CaSO_4$. The following graph shows the relationship between concentration and conductivity for $CaSO_4$, which was determined by finding the conductance for four $CaSO_4$ solutions of known concentration. Using the graph, estimate the concentration of a saturated solution that has a conductivity of 2.5×10^3 μS/cm and then calculate the experimental K_{sp} for a saturated solution of $CaSO_4$:

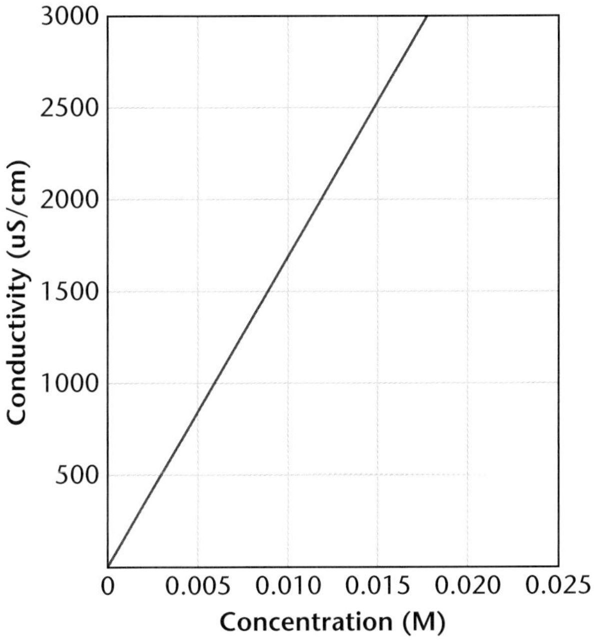

A. 2.25×10^{-4} M^2
B. 1.5×10^{-2} M^2
C. 3×10^{-2} M^2
D. 1.22×10^{-1} M^2

4. In the experiment, a probe was used to measure the conductivities in each solution. The probe generates a potential difference between two electrodes and reads the current that is produced as a voltage. The computer then outputs the conductivity. If several different solutions were all heated from room temperature to 75° Celsius, how would the conductivity of the solutions change and would the K_{sp} be affected?

A. The conductivity would increase and the K_{sp} would increase.
B. The conductivity would decrease and the change in K_{sp} cannot be determined.
C. The conductivity would increase and the change in K_{sp} cannot be determined.
D. The conductivity would decrease and the change in K_{sp} cannot be determined.

5. Instead of using calcium hypochlorite to introduce chlorine into the water, the owner of a water park, Jim, decides to bubble Cl_2 gas into the pool. Will Jim's decision affect the solubility of the plaster that is lining the pools at his water park?

A. Yes, the chlorine gas will increase the solubility of $CaSO_4$ in the plaster as compared with $Ca(OCl)_2$ because it will react with molecules of SO_4^{2-} and shift the equilibrium to the right.
B. Yes, the chlorine gas will increase the solubility of $CaSO_4$ in the plaster as compared with $Ca(OCl)_2$ because Cl_2 will not cause the same common ion effect that occurred with $Ca(OCl)_2$.
C. Yes, the chlorine gas will decrease the solubility of $CaSO_4$ in the plaster as compared with $Ca(OCl)_2$ because the absence of Ca^{2+} from the $Ca(OCl)_2$ will eliminate the common ion effect.
D. No, the chlorine gas will not change the solubility of $CaSO_4$ in the plaster as compared with $Ca(OCl)_2$.

6. $Ca(OCl)_2$ contributes OCl^- to the water, which acts to kill bacteria by destroying enzymes and contents of the cells through oxidation. In its ionic form, OCl^- exists in the following equilibrium:

$$HOCl \longleftrightarrow H^+ + OCl^-$$

In order for cleaning to occur properly, the pH must be at the right level to allow enough of the oxidizing agent, HOCl, to be present. If the pH is raised by the addition of sodium carbonate to the water, what will happen to the oxidizing power of the HOCl?

A. The higher pH will break the HOCl compound into single atoms and will eliminate its oxidizing power.
B. The pH cannot be raised due to the buffering system in the pool, and thus the oxidizing power of the chlorine will remain the same.
C. Fewer H^+ ions will be present and the reaction will shift right. This will decrease the number of HOCl molecules and thus decrease the oxidizing power of chlorine.
D. A high pH will lower the concentration of H^+ by associating H^+ with OCl^-. This will increase the number of HOCl molecules and increase the oxidizing power of chlorine.

7. Due to changes in climate and poor management of ion content in the water, the swimming pool has now become supersaturated with calcium sulfate. What combination of events could have caused this to occur?

A. Cooling of the pool followed by addition of calcium sulfate
B. Warming of the pool followed by addition of calcium sulfate
C. Addition of calcium sulfate followed by cooling of the pool and then subsequent warming of the pool
D. Warming of the pool followed by addition of calcium sulfate and then cooling of the pool

8. Water "hardness" refers to the content of calcium and magnesium in water. When referring to swimming pools, water hardness mainly refers to calcium. One way to measure the balance of ions is to use the Langelier saturation index. The Langelier saturation index is derived from a combination of the following two equilibrium equations. Which of the following accurately expresses the combination of the two equilibrium equations in terms of $[H^+]$?

$$HCO_3^- \longleftrightarrow H^+ + CO_3^{2-} \quad pK_{a2} = 10.33$$

$$CaCO_3 \longleftrightarrow Ca^{2+} + CO_3^{2-} \quad pK_{sp} = 8.35$$

A. $[H^+] = \left(\frac{K_{sp}}{K_{a2}}\right) \times [Ca^{2+}][HCO_3^-]$

B. $[H^+] = \left(\frac{K_{a2}}{K_{sp}}\right) \times [Ca^{2+}][HCO_3^-]$

C. $[H^+] = \left(\frac{K_{sp}}{K_{a2}}\right) \times \left(\frac{[Ca^{2+}]}{[HCO_3^-]}\right)$

D. $[H^+] = \left(\frac{K_{sp}}{K_{a2}}\right) \times \left(\frac{[HCO_3^-]}{[Ca^{2+}]}\right)$

9. Phenol red is the most widely used indicator to determine the pH of water in swimming pools. The pKa_2 of phenol red is equal to 7.96. The acidic form of phenol red appears yellow and the basic form of phenol red appears red. In addition, the absorptivity (how strongly a species absorbs light) of the basic form is around three times greater than the acidic form. The color-changing region is indicated by an orange color. Due to the difference in absorptivity between different forms of phenol red, at what pH would the color change (to orange) be most likely to occur?

A. pH of 4
B. pH of 7.5
C. pH of 8.5
D. pH of 11

PASSAGE II (QUESTIONS 10–17)

Hydrogen is the first element of the periodic table. It contains one proton and one electron. According to one early model of the hydrogen atom developed in the early 20th century by Niels Bohr, that electron is found in any one of an infinite number of energy levels. These energy levels are sometimes called quanta, in that they can be described by a principal quantum number, n, that always has an integer value. As the electron moves from one energy level to another ($n = 1$ to $n \rightarrow 8$, or vice versa) it absorbs or emits some discrete quantity of energy accordingly. This quantity is directly proportional to the frequency of the light radiation that results from the energy change.

It took some time for atomic physicists to arrive at Bohr's conclusions. They struggled to reconcile empirical data about light radiation from hydrogen atoms with their understanding that light photons moved and behaved as particles according to Newtonian mechanics. One discovery that led to Bohr's quantum mechanics was a new quantitative interpretation of light emissions from hydrogen atoms. Hydrogen atoms emit light in characteristic patterns known as line spectra. These patterns are noncontinuous but predictable. In the early 1880s, Theodore Balmer derived a mathematical relationship between the energy emissions of a hydrogen atom and the wavelengths of light they radiated during transitions:

$\lambda = B[m^2/(m^2 - 2^2)] = B[m^2/(m^2 - n^2)]$, where B = 364.56 nm, $m > 2$, λ is the wavelength, n is equal to 2.

The spectrum he used, which is now known as the Balmer series, is illustrated below:

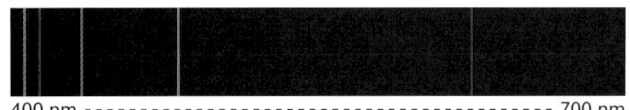

The Rydberg equation is a more general version of this equation that applies to all possible energy level transitions in a hydrogen atom. Physicists used the Rydberg equation to detect other series of energy transitions in other regions of the light spectrum. One such series is the Lyman series, which accounts for transitions from excited states to $n = 1$, the ground state.

10. What is the proper electron configuration of hydrogen in its elemental state?

A. $1s^0$
B. $1s^1$
C. $1s^2$
D. None of the above

11. If an electron is promoted from n = 2 to n = 5, as Balmer observed, which of the following possibilities best describes the source of the line spectra observed?

A. A photon is absorbed.
B. A photon is emitted.
C. An electron is absorbed.
D. An electron is emitted.

12. What region of the light spectrum corresponds to the characteristic emissions in the Balmer series?

A. UV
B. Visible
C. Infrared
D. X-ray

13. One Balmer spectral line, the n = 3 to n = 2 transition, is a common reference point in astronomy for hydrogen gas emissions. The characteristic wavelength of this emission in the scientific literature is 656.3 nm. What color is this light emission?

A. Red
B. Blue-green
C. Violet
D. The emission is not in the visible spectrum.

14. What name best describes the absorption line spectrum pictured below?

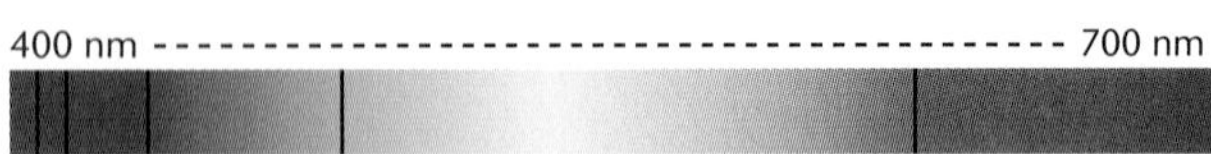

A. Lyman series
B. Balmer series
C. Bohr series
D. None of the above

15. Suppose a scientist tried to obtain a Balmer series with a sample of deuterium. How would this sample change the appearance of the emissions in the line spectrum?

A. Fewer emission lines
B. More emission lines
C. Same number of emission lines with split peaks
D. Same number of emission lines without split peaks (that is, no change in appearance)

16. At high resolution, some of the emissions in the Balmer series appear as doublets. Which of the following best explains this result, which was not predicted by any of the models in the passage?

A. The models in the passage do not account for relativistic effects.
B. The models in the passage do not account for high wavelengths.
C. The models in the passage do not account for the atomic number.
D. The models in the passage do not account for other particles in the atom.

17. When n > 6, the Balmer series features violet light emissions at wavelengths outside the range of the visible spectrum. Which of the following best accounts for this finding?

A. Energy levels are narrower as n → 1 and wider as n → 8.
B. Energy levels are wider as n → 1 and narrower as n → 8.
C. Energy differences between levels are larger as n → 1 and smaller as n → 8.
D. Energy differences between levels are smaller as n → 1 and larger as n → 8.

QUESTIONS 18–22 ARE NOT BASED ON A DESCRIPTIVE PASSAGE.

18. Which of the following pairs of particles would be accelerated in a particle accelerator?

A. Gamma ray and neutron
B. Gamma ray and beta particle
C. Beta particle and neutron
D. Alpha and beta particles

19. What volume of 0.5 M KOH would be necessary to neutralize 15 mL of 1 M nitrous acid?

A. 15 mL
B. 30 mL
C. 45 mL
D. 60 mL

20. Why does high, but not low, pressure cause a deviation from the ideal gas law?

A. Higher pressure decreases the interatomic distance to the point where intermolecular forces reduce the volume below that predicted by the ideal gas equation.
B. Low pressure increases the atomic radius of a gas making it more stable whereas high pressure compresses the gas particles decreasing their stability.
C. Low pressure does cause a significant deviation from the ideal gas law because the increased interatomic distance means that no particles ever collide.
D. Low pressure does cause a significant deviation because a low pressure implies a reduction in temperature via Charles's law, which increases the power of intermolecular forces.

21. What type of molecular geometry is NOT able to result in a nonpolar structure?

A. Bent
B. Diatomic covalent
C. Trigonal planar
D. Square planar

22. A parent and daughter nucleus are isotypes of the same element. Therefore, the ratio of alpha to beta decays that produced the daughter nucleus must be which of the following?

A. 2:3
B. 2:1
C. 1:2
D. 1:1

PASSAGE III (QUESTIONS 23–30)

Many new consumer electronics and electric cars utilize a type of rechargeable battery that extracts its power from the movement of a lithium ion (Li^+) between the cathode and the anode of a galvanic cell. In most cases, the anode is composed of graphite, the cathode is composed of a CoO_2^- complex, and the electrolyte contains a lithium salt in an organic solvent. Following are the half-reactions, where $Li_{1-x}CoO_2$ is the simplest form of the chemical formula $Li(CoO_2)_{1/(1-x)}$ (which represents a complex of one lithium ion with several metal oxide molecules):

$$LiCoO_2 \leftrightharpoons Li_{1-x}CoO_2 + xLi^+ + xe^- \quad \text{(cathode)}$$
$$xLi^+ + xe^- + 6C \leftrightharpoons Li_xC_6 \quad \text{(anode)}$$

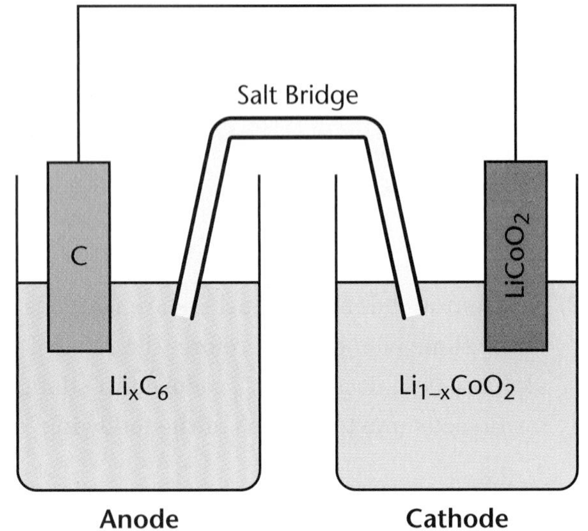

The value of x is equal to the following ratio:

$$\frac{\text{(Present potential energy of the battery)}}{\text{(Original potential energy of the battery)}}$$

When the battery is fully charged, x equals 1. When the battery is fully discharged, x equals 0.

To study the change in a battery's performance over time, a scientist repeatedly charged and discharged cell 1 while leaving cell 2 intact. After several cycles of charging and discharging, the energy-storage capacity of cell 1 deteriorated significantly faster than the capacity of cell 2. Upon further testing, cell 1 was found to contain approximately equal concentrations of lithium oxide and cobalt(II) oxide. The constituents of cell 2 were not analyzed. The scientist hypothesized that the deterioration of cell 1 was caused primarily by the conversion of integral cell components into lithium oxide and cobalt(II) oxide.

23. What is the net overall equation for the cell?

A. $LiCoO_2 + 6C \leftrightharpoons Li_xC_6 + Li_{1-x}CoO_2$
B. $LiCoO_2 + xLi^+ + 6C \leftrightharpoons Li_xC_6 + Li_{1-x}CoO_2$
C. $Li^+ + 6C \leftrightharpoons Li_xC_6$
D. $LiCoO_2 + xLi^+ \leftrightharpoons Li_{1-x}CoO_2$

24. Which of the following is true about the overall potential of the cell when the battery is in use after a complete charge?

A. $E°_{cathode} + E°_{anode} < 0$
B. $E°_{cathode} + E°_{anode} > 0$
C. $E°_{cathode} + E°_{anode} < 1$
D. $E°_{cathode} + E°_{anode} > 1$

25. Which of the following identifies the oxidized and then the reduced species in the forward reaction.

A. Oxidized: Li^+/Reduced: Co^{4+}
B. Oxidized: C/Reduced: Li
C. Oxidized: $C^{x/6}$/Reduced: Co^{4+}
D. Oxidized: Co^{3+}/Reduced: C

26. Which of the following is true about the equilibrium constant of the reaction?

A. The forward reaction exhibits a positive $E°_{cell}$, which suggests a spontaneous process. Because discharging is spontaneous and charging is not, K_{eq} is high during discharging.
B. An increasing value of x will push the cathode reaction to the left and the anode reaction to the right; therefore, charging and discharging will have no net effect on K_{eq}.
C. Discharging is a spontaneous reaction, which requires reduction to occur at the cathode and oxidation to occur at the anode. Because this is only true for the reverse reaction, K_{eq} is low during discharging.
D. Based on the information in the passage, is impossible to predict the effects of charging and discharging on K_{eq}.

27. A certain battery is equipped with a mechanism that calculates its remaining energy by approximating the concentration of various lithium-cobalt-oxygen complexes. The analysis finds that the predominant species in the battery are $LiCoO_2$ and $Li(CoO_2)_2$. If the battery originally stored 100 J of potential energy, how much does it currently store?

A. 100 J
B. 50 J
C. 33 J
D. 0 J

28. Which of the following lithium species carry an oxidation number of +1?

I. Li from $LiCoO_2$
II. Li from $Li_{1-x}CoO_2$
III. Li from Li_xC_6

A. I only
B. II only
C. I and III only
D. I, II, and III

29. Which of the following best explains the appearance of lithium oxide and cobalt(II) oxide in cell 1?

A. A small number of lithium ions occasionally combined with $LiCoO_2$ to produce lithium oxide and cobalt(II) oxide.
B. Because of the energy released by the system, a few $LiCoO_2$ molecules decomposed into lithium oxide and cobalt(II) oxide every time the battery was used.
C. Various constituents of the cell combined with environmental oxygen to produce lithium oxide and cobalt(II) oxide.
D. Various constituents of the cell combined with water to produce lithium oxide and cobalt(II) oxide.

30. If the scientist's hypothesis is correct, which of the following methods would be most likely to effectively measure the deterioration in the energy-storage capacity of a cell (like the one in cell 1)?

A. Determining the value of x for a fully charged battery
B. Determining the value of x for a fully discharged battery
C. Measuring the concentration of cobalt(II) oxide in a fully discharged battery
D. Measuring the concentration of Li_xC_6 in a fully charged battery

PASSAGE IV (QUESTIONS 31–37)

Water is the most abundant liquid on Earth, covering over three-fourths of its surface. Compared with other liquids, it is quite extraordinary. Its chemical structure and resulting phase change properties made the chances for the evolution of life on earth a possibility. Due to their polarity, water molecules have the ability to form hydrogen bonds with one another and with other polar substances. As a result of these forces, water forms a crystalline lattice in its solid state, as depicted by the illustration below. The larger circles represent oxygen and the smaller circles represent hydrogen in the lattice.

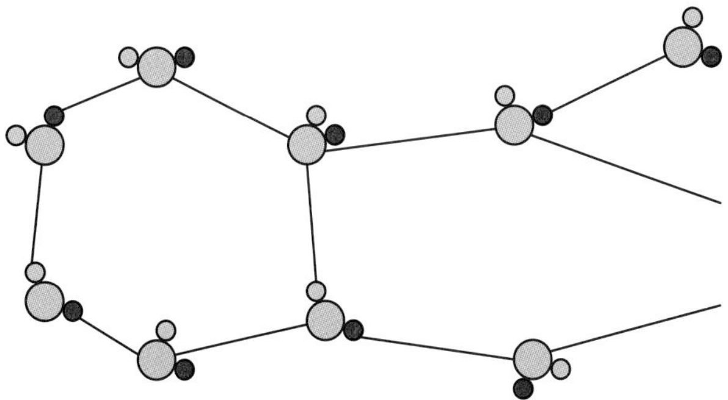

Ammonia is very similar in structure to water. Because of this similarity, many biologists have wondered whether ammonia would be a suitable substitute for water in living systems. The ammonia molecule is composed of hydrogen atoms covalently bonded to nitrogen. As the oxygen in the water molecule has a slightly negative charge, so does the nitrogen atom in ammonia. Some scientists have argued that ammonia-based life could evolve on other planets in a similar manner as life developed on Earth. Others argue that ammonia's heat of vaporization, 295 cal/g, is low compared with water, making it an unlikely candidate for the evolution of life. Modern science agrees that ammonia-based life on other planets will probably not be found to have evolved, if it exists, in the same manner as life on Earth.

31. One could infer from the passage that no form of life based on ammonia has yet been found because its

A. evaporation rate would be too high.
B. condensation rate would be too high.
C. rate of deposition would be too high.
D. rate of sublimation would be too low.

32. Had water not formed a crystalline lattice upon freezing and instead followed the common phase change pathways of most other compounds, one could logically infer that

A. life could not have evolved in a liquid environment.
B. life would have evolved in a gaseous environment.
C. soils would hold greater amounts of liquid water.
D. soils would hold greater amounts of gaseous water.

1. When the water molecules shown in the previous illustration undergo sublimation, what best explains this phenomenon?

A. The attractive forces between the water molecules overcome the kinetic energy that keeps them apart.
B. The kinetic energy of the water molecules overcomes the attractive forces that keep them together.
C. The hydrogen bonds between the water molecules form at a more rapid rate in the solid phase.
D. The hydrogen bonds between the water molecules form at a more rapid rate in the liquid phase.

34. A change in which intrinsic property of water would most affect its polarity?

A. Atomic electronegativity
B. Chirality
C. Intermolecular forces
D. Solubility

35. How would one explain the negative slope of the water-solid equilibrium line in the phase diagram for water, shown below?

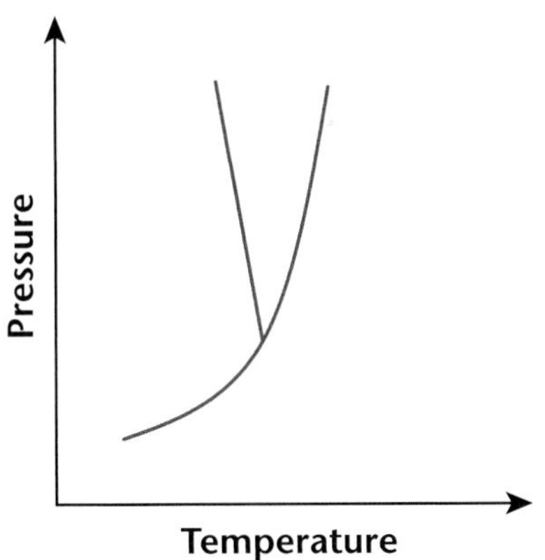

A. Water is more dense at 4° Celsius than at 0.
B. Water's solid lattice collapses under pressure.
C. The triple point determines the slope of the phase-change line.
D. Liquid water is less dense than ice.

36. According to the passage, which of the following is true about a molecule of water undergoing evaporation?

A. The water molecule has more energy than an ammonia molecule.
B. Water evaporation is faster than an ammonia evaporation.
C. The water molecule has less energy than an ammonia molecule.
D. Both A and B

37. What would the addition of an ionic compound do to the lattice structure shown in the illustration above?

A. Collapse the structure
B. Enhance cohesive forces in the structure
C. Enhance crystallization
D. Both B or C

PASSAGE V (QUESTIONS 38–45)

There are many elements in the periodic table that play an integral role in the everyday functions of the human body. While the most obvious of these are carbon, hydrogen, nitrogen, and oxygen, we also have various essential uses for phosphorus. Its physical and chemical properties have made it the perfect candidate to play a role in the molecule that acts as the body's primary location for short-term storage of energy, adenosine-5′-triphosphate (ATP).

Some metabolic syndromes can cause a phosphate ion to be drawn from the blood into the bones and teeth, where the majority of phosphorus exists. The ensuing deficiency of phosphate in the blood can lead to dysfunction of the brain and muscle tissue, which can cause death in severe cases. Scientists are attempting to cure this disease by designing a biologic molecule whose properties and actions are similar to those of phosphate. One way to do this is to find an element that has similar physical and chemical properties to phosphorus.

38. Which of the following is most likely to act as a stronger reducing agent than phosphorus?

A. Na
B. Cs
C. O
D. Bi

39. Which of the following, on average, have more space between two nuclei placed side-by-side than phosphorus?

I. K
II. Pb
III. F

A. I only
B. I and II
C. II and III
D. I, II, and III

40. Which of the following is NOT a property of phosphorus, according to the classifications of types of elements?

A. Brittle in the solid state
B. Poor electrical conductivity
C. Does not show much luster
D. Is generally malleable

41. Which of the following is the correct electron orbital configuration of phosphorus?

A. $1s^2 2s^2 3s^2 2p^6 3p^3$
B. $1s^2 2s^2 2p^6 3s^2 3p^3$
C. $1s^2 2s^2 2p^6 3p^5$
D. $1s^2 2s^2 2p^6 3s^2 3d^{10} 3p^6$

42. Which of the following statements is true about the density of alkali metals and alkaline earth metals?

A. Alkaline earth metals are less dense because they contain unfilled subshells.
B. Alkaline earth metals are less dense because their nuclei contain fewer neutrons.
C. Alkali metals are less dense because they contain fewer orbitals.
D. Alkali metals are less dense because they have a loosely bound electron in their outer shell.

43. Which of the following is NOT a correct characterization of the properties of halogens?

A. At room temperature, halogens naturally exist only in the gaseous and liquid states.
B. Halogens are highly likely to react with alkali metals.
C. Halogens can form stable ionic crystals with alkaline earth metals.
D. In their neutral form, halogens always have an outer shell of p^5.

44. Which of the following contributes most to the malleability shown by transition elements?

A. Natural softness as compared to other metals
B. High electrical conductivity
C. Loosely held d-electrons
D. High melting points

45. Which of the following best explains why scientists closely examine metalloids when trying to find a biologic to replace phosphorus?

A. Phosphorus is a metalloid.
B. Metalloids often behave as semiconductors.
C. Some metalloids exhibit similar bonding capabilities to phosphorus.
D. Metalloids exhibit flexibility in their properties so they can be manipulated easily.

PASSAGE VI (QUESTIONS 46–52)

Aerobic and anaerobic bacteria undergo different types of metabolism, and the properties of their metabolisms are unique. Some anaerobic bacteria are methane-producing bacteria. These bacteria have been studied to determine the relevance of their potential use in generating biological energy or "biogas."

These methane-producing bacteria typically feed off of animal manure or other natural waste. In the process of utilizing animal waste, manure is collected from different types of animals including swine and cows. The manure is separated by phase and contains proteins, carbohydrates, and fats; bacteria then break down components into fatty acids.[1]

"Methanogens" are the particular type of anaerobic bacteria that undertake the final steps of breaking down the fatty acids into simple products: methane and carbon dioxide. A common reactant is acetic acid, which breaks down according to the following reaction shown below:

$$CH_3COOH \longrightarrow CH_4 + CO_2$$

Other fatty acids can be used as substrates for these methane-generating reactions, including propionate and butyrate. Methanogenic bacteria can also convert carbon dioxide and hydrogen gas to form methane and water. At the end of this process, which typically takes place at 95° Celsius, methane can be used to generate energy as an alternative to fossil fuels.

46. What type of reaction is presented in the passage?

A. Combination reaction
B. Single-displacement reaction
C. Decomposition reaction
D. Combustion reaction

47. If the reaction begins with 120 grams of acetic acid, what is the theoretical yield, in grams, of methane?

A. 32.05 grams
B. 64.1 grams
C. 40.92 grams
D. 29.12 grams

48. What piece of evidence would support the passage's argument that the decomposition of fatty acids can create energy serving as an alternative to fossil fuel?

A. Anaerobic bacteria can break down fatty acids efficiently at room temperature.
B. Methane gas can be compressed and transported.
C. The reaction generates gaseous products.
D. The reaction is exothermic.

49. What formula best demonstrates how to calculate the number of grams of acetic acid necessary to produce 88.02 grams of carbon dioxide?

A. $\frac{(88.02 \text{ grams})(\text{molecular weight } CH_3COOH)}{(\text{molecular weight } CO_2)}$

B. $\frac{(88.02 \text{ grams})(2 \text{ moles } CH_3COOH)(\text{molecular weight } CH_3COOH)}{(\text{molecular weight } CO_2)(1 \text{ mole } CO_2)}$

C. $\frac{(\text{molecular weight } CH_3COOH)}{(88.02 \text{ grams})(\text{molecular weight } CO_2)}$

D. $\frac{(2 \text{ moles } CH_3COOH)(\text{molecular weight of } CO_2)(\text{molecular weight } CH_3COOH)}{(88.02 \text{ grams})(1 \text{ mole } CO_2)}$

[1]Information for this entire passage taken primarily from:
www.thepigsite.com/articles/4/waste-and-odor/914/manure-to-energy-the-utah-project ($C_6H_{13}O_5 + xH_2O \rightarrow COOH\text{–}(CH_2)_n\text{–}CH_3 \rightarrow 4CH_4 + 2CO_2$)
With contributions from:
extension.missouri.edu/xplor/agguides/agengin/g01881.htm ($H_2 + CO_2 \rightarrow H_2O + CH_4$)
books.google.com/books?id=ndPuyf4BsXYC&pg=PA26&lpg=PA26&dq=methane+and+bacteria+equation&source=web&ots=sbBVmswSMF&sig=6pQeW_uEd6WiSvcgPuHf_YdYQ4M&hl=en&sa=X&oi=book_result&resnum=5&ct=result
$CH_3COOH \rightarrow CH_4 + CO_2$ $CO_2 + 4H_2 \rightarrow CH_4 + 2H_2O$

50. One form of acetic acid, which is typically used as a salt, is called acetate. Sodium acetate can react with other chemical compounds in solution, an example of which is demonstrated below. What is the correct net ionic equation for this reaction?

A. $Na^+ + CH_3COO^- + Cl^- + CH_3CH_2CH_2^+ \longrightarrow CH_3COOCH_2CH_2CH_3 + Na^+ + Cl^-$

B. $CH_3COO^- + Cl^- + CH_3CH_2CH_2^+ \longrightarrow CH_3COOCH_2CH_2CH_3 + Cl^-$

C. $CH_3COO^- + CH_3CH_2CH_2^+ \longrightarrow CH_3COOCH_2CH_2CH_3$

D. $CH_3COO^- + CH_3CH_2CH_2Cl \longrightarrow CH_3COOCH_2CH_2CH_3 + Cl^-$

51. As described in the passage, methanogenic bacteria can utilize hydrogen gas to produce methane. At standard temperature and pressure, if there are 3 liters of hydrogen gas and 2 liters of carbon dioxide available to the bacteria, what would be the theoretical yield, in moles, of methane?

A. 0.134 moles
B. 0.0893 moles
C. 0.067 moles
D. 0.268 moles

52. What is the percent yield if 8.02 g of methane is formed from the reaction of 50 liters of hydrogen gas, with excess carbon dioxide at standard temperature and pressure?

A. 86.2%
B. 14.4%
C. 43.1%
D. 64.7%

PRACTICE SECTION 3

Time—70 minutes

QUESTIONS 1–52

Directions: Most of the questions in the following General Chemistry Practice Section are organized into groups, with a descriptive passage preceding each group of questions. Study the passage, then select the single-best answer to the question in each group. Some of the questions are not based on a descriptive passage; you must also select the best answer to these questions. In you are unsure of the best answer, eliminate the choices that you know are incorrect, then select an answer from the choices that remain.

Period	1 IA 1A	2 IIA 2A	3 IIIB 3B	4 IVB 4B	5 VB 5B	6 VIB 6B	7 VIIB 7B	8	9 VIII -- 8	10	11 IB 1B	12 IIB 2B	13 IIIA 3A	14 IVA 4A	15 VA 5A	16 VIA 6A	17 VIIA 7A	18 vIIIA 8A
1	1 H 1.008																	2 He 4.003
2	3 Li 6.941	4 Be 9.012											5 B 10.81	6 C 12.01	7 N 14.01	8 O 16.00	9 F 19.00	10 Ne 20.18
3	11 Na 22.99	12 Mg 24.31											13 Al 26.98	14 Si 28.09	15 P 30.97	16 S 32.07	17 Cl 35.45	18 Ar 39.95
4	19 K 39.10	20 Ca 40.08	21 Sc 44.96	22 Ti 47.88	23 V 50.94	24 Cr 52.00	25 Mn 54.94	26 Fe 55.85	27 Co 58.47	28 Ni 58.69	29 Cu 63.55	30 Zn 65.39	31 Ga 69.72	32 Ge 72.59	33 As 74.92	34 Se 78.96	35 Br 79.90	36 Kr 83.80
5	37 Rb 85.47	38 Sr 87.62	39 Y 88.91	40 Zr 91.22	41 Nb 92.91	42 Mo 95.94	43 Tc (98)	44 Ru 101.1	45 Rh 102.9	46 Pd 106.4	47 Ag 107.9	48 Cd 112.4	49 In 114.8	50 Sn 118.7	51 Sb 121.8	52 Te 127.6	53 I 126.9	54 Xe 131.3
6	55 Cs 132.9	56 Ba 137.3	57 La* 138.9	72 Hf 178.5	73 Ta 180.9	74 W 183.9	75 Re 186.2	76 Os 190.2	77 Ir 190.2	78 Pt 195.1	79 Au 197.0	80 Hg 200.5	81 Tl 204.4	82 Pb 207.2	83 Bi 209.0	84 Po (210)	85 At (210)	86 Rn (222)
7	87 Fr (223)	88 Ra (226)	89 Ac~ (227)	104 Rf (257)	105 Db (260)	106 Sg (263)	107 Bh (262)	108 Hs (265)	109 Mt (266)	110 --- ()	111 --- ()	112 --- ()		114 --- ()		116 --- ()		118 --- ()

Lanthanide Series*	58 Ce 140.1	59 Pr 140.9	60 Nd 144.2	61 Pm (147)	62 Sm 150.4	63 Eu 152.0	64 Gd 157.3	65 Tb 158.9	66 Dy 162.5	67 Ho 164.9	68 Er 167.3	69 Tm 168.9	70 Yb 173.0	71 Lu 175.0
Actinide Series~	90 Th 232.0	91 Pa (231)	92 U (238)	93 Np (237)	94 Pu (242)	95 Am (243)	96 Cm (247)	97 Bk (247)	98 Cf (249)	99 Es (254)	100 Fm (253)	101 Md (256)	102 No (254)	103 Lr (257)

PASSAGE I (QUESTIONS 1–8)

The blood-brain barrier is a unique part of the human nervous system. Endothelial cells lining blood vessels in the central nervous system are more tightly attached to one another than in other parts of the human body. As a result, there is limited permeability of both small and large molecules from the circulation into the cerebrospinal fluid (CSF).

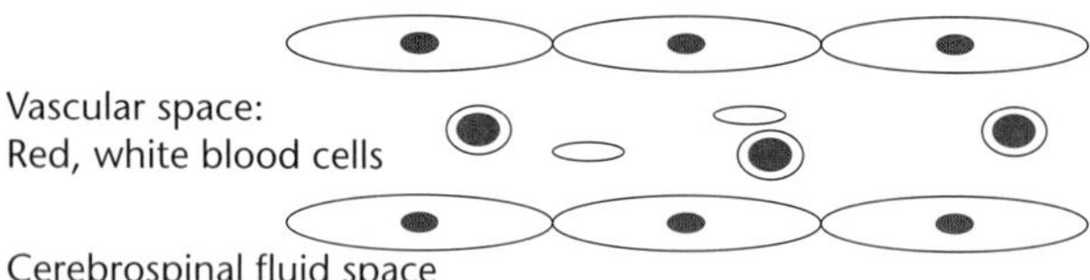

These tightly sealed endothelial cells have both advantages and disadvantages in the human system. The central nervous system is a fragile, essential part of the human body, and the endothelial cells serve as a barrier. Multiple characteristics of any given molecule affect its permeability: its polarity, size, weight, charge, and degree of protein binding in the blood. Nonpolar molecules pass more effectively from the bloodstream into the CSF. Smaller particles, such as water, and small, charged particles will also move with varying ease across this barrier. Water moves freely, but charged ions can take hours to equilibrate between the systemic circulation and the cerebrospinal fluid.

When disease afflicts the central nervous system it is necessary to deliver drugs to the cerebrospinal fluid for delivery into the tissues of the brain and spinal cord. On the other hand, some extremely effective chemotherapeutic agents, such as cisplatin, are beneficial when they do not cross the blood-brain barrier because they are neurotoxic when they penetrate the central nervous system. Alternatively, when beginning general anesthesia for a surgical procedure it is essential that anesthetic agents penetrate from the systemic circulation into the cerebrospinal fluid to alter consciousness and systemic muscle tone during the procedure.

1. Based on the passage, which of the following characteristics would be essential for any pharmaceutical intended for use as a general anesthetic?

A. The molecule should be nonpolar.
B. The molecule should be directly delivered to the CNS without going through the systemic circulation first.
C. The molecule should be polar.
D. The molecule should be slow-acting.

2. What can be logically inferred from the passage about charge and its effect on a molecule's permeability of the blood-brain barrier?

A. Charged molecules are more likely to associate with one another tightly in the blood stream, inhibiting diffusion into the cerebrospinal fluid.
B. Uncharged molecules are more likely to be able to diffuse between endothelial cells.
C. Uncharged molecules are less likely to be transported through endothelial cells.
D. Charged molecules are more soluble in the bloodstream than in the cerebrospinal fluid.

3. What can be logically inferred from the passage about the role of the blood-brain barrier in supporting human life?

A. A permeable central nervous system is essential in allowing diffusion of nutrients from the peripheral circulation into the CNS.
B. The micro-environment of the CNS is similar to that of the systemic circulation.
C. The blood-brain barrier limits the flow of damaged or infected cells from the cerebrospinal fluid into the systemic circulation.
D. The blood-brain barrier adaptively protects the CNS from toxins or other possible insults originating in the systemic circulation.

4. Based on the information in the passage, what type of intermolecular force has the most influence on molecules that pass easily through the blood-brain barrier?

A. Ion-dipole interactions
B. Dipole-dipole interactions
C. Hydrogen bonding
D. Dispersion forces

5. Which of the following statements are NOT true when relating formal charge with permeation across the blood-brain barrier?

I. A formal charge of zero guarantees permeability through the blood-brain barrier.
II. A negative formal change on one or more atoms in a molecule will improve its permeability of the blood-brain barrier.
III. Two molecules, both with formal charges of zero, will be equally permeable through the blood-brain barrier.

A. I only
B. III only
C. II and III only
D. I, II, and III

6. Cisplatin, a commonly used chemotherapeutic agent, is $PtCl_2(NH_3)_2$. What type of bond forms between each of the NH_3 groups and the central platinum?

A. Coordinate covalent bond
B. Polar covalent bond
C. Nonpolar covalent bond
D. Ionic bond

7. Phenytoin, shown below, is an anti-seizure medicine. It is one of many drugs that is actively transported *out* of the central nervous system by cellular transporters. What would be the best estimate of the geometry around the central carbon to which the arrow points?

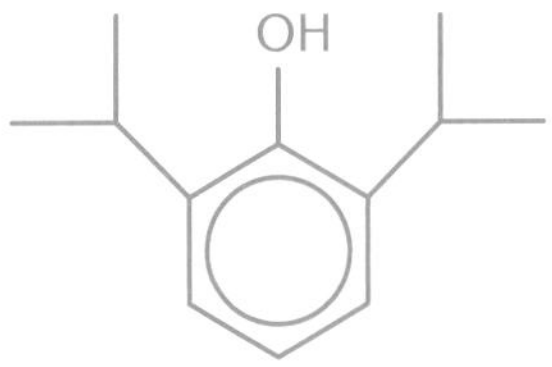

OH

A. Square planar
B. Tetrahedral
C. Trigonal pyramidal
D. Octahedral

8. Which of the following best describes the relationship between resonance structures and molecular polarity?

A. The most stable resonance structures maximize polarity.
B. If a molecule has more than one important resonance structure, it is more likely to be a polar molecule than another molecule without such resonance structures.
C. The most important resonance structures spread out and minimize formal charge.
D. Resonance structures will counterbalance the natural polarity of a bond.

PASSAGE II (QUESTIONS 9–16)

The human body is a dynamic system that has to deal with significant environmental threats on a daily basis. One type of threat is from the effects of reactive oxygen species (ROS). ROS are ions or small molecules containing oxygen that have unpaired valence shell electrons. The superoxide anion, O_2^-, is a toxic threat, becoming lethal at intracellular levels of just 1 nM. It spontaneously forms O_2 and H_2O_2, but is also able to react with NO to form peroxynitrite. Peroxynitrite can cause extreme cellular damage. The enzyme NADPH oxidase produces the superoxide anion in the body to combat invading microorganisms. Because of the threat that it poses in such small quantities, the body has developed ways to dispose of this chemical.

The superoxide anion puts the concept of compartmentalization is on display. It would be a waste of energy to both produce and destroy superoxide in the same cell, so it is only produced in phagocytes (immune cells that ingest infectious agents), and is broken down in any other cell of the body. In two steps, the enzyme superoxide dismutase (SOD) uses iron or other metals to create oxygen and hydrogen peroxide from superoxide and hydrogen ions:

Step 1: $Fe^{3+} - SOD + O_2^- \rightarrow Fe^{2+} - SOD + O_2$
Step 2: $Fe^{2+} - SOD + O_2^- + 2H^+ \rightarrow Fe^{3+} - SOD + H_2O_2$

A graduate student at a local university was given the task of determining the kinetics of this reaction. Her results are shown in table 1 below:

Trial	$[H^+]_{initial}$ (M)	$[O_2^-]_{initial}$ (M)	$r_{initial}$ (M/sec)
1	1	1	2.04
2	1	2	7.98
3	4	1	8.09

The potential energy diagram for the reaction is shown in figure 1 below:

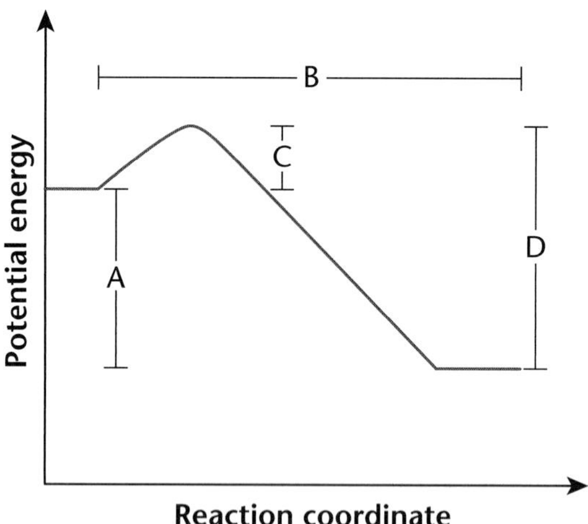

FOR QUESTIONS 9–14, ASSUME BOTH STEPS OF THE REACTION ARE IRREVERSIBLE.

9. What is the order of H^+ in Step 2 of the above reaction?

A. 0
B. 1
C. 2
D. 3

10. What is the rate of step 2 of the reaction if the following concentrations of reactants exist? Assume the rate constant, k = 0.50.

$$[H^+] = 2\text{ M}, [O_2^-] = 2\text{ M}$$

A. 2.5 M/sec
B. 4 M/sec
C. 8 M/sec
D. 10 M/sec

11. What function might Fe^{2+}–SOD play in the overall reaction?

A. A substance used to create a product in the reaction
B. A substance that is created in the reaction
C. A substance that increases the rate of the reaction
D. A short-lived, unstable molecule in the reaction

12. Which of the following is NOT true when describing the kinetics of the previous overall reaction?

A. The rate of the reaction is proportional to the number of collisions between reacting molecules.
B. In some effective collisions, all of the colliding particles do not have enough kinetic energy to exceed activation energy.
C. A transition state is formed when old bonds are breaking and new bonds are forming.
D. The activated complex has greater energy than either products or reactants.

13. What section of the diagram in figure 1 represents the forward activation energy?

A. A
B. B
C. C
D. D

14. What section of the diagram in figure 1 represents the enthalpy change during the reaction?

A. A
B. B
C. C
D. D

FOR QUESTIONS 15–16, ASSUME BOTH STEPS OF THE REACTION ARE REVERSIBLE.

15. What is the equilibrium constant for the overall reaction in the passage? Will an increase in pressure raise or lower the equilibrium constant? Assume $[O_2^-] = 3$ M, $[H^+] = 1$ M, $[H_2O_2] = 1$ M, $[O_2] = 2$ M.

A. 0.22; raise
B. 0.27; lower
C. 2.2; raise
D. 2.7; lower

16. What would best explain the equilibrium shift to the right in reaction 2?

A. Increase in volume
B. Addition of product
C. Increase in pressure
D. Decrease in temperature

QUESTIONS 17–21 ARE NOT BASED ON A DESCRIPTIVE PASSAGE.

17. Latent heat flux is the loss of heat by the surface of a body of water caused by evaporation. To determine the latent heat flux over the Atlantic Ocean, one would need to know

A. ΔH_{fusion} of water.
B. $\Delta H_{vaporization}$ of water.
C. $\Delta H_{sublimation}$ of water.
D. $\Delta H_{ionization}$ of water.

18. A particle is constrained to move in a circle with a 10-meter radius. At one instant, the particle's speed is 10 meters per second and is increased at a rate of 10 meters per second squared. What is the angle between the particle's velocity and acceleration vectors?

A. 0°
B. 30°
C. 45°
D. 60°

19. What compound would not be considered an electrolyte?

A. AgCl
B. CaO
C. LiI
D. HBr

20. Aluminum has a lower electronegativity than iron, but reacts extremely slowly with oxygen in moist air because of a hard, protective aluminum oxide coat that protects all exposed surfaces. Under which of the following conditions would aluminum be more readily eroded?

A. Immersed in a solution of HCl
B. Immersed in a bath of hot sodium metal
C. Immersed in a solution of NH_3
D. Immersed in a solution of NaOH

21. Two gases, X and Y, are combined in a closed container. At STP, the average velocity of a gas A molecule is twice that of a gas B molecule. Gases A and B are most likely which of the following?

A. He and Ar
B. He and Kr
C. Ne and Ar
D. Ne and Kr

PASSAGE III (QUESTIONS 22–29)

Dry ice forms when carbon dioxide gas is cooled to –78° C at atmospheric pressure. After becoming solid, it reforms gas when heat is added as shown in the reversible reaction below:

CO_2 (solid, –78°C) + heat (120kJ/mol) ↔ CO_2 (gas, 25°C)

An experiment was done to test the change, over three days, in a block of dry ice placed in a rigid container at room temperature at 1 atmosphere of pressure. The container was closed to the outside environment for the duration of the experiment. The only components in the container were the dry ice and air (g). No liquid in the container was detected over the three-day period. The apparatus and results of the experiment are shown in Figure 1 below.

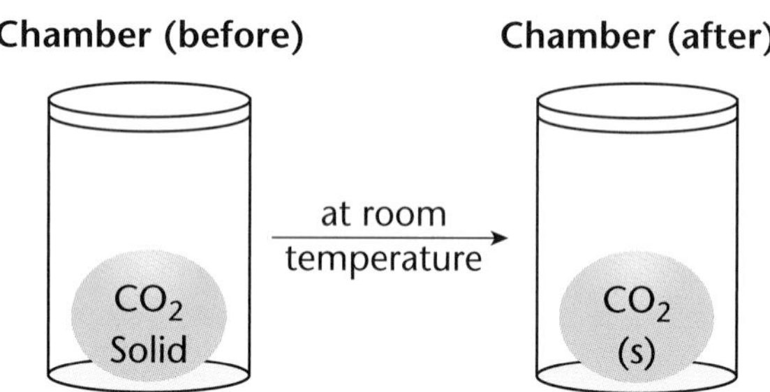

As a solid carbon dioxide has many uses, not the least of which is cooling its surroundings. This transfer of energy is a main method by which coolants operate in many mechanical devices. The phase diagram for carbon dioxide is a major reason for its unique behaviors. The phase diagram for carbon dioxide is shown in Figure 2 below.

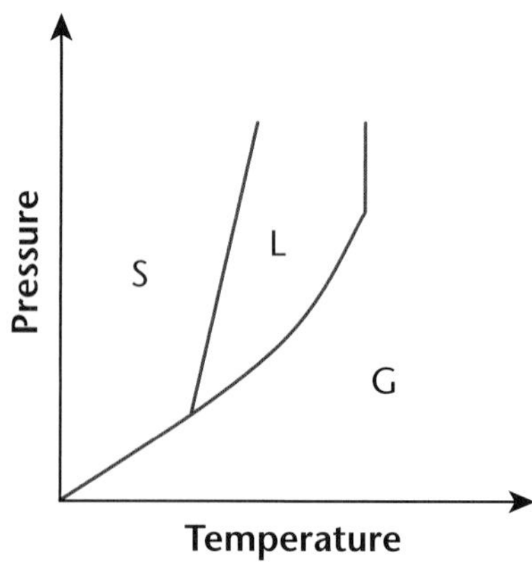

22. Which of the following best describes the equation in the passage?

A. Evaporation
B. Condensation
C. Deposition
D. Sublimation

23. Referring to Figure 2, if liquid carbon dioxide were subject to increasing pressure at a constant temperature, it would

A. become solid.
B. become gaseous.
C. gain kinetic energy.
D. lose kinetic energy.

24. It can be inferred from the results of the experiment that the air in the container

A. lost kinetic energy.
B. gained kinetic energy.
C. gained volume.
D. lost volume.

25. When the dry ice molecules shown undergo phase changes, which of the following is a likely cause?

A. The attractive forces between the carbon dioxide molecules overcome the kinetic energy that keeps them apart.
B. The kinetic energy of the carbon dioxide molecules overcomes the attractive forces that keep them together.
C. The hydrogen bonds between the carbon dioxide molecules form at a more rapid rate in the solid phase.
D. The hydrogen bonds between the carbon dioxide molecules form at a more rapid rate in the liquid phase.

26. The process shown in the experiment from the passage was

A. endothermic, and the dry ice gained potential energy.
B. endothermic, and the dry ice lost potential energy.
C. exothermic, and the dry ice gained potential energy.
D. exothermic, and the dry ice lost potential energy.

27. If the experiment from the passage were allowed to continue until all the carbon dioxide changed phase, one could logically predict that the air in the container would have

A. increased in pressure.
B. decreased in volume.
C. become a solid.
D. increased in temperature.

28. In the heating/cooling curve for carbon dioxide shown below, what represents the location of the phase change described in the passage?

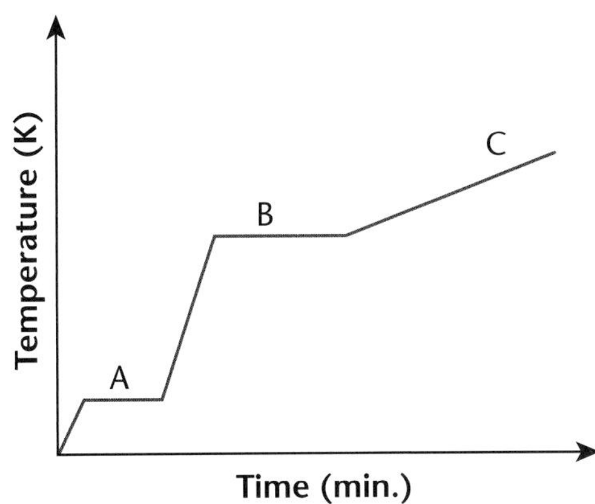

A. A
B. B
C. C
D. None of the above

29. In the phase diagram for carbon dioxide shown below, what represents the phase change shown in the experiment in the passage?

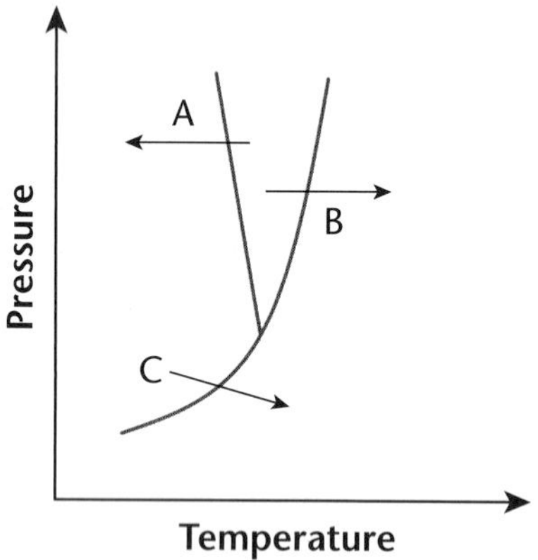

A. A
B. B
C. C
D. None of the above

QUESTIONS 30–36 ARE NOT BASED ON A DESCRIPTIVE PASSAGE.

30. Which of the following will result in a negative free energy change for a reaction?

A. The enthalpy change is negative.
B. The entropy change is positive.
C. The enthalpy change is negative and the entropy change is negative.
D. The enthalpy change is negative and the entropy change is positive.

31. Compared to the atomic radius of calcium, the atomic radius of gallium is

A. larger, because increased electron charge requires that the same force be distributed over a greater number of electrons.
B. smaller, because gallium gives up more electrons, decreasing its size.
C. smaller, because increased nuclear charge causes the electrons to be held more tightly.
D. larger, because its additional electrons increases the volume of the atom.

32. Under which conditions would water vapor demonstrate behavior closest to an ideal gas?

A. High pressure, low temperature
B. Low pressure, low temperature
C. High pressure, high temperature
D. Low pressure, high temperature

33. If the pressure of an ideal gas in a closed container is halved while the volume is held constant, the temperature of the gas

A. decreases by a factor of 2.
B. decreases by a factor of 4.
C. remains the same.
D. increases by a factor of 4.

34. "Greenhouse gases" are gases that will absorb IR radiation and trap energy between the Earth and the atmosphere. CO_2 and H_2O both strongly absorb radiation and are thus considered greenhouse gases, while N_2 and O_2 do not. One quality of greenhouse gases is that

A. they are composed of polar molecules.
B. they have a permanent dipole moment.
C. they experience hydrogen bonding.
D. they have polar covalent bonds.

35. What element contains unpaired electrons in its most common ionized state?

A. Fluorine
B. Aluminum
C. Zinc
D. Iron

36. Which of the following is the correct electron configuration for chromium in the ground state?

A. $[Ar]3d^4 5s^2$
B. $[Kr]4d^5 5s^1$
C. $[Ar]4s^1 4p^5$
D. $[Ar]3d^5 4s^1$

PASSAGE IV (QUESTIONS 37–45)

Decompression sickness involves symptoms that arise from exposure to a rapid decrease in ambient pressure. Decompression sickness can occur in multiple scenarios of decreased pressure and is most prevalent when divers return to the surface of water after a deep dive. If a diver ascends quickly and does not carry out decompression stops, gas bubbles can form in the body and create a multitude of adverse symptoms.

A diver experiences an increase in pressure when submerged many feet under water. Inert gases in the high-pressure environment dissolve into body tissues and liquids. When a diver comes back to the water's surface and the pressure decreases, the excess gas dissolved in the body comes out of solution. Gas bubbles form if inert gas comes out of the body too quickly. These bubbles are unable to leave through the lungs and subsequently cause symptoms such as itching skin, rashes, joint pain, paralysis, and even death.

At sea level the pressure exerted on one square inch is equal to 14.7 pounds, or 1 atm. In water, an additional 1 atm of pressure is exerted for every 33 feet (about 10 m) below sea level. In addition to the decompression sickness, there are other conditions of which divers must be aware that arise from specific gases as a result of the high-pressure environment. For example, increased concentrations of nitrogen in the body lead to nitrogen narcosis. A diver with nitrogen narcosis feels intoxicated and experiences loss of decision-making skills due to nitrogen's anesthetic quality. The table below provides a list of gases and their corresponding solubility constants in water at 298 K.

Gas	k (M torr^{-1})
CO_2	4.48×10^{-5}
O_2	1.66×10^{-6}
He	5.1×10^{-7}
H_2	1.04×10^{-6}
N_2	8.42×10^{-7}

37. What theory could be used to determine the amount of oxygen that is dissolved in water at sea level?

A. Henry's law
B. Boyle's law
C. Raoult's law
D. Le Châtelier's principle

38. What is the solubility (g/L) of N_2 in water (25° C) when the N_2 partial pressure is 0.634 atm?

A. 3.19×10^{-1} g/L
B. 1.5×10^{-2} g/L
C. 1.14×10^{-2} g/L
D. 1.5×10^{-5} g/L

39. Helium is mixed with oxygen in the scuba tanks of divers in order to dilute the oxygen. Why is helium chosen over other gases for this purpose?

A. It is not a diatomic gas.
B. It is less soluble in aqueous solutions and so does not dissolve in body tissues and fluids.
C. It can react with other gases that may dissolve in the body to reverse gas bubble formation.
D. It is present only in trace amounts in water.

40. A scuba tank is filled with 0.32 kg O_2 that is compressed to a volume of 2.8 L. If the temperature of the tank equilibrates with the water at 13° Celsius, what is the pressure inside the tank?

A. 111 atm
B. 83.9 atm
C. 54.6 atm
D. 290 atm

41. Which of the following would you recommend for a diver suffering from decompression sickness?

A. Administration of helium gas
B. Administration of a gas and air mixture, which contains 50 percent nitrous oxide
C. Confinement in a hypobaric chamber
D. Confinement in a hyperbaric chamber

42. The underwater environment in the world's oceans is rapidly changing. Recent years have seen drastic shifts in the ecosystem due to human activity and its impact on the environment. Many populations of fish that rely heavily upon oxygen are declining at extraordinary rates, whereas other ocean species that can survive in oceanic regions of oxygen-depletion are on the rise. What is the most likely explanation, based on scientific theory, for the decline in dissolved oxygen in the world's oceans?

A. Carbon dioxide pollution has increased ocean acidity.
B. A new species of predator shark preys on fish in oxygen-rich regions.
C. The average temperature of the oceans is rapidly increasing.
D. Increased rainfall has added water to oceans without adding more oxygen.

43. A scuba tank contains 0.38 kg of oxygen gas under high pressure. What volume would the oxygen occupy at STP?

A. 0.27 L
B. 35 L
C. 266 L
D. 11 L

44. At 1 atm, the solubility of pure nitrogen in the blood at normal body temperature (37 °C) is 6.2×10^{-4} M. If a diver is at a depth where the pressure is equal to 3 atm and breathes air (78% N_2), calculate the concentration of nitrogen in the diver's blood.

A. 1.3×10^{-3} M
B. 1.4×10^{-3} M
C. 1.5×10^{-5} M
D. 1.9×10^{-3} M

45. Consider two scuba tanks at sea level and 25 °C. Tank 1 is filled with oxygen, and tank 2 is filled with a mixture of oxygen and helium. Will there be a difference in the root-mean-square velocities between these two tanks?

A. Yes, tank 2 has a higher root-mean-square velocity.
B. Yes, tank 1 has a higher root-mean-square velocity.
C. No, they will have the same root-mean-square velocity.
D. The root-mean-square velocity cannot be calculated for the tanks.

PASSAGE V (QUESTIONS 46–52)

Sodium fluoride is used in toothpastes to reduce the virulence of bacteria that cause *dental caries*, also known as cavities. Most U.S. residents are exposed to sodium fluoride, and its use has been correlated with a decline in the incidence of dental caries in most of the population. Although there is debate over the mechanism by which sodium fluoride acts to reduce dental caries, it has been established that the fluoride ion is the main contributor to its efficacy.

Fluoride is the ionic form of the element fluorine. The fluoride ion has a high degree of electronegativity and so holds a negative charge in solution. It thus forms relatively stable bonds with positive ions such as H^+ and Na^+. Fluoride inhibits carinogenic bacteria from metabolizing carbohydrates and thus prevents subsequent production of acid in the oral cavity. The decrease of acidity reduces erosion of tooth enamel, which would otherwise lead to fissures and irregular surface changes in the tooth.

In a variety of laboratory studies, certain types of *Streptococci* bacteria, a main culprit in the formation of caries, are adversely affected when exposed to fluoride ion concentrations of varying levels. In particular, it was found that *Streptococcus sobrinus*, the more virulent species of the *Streptococci*, produces less acid when exposed to fluoride than *Streptococcus sobrinus*, the less virulent form. The reasons for the link of reduced acid production to fluoride levels are still unclear.

46. Based on the passage, which of the following can be definitively stated about the action of fluoride ions on oral health?

A. F- prevents bacteria from forming dental caries.
B. F- kills populations of bacteria that cause dental caries.
C. F- is related to killing populations of bacteria that form dental caries.
D. F- is related to less acid production and reduces the risk of dental caries.

47. Based on the passage, what is a possible mechanism by which fluoride could act upon *Streptococci* bacteria to reduce their production of acid?

A. Fluoride adds enamel to the developing tooth structure.
B. Fluoride fills and closes fissures within the enamel topography.
C. Fluoride adds electrons to bacterial respiration reactions.
D. Fluoride pulls electrons from bacterial respiration reactions.

48. What property contributes to the high electronegativity found in the fluorine atom?

A. Small atomic radius
B. Small number of protons in the nucleus
C. Large number of electrons in the orbit
D. Large number of electron shells in the orbit

49. Which of the following is the correct electronic structure notation for fluoride?

A. $1s^2 2s^2 2p^5$
B. $1s^2 2s^2 2p^4$
C. $[He]2s^2 2p^6$
D. $[Ne]2p^6$

50. According to Heisenberg, what can be accurately, quantitatively determined in a neutral atom when the location of the electron is found?

A. Electron momentum
B. Velocity of electron
C. Mass of electron
D. None of the above

51. What is the effective nuclear charge on the outermost electron in fluoride?

A. 0
B. –1
C. +1
D. +1/2

52. What electrons are most available for bonding in the fluoride ion?

A. 3s
B. 2p
C. 1s
D. 2s

Answers and Explanations

CHAPTER PRACTICE QUESTIONS

CHAPTER 1: ATOMIC STRUCTURE

1. A

The material is ferromagnetic (A). Ferromagnetism refers, loosely, to the ability of a surface to attract an external magnetic field. It is characteristic of iron (Fe), from which it derives its name. More specifically, paramagnetism describes the tendency of electrons to align with the same spin in the presence of a strong magnetic field. Strongly paramagnetic materials, including transition metals, are usually called ferromagnetic. Transition metals like iron are characterized by a "sea" of electrons moving freely about the surface, which makes it easier for all these electrons to align in one direction. (This electron "sea" is an imprecise model, but good enough for thc MCAT.) It is harder for more stable elements (e.g., oxygen, halogens, noble gases) to align their electrons in one orientation because their orbitals are nearly filled; these substances are known as diamagnetic. This particular problem requires a qualitative assessment of this unknown substance's magnetic properties. The electrons in the figure are aligned in a very regular arrangement, so the surface is either paramagnetic or ferromagnetic. While ferromagnetic substances are also paramagnetic (B), large networks of aligned electrons are characteristic of ferromagnetic compounds only. The individual dipole moments of a diamagnetic substance (C) do not align in any organized pattern.

2. A

The 3d subshell is more stable when full, so it will fill with 10 electrons before any fill the 4s subshell. The 4s subshell then fills later, as it indicates an energy level further from the nucleus. (D) accounts for fewer electrons than those actually present in Zn^{2+}.

3. B

Quantum number ℓ, for angular momentum, cannot be higher than n – 1, ruling out (A). The m_l number, which describes the chemical's magnetic properties, can only be an integer value between $-\ell$ and ℓ, and cannot be equal to 1 if $\ell = 0$, ruling out (C) and (D).

4. C

If you did not know this formula by heart, you can calculate it using your knowledge of the four quantum numbers. For the s shell, the principal quantum number is n = 0; n = 1 for the p shell; and n = 2 for the d shell. (Larger values of n suggest higher energy levels further from the nucleus of the atom, as we know energy is quantized—that is, it differs by discrete amounts—between shells.)

5. B

4l + 2 describes the number of electrons in terms of the azimuthal quantum number l, which ranges from 0 to n – 1, where n is the principal quantum number. (C) resembles the equation which describes the maximum number of electrons in an energy level, which is equal to $2n^2$. Note that this equation is in terms of the principal quantum number n rather than the azimuthal quantum number l.

6. D

Sulfur is diamagnetic, as opposed to ferromagnetic (iron, cobalt) or paramagnetic (hydrogen). Ferromagnetism refers, loosely, to the ability of a surface to attract an external magnetic field. It is characteristic of iron (Fe), from which it derives its name. More specifically, paramagnetism describes the tendency of valence electrons to align with the same spin in the presence of a strong magnetic field. Strongly paramagnetic materials, including transition metals, are usually called ferromagnetic. Transition metals like iron are characterized by a "sea" of electrons moving freely about the surface, which makes it easier for all these electrons to align in one direction. (This electron "sea" is an imprecise model, but good enough for the MCAT.) It is harder for more stable elements (e.g., oxygen, halogens, noble gases) to align their electrons in one orientation because their orbitals are nearly filled; these substances are known as diamagnetic. Sulfur has a similar atomic structure to oxygen, so it is also diamagnetic.

7. D

The problem requires the MCAT favorite equation E = hf, where $h = 6.626 \times 10^{-34}$ (Planck's constant) and f is the frequency of the photon. (Memorize Planck's constant!) One can calculate the frequency of the photon using the provided wavelength, 500 nm, with the equation $f = c/\lambda$, where $c = 3 \times 10^8$ m/s, the speed of light. Here, $f = (3 \times 10^8 \text{ m/s})/500 \times 10^{-9}$ m, or $6 \times 10^{14}\ s^{-1}$ ($1 \text{ Hz} = 1\ s^{-1}$). That leads to E = hf, or $E = (6.626 \times 10^{-34}) \times (6 \times 10^{14} \text{ Hz}) = 3.98 \times 10^{-19}$ J. (Don't worry about memorizing the units of Planck's constant—energy is always in joules). But the problem includes an additional trick, in that the answer must account for a mole of photons. The E = hf equation works for a single photon only. Thus the answer must account for this using Avogadro's number, i.e., 6.022×10^{23} photons. Multiply 3.98×10^{-19} J/photon $\times\ 6.022 \times 10^{23}$ photons = 2.39×10^3 J total.

8. B

(C) and (D) are out of scope. There is not enough information to determine how the velocity of the electron will change. There will be some energy change, however, as the electron must lose energy to return to the minimum energy ground state. That will require emitting radiation in the form of a photon (B). Absorbing a photon (A) is opposite.

9. A

Recall that the superscript (i.e., the A in ^AC) refers to the mass number of an electron, which is equal to the number of protons plus the number of neutrons present in an element. (Sometimes a text will list the atomic number, Z, or total number of protons, under the mass number A.) According to the periodic table, carbon contains 6 protons, i.e., its atomic number Z = 6. An isotope contains the same number of protons and a different number of neutrons as the element. Carbon is most likely to have an atomic number of 12, for 6 protons and 6 neutrons. It cannot have 6 protons and 0 neutrons, or it would likely collapse under the stress of the positive charge. That means (A) is an impossible isotope. (B), (C), and (D) are all possible isotopes, as reflected by the atomic number A of carbon, which is usually reported as just under 13 amu. Carbon-12 and carbon-14 (as in 6 protons, 8 neutrons, the isotope used in carbon-14 radioactive dating) are carbon's most common isotopes.

10. C

Make sure to read the question carefully: (A) and (D) (opposite) violate the Heisenberg uncertainty principle, which states that you cannot know the position and momentum of a particle simultaneously. The Heisenberg uncertainty principle refers explicitly to particle position and momentum, but momentum depends on velocity (recall from Newtonian mechanics that $p = mv$), so you can calculate its momentum and its velocity at the same time. (B), which pairs position and velocity, is a distortion, as a known velocity implies a known momentum.

11. C

Orbital shapes such as that in the figure are derived from a wave function, which estimates the probability that an electron will be found within the illustrated space at a given moment in time. The electron is more likely to be found in its more dense regions of space. Here, it is best to rely on qualitative experience with orbital pictures, though quantum numbers also suggest orbital shape. The s-orbital is spherical, and p-orbitals are like s-orbitals split by a central plane in one dimension (x, y, or z) where no electron will be found. This plane creates an overall lobed or "bowling pin" shape, and is known as a nodal plane (for the node of the wave function, or for "no electron," for MCAT purposes). Two nodal planes in two different directions split the d-orbital, and three nodal planes in three directions split the f-orbital. This image suggests two splits, for four total lobes, indicating a d-orbital.

12. B

If an electron falls from a higher energy level to a lower energy level, it emits a photon of a specific wavelength. That is, the transition emits light energy. That rules out (A) and (D), which are opposite. As an electron moves from $n = 1$ to outer energy levels, there is less difference in the energy levels. In other words, there is a larger energy difference between $n = 2$ and $n = 3$ than there is between $n = 3$ and $n = 4$. Though the transition in (C) would absorb energy, the transition in (B) would require absorbing more energy because it must compensate for a larger energy difference.

13. A

The MCAT covers qualitative topics from the Atomic Structure unit more often than its quantitative topics. It is critical to be able to distinguish the fundamental principles that determine electron organization, which are usually known by the name of the scientist who discovered them. The Heisenberg uncertainty principle (B) refers to the momentum and position of a single electron, and the Bohr model (C) was an early attempt to describe the behavior of the single electron in a hydrogen atom. (D) is a tempting distortion, but (A) is more complete. Nitrogen, the smallest element with half-filled p subshell, is often used as an example of Hund's rule in general chemistry textbooks. Hund's rule is really a corollary of the Pauli exclusion principle, in that the Pauli exclusion principle suggests that each orbital contains two electrons of opposite spin. Additional electrons must fill new orbitals so the compound remains stable in its ground state.

14. C

The Thomson model (1904) was the early "plum pudding" idea of the atom. The Rutherford model (1911) is most like the stick and ball drawings familiar from nuclear physics (or biohazard symbols). The Bohr model of the hydrogen atom came later in the early 20th century and accounted for quantized energy levels. A basic understanding of the chronology of atomic theory will increase your understanding of the underlying physical principles that the MCAT will likely test.

15. A

This problem requires distinguishing the atomic number from the mass number. Here, the mass number is equal to the number of protons plus the number of neutrons. Usually the number of neutrons is calculated by subtracting the atomic number, or the number of protons listed on the periodic table, from the mass number. If the atom is uncharged, the number of protons is the same as the number of electrons. A Cs^{+} cation has one fewer electron than the uncharged species. Here it is simplest to use the atomic number from the periodic table, 55, and subtract one, for a total of 54 electrons. (A) is the uncharged species, (C) is the number of neutrons, and (D) is the mass number.

16. B

Set up a system of two algebraic equations, where x and y are the percentages of H (mass = 1 amu) and D (mass = 2 amu) respectively. Your setup should look like the following:

$x + y = 1$ (proportion H(x) + proportion D(y) in whole, i.e., $x\% + y\% = 100\%$)

$1x + 2y = 1.008$ (the total atomic mass).

Substitute one variable for the other so the atomic mass is in terms of one variable (e.g., $1 - y = x$), then solve for the other percentage ($[1 - y] + 2y = 1.008$; simplifies to $0.008 = y$, or 0.8% D). That, plus 99.2% H makes 100%. These isotope calculations are straightforward if you have memorized the method, so they are an MCAT favorite. Remember to convert from proportions to percentages.

17. A

The answer choices refer to the magnetic spin of the two electrons. The quantum number m_s repre-sents this property, as a measure of the electrons' relative intrinsic angular momentum. These electrons' spins are parallel, in that their spins are aligned in the same direction (i.e., $m_s = +½$ for both species. This implies that (B) and (C) are opposite. They would suppose that $m_s = +½$ for one electron and $-½$ for the other. Paired (D) refers to electrons of opposite spin in the same orbital.

18. B

Cr, Fe^{2+}, and Co^{3+} all have 24 total electrons. They are isoelectronic, in that they have the same number of total electrons. Under standard electron configuration rules, this total might suggest an overall configuration $1s^22s^22p^63s^23p^64s^23d^4$. In fact, the 3d subshell fills first, as it is lower in energy than the 4s subshell, so the configuration is actually more like $[Ar]4s^03d^6$. In fact, this arrangement is not precise in the case of Cr. (Keep in mind that electron configuration is an imprecise atomic model.) If the subshells are "filling up," the 3d shell attains maximum stability if it is half-filled with 5 unpaired d electrons of parallel spin (Hund's rule). In rare cases, one and only one electron is "promoted" to achieve maximum stability in the orbitals, i.e., $[Ar]4s^13d^5$. For the isoelectronic cations, electrons are actually removed from previously filled larger neutral atomic species. Neutral Fe has 26 electrons, or $[Ar]4s^03d^8$, and Co has 27, or $[Ar]4s^03d^9$. You cannot promote one electron in either of these atomic arrangements and benefit from Hund's rule in the 3d subshell. Thus, its valence electrons "stay put," so to speak, where they already are. For Fe^{2+} and Co^{3+}, this means that the configuration is actually $[Ar]4s^03d^6$, While Mn^{+} is isoelectronic to the other answer choices, it is actually extremely unlikely in nature; Mn^{2+} and Mn^{4+} are far more common. Neutral Mn is $[Ar]4s^03d^7$, which makes Mn^{2+}, or $[Ar]4s^03d^5$, unusually stable, and Mn^{+}, or $[Ar]4s^03d^6$ unstable. (You cannot promote if you are removing electrons to form cations, only if you are "filling up.") Electron configuration in the transition metals can be confusing, but is essential practice for Test Day.

19. D

Electrons are assumed to be in motion in any energy level, even in the ground state. The electron's principal quantum number, or energy level, is n = 1. It must be an integer value in both the ground and excited states. This number gives a relative indication of the electron's distance from the nucleus, so it must have the smallest radius of all the energy levels. The further the electron moves from the nucleus, the greater energy it needs to overcome its attractive forces.

20. C

High pressure is unlikely to excite an electron out of the ground state unless it causes an extreme change in temperature, which would add enough energy to the system to promote the electron.

CHAPTER 2: THE PERIODIC TABLE

1. B

First recall that the periodic table is organized with periods (rows) and groups (columns). This method of organization allows elements to be organized such that some chemical properties can be predicted based on an element's position in the table. Groups (columns) are particularly significant because they represent sets of elements with the same outer electron configuration. In other words, all elements within the same group will have the same configuration of *valence electrons*, which in turn will dictate many of the chemical properties of those similar elements. Although (A) is true, it does not explain the similarity in chemical properties as effectively as (B); most other metals—similar to lithium and sodium or not—produce positively-charged ions. (C) is not true, because periods are rows and lithium and sodium are in the same column. Finally, although lithium and sodium have relatively low atomic weights (D), their chemical properties are better explained by their valence electron configurations.

2. A

This question assesses understanding of a key periodic trend: atomic radii. As one moves from left to right across a period (row), atomic radii decrease. This occurs because, as more protons are added to the nucleus and more electrons are added within the same shell, there is no increased shielding between the protons and electrons (though there is increased attractive electrostatic force). This effect decreases the atomic radius. In contrast, as one moves from top to bottom down a group (column), extra electron shells have accumulated, despite the fact that the valence configurations remain identical. These extra electron shells provide shielding between the positive nucleus and the outermost electrons, decreasing the electrostatic forces and increasing the atomic radius. Because carbon and silicon are in the same group, and silicon is further down the period table, it will have a larger atomic radius because of its extra electron shell. (C) and (D) are incorrect because all elements in the same group have the same number of valence electrons.

3. C

The number of valence electrons (item I) does have an impact on the atomic radius. As one moves across a period (row) and valence electrons are added, along with protons in the atom's nucleus, the electrons are more strongly attracted to the central protons. This attraction tightens the atom, shrinking the atomic radius. The number of electron shells is also significant, as demonstrated by the trend when moving down a group (column). As more electron shells (item II) are added which separate the positively charged nucleus from the outermost electrons, the electrostatic forces are weakened and the atomic radius increases. The number of neutrons (item III) is irrelevant.

4. C

Ionization energy is related to the same set of forces that explain atomic radius, as well as the rules governing maintenance of a full valence shell octet. The first set of rules dictates that the stronger the attractive forces between the outer electron (the electron to be ionized) and the positively charged nucleus, the more energy will be required to ionize. As a result, strong attractive forces, which make the atomic radius smaller toward the right of a period or the top of a group, will also increase the first ionization energy. With this information alone, one could guess that the ionization energy for beryllium (Be) should be higher than that for Li (lithium), eliminating (C) and (D). Secondly, the first ionization energy is always lower than the second ionization energy. This property holds true for the same reasons previously discussed. For example, once removing one electron from beryllium, the ion is Be^{+1}, which has one more proton in its nucleus than it has electrons surrounding it. Thus, there is a heightened electrostatic force between the positive nucleus and the now less-negative electron cloud, meaning that all remaining electrons will be held more tightly than that first electron. Removing a second electron will be more difficult than the initial electron removal, making the second ionization energy higher than the first. To quantify these differences, the first ionization energy for Li is 520.2 kJ/mol, the first ionization energy for Be is 899.5 kJ/mol, and the second ionization energy for Be is 1757.1 kJ/mol.

5. D

Selenium is to the right of the diagonal line that separates metals and nonmetals, but it is not adjacent to this line and thus is not a metalloid. In its period, Ge is the rightmost metal, while As is a metalloid. Se is the only nonmetal in the fourth period, and to its right is the halogen, Br. Alkali metals are in the first column, Group IA, of which Se is not a member.

6. C

The trend in the periodic table demonstrated by the figure is correct for increasing electronegativity and first ionization energy. Electronegativity describes how strong of an attraction an element will have for electrons in a bond. A nucleus with a stronger electrostatic pull due to its positive charge will have a higher electronegativity; this is represented with an arrow pointing right because nuclear charge increases toward the right side of a period. This mirrors the trend for ionization energies, since a stronger nuclear pull will also lead to an increased first ionization energy (the forces make it more difficult to remove an electron). The vertical arrow can be explained by the size of the atoms. As size decreases, the proximity of the outermost electrons to the positive inner nucleus increases, making the positive charge more effective at attracting new electrons in a chemical bond; this leads to higher electronegativity. Similarly, the more effective the positive nuclear charge, the higher the first ionization energy. Thus, items I and III follow the trends. Atomic radius (item II) follows the opposite trend.

7. C

Although metals have high melting points (D), the most significant property contributing to their ability to conduct electricity is the fact that they have valence electrons that can move freely (C). Metals have large atomic radii and low ionization energies, as well as low electronegativity, all of which contribute to the ability of their outermost electrons to be easily removed. Because electricity is carried by currents of electrons, this free movement of outer electrons is the most important characteristic in making them good conductors. Although it is important that metals are malleable (A) and maybe even more important that they have ductility (they can be easily made into wires), (C) is still the best answer explaining their ability to conduct electricity effectively.

8. B

This group of elements—the alkaline earth metals—is chemically important because its constituents form divalent cations, or ions with a +2 charge. All of the elements in Group IIA have two electrons in their outermost *s* orbital, making their outermost shell have much less than a complete octet. Because loss of these two electrons would then leave a full octet as the outermost shell, becoming a divalent cation is a stable configuration for all of the alkaline earth metals. Although some of these elements might have metallic properties, including conduction, the best conductors in the periodic table are the metals, not Group IIA, so (A) is incorrect. (C) is incorrect because, although forming a divalent cation is a stable configuration for the alkaline earths, the second ionization energy is still always higher than the first due to the increased positive nuclear charge when compared with the outer negative charge from the electrons. (D) is incorrect because atomic radii increase when moving down a group of elements since the number of electron shells increases.

9. C

A few of the solutions are simple to eliminate. Both aluminum and silicon are in the third period, so (A) is incorrect. Silicon is a metalloid while aluminum is a metal (D); in the periodic table, they're on opposite sides of the diagonal line that separates these two groups of elements. Both (B) and (C) are true; however, (C) better describes the difference in reactivity. Metalloids are an unusual set of elements within the periodic table with widely varying physical and chemical properties, which make them definitively different from the elements to their left (the metals) and those to the right (the nonmetals). The metalloids can have widely different densities, boiling points, melting points, appearance, and conductivities. Additionally, many of the metalloids will react differently with different elements and have chemical properties quite different from elements nearby in the periodic table.

10. C

First eliminate (B) and (D) because they represent the notation for periods, not groups. All groups are named with Roman numerals and then use the letters A or B to indicate whether they are representative elements (s or p as outermost orbitals) or nonrepresentative elements (d- or f- orbitals outermost). Next, the correct trend for increasing electronegativity moves from left to right across the periodic table, making (C) correct. This trend occurs because, when moving to the right across the periodic table, electrons are added to the same outermost valence shell, and protons are added to the nucleus. Because there are no new electron shells between the nucleus and the outer electrons, there is no increase in shielding when moving across the periodic table. This means that there is now a stronger electrostatic force between the positive nucleus and the negative outermost electrons, which decreases the atomic radius and increases the attractive forces for new electrons.

11. B

Iron, Fe^{2+}, is a transition metal. Transition metals can often form more than one ion—iron, for example, can be Fe^{2+} or Fe^{3+}. The transition metals, in these multiple different states, can often form hydration complexes, or complexes with water. Part of the significance of these complexes is that when a transition metal can form a complex, its solubility within this complexed solvent will increase.

Although other ions, such as (A) or (C), can dissolve readily in water, they do not typically form complexes with water. S^{2-} (D) is not a transition metal, so it is unlikely to form a complex with water.

12. D

This question is simple if you recall that periods are the horizontal rows of the periodic table, while columns are the vertical groupings. Within one period, an additional valence electron is added with each step toward the right side of the table (D).

13. B

This question requires knowledge of the trends of electronegativity within the periodic table. Electronegativity increases as one moves from left to right across periods, i.e., when protons are added to the nucleus and additional electrons are added to the same valence shell. Electronegativity *decreases* as one moves down the periodic table, because there are more electron shells separating the nucleus from the outermost electrons. The noble gases, however, also have extremely low electronegative since they already have full valence shells and do not have an affinity for holding on to additional electrons. The most electronegative atom in the periodic table is fluoride. Remembering this fact will guide you to recall the electronegativity trend, and might help you quickly identify the answer choice closest in proximity to fluoride. (B) chlorine is the most electronegative here. Though I (D) will be fairly electronegative, its higher atomic radius and position further down on the periodic table makes it less electronegative than Cl. Mg and Li (A) and (C) are elements with very low electronegativity; because they have only two and one valence electrons, respectively, they are more likely to lose these electrons in a bond than to gain electrons, since the loss of electrons would leave them with a full octet. This propensity to lose/not hold tightly electrons in a bond defines low electronegativity.

14. B

Electron affinity is related to several factors, including atomic size (radius) and filling of the valence shell. As atomic radius increases, the distance between the inner protons in the nucleus and the outermost electrons increases, thereby decreasing the attractive forces between protons and electrons. Additionally, as more electron shells are added from period to period, these shells shield the outermost electrons increasingly from inner protons. As a result, increased atomic radius will lead to lower electron affinity. Since atoms are in a low-energy state when their outermost valence electron shell is filled, atoms needing only 1–2 electrons to complete this shell will have high electron affinities. In contrast, atoms with already full valence shells—with a full octet of eight electrons—will have very low electron affinity since adding an extra electron would require a new shell. It is clear that (C) and (D) will likely have lower electron affinities than (A) and (B) because there is an extra electron shell "shielding" the nucleus from the outer electrons. (A)'s valence electron shell is already full with a complete octet, granting it extremely low electron affinity. (B) has one electron missing from its outermost shell, as does (D). This valence electron configuration is conducive to wanting to accept electrons readily or to having a high electron affinity. (B) is the configuration of chlorine, while (D) is bromine. (B) is a better answer than (D), however, because the additional shell of electrons shielding the nucleus in (D) will decrease its electron affinity when compared with (B).

15. C

Electronegativity is a property that describes an atom's attraction for bonding electrons. Highly electronegative atoms pull bonding electrons closely; atoms with low electronegativity, meanwhile, hold bonding electrons loosely. In an atom with a large atomic radius, the distance between the outermost electrons, used in bonding, and the central nucleus with a positive charge, is large. This increased distance means that the positively charged nucleus has little ability to attract new, bonding electrons toward it. In comparison, if the atomic radius is small, the force from the positively charged protons will have a stronger effect, because the distance through which they have to act is decreased. Atomic radius decreases when moving from left to right across periods in the periodic table (A). Atomic radius alone does not give enough information for one to ascertain the second ionization energy (B); it is significant to also consider the valence electron configuration. Finally, there is insufficient information for (D).

16. D

The effective nuclear charge refers to the strength with which the protons in the nucleus can "pull" additional electrons. The effective nuclear charge helps to explain electron affinity, electronegativity, and ionization energy. In Cl, the nonionized chlorine atom, the nuclear charge is balanced by the surrounding electrons, so without knowing the exact number, it is balanced: $17^+/17^-$. The chloride ion, in contrast, has a lower effective nuclear charge, because there are more electrons than protons: $17^+/18^-$. Next, elemental potassium also has a "balanced" effective nuclear charge: $19^+/19^-$. Finally, K^+, ionic potassium, has a higher effective nuclear charge than any of the other choices, because it has more protons than electrons: $19^+/18^-$. Thus, the potassium ion (D) is the correct answer.

17. D

Ionic bonds are bonds formed through unequal sharing of electrons. These bonds typically occur because the electron affinities of the two bonded atoms differ greatly. For example, the halogens have a high electron affinity because adding a single electron to their valence shell would create a full outer octet. In contrast, the alkaline earth metals have a very low electron affinity and are more likely to be electron donors because the loss of one electron would leave them with a full outer octet. This marked difference in electron affinity is the best explanation for the formation of ionic bonds between these two different groups. Because the halogens have high electron affinity and the alkaline earth metals have low affinity, so (A) is incorrect, as is (B) because in ionic bonding electrons are not shared equally. Although (C) is correct because atomic radius decreases when moving to the right across a period, this is not the best explanation for formation of ionic bonds.

18. C

In the first period, all elements have only an s-orbital. Beginning in the second period, elements have a 2s- and a 2p-orbital. In the third period, there are 3s-, 3p-, and 3d-orbitals. However, the 3d-orbital is not filled until the fourth period of the table, in which one encounters the first set of transition elements. Despite the fact that it is unfilled in the third period, these elements still have a 3d-orbital, and some elements utilized unfilled spaces in this orbital for bonding.

19. D

Transition metals such as silver have the ability to form different types of complexes, including hydration complexes with water and complexes with other compounds. Formation of a complex with the transition metal ion will increase the ability of the solute to dissolve into solution. Because the AgBr does not dissolve readily in beaker A, it is unlikely that any complex is being formed. Even if a complex were being formed in that beaker, it has minimal, if any, effect on dissolving AgBr and thus does not explain the phenomenon observed. (A) is incorrect. However, because AgBr dissolves more quickly in beaker B, it is reasonable to consider that silver could form a complex with the solvent, ammonia

(D). Though there might be hydrogen bonding between water and bromide, (C), this would not explain why beaker A dissolves more slowly than B. (B) is irrelevant; the type of bond between Ag and Br would be the same in both beakers and would not explain the different rates of dissolution between the two beakers.

CHAPTER 3: BONDING AND CHEMICAL INTERACTIONS

1. B

Carbon monoxide, CO, has a double bond between carbon and oxygen, with the carbon retaining one lone pair, and oxygen retaining two lone pairs. The most important thing to know here is the definition of a polar covalent bond. This type of bond forms when the difference in electronegativity between two bonded atoms is great enough to cause electrons to move disproportionately toward the more electronegative atom, but not great enough to form an ionic bond. This is the case for CO. Oxygen is more electronegative than CO, and thus will cause a polarity of the bond, with the negative charge disproportionately carried on the oxygen, leaving the carbon atom slightly positive. The bond is not ionic, because this type of bond happens with large differences in electronegativity, typically between atoms in the first 1 or 2 columns of the periodic table when bonded to atoms like halogens. Nonpolar covalent bonds occur when there is no difference in electronegativity between the two bonded atoms, such as the carbon-carbon bond in CH_3–CH_3. Coordinate covalent bonding occurs when a Lewis acid and Lewis base bond through donation of a lone pair from Lewis base to Lewis acid.

2. B

Here you must understand the contribution of resonance structures to average formal charge. In (B) CO_3^{2-}, there are three possible resonance structures. Each of the three oxygen atoms carries a formal charge of –1 in two out of the three structures. This averages to approximately –2/3 charge on each oxygen atom, which is more than that in any of the other answer choices. To prove this, we can estimate the formal charges on each oxygen atom in (A), (C), and (D). There are no formal charges in H_2O, which has no resonance structures. In ozone, O_3, there are two possible resonance structures. The central oxygen carries a positive charge in both structures, and each outer oxygen carries a negative charge in one of the two possible resonance structures. This leaves an average charge of –1/2 on the two outer oxygens, which is less than the –2/3 in CO_3^{2-}. Finally, CH_2O has no resonance structures and therefore no formal charge on oxygen.

3. C

The two most important contributing resonance structures are items I and II. Resonance structures are representations of how charges are shared across a molecule. In reality, the charge distribution is an average of contributing resonance structures. The most stable resonance structures are those that minimize charge on the atoms in the molecule; the more stable the structure, the more it will contribute to the overall charge distribution in the molecule. Both structures in I and II have one negative charge on one of the two oxygens, and one positive charge on the central nitrogen atom. Structure III would not be an important resonance structure because it distributes two negative charges, one on each oxygen atom, and two positive charges, both on the nitrogen atom. Due to this distribution of formal charges, it is a less stable configuration and thus not an important resonance structure for NO_2.

4. E

The key to answering this question is to understand the types of intermolecular forces that occur in each of these molecules. Kr (III) is a noble gas, so the only IMFs present are dispersion forces (also called London forces), which are the weakest type of IMFs. This means that these molecules are held together extremely loosely, and will be the easiest to transition from the organized liquid phase to the disorganized gaseous phase, because they are not held tightly together. Acetone (I) is a polar molecule, and as such it has the benefit of dipole-dipole forces, which are stronger than dispersion forces. In dipole-dipole forces, these polar molecules will be arranged such that the positive and negative ends of molecules associate with each other, holding these molecules more closely together than in nonpolar compounds. Next, the intermolecular forces present in isopropyl alcohol (IV) include hydrogen bonding. In hydrogen bonding, an electronegative atom (i.e., oxygen or nitrogen) is bound to hydrogen, and the highly electronegative atom strips hydrogen of its electrons, leaving hydrogen as a predominantly positive atom, allowing it to interact with nearby partial negative charges. These forces are even stronger than dipole-dipole interactions. Finally, the strongest interaction is a compound with an ionic bond, such as potassium chloride (II). In this compound, the intermolecular forces are so strong that they have formed an ionic bond between two atoms with disparate electronegativities; this type of molecule would have the highest boiling point.

5. C

First check each atom involved to be sure that it follows electron configurations as you would expect. Each of the fluorides should have a full octet, including three lone pairs on each fluoride, with one shared pair bonding the fluoride to the central chloride. All of these are correct. If the chloride did not have any lone pairs, it would have a formal charge of +3. Because chloride is in the third period, all elements in or beyond the third period have d-orbitals, which can accommodate extra electrons. Thus, by adding two pairs of electrons as lone pairs on the central chloride, the central chloride will end up with: FC = 7 – ½(8) – 4 = –1, a formal charge of negative one, by following the equation:

Formal charge = V (valence electrons in the free atom) $-\frac{1}{2}$ $N_{bonding}$ (electrons shared in bonds) – $N_{nonbonding}$ (lone pairs/free electrons)

Because all the fluoride atoms have formal charges of zero, the entire molecule must have a charge of –1.

6. C

The central atom in CO_3, carbon, has no lone pairs. It has three resonance structures with each of its bonds to oxygen, thus carrying partial double-bond character, and it has no further orbitals used for bonding or use for carrying lone pairs. This makes CO_3's geometry trigonal planar. Alternatively, ClF_3 also has three bonds, one to each of three fluoride atoms. However, chloride still maintains two extra lone pairs (without which the formal charge on the central chloride atom is +4; with the two lone pairs it is zero, a more stable configuration). These lone pairs each inhabit one orbital, meaning that the central chloride must organize five items about itself: three bonds to fluorides and two lone pairs. The best configuration for maximizing the distance between all of these groups is trigonal bipyramidal. Although (A) and (B) are true, they do not account for the difference in geometry. (D) is incorrect; CO_3 has no lone pairs on its central atom, while ClF_3 has two lone pairs.

7. A

Try drawing the structure of each of these molecules and then considering the electronegativity of each bond as it might contribute to an overall dipole moment. HCN (A) is correct because it is linear in structure, and nitrogen is more electronegative than carbon, which is more electronegative than hydrogen. This would cause a strong dipole moment in the direction of the nitrogen, with the strongest delta-minus charge over the nitrogen atom. H_2O is bent, and oxygen is more electronegative than hydrogen, thus creating a dipole moment in the direction of the two oxygen atoms. However, due to the bent configuration, the dipole moment is of a smaller magnitude than that of HCN. Sulfur dioxide has a similar bent configuration, and has even less of a difference in electronegativity between sulfur and oxygen than that of the hydrogen and oxygen atoms in water. Thus, SO_2 (D) does not exceed the dipole moment of HCN. CCl_4 (C) has a tetrahedral geometry, so while each individual C–Cl bond is polarized, with the more electronegative chloride atom carrying the slightly negative charge, the orientation of these bonds causes the polarizations to cancel each other out, yielding no overall dipole moment.

8. D

Bond lengths decrease as the bond order increases, and they also decrease in a trend moving up the periodic table's columns or to the right across the rows. In this case, because both C_2H_2 and NCH have triple bonds, we cannot compare the bond lengths based upon bond order. We must rely on one of the other two periodic trends. Bond length decreases when moving to the right along rows because more electronegative atoms have shorter radii as a result of their increased electronegativity. The nitrogen in NCH is likely to hold its electrons closer, in a shorter radius, than the second carbon in C_2H_2. (A) is incorrect; a bond between similar atoms is longer than a bond between two different atoms. (B) is incorrect; there are no significant resonance structures contributing to the character of either triple bond. (C) is incorrect because although carbon is more electronegative than hydrogen, the C–H bond is not the triple bond and thus makes little, if any, contribution to the length of the carbon-carbon triple bond.

9. C

When hydrogen bonds to a strongly electronegative atom such as nitrogen or oxygen, the electronegative atom disproportionately pulls the shared pair in the covalent bond toward itself. Because hydrogen has no lone pairs, the movement of the shared pair further away from the center of the hydrogen atom leaves the hydrogen atom with a partial positive character. This allows the hydrogen atom to have strong interactions—hydrogen bonds—with nearby negative or partial-negative charges. (A) is not true; hydrogen has little electronegativity and does not hold its valence electrons closely. (B) is true, and the fact that hydrogen has no lone pairs is somewhat relevant to the character of hydrogen bonding, though this doesn't explain as well as (C) the forces of hydrogen bonding. (D) is not correct; although these bonds are highly polarized, they are not ionic.

10. D

First you must recall that ammonium is NH_4^+, while ammonia (commonly confused) is NH_3. It helps to associate the suffix *-ium* with a charged form of the molecule. Once you remember that ammonium is NH_4^+, you can eliminate all of the answer choices that refer to three—not four—bonds (A) and (C). Next, it helps to recall that ammonium is formed by the association of NH_3 (uncharged, with a lone pair on the nitrogen) with a positively charge hydrogen cation (no lone pairs). In other words, NH_3 is a Lewis base, while H^+ is a Lewis acid. This type of bonding between Lewis acid and base is a coordinate covalent bond. Thus, we know that there is one coordinate covalent bond in this molecule, making (D) the answer. You can confirm this by knowing that there are three polar covalent bonds in NH_3, each between nitrogen and hydrogen, because nitrogen is more electronegative than hydrogen. (B) is incorrect because the final bond between N–H in NH_4^+ is a coordinate covalent bond, not a polar covalent bond.

11. D

All atoms in the third period and above in the periodic table have d-orbitals, which can hold extra electrons. They are not limited by the typical eight valence electrons of s- and p-orbitals, which hold two and six electrons, respectively. The octet rule can also be violated by having subvalent atoms, as with hydrogen or boron atoms, both of which are typically surrounded by fewer than eight electrons. (A) and (B) are irrelevant. (C) recognizes that an extra orbital can allow expansion, but the f-orbitals are not primarily responsible for expansion beyond the octet.

12. C

All of the listed types of forces dictate interactions among different types of molecules. However, noble gases are entirely uncharged, without polar covalent bonds, ionic bonds, or dipole moments. The only listed forces which could relate to noble gases could be (A) van der Waals or (C) dispersion. Of these two, van der Waals is a more general name for both dispersion and dipole-dipole interactions, whereas dispersion refers specifically to a type of interaction which occurs among all bonded atoms due to the unequal sharing of electrons at any given moment in the electron's orbit. Therefore, without even understanding how these forces relate to phase change, you should be able to appreciate that (C) is most likely correct. More specifically, dispersion forces result from the fact that spinning electrons at any given moment in time are shared unequally between the two atoms between which they form a bond. This unequal sharing allows for instantaneous partial positive and partial negative charges within the molecule, allowing some of the partial charges to provide attraction to their opposite partial charges on nearby molecules. Without these interactions, although small, there would be no attraction at all between molecules of noble gases. Without any attraction, noble gases would be unable to liquefy. Thus, you have confirmed that (C) is in fact correct.

13. B

The key to this question is to understand the pattern of filling for s- and d-orbitals among the transition metals. The d-orbitals will fill first, with one electron in each of the 5 d-orbitals (one of each spin type). After there is one electron in each of the 5 d-orbitals, it takes less energy to put the next electron into the s-orbital than it would to add the same electron to one of the d-orbitals that is already inhabited. Thus, first the d-orbitals will fill for the first five electrons, followed by the sixth electron going into the higher-energy s-orbital, and then the filling of the d-orbitals will continue one at a time. For chromium, atomic number 24, the shorthand allows for designation of the preceding noble gas configuration for Argon (Ar – 18). The next orbitals to be filled for chromium, in the fourth row, are the 3 d-orbitals, up to its first five electrons, with the final electron going into the 4s1 position.

14. A

In this Lewis diagram, the PO_4^{3-} molecule has an overall formal charge of –3. The four oxygens each would be assigned a formal change of –1, based on the following formula:

formal charge = V (valence electrons in the free atom) $-\frac{1}{2}$ $N_{bonding}$ (electrons shared in bonds) – $N_{nonbonding}$ (lone pairs/free electrons).

For each oxygen we calculate: FC = 6 $-\frac{1}{2}$ (2) – 6 = –1. For the central phosphorus, we can assume that with a total formal charge of -3 and four oxygens with a charge of –1 each, the phosphorus must have a formal charge of +1. Alternatively, one could calculate its formal charge:

$$FC = 5 - \frac{1}{2}(8) - 0 = +1$$

Finally, this molecule is actually more complex than the drawn Lewis diagram; it has multiple resonance structures, in each of which the phosphorus forms a double bond with one oxygen, giving that oxygen atom and the central phosphorus each a formal charge of zero. There are four such resonance structures. Thus, the oxygens in fact have formal charges between –1 (in four out of the five structures) and zero (in the one favorable configuration in which it shares a double bond), while the phosphorus has a charge of zero in four out of five of the configurations and a change of +1 in one configuration. This further corroborates that the central phosphorus has the most positive formal charge. It is clear that the atoms do not share the charge equally (B), nor do the four oxygens share the highest charge (C) (they actually share the lowest (most negative) charge). The geometry of this molecule is not trigonal pyramidal, but rather tetrahedral (D).

15. D

Calcium chloride is a molecule formed by ionic bonding. Ionic bonding is a very strong type of bond, with strong intermolecular and electrostatic forces. As a result, ionic compounds have very high melting and boiling points due to the amount of energy required to break down these high-energy interactions. (A) is incorrect; covalent compounds would be more likely to have low boiling points. These electrostatic forces also cause liquid and aqueous states of ionic compounds to be good conductors of electricity, the opposite of (B) and (C). A covalent compound, alternatively, would not conduct electricity in the liquid or aqueous states. Finally, although ionic compounds can conduct electricity well in both the liquid and aqueous phases, they form strong crystal lattices in the solid state, matching positive and negative charges on adjacent molecules, making them poor conductors of electricity in the solid state.

16. C

The reaction in this question shows a water molecule, which has two lone pairs of electrons on the central oxygen, combining with a free hydrogen ion, without any outer electrons. The resulting molecule, H_3O^+, has formed a new bond between H^+ and H_2O. This bond is formed by sharing one of the lone pairs on the oxygen with the free H^+ ion. This is essentially a donation of a shared pair of electrons from a Lewis base (H_2O) to a Lewis acid (H^+, electron acceptor). The charge in the resulting molecule is +1, and is mostly present on the central oxygen, which now only has one lone pair and three shared pairs in bonds, resulting in only five valence electrons. This type of bond, formed from a Lewis acid and Lewis base, is called a coordinate covalent bond. Although this bond is formed between a hydrogen atom and an oxygen atom, (D) is not as good a selection as (C).

17. B

NH_3 has three hydrogen atoms bonded to the central nitrogen, and one lone pair on the central nitrogen. These four groups—three atoms, one lone pair—lead NH_3 to be sp^3 hybridized. By hybridizing all three p-orbitals and the one s-orbital, four groups are arranged about the central atom, maximizing the distance between the groups to minimize the energy of the configuration. This property of NH_3's hybridization leads to its tetrahedral geometry. In contrast, BF_3 has three atoms, but no lone pairs, leading to sp^2 hybridization. This hybridization leads to a trigonal planar geometry. (A) is incorrect; although BF_3 has three bonded atoms and no lone pairs, its geometry is trigonal planar not pyramidal. Although NH_3 has one lone pair (C), that does not provide a strong explanation for the geometrical differences between the two molecules. Although (D) is true, the polarity of the molecules does not explain their geometry; rather, the molecules' different geometries contribute to the overall polarity of the molecules.

18. B

Beryllium is an unusual element in that it does not obey the octet rule. Most atoms require that they have eight outer electrons—the "octet rule." However, some atoms can have fewer than eight valence electrons (sub-octet) or more than eight outer electrons. Beryllium, like hydrogen, boron, and aluminum, can have fewer than eight outer electrons. As a result, when bonding with chloride, beryllium is likely to form only two bonds, using its own two outer valence electrons and one from each chloride to form $BeCl_2$, as drawn in (B). (A) completes the octet for beryllium with two lone pairs, which would be a much less likely configuration. Similarly, (C) and (D) complete beryllium's octet inappropriately. (D) is even less correct because there are too many electrons around each chloride—10 each, due to the double bonds— and chloride should not exceed the octet rule.

19. B

This question requires an understanding of the trends that cause higher or lower bond energies. Bonds of high energy are those that are difficult to break. These bonds tend to have more shared pairs of electrons, and thus cause a stronger attraction between the two atoms in the bonds, which is described in (B). This stronger attraction also means that the bond length of a high-energy, high-order bond (i.e., triple bond) is shorter than that of its lower-energy counterparts (i.e., single or double bonds). (A) is incorrect; bond energy increases with *decreasing* bond length. A high-energy bond, i.e., a triple bond, requires more energy to be broken; thus (C) is incorrect.

20. A

Polarity is dependent on the vector sum of dipole moments. Dipole moments describe the relationship of shared electrons between two bonded atoms. If there is a dipole moment between two atoms, then the electrons in their shared bond are preferentially centered on one atom (typically the more electronegative of the two). For example, in a carbon-nitrogen bond, the dipole moment would be in the direction of the nitrogen atom, indicating that it has a partial negative charge. The polarity of a molecule is then defined as the vector sum of these dipole moments in the molecule's three-dimensional configuration. For example, although individual carbon-chloride bonds have dipole moments with a partial negative charge on chloride, the molecule CCl_4 has a tetrahedral configuration and thus the three polarized bonds cancel each other out for no net dipole moment, creating a nonpolar molecule. (B) is incorrect since molecular geometry is an essential aspect of determining molecular polarity. It is possible for a molecule to contain at least one nonpolar bond and yet be a polar molecule (D). $CH\text{–}_3Cl$, for example, has three non-polar bonds (C–H bonds) and one polar bond. In its tetrahedral arrangement, the one polar bond between C–Cl will have a dipole moment, creating a net polarity of the molecule in the direction of the chloride atom.

HIGH-YIELD SIMILAR QUESTIONS

Melting Points

1. Alkanes with even numbers of carbons.
2. Neopentane will melt higher, because of its greater symmetry.
3. Phenol will melt higher

Boiling Points

1. Eliminate the alcohol's ability to be a hydrogen bond donor by alkylating the oxygen to produce an ether.

2. Displace the chlorine with water or ammonia to give an alcohol or amine, respectively.

CHAPTER 4: COMPOUNDS AND STOICHIOMETRY

1. D

Ionic compounds are comprised of atoms held together by ionic bonds. Ionic bonds associate charged particles with very different electronegativities, for example, sodium (Na^+) with chloride (Cl^-). In ionic bonds, "shared" electrons are disproportionately located on the more electronegative atom. These bonds are different in character from covalent bonds, which result in an equal sharing of electrons between two atoms. As a result, ionic compounds are not formed from true molecules, as are covalent compounds. (A) and (B) describe covalent compounds; their smallest unit is a molecule, which is typically described in terms of molecular weight and moles. In contrast, ionic compounds are made of three-dimensional arrays of their charged particles, as indicated in (D). Ionic compounds do not share electrons equally (C); equal sharing occurs in covalent bonds.

2. A

Of the compounds listed, only (A) and (C) are ionic compounds, which are measured in "formula weight." (B) and (D) are covalent compounds and thus measured in "molecular weight." When estimating the formula weight for the above compounds, (A) is potassium (39.0983) plus chloride (35.453), which has a total weight of 74.551, which is correctly between 74 and 75. Although (B) is also between 74 and 75 (4 carbons: $4 \times 12.0107 = 48.028$ plus 10 hydrogens: $10 \times 1.00794 = 10.0794$ plus one oxygen (15.994) equals a total of 74.101), this is a covalent compound. Moreover, this would be its molecular weight, not its formula weight.

3. B

It is helpful to know the molecular weight of one mole of H_2SO_4, which is found by adding the molecular weight of the atoms that constitute the molecule: 2 × (molecular weight of hydrogen) + 1 × (molecular weight of sulfur) + 4 × (molecular weight of oxygen) = $2 \times 1.00794 + 32.065 + 4 \times 15.9994 = 98.078$. Next, you must understand what "gram-equivalent weight" means. Gram equivalent weight is equal to the molar mass of a compound divided by the number of hydrogens used per molecule, which for H_2SO_4 is two hydrogens per molecule. Thus, the gram equivalent weight is simply 98.078 g/mole divided by two, or 49.039 g/mole.

4. C

An empirical formula is a formula that represents a molecule with the simplest ratio, in whole numbers, of the atoms/elements comprising the compounds. In this case, given the empirical formula CH, any molecule with carbon and hydrogen atoms in a 1:1 ratio would be accurately represented by this empirical formula. Benzene, C_6H_6 (A) and ethyne, C_2H_2 (B), and (D) with eight carbon atoms and eight hydrogen atoms, can all be expressed with CH. (C) is the only choice that cannot, since it has only three carbon atoms and four hydrogens. Both its molecular and empirical formulas would be C_3H_4, because that represents the smallest whole number ratio of its constituent elements.

5. A

This question is relatively simple if you understand to what percent composition refers. The percent composition of any given element within a molecule is equal to the molecular mass of that element in the molecule, divided by the formula or molecular weight of the compound, times 100 percent. In this case, it is clear acetone, C_3H_6O, has a total molecular weight of (12.0107 × 3 + 1.00794 × 6 + 15.994) 58.074 g/mol, of which 12.0107 × 3 = 36.0321 g/mol is from carbon. Thus, the percent composition of carbon is 63.132%. With this calculation serving as an example, you can calculate the percent composition for ethanol (C_2H_6O; MW = 41.023 g/mol) to be 58.556%; for C_3H_8 (MW = 44.096 g/mol) to be 81.713%; and for methanol (CH_4O; MW = 32.036 g/mol) to be 37.491%. Although both acetone (A) and ethanol (B) have percent compositions of carbon close to 63%, acetone is closer. You can estimate from their molecular formulas that the percent composition of carbon would be high in C_3H_8 and low in methanol (CH_3OH), making both of those unlikely solutions.

6. D

This question tests your ability to balance a double-displacement reaction. Calcium has a charge of 2^+, carbonate has a charge of 2^-, aluminum has a charge of 3^+, and finally nitrate has a charge of 1^-. First, it is clear that all of the answer choices undertake the same double-displacement reaction. Next, one must balance the equation so that there are the same number of equivalent moles of each element on both the left and right sides of the equation. In this case, recognizing that one of the products will be aluminum carbonate will combine an ion with a charge of 3^+ with one of a charge of 2^-. In order for this to work, there will have to be 2 aluminum atoms combining with 3 molecules of carbonate for the charge of this molecule to be balanced ($^+6$ and $^-6$ in total). (C) and (D) are the only choices where this is the case. The next step is to balance the reaction. In (D), there are three atoms of calcium on both sides, three molecules of carbonate, two of aluminum on both sides, and six of nitrate on both sizes. Thus, (D) has the correct products and is a balanced equation. (C) is unbalanced, with unequal numbers of multiple atoms/molecules on each side, and it does not have the correct $Ca(NO_3)_2$ product.

7. C

Single displacement reactions are reactions in which one atom/ion within a molecule is replaced by an atom/molecule of another element. Following is an example of a single displacement reaction, in which iron takes the place of copper in the molecule that combines with sulfate:

$$Fe(s) + CuSO_4(aq) \rightarrow FeSO_4(aq) + Cu(s)$$

Many single displacement reactions are in fact redox (reduction/oxidation reactions) reactions, of which the above reaction is one. Single displacement reactions typically change the oxidation states of the participating metals, as demonstrated above, which defines a redox reaction. Neither (A) nor (B) is correct because the number reactants and products is often equivalent in these reactions. Finally, single displacement reactions can have a combination solid and/or aqueous reactants and products (D); they need not have aqueous reactants and solid products.

8. B

This reaction is a classic example of a neutralization reaction, in which an acid and a base react to form water and a new aqueous compound. Although this reaction may also appear to fit the criteria for a double displacement reaction, in which two molecules essentially "exchange" with each other, neutralization reaction is a more specific description of the process. A single displacement reaction is typically a redox (reduction/oxidation) reaction in which one element is replaced in the molecules, making (A) and (D) incorrect.

9. B

You are first given the masses of both reactants used to start the reaction. In order to figure out what will be left over, you must determine which is the limiting reagent and which is present in excess.

First, determine the molecular weight of each of the reactants:

Na_2S = 78.05 g/mol
$AgNO_3$ = 169.9 g/mol

Thus, you are given 0.5 mol Na_2S for the reaction and 0.6669 mol $AgNO_3$. However, you need two molar equivalents of $AgNO_3$ for every mole of Na_2S, so $AgNO_3$ will be the limiting reagent (there must be two moles of it for every mole of the other reagent). Next, determine how much of the Na_2S will be left over by determining how much will be used if it reacts with all of the $AgNO_3$:

$[(1 \text{ mol } Na_2S)/(2 \text{ mol } AgNO_3)] \times 0.6669 \text{ mol } AgNO_3 = 0.3334 \text{ mol } Na_2S$

Then, subtract this amount of reagent used from the total available:

$0.5 \text{ mol } Na_2S - 0.3334 \text{ mol } Na_2S = 0.1666 \text{ mol excess } Na_2S$

Finally, determine the mass that this represents:

$0.1666 \text{ mol excess } Na_2S \times 78.05 \text{ g/mol } Na_2S = 13 \text{ g } Na_2S$

(A) and (D) are incorrect because there will be no remaining $AgNO_3$. One might incorrectly arrive at (A) if he did not convert to using two moles $AgNO_3$ per mole Na_2S.

10. A

Try to come up with your own answer before looking at the choices. First, begin with some give mass, of $KClO_3$, X grams. In order to convert that to a product, we must convert to moles. Thus far you would have:

$$(\text{grams } KClO_3 \text{ consumed}) \times \frac{\text{mol } KClO_3}{\text{g } KClO_3} = \frac{(\text{grams } KClO_3 \text{ consumed})}{(\text{molar mass } KClO_3)}$$

This first step eliminates (C).

Next, we must convert the number of moles of $KClO_3$ to the number of moles of oxygen, according to the balanced equation presented in the question stem:

$$\text{mol } KClO_3 \times \frac{3 \text{ moles } O_2}{(2 \text{ moles } KClO_3)}$$

Putting both steps together, the equation thus far is:

$$\frac{(\text{grams } KClO_3 \text{ consumed})(3 \text{ moles } O_2)}{(\text{molar mass } KClO_3)\ (2 \text{ moles } KClO_3)}$$

This second step eliminates (B), because it does not use the correct molar ratio between $KClO_3$ and O_2. The final step is to convert the number of moles of oxygen to a mass, in grams of O_2. Because at this point in our equation the number of moles is in the numerator, and we want the number of grams of oxygen in the numerator, one can multiply, not divide, by the molar mass of oxygen.

11. C

In the reaction here, there is a single displacement (II), with the silver in silver oxide being replaced by the aluminum to form aluminum oxide. This single displacement reaction also necessitates a transfer of electrons in a reduction/oxidation reaction or "redox" reaction. Therefore, items II and III are correct. A double displacement reaction typically takes two compounds and causes two displacements, and only one occurs in the reaction given here. A combination reaction typically takes two atoms or molecules and combines them to form one product, usually with more reactants than products.

12. D

Begin by converting the grams of glucose reacted to moles of glucose:

$$\frac{10 \text{ grams glucose}}{(180.2 \text{ grams/mol glucose})} = 0.05549 \text{ moles glucose}$$

Next, convert the number of moles of glucose into the number of moles of water to be produced:

$$(0.05549 \text{ moles glucose}) \times \frac{(6 \text{ moles water}}{(1 \text{ mole glucose})} = 0.333 \text{ moles water}$$

Next, convert the moles of water to the number of grams of water:

$$0.333 \text{ moles water} \times \frac{(18.02 \text{ g})}{(\text{mol water})} = 6.001 \text{ grams water}$$

Finally, convert the number of grams of water into the number of milliliters by using the density of water. Don't get hung up with the exact density water would be at a given temperature, such as for a liquid at 4° Celsius, the density of water is 1 g/cm^3. Even at a very high temperature, at 80° Celsius, the density is still close to 1, being 0.9718 g/cm^3. So for the purposes of this question, estimating a density of 1 g/cm^3 is most appropriate, which will yield about 6 milliliters of water.

13. A

The law of constant composition, (A), explains that any sample of any given compound will contain the same elements in the identical mass ratio as described by the compound's formula. In this question, although all of the water samples might be difference in phase or in source, they are all still samples of H_2O and as such will all have a 2:1 ratio of hydrogen atoms to oxygen atoms. Although H_2O, in addition to being the molecular formula for water, is also its empirical formula (B), this does not best explain why all three samples have the same composition. Although the percent composition of hydrogen and oxygen in all samples are the same, percent composition (C) is not as descriptive an answer as (A). Steady-state (D) is irrelevant.

14. C

Single displacement (or oxidation/reduction) and double displacement reactions typically have the same number of reactants and products. For example, single displacement reactions are often of the form (M = metal 1; M′ = metal 2; A = anion):

$$M + M'A \rightarrow M' + MA$$

M takes the place of M′ in combining with an anion. Typically, this is enabled by a process of oxidation and reduction of the involved metals. Double displacement reactions also tend to have the same number of reactants and products, represented by this type of reaction (C = cation 1; C′ = cation 2; A = anion 1; A′ = anion 2):

$$CA + C'A' \rightarrow C'A + CA'$$

The two compounds essentially "swap" anions/cations, beginning and ending with two compounds. Combination reactions typically have more reactants than products, represented by the reaction $A + B \rightarrow C$.

15. D

A net ionic equation represents each of the ions comprising the compounds in the reactants and products as individual ions, instead of combining them as molecules. (A) is not a net ionic reaction. Next, we want to find the simplest of the answer choices, which means that the correct answer does not include any spectator ions, ions that do not participate in reacting and remain the same on both the reactant and product sides of the equation. Here, nitrate, NO_3^-, serves as a spectator ion, and thus would not be included in the simplest net ionic reaction. The only answer choice that eliminates NO_3^- is (D). (B) is incorrect because it is not balanced properly, with only one nitrate in the reactants, and two nitrates in the products.

(C) is further incorrect because copper is not a spectator ion, rather it participates fully in the reaction; thus, it must be included in any net ionic equation, and it is not present in (C).

16. A

The theoretical yield is the amount of product synthesized if all of the reactant is used and goes to product. This question simply asks how much glucose is produced if the limiting reagent is 30 grams of water. First, calculate the number of moles of water represented by 30 grams by dividing by the molecular weight of water (18.01g/mol), which yields 1.666 moles of water. Next, convert to the equivalent number of moles of glucose:

1.666 moles water × (1 mole glucose)/(6 moles water) = 0.2776 moles glucose

Finally, calculate the number of grams of glucose that are equal to 0.2776 moles by multiplying by the molecular weight of glucose (180.2 grams/mol glucose), which results in 50.02 grams of glucose produced. (B) would result from failing to convert via the 1:6 ratio of glucose:water. (C) would result from assuming 1 mole of water. (D) would result from multiplying by 6 instead of 1/6 when calculating the molar equivalents of glucose.

17. B

First, note that this is a net ionic equation, and that to answer this question one must work backward from the amount of product back to the reactant with its spectator ions. To do so, one must consider not just Fe^{3+}, which is shown in the net ionic equation, but actually iron sulfate, $Fe_2(SO_4)_3$, the original compound. The sulfate ion is not shown because it is a spectator ion; spectator ions are not included in net ionic equations. First, calculate the number of moles of $Fe_2(SO_4)_3$ per mole $FeSCN^{2+}$. The fully balanced equation would have two moles of $FeSCN^{2+}$ per mole $Fe_2(SO_4)_3$, so all that needs to be calculated is how many grams of $Fe_2(SO_4)_3$ are in one mole, which is the same as its molecular weight:

(2 × iron) + (3 × sulfur) + (12 × oxygen) = (2 × 55.85 g/mol) + (3 × 32.06) + (12 × 15.999)

= (111.7 g/mol) + (96.18 g/mol) + (191.99 g/mol) = 399.9 grams/mole $Fe_2(SO_4)_3$

CHAPTER 5: CHEMICAL KINETICS AND EQUILIBRIUM

1. D

Based on the information provided, the rate is directly proportional to the concentration of the first reactant; when the concentration of the reactant doubles, the rate also doubles. Because the reaction is third-order, the sum of the exponents in the rate law must be equal to 3. Therefore, the rate law is defined as follows:

$$\text{Rate} = k\,[\text{reactant 1}]\,[\text{reactant 2}]^2$$

Reactant 1 has no exponent because its concentration is directly proportional to the rate. For this reason, the concentration of reactant 2 must be squared in order to write a rate law that represents a third-order reaction. When the concentration of reactant 2 is multiplied by ½, the rate will be multiplied by $(\frac{1}{2})^2 = \frac{1}{4}$.

2. A

First draw a potential energy diagram for the system:

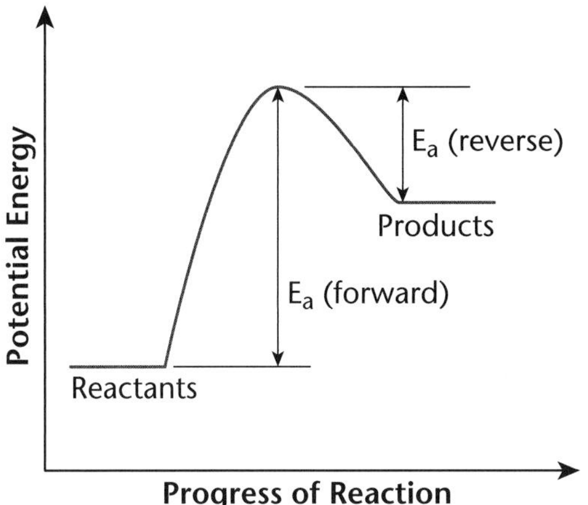

If the activation energy of the forward reaction is greater than the activation energy of the reverse reaction, then the products are higher up on the diagram than the reactants. The overall energy of the system is higher at the end than it was at the beginning, so the net enthalpy change is positive, signifying an endothermic system.

3. C

Recall the ideal gas law, PV = nRT, which states that volume is directly proportional to temperature and inversely proportional to pressure. If the volume of a gas is increased, the pressure will always decrease if the temperature decreases or is held constant; however, it is also possible for a small increase in temperature to be accompanied by a large decrease in pressure.

4. A

When the bottle opens, the volume of the container increases, which causes its pressure to decrease as well. You should have a solid understanding of Le Châtelier's principle, which implies that a decrease in pressure shifts the equilibrium so as to increase the number of moles of gas present; this particular reaction will shift to the left, thereby decreasing the amount of carbonic acid and increasing the amount of carbon dioxide and water. (C) and (D) are distortions; oxygen and nitrogen are not highly reactive and are unlikely to spontaneously combine with CO_2 or H_2CO_3.

5. D

ΔH is always positive for an endothermic reaction (item I is correct) and ΔG is always negative for a spontaneous reaction (item II is correct). Based on these two facts, ΔS can be determined by the free energy equation:

$\Delta G = \Delta H - T\Delta S$, which can be rewritten as:

$$T\Delta S = \Delta H - \Delta G$$

If ΔH is positive and ΔG is negative, $\Delta H - \Delta G$ must be positive. This means that $T\Delta S$ is positive. T (the temperature of the system in Kelvin) is always positive, so ΔS must also be positive. Item III is also correct.

6. C

The K_{sp} of a salt is equal to the product of the concentrations of each ion in the salt in saturated solution. This salt has three A^+ ions and one B^{3-} ion, so K_{sp} is equal to $[A^+][A^+][A^+][B^{3-}] = [A^+]^3[B^{3-}]$. The molar solubility of the salt is equal to the total number of moles of the salt in solution. The molar solubility of the salt is 10 M, thus the A^+ ion is present in a concentration of 30 M (3 A^+ ions per molecule) and the B^{3-} ion is present in a concentration of 10 M (one B^{3-} ion per molecule). These values can be substituted into the K_{sp} expression to yield $K_{sp} = [30\ M]^3[10\ M] = 3^3 \times 10^3 \times 10^1 = 27 \times 10^4 = 2.7 \times 10^5$.

7. B

Adding sodium acetate increases the number of acetate ions present. According to LeChâtelier's principle, this change will push this reaction to the left, resulting in a decrease in the number of H^+ ions and an increase in pH. This problem can also be solved with the K_a equation, $K_a = [CH_3COO^-]\,[H^+]/[CH_3COOH]$. K_a remains constant at any given temperature and pressure, eliminating (C) and (D).

For K_a to remain unchanged while $[CH_3COO^-]$ increases, $[H^+]$ must decrease or $[CH_3COOH]$ must increase. A decrease in products would require an increase in reactants, and vice versa, so the final effect would be both an increase in $[CH_3COOH]$ and a decrease in $[H^+]$. Again, removing hydrogen ions will increase the pH of the solution.

8. A

Only item I is correct. If the sum of the exponents on each concentration the rate law is equal to 2, then the reaction is second-order. Item I is correct because each of the exponents in this rate law is 1, so their sum is 2. Item II is incorrect because the exponents in the rate law are unrelated to stoichiometric coefficients, so NO_2 and Br_2 could be present in any ratio in the original reaction; this particular reaction actually consumes two moles of NO_2 for every mole of Br_2, which you can also guess based on the fact that NO_2 contains one unpaired electron and Br_2 contains two bromine atoms (each of which also has one unpaired electron). Item III is incorrect because the rate can be affected by a wide variety of compounds. A catalyst, for example, could increase the rate. Any compound that would preferentially react with NO_2 or Br_2 (including strong acids/bases and strong oxidizing/reducing agents) would decrease the concentration of reactants and decrease the rate.

9. C

In the first two trials, the concentration of XH_4 is held constant while the concentration of O_2 is multiplied by 4. Because the rate of the reaction is also increased by a factor of approximately 4, we can write the following equation:

Trial 1: $Rate_1 = 12.4 = k[XF_4 (trial\ 1)]^x [O_2 (trial\ 1)]^y = k(1.00)^x (0.6)^y$

Trial 2: $Rate_2 = 49.9 = k[XF_4 (trial\ 2)]^x [O_2 (trial\ 2)]^y = k(1.00)^x (2.4)^y$

When you divide the bottom equation by the top equation, it simplifies to $4.02 = 4^y$, so y is approximately equal to 1. You can follow a similar procedure to calculate the exponent that goes along with $[XF_4]$. The rate increases by a factor of 4 when the concentration increases by a factor of 2, so the rate is proportional to the square of the concentration. Based on this, we can write the rate law, which is Rate = $k [XF_4]^2 [O_2]$.

10. C

A higher K_a implies a stronger acid. Consider the following theoretical reaction, which defines the K_a of acid HA, $HA \rightleftharpoons H^+ + A^-$. In such a reaction, $K_a = [H^+][A^-]/[HA]$. A K_a near 1 therefore implies that there are enough hydrogen ions present to significantly affect the pH. Weak acids usually have a K_a that is several orders of magnitude below 1. A detailed understanding of K_a is not necessary to answer this question, however. According to the pH scale, which sets the K_a of water at 10^{-7} a compound with a K_a above 10^{-7} is acidic; even if the acid is very weak, it will still cause the pH to drop below 7.

11. D

The rate of a reaction is related to the concentration of reactants, but not to the overall volume of the vessel. If a sample of a certain concentration is increased in quantity, the reaction will not be affected. Adding heat will allow a reaction to reach its activation energy faster, while removal of heat will make it more difficult for the reaction to reach its activation energy, so (A) doesn't apply. Changing the activation energy (by adding a catalyst) is the most common way to significantly increase the rate of a reaction, so (D) does not apply, nor does (C) because almost all reactions have a rate law that includes the concentration of each reactant as a key variable.

12. A

Your first step here should be to write out the balanced equation for the reaction of H_2 and N_2 to produce NH_3 [$N_2 + 3H_2 \rightarrow 2NH_3$]. This means that K_{eq} is equal to $[NH_3]^2/([H_2]^3[N_2])$. Because the volume is 1 L, the value of the amount of each gas (in moles) is equal to the value of the concentration of each gas (in *M*). We can plug these concentrations back into the K_{eq} expression to get $K_{eq} = (.05)^2/([3]^3[1])$, which is equal to (0.0025)/(27). This is approximately equal to 0.0001, and approximations are appropriate for the MCAT.

13. D

A system is exothermic if energy is released. For exothermic reactions, the net energy change is negative and the potential energy stored in the final products is lower than the potential energy stored in the initial reactants. Point E, which represents the energy of the final products, is lower on the energy diagram than point A, which represents the energy of initial reactants. Thus energy must have been released from the overall reaction in this case. While point A is useful for determining the energy of the overall reaction, point B represents the activation energy of the first transition state and point C suggests an intermediate. The difference between points D and E indicates the change in energy from the transition state of the second reaction step to the final products.

14. B

The activation energy of a reaction is equal to the distance on the y-axis from the energy of the reactants to the peak energy prior to formation of products. The activation energy of the first step of the forward reaction, for example, is equal to the distance along the y-axis from point A to point B. The largest energy increase on this graph occurs during the progress between points E and D, which represents the first step of the reverse reaction. The other answer choices are opposite.

15. B

This energy diagram presents a two-step system. The first reaction proceeds from point A to point C and the second reaction proceeds from point C to point E. This means the reactants predominate at point A, the intermediates predominate at point C, and the products predominate at point E. Point B, which is between points A and C, is the energy threshold at which most of the reactant starts to be converted into intermediate, so the reactant and the intermediate will both be present at this point. No product is produced until after point C, so it will not be present in the reaction mixture. Catalysts may be present in the mixture at any point, depending on the nature and the quantity of the catalyst.

16. C

Reaction 2 is simply the reverse of reaction 1. Because K_{eq} of reaction 1 is equal to [products]/[reactants], K_{eq} of reaction 2 must be equal to [reactants]/[products]. This means that K_{eq} for reaction 2 is the inverse of K_{eq} of reaction 1, so the answer is 1/0.1 = 10.

17. A

A negative ΔH value always signifies an exothermic reaction, so the forward reaction produces heat. This means that removing heat by decreasing the temperature is similar to removing any other product of the reaction. According to LeChâtelier's principle, decreasing the amount of a product will stimulate the reaction to produce more products; therefore, removing heat will cause the reaction to shift to the right, causing an increase in the concentrations of C and D as well as a decrease in the concentrations of A and B.

18. C

K_a is equal to the ratio of products to reactants in a dissociated acid. A compound with a K_a greater than 10^{-7} contains more H^+ ions than OH^- ions, which makes it a weak acid (unless K_a is several orders of magnitude higher than 1, which would indicate a strong acid). This means that the compound in the question is acidic and that it is likely to react with a compound that is basic. Of the four choices, NH_3 is the only base.

19. D

Recall that the slow step of a reaction is the rate-determining step. Therefore, the rate is always related to the concentrations of the reactants in the slow step, so NO_2 is the only compound that should be included in the correct answer. The concentration of NO_2 is squared in the rate law because, according to the question, the reaction obeys second-order kinetics.

20. D

The faster a reaction can reach its activation energy, the faster it will proceed to completion. Because this question states that all conditions are equal, the reaction with the lowest activation energy will have the fastest rate. (D) illustrates the smallest difference between the initial and peak potential energies, so that reaction can overcome its activation energy more easily than the other proposed scenarios on the energy diagram.

HIGH-YIELD SIMILAR QUESTIONS

Rate Law from Experimental Results

1. $k = 0.0149\ M^{-1}s^{-1}$
2. Rate = $k[C_5H_5N][MeI]$; $k = 75\ M^{-1}s^{-1}$; this is an S_N2 reaction, because it is second order overall.
3. Rate = $k[Ce^{4+}][Fe^{2+}]$; $k = 10^3\ M^{-1}s^{-1}$.

Rate Law from Reaction Mechanisms

1. Rate = $M\ s^{-1}$, so k_{obs} will be in units of $M^{-3}s^{-1}$.
2. In solution, this should be a simple addition of HX to an alkene, so we would expect the rate law to be rate = $k[HCl][CH_3CHCH_2]$.
3. In the solution phase reaction, the key intermediate would be a carbocation, rather than an excited state of 2–chloropropane.

CHAPTER 6: THERMOCHEMISTRY

1. A

The process is adiabatic. Adiabatic describes any thermodynamic transformation that does not involve a heat transfer (Q). An adiabatic process can be either reversible or irreversible, though for MCAT purposes, adiabatic expansions or contractions refer to volume changes in a closed system without experimentally significant losses or gains of heat. The internal energy of the system changes ($U = -P\Delta V$, where $U = Q - W$, $W = P\Delta V$, and $Q = 0$). An isobaric process (B) is conducted at constant pressure, but the curve is more severe. An isothermal process (C) requires a heat transfer at constant temperature, and there is no heat transfer along an adiabatic curve.

2. A

An adiabatic expansion does not involve a heat transfer, so pressure and volume data provide enough information to answer this question. That rules out (D). For ideal gases undergoing reversible adiabatic processes, PV^γ = constant. $\gamma = C_P/C_v$, the molar specific heats of the ideal gas at constant pressure and constant volume. (C) is out of scope. The problem does not provide an expansion constant for triatomic ideal gases, and you do not have to take into account the question of whether a triatomic gas could approximate "ideal" conditions. That leaves (A) and (B). For an ideal monatomic gas, $\gamma = 5/3$. For an ideal diatomic gas, $\gamma = 7/5$.

3. D

There is not enough information in the problem to determine whether the reaction is nonspontaneous.

(A), (B), and (C) are Distortions. Start with $\Delta G = \Delta H - T\Delta S$. Though the magnitudes of ΔH and ΔS might suggest a spontaneous reaction, the overall free energy is temperature-dependent. If the signs of enthalpy and entropy are the same, the reaction is temperature-dependent. If the signs of these terms are different, you can find the sign of the free energy independent of temperature. The most common thermochemistry questions on the MCAT test your ability to manipulate and interpret the $\Delta G = \Delta H - T\Delta S$ equation. Memorize it.

4. B

Sodium oxidizes easily at standard conditions. No calculation is necessary here. There is enough information to predict the equilibrium constant, eliminating (D). If $K_{eq} < 1$, the reverse reaction is favored, indicating that the forward reaction is non-spontaneous. If $K_{eq} = 1$, the reaction is at equilibrium. If $K_{eq} > 1$, the forward reaction proceeds spontaneously. The question states that the sample spontaneously combusts at room temperature, i.e. 25°C. The answer is (B), $K_{eq} > 1$.

5. C

Combustion involves the reaction of a hydrocarbon with oxygen to produce carbon dioxide and water. The longer the hydrocarbon chain, the more product is formed, and the more heat is released in the process of forming new bonds. (Though this question calls on your understanding of alkane structure, you are unlikely to see a quantitative question in the Biological Sciences section.) Exothermic is synonymous with the most negative overall enthalpy, here the heat of combustion. Isobutane combusts less easily than n-butane because of its branched structure.

6. A

This problem requires a quick calculation. The reaction, a Fischer esterification, is an MCAT favorite. The hydroxyl group leaves acetic acid via nucleophilic attack of methanol on the carbonyl carbon of acetic acid. That means 1 O–H bond breaks (methanol), and 1 C–O bond breaks (hydroxyl on acetic acid to carbonyl carbon). One C–O bond reforms in the products, for the new ester, and 2 O–H bonds form (water). Enthalpy is a state function, meaning its value remains the same regardless of the reaction path, so you could calculate the same result in other ways. That allows us to calculate the overall enthalpy of a reaction with the heats of formation of each chemical involved, a calculation shortcut known as Hess's law. (An element's heat of formation is 0 by convention, as long as it is in its standard state.) The problem provides bond disassociation energies instead of heats of formation, meaning you subtract products from reactants, or for bonds broken minus bonds formed. (A) accounts for this error. (B) is opposite, while (C) and (D) are miscalculations.

7. C

Standard temperature and pressure indicates 0°C and 1 atm. Gibbs free energy is temperature-dependent. If a reaction is at equilibrium, $\Delta G = 0$. (C) is the answer. Note that there is no degree sign next to ΔG in this problem; this indicates a standard state reaction at 25° Celsius.

8. B

The correct answer is (B), using $K_{eq} = e^{-\Delta G°/RT}$ from $\Delta G° = -RT\ln(K_{eq})$. Use $e = 2.7$. R is the gas constant, 8.314 $Jmol^{-1}K^{-1}$, and T = 298 K, because of the standard-state sign. The answer in (A) would have omitted a negative sign; we know from the free energy that the reaction must be spontaneous, so the equilibrium constant should be greater than 1. (C) uses T = 273 K rather than 298 K. (D) substitutes a base-10 logarithm for the natural logarithm. With the base-10 log, use $\Delta G° = -2.303RT\ln(K_{eq})$. Comfort with exponent and logarithm calculations is essential for success on Test Day.

9. D

There is not enough information to determine the energy of this reaction, only its entropy. While it appears that a reaction has taken place, we know only that the molecules have moved, not whether something has caused them to move into a new arrangement. Had the reaction been at equilibrium (C), there would not be this much reorganization between molecules.

10. A

This problem asks you to calculate the free energy of reaction at non-standard conditions, which you can do using the equation $\Delta G = \Delta G° + RT\ln(Q)$. (R is the gas constant, 8.314 $Jmol^{-1}K^{-1}$, and T = 298 K.) Though it's a good idea to memorize this equation for Test Day, you can set up the answer from information in the question stem. (A) is correct. (C) and (D) are distortions; with the base-10 logarithm, you must multiply by a conversion factor of 2.303. Often, the MCAT will test your ability to manipulate logarithms without the use of a calculator. Review this material well before Test Day.

11. C

There is not enough information to deduce anything about reaction temperature, which eliminates (B) and (D). Adiabatic and isothermal processes are necessarily opposite because adiabatic processes do not involve heat transfers. A reaction at constant pressure can be either adiabatic (no heat transfer to change volume) or isobaric (constant pressure, as the word roots imply). That means items I and III are correct.

12. A

This question requires interpreting the equation $\Delta G = \Delta H - T\Delta S$. Endergonic indicates a non-spontaneous reaction, and exergonic indicates a spontaneous one. In contrast, exothermic and endothermic suggest the sign of the enthalpy of the reaction. The problem does not provide enough information to determine the free energy of this temperature-dependent reaction. (A) is the correct answer. Endothermic reactions (B) have a positive enthalpy. (C) and (D) are distortions; the suffix *-gonic* indicates Gibbs free energy and is more commonly seen on the Biological Sciences section of the MCAT.

13. A

Disorder in the vessel increases over the course of the reaction. $\Delta S < 0$ (B) would indicate more molecular organization in the vessel after the reaction took place. (C) is faulty use of detail; S = 0 J/K at absolute zero, and compounds at any temperature above 0 K are dynamic. (D) is tricky. While we cannot make a quantitative determination of entropy from the picture, we can estimate the relative amount of disorder from the beginning to the end of the reaction in the vessel.

14. C

This is a definition question. A spontaneous reaction's free energy is negative by convention. Its equilibrium constant is greater than 1 because it is not at equilibrium and moves in the forward direction. (C) is the correct answer.

15. B

A calorimeter measures specific heat or heat capacity. Though calorimeters often incorporate thermometers, thermometers themselves (A) track only heat transfers, not the specific heat value. Barometers (C) measure change in pressure. Volumetric flasks (D) measure liquid quantities, not the heat capacity of the liquid.

16. C

Memorize the Laws of Thermodynamics; they may be stated in different forms on Test Day. Know the equation and how to rephrase it into a sentence or two. The First Law often confuses students—it refers to the overall energy of the universe, not to the enthalpy of the universe—even though enthalpy is usually substituted for this term in introductory college chemistry experiments. The Third Law (absolute zero) is not an equation.

17. A

Eliminate (C) and (D), which describe the free energy of reaction and cannot be determined from this graph. If the heat of formation of the products is greater than that of the reactants, the reaction is endothermic. We can determine this information by their relative magnitude on the graph; an exothermic graph would reflect products with a lower enthalpy than that of the reactants.

HIGH-YIELD SIMILAR QUESTIONS

Reaction Energy Profiles

1. [B]/[A] = 3.5
2. No, because a catalyst only lowers the activation energy (by lowering $G^{\dagger}$). It doesn't affect the energies of the reactants or products.
3.

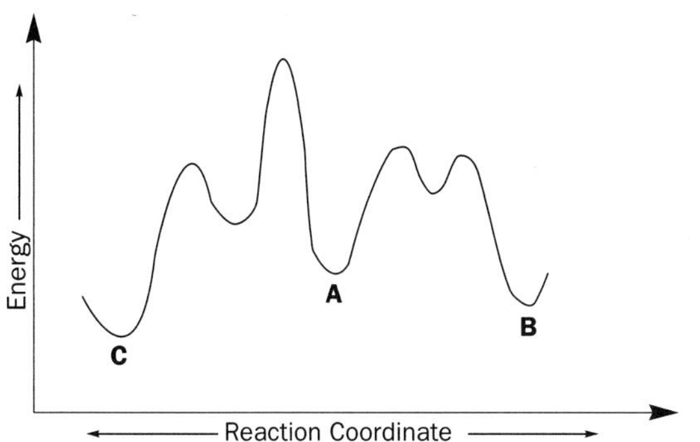

Thermodynamic Equilibrium

1. Reactants are favored
2. 8,688 J/mol; 52,373 J/mol; neither reaction is spontaneous; if $\Delta S > 0$ then $\Delta H > 0$.
3. The student should put flask A on the benchtop, flask E in the cold room, and flask P on the Bunsen burner.

Bond Enthalpy

1. 0.0021 kJ
2. 338.5 kJ/mol
3. 8.53×10^4 kJ/mol

Heat of Formation

1. ΔH_f for ethane
2. –1,255.4 kJ/mol
3. –359.9 kJ/mol

CHAPTER 7: THE GAS PHASE

1. A

One mole of an ideal gas at STP is equal to 22.4 L. The extrapolation of the ammonia graph to zero pressure is extremely close to this value. The slope of the line does not indicate whether the gas is ideal or not, because all gases will deviate at their own rate with increases in pressure. The ammonia gas exhibits ideal behavior at zero pressure even though it deviates at higher pressures.

2. A

The graph shows that gases deviate from ideal behavior at higher pressures, which force molecules closer together and create more intermolecular forces. Similarly, low temperatures cause less space to exist between molecules. Less space also makes the volume of the molecules more significant, causing the gas to lose characteristics of an ideal gas. At high temperatures molecules will move more quickly and exhibit random motion and elastic collisions, which is a property of ideal gases. In an ideal gas it is assumed that there are no intermolecular attractions between gas molecules. At low pressure gas molecules will have more space between them and thus any intermolecular attractions will become negligible.

3. D

Density equals mass divided by volume. The mass of 1 mole of neon gas equals 20.18 grams. At STP, 1 mole of neon occupies 22.4 L. Dividing the mass, 20.18 grams, by the volume, 22.4 L, gives an approximate density of 0.9009 g L^{-1}.

4. C

Graham's law of effusion states that the relative rates of effusion of two gases at the same temperature and pressure are given by the inverse ratio of the square roots of the masses of the gas particles. In equation form, Graham's law can be represented by:

$$\frac{\text{Rate}_1}{\text{Rate}_2} = \sqrt{\left(\frac{M_2}{M_1}\right)}$$

If a molecule has a higher molecular weight then it will leak at a slower rate than a molecule with a lower molecular weight. Both neon and oxygen gas will leak at slower rates than helium because they each have a greater mass than helium.

5. C

The difference between the atmospheric pressure and the pressure from the gas in the flask is equal to 117 mm of mercury. The atmospheric pressure can be seen exerting more force on the mercury compared to the gas in the flask. Therefore, the gas in the flask should have a pressure below 760 torr (760 mm Hg). The difference of 117 mm Hg must be subtracted from 760 mm Hg. So 760 – 117 equals 643 mm Hg, choice (C).

6. B

A hot-air balloon rises because the air inside the balloon is less dense than the surrounding air. We know the air inside is less dense because, according to Charles's law, temperature and volume are directly related. A greater volume creates less density, because D = mass/volume.

7. B

The pressure of the gas is calculated by subtracting the vapor pressure of water from the measured pressure during the experiment: 784 mm Hg – 24 mm Hg = 760 mm Hg, or 1 atm. The ideal gas law can be used to calculate the moles of hydrogen gas. The volume of the gas equals 0.1 L, the temperatures equals 298 K, and R = 0.0821 (L atm/mol K). Solving the equation PV = nRT for n gives 4.09×10^{-3} moles of hydrogen. (A) might result from using 784 mm Hg of the pressure instead of the pressure adjusted for water vapor. (C) and (D) would result from using a pressure in mm Hg instead of converting to atm while using the gas constant R = 0.0821 (L atm/mol K).

8. B

Ideal gases are said to have no attractive forces between molecules. They are considered to have point masses, which take up no volume. Items I and II are correct.

9. C

The first thing to do is balance the given chemical equation. The coefficients, from left to right, are 1, 1, 2. The mass of solid, 8.01 grams, can be converted to moles of gas product by dividing by the molar mass of $NH_4NO_{3(s)}$ (80.06 g) and multiplying by the molar ration of 3 moles of gas product to one mole of $NH_4NO_{3(s)}$. This gives approximately 0.300 moles of gas product. The ideal gas equation can be used to obtain the pressure in the flask. The values are as follows: R equals 0.0821 (L atm/mole K), the temperature in Kelvin is 500 K, and the volume is 10 L. Solving for P in the equation PV = nRT gives a pressure of about 1.23 atm. (B) is three times smaller than correct (C) and would be obtained if the gas moles conversion were not carried out. (D) would result from using 273 K instead of 500 K.

10. D

The partial pressure of each gas after the stopcocks are open can be calculated using $P_1V_1 = P_2V_2$. V_2 is the same for all three gases because the volume with open stopcocks equals 8 L in the system. For each gas, P_1 and V_1 are provided. We must then solve for P_2. The calculation for the various gases, will look like the following:

(2 L) (0.4 atm) = (8 L) (P_{Ne}), i.e. P_{Ne}= 0.1
(2 L) (0.1 atm) = (8 L) (P_{Ar}), i.e. P_{Ar}= 0.025
(4 L) (0.8 atm) = (8 L) (P_{He}), i.e. P_{He}= 0.4

11. A

The average kinetic energy is directly proportional to the temperature of a gas in Kelvin. The kinetic molecular theory states that collisions between molecules are elastic (B). Elastic collisions do not result in a loss of energy (C). The kinetic energy of each gas molecule is not the same (D); varies over a range of kinetic energies.

12. C

At STP, the difference between the distribution of velocities for helium and bromine gas is due to the difference in molar mass ($Rate_1/Rate_2 = \sqrt{(M_2/M_1)}$. Helium has a smaller molar mass than bromine. Particles with small masses travel faster than those with large masses, so the helium gas corresponds to curve B with higher velocities. (A) and (B) inaccurately identify each curve on the graph. (D) is incorrect because the average kinetic energies of the gases cannot be determined with the given information.

13. D

At STP the pressure inside the balloon equals 1 atm. The total number of moles in the balloon equals 0.2 moles plus 0.6 moles, or 0.8 moles. P_{O2} equals the mole fraction of oxygen (0.2/0.8) times the total pressure, 1atm. The partial pressure of oxygen is 0.25 atm.

14. A

The ideal gas law can be modified to include density and determine the temperature of the sun. Solving for T, the equation looks like: T = (P × MW)/(R × D). The density is given in g/cm^3 and must be converted to g/L so the units cancel in the above equation. Because 1 cm^3 equals 1 mL and there are 1,000 mL in 1 L, the density can be multiplied by 1,000 to be converted to g/L.

15. C

Gases are compressible and can conduct electricity but do so very poorly. Because gas particles are far apart from each other and in rapid motion, they tend to take up the volume of their container. Gas particles can flow easily past one another because there is a great deal of space for movement between particles.

16. B

We will use $V_1/T_1 = V_2/T_2$. First we must convert the temperature to Kelvin by adding 273 to get 300 K as the initial temperature. Plugging into the equation and solving for T_2 gives 450 K. Subtracting the initial temperature, 300 K, gives an increase of 150 K. This also corresponds to an increase of 150°C.

17. D

The reaction of two moles of gas, X and Y, to form one mole of gas, XY, will decrease the moles of gas. Because volume and moles of gas are directly related, the volume of gas will decrease and the pistons will move down. The piston does not move up (A) because the gas volume decreases due to less moles of gas that are present. Moreover, there is no way to know from the information given if there is energy given off during the reaction (B). (C) is incorrect because the piston will move down; the decrease in amount of gas in the space under the piston will cause the piston to move.

18. B

The partial pressure of each gas is found by multiplying the total pressure by the mole fraction of the gas. Because 80 percent of the molecules are nitrogen, the mole fraction of nitrogen gas is equal to 0.8. Similarly, for helium the mole fraction is 0.2 because 20 percent of the gas molecules are helium. To find the pressure exerted by nitrogen, multiply the total pressure (150 torr) by 0.8 to obtain 120 torr of nitrogen. To find the pressure exerted by helium, multiply the total pressure by 0.2 to get 30 torr of helium.

19. C

Heating a gas will increase the pressure, and cooling a gas will decrease the pressure at a constant volume. A decrease in volume will increase the pressure, and an increase in volume will decrease the pressure. Heating and increasing the volume will have opposite effects on the pressure of the gas. It is impossible to tell without quantifying if the end result is an increase or decrease in pressure. (C) is the correct choice.

CHAPTER 8: PHASES AND PHASE CHANGES

1. D

Water is the only substance with a negative slope of the solid/liquid equilibrium line shown in the figure. All of the other answer choices have a positive slope in the solid/liquid equilibrium line.

2. C

Solid water has a low density. This low density means that the same mass of water present in a living cell must expand at this lower temperature. This process of increased volume destroys living cells upon freezing by disrupting membrane structures. (B) and (D) are factually incorrect. (A) is true but less relevant to the question about frostbite, which involves frozen water at 0°C.

3. D

The skater increases the pressure on the water molecules while not changing the temperature. This increased pressure causes a phase change from solid to liquid due to the negative slope of the solid/liquid equilibrium line. The other answer choices deal with processes not relevant to the question.

4. A

Intermolecular forces hold molecules closer to one another, which relates to the compound's phase. As the intermolecular forces increase, the amount of heat needed to change phase (such as in vaporization) increases as well, thus showing a proportional, positive relationship between molecular forces and the heat of vaporization.

5. B

This molecule is likely to have unequal sharing of electrons and thus polarity. Polarity often leads to increased bonding because of the positive-negative attractive forces between molecules. More bonding or stronger intermolecular forces both mean higher melting points because more heat is needed to break these interactions to change phase. (A) is nonpolar, making its intermolecular forces weaker than (B) or (C). (D) is only weakly polar, because the geometry of this molecule will make some of the polarized bonds cancel each other out. (C) will have some polarity, but less than in (B) because only one bond is polarized.

6. D

At low pressure there is less force holding the molecules in a more organized state—liquid or solid.

Because temperature is a measure of average kinetic energy of the molecules, an increase in the average kinetic energy increases molecules' movement and thus they move apart from each other, ultimately entering a gaseous state. Increasing pressure or decreasing the temperature (or kinetic energy) both favor more organized states of liquid or solid.

7. A

(A) shows that increased kinetic energy would be necessary to overcome the increased force of pressure holding the molecules within whatever state they're in. In order to maintain the same state at an increased pressure, the temperature must also increase, which would force the line graphing the increasing temperature and changing phase to move up.

8. C

Melting point depresses, making (A) and (B) incorrect. Added solute particles interfere with lattice formation, interrupting the intermolecular forces that would otherwise stabilize the lattice formation. Because these particles do not stabilize the lattice formation, (D) is also incorrect.

9. B

Viscosity implies stronger bonding/intermolecular forces, thus making it harder for molecules to move past one another and flow freely. Those interactions are associated with higher heats required to change phases, and in this question, vaporize. Fusion (C) and critical mass (D) are unrelated to viscosity.

10. D

Tar is the most viscous of the answer choices. With increased viscosity comes increased bonding interactions, which makes it most difficult to cause phase change in a highly viscous substance. As a result, the highest heat of vaporization to break the stronger interactions is required for a highly viscous substance.

11. C

(C) shows movement from the solid to gas phase, which is by definition, sublimation.

12. A

With a positive slop for the solid/liquid equilibrium line, the phase change for solid under increased pressure and constant temperature is to remain solid. This phase change line would need to be negatively sloped, as seen with water, to skate on it. In that case, increased pressure from the skates would move the solid (ice) to a liquid phase (water). This liquid layer enables skating to be possible; otherwise it is like skating on a solid such as dirt.

13. A

In this final stage of the phase change, the particles are already in a gaseous state (the highest-energy phase), and with increasing temperature the particles retain increased kinetic energy. Temperature is the average kinetic energy of the molecules in a substance and so this answer addresses the change in energy shown by a slope in the line. (B) and (C) do not describe the gaseous phase indicated by X's location in the diagram, and (D) is simply incorrect.

14. D

Sweat causes a loss of heat when the high-energy, or hottest, molecules move from liquid to gas and leave the body surface. This evaporation process allows the loss of heat energy, thereby cooling the body (decreasing average kinetic energy). (A) and (B) refer to condensation, which is actually a warming process, instead of evaporation. (C) is incorrect chemically, Because evaporation does not lead to a gain of cooler/low-energy molecules.

15. C

Both items I and II are correct. Dissolved solutes break up the crystalline lattice bonds of a solid and in this phase equilibrium, solutes increase the equilibrium to favor liquid, in which they easily dissolved. As a result, a decreased amount of this solute would favor a solid state (I). Additionally, decreased temperature (II) is a decrease in the average kinetic energy of the molecules, making lower-energy phases (i.e., solid) more likely. Decreasing pressure (III) would actually favor higher-energy phase (i.e., liquid or gas) over solid. Neither (A) alone nor B alone captures all the important variables. (D) is incorrect, as described above, since less pressure means a less force keeping the molecules in the solid lattice-like phase.

16. A

Condensation occurs more on a humid day because there is a greater amount of water in the gaseous phase in the ambient air, which can interact with the human body and transfer heat from these high-energy molecules to the human body. Upon interaction, the initially gaseous water molecules change phase to a liquid (condensation) after losing their heat to the human body. On a dry day there would be few water molecules to cause this transfer of heat, making one feel less hot.

17. A

By definition, condensation is a move from water vapor (clouds) to liquid water (rain).

18. B

Ether (B) has the lowest heat required for vaporization, which by definition determines the boiling point or the lowest temperature required for phase change from liquid to gas. All of the other answer choices have higher heats of vaporization.

HIGH-YIELD SIMILAR QUESTIONS

Partial Pressures

1. P_{O2} = 5 atm; P_{N2} = 1.25 atm; P_{CO2} = 3.75 atm
2. 8
3. 7.5 atm

CHAPTER 9: SOLUTIONS

1. A

The equation $\Delta T_b = k_b \times m_c$ can be used to solve this problem. The change in boiling point is found by subtracting the boiling point of water (the solvent), 100°C, from the elevated boiling point, 101.11°C. Using the given value for k_b we solve for the molality of the solution and get 2.17 moles/kg. Convert to grams by dividing by 1,000 and then multiplying by the volume of the solution, 100 g, to get the moles of solute. To obtain the molar mass, divide the mass of the solute, 70 g, by the number of moles, 0.217 moles, to get a molar mass of 322.58 g/mole. (C) and (D) would result from multiplying 1.11 by the k_b instead of dividing.

2. D

The phases in all three items can make a solution as long as the two components create a mixture that is of uniform appearance (homogenous). Hydrogen in platinum is an example of a gas in a solid. Air is an example of a homogenous mixture of a gas in a gas. Brass and steel are examples of homogeneous mixtures of solids.

3. B

Benzene and toluene are both organic liquids and have very similar properties. They are both nonpolar and are almost exactly the same size. Raoult's law states that ideal solution behavior is observed when solute-solute, solvent-solvent, and solute-solvent interactions are very similar. Therefore, benzene and toluene in solution will be predicted to behave as a nearly ideal solution. (A) states that the liquids would follow Raoult's law because they are different. It is true that the compounds are slightly different but the difference is negligible in terms of Raoult's law. (C) and (D) state that the solution would not obey Raoult's law.

4. A

If the membrane became permeable to water, water molecules would move to the side with the highest solute concentration, according to the principles of osmosis. The left side has a higher concentration of solute because NaCl is dissolved in water. Water will move to this side to attempt to equalize the concentration of solute on both sides. The level on the left will rise because of the excess water molecules and the level on the right will fall because it has lost water molecules. The level would stay the same (B) only if the number of particles dissolved on each side of the membrane were equal. (D) is not possible because it would add volume to the system.

5. D

Step 1 will most likely be endothermic because energy is required to break molecules apart. The strong ionic forces in the crystal must be overcome to separate individual molecules and ions. Step 2 is also endothermic because the intermolecular forces in the solvent must be overcome to allow incorporation of solute particles. Step 3 will most likely be exothermic because polar water molecules will interact with the dissolved ions and release energy.

6. C

CaS will cause the most negative $\Delta S°_{soln}$ because the Ca^{2+} and S^{2-} ions have the highest charge density compared to the other ions. All of the other ions have a charge with a value of 1, whereas Ca^{2+} and S^{2-} have charges with an absolute value of 2. When comparing ions with the same value of charge, the size of the ions must be taken into account. Ions that are smaller will have a higher charge density. For example, LiK will have a higher charge density than KCl. It follows that the $\Delta S°_{soln}$ is more negative for LiK than for KCl.

7. D

A non-electrolyte solution will not dissociate into ions in solution. Its effective molarity in solution will be the same as the number of moles that were dissolved. On the other hand, an electrolyte like $Mg(NO_3)_2$ will dissociate into three ions (Mg and $2NO_3^-$). The effective molarity, which is important for colligative properties, will be three times the number of moles that were dissolved. Osmotic pressure is a colligative property and will therefore be three times larger for $Mg(NO_3)_2$ compared to a non-electrolyte. The molarity of $Mg(NO_3)_2$, 0.02 M, is also two times larger than the non-electrolyte solution (0.01 M). The osmotic pressure will have to be multiplied by three and then by two, which equals multiplication by six. 15 mm Hg × 6 equals 90 mm Hg.

8. A

Vitamin A is hydrophobic and is therefore fat-soluble. It will accumulate in fat for storage purposes and will be released when it is needed. Consuming too much of it will cause a large accumulation and thus hypervitaminosis. Unlike vitamin C, it will not be readily excreted in urine. Vitamin C is hydrophilic and will dissolve in the body's aqueous solutions, leading to regular excretion in the urine. It can be consumed regularly in large amounts and will not build up in the body. Though vitamin A is larger (B), its hydrophobicity is what accounts for its ability to be stored in body fat. Attached methyl groups on a compound are not toxic to a cell (C). Interactions with membrane lipids can occur but there is no evidence that this disrupts transport across the membrane (D).

9. B

The mass percent of a solute equals the mass of the solute divided by the mass of the total solution. To find the mass of the solution, we must find the mass of the solvent, water. Multiplying the volume of the solution by the density gives us a mass of 292.5 grams of water. Adding 3 grams of sugar yields a solution with a mass of 295.5 grams. Next, we divide 3 grams of sugar by 295.5 grams and multiply by 100 to get a percentage. (C) might result from dividing by the mass of the solvent rather the solution.

10. A

Mixtures that have a vapor pressure higher than predicted by Raoult's law have stronger solvent-solvent and solute-solute interactions than solvent-solute interactions. The particles do not want to stay in solution and evaporate more readily, causing a higher vapor pressure than an ideal solution. Two liquids that have different properties, like hexane (hydrophobic) and ethanol (hydrophilic, small), would not have many interactions with each other to cause positive deviation, so (A) is correct. Acetone and water (B) and isopropanol and methanol (C) would not show significant deviation from Raoult's law; due to their similar properties, the molecules are neither attracted to nor repelled from each other. Nitric acid and water (D) would interact well with each other and cause a negative deviation from Raoult's law. The liquids, when attracted to each other, would prefer to stay in liquid form and would have a lower vapor pressure than predicted by Raoult's law.

11. A

Dissolution is governed by enthalpy and entropy, which are related by the equation $\Delta G^\circ_{soln} = \Delta H^\circ_{soln} - T\Delta S^\circ_{soln}$. The cooling of the solution indicates that there is a decrease in enthalpy. The only way the solid can dissolve is if the increase in entropy is great enough to overcome the decrease in enthalpy. It is stated in the question stem that KCl dissolves (B). ΔS°_{soln} must be positive in order for KCl to dissolve (C). (D) is irrelevant and also misstates boiling point depression instead of elevation.

12. D

The equation to determine the change in boiling point of a solution is as follows: $\Delta T_b = m_b(K_b)$. m_b is the molality of the solution and K_b is the boiling point elevation constant. In this case, the solvent is always water so K_b will be the same for each solution and the exact value of K_b is not needed to answer the question. Sucrose will produce the solution of highest molality (moles per kilograms solvent) of all four choices. Although (A) and (C) will dissociate into ionic species, the amount of moles dissolved in not large enough to yield as many particles in solution as sucrose. 0.1 mol of acetic acid, (B), is a very weak acid and only a few molecules will actually dissociate.

13. C

The solubility of gases in liquids is directly proportional to the atmospheric pressure. Therefore, we should expect a decrease in solubility with the decreased pressure in Denver. It must be known that at sea level the atmospheric pressure is equal to 1 atm, where the solubility is 1.25×10^{-3} M. We multiply this number by the new pressure over the old pressure (0.8/1) to get a solubility of 1×10^{-3} M. If you accidentally divided by the ration you would get the answer in (A), and if you just subtracted 0.02 from the solubility you would get (B).

14. C

30 ppb of Pb^{2+} is equivalent to 30 grams of Pb^{2+} in 10^9 grams of solution. We can divide by the molar mass of Pb^{2+}, 207 g/mole, to get moles of Pb^{2+} per

mass of solution. The density of water, 1,000 g/L, can be used to obtain the molarity of the Pb^{2+} in the water, 1.4×10^{-7} M. (B) might result from forgetting to multiply by the density of water.

15. C

All items but III are correct. An electrolyte is a molecule that dissociates into free ions and behaves as an electrically conductive medium. NaF (item I) is an electrolyte because it dissociates to form the ions Na^+ and F^-. Glucose (item II) is a nonelectrolyte because it is a ring structure which dissolves but does not dissociate. CH_3OH (item III) will not ionize in solution and so is not an electrolyte. Acetic acid (item IV) is a weak acid and also a weak electrolyte because it will partially ionize in solution.

16. D

A colligative property depends solely upon the number of molecules and disregards the identity of the molecules. (A), (B), and (C) are properties based on the composition of a solution determined by the number of molecules that are dissolved in the solution. The entropy of dissolution (D) will depend on the chemical properties of the substance, such as charge density and electron affinity. Therefore, the entropy of dissolution is not a colligative property.

17. A

The K_{sp} equation can be written as $[Ag^+][Br^-] = 7.7 \times 10^{-13}$. Because there is a 0.001 M solution of NaBr, the effective concentration of Br^- will be 0.001 M. Substituting this value for $[Br^-]$ in the K_{sp} equation and solving for $[Ag^+]$ gives a concentration of 7.7×10^{-10} M Ag^+. This value can be converted to g/L by multiplying by the molar mass of silver, 107.9 grams/mole. The solubility of Ag^+ is the same as the compound AgBr because there is one molecule of Ag^+ for every molecule of AgBr.

18. B

Formation of complex ions between silver ions and ammonia will cause more molecules of solid AgCl to dissociate. The equilibrium is driven toward dissociation because the Ag^+ ions are essentially being removed from solution when they complex with ammonia. This rationale is based upon Le Chatelier's principle, stating that when a chemical equilibrium experiences a change in concentration, the system will shift to counteract that change. (A) is incorrect because the complex ions may interact with AgCl but this is not the major reason for the increased solubility. (C) and (D) are incorrect because the solubility of AgCl will increase, not decrease.

19. D

Detergents contain a long hydrophobic chain with a polar functional group on one end. The long hydrophobic chains can surround grease and oil droplets, while the polar heads face outward and carry the particles in a solution of water. If a molecule ionizes into two parts, both parts will also be ionic, so (B) is incorrect. (C) is incorrect because, although multiple detergent molecules form a sphere-like shape with oil or grease droplets enclosed, the individual molecules themselves do not circularize.

HIGH-YIELD SIMILAR QUESTIONS

Normality and Molarity

1. 0.25 L of the 4 M solution; 1 L of the 4 N (with respect to H^-) solution
2. The product would be(±)–7–amino–2–heptanol. The reduction would require 0.375 L of th 2 M solution and 1.5 L of the 2 N (with respect to H^-) solution.
3. 1.2 L of the 2.5 M solution; 1.2 L of the 2.5 N (with respect to H^-) solution.
4. Additional question: With respect to H^+, is a 1 M solution of H_2SO_4 slightly greater than

1 N or slightly less than 1 N? What about with respect to HSO_4^-? Ans: Actually, 1 M H_2SO_4 = 2 N H_2SO_4, and 1 M HSO_4^- = 1 N HSO_4^-. Normality with respect to a particular species—in this case H^+—is calculated based on the maximum number of H^+'s the molecule could potentially donate, not how many it actually donates; thus, knowing an acid's strength is irrelevant to calculating its normality.

Molar Solubility

1. Shown in step 5
2. Solve for molar solubility as shown in step 5; substance with highest value is most soluble
3. Decreasing pH decreases sulfate ion concentration, leading to greater dissolution of the sulfate salt.

CHAPTER 10: ACIDS AND BASES

1. D

A Brønsted-Lowry base is defined as a proton acceptor. The other answer choices can accept a proton, while (D) cannot.

2. C

The equation for pH is pH = $-\log[H^+]$. If $[H^+] = 1 \times 10^{-2}$ M, as the question notes, pH equals 2.

3. A

(A) is correct. Acids ending in *–ic* are derivatives of anions ending in *–ate*, while acids ending in *–ous* are derivatives of anions ending in *–ite*. ClO_3^- is named chlorate because it has more oxygen than the other occurring ion, ClO_2^-, which is named chlorite.

4. C

Members of the IA and IIA columns on the periodic table combined with OH^- are always strong bases. This means (A), (B), (D) are strong bases. (C) is the weakest of the choices.

5. B

The purpose of a buffer is to resist changes in the pH of a reaction. They will not affect the kinetics of a reaction. (D) is on the right path, but the wording is too strong because buffers work only to resist changes in pH over a small range, which is what (B) indicates.

6. C

The question is asking for pH, but because of the information given, we must first find the pOH and then subtract it from 14 to get the pH. The equation for pOH is:

$$pOH = pK_b + \log\frac{[\text{conjugate acid}]}{[\text{weak base}]}.$$

When the given values are substituted into this equation, and the Kaplan methods for estimating logarithms are used, we find that the pOH = 4.45, so the pH = 14 – 4.45 = 9.55.

7. A

The first pK_a in this curve can be estimated by eye. It is located between the starting point (when no base had been added yet) and the first equivalence point. This point is approximately at 7-8 mL added, which corresponds to a pH of approximately 1.9.

8. C

The second equivalence point is the midpoint of the second occurrence of a very quick increase in slope. This corresponds to approximately pH = 5.9.

9. B

The value of the second pK_a is notable because it is found in a slightly different way from the first pK_a. It is located at the midpoint between the first and second equivalence points. In this curve, that corresponds to pH = 4.1.

10. B

Gram equivalent weight is the weight (in grams) that would release one acid equivalent. Because H_3PO_4 contains three acid equivalents, we find the gram equivalent weight by dividing the mass of one mole of the species by 3. (B) is correct.

11. A

This question requires application of the following knowledge:

$$K_a = \frac{[H^+][X^-]}{HX}$$

We know that if HX is to dissociate, then $[H^+] = [X^-]$. We can substitute y for both of these values and plug in K_a and [HX]; we then solve for y (representing $[H^+]$). When we do this, we find that $[H^+]$ is 8.0×10^{-3} M.

12. D

An amphoteric species is one that can act as an acid or a base depending on the environment, which means it can also act as an oxidizing or reducing agent depending on the environment, so (A) and (B) are true. (C) is true because, by definition, an amphoteric molecule must contain a proton. (D) is false, and thus the correct answer, because an amphoteric species can be polar or nonpolar in nature.

13. C

The solution to this question is found by using the equation pOH = $-\log[OH^-]$. We must use the Kaplan strategy for estimating logarithms to figure that the pOH is closer to 5 than it is to 4, so we know pOH = 4.5–5. We can then surmise that pH = 9.0–9.5, and because (C) is the only one within that range, it must be correct.

HIGH-YIELD SIMILAR QUESTIONS

pH and pKa

1. The pH would be about 8.85 if the concentration of acetate were halved; if it were doubled, 9.15. (You should be able to predict that the pH would have to go down if there were less acetate and up if there were more.)
2. pH = 13
3. The pH would be 2.87.

Titrations

1. The pH would be approximately 12.2.
2. The pH would be 12.9 (compare this to the pH of 4.72 at the half equivalence point!).
3. The pH would be about 4.4.

CHAPTER 11: REDOX REACTIONS AND ELECTROCHEMISTRY

1. C

In an electrolytic cell, an ionic compound is broken up into its constituents; the cations (positively charged ions) migrate toward the cathode and the anions (negatively charged ions) migrate toward the anode. Electrons are transported from the anode to the cathode in order to balance the charge, meaning that item III will be correct for all electrolytic cells. Because this cell is loaded with water, the ions involved are H^+ and O^{2-}. The cation, H^+, is transported to the cathode, so item I is also correct.

2. A

In a galvanic cell, oxidation occurs at the cathode and reduction occurs at the anode. In this example, Cu is being oxidized. Because the standard reduction potential is +0.52 V, the standard oxidation potential is −0.52 V. The potentials of the half-reactions in a feasible galvanic cell must add up to a value greater than 0, so we can answer this question by simply comparing the oxidation potential of copper to the reduction potentials of the other metals. Mercury has a reduction potential of 0.85 V, which is enough to outweigh the potential contributed by copper (–0.52 V). Zinc and aluminum both have negative reduction potentials, so the overall potential of the cell will be even lower than that of copper. Therefore, mercury is a viable option, while zinc and aluminum are not.

3. A

The oxidizing agent is the species that is reduced in any given equation. In this problem, the two H^+ ions from H_3N are reduced to one neutral H_2 atom. H_3N is not the reducing agent because the H^+ ions and the N^{3-} ions are independent of one another in solution.

4. B

First, we must calculate the oxidation state of chromium in $Cr_2O_7^{2-}$. Because oxygen always carries a –2 charge, the total charge from the O_7 is –14; this means that the Cr_2 contributes a total charge of +12. To reduce the +12 charge to a +4 charge (the charge from the two chromium atoms that are produced in the reaction), 8 electrons are required.

5. A

If a reaction represents a spontaneous process, then the overall potential must be positive. Both half-reactions currently describe a reduction process, so one of the two must be reversed to form an oxidation-reduction system. The only way to create a spontaneous oxidation-reduction system is to reverse the reaction involving O_2 to produce a positive net potential. To balance the reaction, the number of electrons must first be equivocated by doubling all of the quantities in reaction 2. The two reactions are then added together and duplicate instances of H^+, e^-, and H_2O are eliminated from both sides. This yields the reaction in (A).

6. B

It is important to note here that the potential of a half-reaction remains constant even when the reaction is multiplied by a coefficient. $E°_{reaction1}$ is given as 1.23 and $E°_{reaction2}$ is –1.46 (because reaction 2 must be reversed in order to produce the system in question). $E°_{cell}$ is the sum of these individual E° values, which is equal to –0.23.

7. D

In an electrolytic cell, electricity simply provides the energy to induce a reaction. The actual electrons come from within the molecule that is being electrolyzed. In this case, the positively charged sodium ion gains an electron from the negatively charged chloride ion, thereby creating two neutral atoms.

8. C

In the oxidation-reduction reaction of a metal with oxygen, the metal will be oxidized (donate electrons) and oxygen will be reduced (accept electrons). That means (B) and (D) can be eliminated. A species with a higher reduction potential is more likely to be reduced, and a species with a lower reduction potential is more likely to be oxidized. Based on the information here, iron is oxidized more readily than copper, which means that iron has a lower reduction potential.

9. A

To answer this question, you must know that a hydride ion is comprised of a hydrogen nucleus with two electrons, thereby giving it a negative charge and a considerable tendency to donate its extra electron. This means that $LiAlH_4$ is a strong reducing agent.

10. D

Even if you do not memorize the equation $\Delta G = -nFE°_{cell}$, you should understand that Gibbs free energy can be calculated from $E°_{cell}$ and the number of moles.

11. B

The salt bridge contains inert electrolytes. (A), (C), and (D) are all ionic electrolytes, but (B) is a covalent compound. This makes it unlikely for SO_3 to be found in a salt bridge.

12. D

In NaClO (sodium hypochlorite), sodium carries its typical +1 charge and oxygen carries its typical –2 charge. This means that the chlorine atom must carry a +1 charge in order to balance the overall –1 charge; although this is atypical, it is not uncommon (NaClO, for instance, is the active ingredient in household bleach).

13. A

If an electrolytic cell is producing hydrogen and oxygen, it must be breaking up water or hydrogen peroxide. Hydrogen peroxide, however, does not maintain a pH of 7, so we can be sure that the cell is filled with water. Because a water molecule contains two hydrogen atoms for every oxygen atom, the cell will produce twice as much hydrogen as oxygen.

14. C

An increased current will mean that more electrons are transported from the anode to the cathode, thereby driving the electrolytic cell to produce more products. An increase in resistance (A) will decrease the number of electrons in the system, thereby producing the opposite of the desired effect. The amount of electrolyte (B) will affect only the amount of final product; it does not limit the rate. The pH (D) is relevant only to an electrolytic reaction if the reaction involves acids and bases.

15. D

A strong oxidizing agent will be easily reduced, meaning that it will have a tendency to gain electrons. Atoms usually gain electrons if they are one or two electrons away from filling up their valence shell. (A) has a full 4s orbital, meaning it can gain an electron only if it gains an entire p subshell. (B) has a half-full d orbital, so it is unlikely to gain electrons unless it can fill up the entire orbital. (C) has only a single electron in the outer shell, which will probably be lost upon ionization. (D) is the only answer choice that can fill up its outer shell by gaining just one electron.

HIGH-YIELD SIMILAR QUESTIONS

Balancing Redox Reactions

1. Zirconium is being reduced (Zr^{4+} to Zr^{0}), and therefore is the oxidizing agent. Sulfur is being oxidized (S^{4+} to S^{6+}) and is the reducing agent.
2. The balanced equation is:
   $2\ PbSO_4(s) + 2\ H_2O(\ell) \rightarrow$
   $Pb(s) + PbO_2(s) + 2\ SO_4^{2-}(aq) + 4\ H^+(aq)$.
3. The balanced equation is:
   $Zn(s) + 2\ H_2O(\ell) \rightarrow Zn^{2+}(aq) + H_2(g) + 2\ OH^-(aq)$.
   The amalgam must be kept dry because on reacting with water in basic solution, hydrogen gas is generated. The expansion of the gas would potentially cause the tooth or crown to crack painfully and leave the dentist with one angry patient!

Electrochemical Cells

1. Placing a battery of greater than 2.25 V in the circuit (with the positive terminal connected to the cathode of the galvanic cell setup) would cause the current to flow the other way.
2. The cell potential would be about 2.24 V. Changing the amount of zinc metal wouldn't

affect this value (as long as some zinc metal is present), since as a solid it is not incorporated into the reaction quotient.

3. About 6.3 g of $KMnO_4$ would be necessary.

The Nernst Equation

1. $[Br^-] = 3.7 \times 10^{-13}$
2. $K_{eq} = e^{876}$. Clearly, permanganate is a very strong oxidizing agent!
3. The pK_a of acetic acid is approximately 4.74.

PRACTICE SECTIONS

PRACTICE SECTION 1

ANSWER KEY

1. A	19. C	37. B
2. C	20. C	38. A
3. D	21. A	39. C
4. A	22. C	40. D
5. B	23. D	41. C
6. D	24. A	42. B
7. C	25. C	43. A
8. C	26. D	44. A
9. B	27. B	45. C
10. B	28. A	46. B
11. D	29. B	47. B
12. B	30. A	48. C
13. D	31. B	49. B
14. A	32. C	50. A
15. A	33. D	51. D
16. B	34. C	52. C
17. C	35. A	
18. B	36. C	

PASSAGE I

1. A

There are two concepts involved here. The first is that both of these species are strong acids, so they will fully ionize in solution; the bivalent species has two H^+ ions for every one H^+ ion of the monovalent species, so it will produce a more acidic solution. Second is the idea that a more acidic solution will have a lower pK_a.

2. C

It is given in the passage that the pH of normal rain is 5.2, so this problem is simply asking you to convert pH = 5.2 into $[H^+]$. Using the Kaplan logarithm estimation procedure on the answers, it is clear that the only concentration that will produce a pH of 5.2 is (C).

3. D

It is important to know that every Arrhenius acid is also a Brønsted-Lowry acid, and that every Brønsted-Lowry acid is also a Lewis acid (the same idea applies for bases). This means that (B) and (C) can be eliminated. Sulfuric acid produces protons, so it is qualified as an Arrhenius acid, and we then know it can be called a Brønsted-Lowry or Lewis acid as well. All of the items are correct.

4. A

We are able to tell that HCO_3^- is a buffer because it can either donate or accept a proton. Being able to donate a its remaining H^+ allows it to act as an acid, while its overall negative charge allows it to act as a base and accept an H^+. (A) is correct because HCO_3^- will accept a proton from the acid introduced to the blood stream, and act as a buffer. (B) is incorrect because while it will act as a buffer, it will accept an H^+ ion, not donate an H^+ ion. (C) is incorrect because HCO_3^- does act as a buffer. (D) is incorrect because there is enough information.

5. B

Write down the steps as you go. First, we need to figure out what the original $[H^+]$ is in the rain. Because H_2SO_4 is bivalent, we double its concentration to find its contribution to the total $[H^+]$, which is 4.0×10^{-3} M. We then add this to 3.2×10^{-3} M to get $[H^+]_{rain} = 7.2 \times 10^{-3}$ M. If we divide this number by 4 (the factor by which the volume decreased, use $V_1C_1 = V_2C_2$), we get $[H^+]_{rain+pure} = 1.8 \times 10^{-3}$ M. Finally, we can use Kaplan's logarithm estimation strategy to find that the pH is just below 3, so 2.8 is the answer.

6. D

A conjugate base is an acid that loses a proton. (D) shows an acid and a molecule that has lost a molecule of H_2O, so it is not an acid/conjugate base pair. The other choices show an acid and conjugate base that has one less proton.

7. C

This question tests your ability to actively read the passage and synthesize the information presented. The student would likely agree with (A) because pollution is a major cause of acid rain, and industrialization over the past 150 years has greatly increased pollution levels. The student would likely agree with (B) because, as shown in the passage, radicals are integral in the formation of acid rain. The student would likely disagree with (C) because more acid content in water would increase the conductive capacity of water. The student would likely agree with (D) because while rain is naturally acidic, acid rain contains dangerous levels of acid.

8. C

The first pK_a in this curve can be estimated by eye. It is located between the starting point (when no base had been added yet), and the 1st equivalence point. This point is at pH of approximately 6.3. The value of the second pK_a is notable because it is found in a slightly different way than the first pK_a. It is located at the midpoint between the first and second equivalence points. In this curve, that corresponds to pH = 10.3

9. B

Equivalence points are at the midpoint of the quickly escalating slope range. In this titration curve, the value of the first equivalence point is 7.8 and the value of the second is 12.0.

PASSAGE II

10. B

Many MCAT Physical Sciences questions include dimensional analysis calculations. If you do not know the specific heat of water from memory, you'll want to know this constant on Test Day! (It is reported in paragraph 1.) The correct answer is (B). (A) is tempting, as it has the same magnitude as the specific heat of water in $Jg^{-1}K^{-1}$. You will need to convert (A) from grams to moles using the molecular mass of pure water, 18 g/mol. (C) and (D) differ from (B) and (D) by factors of 1,000, a frequent source of error in thermochemistry problems (using kJ rather than J).

11. D

This is a discrete question which draws on information from the passage. The passage does not provide an explicit comparison of intensive and extensive physical properties. You can infer from paragraph 1, however, that intensive properties do not depend on the amount of substance present in the measurement, and that extensive properties do. While viscosity is irrelevant to this specific experiment, it is an intensive property of a liquid. Mass, heat, and enthalpy are all extensive properties. (Heat is an extensive property; temperature is an intensive property.) The correct answer is (D).

12. B

Use a calorimetry equation to determine the heat capacity of the calorimeter. This set-up requires referring to table 1, which describes how the student calibrated the instrument. The equation must account for all heat inputs and outputs in the closed system. In short, the heat lost by one part of the system must be gained by another part of the system. Here, the cold water heats up, and the hot water cools. That transition is summarized by the equation $m_{hot}C_{H20}(T_f - T_{i,, hot}) = m_{cold}\ C_{H20}(T_f - T_{i, cold}) + K_{cal}\ (T_f - T_{i, cold})$. Use the density of pure liquid water, 1 g/mL, to convert the volumes of hot and cold water to mass quantities. (B) is the answer. (A) is the specific heat of water, not the heat capacity of the calorimeter. (C) results from reversing the sign of the hot water temperature change, which obtains a negative heat capacity value. (D) is off by a factor of 1,000, using water specific heat in kg.

13. D

While it is true that mercury is much more dense than alcohol, the thermometer content should not make a difference in the student's results within this temperature range (A) and (B). There is no information to suggest the relative precision of the instruments (C). (Had the question asked about a digital thermometer, this would be relevant.) (D) is correct. There should be negligible differences in the ΔT obtained by each respective thermometer, though initial and final temperature measurements may vary slightly for each instrument.

14. A

Styrofoam is an excellent, though imperfect, insulator. Calibration accounts for heat loss to the calorimeter. The amount of water is irrelevant in a specific heat measurement, and that the calibration is supposed to account for the properties of the styrofoam (B). Calibration (C) accounts for a heat transfer, not a temperature change. The water temperature equilibrates in order to calibrate the thermometer, but that doesn't suggest anything about the reaction of other calorimeter contents inside (D).

15. A

The addition of salt ions to pure water disrupts hydrogen bonding between water molecules. When an aqueous solution is more disordered, there are weaker forces between component molecules. Compared to a highly stable hydrogen bond network like water, the salt water solution is disordered enough that its intermolecular bonding is much easier to break, lowering its specific heat.

16. B

Pressure must remain constant; paragraph 3 implies that bomb calorimeters are useful because they maintain constant pressure. Though specific heat is an intensive quantity, it is important to keep track of mass for the overall calorimetry calculation, which can involve different substances with different heat capacities. Heat should not enter or exit the system in a precise measurement. Items I and III are correct so the answer is (B).

17. C

Bomb calorimeters operate at high pressure, so they can accommodate temperature changes in a gas. Coffee cup calorimeters are no longer useful when the water boils. (A), (B), and (D) are distractors. Saltwater (A), as an aqueous ionic solution, is analogous to the fruit punch solution described in the passage. While ethanol (B) boils at a lower temperature than water, its structure is highly similar to that of pure water and it is relatively stable at room temperature. Coffee cup calorimeters can measure the specific heat of a metal like copper (D) if it is placed in water.

QUESTIONS 18–21

18. B

For every 2 mol of HCl 1 mol of hydrogen gas is produced (assuming excess magnesium). Multiplying both sides of the ratio by 1.5 means that 3 mol HCl under the same conditions should produce 1.5 mol hydrogen gas. At STP, 1 mol of a gas (assuming it to be ideal) occupies 22.4 L so 1.5 mol HCl should occupy 33.6 L.

19. C

Savvy test takers will note that (A) and (D) can be eliminated because the answer is internally inconsistent; favoring a reaction almost always means increasing its rate. To decide between (B) and (C), reason via Le Châtelier's principle. The stress is heat. An endothermic reaction requires heat and so is more likely to consume the heat (i.e., reduce the stress) than an exothermic reaction, which will add to the stress by producing heat.

20. C

By definition, gamma radiation is a stream of energy that in addition to creating the Hulk has neither mass nor charge. No such thing as delta radiation (D) has been defined. Alpha particles and beta particles have both charge and mass.

21. A

Rust, or corrosion, is the oxidation of a substance when it comes into contact with both water and oxygen. (B) can be eliminated because, if true, this would enhance the reactivity of Al or Zn. (C) can be eliminated because reducing agents are oxidized and so that would make Al or Zn more likely to rust. (D) is incorrect because, because Al, Zn still rust, they are oxidized and so function as reducing agents. Self-protective oxides (a common way of finding alkali metals as well) prevent further oxidation by complexing the atom with oxygen.

PASSAGE III

22. C

Compound C is shown to promote the reaction without affecting the overall yield of product. It is not consumed or produced in the net reaction, either. This is enough information to identify compound C as a catalyst, which decreases the activation energy of a reaction by definition. In this case, (C) is more likely than (D). Step 1 of the reaction is the fast step and step 2 is the rate-determining, slow step. Even though the catalyst may have an effect on the fast step, its primary purpose is to speed up the slow step. The bulk of the energy input in the overall reaction is in step 2. The catalyst decreases the activation energy, so it is likely to have its primary effect on the step that requires the greatest energy input.

23. D

To answer this question, you must apply Le Châtelier's principle, which states that adding a compound to a system will shift the system reaction such that less of that compound is produced. Adding compound A decreases the overall yield of the system. This change pushes the equilibrium in step 1 to the left to produce more of compound AB and less of compound A. Unbound compound B is not involved in any step of the reaction, so adding it will have no effect on any of the steps. Compound C is a catalyst; increasing the concentration of a catalyst may increase the rate of the reaction, but will not affect the equilibrium constant at any given temperature. The correct answer is (D), as compound D is present on the left side of step 2. Adding more of Compound D will push the reaction to the right, increasing the amount of product.

24. A

In terms of concentration, K_{eq} is equal to [products]/[reactants]. An increased concentration of products signifies an increased equilibrium constant, so K_{eq} of this reaction will increase along with the equilibrium concentration of BD. The data suggest that this concentration increases with increasing reaction temperature, but the concentration starts to stabilize after the temperature reaches approximately 100°C. Only (A) contains a graph demonstrating a K_{eq} which initially increases with temperature but starts to level off around 100°C. (B) shows a graph which follows the opposite of the correct path. (C) suggests that the equilibrium constant rises faster and faster as temperature increases, which is incorrect. (D) represents an equilibrium constant that does not change with temperature.

25. C

If a reaction is first-order with respect to each of the reactants, the overall rate is directly proportional to the concentration of each reactant. Doubling the concentration of compound A will double the rate of the reaction. In this new experiment, the concentration of compound A is twice as high as the concentration used in the first experiment, so the rate of formation is also twice as high.

26. D

The data in the two tables shows that the second experiment, which omitted the catalytic compound C, was significantly slower than the first at every temperature except 150°C. Recall that under normal circumstances, a catalyst will speed up a reaction by decreasing its activation energy, thereby allowing the reaction to reach its activation energy more easily. Consequently, increasing the amount of heat will also help the reaction achieve its activation energy. In this particular experiment, the catalyzed experiment was not much faster than the uncatalyzed experiment at 150°C. This suggests that the reaction reached its activation energy without the help of a catalyst at this temperature range.

27. B

Single-replacement reactions involve the direct replacement of one constituent of a molecule with another constituent molecule. In this case, compound C replaced compound A to turn AB into BC. Double replacement reactions, on the other hand, involve the replacement of two different species. An example of such a reaction is AB + CD $\rightarrow$ AC + BD. Combination reactions require two or more molecules to combine into one molecule, as in step 2. Decomposition reactions require one molecule to break down into two or more molecules, as in step 3.

28. A

Gases are highly compressible, while solids and liquids are not. For this reason, changes in pressure will not have a substantial effect on solids and liquids. An increase in pressure will push the reaction toward the side with less gas molecules, while a decrease in pressure will do the opposite. Becasue step 1 is the only part of the reaction mechanism that involves gases, it is also the only part that will be affected by a change in pressure.

29. B

This system starts out with two gases (AB and C) and one solution (D) and ends with one gas (A) and two solutions (BD and C). Gases have higher average kinetic energies than solutions do, so they are more disordered (i.e., they have a higher overall entropy, which is a thermochemical measure of the relative disorder in a system). The entropy of the products is lower than the entropy of the reactants, so ΔS for the overall reaction is negative. Based on the information given, it is impossible to determine whether ΔH is positive or negative. Although heat is added to stimulate the reaction, the passage does not specify how much heat is released at the end. ΔG is typically calculated from ΔH and ΔS. ΔH is not known, so ΔG is also impossible to determine.

PASSAGE IV

30. A

Newlands's table suggests that platinum is heavier than gold. According to the modern periodic table, gold is heavier than platinum. (B), (C), and (D) represent pairs of elements that were arranged correctly by Newland.

31. B

Periods 2 and 3 of the periodic table, which contain only elements in the s-block and the p-block, are the only periods that actually contain exactly eight elements. If most of the elements in the d-block and the f-block were discovered, it would become obvious that elements do not occur in matching octaves. (A) is incorrect because the discovery of all of the s-block and p-block elements would create more matching octaves (although the theory would have to be modified to accommodate the noble gases). (C) is incorrect because the law of octaves does not exclude the possibility of electrons, as long as the electrons are not organized as in Bohr's theory. (D) is incorrect for the same reason as (C).

32. C

Mendeleev's table was organized in terms of atomic mass rather than atomic number. Item I did require modification because it was subsequently discovered that an element is characterized by its number of protons (rather than its mass). Item II did not require direct modification of the table and the existing entries were left intact; the only change was the knowledge that future entries would be organized according to their outer orbitals. Item III only strengthened Mendeleev's original model, since the discovery of gallium fulfilled his prediction that two elements exist between zinc and arsenic. Items II and III did not require modification, so (C) is the answer.

33. D

The passage states that Newlands's table contains all of the elements that had been discovered at the time. Because his table contains no noble gases, we can assume that they had not been discovered. The table contains uranium, which is an f-block element (A), and several instances of halogens and metalloids (B) and (C) are evident throughout the table.

34. C

An element's first ionization energy, which is defined as the tendency of the element to donate an electron, decreases with increasing atomic number within a period. Because Mendeleev's predicted element had a higher atomic number than calcium, it is less likely to lose an electron. Atomic radius and ionic radius (A) and (B) both decrease with increasing atomic number. Electronegativity increases with increasing atomic number (D).

35. A

Atomic radius increases as an element gains energy levels and decreases as an element gains protons and electrons; you should know that the largest elements are those that have more energy levels and are found near the bottom of the periodic table. Uranium is the only element on Newlands's table that has seven energy levels, meaning it has the largest atomic radius.

36. C

If Mendeleev had created his table in response to Newlands's theory, then Mendeleev would clearly never have made his breakthrough without Newlands's contribution; if this were the case, it's reasonable to say that Mendeleev simply modified the law of octaves, which was eventually refined to produce the modern version. (A) is incorrect because it does not suggest that Newlands had any impact on the development of today's periodic table. (B) also makes it unlikely for Newlands to have made a direct contribution to the evolution of the system, because Mendeleev only learned about Newlands's work after he had already invented his own table. (D) clarifies the fact that Mendeleev was the first person to publish the modern periodic table and does not suggest that Newlands made any contribution to these findings.

PASSAGE V

37. B

This is a simple ideal gas law question. Using the equation PV = nRT, we are able to substitute: (1 atm)(V) = (1 mol)(R)(318 K), which simplifies to 318*R*. The answer does not need to be simplified past 318*R* (you are not allowed to use a calculator during the exam and multiplication by R takes too much time by hand).

38. A

This question tests your knowledge of the ideal gas law. The law shows that volume and temperature have a direct linear relationship (PV = nRT), meaning that as volume increases, so must T (assuming isobaric conditions). (B) shows an indirect linear relationship, (C) an exponential one, and (D) a logarithmic one.

39. C

In Experiment 2, we see that V_1 has been halved. So using the knowledge that temperature has been held constant, we know that the pressure must be double what it originally was to maintain the ideal gas law. So the right answer is 2 atm. The other choices all would violate the ideal gas law.

40. D

The "a" in the van der Waals equation accounts for the attractive forces between gas molecules. The "b" in the equation accounts for the actual volume that the molecules occupy (B). It isn't necessary to memorize the van der Waals equation for Test Day, but do know what "a" and "b" correct for in the equation.

41. C

The key here is realizing that 64 g O_2 is 2 mol O_2. Substituting the values given into this law, we get: (2 atm)(3 L) = (2 mol)(R)(T). This simplifies to 3/*R* K.

42. B

Dalton's law of partial pressures says that a gas's molar fraction multiplied by the total pressure gives the partial pressure supplied by that specific gas. This question asks specifically about 1.5 mol of NO, out of a total of 3 mol, which means that NO has a molar fraction of $X_{NO} = 0.5$. Solve for P using the ideal gas law: (2 L)(P) = (3.0 mol)(R)(300 K), P = 450*R* atm. This value multiplied by X_{NO} comes to 225*R* atm.

43. A

This question simply tests your knowledge of the conditions under which the ideal gas law is most relevant. The reference to experiment 1 is included just to mislead you. It is necessary to know only that the gases act closest to ideal when they are at high temperatures and low pressures.

44. A

At first glance this question looks extremely simple, yet you must realize that if the center divider is receiving different pressures from each side, it will move until pressure from both sides is equal. When the experimenter reduced the molar concentration in V_2 by half, the pressure was reduced on the V_2 side of the divider, leading to the expansion of V_1. It is important to note that (B) and (D) are incorrect because the question explicitly states that the cylinder is allowed to re-equilibrate with the new molar concentrations.

PASSAGE VI

45. C

An oxidation-reduction reaction requires a transfer of electrons from one atom to another. This reaction simply involves the neutralization of a strong acid by a weak base; no electrons are transferred and all of the oxidation numbers stay constant throughout the reaction.

46. B

The conjugate base of a Brønsted-Lowry acid is the product that does NOT include the H^+ ion that came from the acid. Even if you did not know this definition, there is a hint to this answer in the passage; because the products in reaction 1 contain a salt and an acid, it is clear that the salt is not the conjugate acid in neutralization reactions. Based on this information, you should be able to determine that the conjugate base is $MgCl_2$. You can determine the percent composition of the cation (Mg^{2+}) in this salt by dividing the molecular weight of the cation (24.3 g/mol) by the molecular weight of the molecule (95.2 g/mol). It should be obvious that 24.3/95.2 is approximately equal to 25/100, which equals 25%.

47. B

The passage states that efficacy is equal to the number of moles of HCl that can be neutralized by one gram of antacid. This means that the most effective antacids are those with the maximum neutralization capacity per gram. Because CO_3^{2-} can neutralize two H^+ ions, $Al_2(CO_3)_3$ has the capacity to neutralize six HCl molecules. Similarly, each of the other answer choices can neutralize three HCl molecules. (C) and (D) can be eliminated because they have the same neutralization capacity as $Al(OH)_3$, but are significantly heavier molecules. To decide between (A) and (B), consider that $Al_2(CO_3)_3$ has a molecular weight of 234 g/mol, while $Al(OH)_3$ has a molecular weight of 78 g/mol. Because $Al_2(CO_3)_3$ can neutralize only twice as many molecules as $Al(OH)_3$ but has nearly three times the weight, it is clear that $Al(OH)_3$ has the best per-weight efficacy.

48. C

The passage states that $NaHCO_3$ is an antacid, (A) is incorrect. The reaction suggested in (C) and (D), where H_2CO_3(aq) decomposes to produce H_2O (l) and CO_2 (g), is a common reaction that recurs every time H_2CO_3 is present in aqueous solution. Because nearly all the CO_2 is in gas form, it does not significantly affect the pH of the solution; this means that there are no acids left to decrease the pH and, therefore, $NaHCO_3$ is an effective antacid.

49. B

The limiting reagent is the reactant that is completely used up during the reaction while the other reactant still remains. Antacids are alkaline, so if the pH is below 7, there must not have been enough antacid to neutralize all of the HCl. This means that the progress of the reaction was limited by the amount of antacid.

50. A

The passage states that the student initially tested 1 gram of antacid along with 100 mL of 0.1 M HCl. Magnesium hydroxide, $Mg(OH)_2$, has a molecular weight of about 58 g/mol; because the answer choices are all very rough approximations, we can estimate the weight as about 50 g/mol in order to make the calculations easier. At this mole-cular weight, 1 gram of antacid is approximately equal to (1g)/(50g/mol) = 0.02 mol. 100 mL of 0.1 M HCl is equal to (0.1 L) × (0.1 mol/L) = 0.01 mol. Because each molecule of $Mg(OH)_2$ has two OH^- ions, only half a mole of $Mg(OH)_2$ is required to neutralize a mole of acid; therefore, only 0.005 moles of antacid is used up. The student started with 0.02 moles of antacid, so he is now left with 0.02 – 0.005 = 0.015 moles. To convert back to grams, we multiply 0.015 moles by 50 g/mol to get 0.75 g—which is equal to 750 mg.

51. D

A stronger antacid can neutralize the same amount of acid while using a smaller quantity of reactant. This means that more reactant will be left over after the neutralization is complete. Often, this leftover reactant will present itself in the precipitate (some antacids, however, will dissolve in the solution; this is why the student's logic was flawed). (A) is incorrect because the question states that the antacid is present as an excess reagent; increasing the amount of an excess reagent does not increase the amount of product unless more of the limiting reagent becomes available. (B) is incorrect for the same reason.

52. C

Sodium and potassium (and the rest of the alkali metals) form soluble salts, while aluminum, magnesium, and calcium do not; however, you do not need to know this fact in order to answer this question. The increased solubility of the compounds in group B caused the unreacted material to dissolve in solution, so the student was unable to detect any of the starting compound in the precipitate. The compounds in group A are sparingly soluble, so stronger antacids left a larger amount of unreacted solid. The alkalinity of the compound has no bearing on its ability to precipitate (A); also, you should know that strong bases containing sodium and potassium (i.e., NaOH and KOH) are just as alkaline as their counterparts which contain magnesium, calcium, and aluminum. (B) and (D) are accurate statements, but do not explain the student's results as well.

PRACTICE SECTION 2

ANSWER KEY

1. B	19. B	37. A
2. D	20. A	38. C
3. A	21. A	39. B
4. C	22. C	40. D
5. B	23. A	41. B
6. C	24. B	42. D
7. D	25. D	43. A
8. B	26. C	44. C
9. B	27. B	45. C
10. D	28. D	46. C
11. A	29. A	47. A
12. B	30. C	48. B
13. A	31. A	49. A
14. B	32. A	50. D
15. C	33. B	51. C
16. A	34. A	52. C
17. C	35. B	
18. D	36. D	

PASSAGE I

1. B

The dissociation reaction tells us that the coefficients for both products are equal to 1. We use this information to write the solubility equation. The solubility equation for the dissociation of $CaSO_4$ is the following:

$$4.93 \times 10^{-5} = [Ca^{2+}][SO_4^{2-}]$$

Because Ca^{2+} and SO_4^{2-} have a one-to-one ratio they can be replaced by the variable "x" to solve for their concentration. Solving the equation $4.93 \times 10^{-5} = (x)^2$, we obtain a concentration of 7.02×10^{-3} M for each ion. Because one mole of ion is equivalent to one mole of salt, this is the concentration of $CaSO_4$ needed to equal the K_{sp}, at which point the solution is saturated. The concentration of $CaSO_4$ ions,

7.02×10^{-3} M, can be multiplied by the volume, 3.75×10^5 L, to obtain a value of 2.63×10^3 moles. Converting moles of $CaSO_4$ to grams is accomplished by multiplying by the molar mass of $CaSO_4$, 136.14 grams/mole, to give a mass of 3.58×10^5 grams needed to reach saturation. (A) is the number of moles, not grams, of $CaSO_4$.

2. D

One way to solve this problem is to calculate the Ca^{2+} concentration for one mole of each compound using the K_{sp} and chemical equilibrium equation. Looking at the answer choices, (C) can be ruled out immediately because of the extremely small K_{sp}, which indicates that very few of the salt ions will dissolve. The other K_{sp} values are comparable for (A), (B), and (D). Remember to raise the ion to the power of its coefficient when setting up the equilibrium equation. For example, the equilibrium equation for the correct (D) would be $K_{sp} = 6.47 \times 10^{-6} = [Ca^{2+}][IO_3^-]^2$. The concentration of calcium for each of these answer choices, respectively, equals 6.93×10^{-5} M, 2.14×10^{-4} M, and 1.17×10^{-2} M. (D) has the highest concentration of Ca^{2+} at 1.17×10^{-2} M.

3. A

The concentration of a saturated solution of $CaSO_4$ is equal to approximately 0.015 M, according to the graph. This number was found by determining the corresponding concentration for a conductivity value of 2500 μS/cm. The concentration of $CaSO_4$ is equal to the concentration of both Ca^{2+} and SO_4^{2-} ions in solution according to equation 1 because the coefficients are all 1. Therefore, the $K_{sp} = [Ca^{2+}][SO_4^{2-}] = (.015\ M)^2$, which equals $2.25 \times 10^{-4}\ M^2$. The concentration of $CaSO_4$ must be square to obtain the K_{sp}, so (B) is incorrect. (C) doubles, not squares, the concentration. (D) might be obtained if you had taken the square root, not squared, the concentration.

4. C

As temperature increases in a solution, movement of molecules and ions increase. This will increase the current between the electrodes in the probe and increase the value of conductivity. Temperature's effect on the solubility product constant cannot be determined without further information. Although many salts have a higher solubility with higher temperatures, not all salts share this property. The only sure way to determine the relationship is by experimentation. An increase in temperature would increase the conductivity, not decrease it, so (B) and (D) is incorrect. (A) is incorrect because it is impossible to determine the relationship between temperature and K_{sp}.

5. B

The common ion effect is when an ion is already present in the solution and affects the dissociation of a compound that contains the same ion. In this case, $Ca(OCl)_2$ contains calcium and will cause the reaction in equation 1 to shift to the left due to Le Châtelier's principle. If there is no $Ca(OCl)_2$ and therefore no extra Ca^{2+} present in solution, more $CaSO_4$ will dissociate. (C) is the opposite (A) is misleading because chlorine gas will not react with SO_4^{2-}. (D) is incorrect because changing from $Ca(OCl)_2$ to chlorine gas will remove the common ion effect and cause more dissociation of $CaSO_4$.

6. C

An increase in pH means that fewer H^+ ions are present in solution. Lowering the concentration of H^+ will shift the equilibrium in equation 2 to the right, and fewer HOCl molecules will be in solution. Because the HOCl molecules can oxidize harmful agents, the oxidizing power has been reduced as a result of the pH increase. An increase in pH will not break the HOCl compound (A), though over time it will break down. Although salts do act as buffers (B), it is still possible to change the pH of the pool. As for (D), an increase in pH will decrease $[H^+]$ and thus result in fewer H^+ ions available to associate with OCl^-.

7. D

To make a supersaturated solution you must first heat the solution, which allows additional salt to dissolve. (While not all salts have a higher solubility at higher temperatures, this statement holds true for the majority of salts; an increase in temperature will generally increase the solubility of a collection of salts.) This occurs because at higher temperatures, the K_{sp} generally increases. The solution can then be cooled and the salt will remain dissolved, creating a supersaturated solution.

8. B

Using the top equation we can write the following:

$$K_{a2} = \frac{([H^+][CO_3^{2-}])}{[HCO_3^-]}$$

We can manipulate the equation to solve for $[H^+]$, where $[H^+] = \frac{(K_{a2}[HCO_3^-])}{[CO_3^{2-}]}$.

Using the bottom equation we can write the following: $K_{sp} = [Ca^{2+}][CO_3^{2-}]$

We can rearrange this equation to solve for $[CO_3^{2-}]$, which can then be substituted into the top equation:

$$[CO_3^{2-}] = \frac{K_{sp}}{[Ca^{2+}]}$$

Substituting into the top equation gives:

$$[H^+] = \left(\frac{K_{a2}}{C_{sp}}\right) \times [Ca^{2+}][HCO_3^-]$$

The K_a equation includes the reactant in the denominator because the reactant is aqueous (in contrast to the K_{sp} equation which doesn't include the reactant in the denominator). The K_{sp} reactant is a salt in its solid form; solids are not included in equilibria equations.

9. B

The color change will occur slightly before the pK_a of phenol red is reached. This is because the basic form, which is prevalent above the pK_a, has a higher absorptivity than the acidic form. This means that the basic form will absorb light more strongly than the acidic form. At the pK_a the basic and acidic forms are equal (definition of pK_a), but because of the higher absorptivity of the basic form the color will begin to change when there still is more acidic than basic molecules of phenol red. (C) and (D) are above the pK_a value, after the color change has occurred. (A) is under the pK_a but is too low. At pH 4, acidic molecules heavily dominate the solution so the absorptivity difference between acidic and basic forms does not come into play.

PASSAGE II

10. D

Hydrogen is diatomic in its elemental state, i.e., H_2 (g). The passage refers to the fact that each gaseous hydrogen atoms has a single electron, for two total electrons in H_2, but the proper electron configuration of a diatomic substance requires using the bonding-antibonding model from molecular orbital theory. None of the choices are that specific, so they are not correct. (A) is a distortion; substances in their elemental state are presumed to keep their electrons in the ground state. (B) is a distortion. as well; hydrogen is diatomic in its elemental state, meaning two electrons.

11. A

(B) is opposite; light is absorbed when the electron moves away from the nucleus. While electrons make the energy transitions, the energy transitions result in light radiation, not the emission of the electron itself, so (C) and (D) are incorrect.

12. B

The Lyman series transitions occur in the UV range (λ = 200 – 400 nm). The Balmer series corresponds to four visible wavelengths (λ = 400 – 700 nm), though the Balmer constant itself is in the UV range. Both the infrared and x-ray ranges of the light spectrum (C) and (D) fall far outside the transitions which characterize these spectra. Infrared rays are low-energy and have higher wavelengths, while x-rays are high-energy and have very short wavelengths. It is not necessary to memorize the specific wavelengths in different kinds of radiation as long as you have a general sense of differences in magnitude.

13. A

If you ignore the digression about astronomy, the question is straightforward and does not require referring back to the passage. It simply asks what color of visible light corresponds to 656.3 nm. The visible light spectrum covers 400–700 nm. Using the ROYGBIV mnemonic and prior knowledge that infrared wavelengths are longer than visible wavelengths, you know that red is on the 700 nm end, and that violet is on the 400 nm end.

14. B

This image is an absorption spectrum, in contrast to the emission spectrum presented in the passage. Think of it as the inverse of the emission spectrum. We cannot tell from the passage what a Lyman or Bohr series looks like.

15. C

Deuterium is "heavy" hydrogen, with one neutron, one proton, and one electron. The Balmer series concerns only electron transitions, so there will be no change in the number of peaks. In other words, there will be the same number of peaks, but with more splitting; the nucleus is heavier, which will slow down the transitions. This effect is visible at high resolutions.

16. A

A full explanation is out of the scope of the MCAT Physical Science section, but you should know from general physics that Bohr's model was incomplete because it didn't incorporate the theory of relativity. We know from the question stem and equation that the Balmer series works only for wavelengths related to the quantized energy levels (B). Though it is not stated explicitly in the passage, Bohr's quantitative model incorporates atomic number (C) (more detail is unnecessary for now; in short, it affects the atomic radius). Hydrogen atoms have only one electron (D), and we have no indication that other particles are involved.

17. C

According to Bohr's model, the energy differences between quantized energy levels become progressively smaller the further away the electron moves from the nucleus. Textbooks will sometimes describe this concept as if the energy levels themselves are "narrowing." (If energy levels are depicted as rings around a nucleus, they will appear to be closer together as you move further from the nucleus.) Read carefully. (B) describes a drawing like this one, but the graphical representation of this concept does not really explain the difference in energy. We do not have enough information in the passage to determine whether the energy levels themselves are a greater or smaller distance apart. (A) is the opposite of (B), intended to stump readers who might not read through to (C) and (D). Because (C) refers directly to energy differences between energy levels, it is more accurate. (Remember $E = hf = h \times$ [speed of light/wavelength].) (D) is its opposite.

QUESTIONS 18–22

18. D

Only (D) gives a response where both kinds of particles have a mass. Neither neutrons nor gamma rays have mass and so they are unchanged by the actions of a particle accelerator. The dependence on mass arises because a particle accelerator works by means of high-energy ideally elastic collisions. Also, if there is no mass, both kinetic energy and momentum are undefined.

19. B

A solution is available here which doesn't require an equation. Both the acid and base are monoprotic, thus there are no multiple dissociations. Notice that the acid is twice as concentrated as the base. Thus, double the amount of base will be needed to neutralize the acid or 2×15 mL = 30 mL. If you forgot this factor of 2, you might have chosen (A), and if you squared the 2 out of uncertainty (only in physics do you square things when in doubt) you might have chosen (D). C is the total volume of the solution, not the volume just of the base.

20. A

The ideal gas theory assumes that the particles have large interatomic distances and a relative absence of intermolecular forces. This is more true at lower pressures than at higher ones, thus eliminating (C) and (D). (B) implies that high pressure squishes the molecules. According to the kinetic theory of gases, individual atoms are treated as incompressible point properties. The main effect of the pressure is to reduce the interatomic distance, not the intra-atomic distance (i.e., the atomic radius).

21. A

Molecules can only be nonpolar if they have total symmetry around the central atom. Bent molecules lack this symmetry (think of a molecule of water with two lone pairs of electrons and two hydrogen atoms extending from the central oxygen atom) and so a dipole is created which causes polarity in the molecule. A diatomic covalent (B) molecule (such as H_2 or O_2) is perfectly symmetrical. (C) and (D) are incorrect because, although dipoles can exist in these configurations, symmetrical arrangements are also possible.

22. C

Isotypes of the same element have the same number of protons. Alpha decay results in the loss of two protons and two neutrons, while beta decay (β- decay) causes the gain of one proton. Thus, two beta decays must occur for each alpha decay to ensure that the number of protons in the daughter nucleus is equal to the number of protons in the parent nucleus. The answer is (C), 1:2.

PASSAGE III

23. A

In order to balance the equation, we must first combine the half-reactions. This requires writing all of the products and all of the reactants for both reactions in one equation:

$LiCoO_2 + xLi^+ + xe^- + 6C \leftrightharpoons Li_{1-x}CoO_2 + xLi^+ + xe^- + Li_xC_6$

If a certain compound/particle is on both the left and the right sides of the equation, then it is appearing as both a reactant and a product. Since there is no net change in that specific species, we can omit it from the net reaction; for this reason, we can eliminate the terms "xLi^+" and "xe^-" from both sides of this equation. This leaves us with (A) as the correct choice.

24. B

You should know that the overall potential of a galvanic cell ($E°_{cell}$) is equal to the sum of the potentials at the cathode and the anode. The overall potential of a discharging cell is always positive, but not necessarily greater than 1; for this reason, (B) is the only viable option. You can also arrive at this conclusion by realizing that the reaction in a battery is always spontaneous, since the battery must supply energy. Spontaneous reactions always have a negative ΔG, which you can plug into the free energy equation ($\Delta G = -nFE°_{cell}$). To get a negative ΔG from the free energy equation, you must have a positive $E°_{cell}$.

25. D

The first thing to note here is that lithium acts as an electrolyte in this reaction, meaning that it is not oxidized or reduced; that rules out (A) and (B) immediately. By definition, reduction happens at the cathode and oxidation happens at the anode. However, because this is a reversible reaction (which you should know based on the fact that the reaction is at equilibrium), we cannot use these definitions to distinguish between the species that is oxidized and the species that is reduced. The easiest way to answer this question is by noting that the carbon in the anode is neutral on the left side of the forward reaction and is negatively charged on the right side. This means that carbon is reduced, allowing us to select (D) as the correct answer. You can verify this by checking the cathode side: Because the cathode is made of CoO_2^-, in which Co has a +3 charge (since oxygen almost always carries a −2 charge, two oxygen atoms add up to a −4 charge; to create an overall −1 charge, Co must be +3), Co^{3+} must be oxidized in the conversion of $LiCoO_2$ to $Li_{1-x}CoO_2$. The product of this reaction, because it contains less +1 charge from lithium, must contain a more positive charge from cobalt (further confirming that the cobalt is reduced).

26. C

Because of the complexity of this question, the first step should be to eliminate as many choices as possible. There is no indication in the passage that $E°_{cell}$ is positive for the forward reaction (A). The assumption about reaction kinetics in (B) is correct, but it's likely that the effect of a change in x will be different for each reaction. One reaction will shift to the left and the other will shift to the right, but the shifts will not be exactly identical to one another; therefore, K_{eq} will change and (B) is incorrect. A galvanic cell gradually discharges while transporting electrons from the anode, where oxidation occurs, to the cathode, where reduction occurs. In the forward reaction, oxidation occurs at the anode and reduction occurs at the cathode. This means that the forward reaction does not represent a discharging cell, so the reverse reaction must be favored when the battery is in use. Because the reverse reaction takes precedence over the forward reaction, K_{eq} is low when the cell is discharging.

27. B

$LiCoO_2$ is usually present in the battery since it is on the left side of the cathode reaction. The presence of the $Li(CoO_2)_2$ complex is more important for this question. It is clear that $Li(CoO_2)_2$ a form of the $Li(CoO_2)_{1/(1-x)}$ complex, so we can calculate x by writing the equation $1/(1-x) = 2$. Simple algebra yields the fact that ½ of the battery's initial energy is remaining. Because the initial energy was equal to 100 J, the current energy equals 50 J.

28. D

According to the passage, the system contains only lithium as a salt in a solvent. Because it is not part of the cathode or the anode, it always retains its +1 charge. All three items are correct.

29. A

When atoms or molecules are in close proximity for an extended period of time, there is a substantial probability that they will interact with one another. The reaction suggested in (A) would require reduction of Co^{3+} to Co^{2+}, which is not unlikely to occur in small quantities. Though the passage does not directly indicate that this was the mechanism of production of lithium oxide and cobalt(II) oxide, it is more likely than any of the other answer choices. It would be incorrect to dismiss the possibility of decomposition, but the reaction suggested in (B) ($LiCoO_2 \rightarrow Li_2O + CoO$) is stoichiometrically impossible. (C) is incorrect because interaction with environmental oxygen would affect cell 2 just as much as it would affect cell 1. (D) is incorrect because we have no evidence suggesting that any water is present in the system; the passage clarifies that organic solvents are used.

30. C

The scientist believes that battery deterioration is caused primarily by the formation of cobalt(II) oxide and lithium oxide in equal quantities. Therefore, increased amounts of cobalt(II) oxide suggest a decrease in battery capacity. (A) and (B) are incorrect because x is a ratio that is unaffected by the energy storage capacity of a cell. (D) is incorrect because, although a decrease in concentration of Li_xC_6 would suggest a decrease in cell capacity, most of the deterioration is caused by the conversion of $LiCoO_2$ to Li_2O and CoO_2.

PASSAGE IV

31. A

Ammonia's heat of vaporization is given in the data and described as low compared with that of water. Thus, its evaporation rate must also be high compared to that of water so life could not have evolved in a liquid ammonia environment as life on earth evolved in a liquid water environment. The phases in (B), (C), and (D) would matter less for life's evolution from a liquid environment; they are also incorrect applications of the data from the passage.

32. A

Solid water would have been most dense if it were like other substances, and thus sunk to the bottom of any liquid system. Liquid systems would have been frozen from the bottom up, and life could not have evolved in the liquid phase of a watery environment. (B), (C), and (D) do not address this "what-if" scenario.

33. B

It is the kinetic energy of the molecules that moves them further apart to allow a phase change from solid to gas, as described in the question. The same process would dictate a phase change from solid to liquid, or liquid to gas.

34. A

The electronegativities of the atoms comprising a molecule determine the polarity of that molecule. None of the other choices will make as significant a contribution. (C) is the next most logical but is less correct because forces emanate from the intrinsic nature of electronegativity within the water molecule, not between.

35. B

The crystalline lattice formed for a water-solid uniquely collapses under pressure to become a liquid. (A) is a true statement, though it doesn't directly address the question.

36. D

Both (A) and (B) are true. Water has a higher heat of vaporization than ammonia and therefore evaporates at a higher temperature. Temperature is a measurement of average kinetic energy, so high temperature means higher average kinetic energy; the molecules are also moving faster.

37. A

Ions dissolved in the lattice break existing intermolecular attractive forces. This process interferes with the formation of a crystal lattice in ice, which explains why ice melts when salt is added.

PASSAGE V

38. C

Asking for the strongest reducing agent is equal to asking for the element with the highest electronegativity. Electronegativity increases as we move from the left to the right and from the bottom to the top of the periodic table. Therefore, you are looking for an element that is above and to the right of phosphorus. (C), oxygen, fits this description.

39. B

You're being asked which elements have a larger atomic radius than phosphorus. Atomic radius increases from right to left and from top to bottom of the periodic table. Therefore, you are looking for elements that are below and to the left of phosphorus. Both K and Pb fit this description, so B is the correct answer.

40. D

To answer this question, you must know that phosphorus is a nonmetal. The other answer choices describe properties of nonmetals. (D) describes a property of metals, so it is the correct answer.

41. B

(B) is the correct full electron configuration. (C) places the 3s-electrons in the 3p-orbital. (D) is incorrect because phosphorus does not have a 3d-orbital.

42. D

(A) and (B) are incorrect because alkaline earth elements are generally more dense than alkali metals. (C) is incorrect because alkali metals contain the same number of orbitals as the alkaline earth element in the corresponding row. (D) is a true statement.

43. A

Halogens can naturally exist in the gaseous, liquid, and solid states (iodine).

44. C

(A), (B), (D) are all true properties of transition elements, but they do not greatly contribute to the malleability shown by these elements. Their malleability can be attributed mostly to the loosely held d-electrons.

45. C

(A) is incorrect because phosphorus is not a metalloid. Metalloids do often behave as semiconductors (B) but it is not relevant here. (C) is correct because both arsenic and antimony are in the same group as phosphorus and they have similar properties.

PASSAGE VI

46. C

The reaction presented in the passage, beginning with acetic acid and forming methane and carbon dioxide, is a decomposition reaction. It begins with one reactant and ends with two products, which is typical of a decomposition reaction. A combination reaction (A) would have been the opposite: more reactants than products. A single displacement reaction (B) typically is an oxidation/reduction reaction, which is not demonstrated in this question. A combustion reaction (D) is catalyzed by oxygen and results in carbon dioxide and water as products.

47. A

First, calculate the molecular weight of acetic acid, CH_3COOH, which is 60.05 g/mol. Next, recognize that there is a 1:1 molar ratio between this reactant and the product, methane. By beginning with 120.0 grams of acetic acid and dividing by the molecular weight, this yields 1.998 moles of acetic acid and should produce the same number of moles of methane. The molecular weight of methane is 16.04 g/mol. By multiplying this molecular weight by the number of expected moles yield, 1.998, the theoretical yield expected if all of the acetic acid were decomposed would be 32.05 grams of methane product.

48. B

A key issue here in harnessing a gaseous product is its phase and transport, so (B) is correct. If compressible, then methane would take up significantly less volume and be easier to transport, making it more likely to be efficient as a common energy source. The passage states that this reaction typically takes place at a temperature well above room temperature. Even if (A) were true, it doesn't support an argument toward using methane gas as a major energy source. While (C) is true, the production of gas challenges, more than supports, the passage's argument of making clean energy. Finally, whether or not the reaction is exothermic, the energy source is the product, methane gas, so (D) presents an irrelevant piece of information.

49. A

To build the equation necessary to answer this question, begin with 88.02 grams of CO_2 in the numerator. Next, convert this to moles of CO_2 by dividing by grams per mole. This eliminates (D), since 88.02 grams is in the denominator and the molecular weight of CO_2 is in the numerator. (C) is also out with 88.02 grams in the denominator. Next, recognize that there is a 1:1 ratio of CO_2 to CH_3COOH, making it unnecessary to convert the number of moles. This eliminates (B), which incorrectly uses a 1:2 ratio. The only choice remaining is (A), which correctly ends by multiplying by the molecular weight of acetic acid; this would yield the number of grams of acetic acid necessary for the proposed reaction.

50. D

The net ionic equation shows all aqueous ions that productively participate in the reaction, eliminating all spectator ions. The only true spectator ion in this equation is sodium, so it should not be present in a net ionic equation, which proves that (A) is incorrect. Next, $CH_3CH_2CH_2Cl$ has a covalent bond between the carbon and chloride atoms, meaning that it is unlikely to ionize in solution; chloride, thus, should not be represented as an ion on the reactant side of the equation, as it is in (A) and (B). Finally, (D) correctly keeps the reactant as one molecule and has the chloride ion written as a product.

51. C

The first step in this question requires you to consider the correctly balanced equation for converting CO_2 and H_2 to CH_4 and H_2O (the reactants and products specified in the passage and in the question stem):

$$CO_2 + 2\ H_2 \rightarrow CH_4 + 2\ H_2O$$

The correctly balanced equation uses the molar ratio of 1 CO_2 : 2 H_2 : 1 CH_4 : 2 H_2O. Next, recall that according to the ideal gas law, one mole of an ideal gas has a volume of 22.4 L at standard temperature and pressure (STP). From this, one can calculate that there are 0.134 moles of hydrogen gas and 0.0893 moles of carbon dioxide available as reactants. Then, calculate the molar equivalents of each, since 2 moles of hydrogen gas are required per mole of CO_2. Thus, there are 0.0670 molar equivalents available of hydrogen gas per 0.0893 moles CO_2, meaning that the hydrogen gas is the limiting reagent. Finally, because there is only one mole of methane produced per one mole of hydrogen gas used, there will be 0.0670 moles of methane produced. (A) does not correct for the 2:1 molar equivalency of H_2:CH_4. (B) uses carbon dioxide as the limiting reagent. (D) reverses the molar ratio of H_2:CH_4, thus multiplying 0.134 moles by 2 instead of dividing.

52. C

Begin by calculating the theoretical yield of methane, which is the amount (in either grams or moles) of methane expected to be produced if all the hydrogen were fully consumed by the following formula:

$$CO_2 + 2\,H_2 \rightarrow CH_4 + 2\,H_2O$$

Recall that at STP, one mole of gas has a volume of 22.4 liters, which allows one to calculate that there are 2.32 moles of hydrogen gas given to react. Next, use the balanced equation for converting CO_2 and H_2 to CH_4 and H_2O (the reactants and products specified in the passage and in the question stem). The correctly balanced equation uses the molar ratio of 1 CO_2 : 2 H_2 : 1 CH_4 : 2 H_2O. Thus, with 2.32 moles of hydrogen gas, one would expect to form one mole of methane per two moles of hydrogen gas, or 1.16 moles of methane product. Finally, multiply by methane's molecular weight, 16.04, which results in 18.6 grams of methane; this is the theoretical yield. However, the question stem states that only 8.02 grams of methane were produced. Thus, the percent yield is calculated by dividing the actual yield (8.02 grams) by the theoretical yield (18.6 grams) and multiplying by 100 percent, which results in a percent yield of 43.1 percent.

PRACTICE SECTION 3

ANSWER KEY

1. A	19. A	37. A
2. B	20. A	38. C
3. D	21. D	39. B
4. D	22. D	40. B
5. D	23. A	41. D
6. A	24. A	42. C
7. B	25. B	43. C
8. C	26. A	44. B
9. B	27. A	45. A
10. B	28. D	46. D
11. C	29. C	47. D
12. B	30. D	48. A
13. C	31. C	49. C
14. A	32. D	50. D
15. A	33. A	51. A
16. C	34. D	52. B
17. B	35. D	
18. C	36. D	

PASSAGE I

1. A

For a molecule to pass from the systemic circulation to the central nervous system, it must pass between the tightly sealed endothelial cells or through the endothelial cells. Unless a medication has a transporter to cross the cell membrane twice, it is more likely to diffuse between endothelial cells, despite their tightly sealed spaces. Because cell membranes are composed primarily of nonpolar lipid molecules, it will be easiest for a lipophilic, or nonpolar compound to diffuse into the CSF. Although (B) does describe a method for delivering drugs to the CNS, a nonsystemic route would be inefficient for a process as routine as general anesthetic administration; (A) is a better option. (C) is incorrect, because nonpolar or lipophilic molecules will penetrate more effectively than will a polar molecule. (D) is irrelevant; furthermore, a slow-acting general anesthetic would be impractical when physicians are aiming to minimize time under anesthesia and maximize patient comfort.

2. B

The key to understanding the blood-brain barrier is that the endothelial cells are tightly sealed, prohibiting free passage of molecules, unlike the leaky capillary systems of the peripheral circulation. The molecules that are most likely to still move between these cells and enter the CSF are those that are uncharged and not repelled by the hydrophilic cell membranes. Even though charged particles might associate closely with one another (A), this doesn't affect their passage through the blood-brain barrier. (D) is incorrect because the passage relates no information about the differential solubilities of charged molecules in the bloodstream versus CSF.

3. D

The blood-brain barrier, as described in the passage, provides a tight seal between the systemic circulation and the more sensitive central nervous system. As a result, this barrier can serve to protect the central nervous system from potentially damaging substances that can more readily enter the systemic circulation, and then be filtered before entering the CNS. (A) is incorrect because the blood-brain barrier's adaptive seal is not designed for maximizing nutrient transport; in fact, it limits transport/transfer between two systems. (B) is incorrect because this barrier necessarily means that many molecules and particles cannot pass between the CNS and systemic compartments, thus making these two micro-environments different. (C) is incorrect because the blood-brain barrier's main role is not to limit movement of particles or agents from CSF to the systemic circulation, but rather to limit flow in the other direction because the systemic circulation is more readily contaminated.

4. D

According to the passage, molecules most likely to cross the blood-brain barrier are hydrophobic or nonpolar. Thus, ion-dipole and dipole-dipole interactions (A) and (B) are unlikely to be the most important forces governing intermolecular interactions among these molecules (because they require charge and/or polarity). Although hydrogen bonding (C) might have a role in these molecules, hydrogen bonds, because they occur between atoms in otherwise polarized bonds (a hydrogen with a partial negative charge and a lone pair or otherwise electronegative atom with a negative charge), would be unlikely to facilitate transport in a hydrophobic environment. Dispersion forces (D) refer to the unequal sharing of electrons that occurs among nonpolar molecules as the result of rapid polarization and counterpolarization; these are likely to be the prevailing intermolecular forces affecting molecules that move easily through the blood-brain barrier.

5. D

All three items are false. A polar molecule can still have a formal charge of zero, because the molecule's formal charge is the sum of the formal charges of the individual atoms. Each atom could individually still have a positive or negative formal charge, calculate by the formula:

FC = Valence electrons – ½ bonding electrons – nonbonding electrons

Thus, a molecule with a formal charge of zero could have multiple polarized bonds and/or multiple atoms with positive/negative formal charges, making it unlikely to permeate through the nonpolar blood-brain barrier. Similarly, having a negative formal charge on the molecule overall would be unfavorable to move through a nonpolar barrier. Finally, two molecules, both with formal charges of zero, could have very different characteristics, making them more or less likely to permeate the blood-brain barrier. For example, one compound could be comprised entirely of nonpolar bonds, with all atoms of formal charge of zero, both of which would make it favorable to pass through the blood-brain barrier. Size also plays a key role, as large molecules do not readily pass through the barrier. A separate molecule with a formal charge of zero could, as described above, contain positive or negative formal charges on different atoms and/or have polar bonds, making it pass through the barrier less readily.

6. A

In cisplatin, a molecule with square planar geometry, two chloride atoms and two ammonia molecules each are bonded directly to the central platinum, without any remaining lone pairs on the central platinum. The NH_3 groups bond to the central platinum by donating a lone pair of electrons into an unfilled orbital of the platinum atom. As such, NH_3 is acting as a Lewis base, and platinum is acting as a Lewis acid, and they form a coordinate covalent bond. A polar covalent bond (B) is not formed from this type of donation of a lone pair; an example of a polar covalent bond would be the N–H bonds in the NH_3 group, with partial negative charge on the nitrogen and partial positive charge on the hydrogen. In (C) and (D), the Pt–N bond is formed by a Lewis acid/base relationship, which is not the case for a nonpolar covalent bond or ionic bond.

7. B

Although the geometry of this carbon atom is likely to be changed somewhat by the ring strain on the adjacent ring structures, it is still most likely to approximate a tetrahedral geometry. This carbon is bonded to four groups: the two phenol groups, a nitrogen, and the additional carbon atom in the adjacent carboxyl group. The tetrahedral geometry (B) maximizes the space among these four groups. Octahedral geometry (D) typically refers to a central atom surrounded by six groups, not four.

8. C

Resonance structures serve to spread out formal charge. The most important resonance structures minimize or eliminate the formal charge on individual atoms. As a result, polarity in any single bond might be minimized. (A) is essentially the opposite of this argument. (B) is incorrect; it is possible for molecules with or without resonance to be polar, and this is too broad of a generalization to be true. (D) is incorrect because polar bonds will intrinsically place a partial negative charge on the more electronegative atom. Important resonance structures would likely further accentuate this inclination, placing extra electrons on more electronegative atoms. Counteracting this effect and essentially "removing" electrons from highly electronegative atoms to counterbalance the natural polarity of the bond would form an extremely high-energy, unfavorable, and thus unimportant, resonance structure.

PASSAGE II

9. B

The order of this reaction can be determined by the equation $r = k[A]_x[B]_y$. You must divide r_3 by r_1 to get: $\frac{8.09}{2.04} = \frac{k(4.00)^x(1.00)^y}{k(1.00)^x(1.00)^y}$. This simplifies to $4 = 4^x$, so $x = 1$. This means that H^+ is a first-order reactant.

10. B

The equation for the rate of a reaction is:

$$\text{Rate} = k[\text{reactant}_1]^{\text{order1}}[\text{reactant}_2]^{\text{order2}}$$

Using the equation for determining order of a reactant detailed in the explanation for the answer to question 9, we find that O_2 is second order. Substituting the information into the equation for the rate of a reaction leads to:

$$\text{Rate} = (0.5)[2.0\ M]^1[2.0\ M]^2$$

Simplifying this equation allows us to determine that the rate is 4 M/sec.

11. C

(A) is incorrect because it describes a reactant, and Fe^{2+} – SOD is not a reactant. (B) is incorrect because it describes a product, and Fe^{2+} – SOD is not a product. (C) is correct because it describes a catalyst, which is exactly the role Fe^{2+} – SOD plays. (D) describes a transition state, and is incorrect because transition states are temporary states of highest energy of the conversion of reactant to product.

12. B

(A) is true because particles must collide to react, and thus the rate of reaction is both dependent on and proportional to the number of particles colliding. (B) is not true (making it the correct answer) because all the colliding particles must have enough kinetic energy to exceed activation energy if a collision is to be effective. (C) is the accurate definition of a transition state. (D) is true because "activated complex" is another name for "transition state," which by definition has greater energy than both reactants and products.

13. C

Section C shows the energy that must be put into the reaction to drive it in a forward direction. Section A in the diagram represents the change in enthalpy; it shows the difference between the starting and the final energy values. Section B does not represent any specific energy value. Section D represents the reverse activation energy. It is much greater than the forward activation energy because the reactant is starting at a much lower level of energy, yet must still reach the same amount of total energy to proceed with the reaction.

14. A

Section A is correct because it shows the difference between the starting and the final energy values.

15. A

The equation to determine the equilibrium constant for a reaction aA + bB = cC + dD is $K_c = ([C]^c[D]^d)/([A]^a[B]^b)$. For this reaction, $K_c = ([2]^1[1]^1/([3]^2[1]^2 = 2/9 = 0.22$. When the corresponding values are plugged into the equation, $K_c = 2/9$, or 0.22.

16. C

(C) is correct because an increase in pressure will cause an equilibrium to shift toward the side of the reaction with fewer moles of gas, which in this case is the right side of the equation. An increase in volume (A) would have no effect or would cause a decrease in pressure, shifting the equilibrium to the left. An addition of product (B) would also cause a shift to the left. A temperature decrease (D) would most likely cause a shift to the left due to fewer numbers of collisions between particles, assuming kinetic energy is proportional to temperature.

QUESTIONS 17–21

17. B

The question says that latent heat flux is caused by evaporation. Therefore, simply identify which value of ΔH is related to this phase change. Vaporization is another way of saying evaporation, so (B) is correct. Fusion (A) refers to the change from a solid to a liquid, and sublimation (C) refers to the change from a solid to a gas. Ionization (D) is unrelated to a phase change.

18. C

The centripetal acceleration is equivalent to the tangential velocity squared divided by the radius or [$(10\text{ m/s})^2$ divided by 10 m = 10 m/s^2]. Because the tangential acceleration vector is parallel to the tangential velocity vector, and the centripetal acceleration is perpendicular to the direction of velocity, the vector sum will provide the angle between the velocity and acceleration vectors. Because the tangential acceleration is equivalent to the centripetal acceleration, the velocity and acceleration vectors are 45° apart.

19. A

The question requires you to know the solubility rules. Because an electrolyte must dissociate into its component ions in water, look for the substance that will not dissolve. The answer is (A), silver chloride (AgCl), which is insoluble in water. All of the other compounds will readily dissociate into their constituent ions.

20. A

(A) is correct. Because aluminum oxide is alkaline, immersion in an acidic solution would readily strip away the protective coating and allow the acid to oxidize the metal below.

21. D

How can you relate the average velocities of gases at the same temperature? Two gases at the same temperature will have the same average molecular kinetic energy. Because two gases at the same temperature will have the same average molecular kinetic energy, $(1/2)m_A v_A^2 = (1/2)m_B v_B^2$, which gives $m_B/m_A = (v_A/v_B)^2$. Since $v_A/v_B = 2$, we have $m_B/m_A = 4$. Only (D) lists two gases with a mass ratio around 4:1 (krypton 83.3g/mol and neon 20.2 g/mol).

PASSAGE III

22. D

The solid block becomes smaller in the experiment and so must move from the solid phase to the gaseous phase, sublimation. The other answer choices require a liquid phase, which is not valid because the experimental results demonstrate that no liquid was detected when the solid shrunk in size.

23. A

The solid/liquid equilibrium line is sloped positively and so the phase change from liquid to solid at a constant temperature is the only correct possible phase change. (B) is wrong because the gas phase is not possible as pressure increases; the liquid would change to gas, however, if the temperature were increased while maintaining constant pressure. (C) and (D) are illogical because kinetic energy is equivalent to temperature. Because temperature is constant according to the question stem, there is no kinetic energy change.

24. A

You must deduce from both the experimental results and the chemical equation that the volume does not change. The volume does not change because it is described as a rigid container, and no change in volume is described in the experimental results. As a result, the dry ice must absorb energy from its surrounding (the air in the container) in order to change phase. Because the total energy must remain constant, the air initially present in the container must lose an equivalent amount of kinetic energy.

25. B

The chemical equation shows that the dry ice absorbs heat from its environment to change into a gas, requiring it to overcome the intermolecular forces that organize it in the solid form. (C) and (D) refer to hydrogen bonds, which are not present in carbon dioxide.

26. A

The chemical equation shows that the heat of room temperature ambient air must be absorbed to change the carbon dioxide from solid to gas. This use of heat defines an endothermic reaction, which must therefore characterize the reaction occurring in the container. (C) and (D) refer to an exothermic reaction, which would release heat. (B) is incorrect since an endothermic reaction absorbs/uses heat, which increases the energy of some of the molecules in the reaction; thus, the potential energy should not decrease.

27. A

The air gains dry ice molecules and these exert a pressure on the container, according to the equation PV = nRT, where n represents the number of moles of gas. (B) is the opposite; its volume would increase, according to the same equation if possible. However this experiment takes place in a rigid container, preventing any change in volume. (C) is incorrect because the question clearly states that the solid changes phase. Air temperature decreases with this endothermic reaction, absorbing heat to change from a solid to gas carbon dioxide (D).

28. D

None of the choices shows a substance moving from the solid directly to the gas phase in the process of sublimation. (A) and (B) show fusion and evaporation, respectively, but not sublimation. (C) indicates the heating of a gas; in the experiment, the carbon dioxide solid is increased in its kinetic energy; the gas is not being heated.

29. C

(C) indicates change from a solid to a gas as described in the passage for dry ice, which is called sublimation.

QUESTIONS 30-36

30. D

Because $\Delta G = \Delta H - T\Delta S$ can be used to relate free energy to enthalpy and entropy, and T is always positive, a negative ΔH (enthalpy) and a positive ΔS (entropy) will always give a negative ΔG value; that is, the reaction will occur spontaneously. (D) is correct.

31. C

Moving from left to right across the periodic table, atomic radii will decrease. Because calcium is on the left side of the table and gallium is on the right, in the same period, gallium should have a smaller atomic radius. As stated in (C), this is due to the greater number of protons in the nucleus holding the electrons more tightly.

32. D

The major forces that cause gases to deviate from ideal behavior are intermolecular attractions and the volume of the gas molecules. These factors are minimized when gas molecules are far apart and moving quickly, which occurs at low pressures and high temperatures, (D).

33. A

The question says that this gas is ideal, so use PV = nRT. The ideal gas law shows that P is directly proportional to T. So with volume held constant, if pressure is reduced by a factor of 2, temperature will also be reduced by a factor of 2. (A) is correct.

34. D

Though this question begins by telling you about greenhouse gases, it ultimately asks you to identify similarities between CO_2 and H_2O which N_2 and O_2 lack. CO_2 is not a polar molecule; its linear geometry allows the opposing dipole moments to cancel out, so (A) is incorrect. Because its dipole moments cancel, (B) is incorrect. Furthermore, it lacks hydrogen atoms and is therefore incapable of hydrogen bonding, so (C) is incorrect. However, both CO_2 and H_2O have polar bonds, while N_2 and O_2 both have diatomic, nonpolar covalent bonds between two atoms of the same element.

35. D

Fluorine (A) is not a transition metal, so its ionized counterparts will have an valence octet of electrons implying no unpaired electrons. (B), (C), (D) are all transition metals; however (B) and (C), commonly oxidize to the 2 and 3 positive states, respectively, which fill their d subshells. Iron (D) commonly oxidizes to the 2 positive state, which gives one extra s-subshell electron. This unpaired electron helps to give iron its magnetic properties and explains why iron in the body is further oxidized to the 3 positive state (to avoid inductive currents that could damage protein structure).

36. D

Chromium is an exception to the general rule that the 3d-subshell is filled completely before the 4s-subshell. The 3d-subshell partially fills, then the 4s-subshell fills completely and finally the 3d-subshell finishes filling. (B) is incorrect because the nearest noble gas to Cr is Ar not Kr.

PASSAGE IV

37. A

Henry's law states that the amount of gas dissolved in a liquid is directly proportional to the partial pressure of the gas in equilibrium with the liquid. Therefore, Henry's law can be used to calculate the concentration of oxygen in water using the partial pressure of oxygen in air. Boyle's law (B) deals with the relationship between the pressure and volume of gases but does not address concentration of gases in water. Raoult's law (C) pertains to the vapor pressure of a mixture of liquids, not a gas dissolved in a liquid. Le Châtelier's principle (D) addresses changes to an equilibrium state and cannot stand alone to explain the equilibrium between a gas in air and in solution.

38. C

We can use the solubility constant for nitrogen provided in the passage, 8.42×10^{-7} M/torr, to solve this question. Because the units in the constant are in torr, we first convert 0.634 atm to torr by multiplying by 760 torr/1 atm. The partial pressure of nitrogen equals 481.8 torr. Multiplying the pressure by the constant 8.42×10^{-7} M/torr gives us 4.06×10^{-4} M nitrogen. The units for the answer are in g/L, so we multiply by the molar mass of nitrogen, 28 g/mole, to get our answer of 1.14×10^{-2} g/L.

39. B

The solubility constants provided in the passage can be used to determine that helium is the least soluble gas. A soluble gas is not desired because we want to minimize gas bubbles in the body. Moreover, helium is an inert gas, meaning it does readily react with other gases. Whether helium is diatomic (A) has no bearing on its use in scuba tanks. Many gases are present in trace amounts in the water (D), so this fact alone could not account for the use of helium in scuba tanks.

40. B

This is a classic ideal gas law problem using PV = nRT. You are given the volume, then must convert the temperature to degrees Kelvin to obtain a useable temperature and must convert the mass of oxygen to moles to find *n*. P equals 2.80 L. T equals 273.15 + 13.0 = 286.15 K. The mass, 0.320 kg, equals 320 grams. We divide the mass by the molar mass of oxygen, 32 g/mole, to obtain the moles of oxygen, 10 moles. R equals 0.0821 L atm/(mole K). Plugging in these numbers to the equation, PV = nRT. Solving for P gives a pressure of 83.9 atm.

41. D

Immediate isolation in a hyperbaric chamber is the most effective and common treatment for those suffering from severe decompression sickness. The chamber recreates a high-pressure environment to allow gas bubbles to dissolve back into body fluids and tissues. The chamber can be brought back to normal pressure slowly in order to allow the body to adjust to the decreased pressure. Helium gas administration (A) or gas and air mixture (B) would not rid the body of excess gas bubbles. In fact, it might increase the gases bubbles and make symptoms worse. A hypobaric chamber (C) would certainly make symptoms worse because it decreases the pressure below 1 atm.

42. C

The solubility of gas in liquids decreases with an increase in liquid temperature. The warming of oceans has resulted in less dissolved oxygen and many oxygen-depleted "dead zones." It is true that carbon dioxide has increased ocean acidity (A), but acidity alone cannot account for decreased oxygen levels. A predator shark may explain why certain fish are dying off (B), but it would not explain the decrease in oxygen. If rainfall did increase water levels in the ocean (D), the oxygen levels would equilibrate (as per Henry's law) between the ocean and atmosphere to allow more dissolved oxygen in the oceans.

43. C

This is a PV = nRT problem. Find the moles of oxygen by converting 0.38 kg to grams and dividing by the molar mass of oxygen, 32.g/mole. The number of moles equals 11.875. STP indicates a temperature of 273.15 K and a pressure of 1 atm. R equals 0.0821 (L atm/mole K). Plugging these numbers into PV = nRT and solving for V gives a volume of 266 L.

44. B

Multiplying the amount of nitrogen gas in the air by the solubility constant of nitrogen will give the amount of nitrogen that is dissolved in the diver's blood. The solubility constant for nitrogen can be obtained by dividing the solubility of nitrogen, 6.2×10^{-4} M, by 1 atm to get 6.2×10^{-4} M/atm. The amount of nitrogen in the air can be obtained by finding the partial pressure of nitrogen. The total pressure, 3 atm, is multiplied by the percentage of nitrogen in the air, 78 percent, to get a partial pressure of nitrogen equal to 2.3 atm. Finally, we multiply 2.3 atm of nitrogen by the solubility constant to obtain a value of 1.4×10^{-3} M for the concentration of nitrogen in the diver's blood.

45. A

The root mean square velocity (v_{rms}) can be calculated by taking the square root of ($3RT/M_m$). This equation tells us that the v_{rms} increases when molar mass decreases. Tank 2 contains a mixture of helium and oxygen; the helium will lower the average molar mass of the gas molecules because it has a lower molar mass compared to oxygen. The v_{rms} of tank 2 will therefore be higher. Tank 1, which contains only oxygen, will have a higher molar mass and a lower v_{rms} value.

PASSAGE V

46. D

F- is related to less acid production and reduces the risk of dental caries, choice (D). The fluoride ion is related to acid production and reduces the risk of dental caries, according to the passage. Fluoride has not been proven to directly cause or even be related to bacterial death (B, D), nor has it directly been proven to stop bacteria from forming dental caries (A). However, fluoride is related to/correlated with acidity reduction and dental caries reduction. The other choices imply relationships and causations not inferred from the passage.

47. D

The high electronegativity of fluorine means that it is inclined to hold onto or pull electrons. (C) is the opposite of this atomic property because fluorine would not easily give off electrons. While the passage discusses fissures as a cause of caries (A) and (B), it does not infer that fluoride is involved directly with its filling or repair.

48. A

You must deduce from the definition of electronegativity that in order for the nucleus to pull on the orbital electrons, it should be closer to the electrons; therefore, a smaller radius is desirable. (B), (C), and (D) all contribute to a decrease in electronegativity because the distractors either favor a larger size of the atom with more electron shells or a smaller positive core of the protons that are responsible for the electronegative attraction in the first place.

49. C

The fluoride ion has the atomic structure of the element fluorine, which would be $1s^22s^22p^5$, with an additional electron to make it an anion with a charge of negative one. Using [He] at the beginning of the notation accurately reflects the fact that F^- has the same structure as helium, but with the additional shells as noted. (A) is incorrect because this is the notation for the element fluoride, not the ion. (B) is the structure for oxygen. (D) is incorrect because when using the notation [Ne], one implies that the atom has the structure of that noble gas, with additional shells. [Ne] comes after fluorine in the periodic table, and it would not be correct to add a level 2 shell after completing that shell in [Ne].

50. D

(D) is correct because Heisenberg's uncertainty principle states that the momentum (m and v) cannot be determined exactly and quantitatively if the location of an electron in an atom is known and conversely, the location cannot be known if the momentum is known. One could get a qualitative measurement of momentum, since the measurement is still possible, but simple becomes less accurate as the accuracy of the measurement of position increases. (A), (B) and (C) all violate this principle, as the location is stated to be known in the stem of the item.

51. A

The effective nuclear charge is calculated by the following equation: $Z_{eff} = Z - S$, where Z is the atomic number (the number of protons in the nucleus), and S is the average number of electrons between the nucleus and the electron in question. Because fluorine's atomic number is 9 and there are 9 electrons in this element, the outermost electron in fluorine (not an ion), would have a Z_{eff} of the following: $Z_{eff} = 9 - 8 = +1$. However, in the fluoride anion, an additional electron has been added, so the $Z_{eff} = 9 - 9 = 0$. (B) would require an additional electron between the nucleus and the outermost electron, and (D) is impossible because no protons/electrons would allow a calculation of ½ of a unit of charge.

52. B

(B) is correct because the highest electron shells, or orbitals, are most loosely held by the nucleons and thus are most available for bonding. 3s is higher than any other level (A), but it is unoccupied in the fluoride ion. (C) and (D) are lower energy levels/orbitals than 2p.

INDEX

T

U

V

W

X

Y

Z